AO TRAUMA

Stefan Rammelt, Michael Swords, Mandeep S Dhillon, Andrew K Sands

Manual of Fracture Management
Foot and Ankle

Manual of Fracture Management—Foot and Ankle Stefan Rammelt, Michael Swords, Mandeep S Dhillon, Andrew K Sands

AO TRAUMA

Stefan Rammelt, Michael Swords, Mandeep S Dhillon, Andrew K Sands

Manual of Fracture Management
Foot and Ankle

Includes more than 1,650 x-rays, clinical photographs, and illustrations

Library of Congress Cataloging-in-Publication Data is available from the publisher.

Hazards

Great care has been taken to maintain the accuracy of the information contained in this publication. However, the publisher, and/or the distributor, and/or the editors, and/or the authors cannot be held responsible for errors or any consequences arising from the use of the information contained in this publication. Contributions published under the name of individual authors are statements and opinions solely of said authors and not of the publisher, and/or the distributor, and/or the AO Group.

The products, procedures, and therapies described in this work are hazardous and are therefore only to be applied by certified and trained medical professionals in environments specially designed for such procedures. No suggested test or procedure should be carried out unless, in the user's professional judgment, its risk is justified. Whoever applies products, procedures, and therapies shown or described in this work will do this at their own risk. Because of rapid advances in the medical sciences, AO recommends that independent verification of diagnosis, therapies, drugs, dosages, and operation methods should be made before any action is taken.

Although all advertising material which may be inserted into the work is expected to conform to ethical (medical) standards, inclusion in this publication does not constitute a guarantee or endorsement by the publisher regarding quality or value of such product or of the claims made of it by its manufacturer.

Legal restrictions

Distribution by Georg Thieme Verlag, Rüdigerstrasse 14, 70469 Stuttgart, Germany, and Thieme New York, 333 Seventh Avenue, New York, NY 10001, USA

Cover photograph: Thomas Albrecht, DGPh; Stefan Rammelt.

ISBN: 9783132434585
e-ISBN: 9783132434592

2 3 4 5 6

Foreword

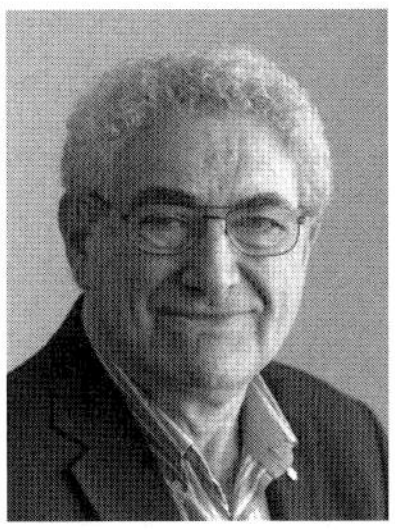

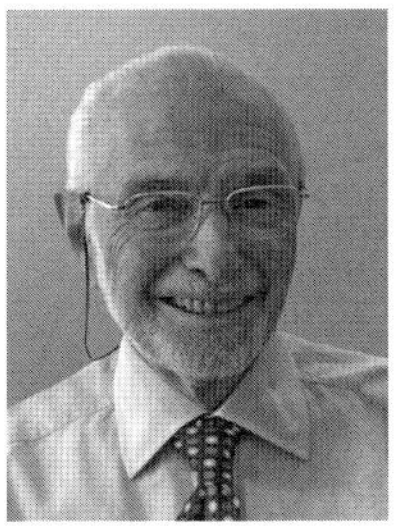

Marvin Tile, CM, MD, BSc (Med), FRCSC
Professor Emeritus
Surgery University of Toronto
Orthopedic Surgeon, Sunnybrook HSC
Canada
AO Foundation Past President

Joseph Schatzker CM, MD, BSc, FRCSC
Professor Emeritus
Orthopedic surgeon active staff
Sunnybrook Hospital, University of Toronto
Canada
AO Foundation Past President

In 1958, a group of Swiss general and orthopedic surgeons met in Biel, Switzerland and founded an organization devoted to the study of internal fixation of fractures; thus was born the AO (Arbeitsgemeinschaft für Osteosynthesefragen). At that time, the concept of internal fixation of fractures was well known but rarely recommended because of the many risks and concerns, especially infection.

In 1907, an early comprehensive manual *L'Intervention Operatioire* was published by Albin Lambotte in Brussels, Belgium.

In 1949, Robert Danis at the University of Brussels, published his book, *Théorie et pratique de l'ostéosynthèse*. He introduced the concept of anatomical reduction of fractures, stable fixation, primary bone healing ("soudure autogene"), and early mobilization of the injured limb. Danis had a major influence on Maurice E Müller, one of the AO founders, which led to the founding of AO in 1958.

Müller quickly realized the important principles espoused by Danis but was hampered by the lack of appropriate equipment and implants to apply those principles. The AO founders made it happen by closely collaborating with two Swiss companies and developing the implant systems to fulfill the principles. With this AO system, it became possible to achieve stable fixation, allow early motion and restoration of limb function. The timing was right for the AO principles of internal fixation, with control of sepsis, improved critical care of the traumatized patient, improved metallurgy, and better soft-tissue handling during surgery.

We were trained in the principles of internal fixation of fractures by our mentors in Toronto but immediately recognized the important contribution of the AO group after meeting founder and innovator Müller; in St Gallen in 1965 (Tile), and in Toronto in 1966 (Schatzker), followed by a research fellowship with him in Berne, Switzerland in 1967. Our close collaboration with AO resulted in teaching the earliest AO courses in North America, in research and book publications, and the Presidency of the AO Foundation of Tile (1992–1994) and Schatzker (1998–2000).

Education has always been a pillar of the AO and a key to their continuing success. The first publication, *Techniques of Internal Fixation of Fractures* by Müller et al, was published in 1965 and discussed the principles in depth; this was followed by the *Manual of Internal Fixation of Fractures* in 1969 describing the techniques in detail.

To ensure good patient outcomes, surgeons could only obtain the equipment by attending courses or spending time in an AO fellowship. The early equipment was basic and most fractures could be managed with it.

In the first decade, the principles were considered radical, therefore challenged and not accepted in many parts of the world, but with well-trained young surgeons publishing improved patient outcomes, they soon became conventional wisdom.

With specialization of trauma surgeons came the need for more specialized equipment and implants; hence the need for more detailed manuals, such the *Manual of Fracture Management—Wrist* and now, this important contribution on foot and ankle trauma: the *Manual of Fracture Management—Foot and Ankle*. Trauma to the distal tibia, the ankle and the foot bones are common in polytrauma as well as more isolated trauma to that anatomical region and are too often a source of continuing and significant disability.

This book deserves a place in the library of all surgeons managing foot, ankle, and distal tibial trauma. The text is arranged in a case-based format, is comprehensive and very well organized. Each case study discusses general considerations of that specific injury, decision making about open or closed treatment, preoperative planning, surgical approaches, risks and complications, alternative techniques, and rehabilitation. The book is beautifully illustrated, and the tips on each case valuable to the reader and written by acknowledged experts in that field. The 644 pages "cover the waterfront" and will become an essential manual for all surgeons dealing with operative care of fractures.

This book is a logical extension of the education process started by the AO Group in 1958 and furthers the importance of the education pillar to improve patient outcomes in this important anatomical area of trauma.

Marvin Tile
Joseph Schatzker

Dedication

We would like to dedicate this book to our AO teachers and colleagues.

Through the years, we discussed and improved the AO techniques which have led to better treatment of foot and ankle injuries. We have been blessed to work with many skilled surgeons throughout the world who donated their time, knowledge, and enthusiasm to AO events, courses, and committees. Listing them all would invariably lead to omissions. Luckily, several of them agreed to contribute their cases and ideas to this book.

Specifically, we dedicate this book to two persons who shaped the AO foot and ankle world as it is today and whose thoughts you will find throughout this book.

We would like to honor Hans Zwipp who was instrumental in spreading the AO principles through Europe and to the rest of the world. He has been a friend, mentor, and a true AO leader.

We share a special note of appreciation to Sigvard T Hansen Jr. He was the pioneer who brought the AO principles of rigid internal fixation to the foot. He was instrumental in championing functional and structural salvage of foot and ankle injuries and their reconstruction after injury. He is truly a friend to all and the man who brought all of us throughout the world together under the AO banner.

Preface

The human foot is a unique and delicate structure. Phylogenetically, it is the youngest part of our locomotor system and can be affected by atavistic traits. The ankle cannot be separated from the foot as it is instrumental in converting the vertical forces from the leg to the horizontal or uneven ground for standing, walking, running, and jumping. It is evident, that even slight deviations from the physiological axial alignment and any step-off in a weight-bearing joint will potentially have serious consequences for the affected patient. Therefore, restoring alignment, joint congruity and stability is of utmost importance in the treatment of foot and ankle injuries.

There was a time when it was commonly said that a person who sustained a severe foot or ankle injury was "done" as far as being able to be a productive member of the society. It has also been shown that in a multiply-injured person, after the life-threatening injuries are dealt with, it is the foot and ankle injuries that lead to the most prolonged disability. Still, foot and ankle fractures are overlooked in many patients either due to concomitant injuries or lack of knowledge of the signs of subtle but potentially disabling injuries.

Foot and ankle surgery has advanced considerably over the last few decades. Earlier treatment using casting, traction, pinning, and late bracing to bring a deformed foot straight to the ground, became early anatomical reduction and rigid internal fixation. This allowed functional aftertreatment which maximized function after foot and ankle injuries. A wide range of pedicled and free flaps using microvascular techniques have greatly enhanced the options for the treatment of, for example, open fractures and dislocations with serious soft tissue injury. However, although we can technically do everything surgically, we should not be tempted to use the full armamentarium in every case. Evaluation begins with the whole patient, taking into consideration their functional demands and comorbidities, in the process of obtaining the best individual result.

Although diagnostic techniques have greatly improved, a thorough clinical evaluation and knowledge of the correct projections and findings in plane x-rays, forms the basis of making the correct diagnosis—best practice is not to obtain a magnetic resonance image before touching the foot of the patient.

This book provides a step-by-step approach to the evaluation and management of a wide range of fractures, dislocations, and soft-tissue injuries to the foot and ankle. Based on the principles of AO teaching and learning that, like the surgical techniques, have evolved over the recent years, assessment and treatment of injuries from the tibial pilon to the toes is presented in a case-based manner.

It is our hope that this book helps patients worldwide receive better care and return to a more functional life. We also sincerely hope that the provided cases and solutions stimulate discussions and lead to further improvement of patient management and surgical techniques. This would truly reflect the AO spirit to which the contributors to this book are committed.

The Editors

Acknowledgments

Production and publication of the *Manual of Fracture Management —Foot and Ankle* would not have been possible without the dedication and support of an extensive list of contributors. From AO surgeons donating their time within the various education committees and working groups, to our many colleagues that volunteered case notes and images, to the staff within our own medical practices, and to the teams at AOTrauma and AO Education Institute, we thank you for assisting us to develop this worthwhile publication.

While there are many people to thank, we would especially like to mention these individuals:

- Members of the AOTrauma Education Commission for recognizing the importance and significance of this educational opportunity and for approving the development of this publication.
- Urs Rüetschi and Robin Greene from the AO Education Institute for their guidance and expertise as well as for enabling extensive resources and staff to prepare this publication and make it into the best publication possible.
- The many distinguished colleagues from around the world who provided chapters despite their busy schedules.
- Marvin Tile and Joseph Schatzker for writing the Foreword to this book.
- Jecca Reichmuth, for the successful planning and management of this book project, as well as her guidance, support, and expertise throughout the production process.
- Carl Lau, Manager Publishing who ensured that the Publishing team were available to provide their professional support.
- Roman Kellenberger, the graphic designer responsible for the exclellent layout of this book.
- Marcel Erismann for the splendid illustration work.
- And finally, to our own families for their encouragement and never-ending support for our involvement with the AO Foundation's many activities—courses, committees, task forces—which culminated in this book project. Without their kind understanding, this venture would not have come to fruition.

Stefan Rammelt
Michael Swords
Mandeep S Dhillon
Andrew K Sands

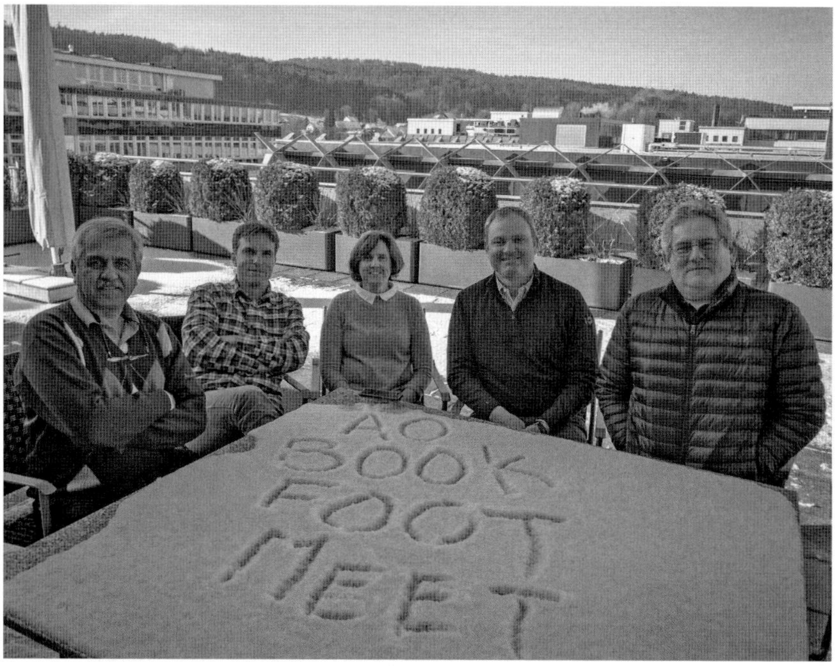

Editorial book meeting, January 2019, Dübendorf, Switzerland

Online Educational Content

Abundant online educational offerings from across AO are accessible through the QR codes printed on each chapter title page. Also included are the journal references linked to PubMed. Using a QR code scanner on a mobile device, readers will be taken to specific chapter microsites that contain this chapter-specific content.

Links to supplemental AO educational content include:

- AO Surgery Reference
- Webinars and webcasts
- Lectures
- Teaching videos
- AO/OTA Fracture and Dislocation Classification

As the array of online AO educational resources evolves and develops, the AO offerings in the chapter microsites will be reviewed and updated by the book editors. This will ensure that readers are linked to the latest in AO education.

Contributors

Editors

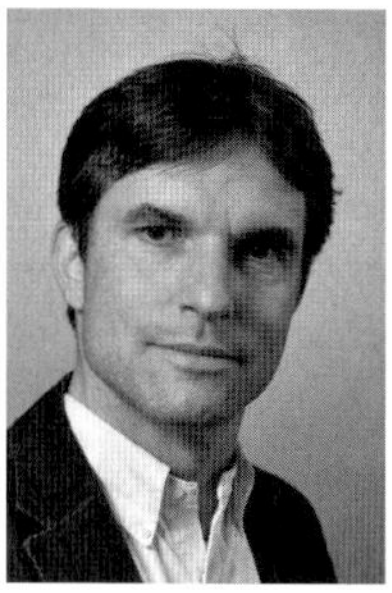

Stefan Rammelt, Prof Dr med
UniversitätsCentrum für Orthopädie und Unfallchirurgie
Universitätsklinikum Carl Gustav Carus
Fetscherstr 74
01307 Dresden
Germany

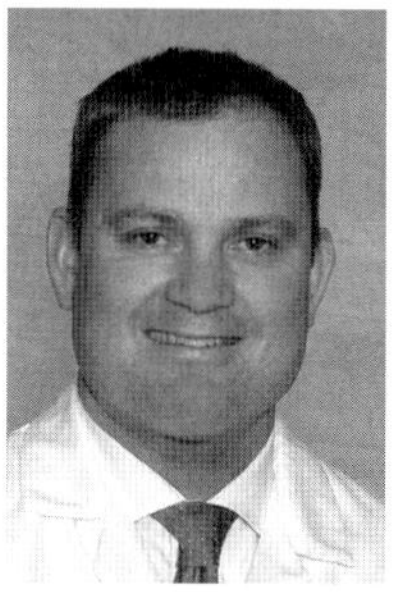

Michael Swords, DO
Michigan Orthopedic Center
Chair, Department of Orthopedic Surgery
Director of Orthopedic Trauma
Sparrow Hospital
Lansing, Michigan
USA

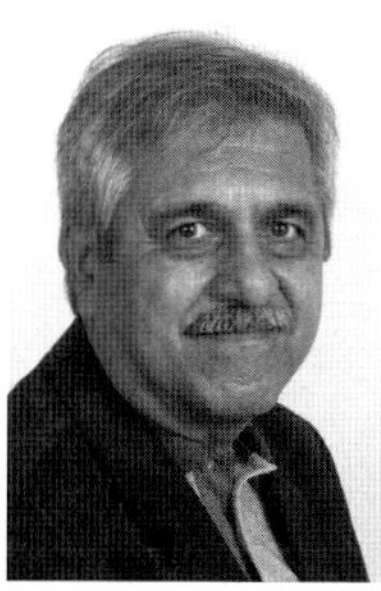

Mandeep S Dhillon, MBBS, MS, FAMS, FRCS
Professor and Chair, Department of Orthopaedic Surgery
Chair, Dept of Physical Medicine and Rehabilitation
Post Graduate Institute of Medical Education and Research, Sector 12
Chandigarh 160012
India

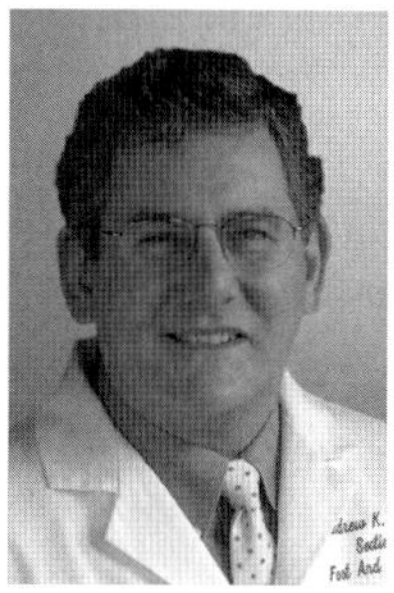

Andrew K Sands, MD
Clinical Associate Professor of Orthopedic Surgery
Weill Cornell Medical College
Chief, Foot & Ankle Surgery,
Downtown Orthopedic Associates
NYP-Lower Manhattan Hospital
170 William Street
Department of Orthopedics
New York, NY 10038
USA

Authors

Arun Aneja, MD, PhD
Assistant Professor of Orthopedic Surgery
University of Kentucky Medical Center
Orthopaedic Surgery
740 South Limestone
K401 Kentucky Clinic
Lexington, KY 40536-0284
USA

Mathieu Assal, MD, PD
President, Swiss Foot & Ankle Society
FMH chirurgie orthopédique et traumatologie
Clinique La Colline
Avenue de Beau-Séjour 6
1206 Genève
Switzerland

Jan Bartoníček, Prof MUDr, DrSc
Head of Department of Orthopaedics
Central Military Hospital Prague
UVN Praha
U Vojenské nemocnice
169 02 Prague 6
Czech Republic

Omkar Baxi, MD
Orthopedic Surgery Resident
Rutgers New Jersey Medical School University Hospital
140 Bergen St, Suite D-1610
Newark NJ 07103
USA

Marschall Berkes, MD
Assistant Professor
Washington University School of Medicine
660 S Euclid Ave
Campus Box 8233
St Louis MO 63110
USA

Candice Brady, DO
Orthopedic Surgeon
400 Camarillo Ranch Road
Unit 101
Camarillo, CA 93012
USA

Richard E Buckley, MD, FRCS
Professor
Foothills Medical Center NW
0490 Ground Floor, McCaig Tower
3134 Hospital Drive
Calgary, AB T2N 5A1
Canada

Devendra K Chouhan, MD
Associate professor
Department of Orthopedics
Post Graduate Institute of Medical Education & Research (PGIMER)
Sector 12
Chandigarh 160012
India

Chrea Bopha, MD
University of Mississippi Medical Centre
2500 North State St
Jackson, MS 39216
USA

David Ciufo, MD
University of Rochester Medical Center
601 Elmwood Ave
Department of Orthopaedics
Box 665
Rochester, NY 14642
USA

Georgios Datsis, MD, PhD, FEBOT
Consultant Orthopaedic Foot & Ankle Surgeon
Cretan Foot Clinic Private Practice
59 Kapodistriou
Rethymno 74100
Greece

Mandeep S Dhillon, MBBS, MS, FAMS, FRCS
Professor and Chair, Department of Orthopaedic Surgery
Chair, Dept of Physical Medicine and Rehabilitation
Post Graduate Institute of Medical Education and Research, Sector 12
Chandigarh 160012
India

Juan Bernardo Gerstner Garces, MD
Head, Foot and Ankle Surgery
Centro Medico Imbanaco de Cali
Carrera 38#5A-100 Cons 233A
Cali
Colombia

Matthew L Graves, MD, FACS, FAOA
Hansjörg Wyss AO Medical Foundation Chair of Orthopaedic Trauma
Vice Chair, Professor, Residency Program Director
Department of Orthopaedic Surgery
University of Mississippi Medical Center
2500 North State Street
Jackson, MS 39216
USA

Christopher E Gross, MD
Department of Orthopaedics and Physical Medicine
96 Jonathan Lucas Street
MSC 622, Suite 708
Charleston, SC 29425
USA

Jens Anthony Halm, MD, PhD, FEBS (Trauma)
Amsterdam UMC, location AMC
Meibergdreef 9
1105 AZ Amsterdam
Netherlands

Kartik Hariharan, MB Bch, FRCS(I) FRCS(Orth)
Consultant Orthopaedic and Foot and Ankle Surgeon
Aneurin Bevan University Health Board
Royal Gwent Hospital
Cardiff Road
Newport South Wales NP26 3AD
United Kingdom

Michaël Houben, MD
Resident Orthopedic Surgery
MUMC+ Maastricht Netherlands
P. Debyelaan 25
6229 HX Maastricht
Netherlands

Konrad Kamin, Dr med
Consultant
UniversitätsCentrum für Orthopädie und Unfallchirurgie am Universitätsklinikum Carl Gustav Carus
Fetscherstr. 74
01307 Dresden
Germany

John Ketz, MD
Assistant Professor
University of Rochester Medical Center
601 Elmwood Ave
Department of Orthopaedics
Box 665
Rochester, NY 14642
USA

Lubomír Kopp, MD, PhD
Deputy to the head surgeon,
Head of Arthroscopic Centre
Clinic of Trauma Surgery
Masaryk Hospital
Sociální péče 3316/12A
400 11 Ústí nad Labem-Severní Terasa
Czech Republic

Steven J Lawrence, MD
Retired Professor of Orthopedic Surgery
Former Head of Foot and Ankle Orthopedic Surgery
University of Kentucky Medical Center
740 South Limestone
Lexington, KY 40536
USA

Keun-Bae Lee, MD, PhD
Professor, Chairman of Department of Orthopaedic Surgery
Director of Foot and Ankle Service
Director of Orthopaedic Trauma Service
Director of Biomedical Research Institute at CNUH
Chonnam National University Hospital (CNUH)
Republic of Korea

Sheldon Lin, MD
Associate Professor
Chief Foot Ankle Division
Department of Orthopaedics
Rutgers New Jersey Medical School
90 Bergen Street, Suite 7300
Newark, NJ 07101
USA

May Fong Mak, FRCSEd (Orth)
Consultant Orthopaedic Surgeon
Department of Orthopaedics
Waikato Hospital
Waikato District Health Board
Pembroke Street
Hamilton 3240
New Zealand

Jitendra Mangwani, MS (Orth), FRCS (Trauma and Orth)
Consultant Orthopaedic Foot and Ankle Surgeon
University Hospitals of Leicester
Honorary Fellow, University of Leicester
Infirmary Square
Leicester LE1 5WW
United Kingdom

Arthur Manoli II, MD
Clinical Professor
Departments of Orthopaedic Surgery,
Wayne State University
Detroit, MI 48201
Michigan State University
College of Osteopathic Medicine
East Lansing, MI 48824
USA

Khairul Faizi Mohammad, BMedSci (Hons), BMBS (Nottingham), MRCS(Edin), MSOrth (UKM)
Consultant Orthopaedic Foot and Ankle Surgeon
Pantai Hospital
Kuala Lumpur Foot Ankle Clinic
Suite 3.21, Pantai Hospital Cheras
No1 Jalan 1/96a, Taman Cheras Makmur
56000 Kuala Lumpur
Malaysia

John W Munz, MD
Associate Professor, Department of Orthopedic Surgery–UT Health
Orthopedic Trauma Service
Walter R. Lowe, MD, Professorship
Memorial Hermann-Texas Medical Center
6400 Fannin Street
Houston, TX 77030
USA

Petr Obruba, MUDr, PHD
Senior Consultant
Masaryk's Hospital Ústí nad Labem
Klinika úrazové chirurgie
Masarykova nemocnice
Sociální péče 3316/12A
401 13 Ústí nad Labem
Czech Republic

Vinod Kumar Panchbhavi, MD, FACS Prof
Chief, Division of Foot & Ankle Surgery
Director, Foot & Ankle Fellowship Program
Department of Orthopedic Surgery
301 University Blvd
Galveston, TX 77555-0165
USA

Selene G Parekh, MD, MBA, FAOA
Professor, Department of Orthopaedic Surgery
Duke University
3609 SW Durham Drive
Durham, NC 27707
USA

Sampat Dumbre Patil, MBBS, D(Ortho), DNB(Ortho), MNAMS
Director, Orthopedic Department
Consultant Orthopedic and Foot & Ankle Surgeon
Sahyadri Super Speciality Hospital
Hadapsar
Pune, Maharashtra
India

Martijn Poeze,MD, PhD, MSc
Professor of Trauma Surgery
Maastricht University Medical Center
P. Debyelaan 25
6202 AZ Maastricht
Netherlands

Sharad Prabhakar, MBBS, MS (Ortho)
Additional Professor
Post Graduate Institute of Medical Education and Research
Department of Orthopedics
Sector 12
Chandigarh
India

Stefan Rammelt, Prof Dr med
UniversitätsCentrum für Orthopädie und Unfallchirurgie
Universitätsklinikum Carl Gustav Carus
Fetscherstr 74
01307 Dresden
Germany

Andrew Sands, MD
Clinical Associate Professor of Orthopedic Surgery
Weill Cornell Medical College
Chief, Foot & Ankle Surgery,
Downtown Orthopedic Associates
NYP-Lower Manhattan Hospital
170 William Street
Department of Orthopedics
New York, NY 10038
USA

Tim Schepers, MD, PhD
Trauma Surgeon
Amsterdam UMC
Trauma Unit, Location AMC
Meibergdreef 9
1105 AZ Amsterdam
Netherlands

Rajiv Shah, MBBS, MS
Director, Foot & Ankle Orthopaedics
Sunshine Global Hospital
Behind ICICI bank, near Shreyas School
Manjalpur 390011
Vadodara, Gujarat State
India

Shivam Shah, MBBS
Orthopaedic Resident
SSG Hospital, Vadodara
Department of Orthopaedics
Sir Sayajirao General Hospital
Vadodara
India

John R Shank, MD
Orthopaedic Surgeon
Colorado Center of Orthopaedic Excellence
2446 Research Pkwy #200
Colorado Springs, CO 80920
USA

Siddhartha Sharma, MD, FRCS (Ed)
Assistant Professor
Postgraduate Institute of Medical Education and Research
Department of Orthopaedics
Sector 12
Chandigarh 160012
India

Michael Swords, DO
Michigan Orthopedic Center
Chair, Department of Orthopedic Surgery
Director of Orthopedic Trauma
Sparrow Hospital
Lansing, Michigan
USA

Kar Hao Teoh, Dip SICOT, FEBOT, FRCS (T&O)
Consultant Foot and Ankle Surgeon
Department of Trauma & Orthopaedics
Princess Alexandra Hospital
Hamstel Rd, Harlow, CM20 1QX
United Kingdom

Matthew Tomlinson, MB ChB, FRACS
Clinical Director, Deptartment of Orthopaedic Surgery
Middlemore Hospital
Counties Manukau Health
100 Hospital Road
Otahuhu
Auckland 1640
New Zealand

Joseph Tracey, MS
Research Fellow
Medical University of South Carolina
96 Jonathan Lucas Street CSB. 708
Charleston, SC 29425
USA

Georgina Wright, MD
Consultant Orthopaedic Surgeon
Colchester General Hospital
Turner Road
Colchester CO45JL
United Kingdom

Michael Yeranosian, MD
Resident Orthopaedic Surgeon
Rutgers New Jersey Medical School
140 Bergen St, Suite D-1610
Newark, NJ 07103
USA

Abbreviations

2D	two-dimensional
3D	three-dimensional
ADTA	anterior distal tibial angle
AITFL	anterior-inferior tibiofibular ligament
AP	anteroposterior
ATA	anterior tibial artery
ATFL	anterior tibiofibular ligament
CAM	controlled-ankle-motion
CS	compartment syndrome
CT	computed tomography(ic)
DVT	deep vein thrombosis
EHB	extensor hallucis brevis
EHL	extensor hallucis longus
ELA	extended lateral approach
FCS	foot compartment syndrome
FDL	flexor digitorum longus
FHL	flexor hallucis longus
FHB	flexor hallucis brevis
I&D	irrigation and debridement
IP	interphalangeal
IT	intertarsal
LCP	locking compression plate
MAP	mean arterial pressure
MCS	medial clear space
MIO	minimally invasive osteosynthesis
MIPO	minimally invasive plate osteosynthesis
MRI	magnetic resonance imaging
MT	metatarsal
MTP	metatarsophalangeal
NWB	nonweight bearing/nonweight-bearing
OR	operating room
ORIF	open reduction and internal fixation
PA	peroneal artery
PA	pronation-abduction
PTA	posterior tibial artery
PER	pronation-external rotation
PIP	proximal interphalangeal
PTT	posterior tibial tendon
RIA	reamer-irrigator-aspirator
ROM	range of motion
SER	supination-external rotation
SPN	superior peroneal nerve
TCS	tibiofibular clear space
TMT	tarsometatarsal
TN	talonavicular
VA	variable angle
VA LCP	variable angle locking compression plate
VAL	variable angle locking
WB	weight bearing/weight-bearing

Malleoli

Calcaneus

Metatarsals

Phalanges and sesamoid

Appendix

1 Introduction

Introduction

1 General considerations in foot and ankle surgery

Andrew K Sands, Michael Swords, Mandeep S Dhillon, Stefan Rammelt

1 Anesthesia

There are several options for anesthesia for foot and ankle procedures. Many procedures are performed with patients under general anesthesia. If there is an associated head trauma or pulmonary injury, anesthesia modifications may be required. Reduction of displaced injuries requires adequate relaxation. Often the best combination for pain relief both during surgery and in the postoperative period is general anesthesia plus a regional block. When the regional block is performed immediately before the surgical procedure, less narcotic is necessary as part of the general anesthesia that decreases the risk of adverse side effects. If an accurate assessment of pain or neurological status is required, such as in suspected compartment syndrome, then regional anesthesia should be avoided.

Spinal, epidural, and combined spinal-epidural are all effective means of anesthesia for surgical procedures in the lower extremity. The use of short-acting agents prevents delay in the ability to ambulate. In emergency situations regional techniques are useful in patients with contraindications to general anesthesia, such as critical medical conditions or recent meal intake. Spinal anesthesia is contraindicated in patients with spinal disorders and in those taking anticoagulant agents.

Regional blocks can be used as the sole means of anesthesia for numerous foot and ankle surgical procedures. Some sedation is helpful when regional block without general anesthesia is used.

Appropriate supervision of blood pressure is an important aspect of anesthesia management. A good working relationship with the anesthesiology providers allows for appropriate control of the pressure throughout the procedure, especially at the end of surgery if allowing the pressure to rise might result in excessive bleeding when the tourniquet is released. The patient must be kept sufficiently sedated until the postoperative splint is in place and secured. Allowing the patient to awaken too early with excessive motion can compromise the surgical repair. To prevent such a situation good communication with anesthesia providers is paramount.

At the end of the procedure, supplemental medication may be given to assist with the patient transitioning from the operating room (OR) to the next phase of care. Options include standard local anesthetic at the surgery site, liposomal bupivacaine if available, antiinflammatory medication, or narcotic medication. A patient-controlled anesthesia pump allows for additional intravenous delivery of pain medicine on demand.

2 Antibiotics

The use of single-dose antibiotics in the immediate preoperative phase is current standard of practice in most countries. Usually, orthopedic surgery routine antibiotic prophylaxis is considered the standard of care. Patients who receive appropriate antibiotic prophylaxis are about half as likely to acquire a surgical site infection compared with those without chemoprophylaxis. A systematic analysis of randomized controlled trials provided evidence that antibiotic prophylaxis reduces subsequent infection after open fractures and that courses as short as 1 day are as effective as courses of 3–5 days.

For several reasons, the incidence of surgical site infections in foot and ankle surgery is higher than in other orthopedic subspecialties. The incidence rises further with individual risk factors like complicated diabetes mellitus. If postoperative antibiotics are administered, they should be discontinued within 24 hours.

Antibiotics are given intravenously within 60 minutes before the incision. In practice, they are administered by the anesthesiologist. Confirmation of administration of the preoperative antibiotic should be included as part of the preoperative time-out. The amount given is based on patient body mass index and duration of surgery.

If antibiotics are given in the emergency department because of an open injury, then they might not be needed in the OR again if administered within 60 minutes of the surgical incision. After initial debridement and irrigation of open fractures and wounds, antibiotics are continued until secondary wound closure but not beyond 72 hours from the surgery.

The standard antibiotic used for foot and ankle surgery is 2 g of first-generation cephalosporin given intravenously, with a higher dose administered in the morbid obese population. For patients with true allergy, 900 mg of clindamycin is given. For procedures lasting several hours, a repeat dose of the same antibiotic should be considered after 3 hours of surgery.

Administering antibiotics when uisng external fixation is controversial. Most surgeons use the standard prophylactic protocol as outlined above when an external fixator is being applied. The routine uses of ongoing suppressive oral antibiotics when an external fixator is in place is controversial.

3 Patient positioning

Proper patient positioning is essential for a successful surgery (**Fig 1-1**–**Fig 1-3**). Hence, preplanning is imperative when deciding the necessary approaches. The operating surgeon is responsible for correct patient positioning. Proper airway management and intravenous access is established by the anesthesia team. Adequate cushioning of bony prominences (elbow, pelvis, knee, ankle) of both the operative and nonoperative limb is important to avoid skin lesions from local pressure. The patient must be properly secured to the operative table, particularly when tilting of the table is intended. With the patient supine, a bump placed under the ipsilateral pelvis is helpful to bring the foot in a neutral position.

A ramp can be placed under the operative leg. This elevates the operative site out of the plane of the other leg, which allows unobstructed C-arm images. A towel bump may also be added to further elevate the foot. The towel bump is also helpful in unweighting the heel that may help in ankle trauma reduction. Care must be taken while positioning to prevent neuropraxia or stretch injury to the peripheral nerves. Special attention must be taken when the patient is in the lateral decubitus position to pad the peroneal nerve of the down leg (**Fig 1-3**).

In each chapter, specific positioning aids and variants of these standard positions are described.

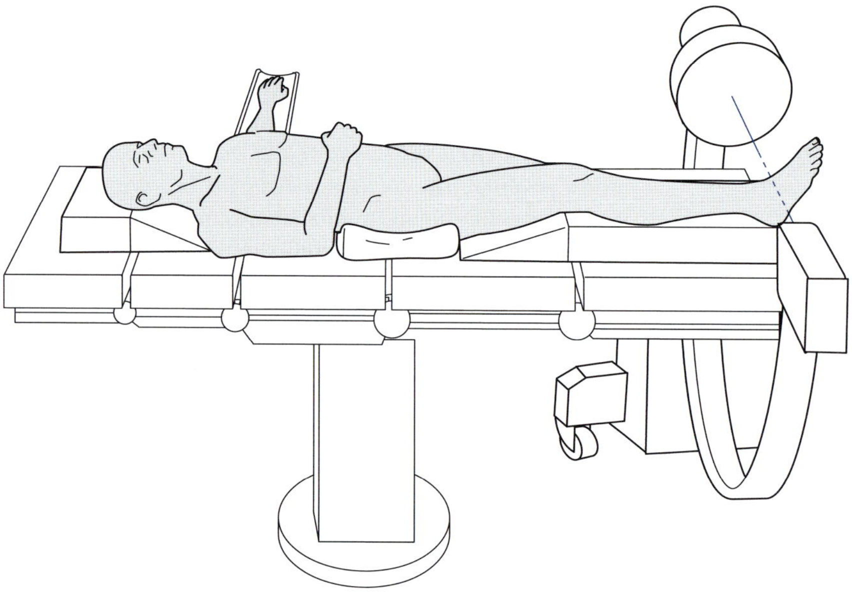

Fig 1-1 Supine position. Sheets/ blankets or a wedge raise the ipsilateral hip to avoid excessive external rotation of the leg. A foam ramp lifts the leg out of the plane of the other leg allowing for lateral imaging.

4 Imaging

Positioning

The C-arm is positioned from the foot of the bed/ipsilateral to the operative side allows the surgeon to directly manipulate the C-arm and leg to obtain all needed views. A mini-C-arm is useful for most foot and ankle procedures.

For flat panel display the panel can be placed on the bed, for AP and mortise views with rotation of the leg cautiously done from the proximal tibia. For the lateral view the heel can be placed on a towel bump (additionally, the operative leg is also elevated on the foam ramp). The C-arm is then rotated parallel to the floor allowing for unobstructed lateral views.

For an AP (dorsal-plantar) view of the foot, the C-arm can be manipulated so that the flat stage is under the sole of the foot and the radiation source is aimed inferiorly from an area just inferior to the knee. Alternatively, the stage can be placed flat on the table and the knee flexed to allow the foot to sit on the stage.

For a large C-arm (including 3D imaging), the stage should be placed under a radiolucent operative table.

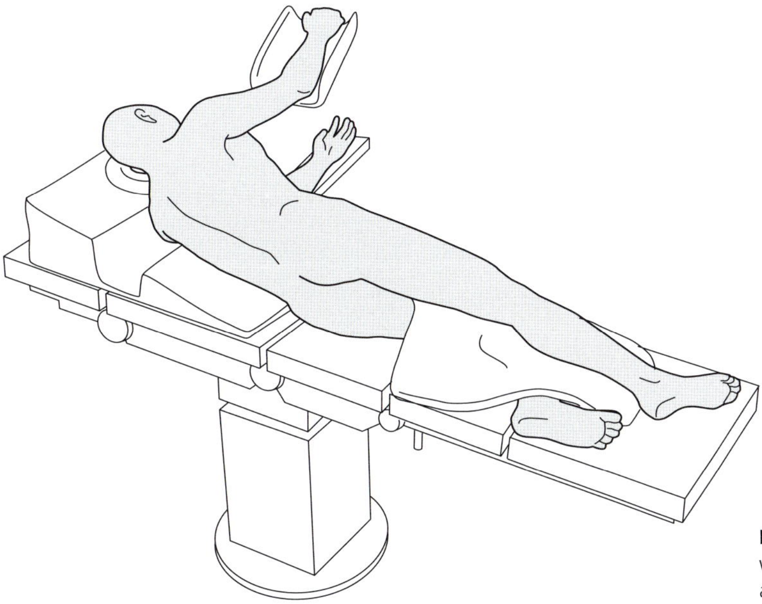

Fig 1-2 Lateral decubitus positioning with protective brachial plexus axillary roll and protective padding between the legs.

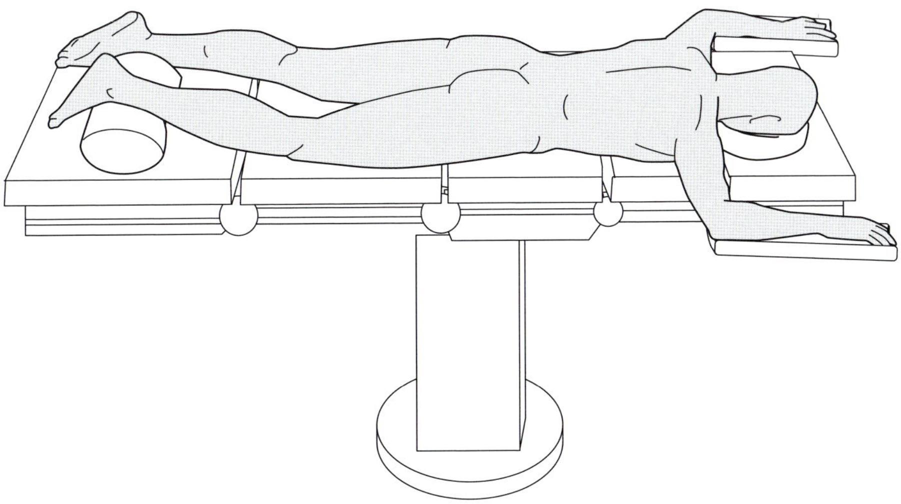

Fig 1-3 In the prone position, proper positioning must include checking the breasts and peroneal areas.

Safety

In general, lead shielding should be worn covering the body and pelvis of all members of the surgical team. Thyroid shields and leaded glasses should also be worn. For foot and ankle surgery, the patient is protected with a lead shielding under the body and pelvis.

In the case of the mini-C-arm, the safe distance is 50 cm. With large C-arms, the safe zone starts at 2 m (**Fig 1-4**). Staff members in the OR standing well within the safe zone are not necessarily required to wear radiation safety devices (**Fig 1-5**). Surgeons should keep their hands out of the field by using longer handled instruments and retractors.

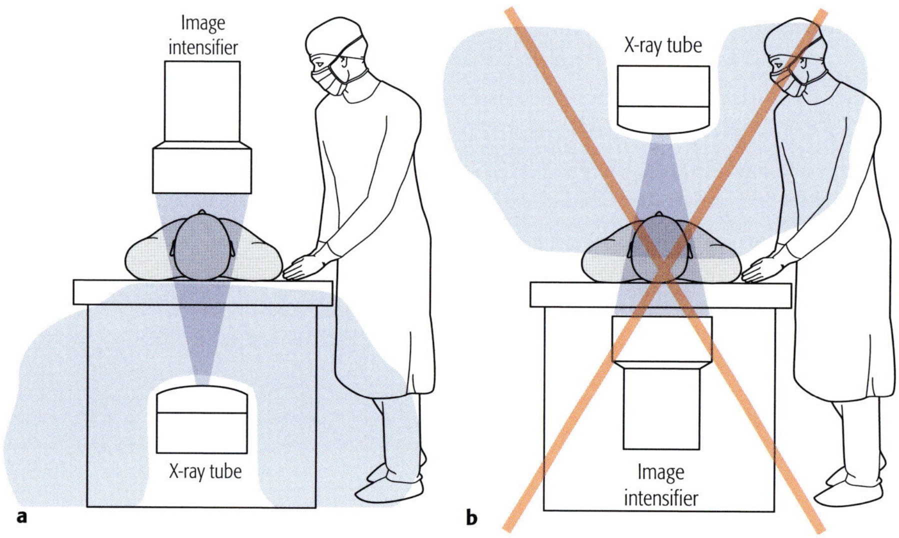

Fig 1-4a–b Positioning of the C-arm (image intensifier).
- **a** Minimize the distance between the image intensifier and the patient.
- **b** Positioning the x-ray tube above the patient creates higher doses of radiation exposure due to reflected and scattered radiation.

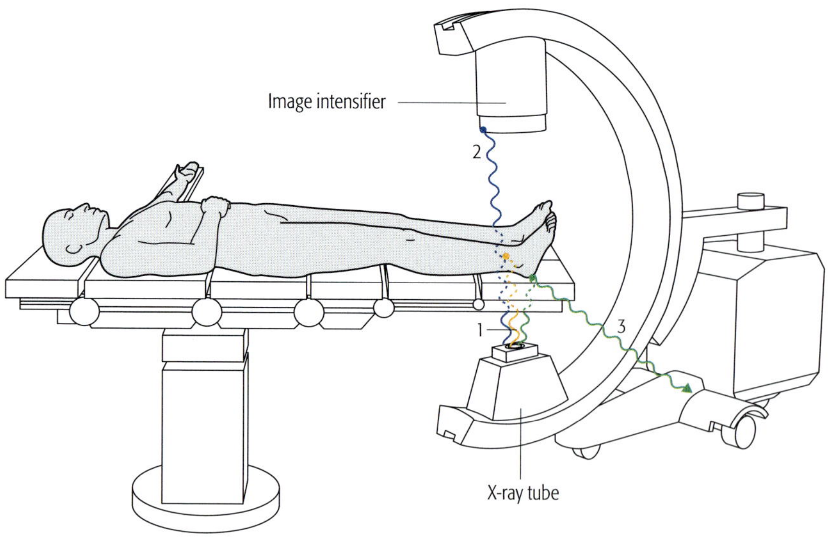

Fig 1-5 The x-ray tube generates radiation (1). After passing through the patient, the transmission (2) reaches the image intensifier. Scatter (3) is reflected from the patient and exposes the surgical team.

5 Skin preparation

Presurgical cleaning has been shown to enhance surgical skin preparation and lower the rates of surgical site infection. The patient may be given the prepackaged scrub sink sponges to use on the surgical site the night before and the morning of surgery. Alternatively, a footbath in chlorhexidine scrub solution before regular preoperative skin antisepsis in the OR significantly reduces the number of bacteria in the nailfolds, the web spaces, and at the site of surgical incision.

Decolonization with mupirocin ointment is recommended in nasal carriers of *Staphylococcus aureus* undergoing elective orthopedic surgery. Shaving the surgical site prior to surgery is strongly discouraged at any time. If absolutely necessary, hair should be removed only with a clipper.

The surgical site is disinfected with alcohol-based sticks containing chlorhexidine and then draped free for foot and ankle surgery. Several studies have confirmed higher infection rates following orthopedic procedures of the foot and ankle compared with procedures involving other areas of the body, which is most likely because of difficulty eliminating bacteria from the forefoot before surgery. There is evidence from high-quality studies that chlorhexidine in alcohol provides better preparation than povidone-iodine. Antimicrobial sealants should not be used after surgical site skin preparation

6 Tourniquet use

The tourniquet is typically placed at the top of the thigh. Leg or ankle tourniquets may be used with distal regional anesthesia. Caution should be taken to prevent extremely high unrecognized pressure under the cuff with resulting soft tissue crushing.

The tourniquet is applied over a cotton roll or fabric layer and the length chosen should be 1.5 times the diameter of the leg. Care must be taken to ensure that any irritating surgical preparation material does not seep into the protective material under the cuff, as it may cause skin irritation in the upper aspect of the thigh or perineum. Care must also be taken with inspection and manipulation to make certain the external genitalia are not incorporated under the cuff.

The pressure is set to 100 mm Hg over the mean arterial pressure (MAP). In older patients with calcification showed on x-ray, higher pressures may be used. If possible, the cuff should not be inflated and the surgery performed without tourniquet inflation. If anesthesia can safely maintain a lower MAP, then surgery without a tourniquet is possible.

Advantages of surgery performed with a tourniquet:

- Improved visualization of the surgical site both during dissection and during the procedure (particularly joint reduction)
- Decreased blood loss during the procedure

Advantages of surgery performed without a tourniquet:

- Less cuff irritation to the patient and a decreased need for anesthetic drugs
- Less reactive blood inflow when the tourniquet is deflated with less resultant blood loss

If the tourniquet is inflated, the maximum tourniquet time must not exceed 120 minutes. For longer lasting procedures the cuff is deflated, and surgery may continue. The use of direct pressure with lap pads, cautery, or commercially available hemostatic agents can assist with hemostasis once the cuff has been deflated. If additional time is required, or if the cuff is needed to control bleeding, then it may be reinflated after 20 minutes of being deflated. Longer tourniquet times may lead to increased risk of tourniquet-related nerve palsy.

7 Instruments and implants

Several useful instruments for fragment manipulation and fracture reduction in the foot and ankle are depicted in **Fig 1-6**. Screws and plates used around the foot and ankle are necessary in various sizes and shapes to accommodate the varied anatomy encountered (**Fig 1-7**). Specific implants for the different anatomical areas are described in the respective chapters. Surgeon preference will dictate the choices made. For the screws, larger shafts with smaller heads give increased strength and resistance to bending and torque that are more problematic in the foot, as it is not axially aligned. The smaller heads are helpful to avoid prominence under the skin since there is less soft-tissue coverage in this region. Countersinking screw heads or the use of headless screws can be considered around the joints. Obliquely inserted screws, as in the midfoot, must be inserted through the pocket hole to prevent dorsal cortex failure

8 Wound closure and dressing

If the wound is amenable to primary closure, the first deep layer (fascia) is closed with absorbable undyed braided material. Dyed suture, especially in the subcutaneous area, may be visible in lighter-skinned people. The subcutaneous layer is closed with interrupted stiches of monofilament absorbable suture. The skin should be closed with minimal tension. The use of absorbable suture makes suture removal in the office unnecessary.

If there is moderate tension in the wound, some form of vertical mattress suture can be used. However, undue tension on the sutures should be avoided.

If tension-free wound closure is impossible at the end of surgery, several options exist:

- The wound can be left open in the subcutaneous area and be covered with collagen-based artificial skin grafting for 3–5 days. After swelling has subsided, delayed primary wound closure is more easily done.
- Placement of a vacuum-assisted device over the wound.
- Skin extension which relieves the tension from the edges, ie, "pie crusting" (multiple small relaxing incisions in a staggered pattern).

The general treatment for open fractures and dislocations of the foot and ankle does not differ substantially from that in other body locations. For the grading of open fractures, the Gustilo-Anderson Classification (see appendix) is the most widely used. Early treatment consists of thorough debridement of all necrotic and devitalized tissue, copious lavage with normal saline and antiseptic (not antibiotic) solutions, reduction of gross deformities, and in most instances minimal internal and external fixation until soft tissue consolidation. Early soft-tissue coverage is essential in minimizing the risk of infection. If necrotic skin or subcutaneous tissue must be debrided at the time of surgery, then secondary skin grafting, local, or free tissue transfer should be considered.

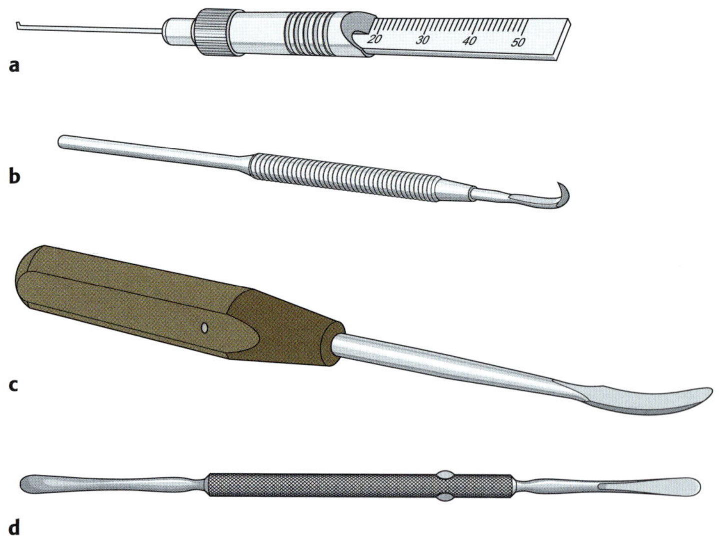

Fig 1-6a–f Instruments.
- **a** Depth gauge.
- **b** Dental scaler.
- **c** The "AO" periosteal elevator is more robust with a bigger tip, but it is unable to get into all the places unlike a dental scaler.
- **d** Small (Freer) elevator.

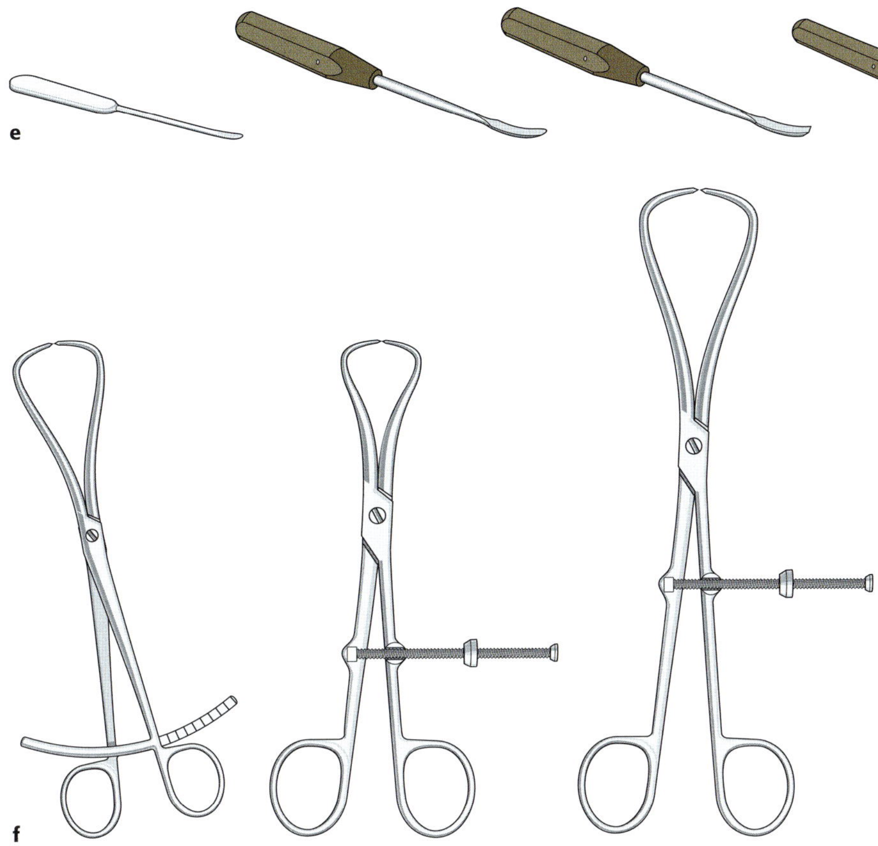

Fig 1-6a–f (cont) Instruments.

e Elevators of various sizes and shapes help approach and retract different areas of injury.

f Point-to-point reduction (Weber) clamps in various sizes. The advantage of this clamp is that the amount of pressure applied can be controlled.

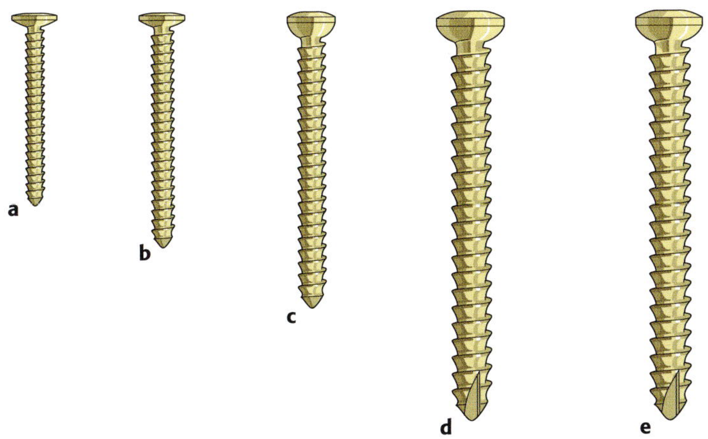

Fig 1-7a–e Frequently used cortex screws for foot and ankle fracture fixation.

a 2.0 mm

b 2.4 mm

c 2.7 mm

d 3.5 mm

e 4.0 mm

Once the wound is closed, it is covered with a nonadherent dressing. Some surgeons will additionally apply an antibacterial ointment to the incision area over the nonadherent dressing. This helps to keep the dressing in place when the outer layers are placed. It is then covered with sterile 4 x 4 and larger absorbent dressings. Next, web roll is wrapped from toes to knee, taking care to avoid wrinkles. If immobilization consists of a boot or postoperative shoe, an elastic wrap can be applied. Excessive compression should be avoided.

To prevent causing pressure points when a plaster splint is applied, it is molded so that it that does not close around the front of the foot and leg. The anterior and dorsal areas should be free of plaster to allow for expansion caused by swelling. The foot and leg are then overwrapped with elastic bandages, making certain all five toe tips are exposed, thus allowing for capillary refill testing. A prefabricated splint can be used as an alternative. It should be well padded.

9 Immobilization, rehabilitation, and weight-bearing precautions

Postoperative immobilization must balance the requirements necessary to prevent loss of fixation, encourage soft-tissue healing, and minimize immobilization of joints.

Loss of motion can result from prolonged immobilization. Long-term disability can occur from immobilization in the incorrect position, particularly equinus. With few exceptions (eg, tuberosity avulsion calcaneal fractures, certain Achilles-tendon procedures) the foot should be immobilized in a plantigrade neutral position (**Fig 1-8**). Range-of-motion (ROM) exercises should be started as soon as possible, as early motion even if nonweight bearing (NWB) allows for better healing of articular cartilage, ligament, and soft-tissue injuries, and helps prevent muscle atrophy of the surgical limb.

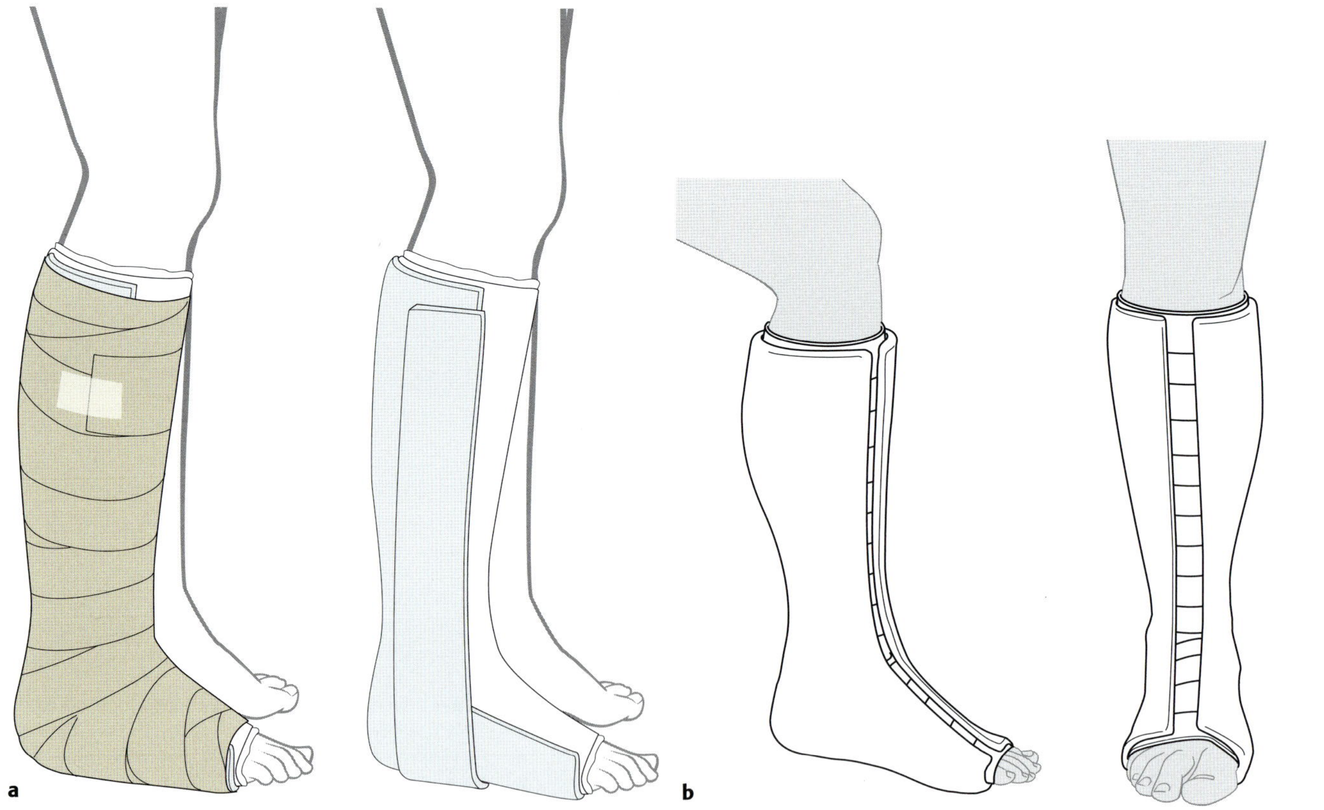

Fig 1-8a–b Postoperative immobilization of the foot and ankle with a 3-sided ("AO") splint (**a**) or below knee split plaster cast (**b**) left open in the front and in neutral position. The splint/cast is removed temporarily for ROM exercises.

Position of the foot, ankle, and leg in the postoperative period

The lower extremity should be kept level on the bed with adequate cushioning under the leg. A well-padded positioning splint can be used to keep the leg and foot in proper position (**Fig 1-9**). If the foot is positioned below the knee, patients feel pain and throbbing pressure. There is no need to elevate the leg above the heart. Excessive elevation can lead to problems with circulation and damage to the extremity, especially in the immediate postoperative period when the blood pressure level is often lower than normal. When sitting in a chair, the leg can be placed onto another chair or should be kept elevated (**Fig 1-10**).

When ambulation starts, the patient should be advised not to attempt to go too far, and to take breaks from ambulation with the foot elevated. This decreases the resultant swelling and throbbing pain. The patient can be switched from a splint to a fracture boot when the swelling has subsided and the wounds are stable.

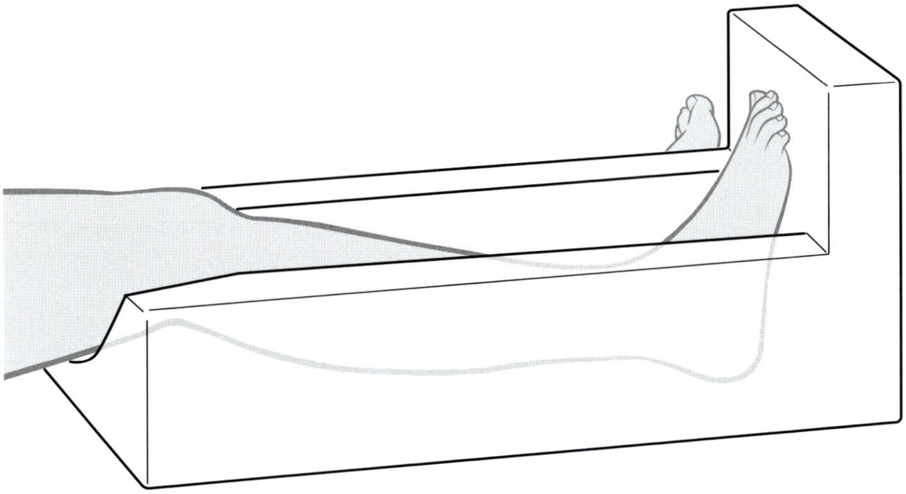

Fig 1-9 Padded device (Volkmann splint) for postoperative positioning and immobilization.

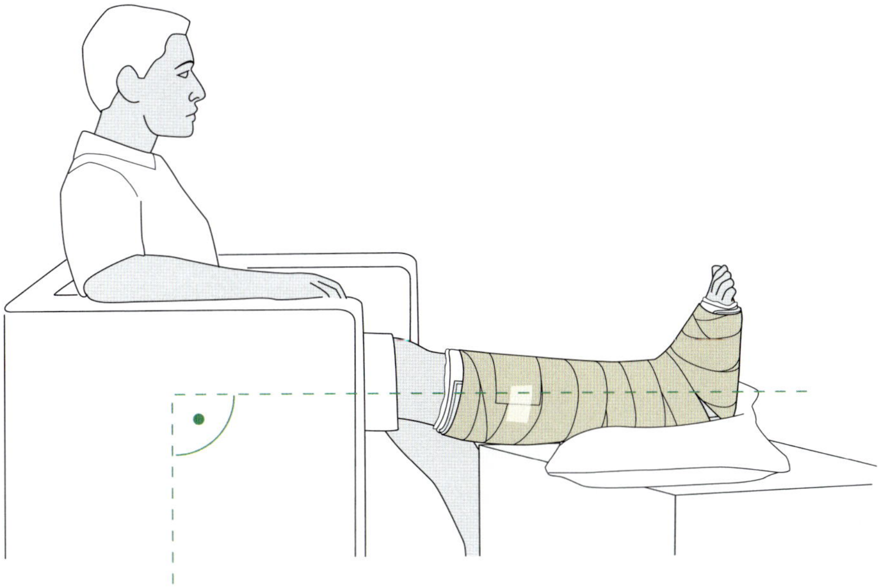

Fig 1-10 Foot position with the patient sitting in a chair.

In an outpatient setting, the 3-sided ("AO") splint (**Fig 1-11**) is removed at the first postoperative visit, usually within 2 weeks. The incisions are assessed for healing. Any non-absorbable sutures are evaluated for removal. The leg is cleaned. At this point the leg is placed into a fracture boot. A posterior splint in neutral can also be used to protect patients during sleep as they are often unwilling to wear the "outside the house" boot (which gets dirty outdoors) in bed. The posterior splint in neutral is left in the house. The boot can be removed for wound care and for ROM exercises. While the patient remains NWB, the boot can be removed and gentle motion can be started as early as possible.

If the surgeon desires, partial weight bearing (WB) of the operated leg with its own weight (typically 15–20 kg) is allowed in compliant patients. This regimen provides a stimulus for bone healing and increases venous return. Patients are instructed to control partial WB with a personal scale. In most cases, early NWB ROM is started but WB is delayed until x-ray evidence of healing occurs, usually at 5–6 weeks postoperatively. If the surgeon desires, gradual transition to full WB is initiated after radiographic evidence of bone healing, typically at 6 weeks after surgery but may be significantly longer depending on the type of injury. The exact timing may vary based on age and bone quality and specific injury and must be catered to the individual case. The patient advances from NWB with crutches, walker, or roll-a-bout device to progressive ambulation using a cane. If the patient is unreliable, or fixation is tenuous, then a short leg fiberglass or plaster cast is sometimes needed.

An individually fitted fiberglass cast shoe with a hard cast sole and soft cast cover (**Fig 1-12**) can be used in compliant patients together with partial WB of 15–20 kg after midfoot procedures. This cast shoe preserves ROM at the ankle, thus reducing the risk of venous thromboembolism.

Surgery on the toes, metatarsals, and some midfoot procedures may allow heel WB with a surgical forefoot-offloading shoe (**Fig 1-13**). This prevents excessive muscle atrophy from occurring and allows ROM at the ankle. A gel heel pad may be inserted into the postoperative shoe to prevent soreness of the heel from the altered gait.

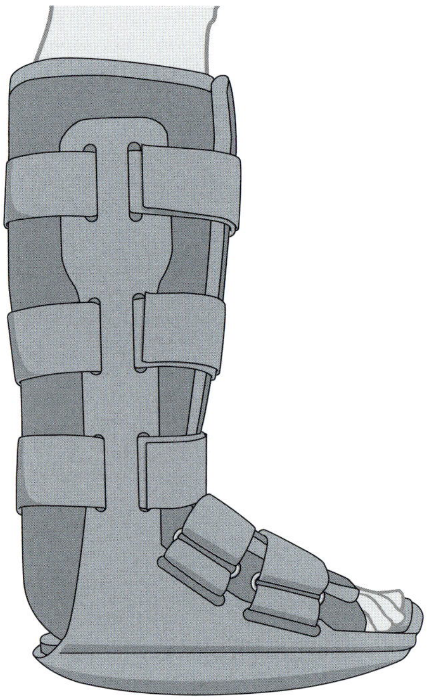

Fig 1-11 Padded, removable foot and ankle boot (controlled-ankle-motion [CAM]) for postoperative rehabilitation.

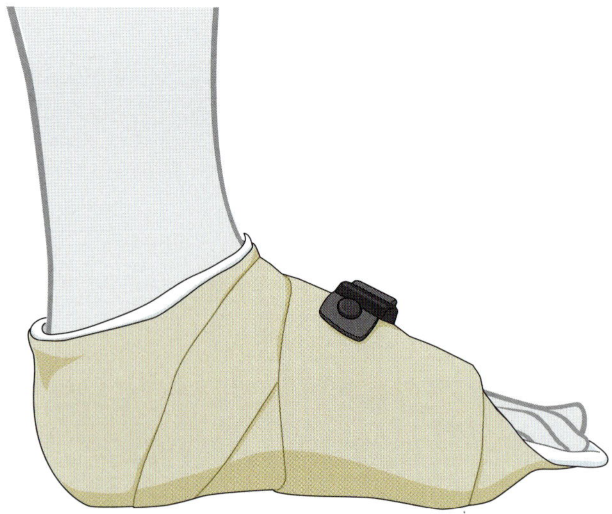

Fig 1-12 Individually fitted, removable cast shoe for rehabilitation after midfoot surgery.

Physical therapy

A good collaboration with physical therapists is paramount for regaining function after foot and ankle procedures. Physical therapy progresses in stages (**Table 1-1**).

Stage 1	• Education and training for altered WB and ROM restrictions as required by the procedure • Patient education should be part of the presurgical program and repeated postoperatively
Stage 2	• Decrease pain and swelling and progress to full WB • ROM exercises when nonambulatory
Stage 3	• Regain full ROM • Gait training
Stage 4	• Regain muscular strength and advance gait training • Muscular balancing
Stage 5	• Proprioception • Sport/activity specific therapy, ie, cutting or jumping

Table 1-1 Stages of physical therapy.

As physical therapy progresses, the foot is placed under increasing load and stress. So long as the progress is slow and gentle, the foot has a chance to adapt to the new stresses. If the physical therapy accelerates too quickly, the patient may have pain or injury or even failure of surgery. Each patient is different and some may return to normal function sooner than others. Secondary gain (litigation) or workers compensation issues may also influence therapy progress.

10 Anticoagulation

The overall incidence of clinically significant extremity deep vein thrombosis (DVT) following foot and ankle surgery is low. Reported rates of DVT range from 0 to 19% depending on the method of detection, the site of surgery, and postoperative immobilization. When looking at isolated lower extremity fractures of the tibia and distal bones, DVT rates range between 10 and 40%. The prevalence of fatal pulmonary embolism, the most dreaded complication from DVT, is below 1% in foot and ankle surgery. The clinical benefit of formal anticoagulation after foot and ankle surgery remains unclear.

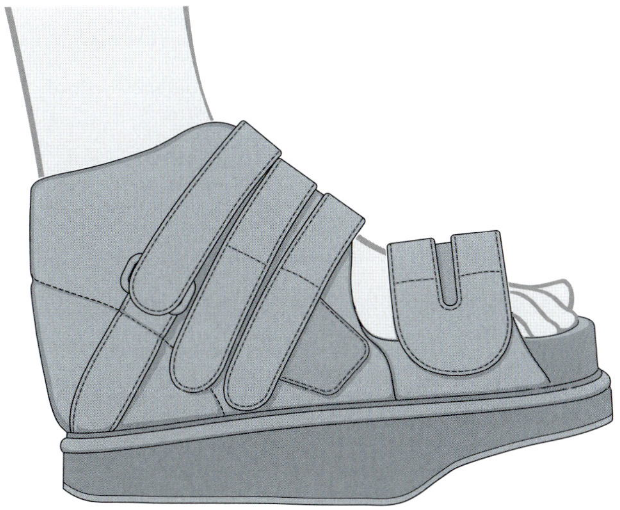

Fig 1-13 Forefoot-offloading shoe for rehabilitation after forefoot surgery.

Due to the low overall incidence of symptomatic thromboembolic events, anticoagulation is a controversial topic in patients with foot and ankle injuries. Many regional, local, and surgeon variations occur. In general, postoperative patients who are immobilized and have altered weight-bearing status are at increased risk for thromboembolic events. While most foot and ankle patients fit this description, there is no consensus on the need for anticoagulation. Additional risk factors include obesity, hormone replacement therapy or contraception, age greater than 50 years, trauma, Achilles tendon rupture, history of thromboembolic events, hypercoagulable states, and surgical procedures lasting more than 60 minutes. Thus, the indication to use anticoagulants is based on an individual risk evaluation of the patient and national guidelines that vary from country to country.

Usually if the surgeon concludes that anticoagulation is indicated for a patient, many options are available, and the choice is influenced by local practice norms. If anticoagulation is used, a low-molecular-weight heparin or one of the newer classes of antifactor-specific medications are the most common options. Aspirin is used by some surgeons as a cheap and low-risk alternative. The duration of therapy is not well established.

Importantly, prevention of thromboembolic events is not restricted to anticoagulative agents. It includes early definitive fracture fixation, physical measures, such as elastic dressings (lymphatic drainage), compression socks, venous pump, early motion, and WB of more than 20 kg, if feasible.

Complications associated with anticoagulation include wound drainage problems, hematoma, and the development of heparin-induced thrombocythemia, and major bleeding complications. However, the reported incidence of these adverse events is low. It is estimated that ten symptomatic DVT events are preventable for one major bleed.

11 Recommended reading

Allegranzi B, Zayed B, Bischoff P, et al. New WHO recommendations on intraoperative and postoperative measures for surgical site infection prevention: an evidence-based global perspective. *Lancet Infect Dis.* 2016 Dec;16(12):e288–e303.

Backes M, Dingemans SA, Dijkgraaf MGW, et al. Effect of antibiotic prophylaxis on surgical site infections following removal of orthopedic implants used for treatment of foot, ankle, and lower leg fractures: a randomized clinical trial. *JAMA.* 2017 Dec 26;318(24):2438–2445.

Bibbo C, Patel DV, Gehrmann RM, et al. Chlorhexidine provides superior skin decontamination in foot and ankle surgery: a prospective randomized study. *Clin Orthop Relat Res.* 2005 Sep;438:204–208.

Brenner P, Rammelt S, Gavlik JM, et al. Early soft tissue coverage after complex foot trauma. *World J Surg.* 2001 May;25(5):603–609.

Chang Y, Kennedy SA, Bhandari M, et al. Effects of antibiotic prophylaxis in patients with open fracture of the extremities: a systematic review of randomized controlled trials. *JBJS Rev.* 2015 Jun 9;3(6).

Dingemans SA, Spijkerman IJB, Birnie MFN, et al. Preoperative disinfection of foot and ankle: microbiological evaluation of two disinfection methods. *Arch Orthop Trauma Surg.* 2018 Oct;138(10):1389–1394.

Galanaud JP, Monreal M, Kahn SR. Epidemiology of the post-thrombotic syndrome. *Thromb Res.* 2018 Apr;164:100–109.

Gillespie WJ, Walenkamp GH. Antibiotic prophylaxis for surgery for proximal femoral and other closed long bone fractures. *Cochrane Database Syst Rev.* 2010 Mar 17(3):Cd000244.

Gustilo RB, Anderson JT. Prevention of infection in the treatment of one thousand and twenty-five open fractures of long bones: retrospective and prospective analyses. *J Bone Joint Surg Am.* 1976 Jun;58(4):453–458.

Hickey BA, Watson U, Cleves A, et al. Does thromboprophylaxis reduce symptomatic venous thromboembolism in patients with below knee cast treatment for foot and ankle trauma? A systematic review and meta-analysis. *Foot Ankle Surg.* 2018 Feb;24(1):19–27.

Hromádka R, Barták V, Popelka S, et al. Ankle block implemented through two skin punctures. *Foot Ankle Int.* 2010 Jul;31(7):619–623.

Jeng CL, Torrillo TM, Rosenblatt MA. Complications of peripheral nerve blocks. *Br J Anaesth.* 2010 Dec;105 Suppl 1:i97–107.

Lachman JR, Elkrief JI, Pipitone PS, et al. Comparison of surgical site infections in ankle fracture surgery with or without the use of postoperative antibiotics. *Foot Ankle Int.* 2018 Nov;39(11):1278–1282.

Modha MRK, Morriss-Roberts C, Smither M, et al. Antibiotic prophylaxis in foot and ankle surgery: a systematic review of the literature. *J Foot Ankle Res.* 2018;11:61.

Ng AB, Adeyemo FO, Samarji R. Preoperative footbaths reduce bacterial colonization of the foot. *Foot Ankle Int.* 2009 Sep;30(9):860–864.

Ohge H, Takesue Y, Yokoyama T, et al. An additional dose of cefazolin for intraoperative prophylaxis. *Surg Today.* 1999;29(12):1233–1236.

Ostrander RV, Botte MJ, Brage ME. Efficacy of surgical preparation solutions in foot and ankle surgery. *J Bone Joint Surg Am.* 2005 May;87(5):980–985.

Patterson JT, Morshed S. Chemoprophylaxis for venous thromboembolism in operative treatment of fractures of the tibia and distal bones: a systematic review and meta-analysis. *J Orthop Trauma.* 2017 Sep;31(9):453–460.

Prince RM 3rd, Lubberts B, Buda M, et al. Symptomatic venous thromboembolism after nonoperatively treated foot or ankle injury. *J Orthop Res.* 2019 Jan;37(1):190–196.

Richey JM, Ritterman Weintraub ML, Schuberth JM. Incidence and risk factors of Smptomatic venous thromboembolism following foot and ankle surgery. *Foot Ankle Int.* 2019 Jan;40(1):98–104.

Tantigate D, Jang E, Seetharaman M, et al. Timing of antibiotic prophylaxis for preventing surgical site infections in foot and ankle surgery. *Foot Ankle Int.* 2017 Mar;38(3):283–288.

2 Distal tibia

Distal tibia

2 Distal tibia/pilon fractures

Michael Swords

1 Introduction

Pilon fractures are rare, accounting for less than 10% of fractures around the ankle. The soft tissue in the distal tibia is unforgiving with poor soft-tissue coverage, increasing the difficulty of fracture management. Pilon fractures are known for comminution, displacement of the articular surface, and soft-tissue injury. Most fractures will require operative fixation due to alteration in joint congruency and overall limb alignment. Definitive operative treatment should be catered to the specific fracture pattern, soft-tissue injury, and patient. Appropriate timing of surgical treatment is essential for successful outcomes.

2 Anatomy and pathomechanics

The distal tibia is a relatively subcutaneous bone. Soft-tissue coverage at the ankle level is minimal, consisting almost entirely of skin and tendon. As a result, injuries in this area must be managed carefully. Open injuries require emergent management and may require free-tissue transfer depending on severity. Due to the subcutaneous nature of the ankle, grossly displaced fragments may lead to soft-tissue necrosis if left displaced.

The medial border of the tibia flares out and terminates in the medial malleolus with the deltoid attachment. The anterolateral surface has the tubercle of Chaput and the attachment of the anterior inferior tibiofibular ligament. The posterior portion of the tibia is the attachment site of the posterior tibiofibular ligament. Laterally the tibia has the incisura fibularis, and the interosseus ligament and membrane. Screws directed from medial to lateral must be measured accurately as the AP x-ray may not accurately reflect screw length.

The extensor tendons of the foot and ankle are contained in the anterior compartment along with the anterior tibial artery and the deep peroneal nerve. Anteriorly displaced fragments may compromise perfusion of the dorsum of the foot by occluding the anterior tibial artery (**Fig 2-1**). The lateral compartment contains the peroneus brevis and longus muscles. The superficial peroneal nerve is vulnerable as it crosses the fibula and moves anterior over the distal tibia and ankle. It must be identified and protected with anterior and anterolateral approaches. The deep posterior compartment contains the flexor hallucis longus (FHL), which originates on the fibula and crosses the posterior ankle to run on the medial side of the foot. The muscle belly and tendon of the FHL must be identified and retracted with posterior approaches. The tibial nerve and the posterior tibial artery are also in the deep posterior compartment between the FHL, the flexor digitorum longus (FDL), and posterior tibialis tendons. The posterior tibial tendon may become entrapped with displaced fractures that exit along the posteromedial border of the tibia, blocking reduction. The Achilles tendon, Kager's fat pad, the gastrocnemius and soleus muscles are in the posterior compartment. The Achilles sheath (peritendineum) is left undisturbed in posterior approaches. The sural nerve transitions from midline at the mid level of the tibia to posterolateral at the level of the ankle.

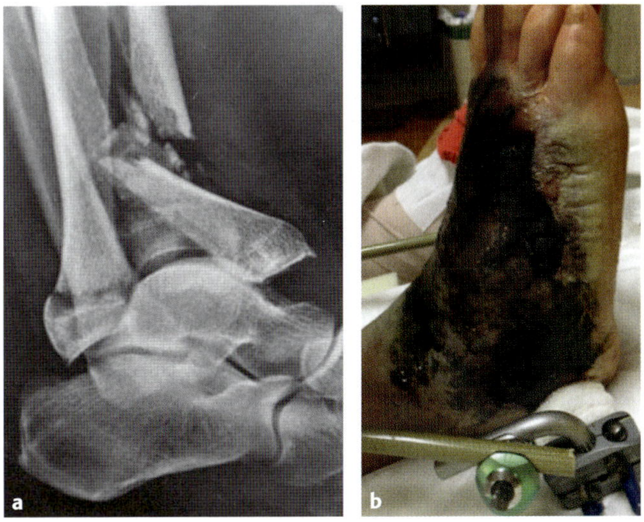

Fig 2-1a–b Lateral x-ray revealing a tibial pilon fracture with severe displacement of the anterior fragment resulting in occlusion of the anterior tibial artery (**a**). The fragment was not addressed urgently resulting in complete necrosis of the skin on the dorsum of the foot (**b**).

Fractures are typically the result of an axial load. Roughly 60–70% will have an associated fibular fracture. The dome of the talus impacts on the articular surface of the tibia resulting in a fracture. Often, a bending component occurs secondarily resulting in failure in tension on one side of the tibia and failure in compression on the other. The amount of comminution and displacement of fracture fragments is directly related to the amount of energy. The fracture pattern seen at the articular level consists of three main fragments: a medial fragment, an anterior or anterolateral fragment, and a posterior fragment (**Fig 2-2**). Comminution generally occurs where the fracture lines meet. Each of the three major fragments may be comminuted and have additional fracture lines.

Preservation of the vascular supply is important. The soft tissues should be handled with care and retracted only as necessary to avoid wound healing problems. Excessive stripping of fragments should be avoided to prevent devascularizing fracture segments.

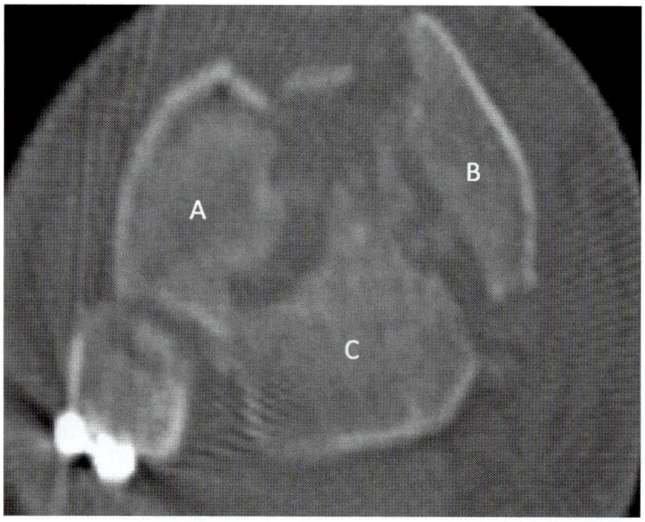

Fig 2-2 Type C pilon fractures typically result in three major articular fragments: anterior (A), medial (B), and posterior (C).

3 Fracture classification

Fractures of the distal end segment of the tibia in the AO/OTA Fracture and Dislocation Classification system are assigned the number 43, which is applicable for pilon fractures. The classification divides the fractures in to three types:

- 43A fractures include extraarticular fractures
- 43B fractures include partial articular fractures of the distal end segment of the tibia
- 43C fractures are complete articular fractures

Each fracture type can be further classified into groups and subgroups to better describe and code the particular injury. Qualifications are also included in the classification at certain levels to further describe fracture line locations with more precision. See the appendix for information on the AO/OTA classification of distal tibial (pilon) fractures.

4 Clinical assessment

The initial evaluation of pilon fractures should be thorough. Examination of sensation should include assessment of the sensory nerve distribution. The deep peroneal, superficial peroneal, sural, and tibial nerve distributions including the medial and lateral plantar nerves should all be evaluated and recorded. Perfusion should be assessed by palpation of the posterior tibial and dorsalis pedis pulses. Capillary refill should be assessed.

The soft tissues must be examined. Most pilon fractures are the result of high-energy injuries resulting from an axial load, such as a fall from height or a motor vehicle collision. These injuries result in significant soft-tissue swelling that will often increase over time. The soft tissues should therefore be regularly monitored and surgical fixation should only be considered when the swelling has resolved allowing safe closure of the wounds. Surgical treatment is typically performed between 5 and 21 days after injury, depending on the severity of the soft-tissue component of the injury.

Imaging

Initial imaging for pilon fractures includes lateral, AP, and mortise ankle views. Full-length x-rays of the tibia are necessary in fractures that extend proximally. X-rays obtained when the overall limb alignment is improved, such as after reduction, are of more benefit in evaluation of the injury.

Intraarticular fractures are best examined with a computed tomographic (CT) scan including sagittal, axial, and coronal planes. This will allow full assessment of the fracture pattern and aid in surgical planning. The necessary surgical approaches as well as fixation construct will be planned from the CT scan. Additional foot x-rays may be needed based on the individual injury being evaluated.

5 Nonoperative treatment

Nonoperative treatment is rare for pilon fractures and is reserved for fracture patterns with minimal displacement and in patients with comorbidities that put them at increased risk during operative treatment. Extraarticular fractures with minimal alteration of the overall alignment of the tibia may also be treated without surgery by cast immobilization. A splint is used until such time as the injury-related swelling has resolved allowing a cast to be applied. Gross alteration of the alignment of the tibia or articular surface may cause problems with limb alignment or stability. Serial x-rays are necessary to ensure articular congruency and limb alignment are maintained over time.

Select intraarticular fractures may also be treated nonoperatively. Fractures with intraarticular involvement with less than 2 mm of articular step-off and less than 3 mm of gap may be considered for nonoperative treatment in low-demand individuals.

Systemic diseases such as dense neuropathy, peripheral vascular disease, poorly controlled diabetes, or noncompliance from substance abuse may be contraindications for surgical treatment as long as the overall limb alignment is acceptable and the articular surface has minimal displacement. In these high-risk populations, limb alignment may be prioritized over articular congruency. This can be accomplished with a circular external fixation device.

6 Operative treatment

Emergent operative treatment is indicated for open fractures, fractures with an associated dislocation, and fractures with soft tissues at risk of breakdown due to gross fracture fragment displacement or malalignment. Current or impending compartment syndrome is also an indication for emergent operative treatment for compartmental releases.

External fixation

Most pilon injuries will be treated with temporizing external fixation at the time of injury to restore limb alignment and length, providing relative stability, while the soft-tissue injury recovers (**Fig 2-3**). This method of staged management

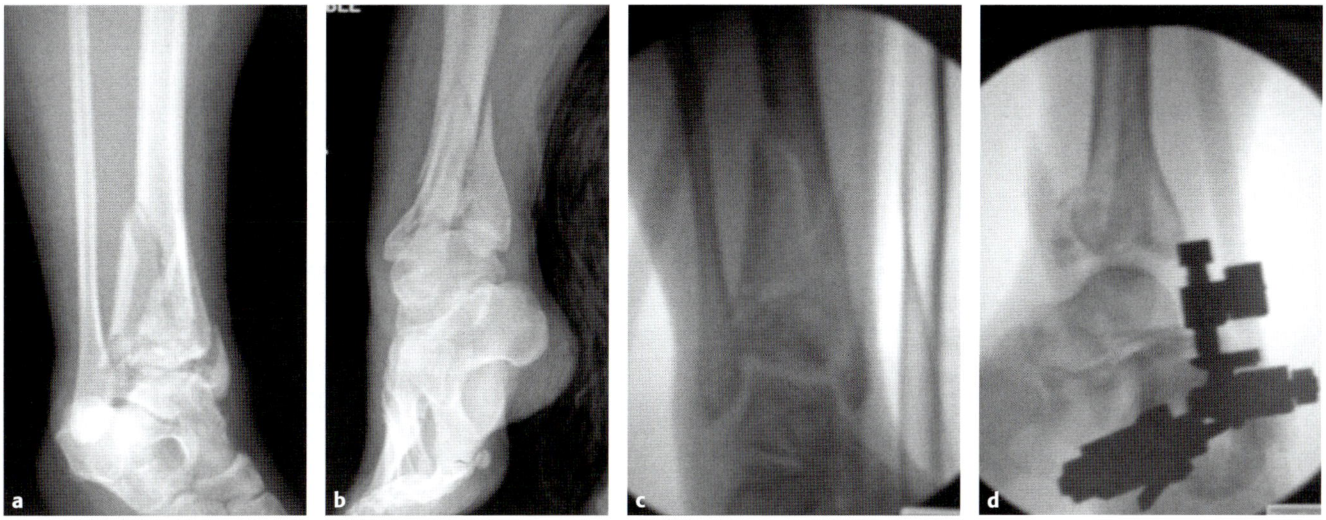

Fig 2-3a–d A highly comminuted intraarticular tibial pilon fracture in a young woman. Injury AP (**a**) and lateral (**b**) x-rays show severe comminution and impaction of the articular surface. The AP (**c**) and lateral (**d**) C-arm images show marked improvement in alignment with the talus centered under the tibia in both views. The distraction device is visible in the lateral C-arm image.

results in lower rates of soft-tissue complications with delayed definitive fixation. The goal of external fixation is to center the talus under the tibia on both AP and lateral x-ray views. Distraction will prevent further injury to the articular cartilage of the talar dome, which may occur from the opposing fractured surface of the tibia. Fixation of the fibula can be performed at the same time as external fixation application or on a delayed basis. Ideally, the individual who will ultimately manage the pilon fracture should also treat the fibular fracture. Poor incision placement and inadequate reduction may complicate care. Appropriate timing of surgical fixation is necessary. Surgical treatment will allow anatomical restoration of the articular injury. This requires direct reduction by open approaches. In general, the external fixator is maintained on the limb until after final fixation has been achieved. The external fixator maintains overall limb alignment while reduction of the articular surface is performed.

Patient positioning

The majority of pilon fractures are treated in the supine position. Select fractures may require additional posterior approaches. Posterior fractures that are partial articular injuries must be treated with posterior approaches.

Supine

The patient is positioned using a beanbag in a supine position on an operating table that is radiolucent distally. The patient is positioned with the feet at the end of the table, allowing the surgeon to move easily around the end of the table as needed to work through any combination of approaches that are necessary. A foam-positioning ramp is placed under the affected leg. Alternatively, pillows or blankets can be used to elevate the affected limb to avoid interference with C-arm imaging. A bump or wedge is placed under the ipsilateral hip to internally rotate the affected leg so it is positioned perpendicular to the floor. A tourniquet is placed on the upper thigh and a nonsterile U-drape placed circumferentially just distal to the tourniquet.

Prone

The patient is placed prone after the airway is secured. Chest rolls are placed under the patient. A small pillow under the lower leg elevates the affected extremity, easing instrumentation and imaging. A bump is placed under the contralateral hip to internally rotate the affected leg so it is positioned perpendicular to the floor. This allows improved ability to obtain C-arm imaging. When imaging the ankle, the C-arm will typically need to be tilted caudad to improve imaging. The leg must be internally rotated to get a mortise view.

C-arm positioning

The C-arm is positioned at the side of the table and opposite the injured extremity. The monitor is placed at the head of the table within view of the surgeon. Occasionally, tilting the C-arm caudad or cephalad 20° will aid in obtaining images of the anterior and posterior portions of the articular surface by accommodating for the curvature of the distal tibial articular surface.

Surgical approaches

Numerous surgical approaches can be used for fixation of pilon fractures. Generally, open surgical approaches are required to directly reduce the articular surface with plates and screws used to maintain the reduction. Most type C pilon fractures will require more than one incision and more than one plate. Historically, it was recommended that incisions be at least 7 cm apart. While this is not the case today, it is still imperative that excessive dissection and undermining of skin flaps should be avoided, as it will increase the risk of wound complications. The single most important factor in avoiding soft-tissue complications related to surgical treatment is appropriately timing the surgical intervention when swelling has resolved.

Alternative approaches for operative management include management with ring external fixation, external fixation for limb alignment, percutaneous screws for articular reduction, and percutaneous screws coupled with intramedullary (IM) nailing.

Anterolateral approach

This approach is useful for management of complete articular injuries, partial articular injuries of the anterior or anterolateral articular surfaces, and for submuscular plating of the tibia. The surgical approach extends over the ankle in line with the fourth metatarsal. The superficial peroneal nerve is at risk and requires identification in the proximal extent of the incision (**Fig 2-4**). The approach results in medial retraction of all of the tendons of the anterior compartment, including the peroneus tertius if present. The incision may be extended distally to address concomitant foot injuries. Proximal extension of the approach is limited by the contents of the anterior compartment. This approach allows direct access to the Chaput tubercle and central comminution. In most situations, direct articular reduction and distal plate fixation will occur through this incision. The plate will be slid under the anterior compartment and proximal screws will be inserted through a small secondary incision or by percutaneous methods. Fixation of the medial portion of the injury is limited with this approach and a second approach to address the medial injury is often necessary in more severe injuries.

Anterior approach

The anterior approach uses the interval between the anterior tibialis and extensor hallucis longus. The dorsal is pedis artery and the deep peroneal nerve are located laterally and over-retraction should be avoided. The neurovascular bundle is at risk both proximally and distally in this approach. The entire anterior portion of the distal tibia is accessible using this approach.

Anteromedial approach

The anteromedial approach can be used for fractures with significant displacement and multiple intraarticular fracture lines involving the central and/or medial portion of the distal tibia including the medial malleolus. The skin incision is made just lateral to the tibial crest and then dissection continues just medial to the anterior tibialis tendon (**Fig 2-5**).

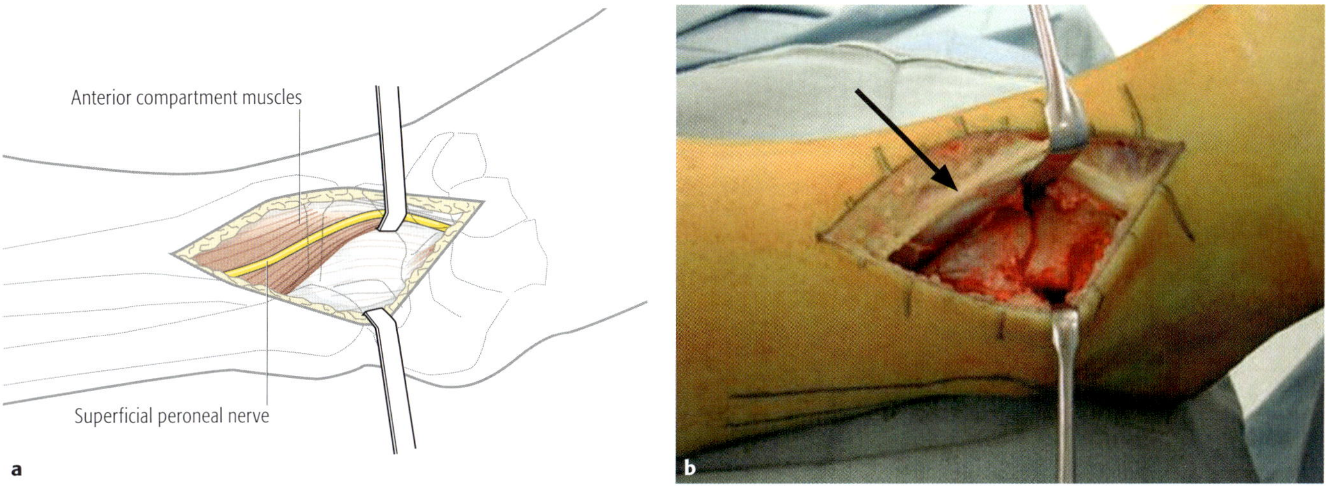

Fig 2-4a–b Anterolateral approach.

a The superficial peroneal nerve must be identified and protected. The extensor retinaculum is opened and the anterior compartment musculature is retracted medially.

b Intraoperative image demonstrating the superficial peroneal nerve (arrow) and anterior compartment musculature being retracted medially. The ankle joint is visible through the open capsule.

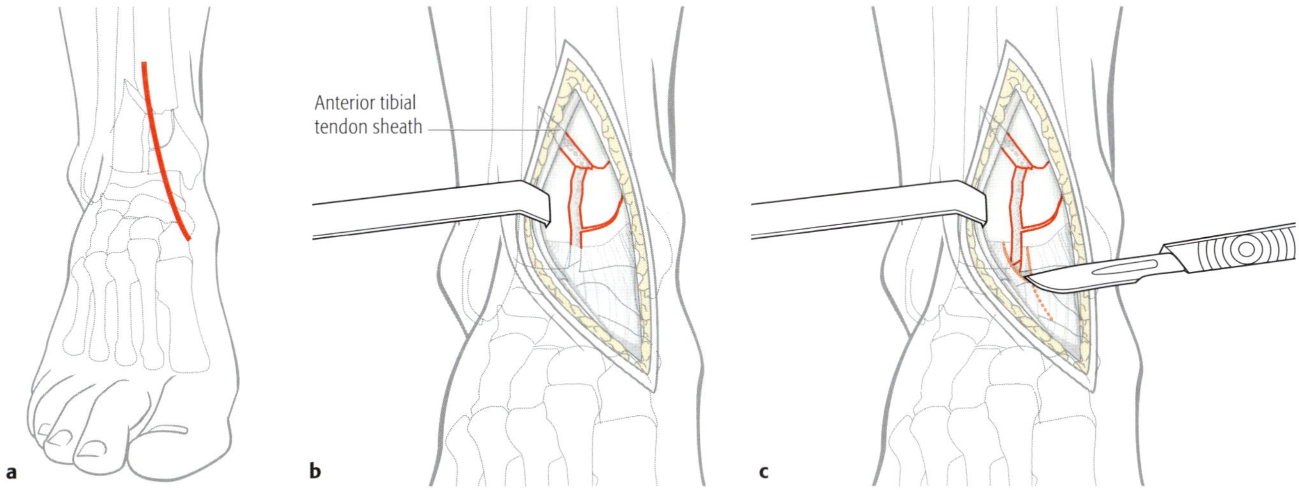

Fig 2-5a–c Anteromedial approach.

a The skin is incised just medial to the anterior tibialis tendon.

b The anterior tibialis is maintained in its sheath as the tendon is retracted laterally as the dissection continues deeper.

c The ankle joint capsule is only opened if necessary. Unnecessary dissection will damage the perforating branches of the anterior tibial artery and may devitalize the anterior fracture fragments.

The sheath of the anterior tibialis tendon is maintained throughout the dissection. The anterior aspect of the distal tibia can be approached between the posterior border of the tendon sheath and the periosteum. Care must be taken to avoid over dissection, particularly when a complementary small anterolateral incision is made to address the Chaput component. Surgery should be performed on a delayed basis when soft-tissue swelling has resolved. Careful handling and closure techniques for soft tissues are necessary to reduce the risk of wound-healing complications. Soft-tissue flaps should be full thickness.

Posteromedial approach

This surgical approach allows for direct reduction and visualization of posteromedial fracture fragments. Placement of an antiglide plate to reduce the shaft component is easily performed with this interval. This incision is also useful in removing the posterior tibialis if it is entrapped in the fracture fragments. The incision is curved from just distal to the tip of the medial malleolus and follows along the posterior edge of the medial tibia (**Fig 2-6**). The deep dissection may be carried out in three different intervals depending on the specific needs of the case. Dissection may be carried out between the posterior border of the tibia and the posterior tibialis tendon. The tendon should be left in its sheath at the level of the medial malleolus or carefully repaired when closing. Alternatively, dissection may be carried between the posterior tibialis and the FDL.

Finally, in select cases the interval between the flexor digitorum longus and flexor hallucis longus may be used. This interval is seldom used, as it requires direct exposure and protection of the neurovascular bundle.

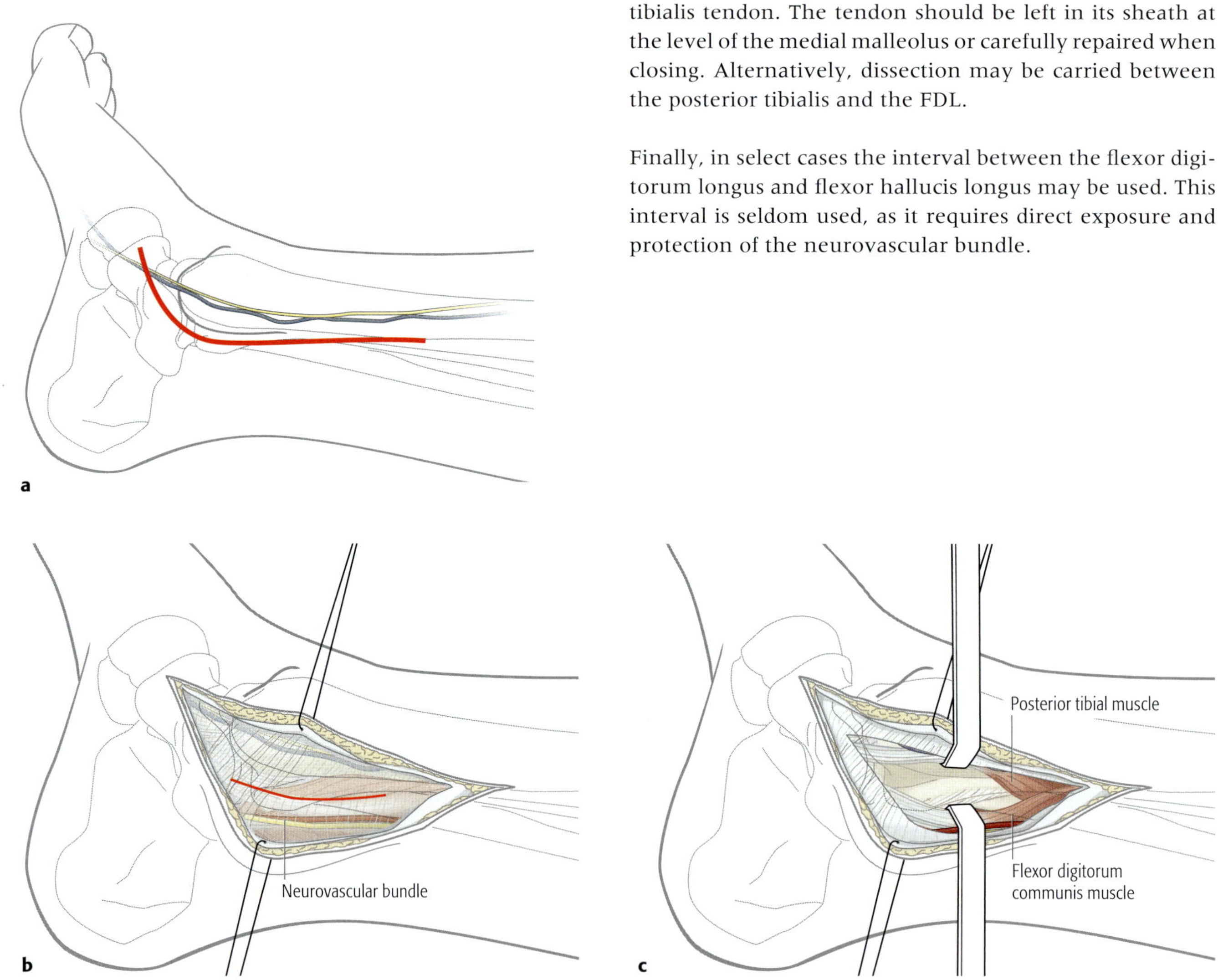

Fig 2-6a–c Posteromedial approach.

a The skin is incised extending from the tip of the medial malleolus then curving gently along the posterior border of the tibia.

b The fascia is incised anterior to the neurovascular bundle along the posterior tibialis tendon.

c Dissection continues between the posterior tibial muscle (which is retracted anteriorly) and the FDL (which is retracted posteriorly). Alternatively, the window between the tibia and the posterior tibial muscle may be used or the interval between the FDL and FHL, which would require dissecting out the neurovascular bundle.

Posterolateral approach

The posterolateral approach allows for direct reduction of the posterior portion of the articular surface. The incision uses the interval between the peroneal tendons and the Achilles superficially. If the fibula is also fractured, it can be approached with this incision as well. The sural nerve is protected in the subcutaneous tissue without direct dissection. The peroneal fascia is opened and the superior peroneal retinaculum is released allowing the peroneals to be retracted medially to expose the fibula. To expose the posterior tibia, deep dissection is carried out medially to the peroneal tendons along the lateral aspect of the FHL muscle belly with the muscle retracted medially (**Fig 2-7**). The entire posterior aspect of the tibia is accessible. The sural nerve is at risk and is generally located above the superficial crural fascia and retracted laterally within the subcutaneous fat. Damage to the peroneal artery or veins may occur at the level of the ankle joint and must be identified.

Percutaneous approach

Some fractures will be treated with a combination of external fixation to restore general limb alignment and percutaneous screws for reduction and stabilization of the articular component of the injury. Select fractures with less severe articular injury can also be treated with screws for the articular surface, and then treated with IM nailing. A CT scan is essential to allow for fragment-specific reduction and fixation. Small incisions are made to introduce elevators, reduction clamps, K-wires, Schanz screws, or any other necessary reduction tools. Once reduced, the articular surface is provisionally stabilized with K-wires and then screws are used to stabilized the articular surface. The screws can be inserted in a lag screw fashion when two solid fragments are present. If substantial comminution is present and there is concern that screws placed in a lag screw fashion will result in over compression of the articular surface, then positional screws should be used.

7 Postoperative care

The patient is instructed to elevate the extremity to prevent wound complications associated with postoperative swelling. Sutures are removed when the wound is healed. Range-of-motion (ROM) exercise is encouraged as soon as the wounds are stable to prevent stiffness of the ankle; usually at around 2–3 weeks postoperatively.

X-rays are taken periodically to assess for union. Weight-bearing progression is allowed once the fracture is healed. Patients with extraarticular injuries treated with an IM device may be able to weight bear as early as 2–3 weeks. Partial articular injuries treated with plate fixation are highly variable in severity and may be able to advance weight bearing any time from 6 to 12 weeks depending on the specific injury. Weight bearing may not be possible prior to 12 weeks for fractures with severe comminution and for complete articular injuries.

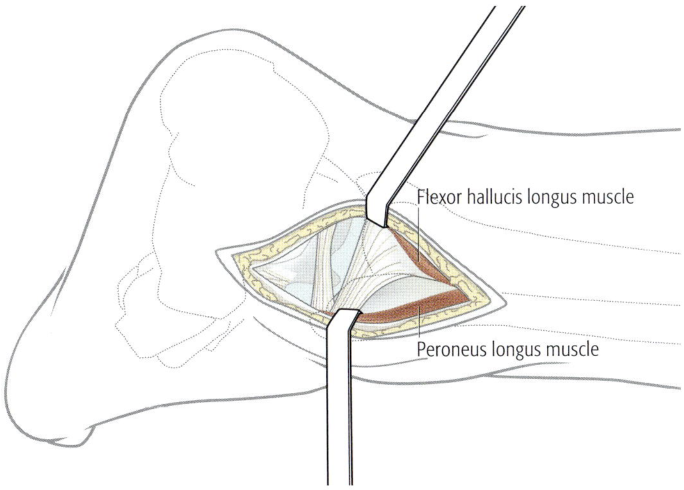

Fig 2-7 Posterolateral approach. The incision is carried down just lateral to the Achilles. The deep interval is between the peroneal tendons and the FHL. The FHL muscle belly is retracted medially. Both the posterior tibia and fibula can be addressed with this single approach.

8 Complications and outcomes

Complications

Complications of pilon fractures can be a result of the injury itself, surgical treatment, or late complications. Surgical treatment of pilon fractures is technically difficult. There is a significant learning curve and improved results occur with surgeon experience. Open fractures are at high risk of soft-tissue complications and may require soft-tissue transfer and prolonged wound management. Necrosis of soft tissues may arise from gross malalignment of fracture fragments if left untreated. Postoperative problems include delayed wound healing and infection. Appropriate surgical timing for when the swelling has resolved is the best prevention for these complications. With staged management, wound complications occur less than 10% of the time. Nonunion is more common in cases with severe metadiaphyseal comminution. Malunion may occur from poor surgical technique, insufficient fixation, or late collapse. Posttraumatic stiffness is common, therefore early ROM exercise is encouraged. Finally, posttraumatic ankle arthritis may occur. This may be a result of articular injury, malalignment, or cartilage death stemming from the initial injury.

Outcomes

Worse outcomes are associated with severe fracture patterns. Operative treatment coupled with malreduction combines the potential of complications of surgical treatment with those related to malreduction including decreased function and development of arthritis. Numerous studies have demonstrated a correlation between fracture severity by the AO/OTA classification and the development of posttraumatic arthritis. The most important factor determining outcome in pilon fractures treated operatively is quality of reduction.

Range of motion is typically not normal after pilon fractures. Reduction in ROM can be expected with studies reporting between 35° and 45° of total ROM on average. Gait analysis has shown decreased load bearing on the heel and under the first metatarsal with a general lateralization of the gait axis on the injured limb. Improvement in function on outcomes scores has shown no improvement beyond a year after injury, while in another study looking at outcomes of pilon fractures, patients self-reported improvement up to 2.4 years on average.

These injuries are severe and result in change in employment in many patients whose occupation requires prolonged walking or standing. The ability to participate in recreational activities is clearly altered after a pilon fracture and most patients are unable to participate in activities involving running.

Nonunion is more likely to occur in cases with infection. Pilon fractures that develop a deep infection, either from an open fracture or as a complication of surgery, have the worst outcomes.

9 Recommended reading

Assal M, Ray A, Fasel JH, et al. A modified posteromedial approach combined with extensile anterior for the treatment of complex tibial pilon fractures (AO/OTA 43-C). *J Orthop Trauma.* 2014 Jun;28(6):e138–145.

Assal M, Ray A, Stern R. Strategies for surgical approaches in open reduction internal fixation of pilon fractures. *J Orthop Trauma.* 2015 Feb;29(2):69–79.

Cole PA, Mehrle RK, Bhandari M, et al. The pilon map: fracture lines and comminution zones in OTA/AO type 43C3 pilon fractures. *J Orthop Trauma.* 2013 Jul;27(7):e152–156.

Hessmann M, Nork S, Sommer C, et al. Distal tibia. In: Colton C, Krikler S, Schatzker J, et al (eds). *AO Surgery Reference.* Available at: www.aosurgery.org. Accessed July 15, 2019.

Jansen H, Fenwick A, Doht S, et al. Clinical outcome and changes in gait pattern after pilon fractures. *Int Orthop.* 2013 Jan;37(1):51–58.

Ketz J, Sanders R. Staged posterior tibial plating for the treatment of Orthopaedic Trauma Association 43C2 and 43C3 tibial pilon fractures. *J Orthop Trauma.* 2012 Jun;26(6):341–347.

Konrath G, Moed BR, Watson JT, et al. Intramedullary nailing of unstable diaphyseal fractures of the tibia with distal intraarticular involvement. *J Orthop Trauma.* 1997 Apr;11(3):200–205.

Korkmaz A, Ciftdemir M, Ozcan M, et al. The analysis of the variables, affecting outcome in surgically treated tibia pilon fractured patients. *Injury.* 2013 Oct;44(10):1270–1274.

Marsh JL, Weigel DP, Dirschl DR. Tibial plafond fractures. How do these ankles function over time? *J Bone Joint Surg Am.* 2003 Feb;85(2):287–295.

Patterson MJ, Cole JD. Two-staged delayed open reduction and internal fixation of severe pilon fractures. *J Orthop Trauma.* 1999 Feb;13(2):85–91.

Penny P, Swords M, Heisler J, et al. Ability of modern distal tibia plates to stabilize comminuted pilon fracture fragments: Is dual plate fixation necessary? *Injury.* 2016 Aug;47(8):1761–1769.

Rubio-Suarez JC, Carbonell-Escobar R, Rodriguez-Merchan EC, et al. Fractures of the tibial pilon treated by open reduction and internal fixation (locking compression plate-less invasive stabilising system): Complications and sequelae. *Injury.* 2018 Sep;49 Suppl 2:S60–s64.

Sands A, Grujic L, Byck DC, et al. Clinical and functional outcomes of internal fixation of displaced pilon fractures. *Clin Orthop Relat Res.* 1998 Feb(347):131–137.

Sirkin M, Sanders R, DiPasquale T, et al. A staged protocol for soft tissue management in the treatment of complex pilon fractures. *J Orthop Trauma.* 2004 Sep;18(8 Suppl):S32–38.

Sommer C, Nork SE, Graves M, et al. Quality of fracture reduction assessed by radiological parameters and its influence on functional results in patients with pilon fractures-A prospective multicentre study. *Injury.* 2017 Dec;48(12):2853–2863.

2.1 Tibial shaft fracture extending into the plafond—plate fixation

May Fong Mak, Mathieu Assal

1 Case description

A 26-year-old man fell from a height of 3 m into a hole sustaining an injury to his right lower extremity. He was initially admitted to a hospital where x-rays revealed a displaced tibial shaft fracture extending into the plafond, with articular involvement (**Fig 2.1-1**).

Clinical examination revealed a closed fracture and an acute compartment syndrome of the leg. The patient underwent an immediate 4-compartment fasciotomy, at the initial hospital, through two longitudinal skin and fascia incisions. At the same time, temporary external fixation for stabilization of bone and soft tissues was applied.

The following day, he was transferred to another hospital for further care. The patient required revision of the external fixator to change the location of the calcaneal pin due to tibial nerve irritation. After external fixation x-rays and computed tomographic (CT) scan with 3D reconstruction revealed a displaced multifragmentary, oblique fracture of the midshaft of the tibia extending into the plafond. None of the anterolateral, medial, and posterior articular fragments were in continuity with the shaft (AO/OTA 43C3.3). Impaction of the distal tibial articular surface was also noted (**Fig 2.1-2** and **Fig 2.1-3**).

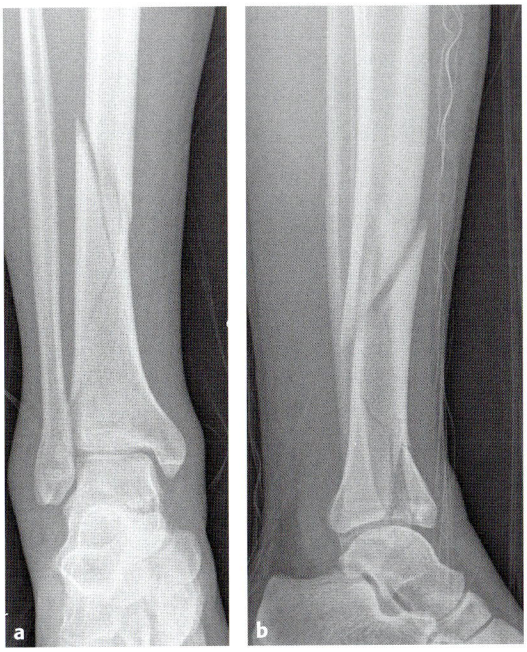

Fig 2.1-1a–b Immediate postinjury x-rays.
a AP view showing the tibial shaft fracture extending into the plafond.
b Lateral view revealing the multifragmentary fracture of the plafond (AO/OTA 43C3.3).

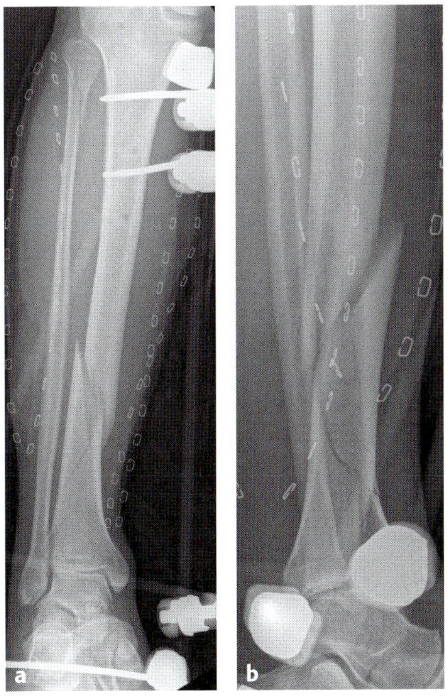

Fig 2.1-2a–b Initial fracture stabilization with spanning external fixator. Fasciotomy wounds are outlined by skin staples.

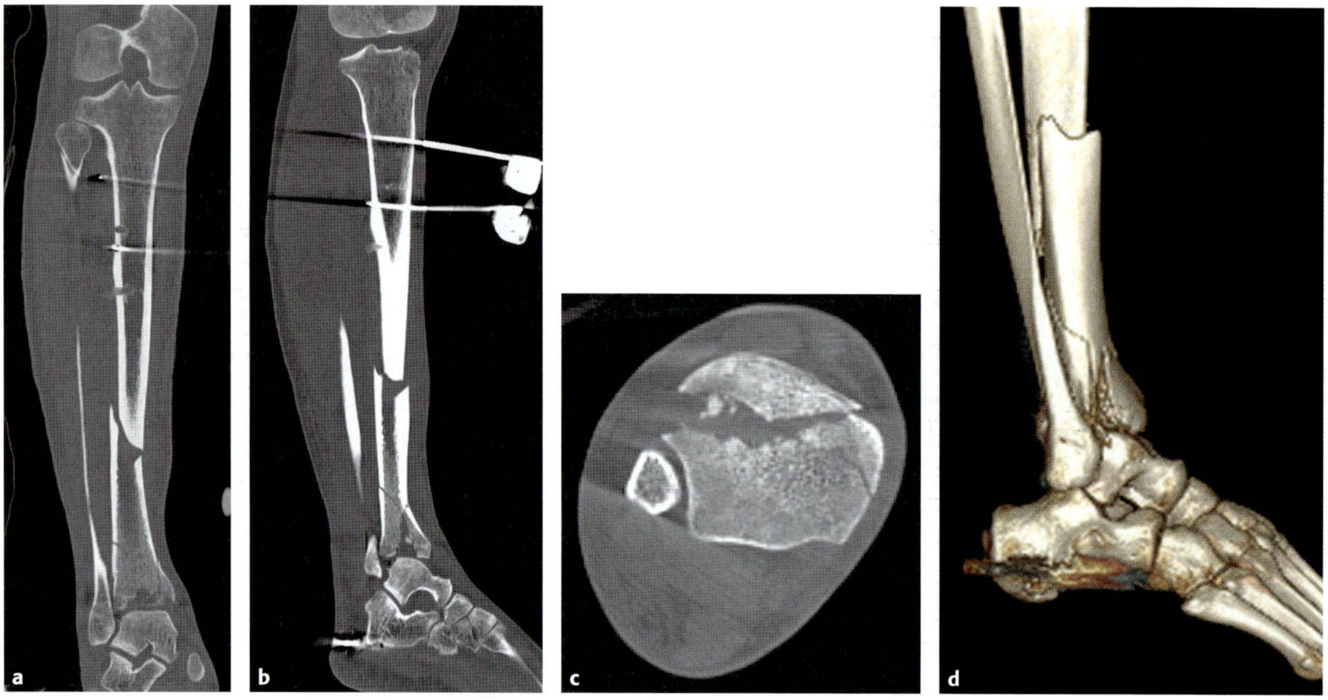

Fig 2.1-3a–d Computed tomographic scans with 3D reconstruction.

a–c Coronal, sagittal, and axial images demonstrating plafond comminution and displacement, particularly of the anterolateral fragment resulting in intraarticular step and gap. There is an incarcerated fragment at the center of the plafond.

d 3D reconstructed image showing the external fracture anatomy and general alignment.

2 Preoperative planning

Indications for surgery

Displaced lower limb fractures require restoration of anatomy, specifically length, alignment, and rotation. Intraarticular fractures require open reduction and internal fixation (ORIF) to restore and support the articular surface.

Approach

When selecting the definitive approach, the preexisting medial and lateral fasciotomy incisions must be considered (**Fig 2.1-4**). For this patient, the entire fracture from shaft to joint was accessed with a single incision, using the extensile approach. This was done by extending the lateral fasciotomy wound distally and medially.

Where possible, the placement of the fasciotomy incisions should be where they will not interfere and indeed facilitate proper ORIF approach. The external fixator should be placed with the pins far enough apart to remain out of the surgical field of definitive surgery.

Plate positioning

In this case due to concerns about medial soft-tissue coverage, a lateral plate was preferred for fixation of the shaft fracture. As an aid for reduction the first step was to anatomically reconnect the shaft to the lateral column of the distal tibia (converting AO/OTA 43C to a 43B). This was performed by use of a 4-hole straight locking compression plate (LCP) placed anteriorly so as not to disturb future plate placement. A long anterolateral plate was then used to buttress the entire fracture. The vertical limb was of sufficient length to overlap the previously applied tibial shaft plate. This avoids creating a stress-riser with a fracture between the plates. Additionally, the plate augments the fixation of the shaft. The medial distal tibia was buttressed with a short low-profile medial plate.

Order of fixation

1. Reduce and stabilize the shaft component of the fracture.
2. Reconstruct the articular surface.
3. Connect the articular surface to the shaft.

External fixator in situ

Surgery was performed with the external fixator left in place to aid in maintaining limb alignment, length, and rotation. The external fixator is prepared into the field in its entirety using betadine paint. This maintains alignment that has been achieved when the external fixator was assembled, aiding in the reconstruction. It also helps in distraction and visualization of the ankle joint. Small adjustments to the external fixator are often necessary during the surgery. Any time a part is removed or adjusted, betadine must be applied to the newly exposed portion of the external fixator as it is not possible to disinfect under the clamps at the beginning of the operative case.

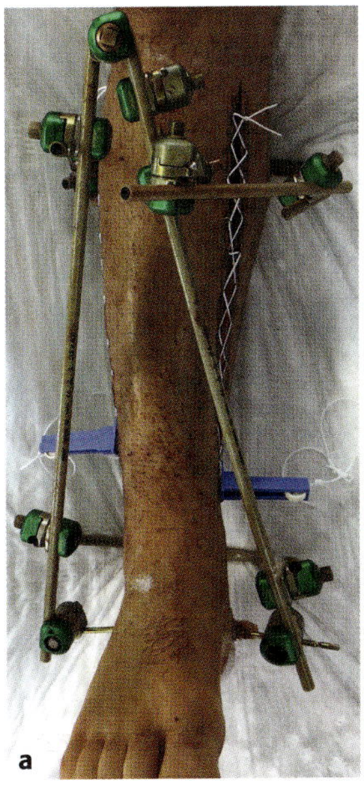

a

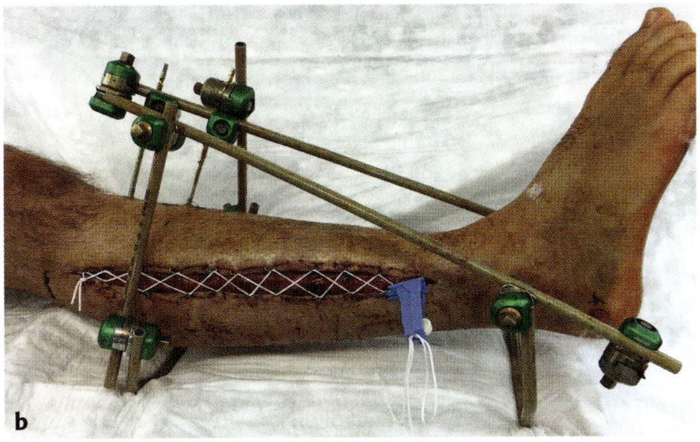

b

Fig 2.1-4a–b Fasciotomy wounds are progressively approximated to achieve primary wound closure using the "shoelace technique".

3 Operating room setup

Patient positioning	• Supine on a radiolucent table. • The patient is positioned so the foot is at the end of the operative table for easy access to the fracture.
Anesthesia options	• General, often supplemented with a regional nerve block
C-arm location	• Positioned on the contralateral side with the monitor placed near the head of the operative table.
Tourniquet	• Used at surgeon's discretion. • Improves the ability to see the joint surface and the reduction.
Tips	• Placing a bump under the ipsilateral hip internally rotates the leg to neutral allowing improved access to the lateral part of the plafond.

For illustrations and overview of anesthetic considerations, see chapter 1.

Equipment

- LCP 3.5 (for fixation of midshaft tibial fracture)
- Anterolateral LCP 2.7/3.5 (for fixation of anterolateral plafond fragment)
- LCP 2.4/2.7 (for fixation of medial plafond fragment)
- K-wires
- Point-to-point reduction (Weber) clamps
- Smooth and sharp elevators

Size of system, instruments, and implants may vary according to anatomy of the fracture and the patient. Conventional compression plates can be used in good bone quality, while locking plates are preferred in osteopenic bone and in fractures with comminution.

4 Surgical procedure

The first step is fixation of the oblique fracture of the tibial shaft, which will restore length, rotation, and alignment. Fixation of the shaft provides a template for reduction and fixation of the plafond articular fragments, which is the second part of the operation.

When selecting the approach, careful consideration must be given to the preexisting fasciotomy wounds and to the width and length of skin bridge, neurovascular damage, excessive soft-tissue stripping, adequacy of soft-tissue coverage especially on the medial side of the tibia, and the strategy for wound closure.

The extensile approach is used as it permits complete and direct visualization of the distal tibial articular surface and planned placement of medial and anterolateral plates. Thus, it provides ideal access for this AO/OTA type C pilon fracture. The lateral incision of the fasciotomy is extended distally and medially and ends 10 mm below the tip of the medial malleolus (**Fig 2.1-5**). The incision is carried out down to the subcutaneous tissue avoiding dissection of the superficial layers. The extensor retinaculum is carefully incised leaving the tibialis anterior tendon undisturbed in its sheath. The full-thickness subcutaneous flap is retracted medially while the tibialis anterior tendon is retracted laterally. The flap is handled atraumatically without strong retraction or the use of forceps. Nylon stay sutures in the skin may be used to retract soft tissues. At the level of the ankle, the capsule is opened longitudinally, exposing the talus. Subperiosteal dissection exposes the distal tibia fracture, and extending the dissection proximally clearly exposes the fractured shaft.

The shaft fracture is first reduced anatomically and fixed using a short straight 4-hole, locking compression 3.5 plate (**Fig 2.1-6**). Retraction of tissues laterally exposes the entire anterolateral articular fragment of Chaput. The anterolateral fragment is reduced and fixed anatomically to the previously fixed shaft with its nondisplaced posterior articular fragment. The external fixator aids in alignment and visualization during this reduction.

Finally, the medial fragment is reduced to the anterolateral and posterior fragments and temporarily stabilized with K-wires. For definitive fixation, the anterolateral fragment and tibial shaft are fixed with a long anterolateral plate overlapping the already applied short tibial shaft plate, and the medial fragment is buttressed with a medial plate. If the plates are longer than the incision, they can be slid proximally deep to the soft tissues, and screws inserted using a minimally invasive technique.

Large metaphyseal defects should be bone grafted. The wounds are closed primarily. The external fixator is left in situ temporarily to facilitate wound healing (**Fig 2.1-7**). In this patient, it was removed after 1 week (**Fig 2.1-8**).

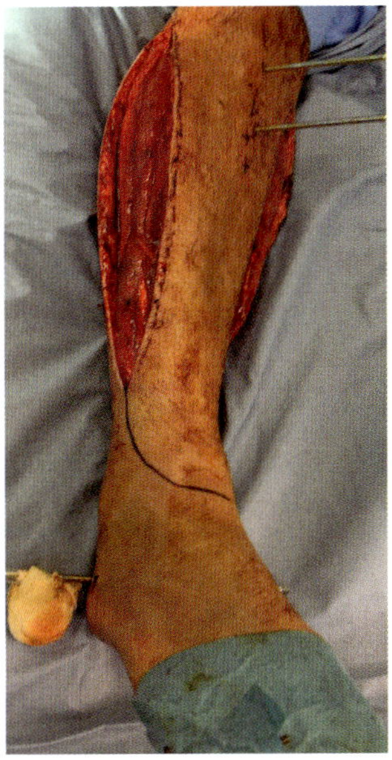

Fig 2.1-5 Distal and medial extension of lateral fasciotomy wound, as marked on skin, to gain access to the plafond.

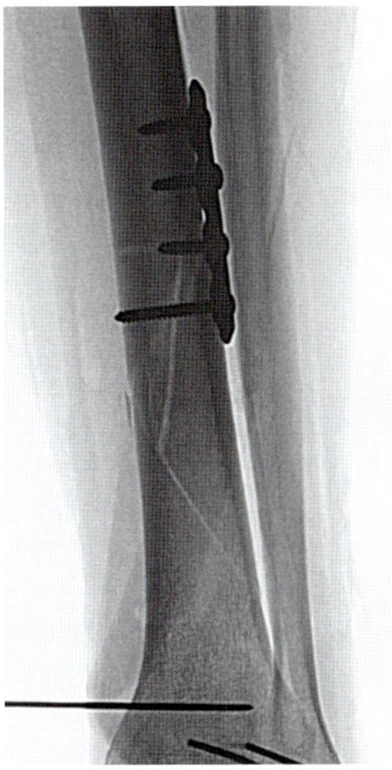

Fig 2.1-6 Plating of the shaft fracture improves limb stability and alignment by converting a segmental fracture into an isolated pilon fracture.

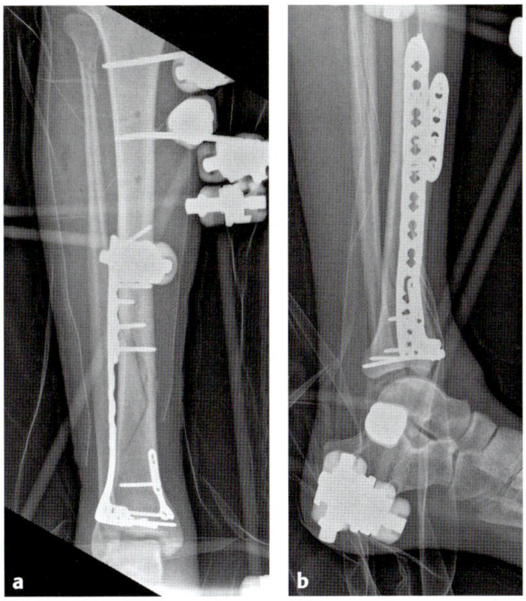

Fig 2.1-7a–b Immediate postoperative x-rays show the external fixator left in place to facilitate soft-tissue healing.
a AP view.
b Lateral view.

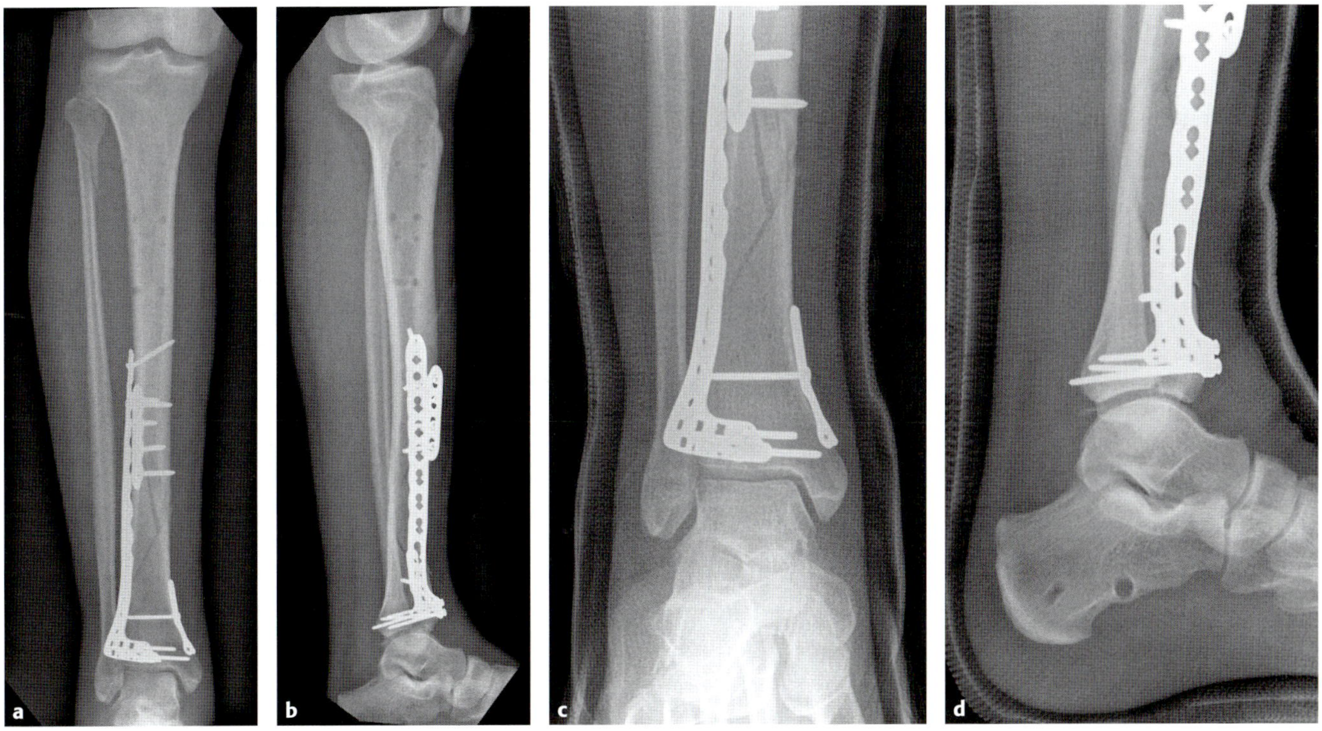

Fig 2.1-8a–d The external fixator was removed 1 week postoperatively (**a–b**) and the ankle was immobilized in a cast (**c–d**).

Principles of fracture fixation

The shaft fracture was anatomically reduced under direct vision and fixed using a straight 4-hole plate. Plates used in fixation of pilon fractures usually function as buttress plates. Therefore, a fracture that is primarily in varus should be buttressed with a medial plate, and conversely, a fracture that is primarily in valgus should be buttressed with an anterolateral plate.

Considerations for shaft fixation

In cases of a tibial shaft fracture that extends into the plafond, fixing the diaphysis before the plafond potentially simplifies the fixation by converting a segmental fracture into an isolated pilon fracture. The timing of initial shaft fixation is controversial. The shaft fracture can be plated at initial surgery when the external fixation is applied or at definitive ORIF. Careful planning is necessary to ensure the hardware and incision will not interfere with definitive fixation of the articular injury.

The authors prefer to initially stabilize both the shaft fracture and the pilon injury temporarily with an external fixator, and fix the shaft and plafond together during definitive ORIF after soft-tissue edema has resolved and preoperative planning has been performed.

In general, posteromedial or anterolateral approaches offer a more robust musculocutaneous soft-tissue cover for the plates, while the medial approach carries a higher risk of wound breakdown and exposed implants due to the thin medial soft-tissue envelope.

5 Pitfalls and complications

Pitfalls

Soft-tissue problems

Soft-tissue problem are a major pitfall when treating pilon fractures, owing to the inherently thin soft-tissue envelope around the distal tibia, the fragility of soft tissues after high-energy trauma, and the necessity for multiple incisions to approach different parts of this complex fracture (**Table 2.1-1**).

Pitfall	Tip
Insufficient resolution of soft-tissue edema	• Wait for wrinkle sign before definitive surgery (may require waiting 14–21 days or more, postinjury)
Rough soft-tissue handling	• Gentle atraumatic retraction • Avoid desiccation of tendons or flap during surgery by repeated irrigation
Inadequate skin bridge between incisions	• Maximize distance between incisions and keep parallel (5 cm)
Contracted and unstable soft tissues	• Early application of the external fixator not only stabilizes the fracture but also stabilizes and prevents contracture of soft tissues while waiting for definitive fixation.
Subcutaneous medial border of tibia	• Plating on the lateral side of the tibial shaft if appropriate where the soft-tissue coverage is more robust

Table 2.1-1 Major pitfalls pertaining to soft-tissue care.

Inadequate fracture visualization

In most articular fractures, visualization of and access to the entire articular surface is often necessary. Selection of an approach that is suboptimal for a fracture pattern may result in excessive traction being used for reduction. An external fixator is frequently used to aid visualization of the articular surface by distracting the tibiotalar joint.

Irreducible or non-fixable articular fragments

Small or comminuted articular surface fragments that are impossible to anatomically reduce or fix are at risk of affecting joint congruency by displacing into the joint as loose fragments. Removal of these fragments is recommended.

Inadequate diagnosis and fixation

A simple extension of a distal tibial shaft spiral fracture into the joint may be overlooked on plain x-rays. Secondary joint displacement may be the consequence.

Complications

Flap necrosis

The incidence of flap necrosis can be decreased through appropriate timing of definitive ORIF, meticulous and gentle soft-tissue handling, and repair of extensor retinaculum to prevent tibialis anterior tendon from bowstringing which exerts pressure on the overlying soft tissues.

Infection

The risk is decreased through a combination of prophylactic antibiotics, extreme care with soft tissues, and reducing duration of surgery.

Loss of fixation

Incidence can be decreased through use of locking plates in comminuted fractures, correct placement of plates, and correct principle of buttress plating.

Malunion

Malunion is decreased by anatomical reduction of articular surface, and functional reduction of tibial length, rotation, and varus/valgus alignment.

In the case of osteoporotic bone or noncompliant patients, the external fixator may be left in place postoperatively for 1–6 weeks as an additional support for the fracture.

Nonunion

Nonunion is best prevented by fixation of shaft fracture in compression, bone grafting of large metaphyseal defects, preserving soft-tissue attachments to fracture fragments, and by providing adequate stability.

Patients should also be advised on nutritional support (ie, multivitamins and calcium) and cessation of tobacco use.

Posttraumatic arthritis

While severity of injury and quality of reduction play a role in the development of posttraumatic arthritis, the most important factor is primary articular cartilage damage that occurs at the time of the initial injury

6 Alternative techniques

Selecting appropriate incisions is dependent on the fracture pattern and the soft-tissue envelope. Traumatized soft tissue, prior incisions, or preexisting scars require incisions to be placed away from the area of concern.

In cases of a tibial shaft fracture extending distally resulting in a nondisplaced intraarticular split of the plafond, the plafond should first be fixed with two percutaneous interfragmentary partially threaded screws. With the articular block restored, the tibial shaft fracture can then be fixed with a standard intramedullary nail.

7 Postoperative management and rehabilitation

In the first 6 weeks, the patient should be maintained on toe-touch weight-bearing with early gentle range of motion (ROM) of the ankle and hindfoot. In the subsequent 6 weeks, the patient should gradually increase to full weight bearing as tolerated in a removable orthosis and increase ROM exercises and gentle resistance training.

After 12 weeks, the patient can begin neuromuscular retraining which focuses on coordination, balance, and gait. Serial postoperative x-rays are done beginning in the immediate postoperative period until 2 years postoperative. X-rays are evaluated for healing in the initial months and for signs of posttraumatic arthrosis beyond 1 year.

Implant removal

Removal of implants is not mandatory but recommended if implants are prominent under the subcutaneous envelope of the distal tibia. Implant removal should be undertaken only after healing is complete, ie, after 12–18 months at the earliest.

This patient showed good radiographic and functional healing at the 6-month postoperative review (**Fig 2.1-9** and **Fig 2.1-10**).

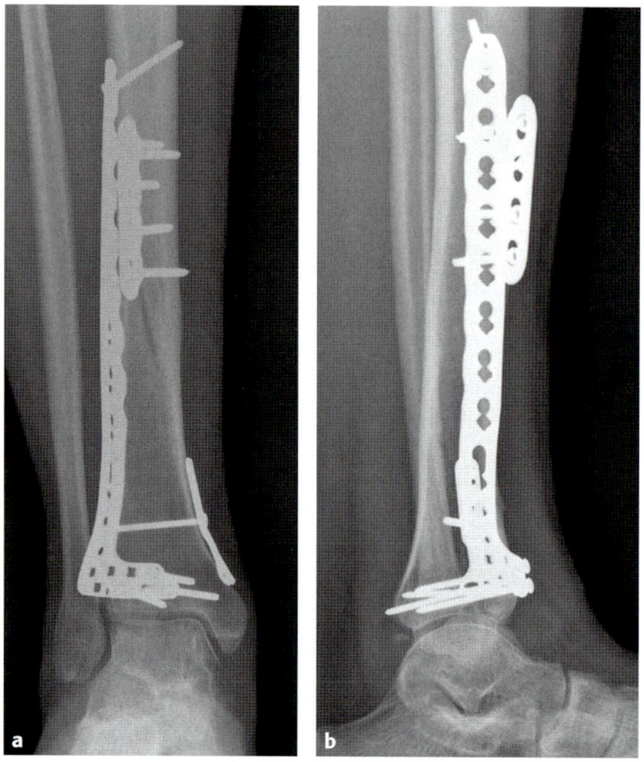

Fig 2.1-9a–b Postoperative x-rays at 6 months showing progress in fracture healing.

a AP view.

b Lateral view.

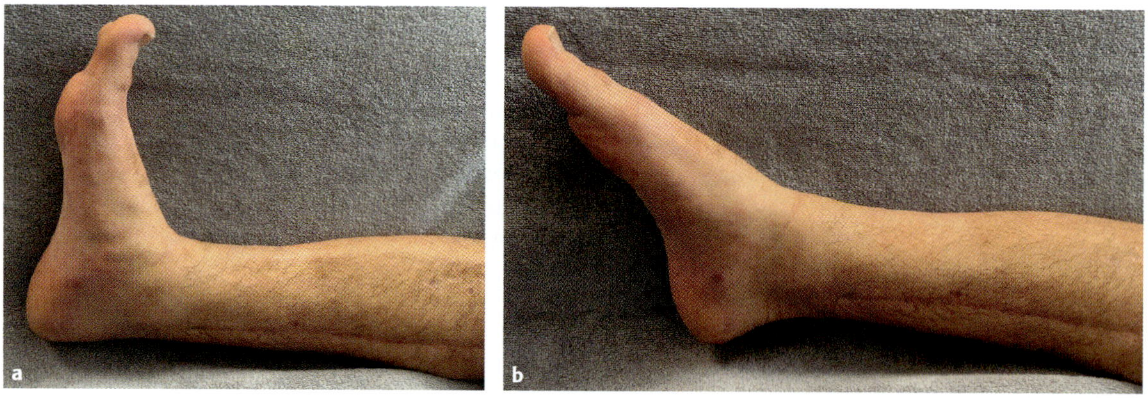

Fig 2.1-10a–b Good functional recovery at 6 months postoperative, demonstrated by active dorsiflexion of 10° and active plantarflexion of 30°.

8 Recommended reading

Assal M, Ray A, Stern R. Strategies for surgical approaches in open reduction internal fixation of pilon fractures. *J Orthop Trauma.* 2015 Feb;29(2):69–79.

Assal M, Ray A, Stern R. The extensile approach for the operative treatment of high-energy pilon fractures: surgical technique and soft-tissue healing. *J Orthop Trauma.* 2007 Mar;21(3):198–206.

Berman SS, Schilling JD, McIntyre KE, et al. Shoelace technique for delayed primary closure of fasciotomies. *Am J Surg.* 1994 Apr;167(4):435–436.

Sands A, Grujic L, Byck DC, et al. Clinical and functional outcomes of internal fixation of displaced pilon fractures. *Clin Orthop Relat Res.* 1998 Feb(347):131–137.

2.2 Metaphyseal fracture with joint involvement

May Fong Mak, Mathieu Assal

1 Case description

A 38-year-old woman was involved in a motor vehicle accident. She experienced immediate pain and noticed her left lower extremity was deformed. In the emergency department, x-rays showed a displaced metaphyseal fracture of the distal tibia with articular involvement (AO/OTA 43C3.3(5b) with a 4F3B fibular fracture), and posterior dislocation of the tibiotalar joint (**Fig 2.2-1**). The fracture was closed.

Temporary ankle-spanning external fixation was used to stabilize the fracture and soft tissues. X-rays taken after external fixation showed improved alignment and allowed for better understanding of the fracture pattern (**Fig 2.2-2**). Computed tomographic (CT) scanning with 3D reconstruction was performed for precise assessment of the fracture pattern of the tibial plafond. The CT revealed displaced fragments with a resultant intraarticular step-off and gap. The distal tibial metaphyseal fracture was multifragmentary. In addition, an associated long oblique fibular fracture was present (**Fig 2.2-3**).

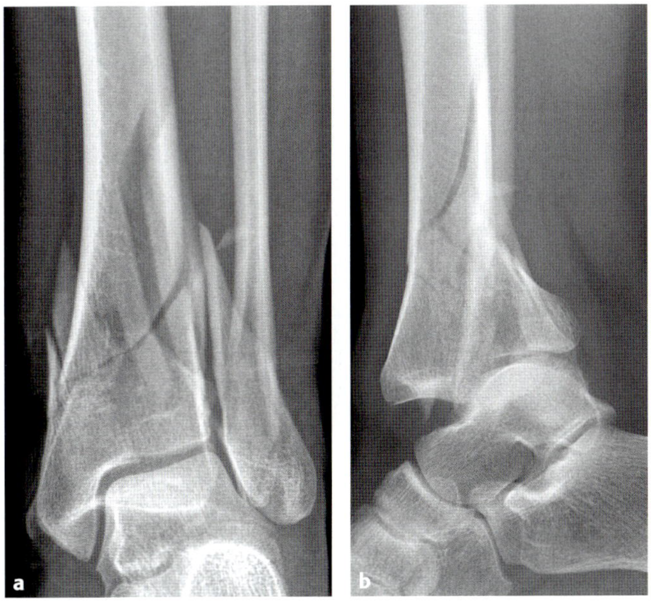

Fig 2.2-1a–b Immediate postinjury x-rays.
a Comminuted pilon fracture (AO/OTA 43C3.3[5b]) with 4F3B fibular fracture (AP view).
b Posterior dislocation of the tibiotalar joint (lateral view).

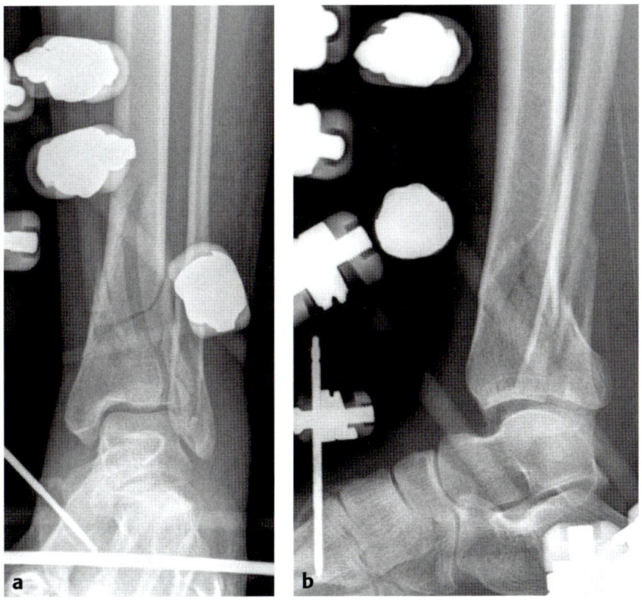

Fig 2.2-2a–b Realignment of fracture through application of spanning external fixator.
a AP view.
b Lateral view.

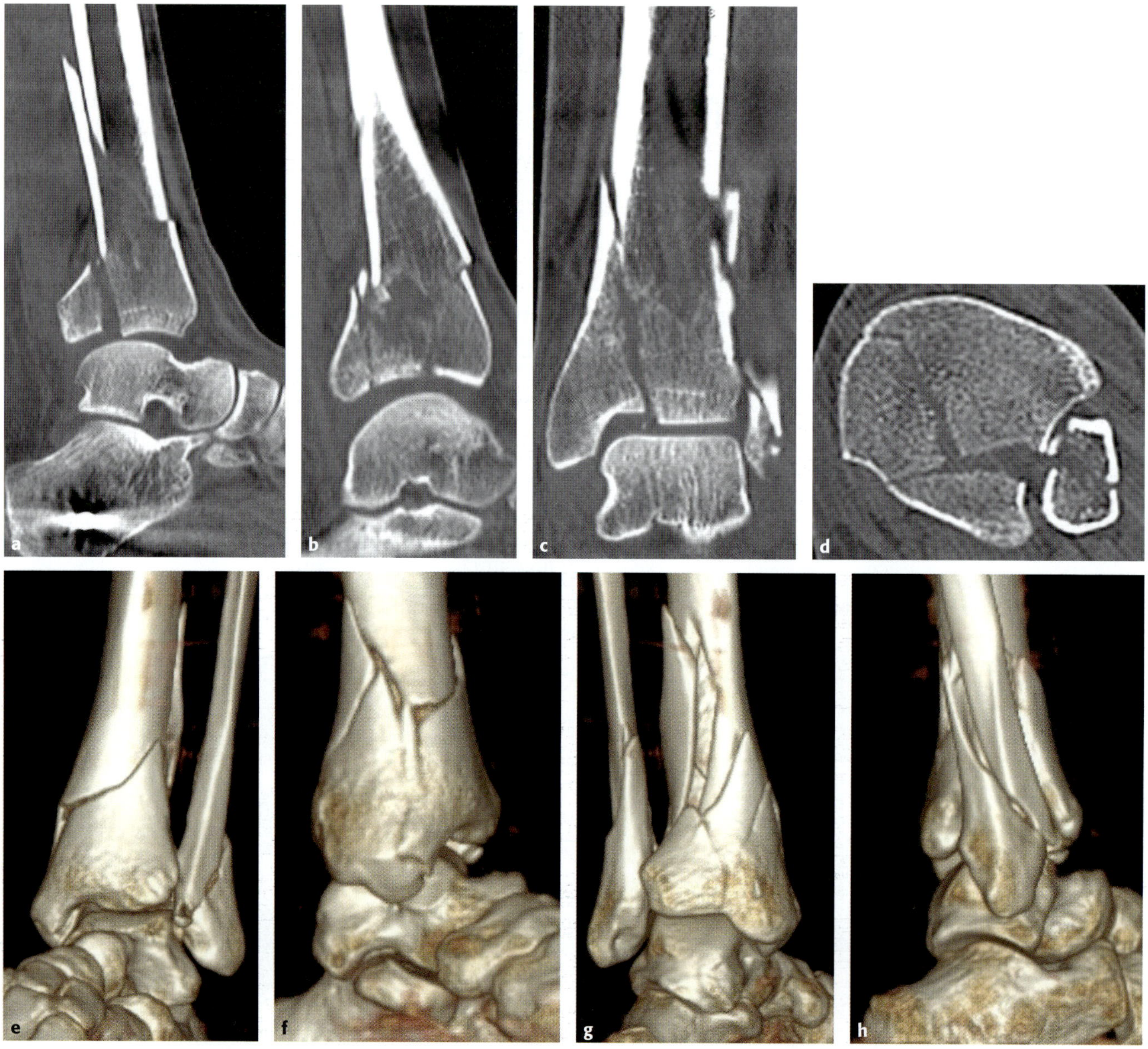

Fig 2.2-3a–h A CT scan with 3D reconstruction.
a–d Sagittal (**a–b**), coronal (**c**), and axial (**d**) images demonstrate displaced posterior, anterolateral, and medial fracture fragments resulting in intraarticular step and gap. The incongruent tibiotalar joint is best appreciated on the sagittal scan.
e–h The 3D reconstructed images show the external fracture anatomy and general alignment.

2 Preoperative planning

Indications for surgery

Displaced intraarticular fractures require open reduction and internal fixation (ORIF).

Principles of fracture fixation

The tibial plafond articular surface injury requires anatomical reduction and stable fixation providing absolute stability. The multifragmentary metaphyseal injury requires reduction to restore length, rotation, and alignment as well as stable fixation providing stability. Fixation of fibula fracture remains controversial but may help to reduce the tibia and provide additional stability, preventing tibia drift into malunion.

Approach

Three separate approaches are required:

- The posterior fragment is accessed by a modified posteromedial approach.
- The anterolateral and medial fragments are approached with a single incision, the extensile approach.
- The fibula is approached with an incision along its posterior margin to increase the width of the soft-tissue bridge.

Plate positioning

When selecting the lengths of the three tibial plates, consideration must be given to their proximal ends which should be at different levels of the tibial shaft to avoid the development of stress fractures. The valgus deformity requires a long anterolateral plate which acts as a buttress.

Order of fixation

1. The posterior tibial fracture is anatomically reduced and fixed.
2. The remaining tibial articular fragments are reconstructed with an anterolateral plate followed by a medial plate.
3. The fibula is the last structure to be fixed (**Fig 2.2-4**).

External fixator in situ

Surgery should be performed with the external fixator left in place, as it can aid in maintaining limb alignment, length, and rotation. It also aids in distraction and thus visualization of the ankle joint.

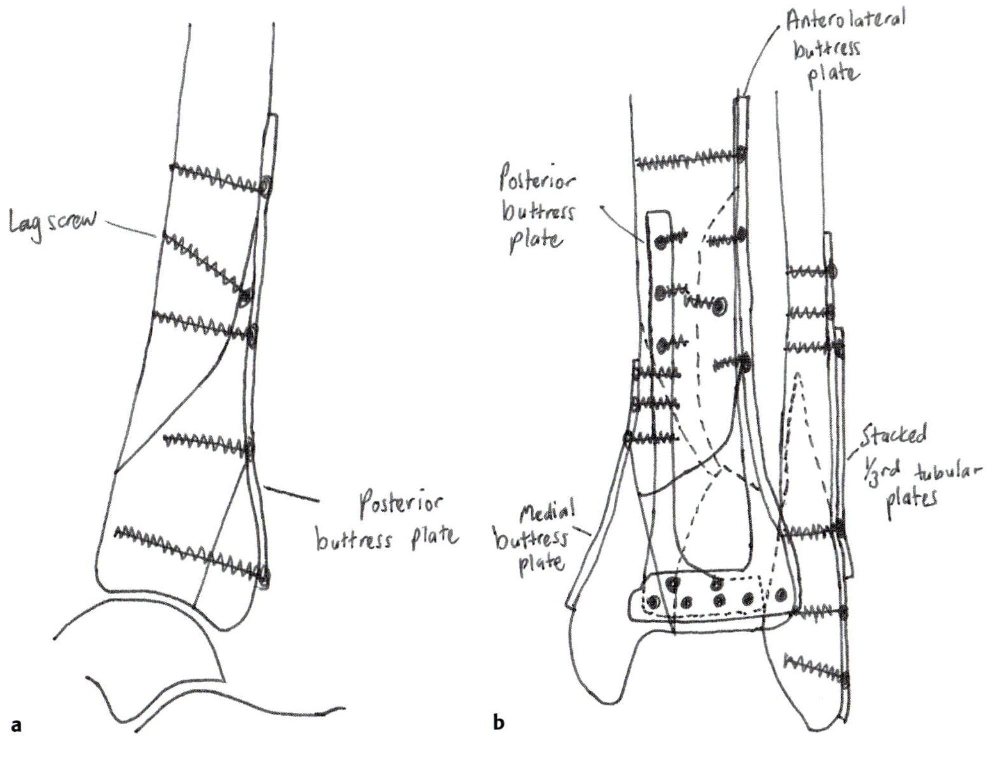

Fig 2.2-4a–b Preoperative plan.
a The posterior tibial fragment is directly reduced and fixed with a buttress plate via modified posteromedial approach.
b The anterolateral and medial fragments are directly reduced and fixed with a longer anterolateral plate and a shorter medial buttress plate via the extensile approach. The fibular fracture is directly reduced and fixed with stacked one-third tubular plates via an incision placed along its posterior margin.

3 Operating room setup

Patient positioning	• This surgery requires a change in patient position from prone to supine. • Prone on a radiolucent table for posterior tibial fragment fixation: – The foot is positioned at the end of the table for improved access. – When this part of surgery is completed, the wounds are closed and covered, and the drapes are removed. • Supine for pilon and fibular fixation and fixation of the anterolateral and medial fragments and fibula fracture.
Anesthesia options	• General, often supplemented with a regional nerve block
C-arm location	• The monitor placed at the head of the operative table. • Posterior tibial fragment fixation: – C-arm from the contralateral side of the table • Pilon fixation and fibular fixation: – C-arm is moved to the ipsilateral side of the operative table
Tourniquet	• Used at surgeon's discretion. • Improves ability to visualize both the joint and the reduction
Tips	• A bump may be placed under the ipsilateral hip to assist in positioning as needed. • The operative limb is placed on an elevating ramp to aid in obtaining clear C-arm images and improve visualisation.

For illustrations and overview of anesthetic considerations, see chapter 1.

Equipment

- Variable angle locking (VAL) distal tibia T-plate or L-plate 2.7 (for fixation of posterior tibial fragment)
- VAL anterolateral plate 2.7/3.5 (for fixation of anterolateral tibial fragment)
- Locking compression plate 2.4/2.7
- One-third tubular plate(s) (for fixation of fibula fracture)
- K-wires
- Point-to-point reduction (Weber) clamps
- Smooth and sharp elevators

Size of system, instruments, and implants may vary according to anatomy of the fracture and the patient. Conventional compression plates may be used in good bone quality, while locking plates are preferred in osteoporotic bone and comminution.

4 Surgical procedure

Posterior tibial fragment fixation

The first step is fixation of the posterior tibial fragment to restore the posterior tibia, onto which the anterolateral and medial fragments will be reduced. The patient is positioned prone.

Prone positioning

With the patient in prone position, it is vital to ensure a sufficiently large bolster is placed beneath the anterior tibia to enable the surgeon to fully flex and extend the patient's ankle. C-arm projections must be adjusted accordingly to allow precise posterior-anterior, mortise, and lateral views of the tibiotalar joint.

The modified posteromedial approach is used as it provides excellent access to center of the posterior aspect of the tibial plafond, so that direct reduction and plating can be performed. The incision is made 1 cm medial to the medial border of the Achilles tendon, starting just proximal to the insertion of the Achilles tendon on the calcaneus, and extending 12 cm proximally. The Achilles tendon is retracted laterally within its sheath.

Next, the transverse intermuscular septum which separates the superficial and deep posterior compartments is cut longitudinally. The tendon and muscle belly of the flexor hallucis longus (FHL) tendon and the tibial nerve are identified, and an interval is developed between them. The FHL is retracted laterally and the tibial nerve is gently retracted medially. The disrupted posterior ankle capsule usually requires further dissection to expose the entire fracture. This approach allows exposure of the entire posterior tibial metaphysis and proximal dissection allows exposure of the diaphysis. An external fixator (or large distractor) is useful to distract the tibiotalar joint to aid in visualization. The fracture is reflected laterally hinging on the intact posterior inferior tibiofibular ligament, cleared of its hematoma, and anatomically reduced to the proximal tibial cortex. The anatomically reduced posterior fragment is provisionally held with K-wires. The large butterfly fragment is fixed with a lag screw. Definitive fixation is achieved with posterior buttress plating. Care must be taken to avoid excessively long posterior to anterior screws so as not to interfere with subsequent reduction of the medial and anterolateral fragments.

Pilon and fibular fixation

In the next part of the surgery the patient is positioned supine, and the extensile approach is used as it permits complete and direct visualization of the tibial articular surface and placement of medial, anterior, anterolateral plates, thus making it ideal for the AO/OTA type C pilon fracture. The incision starts 10 mm below the tip of the medial malleolus and proceeds transversely across the ankle to a point just lateral to the midline and then turns, continuing proximally 10 mm lateral to the tibial crest. Thus, the vertical limb of the incision lies lateral to the tibialis anterior tendon and can be extended as desired. The incision is carried down to the subcutaneous tissue. Care should be taken to avoid unnecessary dissection.

Next, the extensor retinaculum is incised with an attempt to leave the tibialis anterior tendon undisturbed in its sheath. The full-thickness subcutaneous flap is retracted medially while the tibialis anterior tendon is retracted laterally. The flap is handled atraumatically without strong retraction or the use of forceps. The flap can be retracted using nylon stay sutures in the skin. At the level of the ankle, the capsule is opened longitudinally, exposing the talus. Subperiosteal dissection exposes the distal tibia fracture. Retraction of the tissues laterally exposes the entire lateral articular fragment of Chaput. The anterolateral fragment is reduced anatomically onto the previously fixed posterior fragment, then the medial fragment is reduced onto the posterior and anterolateral fragments. It is temporarily stabilized with K-wires.

Fracture fixation principle

Plates used in fixation of pilon fractures usually function as buttress plates. Generally, a fracture that is primarily in varus should be buttressed with a medial plate; and conversely, a fracture that is primarily in valgus should be buttressed with an anterolateral plate.

For definitive fixation, the anterolateral fragment is buttressed with an anterolateral plate and the medial fragment is buttressed with a medial plate. If the plates are longer than the incision, the plates can be slid proximally along the periosteum, and screws inserted using a minimally invasive technique. Large metaphyseal defects should be bonegrafted (**Fig 2.2-5**).

After pilon fracture fixation is completed, the fibula is fixed. Fibular fixation provides greater stability to the construct. The skin bridge must be considered when placing this third incision, aiming to maximize the distance between it and the vertical limb of the extensile approach and the modified posteromedial approach. The fibula is reduced anatomically and plated (**Fig 2.2-6**). In situations of tenuous soft tissue, the fibula can be reduced with a mini-open approach and stabilized with an intramedullary rod or screw inserted retrograde from the distal end of the fibula.

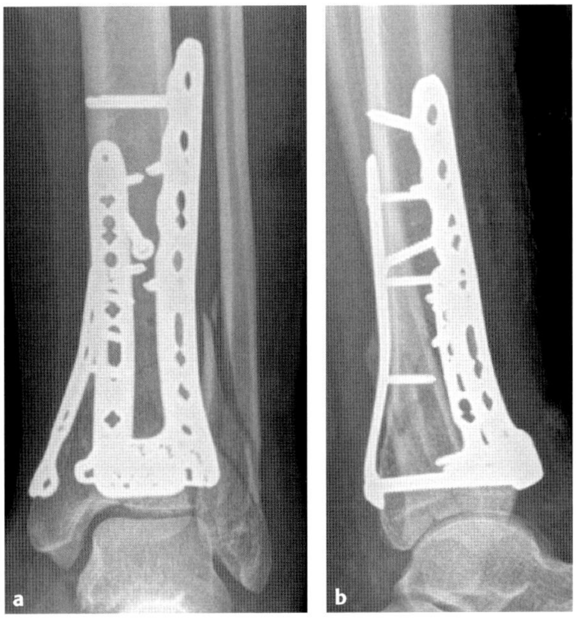

Fig 2.2-5 Intraoperative images.

a Posterior, anterolateral, and medial plates have been applied. Anatomical reduction and stable fixation of the tibial plafond articular surface has been successfully achieved. At this stage, the fibula had not yet been fixed.

b Lateral image shows a well-reduced tibial articular surface and a congruent tibiotalar joint.

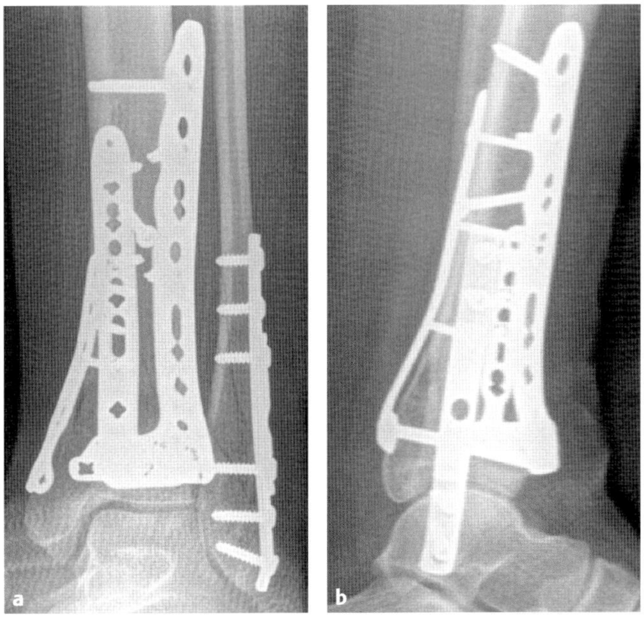

Fig 2.2-6a–b Immediate postoperative x-rays showing restoration of the ankle mortise and distal tibia alignment through anatomical and stable fracture fixation.

a AP view.

b Lateral view.

5 Pitfalls and complications

Pitfalls

Soft-tissue problems

This is a major pitfall when treating pilon fractures, owing to the inherently thin soft-tissue envelope around the distal tibia, the fragility of soft tissues after high-energy trauma, and the necessity for multiple incisions to approach different parts of the complex fracture (**Table 2.2-1**).

Pitfall	Tip
Insufficient resolution of soft-tissue edema	• Wait for wrinkle sign before definitive surgery (may require waiting 14–21 days or more, postinjury)
Rough soft-tissue handling	• Gentle atraumatic retraction • Avoid desiccation of tendons or flap during surgery
Inadequate skin bridge between incisions	• Maximize distance between incisions
Contracted and unstable soft tissues	• Early application of external fixator not only stabilizes the fracture but also stabilizes and prevents contracture of soft tissues while waiting for definitive ORIF.
Posterior plate screws too long and block reduction of anterolateral and medial fracture fragments	• Ensure posterior screws are the correct length.

Table 2.2-1 Major pitfalls pertaining to soft-tissue care.

Inadequate fracture visualization

In C-type fractures, visualization of and access to the entire articular surface is often necessary. Selection of an approach that is suboptimal for a particular fracture pattern may result in excessive traction, skin edge necrosis, difficult access, and poor quality reduction and fixation. An external fixator is frequently used to aid visualization of the articular surface by distracting the tibiotalar joint.

Irreducible or non-fixable articular fragments

Very small or comminuted articular surface fragments that are impossible to anatomically reduce or fix and are at risk of affecting the congruency of the joint or displacing into the joint as loose fragments are better off removed than poorly fixed.

Fibular malreduction

Malreduction of the fibula either occurring during the time of external fixation, or as the first step in definitive ORIF will complicate reduction of the tibial pilon fracture. As such, the sequence of fixation always starts with the tibial pilon fracture and ends with the fibula. Fibular fixation may sometimes be performed in a subsequent surgery if the limb is deemed too swollen after fixation of the tibial pilon fracture. The fibula is fixed to increase stability of the pilon fixation and restore the ankle mortise.

Complications

Flap necrosis

Avoided through appropriate timing of definitive ORIF, meticulous and gentle soft-tissue handling, and repair of extensor retinaculum to prevent tibialis anterior tendon from bowstringing and exerting pressure on the overlying subcutaneous flap.

Infection

Avoided through a combination of prophylactic antibiotics, extreme care with soft tissues, and reducing duration of surgery (**Fig 2.2-7**).

Injury to tibial nerve

Avoided through delicate dissection and gentle retraction.

Loss of fixation

Avoided through use of locking plates in comminuted fractures, correct placement of plates, and correct principle of buttress plating.

Malunion

Avoided through anatomical reduction of articular surface, and functional reduction of tibial length, rotation, and varus-valgus alignment.

Nonunion

Avoided through bone grafting of large metaphyseal defects, preserving soft-tissue attachments to fracture, and providing adequate stability.

Posttraumatic arthritis

This is related to the severity of injury, quality of reduction, and primary articular cartilage damage.

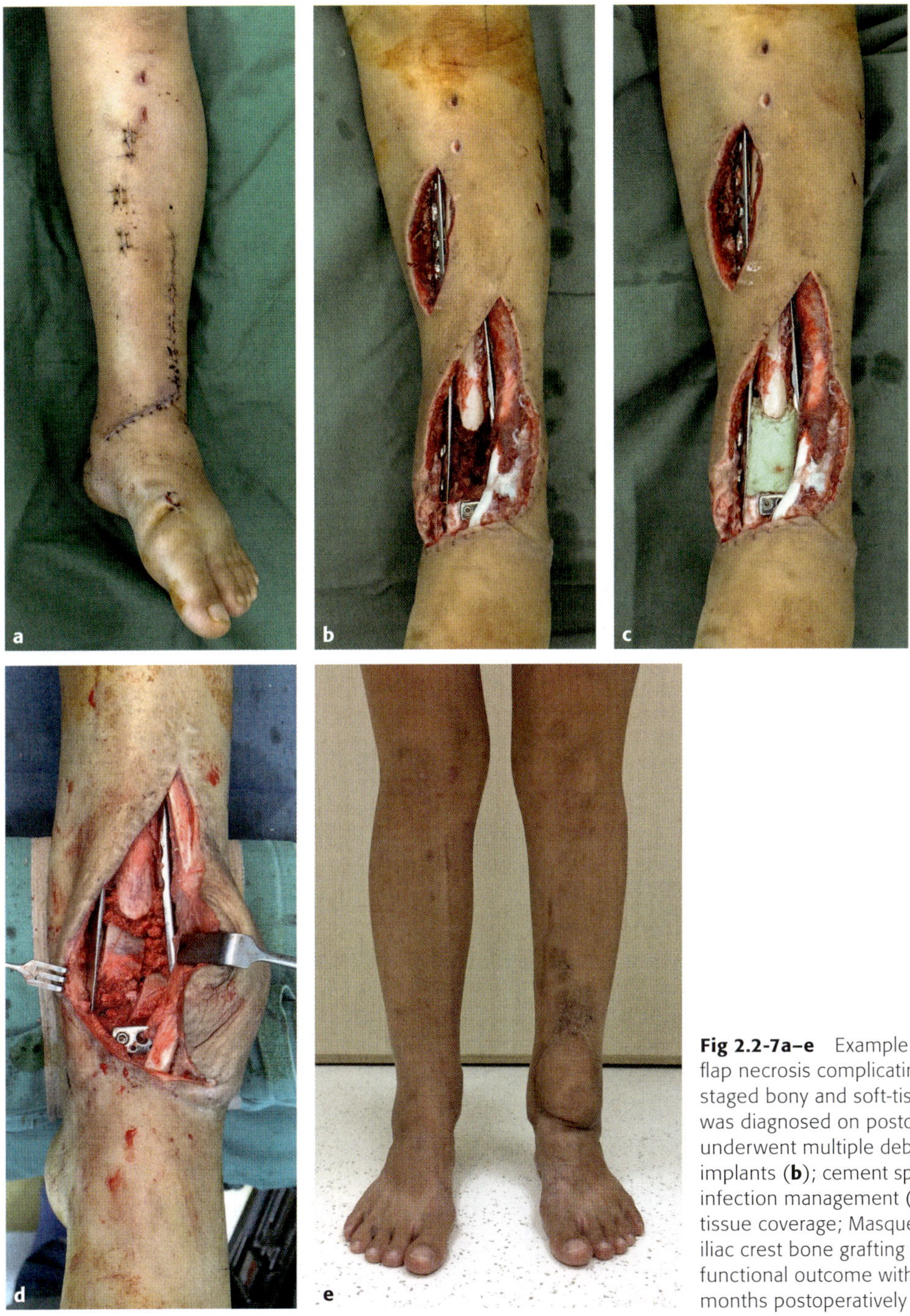

Fig 2.2-7a–e Example from a different case of infection and flap necrosis complicating pilon fracture ORIF, managed with staged bony and soft-tissue reconstruction. An acute infection was diagnosed on postoperative day 3 (**a**). The patient underwent multiple debridement surgeries with retention of implants (**b**); cement spacer implantation for dead space and infection management (**c**); free flap reconstruction for soft-tissue coverage; Masquelet-induced membrane technique and iliac crest bone grafting of the metaphyseal defect (**d**). A good functional outcome with healed fracture and free flap at 15 months postoperatively (**e**).

6 Alternative techniques

Selecting appropriate incisions is dependent on the fracture pattern and the soft-tissue envelope. Traumatized soft tissue, injury wounds, or preexisting scars will require incisions to be placed away from the area of concern.

In patients who are at high risk of developing wound problems (diabetes, arteriosclerosis, smoking), a limited ORIF of the articular block may be performed and the metaphyseal fracture may be definitively treated with a ring fixator.

Nonoperative treatment with late reconstruction of the ankle may also be considered in patients with multisystem disease.

7 Postoperative management and rehabilitation

Postoperatively, the leg is immobilized in a below-knee splint until satisfactory wound healing. After the wounds have healed, start active and passive range-of-motion (ROM) exercises. In the first 6 weeks, the patient should be toe-touch weight-bearing. In the second 6 weeks, the patient should gradually increase to full weight bearing as tolerated in a removable orthosis and continue ankle ROM exercises and gentle resistance training. After 12 weeks, the patient may begin neuromuscular retraining which focuses on coordination, balance, and gait.

Postoperative x-rays are obtained in the at 6 weeks, 12 weeks, 6 months, 1 year, and 2 years. X-rays are evaluated for healing in the initial months and for signs of posttraumatic arthrosis beyond 1 year.

Implant removal

Removal of implants is not mandatory but recommended if implants are prominent under the subcutaneous envelope of the distal tibia. Implant removal should be undertaken only after healing is complete, ie, after 1 year at the earliest. This patient had achieved good radiographic and functional healing at the 1-year postoperative review (**Fig 2.2-8** and **Fig 2.2-9**).

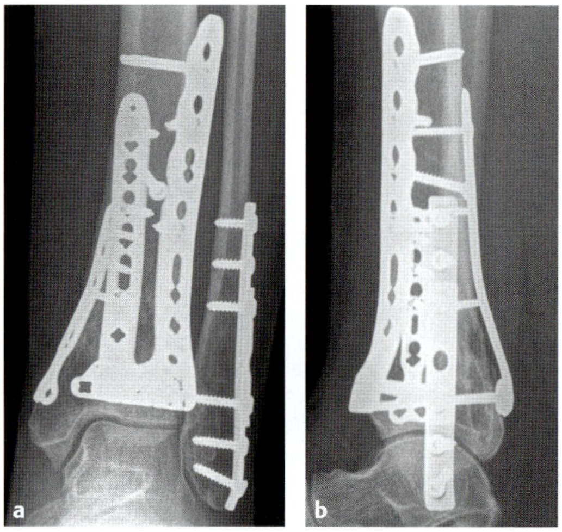

Fig 2.2-8a–b Postoperative x-rays at 1 year showing healed fractures, implants in situ, and limited tibiotalar arthrosis.
a AP view.
b Lateral view.

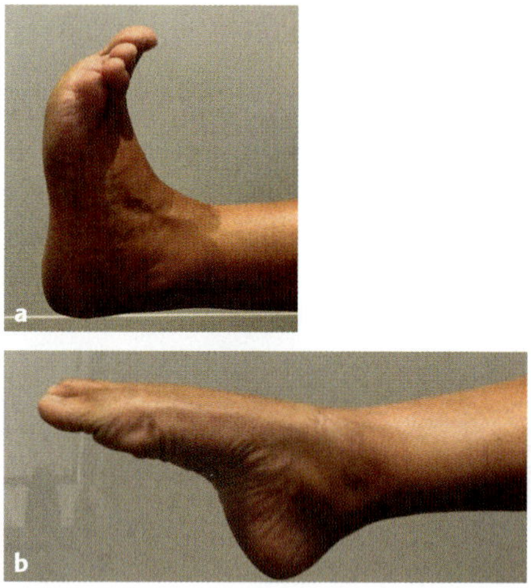

Fig 2.2-9 Good functional recovery at 1 year postoperatively.
a Active dorsiflexion of 10°.
b Active plantarflexion of 35°.

8 Recommended reading

Assal M, Ray A, Fasel JH, et al. A modified posteromedial approach combined with extensile anterior for the treatment of complex tibial pilon fractures (AO/OTA 43-C). *J Orthop Trauma.* 2014 Jun;28(6):e138–145.
Assal M, Ray A, Stern R. Strategies for surgical approaches in open reduction internal fixation of pilon fractures. *J Orthop Trauma.* 2015 Feb;29(2):69–79.
Assal M, Ray A, Stern R. The extensile approach for the operative treatment of high-energy pilon fractures: surgical technique and soft-tissue healing. *J Orthop Trauma.* 2007 Mar;21(3):198–206.
Sands A, Grujic L, Byck DC, et al. Clinical and functional outcomes of internal fixation of displaced pilon fractures. *Clin Orthop Relat Res.* 1998 Feb;(347):131–137.

2.3 Partial articular fracture—plate fixation

May Fong Mak, Mathieu Assal

1 Case description

A 53-year old man injured his right ankle in a motor vehicle accident. Clinical examination revealed a swollen and painful right ankle. It was a closed injury. X-rays revealed a fracture dislocation of the distal tibia with partial articular involvement (AO/OTA 43B3), and associated fracture of the fibula above the level of the syndesmosis (**Fig 2.3-1**). A computed tomographic (CT) scan showed a fracture of the posterior tibial plafond with the fracture line extending from midline of the medial malleolus into the incisura fibularis, with impaction and incarceration of joint fragments (**Fig 2.3-2**).

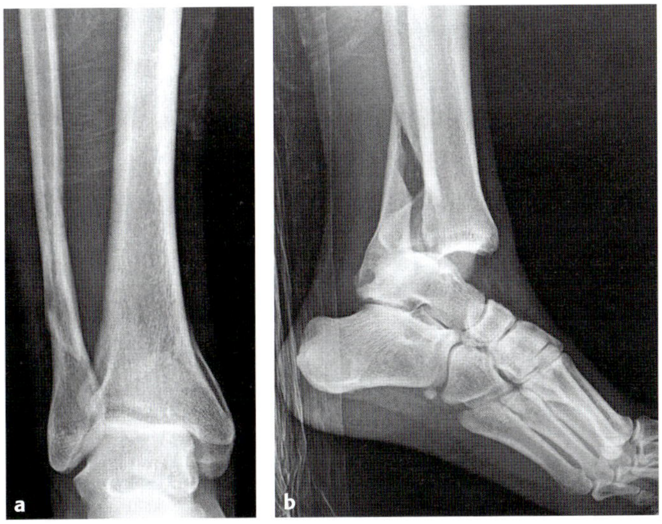

Fig 2.3-1a–b Immediate postinjury x-rays.
a AP x-ray showing the characteristic medial malleolar double contour sign.
b Lateral x-ray showing a displaced partial articular fracture of the posterior distal tibia (AO/OTA 43B3) with tibiotalar dislocation.

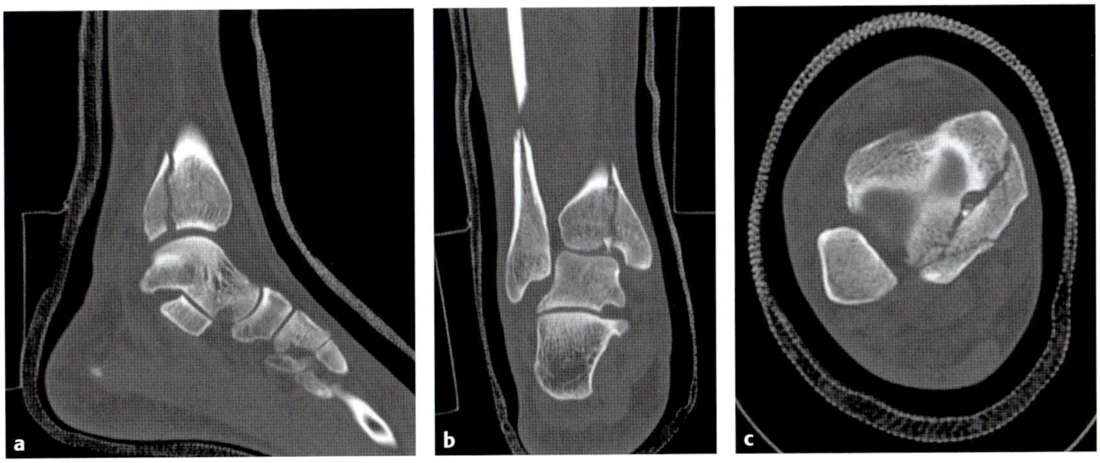

Fig 2.3-2a–c Computed tomographic images.
a Coronal split of the medial distal tibia.
b Incarcerated impacted articular fragment.
c Fracture line extends across the entire width of the posterior distal tibial articular surface.

2 Preoperative planning

Indications for surgery

Displaced lower extremity fractures require restoration of anatomy, specifically length, alignment, and rotation. Displaced intraarticular fractures with loss of congruity of a weight-bearing joint require open reduction internal fixation (ORIF) to restore the articular surface.

If after attempts at closed reduction there is still malalignment of the extremity and displacement of the articular surface, then open treatment should be considered.

Fracture fixation principle

Plates used in fixation of pilon fractures usually function as buttress plates. Posterior pilon fractures generally displace posteriorly and superiorly, with the foot dislocating with the fragment. These fractures should be addressed through posterior buttress plating.

3 Operating room setup

Patient positioning	• This involves a two-stage positioning with repeat draping: – Prone for fixation of the posterior tibial and medial malleolus – Supine for the lateral malleolus • Alternatively, a "sloppy" lateral position with the leg mobile or fixation of the lateral malleolus with the patient prone can be used to avoid repositioning.
Anesthesia options	• General, with regional nerve block
C-arm location	• Positioned for ease of viewing by surgeon
Tourniquet	• Used at surgeon's discretion • Generally, improves visualization of anatomy
Tips	• A headlight improves visualization of both the pertinent anatomy as well as fracture visualization.

For illustrations and overview of anesthetic considerations, see chapter 1.

Equipment

- Locking compression plate 2.4/2.7 (for buttress fixation of posterior tibial plafond fragment)
- 2.4 mm screws (for fixation of the medial malleolus)
- 2.7 mm screws (for fixation of the fibular fracture)
- K-wires
- Point-to-point reduction (Weber) clamps
- Smooth and sharp elevators

Size of instruments and implants may vary depending on the anatomy of the fracture and the patient. In a noncomminuted fracture of the fibula with good bone quality and a large surface area, several independent lag screws may be sufficient for fixation without requiring a neutralization plate.

4 Surgical procedure

The surgical sequence starts with restoration of the distal tibial articular surface through fixation of the posterior column fracture. Next, the coronal split of the medial malleolus is fixed. Subsequently, the fibular fracture is fixed. Finally, the syndesmosis is stressed manually to check for diastasis, and fixed if any instability is present.

Although this sequence differs from that taught by the original AO surgeons who started with fibular fixation, many surgeons choose to address the tibia first as fibular hardware may obscure proper visualization of the plafond.

Posterior tibial and medial malleolar fragment fixation

The first step is fixation of the posterior tibial fragment to restore the articular surface and tibiotalar congruency.

The modified posteromedial approach is used as it provides excellent access to the greatest portion of the distal tibia without excessive traction on the soft tissues. The patient is positioned prone. With the patient in the prone position it is vital to ensure that a sufficiently large bolster is placed beneath the anterior tibia to enable the surgeon to fully flex and extend the patient's ankle. C-arm projections must be adjusted accordingly to allow precise posterior-anterior, mortise, and lateral views of the tibiotalar joint.

The incision is made 1 cm medial to the medial border of the Achilles tendon, starting just proximal to the insertion of the Achilles tendon on the calcaneus, and extending 12 cm proximally. The Achilles tendon is retracted laterally with care to preserve its sheath. Then the transverse intermuscular septum, which separates the superficial and deep posterior compartments, is cut longitudinally. The tendon and muscle belly of the flexor hallucis longus (FHL) tendon and the tibial nerve are identified, and the interval is developed between them. The FHL is retracted laterally and the tibial nerve is gently retracted medially. This approach allows exposure of the entire posterior tibial metaphysis and proximal dissection permits exposure of the diaphysis. The cortical surface of the fracture is exposed. However, in this technique, there is no possibility to visualize the articular surface directly, and the quality of reduction must be assessed by lateral

C-arm views. The surgeon may also use a small scope to assess the articular reduction as well as inserting a small (Freer) elevator into the joint to assess any step-off.

Small, nonfixable fragments are removed. The main articular incarcerated fragment located deep in the joint is approached by separating the main posterior fragments. This fragment is reduced anatomically together with the main posterior fragments, and temporarily held with K-wires. After anatomical reduction of the articular surface has been confirmed, an antiglide plate is fixed with a single screw placed proximal to the fracture. This construct will buttress the whole posterior column at the level of the joint.

The medial malleolus is fixed through the same surgical approach. A point-to-point reduction (Weber) clamp is used to reduce the coronal split of the medial malleolus before three independent screws are placed from posterior to anterior, effectively functioning as lag screws. The tourniquet is deflated and the wound is closed in layers. A temporary dressing is applied.

Fibular fixation

At this point the patient is positioned supine for fixation of the fibular fracture. Alternatively, the fibula can be reduced and fixed via a lateral approach (see chapter 3.7) or a posterolateral approach (see chapter 3.8) with the patient prone. For repositioning of the patient, the temporary dressing is removed, and the limb is again prepared and draped. It may be necessary to place a sandbag or rolled blanket under the ipsilateral hip to internally rotate the leg to neutral rotation for easy access to the fibula. The C-arm can be moved to the other side of the table, but the screen can remain in the same place. Standard preparation and draping is then performed with the patient supine. The tourniquet may be reinflated during surgery.

The fibula is approached through a direct lateral incision. The fracture is anatomically reduced, temporarily reduced with a point-to-point reduction (Weber) clamp, and fixed with two independent screws (**Fig 2.3-3**). A plate may be used as per surgeon preference.

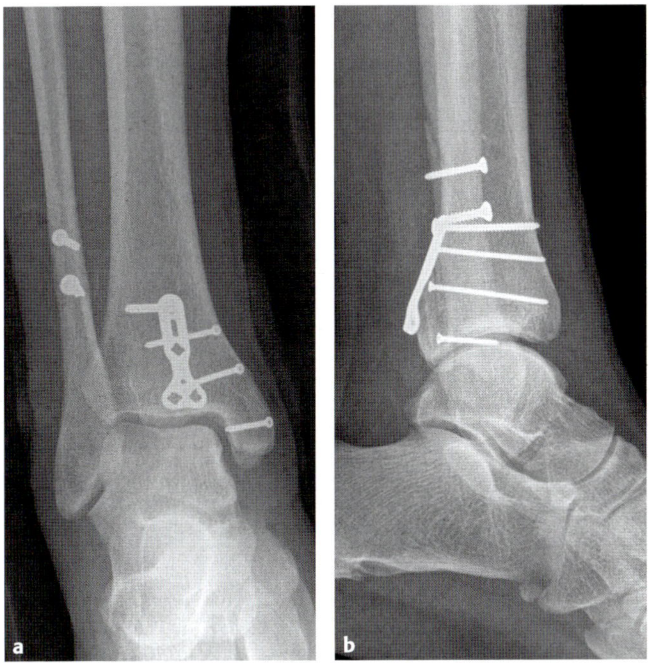

Fig 2.3-3a–b Immediate postoperative x-rays showing an anatomical ankle mortise achieved using a combination of posterior buttress plate and lag screws.

Stress test of the syndesmosis

During the final part of surgery, the Cotton stress test is performed by means of a hook with manual traction on the restored fibula under C-arm imaging. Additional stress is given to evaluate anteroposterior instability. For this patient, the stress test was negative, implying a stable syndesmosis, thus syndesmosis fixation was not performed.

5 Pitfalls and complications

Pitfalls

Soft-tissue problems

This is a major pitfall when treating pilon fractures, owing to the inherently thin soft-tissue envelope around the distal tibia, the fragility of soft tissues after high-energy trauma, and the necessity for multiple incisions to approach different parts of the complex fracture (**Table 1.3-1**).

Pitfall	Tip
Insufficient resolution of soft-tissue edema	• Wait for the wrinkle sign before definitive surgery (may require waiting 9–14 days postinjury). • Early application of the external fixator not only stabilizes the fracture, but also stabilizes the soft tissues which allows the swelling to resolve. • It preserves the length of the fracture.
Rough handling of soft tissue	• Gentle atraumatic retraction, avoid dessication of tendons or flap during surgery.
Inadequate skin bridge between incisions	• Maximize the distance between incisions (5 cm).

Table 1.3-1 The major pitfalls pertaining to soft-tissue care.

Inadequate fracture visualization

In fractures that involve the entire posterior column, where the fracture line extends from the midline of the medial malleolus into the incisura fibularis, access to the entire width of the distal tibia at the level of the joint is necessary. The modified posteromedial approach is useful for this particular fracture pattern. Selection of an approach that is suboptimal may result in excessive traction, skin-edge necrosis, neurovascular traction injury, difficult access, and poor-quality reduction and fixation.

Irreducible or nonfixable articular fragments

Very small or comminuted articular surface fragments that are impossible to anatomically reduce or fix and are at risk of affecting joint congruency or displacing into the joint, as loose fragments are better removed than poorly fixed.

Inability to visualize the articular reduction

It is not possible to directly visualize the articular surface of the distal tibia during fixation of posterior pilon fractures. Reduction is assessed with good-quality intraoperative lateral C-arm views or intraoperative CT scan.

Complications

Soft-tissue complications

Avoided by appropriate timing of definitive ORIF, meticulous and gentle soft-tissue handling.

Infection

Avoided by a combination of prophylactic antibiotics, extreme care with soft tissues, and reduced duration of surgery.

Injury to tibial nerve

Avoided by delicate dissection and gentle retraction.

Malreduction

Avoided by obtaining anatomical reduction.

Loss of fixation

Avoided by correct use of buttress plate and lag screw fixation principles.

Nonunion

Avoided by preserving soft tissue and capsular attachments to the fracture and providing adequate stability.

Posttraumatic arthritis

This is related to the severity of injury, quality of reduction, and articular cartilage damage at the time of the injury.

6 Alternative techniques

Lag screw only fixation

In a posterior pilon fracture that is nondisplaced, noncomminuted, and sustained after a low-energy injury, multiple lag screws providing absolute stability may work as an alternative method to buttress plating. Case selection, however, must be precise.

Intramedullary fixation

Carefully selected B-type fractures that also have a more proximal component can be treated with reduction and screw fixation for the distal tibial articular surface followed by intramedullary fixation of the more proximal injury (see chapter 2.4).

7 Postoperative management and rehabilitation

Postoperatively the limb is placed in a short leg cast and the patient remains nonweight bearing for 6 weeks. If x-rays at 6 weeks demonstrate early healing, the patient is permitted progressive full weight bearing as tolerated in a removable orthosis and should commence ankle range-of-motion exercises and gentle resistance training. After 12 weeks the patient may focus on coordination, balance, and gait. Serial postoperative x-rays are performed up to 2 years postoperative and evaluated for signs of posttraumatic arthrosis.

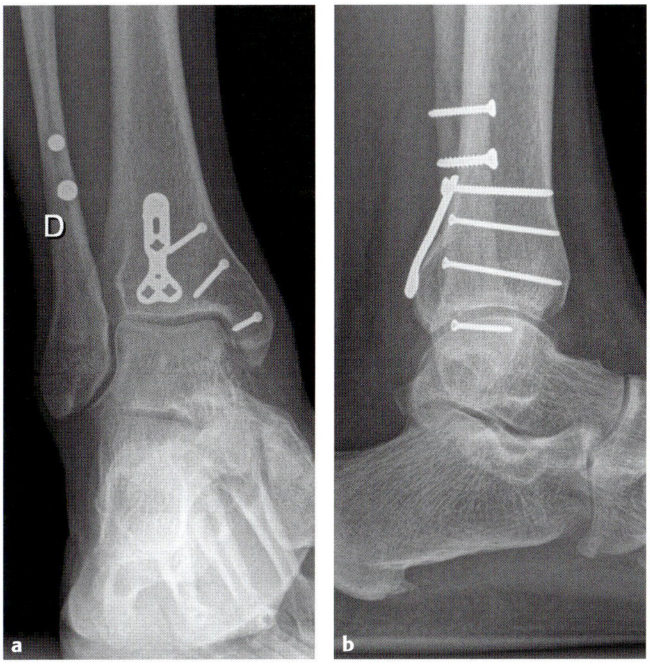

Fig 2.3-4a–b Postoperative x-rays at 6 months show fracture healing without loss of fixation.

Implant removal

Routine removal of implants is not performed unless they are prominent and symptomatic but only after healing is complete, so at 12–18 months at the earliest. This patient showed good radiographic healing at the 6-month postoperative review (**Fig 2.3-4**). He regained full range-of-ankle motion at 6 months postoperative (**Fig 2.3-5**).

In most cases of pilon fracture full motion is not achieved, and patients should be made aware at the time of injury that the goal is to regain functional motion. Very rarely will the patient achieve motion equal to the uninjured side whether the fracture is treated nonoperatively or with ORIF.

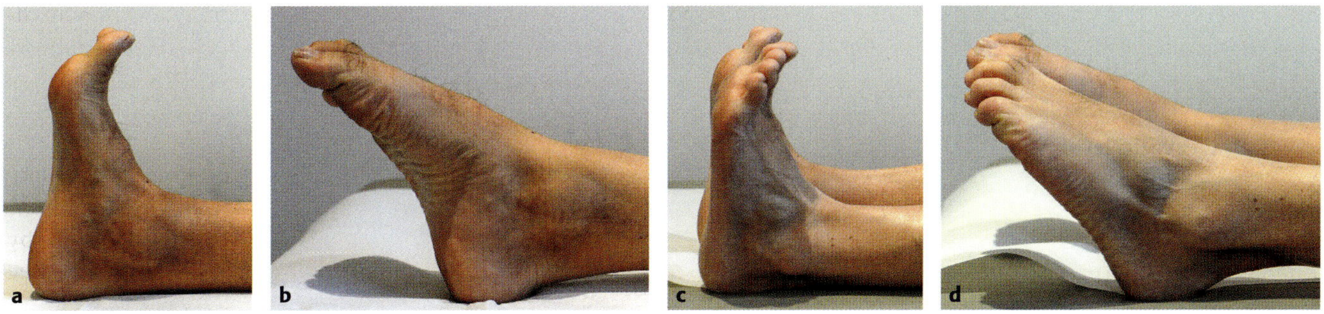

Fig 2.3-5a–d Full range-of-ankle motion at 6 months postoperative.

8 Recommended reading

Assal M, Dalmau-Pastor M, Ray A, et al. How to get to the distal posterior tibial malleolus? A cadaveric anatomic study defining the access corridors through 3 different approaches. *J Orthop Trauma.* 2017 Apr;31(4):e127–e129.

Assal M, Ray A, Fasel JH, et al. A modified posteromedial approach combined with extensile anterior for the treatment of complex tibial pilon fractures (AO/OTA 43-C). *J Orthop Trauma.* 2014 Jun;28(6):e138–145.

Bartoníček J, Rammelt S, Tucek M. Posterior malleolar fractures: changing concepts and recent developments. *Foot Ankle Clin.* 2017 Mar;22(1):125–145.

Cotton FJ. *Dislocations and joint-fractures.* Philadelphia: WB Saunders; 1910.

Sands A, Grujic L, Byck DC, et al. Clinical and functional outcomes of internal fixation of displaced pilon fractures. *Clin Orthop Relat Res.* 1998 Feb(347):131–137.

Switaj PJ, Weatherford B, Fuchs D, et al. Evaluation of posterior malleolar fractures and the posterior pilon variant in operatively treated ankle fractures. *Foot Ankle Int.* 2014 Sep;35(9):886–895.

2.4 Tibial shaft fracture extending into the plafond—intramedullary fixation

Tim Schepers, Jens Anthony Halm

1 Case description

A 25-year-old woman landed forcefully with a twisting motion on her left foot in shallow water while kitesurfing. She had no previous medical history. Her leg was placed in a vacuum splint and she was transported by ambulance to a nearby hospital.

Clinical examination revealed deformity of her left leg. The injury was closed and there were no neurovascular issues or other injuries. Subsequent x-rays taken revealed an AO/OTA 42B diaphyseal fracture of the tibia and fibula (**Fig 2.4-1**). Upon closer inspection, a fracture line was suspected in the ankle joint. Therefore, a computed tomographic (CT) scan of the distal tibia was performed, which revealed an additional nondisplaced fracture of the posterior tibia at the level of the ankle joint (**Fig 2.4-2**).

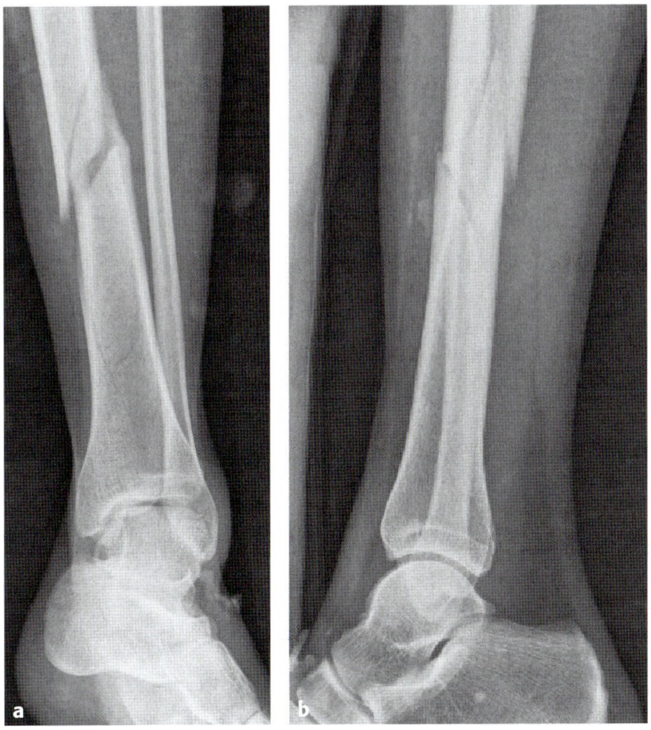

Fig 2.4-1a–b Postinjury x-rays.
a AP view.
b Lateral view.

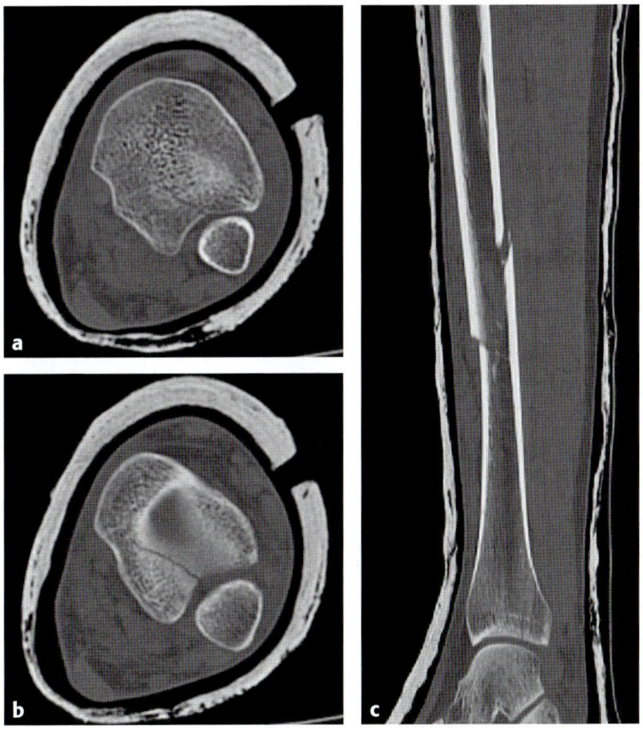

Fig 2.4-2a–c Computed tomographic images.
a Axial view, 5 mm above the pilon.
b Axial view at the level of the pilon.
c Sagittal view.

2 Preoperative planning

Indications for surgery

The surgical indication for a multifragmentary tibial fracture in an adult patient is well established. Nonoperative management may lead to unacceptably high rates of displacement with malunion or nonunion. In addition, prolonged joint immobilization may lead to stiffness. Tibial shaft fractures may be safely managed with an intramedullary (IM) device. While insertion of tibial IM nails has the known side-effect of knee pain, the main advantages of nailing are:

- Little damage to the soft-tissue envelope
- The ability to commence early weight-bearing, range-of-motion (ROM) exercises, and rehabilitation

Based upon the extent of the fracture into the tibial articular surface, a preoperative plan was made (**Fig 2.4-3**). In this case, the ankle joint surface was addressed with a percutaneous screw fixation and stabilization of the tertiary fragment, followed by an IM nail. Failure to stabilize the posterior tibial fracture at the ankle joint can lead to secondary joint displacement through insertion of the IM tibial nail.

3 Operating room setup

Patient positioning	• Supine on a radiolucent operating table with the foot brought to the end of the table
Anesthesia options	• General or spinal: if spinal is chosen, the drug used should be short-acting to allow for monitoring for compartment syndrome post surgery.
C-arm location	• C-arm and monitor on the opposite side of the table to the surgeon
Tourniquet	• A well-padded tourniquet may be applied to the thigh but is probably not needed in most cases. • Use of tourniquet while reaming the IM canal remains controversial.
Tips	• Large point-to-point reduction (Weber) clamps, and positioning triangle are useful for fracture reduction positioning the bent knee bend and during fracture reduction.

For illustrations and overview of anesthetic considerations, see chapter 1.

Equipment list

- Screws and K-wires as per surgeon preference
- Intramedullary nail system with reamers

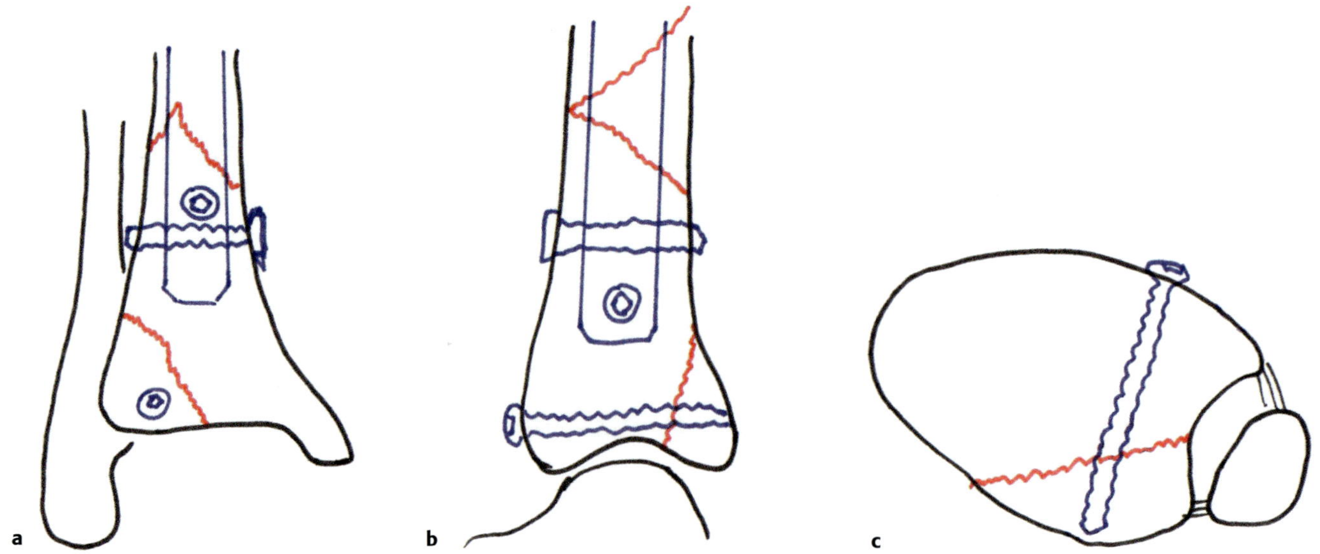

Fig 2.4-3a–c Preoperative plan.
a AP view.
b Lateral view.
c Axial view.

4 Surgical procedure

Following anesthesia and antibiotic prophylaxis the patient is positioned supine. Using the C-arm, a mortise view of the ankle is obtained: the foot in neutral position at the leg and rotated internally 15°. A small anterolateral skin incision is made using the tip of a #15 blade. The incision is deepened using a small clamp until the anterior cortex is reached. The correct position is found using the C-arm and an appropriately sized hole (based on screw size) is drilled into the posterolateral fragment using a drill guide/soft-tissue protection sleeve.

For this patient, a partially threaded screw was used to obtain compression at the fracture. If the fracture is displaced, a reduction clamp placed percutaneously can be used to hold the reduction prior to screw insertion. In this case, the fragment was well aligned, and reduction was not necessary.

Following stabilization of the distal fracture, the leg is flexed at the knee using a triangular stand. A longitudinal midline incision is made over the patellar tendon and the tendon is split. The correct entry point is established using AP and lateral views, and the cortex is opened. A guide wire is inserted and positioned in the center of the distal tibia on both AP and lateral views. The IM canal is reamed 1–1.5 mm larger than the diameter of the chosen tibial nail. In this patient, an 11 mm nail was inserted.

The nail was locked distally with two screws placed using freehand "perfect circles" technique under C-arm guidance. For a simple fracture pattern, one screw may be used proximally, however, for the patient in this case, three proximal screws were inserted. The wounds were irrigated and closed in layers.

5 Pitfalls and complications

Pitfalls

- Although IM nailing is a commonly performed procedure, adequate positioning, with the use of the C-arm, is key to a successful outcome.
- The nail entry point should be chosen precisely, and the guide wire should be in the middle of the tibia, just above the plafond, in the center on both AP and lateral images.
- Improper entry localization or failure to ream in a center (AP)-center (lateral) manner distally may cause malreduction and subsequent malunion of the fracture.
- The surgeon should regularly check for rotation deformity during the procedure. The contralateral leg can be sterile draped into the field for comparison of rotation and alignment.
- For more proximal or distal fractures, use of small incision open reduction and (temporary) small plate fixation allows for a perfect reduction. In addition, more proximal or distal fractures may require additional locking screws through the nail to maintain alignment.

Complications

- Postoperative wound infection and deep medullary infection:
  - The surgeon must check for sequestrum and construct stability. If there is loosening, the implant should be converted to an external frame (**Fig 2.4-4**)
- Screw malpositioning (eg, too long locking screws)
- Insufficient reduction or stabilization of posterior malleolus
- Loss of reduction of the fracture in case of insufficient stability
- Delayed or nonunion
- Anterior knee pain at nail insertion site
- Failure to recognize and treat compartment syndrome
- Injury to tendons, vessels, and nerves at the anterior aspect of the tibia through clamping (if performed) and percutaneous screw insertion

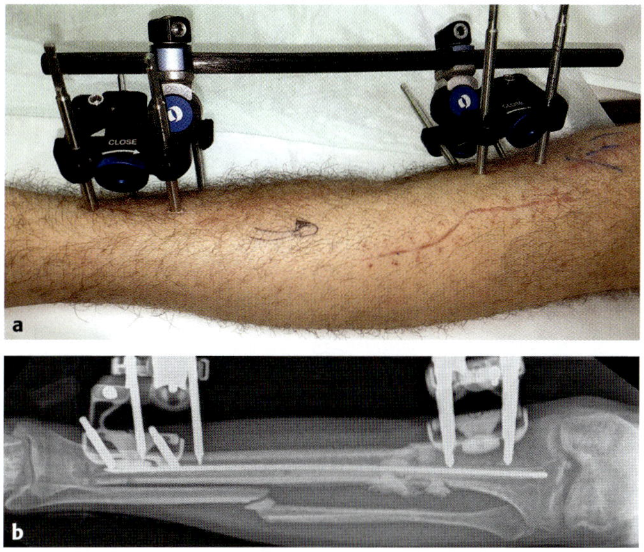

Fig 2.4-4a–b Example from a different case showing unicortical external fixator placement after late infection of the IM nail.
a Unicortical external fixator following removal of an infected IM nail.
b Unicortical external fixator and polymethylmethacrylate nail IM and spacer at fracture site.

6 Alternative techniques

Instead of an IM nail, less invasive plate fixation can be used. This option requires intact anteromedial soft tissues and allows for a lag screw over the fracture if not too comminuted. Plate fixation might be advisable in a case of more severe extension of the fracture line(s) into the plafond (**Fig 2.4-5**).

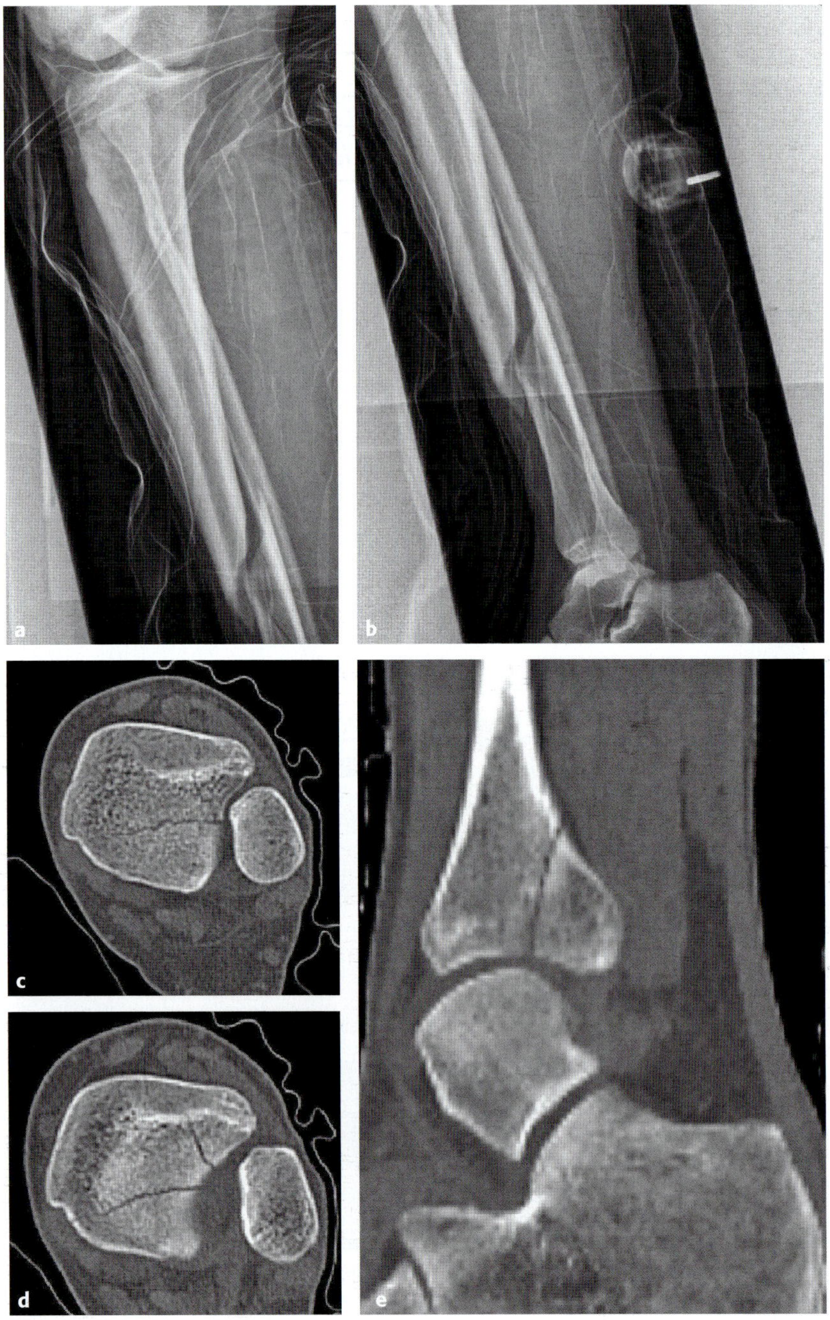

Fig 2.4-5a–i Example of a different case showing treatment with plate fixation.

a–b X-rays in AP (**a**) and lateral (**b**) views show a spiral fracture distal third tibia and proximal fibula. Note the staples at the lateral side used following release of all four compartments via a single lateral incision as this patient also had compartment syndrome of the lower leg.

c–e Axial and sagittal CT scan images at the level of the ankle joint show a more significant injury at the level of the ankle: axial view 5 mm above the pilon (**c**); axial view at the level of the pilon (**d**); sagittal view (**e**).

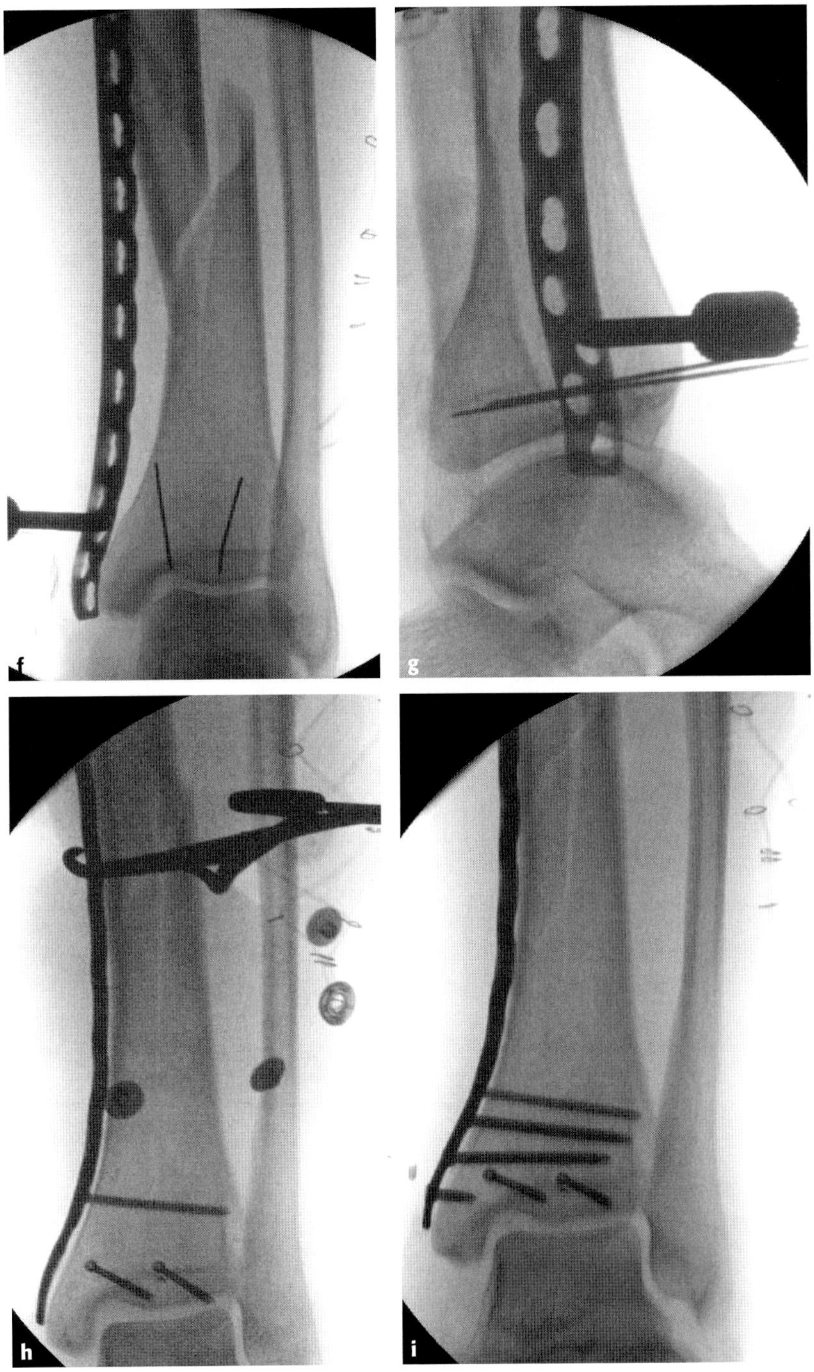

Fig 2.4-5a–i (cont) Example of a different case showing treatment with plate fixation.
f–g Intraoperative AP (**f**) and lateral (**g**) images showing K-wires for cannulated screws.
h–i Distal plate fixation.

7 Postoperative management and rehabilitation

Aftercare is similar to that required for a regular tibial fracture. Early full ROM exercise is allowed, and weight bearing is gradually increased.

Follow-up is at 2 weeks for removal of sutures and after 3 and 6 months for radiographic evaluation.

Implant removal

Intramedullary implants are not routinely removed due to substantial risk of complications and limited benefit in functional outcome. Generally, the IM component of the fixation construct is well tolerated. If symptoms develop it is usually only at the sites of the interlocking screws. These may be removed if they are symptomatic after union is present. If delayed union is present, removal of cross-lock screws may be considered for dynamization of the rod.

This patient healed uneventfully (**Fig 2.4-6** and **Fig 2.4-7**). The nail was removed 1 year after injury at the request of the patient.

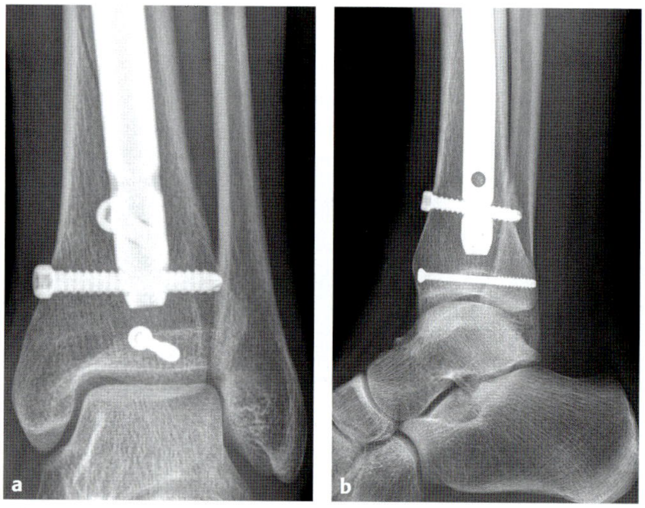

Fig 2.4-6a–b Postoperative x-rays of the ankle in the 25-year-old treated with intramedullary fixation showing adequate reduction.
a AP view.
b Lateral view.

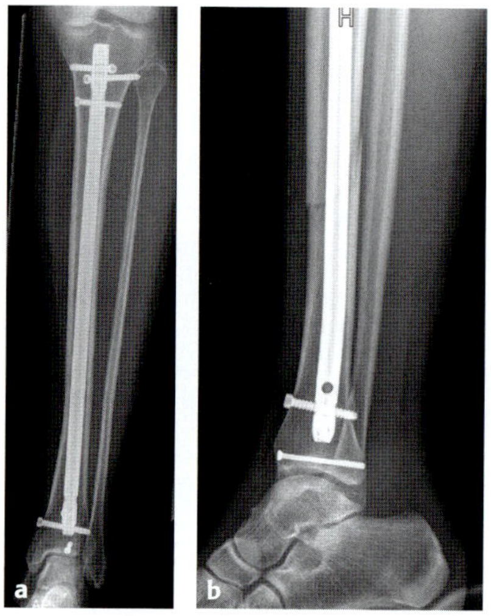

Fig 2.4-7a–b Follow-up x-rays of the 25-year-old treated with intramedullary fixation at 3 months showing maintenance of reduction over time with interval healing of the fracture.
a AP view.
b Lateral view.

8 Recommended reading

Backes M, Dingemans SA, Dijkgraaf MGW, et al. Effect of antibiotic prophylaxis on surgical site infections following removal of orthopedic implants used for treatment of foot, ankle, and lower leg fractures: a randomized clinical trial. *Jama.* 2017 Dec 26;318(24):2438–2445.

Georgiadis GM, Ebraheim NA, Hoeflinger MJ. Displacement of the posterior malleolus during intramedullary tibial nailing. *J Trauma.* 1996 Dec;41(6):1056–1058.

Hou Z, Zhang L, Zhang Q, et al. The "communication line" suggests occult posterior malleolar fracture associated with a spiral tibial shaft fracture. *Eur J Radiol.* 2012 Mar;81(3):594–597.

Hou Z, Zhang Q, Zhang Y, et al. A occult and regular combination injury: the posterior malleolar fracture associated with spiral tibial shaft fracture. *J Trauma.* 2009 May;66(5):1385–1390.

Konrath G, Moed BR, Watson JT, et al. Intramedullary nailing of unstable diaphyseal fractures of the tibia with distal intraarticular involvement. *J Orthop Trauma.* 1997 Apr;11(3):200–205.

Kukkonen J, Heikkilä JT, Kyyrönen T, et al. Posterior malleolar fracture is often associated with spiral tibial diaphyseal fracture: a retrospective study. *J Trauma.* 2006 May;60(5):1058–1060.

Rammelt S, Boszczyk A. Computed tomography in the diagnosis and treatment of ankle fractures: a critical analysis review. *JBJS Rev.* 2018 Dec;6(12):e7.

Robinson CM, McLauchlan GJ, McLean IP, et al. Distal metaphyseal fractures of the tibia with minimal involvement of the ankle. Classification and treatment by locked intramedullary nailing. *J Bone Joint Surg Br.* 1995 Sep;77(5):781–787.

Vallier HA, Cureton BA, Patterson BM. Randomized, prospective comparison of plate versus intramedullary nail fixation for distal tibia shaft fractures. *J Orthop Trauma.* 2011 Dec;25(12):736–741.

2.5 Medial plating and screws

John R Shank

1 Case description

A 65-year-old man fell down a flight of stairs and presented to the emergency department with a chief complaint of left leg pain. Clinically, the patient had significant deformity of his left ankle. The result of neurovascular examination was normal except for swelling. He had a small laceration (< 1 cm) over the fibular fracture where the distal end of the proximal fracture fragment penetrated through the skin. There was no evidence of compartment syndrome. The wound was immediately dressed, and the leg was placed in a splint. Tetanus prophylaxis and intravenous cefazolin were administered. X-rays of the tibia revealed a fracture of the distal third of the tibia and fibula (**Fig 2.5-1**). Computed tomographic (CT) scan was performed by the emergency department, which demonstrated a distal third tibia fracture with extension into the tibial plafond (AO/OTA 43C2.3) (**Fig 2.5-2**). Irrigation and debridement (I&D) of the open fracture and external fixation of the tibia were done (**Fig 2.5-3**). The patient had a previous ipsilateral total knee arthroplasty.

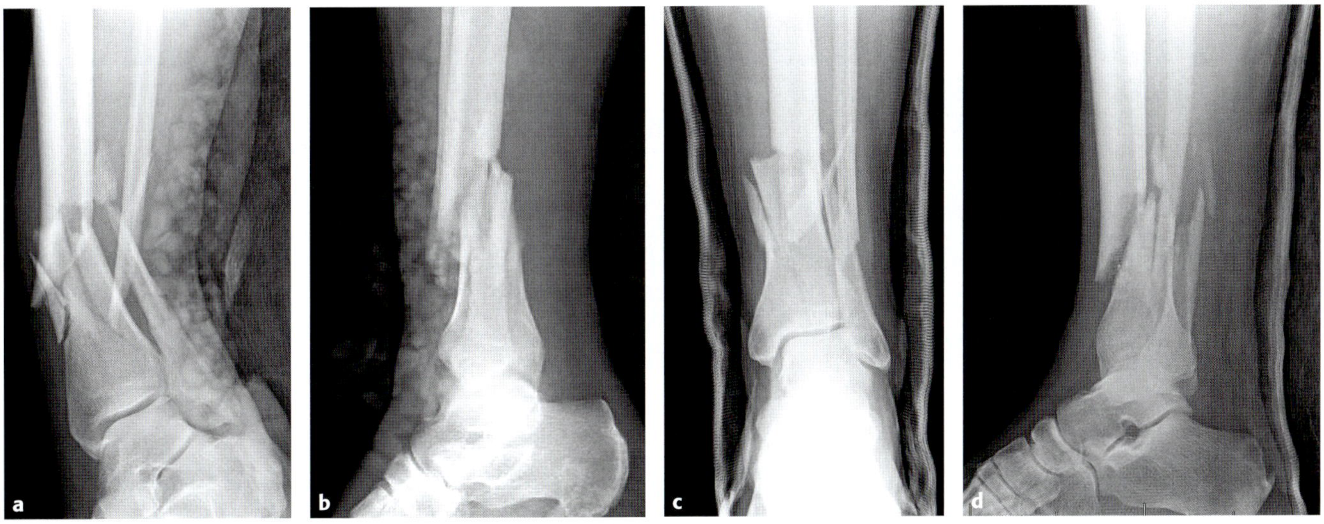

Fig 2.5-1a–d Postinjury images taken in the emergency department.
a–b AP and lateral x-rays obtained at presentation.
c–d AP and lateral x-rays obtained after reduction.

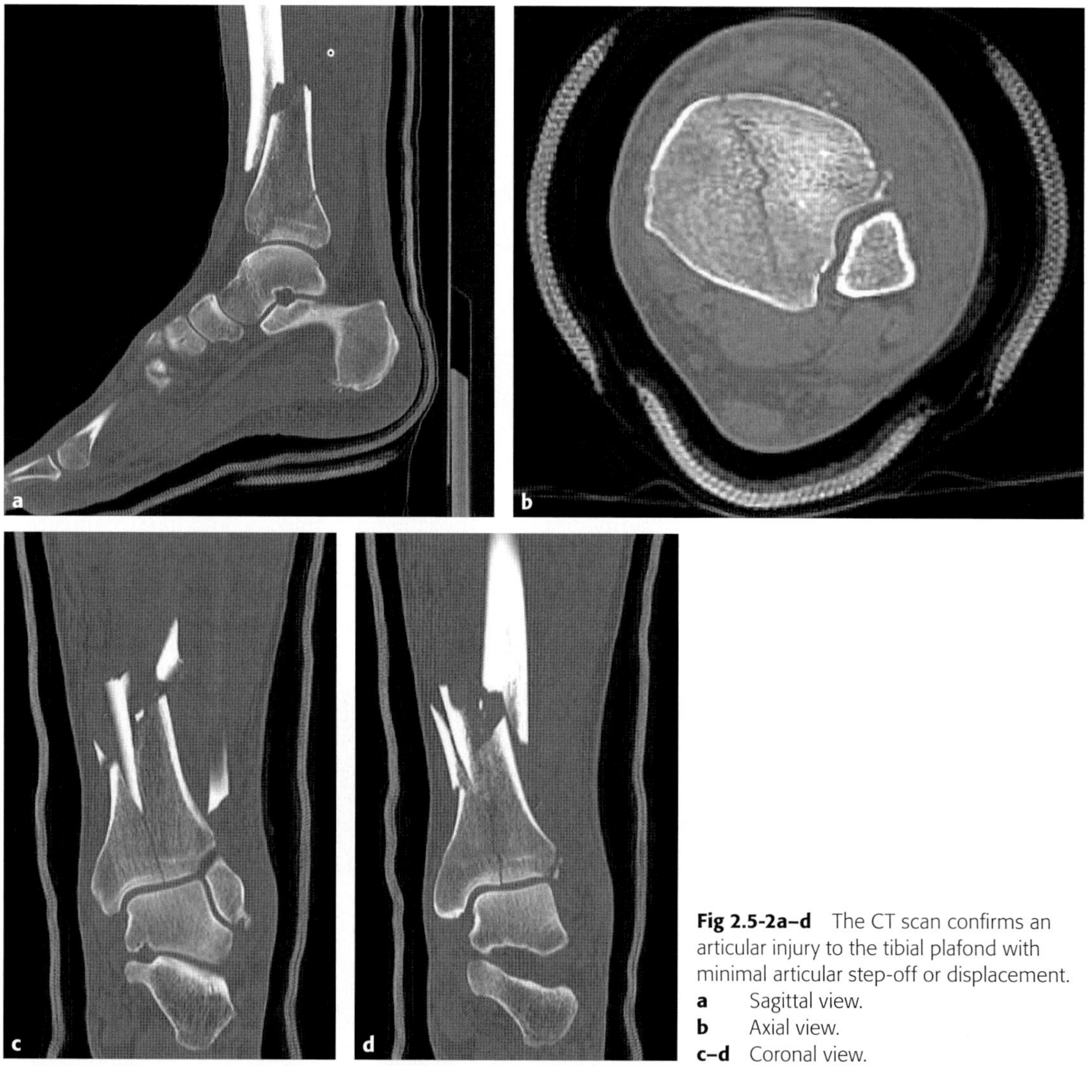

Fig 2.5-2a–d The CT scan confirms an articular injury to the tibial plafond with minimal articular step-off or displacement.
a Sagittal view.
b Axial view.
c–d Coronal view.

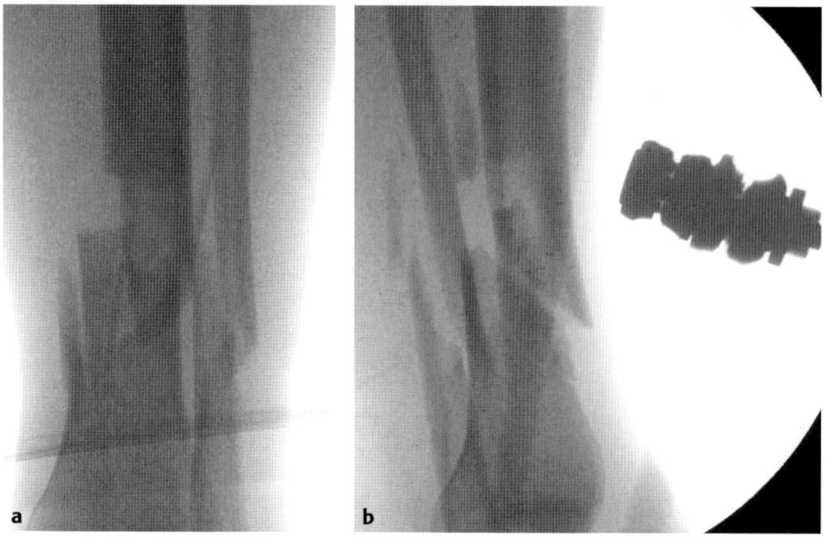

Fig 2.5-3a–b Intraoperative C-arm images taken after I&D and external fixation of the open tibia-fibula fracture.

2 Preoperative planning

Indications for surgery

Surgical treatment of this injury is necessary based on the open nature of the injury. Restoration of length, rotation, and alignment of the tibia and fibula, and reconstruction of the plafond injury cannot be achieved with nonoperative treatment.

Treatment options

A staged approach, with initial irrigation, debridement of the open fracture, and external fixation of the tibia is essential to minimize complications.

Open reduction and internal fixation of the fibula, limited fixation plafond, intramedullary nailing fixation of tibia

This injury ideally could be treated with open reduction and internal fixation (ORIF) of the fibula, limited open reduction of the tibial plafond and intramedullary nailing of the tibia. However, the patient's total knee arthroplasty precludes intramedullary nail fixation.

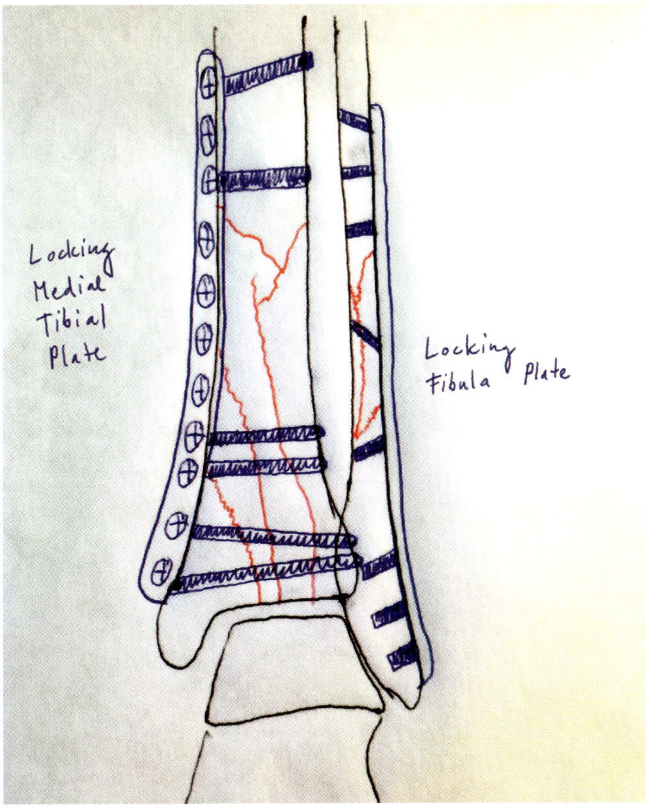

Fig 2.5-4 Preoperative plan.

Open reduction and internal fixation with direct reduction and plate fixation

The goal of surgical treatment is restoration of the diaphyseal-metaphyseal junction of the tibia with anatomical reduction of the articular surface of the ankle to provide bony union and minimize posttraumatic arthropathy.

Based on the x-rays and CT imaging obtained, a posterolateral approach to the fibula and anteromedial approach to the tibia was chosen. Evaluation of the soft-tissue envelope 1 week after external fixation showed that the tissues had recovered sufficiently to allow surgical ORIF. This time allowed the surgeon to formulate an appropriate preoperative plan before proceeding with surgical treatment (**Fig 2.5-4**).

3 Operating room setup

Patient positioning	• Supine
Anesthesia options	• General, spinal, or regional • Avoid regional anesthesia in higher-energy injuries, as it may mask developing compartment syndrome.
C-arm location	• Placed on contralateral side of the table with the monitor at the head of the table.
Tourniquet	• Used at surgeon's discretion • Generally improves visualization
Tips	• Placing the injured leg on an elevating ramp improves imaging and allows unobstructed access to the injured extremity.

For illustrations and overview of anesthetic considerations, see chapter 1.

Equipment

- Headlamp for visualization
- Elevators and dental picks
- External fixator and distractor device
- K-wire set
- Distal tibial plates with small fragment screws
- Locking plates as an alternative

Size of system, instruments, and implants may vary according to anatomy.

4 Surgical procedure

The fibula is approached using a posterolateral approach. Recreating appropriate length, alignment, and rotation is essential and assists in reconstruction of the tibia (**Fig 2.5-5**). This may be done as an isolated surgical procedure or at the time of fixation of the tibia.

Carefully plan the anteromedial tibial approach to minimize wound complications. The incision is performed 1 cm lateral to the tibial crest, extended to the articular surface of the ankle then extended medially, forming an apex prior to the incision curving medially (**Fig 2.5-6**). This approach can be extensile proximally. The fascia over the anterior compartment is released and the anterior compartment muscles are retracted laterally after incising the extensor retinaculum. The saphenous nerve and vessels are carefully protected throughout the approach. Subperiosteal dissection of the tibia is performed, creating a full-thickness flap. The entire anterior articular surface of the ankle from medial to lateral can be exposed through this approach (**Fig 2.5-7**). Application of a distractor allows better restoration of length and aids fracture reduction.

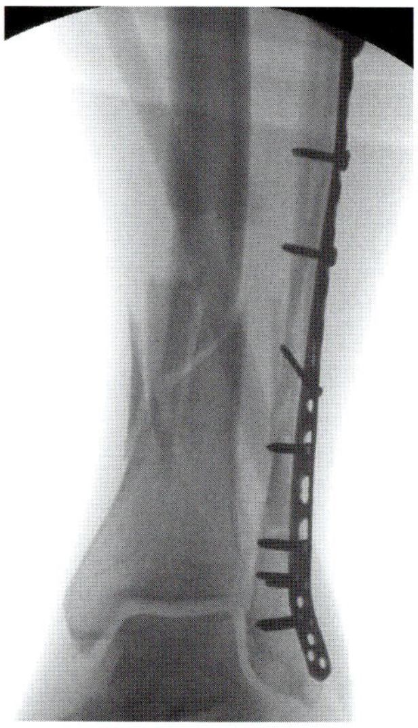

Fig 2.5-5 Intraoperative imaging following fibular reduction and fixation.

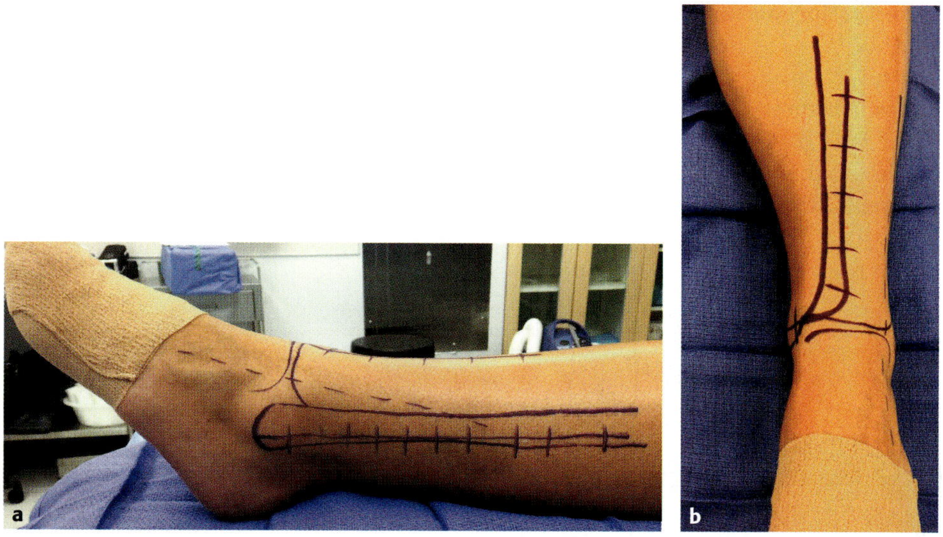

Fig 2.5-6a–b Surgical approaches to the fibula. (Image of a different patient.)
a Posterolateral approach.
b Anteromedial approach.

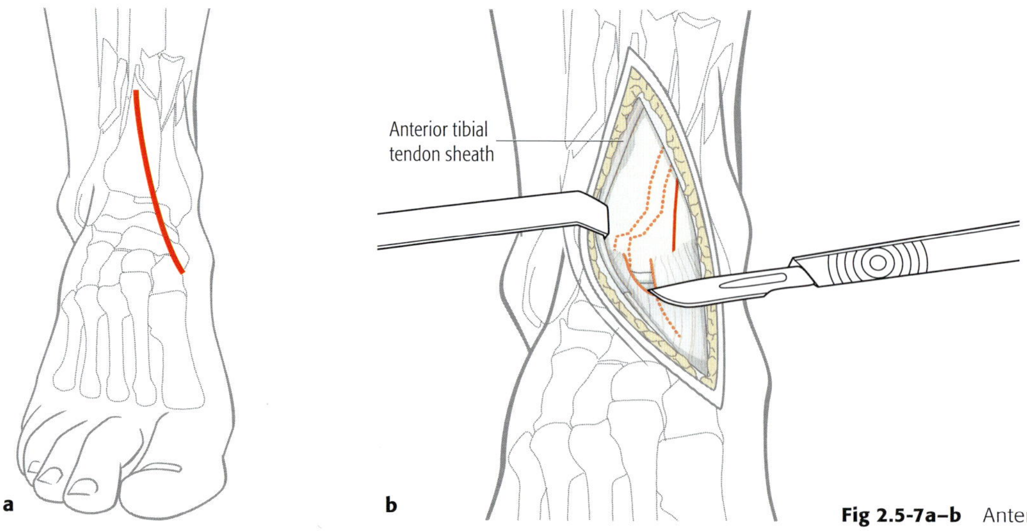

Fig 2.5-7a–b Anteromedial approach.

Distraction for diaphyseal-metaphyseal reduction and reduction of the articular surface with K-wires is performed. For the case presented here, a medial buttress plate was used, with a smaller anterior plate used to bridge the anterior comminution. Bone grafting of metaphyseal or subchondral defects can be performed (**Fig 2.5-8**).

Be careful to ensure that implants are not impinging within the ankle joint. The external fixator can be left in place for several weeks to maintain articular reduction, especially with comminution or in patients with poor bone density. X-rays are performed at regular intervals postoperatively to assess healing (**Fig 2.5-9**).

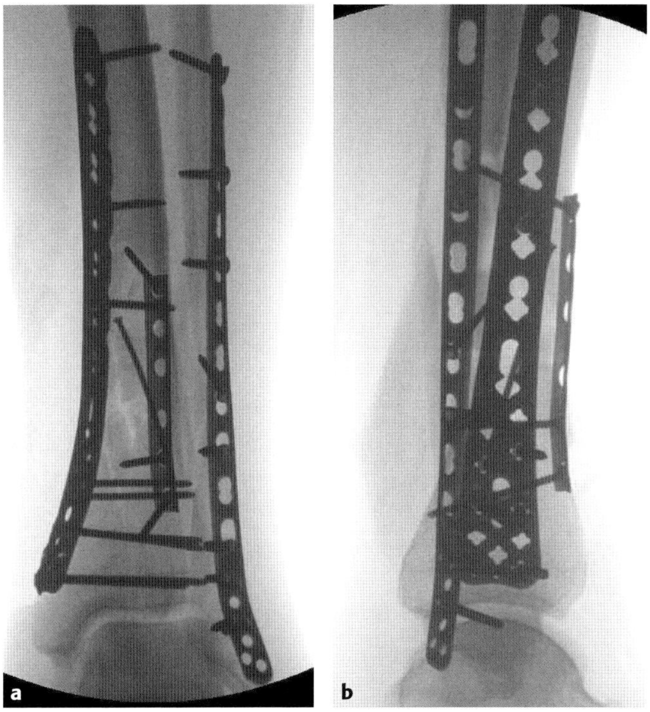

Fig 2.5-8a–b Intraoperative imaging demonstrates reduction of the diaphyseal-metaphyseal junction with anatomical restoration of the articular surface.
a AP view.
b Lateral view.

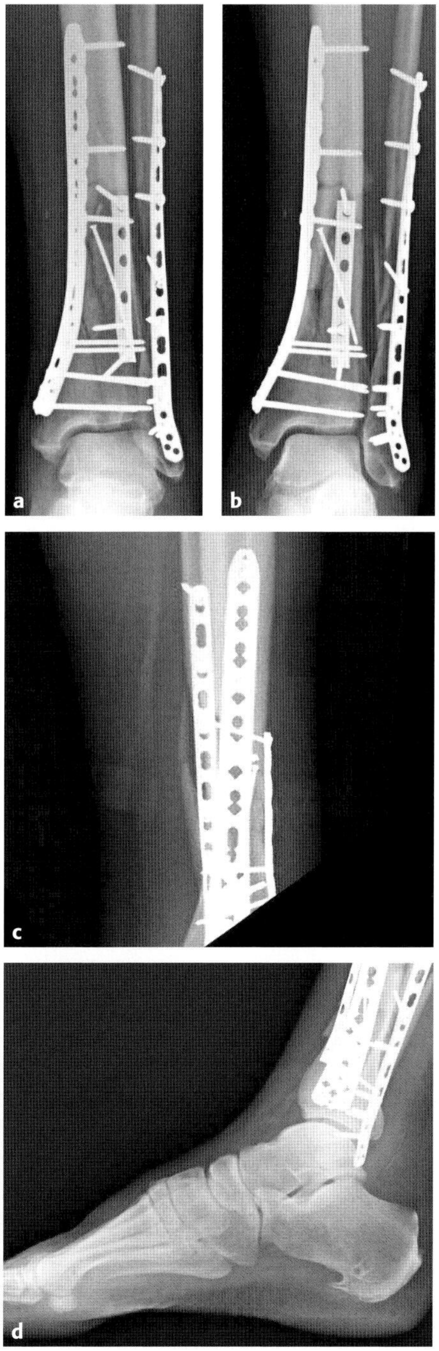

Fig 2.5-9a–c Postoperative x-rays.
a AP view.
b Mortise view.
c Lateral view showing proximal hardware.
d Lateral view of the ankle.

5 Pitfalls and complications

Pitfalls

Inadequate reduction and fixation

The choice of approach is critical in successful reduction and fixation strategies for these injuries. A poorly planned surgical approach may not allow adequate visualization of the articular injury and appropriate fixation. The CT scan is the investigation of choice to formulate a preoperative plan that is appropriate for each unique fracture.

Distractor use

The surgeon should become familiar with a distractor device, whether the older large femoral distractor or the newer rack and pinion device. This instrument becomes a critical tool for visualization and for achieving fracture reduction. Placement of Schanz pins should be well planned according to the fracture pattern.

Irreducible intercalary fragments

Remove small intercalary fragments (ie, < 5 mm in diameter) and fragments without adequate overlying cartilage rather than attempting fixation. These fragments do not contribute to joint congruity and may impede anatomical reduction or may displace into the joint as loose bodies.

Complications

- Injury to the anterior neurovascular bundle
- Injury to the saphenous nerve or vessels
- Intraarticular placement of implants
- Loss of fixation
- Nonunion
- Malunion
- Avascular necrosis
- Posttraumatic arthritis
- Compartment syndrome
- Infection
- Wound complications

6 Alternative techniques

Ideally, intramedullary nail fixation with limited ORIF of the articular surface is used for this fracture. However, the patient's previous ipsilateral total knee arthroplasty precludes this approach. A minimally invasive medial tibial plate could have been used for this distal tibial injury. A thin wire fixator is another treatment option.

7 Postoperative management and rehabilitation

Postoperatively, immobilize the ankle in a splint or fracture brace, with the ankle held at 90°. Always keep the leg elevated. On postoperative day 1 or day 2 remove any applied suction drain. Keep sutures in place for 2–3 weeks, then remove. If the external fixator is retained, remove it several weeks postoperatively with the timing based on fracture severity. Toe range of motion (ROM) is encouraged immediately after surgery, which helps prevent deep vein thrombosis and maintains metatarsophalangeal motion. Start active and passive ROM exercises of the ankle as soon as the external fixator is removed.

Nonweight bearing is recommended for 8–12 weeks postoperatively depending on fracture severity. Standard postoperative x-rays are obtained to ensure fracture union. If uncertain of fracture healing, obtain a postoperative CT scan. An active rehabilitation program is initiated at weight bearing to emphasize ROM, muscular balance, and gait training.

Implant removal

Removal of plates and screws for tibial and pilon fractures can be performed at 1 year if the patient experiences hardware-related pain. Implants can be retained long-term if there is no pain or hardware prominence.

8 Recommended reading

Blauth M, Bastian L, Krettek C, et al. Surgical options for the treatment of severe tibial pilon fractures: a study of three techniques. *J Orthop Trauma*. 2001 Mar–Apr;15(3):153–160.
Chen L, O'Shea K, Early JS. The use of medial and lateral surgical approaches for the treatment of tibial plafond fractures. *J Orthop Trauma*. 2007 Mar;21(3):207–211.
Di Giorgio L, Touloupakis G, Theodorakis E, et al. A two-choice strategy through a medial tibial approach for the treatment of pilon fractures with posterior or anterior fragmentation. *Chin J Traumatol*. 2013;16(5):272–276.
Lee T, Blitz NM, Rush SM. Percutaneous contoured locking plate fixation of the pilon fracture: surgical technique. *J Foot Ankle Surg*. 2008 Nov–Dec;47(6):598–602.
Liporace FA, Yoon RS. An adjunct to percutaneous plate insertion to obtain optimal sagittal plane alignment in the treatment of pilon fractures. *J Foot Ankle Surg*. 2012 Mar–Apr;51(2):275–277.
Paluvadi SV, Lal H, Mittal D, et al. Management of fractures of the distal third tibia by minimally invasive plate osteosynthesis—a prospective series of 50 patients. *J Clin Orthop Trauma*. 2014 Sep;5(3):129–136.
Patterson MJ, Cole JD. Two-staged delayed open reduction and internal fixation of severe pilon fractures. *J Orthop Trauma*. 1999 Feb;13(2):85–91.
Sirkin M, Sanders R. The treatment of pilon fractures. *Orthop Clin North Am*. 2001 Jan;32(1):91–102.

Acknowledgement

Special thanks to Miyoko Green in her assistance with preparation of this chapter.

2.6 Anterolateral plating and medial buttress

John R Shank

1 Case description

A 52-year-old woman fell down a flight of stairs and presented to the emergency department with a chief complaint of right ankle pain and deformity.

The clinical examination revealed significant deformity on the right leg and ankle with no neurovascular deficit, without evidence of open fracture or compartment syndrome. The patient underwent reduction and was immediately splinted.

X-rays of the ankle revealed a multifragmentary articular, epiphyseal distal tibial plafond fracture (AO/OTA 43C3.1) (**Fig 2.6-1**).

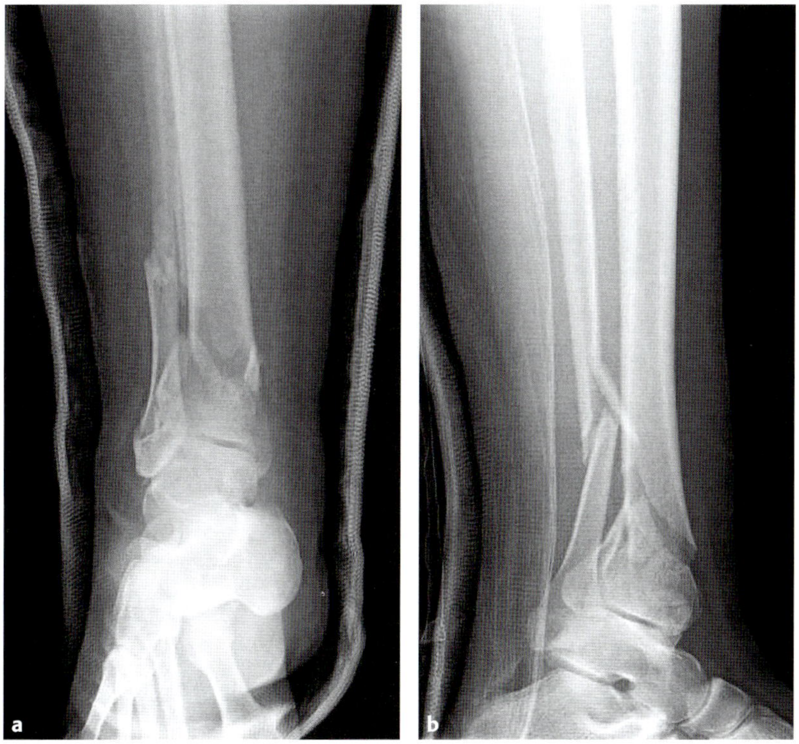

Fig 2.6-1a–b Postinjury images.
a The AP x-ray after splint application demonstrates a comminuted distal tibial and fibula fracture with gross shortening and overall valgus alignment.
b The lateral x-ray after splint application confirms a distal tibial fracture with articular disruption of the tibial plafond with a shortened, comminuted fibula fracture.

External fixation of the tibia and open reduction and internal fixation (ORIF) of the fibular fracture were performed (**Fig 2.6-2**).

A posterolateral approach to the fibula was used for ORIF of the fibular fracture. This incision was used to maximize the distance (skin bridge) between the fibular approach and the incision that would be used to approach the pilon injury. Excessive dissection was avoided. Computed tomography (CT) following external fixation confirmed a complex tibial plafond injury (**Fig 2.6-3**).

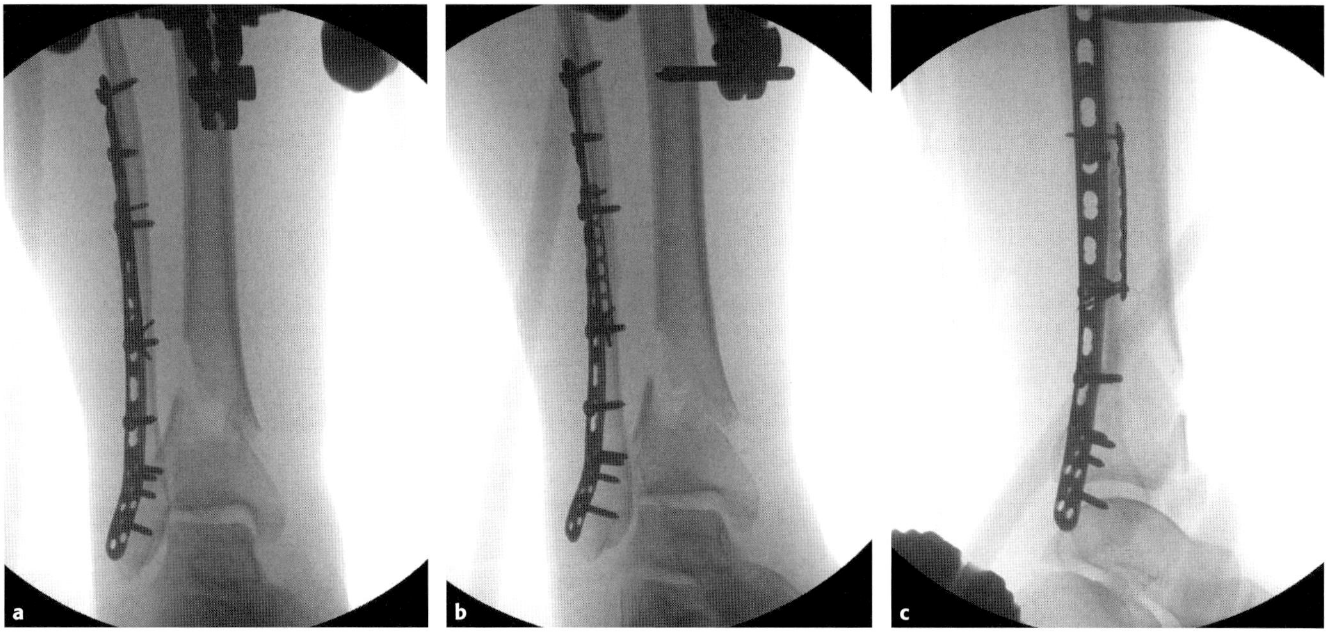

Fig 2.6-2a–b Intraoperative C-arm images.
- **a** AP view.
- **b** Mortise view.
- **c** Lateral intraoperative C-arm images after reduction of the fibula and external fixation of the tibia. A metaphyseal tibial fracture is noted with gross restoration of the articular surface of the ankle.

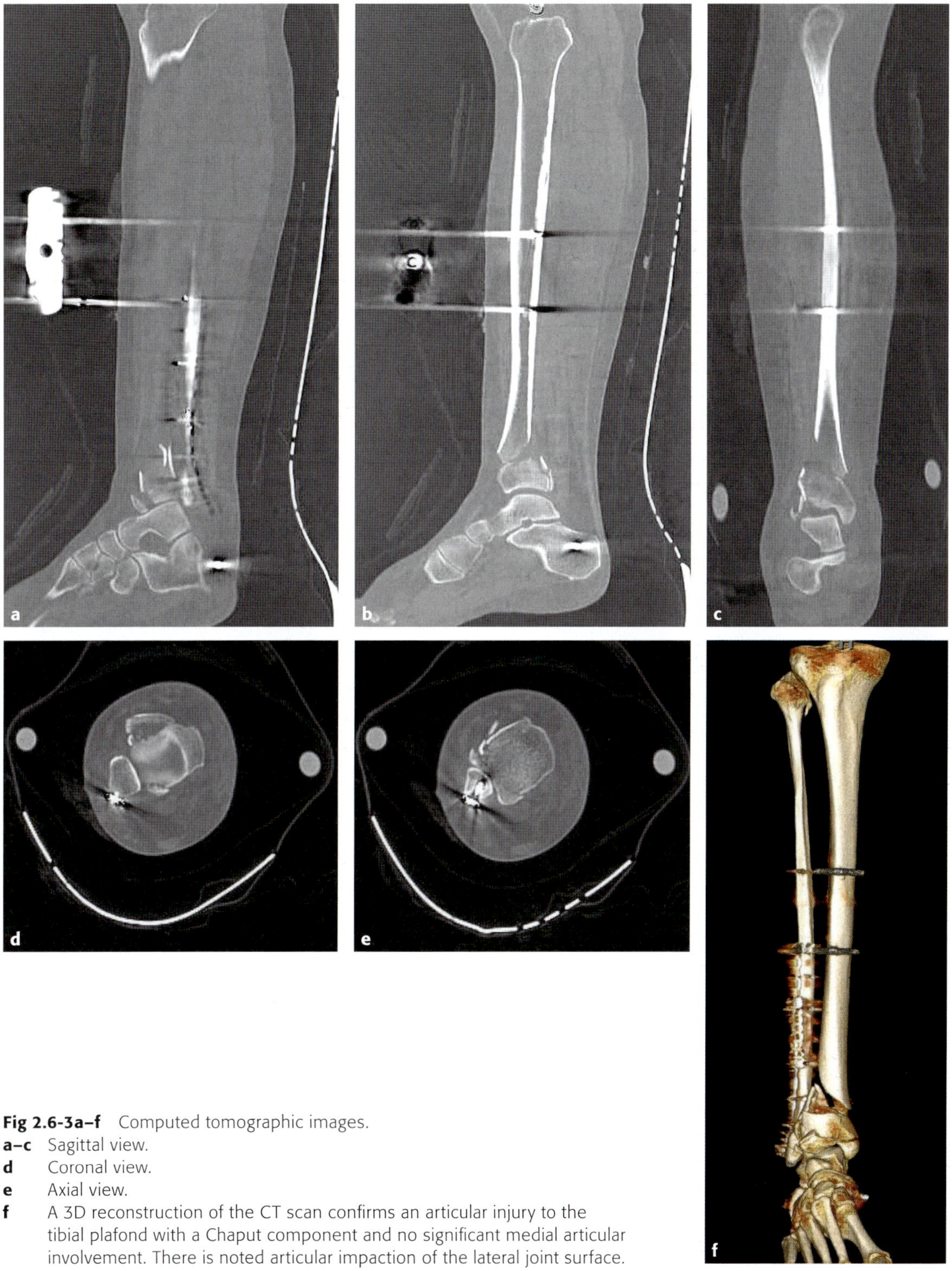

Fig 2.6-3a–f Computed tomographic images.
a–c Sagittal view.
d Coronal view.
e Axial view.
f A 3D reconstruction of the CT scan confirms an articular injury to the tibial plafond with a Chaput component and no significant medial articular involvement. There is noted articular impaction of the lateral joint surface.

2 Preoperative planning

Indications for surgery

Surgery is indicated for this tibial plafond injury to restore articular congruity and alignment of the limb.

Treatment options

Surgical treatment of this injury decreases the incidence of malunion or nonunion occurring. Restoration of length, rotation, and alignment of the tibia and fibula plus reconstruction of the plafond injury cannot be achieved with nonoperative treatment. Thin wire external fixation can be performed, but anatomical articular reconstruction with this method is challenging. A staged approach, with initial external fixation of the tibia and ORIF of the of the fibula, minimizes complications and increases the likelihood of successful management of pilon injuries. The goal is restoration of the diaphyseal-metaphyseal junction of the tibia, with anatomical reduction of the articular surface of the ankle. This aids bony union and minimizes posttraumatic arthropathy.

There are numerous approaches to a pilon injury, with the CT scan being critical in formulating a preoperative plan.

For this patient, the CT scan shows Chaput fragment involvement and a relatively intact medial articular surface. After CT review, an anterolateral approach was chosen for anterolateral plating. A medial buttress plate was also used to provide additional needed stability to the articular reconstruction.

An appropriate preoperative plan should be formulated before proceeding with ORIF (**Fig 2.6-4**).

3 Operating room setup

Patient positioning	• Supine
Anesthesia options	• General, spinal, or regional • Avoid regional anesthesia in higher-energy injuries, as it may mask developing compartment syndrome.
C-arm location	• Placed on contralateral side of the table with the monitor at the head of the table.
Tourniquet	• Used at surgeon's discretion • Generally improves visualization
Tips	• Placing the injured leg on an elevated ramp or blankets improves imaging and access to the limb with surgical instruments. • A padded bump may be placed under the ipsilateral hip to allow additional internal rotation and improved visualization of the anterolateral ankle.

For illustrations and overview of anesthetic considerations, see chapter 1.

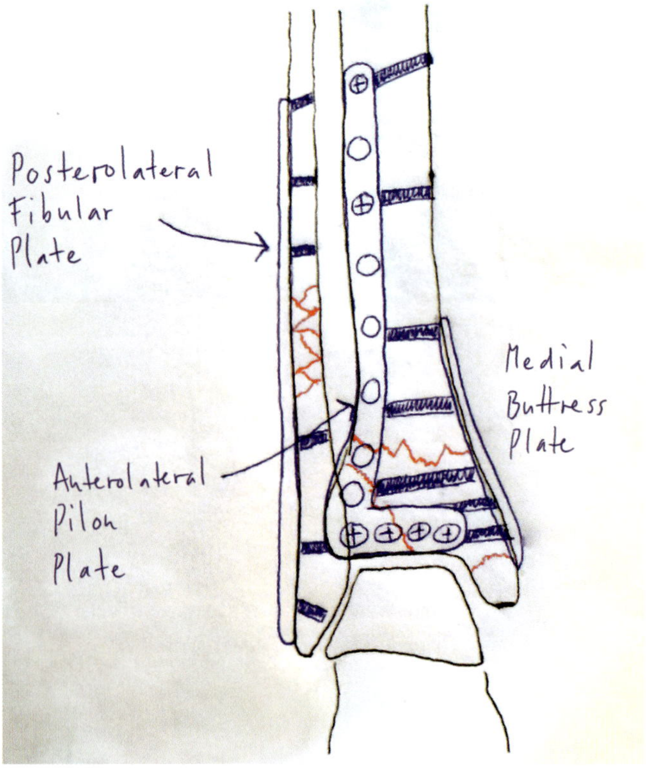

Fig 2.6-4 Preoperative plan.

Equipment

- Headlamp for visualization
- Elevators and dental scalers
- External fixator and femoral distractor
- K-wire set
- Pilon plates with small and minifragment screws
- Locking plates as an alternative
- Bone graft or bone graft harvesting instruments

Size of system, instruments, and implants may vary according to anatomy.

4 Surgical procedure

Carefully plan the anterolateral pilon approach to allow for an appropriate skin bridge with the fibular incision. Mark all anatomical structures including the superficial peroneal nerve (**Fig 2.6-5**). The incision is performed over the lateral distal tibia, in line with the fourth metatarsal distally. This approach can be extensile both proximally and distally. Identify and protect the superficial peroneal nerve throughout the operative procedure.

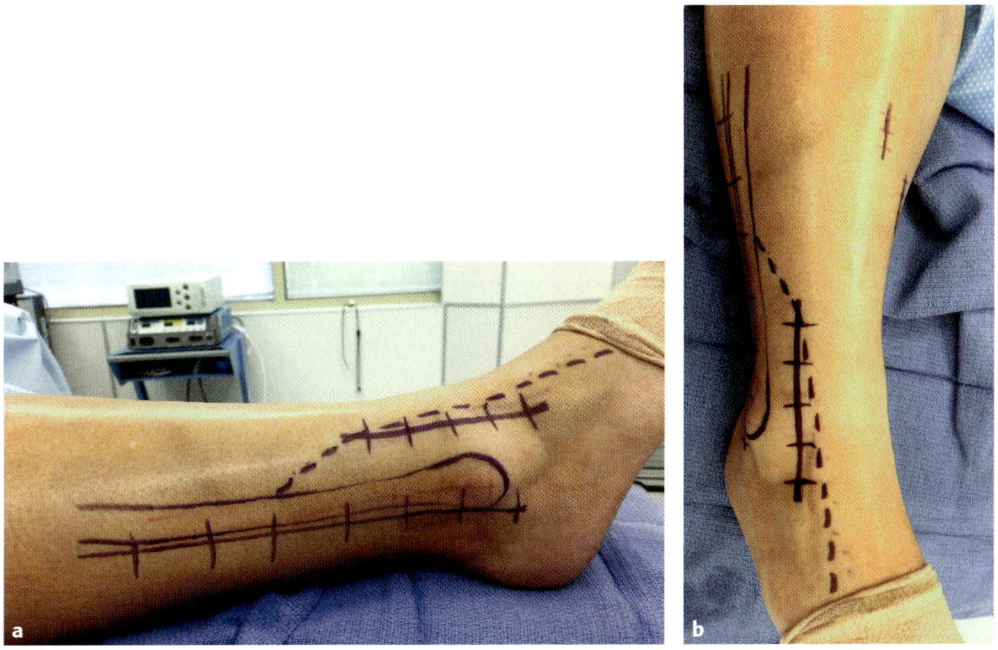

Fig 2.6-5a–b The anterolateral approach to the ankle should respect the posterolateral approach to the fibula allowing an appropriate skin bridge. Identify, isolate, and protect the superficial peroneal nerve throughout the operative procedure. (Image of a different patient.)

The fascia over the anterior compartment is released and the anterior compartment muscles are retracted medially after incising the superior extensor retinaculum (**Fig 2.6-6**). This allows for exposure of the anterolateral surface of the tibia for open reduction and internal fixation. Exposure to the level of the medial shoulder of the distal tibia is possible through this approach. Application of a distractor helps with visualization of the articular surface (**Fig 2.6-7**).

Reduction of the articular surface is made from posterolateral to posteromedial, followed by reduction of the central articular surface and finally the anterior and anterolateral articular surfaces. After the external fixator or distractor has been used to restore length and alignment of the tibia, K-wire fixation is used for provisional articular reduction. The articular surface reduction is performed under direct visualization. In this case, a small medial buttress plate was used to stabilize the diaphyseal-metaphyseal component of the fracture, after temporary reduction of the anterolateral articular surface (**Fig 2.6-8**).

The medial approach is a small medial incision with careful protection of the saphenous nerve and vessels. This can be extended proximally for longer plate fixation or with smaller proximal incisions for a percutaneous screw insertion. Bone grafting of any metaphyseal or subchondral defects can be performed. Plate fixation of the anterolateral surface of the distal tibia is then performed (**Fig 2.6-9**). A separate tibial incision is made for proximal screw fixation into the anterolateral plate.

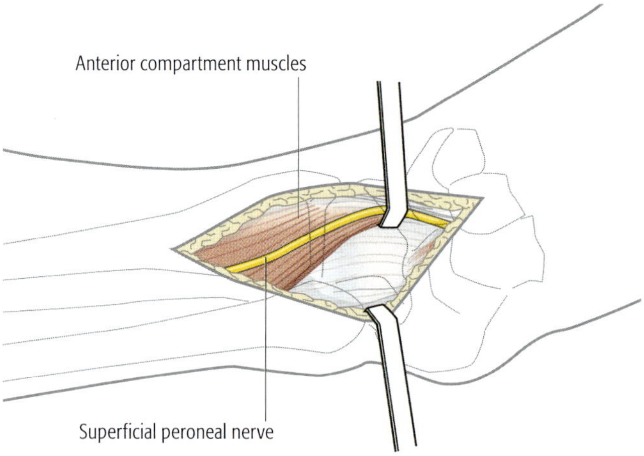

Fig 2.6-6 Anterolateral approach.

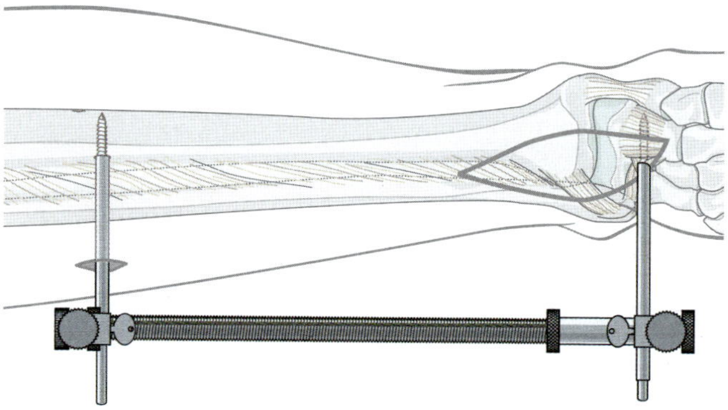

Fig 2.6-7 Femoral distractor.

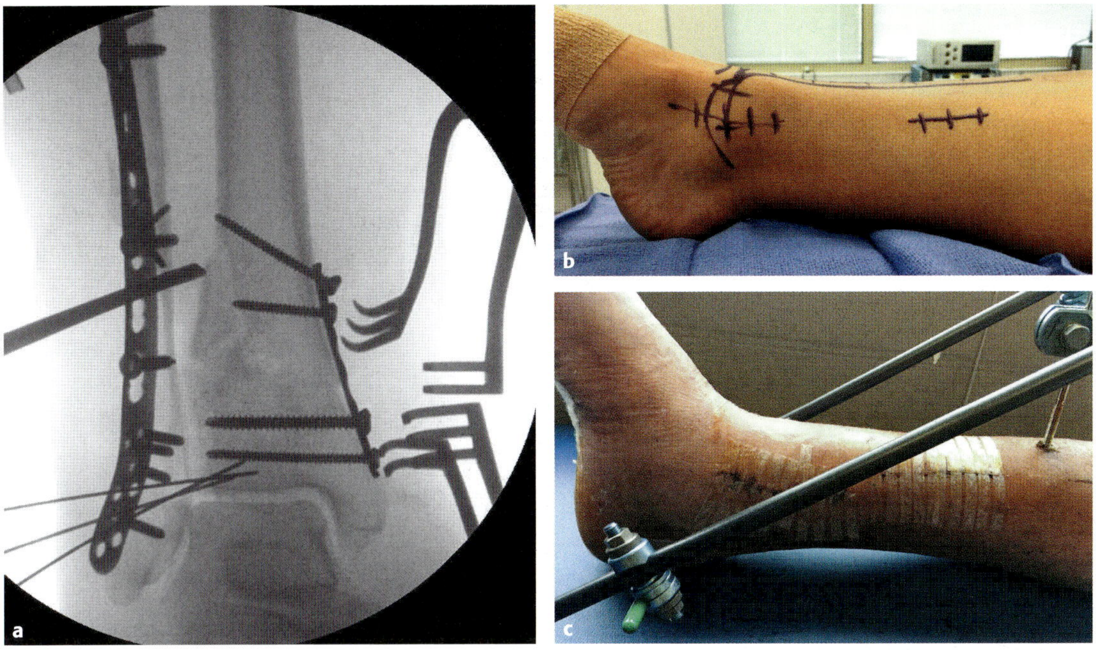

Fig 2.6-8a–c Medial approach.

a A small medial incision is made for medial buttress plate fixation. The plate is relatively short, so it is inserted using a small incision.

b For longer medial plates, a small incision is used to insert the plate and a separate proximal incision is used for screw fixation. (Image of a different patient.)

c Post surgical example of longer medial plate insertion using two incisions

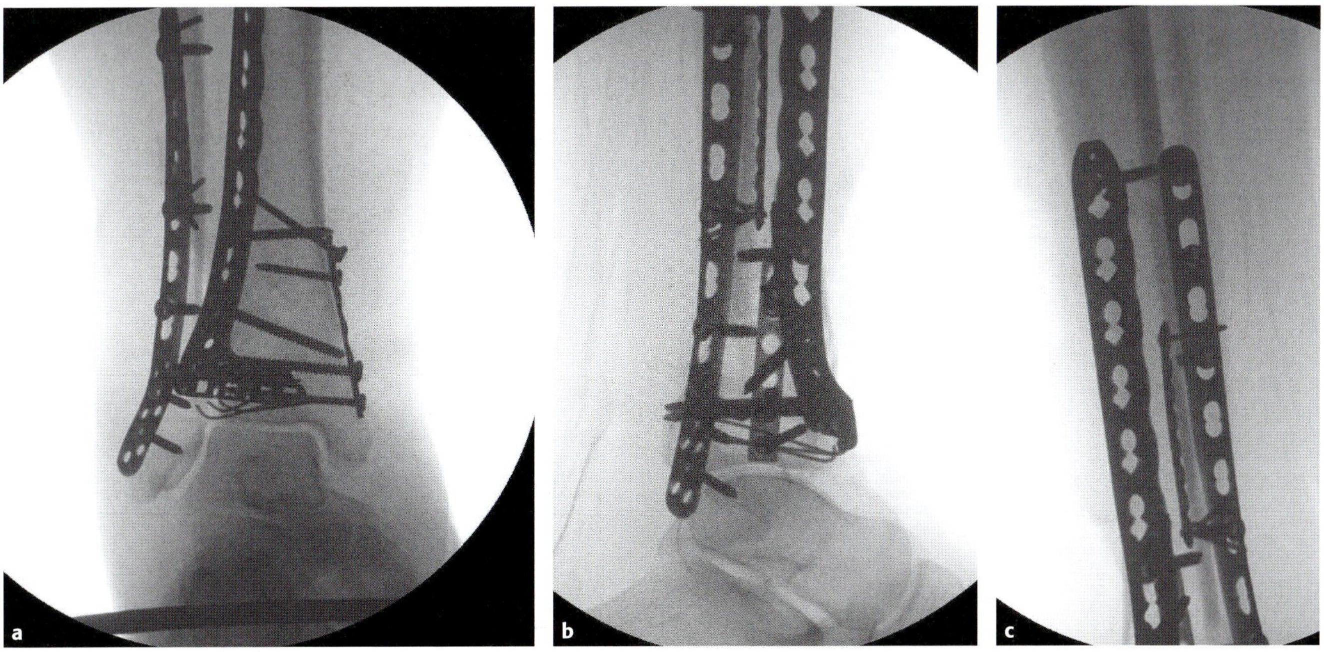

Fig 2.6-9a–d Intraoperative C-arm images showing reduction of the diaphyseal-metaphyseal junction with anatomical restoration of the articular surface. K-wires are retained to maintain articular reduction.

a Mortise view.

b Lateral view.

c Lateral of proximal fixation.

Care should be taken to ensure that implants are not impinging within the ankle joint. The external fixator should be maintained for at least 6 weeks to assist with articular reduction, especially if there is comminution. X-rays are performed at regular intervals postoperatively to assess healing (**Fig 2.6-10**).

5 Pitfalls and complications

Pitfalls

Poor surgical planning

Appropriate location of incisions is necessary for successful management of these complex injuries. If poorly placed, the fibular incision may compromise the ability to use the anterolateral approach.

Inadequate reduction and fixation

The surgeon's choice of approach is critical in successful reduction and fixation strategies of these injuries. A poorly planned surgical approach may not adequately allow for visualization of the articular injury and appropriate fixation. A CT scan is the examination of choice to formulate a preoperative plan that is appropriate for each unique fracture.

Distractor use

The surgeon should become familiar with the femoral (or other type) distractor. This instrument is a critical tool in achieving fracture reduction. Placement of Schanz pins should be planned appropriately according to the fracture pattern.

Irreducible intercalary fragments

Remove small intercalary fragments (ie, < 5 mm in diameter) and fragments without adequate overlying cartilage rather than attempting fixation. These fragments do not contribute to joint congruity and may impede anatomical reduction or may displace into the joint as loose bodies.

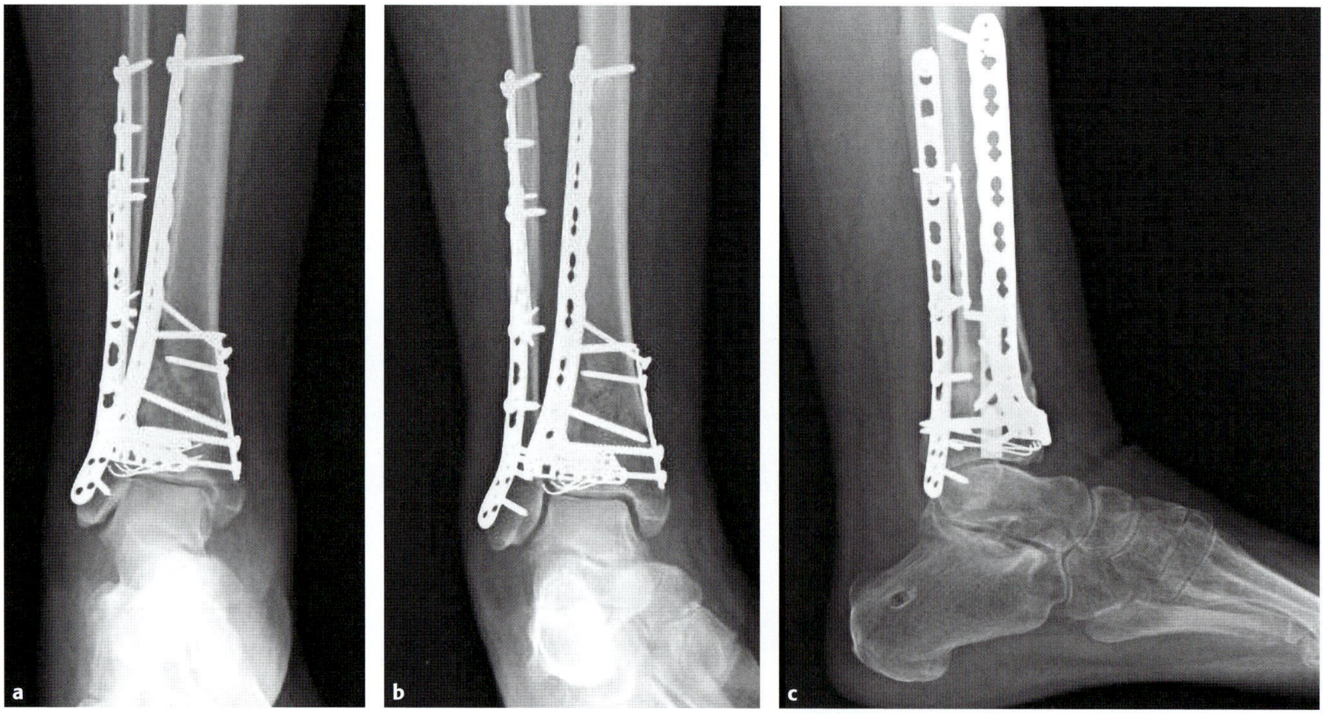

Fig 2.6-10a–c Postoperative x-rays.
a AP view.
b Mortise view.
c Lateral view.

Complications

- Injury to the superficial peroneal nerve
- Injury to the saphenous nerve or vessels
- Intraarticular placement of implants
- Loss of fixation
- Nonunion
- Malunion
- Avascular necrosis
- Posttraumatic arthritis
- Compartment syndrome
- Wound breakdown
- Skin necrosis
- Superficial or deep infection

6 Alternative techniques

Less comminuted injuries can be treated without dual plating. A single anterolateral plate can be used for more simple fracture patterns. A thin wire fixator is another treatment option for surgeons comfortable with this technique.

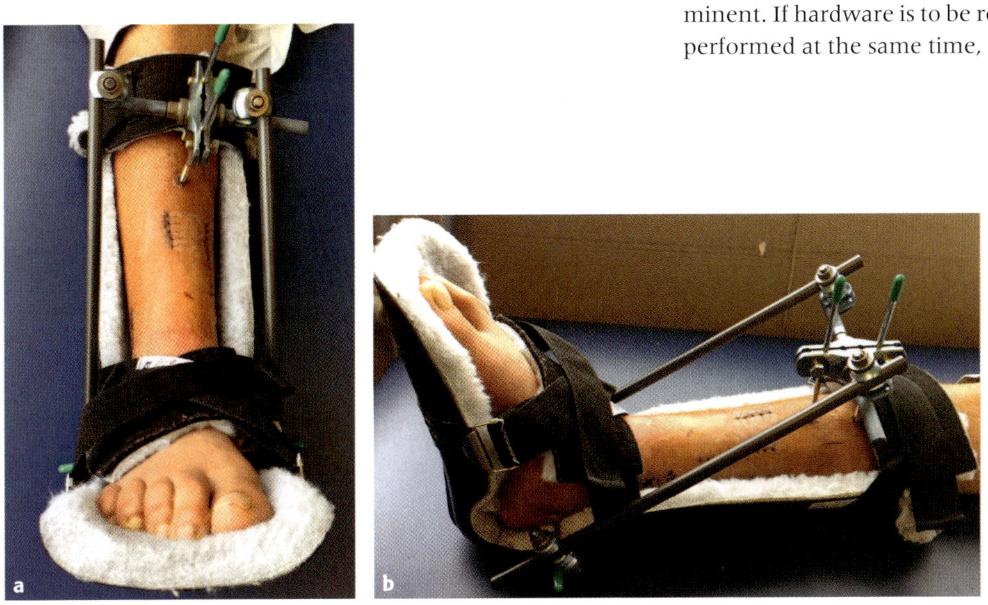

Fig 2.6-11a-b Postoperative splint.

7 Postoperative management and rehabilitation

Postoperatively the ankle is immobilized in a splint or fracture brace with the ankle held at 90° (**Fig 2.6-11**). Always keep the leg elevated. On postoperative day 1 or 2 remove any applied suction drain. Keep the sutures in place for 2–3 weeks, then remove.

The external fixator is removed around 6 weeks postoperatively, with the timing based on fracture severity. Toe motion is encouraged with active and passive range-of-motion (ROM) exercises for the ankle initiated as soon as the external fixator is removed.

Nonweight bearing is recommended for 8–12 weeks postoperatively depending on fracture severity. Standard postoperative x-rays are obtained to ensure fracture union. If uncertain of fracture healing, perform a postoperative CT scan. Initiate an active rehabilitation program at weight bearing to emphasize ROM, muscular balance, and gait training.

For additional information on postoperative care, see chapter 1.

Implant removal

Removal of plates and screws for pilon fractures can be performed at 1 year if the patient experiences hardware-related pain. Implants can be left in place if not bothersome or prominent. If hardware is to be removed, then arthrolysis can be performed at the same time, which may improve motion.

8 Recommended reading

Cole PA, Mehrle RK, Bhandari M, et al. The pilon map: fracture lines and comminution zones in OTA/AO type 43C3 pilon fractures. *J Orthop Trauma.* 2013 Jul;27(7):e152–156.
Deivaraju C, Vlasak R, Sadasivan K. Staged treatment of pilon fractures. *J Orthop.* 2015 Oct;12(Suppl 1):S1–6.
Fisher BE, Nathan ST, Acland RD, et al. The anterolateral incision for pilon fracture surgery: an anatomic study of cutaneous blood supply. *Acta Orthop Belg.* 2011 Jun;77(3):355–361.
Hak DJ. Anterolateral approach for tibial pilon fractures. *Orthopedics.* 2012 Feb;35(2):131–133.
Hickerson LE, Verbeek DO, Klinger CE, et al. Anterolateral approach to the pilon. *J Orthop Trauma.* 2016 Aug;30 Suppl 2:S39–40.
Liu J, Smith CD, White E, et al. A systematic review of the role of surgical approaches on the outcomes of the tibia pilon fracture. *Foot Ankle Spec.* 2016 Apr;9(2):163–168.
Mehta S, Gardner MJ, Barei DP, et al. Reduction strategies through the anterolateral exposure for fixation of type B and C pilon fractures. *J Orthop Trauma.* 2011 Feb;25(2):116–122.
Penny P, Swords M, Heisler J, et al. Ability of modern distal tibia plates to stabilize comminuted pilon fracture fragments: is dual plate fixation necessary? *Injury.* 2016 Aug;47(8):1761–1769.
Yenna ZC, Bhadra AK, Ojike NI, et al. Anterolateral and medial locking plate stiffness in distal tibial fracture model. *Foot Ankle Int.* 2011 Jun;32(6):630–637.

Acknowledgement

Special thanks to Miyoko Green in her assistance with preparation of this chapter.

2.7 Anterior plating

John R Shank, Michael Swords

1 Case description

A 30-year old woman was involved in a motor vehicle accident and presented to the emergency department by ambulance with a chief complaint of severe right ankle pain. Clinically, she had significant deformity. The injury was closed. There was no evidence of compartment syndrome and her neurovascular status was intact.

X-rays of the ankle revealed the following: a multifragmentary pilon fracture, significant articular (plafond) involvement, deformity, and step-off (AO/OTA 43C3.3), and an intact fibula (**Fig 2.7-1**). Computed tomographic (CT) imaging was obtained to better evaluate the fracture anatomy (**Fig 2.7-2**).

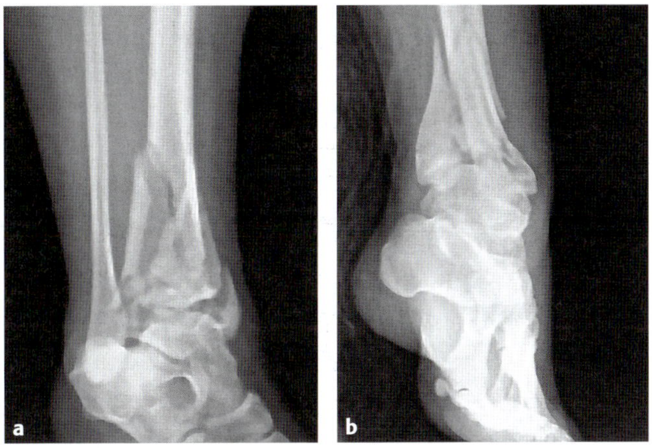

Fig 2.7-1a–b Postinjury x-rays obtained at presentation to the emergency department.
a AP view.
b Lateral view.

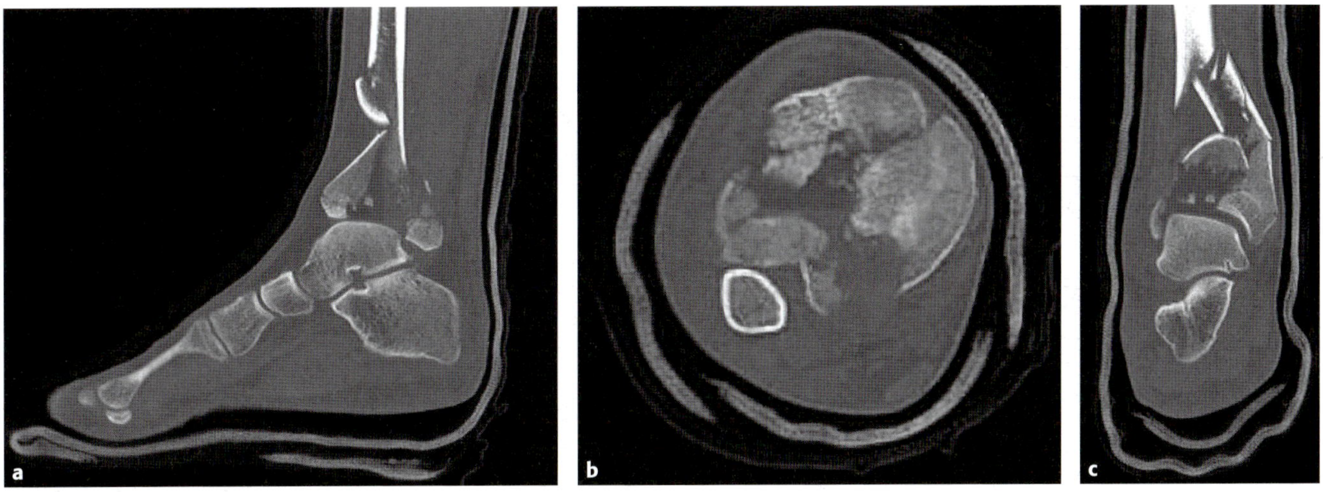

Fig 2.7-2a–c The CT scan confirms a highly comminuted injury with significant involvement of the tibial plafond.
a Sagittal view.
b Axial view.
c Coronal view.

2 Preoperative planning

Indications for surgery

Surgical indications include severe articular comminution, malalignment of the limb, and gross instability resulting from the fracture.

Considerations for surgery

Surgical treatment of this injury is preferable based on the fracture type and pattern. Restoration of length, rotation and alignment of the tibia, and reconstruction of the plafond injury cannot be achieved with nonoperative treatment.

Staged management decreases risk of complications and is ideal for this injury. Initially, external fixation is placed to allow for the soft-tissue envelope to recover from the initial trauma (**Fig 2.7-3**). After swelling decreases with return of soft-tissue skin wrinkles, open reduction and internal fixation (ORIF) can be performed with less complications. The goal of surgical treatment is restoration of the diaphyseal-metaphyseal junction of the tibia with anatomical reduction of the articular surface of the ankle. Accurate reduction and appropriate fixation provide the stability necessary for bony union and reduces the potential for posttraumatic arthritis. For the case presented here, an anterior approach with plate fixation was chosen, based on the findings obtained from x-rays and CT images. The patient had a good soft-tissue envelope 1 week after initial external fixation that allowed ORIF to proceed. An appropriate preoperative plan should be performed before proceeding with surgery (**Fig 2.7-4**).

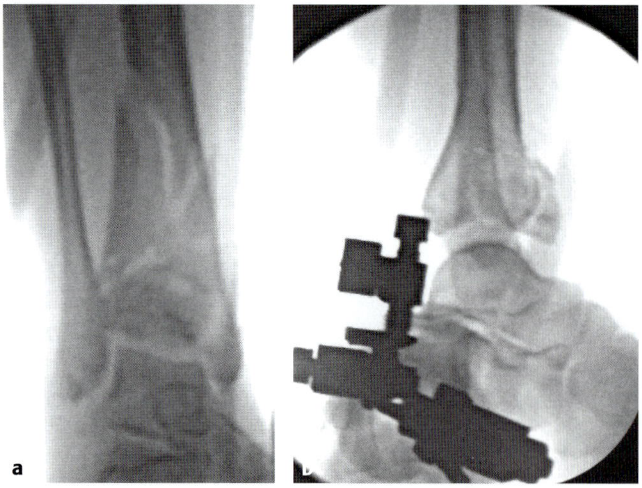

Fig 2.7-3a–b Intraoperative C-arm images during closed reduction and external fixation.
a Mortise view.
b Lateral view.

3 Operating room setup

Patient positioning	• Supine
Anesthesia options	• General, spinal, or regional • Avoid regional anesthesia in high-energy injuries, as it may mask developing compartment syndrome.
C-arm location	• Placed on contralateral side of the table with monitor at the head of the table.
Tourniquet	• Used at surgeon's discretion • Generally improves visualization
Tips	• Placing the injured leg on an elevated ramp or blankets improves imaging and instrumentation of the injured extremity. • A padded bump may be placed under the ipsilateral hip to allow additional internal rotation and improved visualization of the anterior ankle.

For illustrations and overview of anesthetic considerations, see chapter 1.

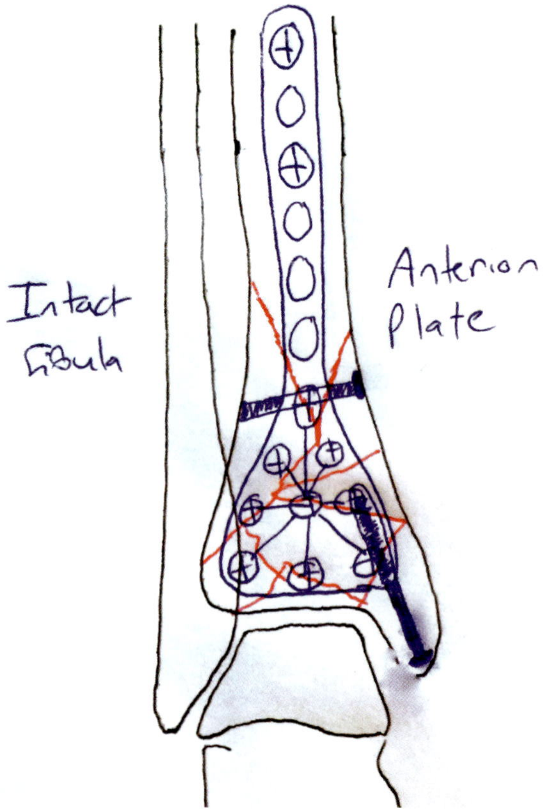

Fig 2.7-4 Preoperative plan.

Equipment

- Headlamp for visualization
- Elevators and dental scalers
- External fixator or femoral distractor
- K-wire set
- Locking anterior distal tibial plate
- Small fragment cortex and locking screws

Size of system, instruments, and implants may vary according to anatomy.

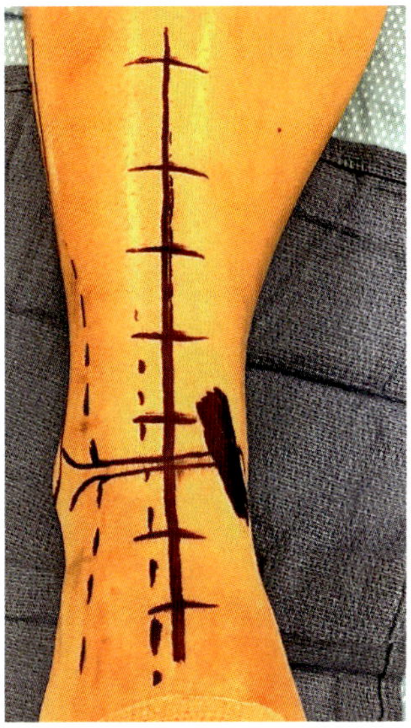

Fig 2.7-5 Anterior approach to the ankle.

4 Surgical procedure

The anterior tibial approach should be carefully to minimize wound complications. The incision is performed lateral to the tibial crest, centrally bisecting the ankle distally (**Fig 2.7-5**). This approach can be extensile proximally and distally. The fascia over the anterior compartment is released and the interval between the tibialis anterior and extensor hallucis longus tendons is developed (**Fig 2.7-6**). Care should be taken to protect the anterior neurovascular bundle and all branches of the deep and superficial peroneal nerves. Subperiosteal dissection of the tibia is performed, creating full-thickness flaps as necessary to provide accurate reduction. Excessive dissection should be avoided, as it may lead to an increased risk of avascular necrosis. The entire anterior articular surface of the ankle from medial to lateral can be exposed through this approach. Application of a femoral distractor can be performed to allow for restoration of length and to improve fracture reduction.

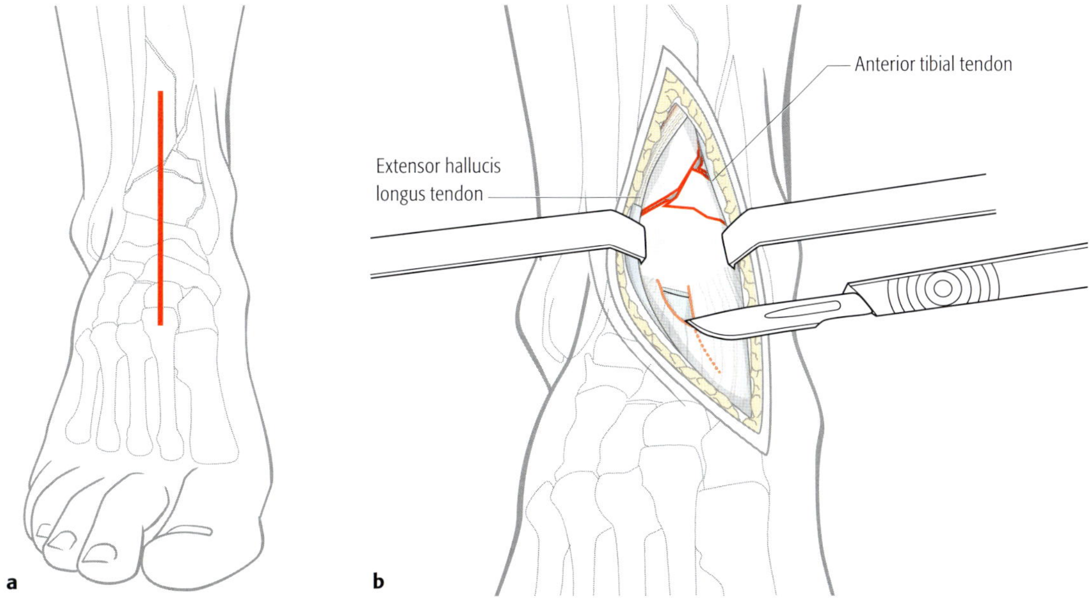

Fig 2.7-6a–b Anterior approach.
a Skin incision for anterior ankle approach.
b Deep dissection is between the tibialis anterior tendon and the extensor hallucis longus tendons.

Reduction of the diaphyseal-metaphyseal junction is performed with distraction and provisional articular reduction is initiated with K-wires. Generally, the external fixator or distractor maintain overall length and alignment while the articular surface is reduced. The articular surface is reduced working from posterior to anterior. Each fragment is held with provisional K-wires until the entire articular surface is reconstructed. Independent lag or positional screws may be placed just proximal to the joint as needed to assist in stabilization. A plate is then selected and used to bridge the diaphyseal-metaphyseal junction and connect the articular surface to the shaft. In this patient, an anterior locking plate was used for fixation (**Fig 2.7-7**). The plate is provisionally secured proximally and distally and confirmed by C-arm imaging. The distal articular block is stabilized with screws through the plate. Final fixation is achieved by adding screws to the shaft portion of the plate. This may be done in open fashion or, more commonly, by using small incisions in a minimally invasive plate osteosynthesis fashion. The talar body injury is treated through the same surgical approach. Bone grafting of any metaphyseal or subchondral defects can be performed if necessary.

Care should be taken to ensure implants do not impinge within the ankle joint. The external fixator should be maintained for approximately 6 weeks to assist with articular reduction and to help hold the overall alignment. X-rays are performed at regular intervals postoperatively to assess healing (**Fig 2.7-8**).

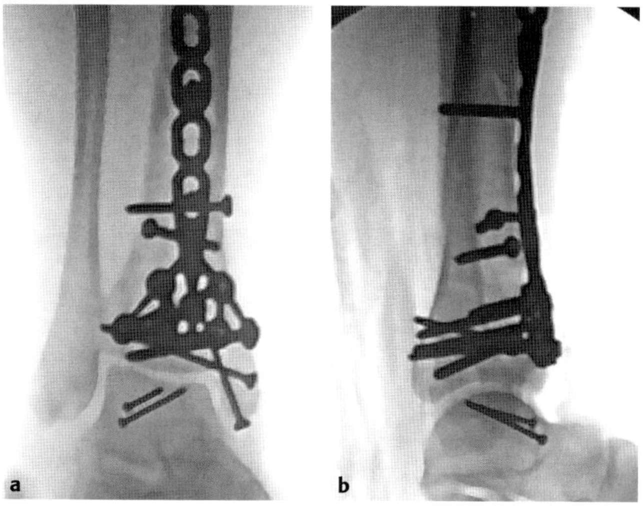

Fig 2.7-7a–b Intraoperative imaging demonstrates reduction of the diaphyseal metaphyseal junction and restoration of the articular surface. (The anterior plate shown in this case is no longer commercially available.)
a Mortise view.
b Lateral view.

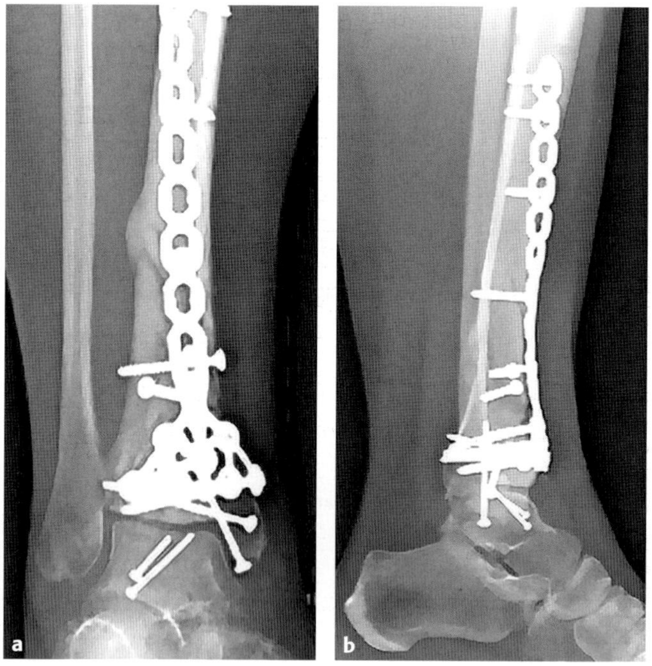

Fig 2.7-8a–b Postoperative x-rays. (The anterior plate shown in this case is no longer commercially available.)
a Mortise view.
b Lateral view.

5 Pitfalls and complications

Pitfalls

Inadequate reduction and fixation

The choice of approach is critical in successful reduction and fixation strategies for these injuries. A poorly planned surgical approach may not adequately allow for visualization of the articular injury and appropriate fixation. A CT scan is the investigation of choice to formulate a preoperative plan that is appropriate for each unique fracture.

Distractor use

The surgeon should become familiar with the distractor, as it is a critical tool in achieving fracture reduction. Placement of Schanz pins should be well planned according to the fracture pattern.

Irreducible intercalary fragments

Small intercalary fragments (ie, < 5 mm in diameter) and fragments without adequate overlying cartilage should be removed rather than attempting fixation. These fragments do not contribute to joint congruity and may impede anatomical reduction or may displace into the joint as loose bodies.

Anterior incision

The anterior approach to the ankle is useful for certain pilon fractures. This incision does not allow for easy precontoured plate application to the anterolateral and medial distal tibial. The anterior approach should be reserved for cases in which a true anterior plate can be used to address the fracture. It is advantageous for conversion to ankle arthrodesis or total ankle arthroplasty, if necessary.

Complications

- Injury to the anterior neurovascular bundle
- Injury to the superficial peroneal nerve
- Intraarticular placement of implants
- Loss of fixation
- Nonunion
- Malunion
- Avascular necrosis
- Posttraumatic arthritis
- Compartment syndrome
- Infection
- Wound complications

6 Alternative techniques

The preferred alternative anterior approaches to pilon fractures of the distal tibia are:

- Anterolateral approach
- Anteromedial approach

Standard precontoured pilon plates can be used with these more traditional approaches. The thin wire fixator is another treatment option if the surgeon is comfortable with the technique. However, the articular reduction is often not as exact with thin wire external fixation techniques.

Primary arthrodesis may be performed in select patients with multiple comorbidities or in select cases when articular reconstruction is not possible.

Small wire fixation works well to reestablish limb alignment but is limited in the ability to restore articular congruity and address impacted articular segments.

7 Postoperative management and rehabilitation

Postoperatively, the ankle is immobilized in a splint or fracture brace, with the ankle held at 90°. If there is a coexisting equinus contracture, then a tendo-Achilles lengthening procedure is needed to achieve proper position. This can be performed in the Achilles tendon by percutaneous lengthening or can be performed as a gastrocnemius recession, depending on what structure is causing the equinus. Equinus testing of the contralateral side may aid in locating the cause of the contracture. Always keep the leg elevated. Remove any applied suction drain on day 1 or day 2 postoperatively. Keep sutures in place for 2–3 weeks and then remove them.

If the external fixator is retained after surgery, it should be removed several weeks postoperatively with the timing based on fracture severity. Toe motion is encouraged immediately with active and passive range-of-motion (ROM) exercises for the ankle, subtalar, and Chopart joints initiated as soon as the external fixator is removed. Nonweight bearing is recommended for 8–12 weeks postoperatively depending on fracture severity. Standard postoperative x-rays are obtained to ensure fracture union. If uncertain of fracture healing, perform a postoperative CT scan. An active rehabilitation program is initiated at weight bearing to emphasize ROM, muscular balance, and gait training.

Implant removal

Removal of plates and screws for pilon fractures can be performed at 1 year if the patient experiences hardware-related pain. Implants can be retained long-term if they are not bothersome.

8 Recommended reading

Assal M, Ray A, Stern R. Strategies for surgical approaches in open reduction internal fixation of pilon fractures. *J Orthop Trauma*. 2015 Feb;29(2):69–79.
Beaman DN, Gellman R. Fracture reduction and primary ankle arthrodesis: a reliable approach for severely comminuted tibial pilon fracture. *Clin Orthop Relat Res*. 2014 Dec;472(12):3823–3834.
Calori GM, Tagliabue L, Mazza E, et al. Tibial pilon fractures: which method of treatment? *Injury*. 2010 Nov;41(11):1183–1190.
Jacob N, Amin A, Giotakis N, et al. Management of high-energy tibial pilon fractures. *Strategies Trauma Limb Reconstr*. 2015 Nov;10(3):137–147.
Liu J, Smith CD, White E, et al. A systematic review of the role of surgical approaches on the outcomes of the tibia pilon fracture. *Foot Ankle Spec*. 2016 Apr;9(2):163–168.
McAlister JE, DeMill SL, Hyer CF, et al. Anterior approach total ankle arthroplasty: superficial peroneal nerve branches at risk. *J Foot Ankle Surg*. 2016 May–Jun;55(3):476–479.
Zelle BA, Gruen GS, McMillen RL, et al. Primary arthrodesis of the tibiotalar joint in severely comminuted high-energy pilon fractures. *J Bone Joint Surg Am*. 2014 Jun 4;96(11):e91.

Acknowledgement

Special thanks to Miyoko Green in her assistance with preparation of this chapter.

2.8 Staged treatment of pilons (posterior to anterior)

John Ketz, David Ciufo

1 Case description

A 47-year-old woman fell 4.6 m from a ladder while cleaning her gutters, landing on her left leg. She immediately experienced pain in her ankle, but had no other injuries. On arrival at the emergency department, there was obvious deformity of the ankle with ecchymosis and swelling but no blisters, tented skin, or open wounds. X-rays of the ankle and leg demonstrated a complete, multifragmentary articular, metaphyseal fracture of the distal tibia (AO/OTA 43C3), with an associated distal fibular fracture (**Fig 2.8-1**). The neurovascular examination was normal.

A closed reduction was performed under intravenous analgesia, and a computed tomographic (CT) scan was obtained for thorough evaluation of the fracture pattern and operative planning.

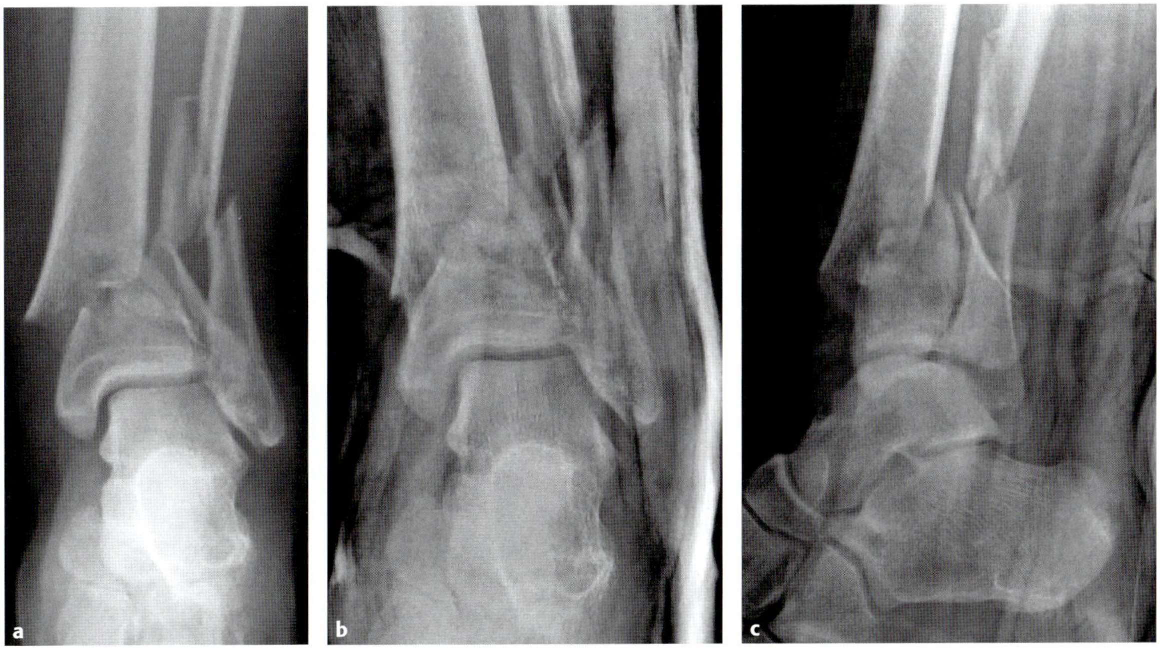

Fig 2.8-1a–c Emergency department x-rays.
a AP ankle x-ray on arrival.
b–c Ankle x-rays after preliminary manipulation and splinting.

2 Preoperative planning

When evaluating a patient with a suspected fracture of the ankle, the extremity should be examined carefully. The soft-tissue injury will dictate operative treatment. Careful attention should be paid to abrasions, fracture blisters or lacerations indicative of an open injury that requires urgent attention. A thorough neurovascular examination should be performed. If there is neurovascular compromise, the injured extremity should be reduced and immobilized in a splint and the neurovascular status rechecked. Once the limb has been stabilized, formal x-rays of the tibia/fibula, ankle, and foot should be obtained and reviewed.

The x-rays will provide significant information about the fracture. Particular attention should be paid to the proximal extent of the fracture, displacement of the posterior malleolus fracture, and the articular involvement. Preoperative planning is crucial. If there is presence of an open fracture, antibiotics should be started on arrival to the hospital and urgent irrigation and debridement with stabilization should be performed. It is important to note that if the open wound is small and not in a plane of a viable approach, smaller formal approaches can be performed to irrigate and debride the fracture along with debridement of the open wound. Larger open wounds limit additional incisions and should be debrided and treated with staged fixation:

- Stage 1: Posterior fixation and external fixator placement
- Stage 2: Anterior fixation

If the soft-tissue envelope allows, limited internal fixation of certain fracture fragments can greatly improve the alignment and stability of the fracture. If this is being considered, a CT scan should be obtained (**Fig 2.8-2**). The CT can provide additional 3D information about the fracture and may provide anatomical detail which allows for early fixation of certain fragments of the fracture. This is particularly true for posterior malleolar fractures. When these fragments are displaced as a result of the injury, they often do not reduce with ligamentotaxis after applying an external fixator. At the time of definitive fixation, the posterior fragment is extremely difficult to reduce indirectly, and open reduction requires significant soft-tissue dissection due to scarring, to mobilize the fragment and reduce it after it has migrated proximally as a result of the injury.

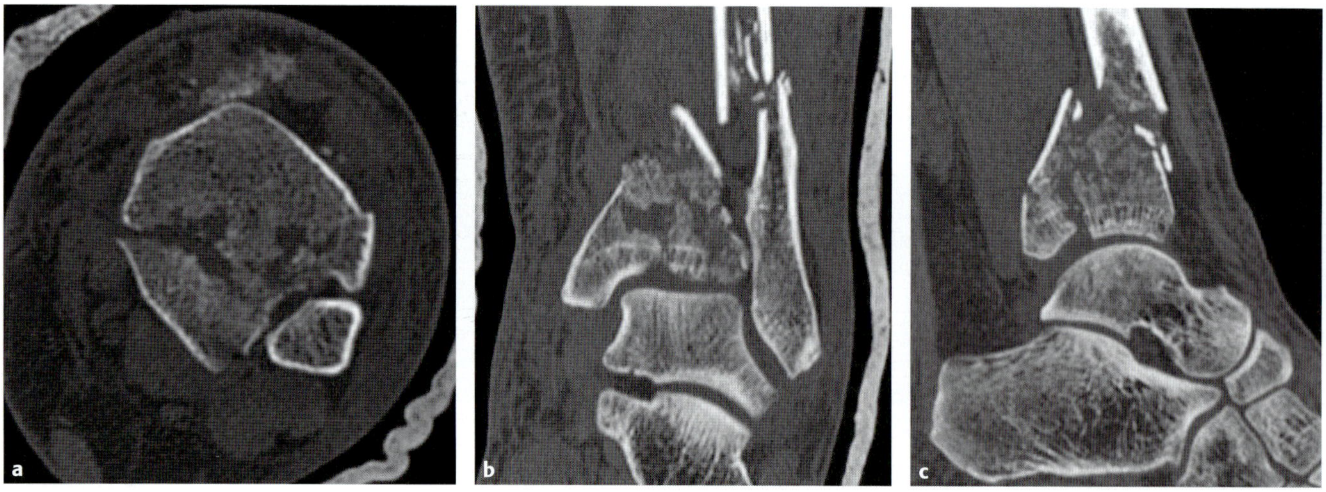

Fig 2.8-2a–c Computed tomographic images revealing articular and metaphyseal comminution and displacement.
a Axial view.
b Coronal view.
c Sagittal view.

3 Operating room setup

Patient positioning	• Stage 1: - Prone - For patients with thoracic injuries preventing prone positioning, consideration should be given to a lateral decubitus position or standard staged fixation. • Stage 2: - Supine
Anesthesia options	• As the patient is going to be placed in the prone position, general anesthesia is required for staged posterior fixation of pilon fractures. This also allows for use of muscle relaxation if needed. • Polytrauma patients may require advanced monitoring for anesthetic needs. • Proper antibiotic selection should be performed based on individual patient allergies.
C-arm location	• On the opposite side of the table from the operative extremity. • Monitor toward the head of the table. • During the procedure the C-arm may need to be canted such that it is perpendicular to the lower leg.
Tourniquet	• Stage 1: - A nonsterile tourniquet is placed high on the thigh. - The patient is then positioned prone, with the foot at the end of a radiolucent table such that it can be dorsiflexed to neutral. - All prominences should be padded well. The leg is draped to allow flexion of the knee. • Stage 2: - The patient is then returned for staged fixation of the anterior components of the injury the patient is positioned supine, with the foot at the end of a radiolucent table. - The leg is draped free.
Tips	• The pins of the external fixator may be used for distraction during reconstruction of the tibial plafond.

For illustrations and overview of anesthetic considerations, see chapter 1.

Equipment

- K-wire
- Absorbable pins
- Minifragment locking plate set
- Small fragment set
- Reduction clamps
- Periosteal elevators
- Large external fixator set

4 Surgical procedure

Stage 1: Posterior fixation and external fixator placement

A posterolateral approach is centered between the lateral aspect of the Achilles and the posterior fibular border (**Fig 2.8-3**). Incision length is determined by the proximal extension of the posterior fragment. Sharp dissection is carried out through the skin and blunt dissection is performed through the subcutaneous tissues. Because the sural nerve is in proximity, it is vulnerable in the superior portion of the incision. Carefully identify and protect the nerve from injury.

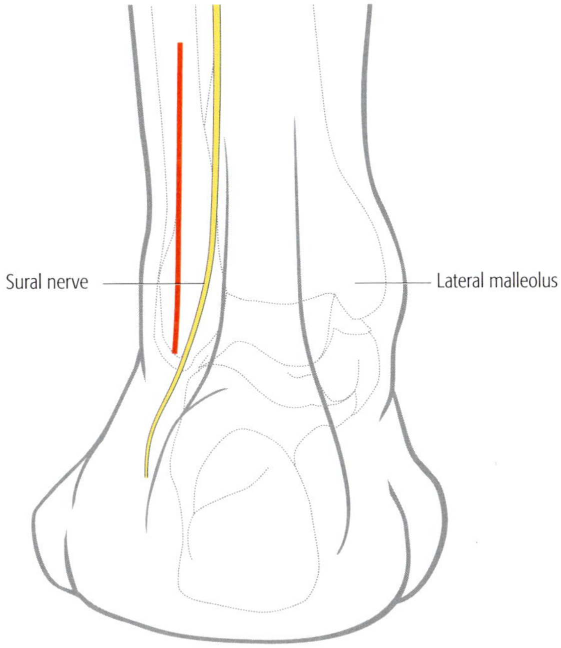

Fig 2.8-3 Incision planning for the posterolateral approach.

The plane of dissection is between the peroneal tendons and the flexor hallucis longus (FHL). Care should be taken proximally as the main branch of the peroneal artery is at risk and care must be taken to avoid injury. Dissection is carried down to the posterior tibia (**Fig 2.8-4a**). As the goal of fixation is to restore the posterior buttress, minimal stripping and excessive dissection should be avoided. The posterior malleolar fracture is identified. During preoperative planning, it is important to determine whether the posterior malleolar fragment is singular or multifragmentary.

For singular fragments, there is often a triangular shape to the proximal portion of the posterior articular fragment that will fit precisely into the shaft component of the fracture allowing accurate reduction.

It is possible to view the articular surface before the posterior piece is reduced. Minute displacement after reduction of the posterior malleolus may not be appreciated on the C-arm views and may only be detected by palpation with a small (Freer) elevator. Alternatively, a small arthroscope can be introduced to assess the reduction. Once this reduction is performed, it can be temporarily stabilized with K-wires. A 3.5 mm tubular or small fragment plate (linear or T-shaped) can then be contoured to the posterior tibia (**Fig 2.8-4b**). Undercontouring can lead to an extension deformity of the articular fragment and overcontouring can flex the fragment and displace it posteriorly. Proximal screws are placed through the plate to stabilize the fragment. When placing the distal screws, they should remain completely within the posterior fragment (typically < 16 mm). If they protrude into the central portion of the fracture, they can block reduction during the second stage (anterior fixation).

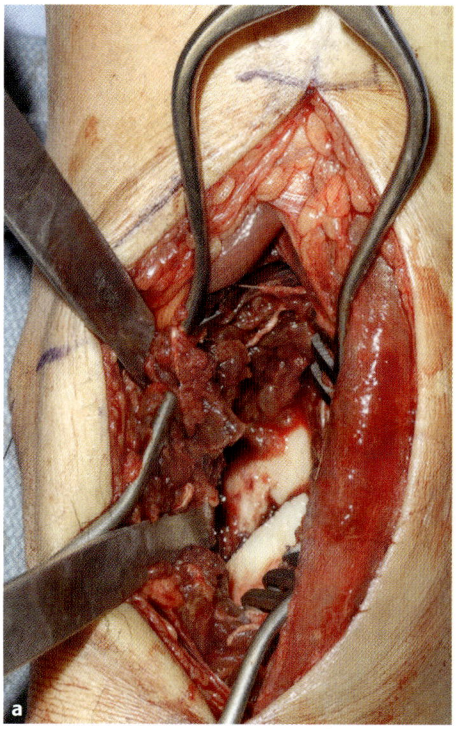

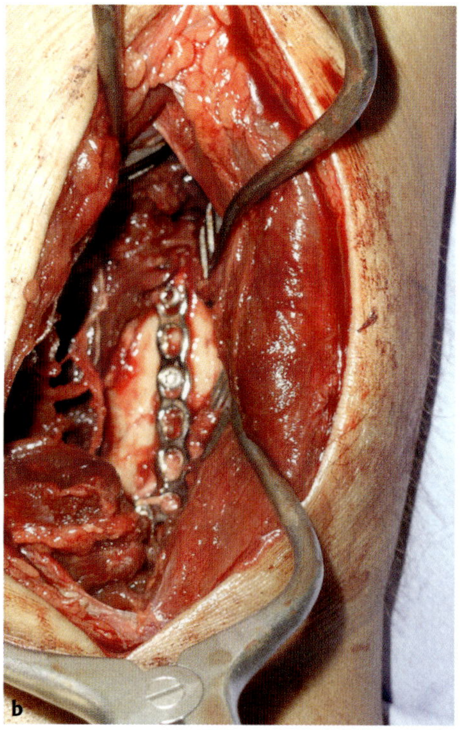

Fig 2.8-4a–b Intraoperative visualization of the posterior malleolar fracture (**a**) and plate placement (**b**).

For multifragmentary pieces, the most proximal fragment should be reduced first using the proximal triangular shape of this fragment as a cortical key if it is available. The fragment is then stabilized with K-wires and the sagittal fracture planes can then be reduced and temporarily stabilized. Lateral C-arm imaging should be obtained to ensure proper alignment of the posterior articular surface. Occasionally, small adjustments may be necessary to improve the reduction if a small articular step off is detected on the lateral C-arm image. This fracture pattern requires a T-plate or precontoured plate that allows for screw placement through each fragment (**Fig 2.8-5**). The proximal screws are placed first and then at least one screw is placed through each fragment as described above.

In cases where there is a proximal diaphyseal extension of the posterior malleolar fragment, a similar antiglide technique can be applied with slight modifications. Stabilization of the posterior diaphyseal fragment can convert an AO/OTA 43C-type fracture to a simpler AO/OTA 43B-type, providing a stable posterior buttress for later reconstruction, as well as providing early stability of length, alignment, and rotation in addition to the external fixator. Depending on the fracture type, a proximal tubular, DCP, or LC/DCP plate can be applied in isolation through a more proximal anterolateral or posteromedial incision, or in addition to a distal plate (as described above) when articular comminution is present (**Fig 2.8-6**).

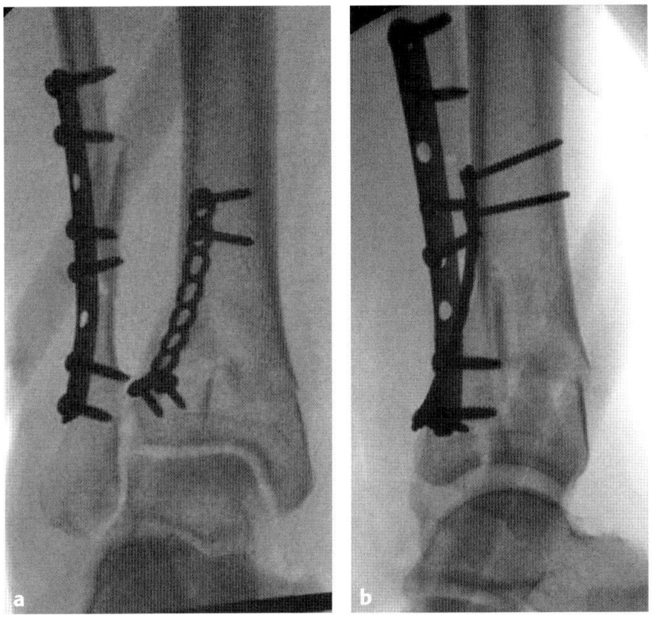

Fig 2.8-5a–b Intraoperative imaging of posterior fixation and external fixator after posterior tibial and fibular fixation.
a Mortise view.
b Lateral view.

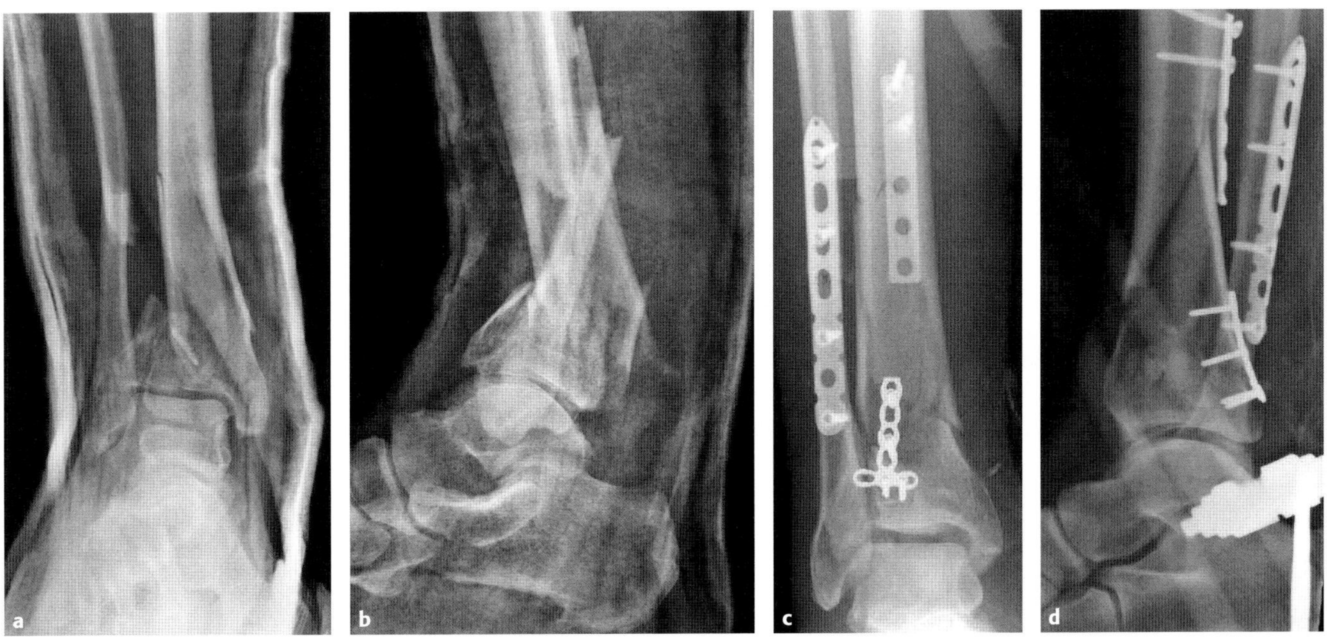

Fig 2.8-6a–d Use of a proximal posterior plate in the setting of diaphyseal extension.
a–b AP and lateral injury images highlighting the proximal extent of fracture.
c–d AP and lateral postoperative x-rays demonstrating the proximal antiglide plate technique.

If a fibular fracture is present, it can also be reduced at this time. Fixation of the posterior malleolus should be performed first. If the fibula is fixed first the fibular hardware may block the imaging of the central portion of the plafond on lateral C-arm images. Dissection is carried out lateral to the peroneal fascia. The peroneal fascia is incised from the posterolateral fibula. The peroneal tendons are mobilized and retracted medially for visualization of the posterior fibula. Alternatively, the peroneal tendons can be retracted laterally and the same interval between the FHL and peroneal tendons may be used to approach the fibula. The fibula is reduced with clamps. This is performed if anatomical reduction with a lag screw and neutralization or antiglide plate is appropriate. In the setting of greater comminution, which is common in this type of injury, a bridge plating technique is performed. It is critical to restore proper anatomical length, alignment, and rotation of the fibula. Malreduction of the fibula, particularly shortening, may create difficulties with staged anterior fixation. C-arm imaging should be used to assist and confirm reduction. The wound is irrigated and closed in a layered fashion, with interrupted 3-0 nylon skin sutures.

After wound closure, the external fixator is placed. The knee is flexed to 90°. Two 5.0 mm half-pins are placed in the tibia proximal to the fracture site, if possible, proximal to the estimated location of the proximal extension of the final anterior plate. A transcalcaneal pin is placed under C-arm guidance and a delta frame is constructed. An additional pin is placed in the first metatarsal or across the cuneiforms to control the foot position and increase stability. Longitudinal traction is applied to obtain appropriate fracture length and rotation and confirmed using the C-arm. Care is taken to place the bars far enough from the skin to accommodate swelling. The tourniquet is then released, and the patient turned supine. A postoperative CT scan is obtained to evaluate posterior fragment reduction and to plan incisions and reduction for anterior fixation (**Fig 2.8-7**). If there is malreduction of the posterior fragments or fibula that will affect definitive fixation, it should be corrected during the following stage.

Stage 2: Anterior fixation

The patient is brought back to the operating room for staged anterior fixation when the soft tissues allow, typically after 10–14 days. The external fixator frame is disassembled but the pins left in place and prepared into the sterile field. The anterior incision is based on fracture fragment orientation seen on the CT scan following external fixation. Options include direct anterior, anterolateral, or the anteromedial incision.

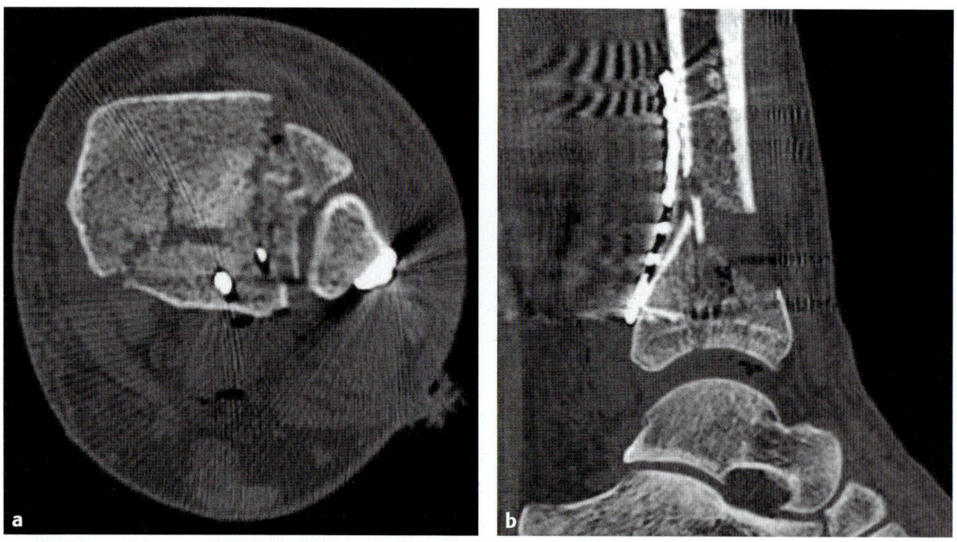

Fig 2.8-7a–b Postoperative CT scan obtained after posterior fixation showing reduction of the articular surface and posterior fragments.
a Axial cut.
b Sagittal cut.

The anterior approach affords complete visualization of the anteromedial and anterolateral tibia and can also be used for future ankle arthroplasty or arthrodesis, if needed (**Fig 2.8-8**). The incision is centered over the ankle lateral to the tibialis anterior tendon. The superficial peroneal nerve should be identified and protected as it crosses the incision distally from the lateral side. The extensor retinaculum is incised in line with the skin incision and dissection is carried out between the tibialis anterior and the extensor hallucis longus (EHL) tendon. The anterior tibial artery and deep peroneal nerve must be identified and protected. They are located deep and slightly lateral to the EHL tendon. The neurovascular bundle will be retracted laterally with EHL, and the tibialis anterior is retracted medially. The ankle capsule will now be in view. If it has not been disrupted by the injury, the capsule can be incised sharply in line with the skin incision at the level of the articular surface and excised.

With the joint exposed, the fragments are identified and cleared of hematoma. Reduction is performed in a posterior to anterior fashion, building from the previously stabilized posterior tibia. Impaction of the posterior joint surface should be addressed first. Fragments can be temporarily stabilized with 1.6 mm K-wires. Smaller osteochondral fragments can be stabilized with absorbable pins; compressed between larger fragments; or by using the "lost K-wire" technique, where the small osteochondral fragment is held in position with a K-wire. The portion of the K-wire extending beyond the bone is cut flush so the remaining portion of the wire is entirely buried in bone. Once the articular surface is temporarily stabilized, the reduction is confirmed with C-arm imaging. Attention is then turned to the metaphyseal component which is reduced to the shaft using a combination of K-wires and clamps.

Initially, the separate articular fragments are stabilized with individual lag screws using either minifragment or small fragment screws. A precontoured anterolateral plate is then used to stabilize the metaphyseal-diaphyseal segment. This can be done in a percutaneous fashion by passing the plate through the anterior incision. A separate anterolateral incision is then made proximally over the plate. Screws are placed proximally and distally through the plate until adequate stability is achieved. C-arm imaging is then used to verify reduction (**Fig 2.8-9**). The external fixator pins are removed, followed by curettage and irrigation of the pin tracts. The wounds are irrigated. Closure is performed in a layered fashion.

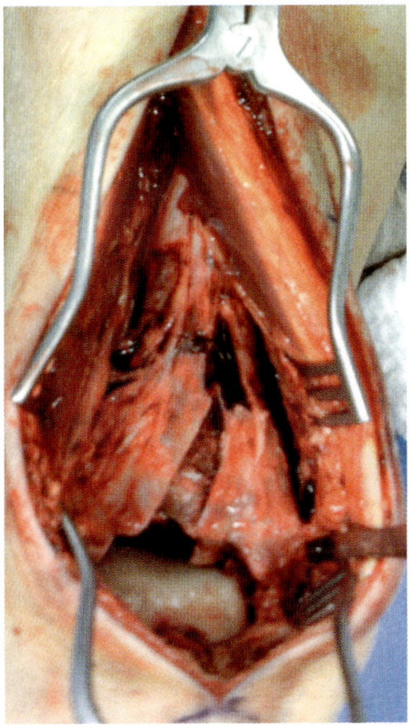

Fig 2.8-8 Exposure after anterior approach to ankle.

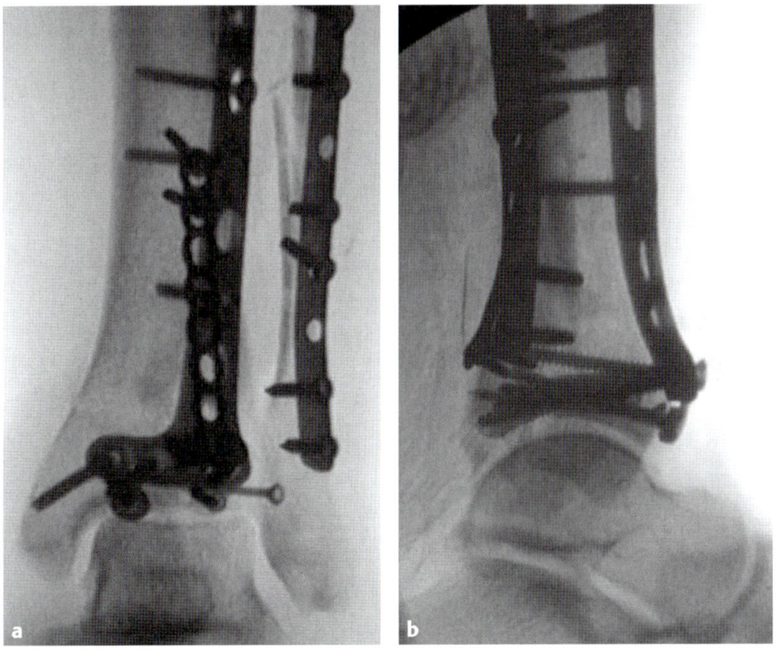

Fig 2.8-9 Intraoperative imaging of the staged anterior fixation showing the reconstruction of the articular surface and fixation to the diaphyseal segment.
a Mortise view.
b Lateral view.

5 Pitfalls and complications

Pitfalls

Inadequate reduction or malreduction

Particularly in cases with significant comminution, reduction of the posterior malleolus can be difficult. Small amounts of residual displacement or impaction can be corrected during the second stage if identified. Significant malreduction of the posterior distal tibia will limit the ability to appropriately reconstruct the anterior tibia during the second stage and should be revised early. This should be evaluated on postoperative CT following external fixation. If the fibula is addressed initially, malreduction can also limit the ability to reduce the fracture during the second stage. In this scenario, revision of the fibula should be performed.

External fixator placement difficulty

Most surgeons have less experience with placement of an external fixator on a patient in the prone position. This may require additional assistance compared to supine placement. This should be planned for, and fixator placement should be verified with the C-arm to ensure adequate positioning and fracture alignment.

Poor patient selection

Proper patient selection is crucial when deciding to perform staged posterior-anterior fixation. Patients should have adequate soft tissues to allow for both stages of treatment. Also, patients with preexisting ankle arthritis may benefit from primary arthrodesis or delayed open reduction and internal fixation (ORIF). This technique requires early presentation to allow for posterior stabilization. After early posterior plating, the soft-tissue swelling and trauma are allowed time to improve before another surgical exposure is performed.

Complications

- Wound healing in the setting of acute trauma
- Late infection necessitating removal of implants requires two approaches
- Injury to the sural nerve (posterolateral), superficial peroneal nerve, or deep peroneal nerve (anterior)
- Ankle stiffness can occur as a result of posterior approach
- Malunion
- Nonunion
- Avascular necrosis
- Posttraumatic arthritis

6 Alternative techniques

Delayed fixation

At times the soft tissues or patient comorbidities may not allow for a posterior-anterior technique. In this scenario, initial external fixation with delayed fixation should be performed. For elderly, low-demand patients, or those with preexisting arthritis, anterior only or small incision approaches to fixation may be the best treatment as it reduces the risk of soft-tissue complications in these patient populations.

Primary arthrodesis

Primary arthrodesis can be used as an alternative technique in case of extensive cartilage loss, comminution, or preexisting ankle arthritis.

Depending on the fracture pattern and the soft tissues, certain pilon fractures can be treated initially with definitive ORIF. Care should be taken when performing immediate ORIF and should be only performed by surgeons who are experienced in treating pilon fractures.

7 Postoperative management and rehabilitation

Stage 1: Posterior and external fixator

Plain x-rays and a CT scan are obtained after the initial posterior fixation to assess fibular and tibial articular reduction for planning of the anterior incision and fixation. The patient can be discharged home after 1–2 days and followed up weekly as an outpatient to assess soft tissues (usually for about 2–3 weeks). Patients should maintain strict nonweight-bearing precautions and lower extremity elevation. Pin care is performed daily.

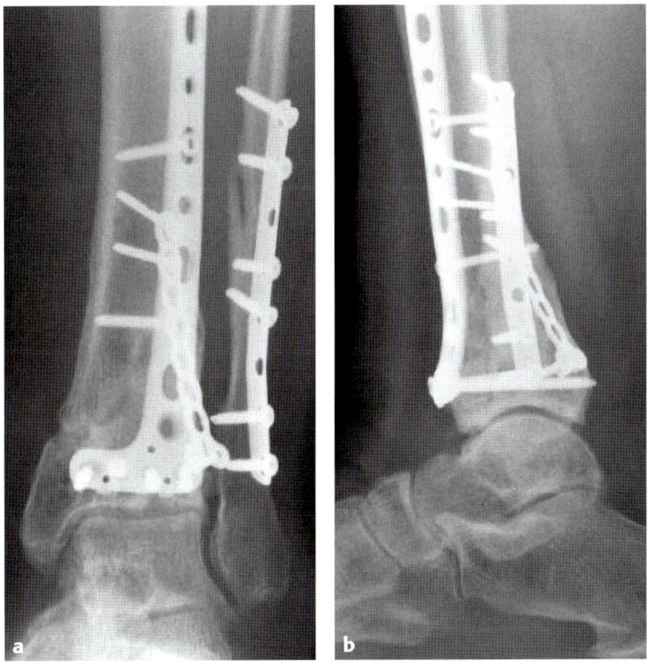

Fig 2.8-10a–b Postoperative imaging at 3-year follow-up demonstrating well-healed fractures, with good articular surface alignment and well-maintained joint space.

a Mortise view.
b Lateral view.

Stage 2: Anterior fixation

A well-padded posterior plaster splint is placed immediately postoperatively. Postoperative x-rays are obtained. The patient is typically discharged after 1–2 days. At 2 weeks, if the soft tissues allow, the patient is transitioned to a removable boot and the sutures are removed. Range-of-motion (ROM) exercises about the ankle, subtalar, and Chopart regions are started at this time. Patients remain nonweight bearing until the fracture demonstrates radiographic healing, usually at 10–12 weeks. The patient is transitioned to a removable ankle brace and therapy is started for ROM and strengthening (**Fig 2.8-10**).

8 Recommended reading

Cole PA, Mehrle RK, Bhandari M, et al. The pilon map: fracture lines and comminution zones in OTA/AO type 43C3 pilon fractures. *J Orthop Trauma.* 2013 Jul;27(7):e152–156.
Dunbar RP, Barei DP, Kubiak EN, et al. Early limited internal fixation of diaphyseal extensions in select pilon fractures: upgrading AO/OTA type C fractures to AO/OTA type B. J *Orthop Trauma.* 2008 Jul;22(6):426–429.
Ketz J, Sanders R. Staged posterior tibial plating for the treatment of Orthopaedic Trauma Association 43C2 and 43C3 tibial pilon fractures. *J Orthop Trauma.* 2012 Jun;26(6):341–347.
Tornetta P 3rd, Gorup J. Axial computed tomography of pilon fractures. *Clin Orthop Relat Res.* 1996 Feb(323):273–276.

2.9 Pilon fracture with compartment syndrome of the foot

Matthew Graves, Bopha Chrea

1 Case description

A 37-year-old man with no significant medical history was admitted to the emergency department after he fell 3.6 m from a deer stand sustaining a closed injury to his left lower extremity. Upon arrival to the hospital, x-rays revealed a left ankle articular pilon fracture (AO/OTA 43C3) with an associated spiral Weber C fibular fracture (**Fig 2.9-1**). Injury x-rays also revealed a valgus, axial-loading injury pattern. His ankle was reduced in the emergency department and placed in a splint. The patient had no history of tobacco use.

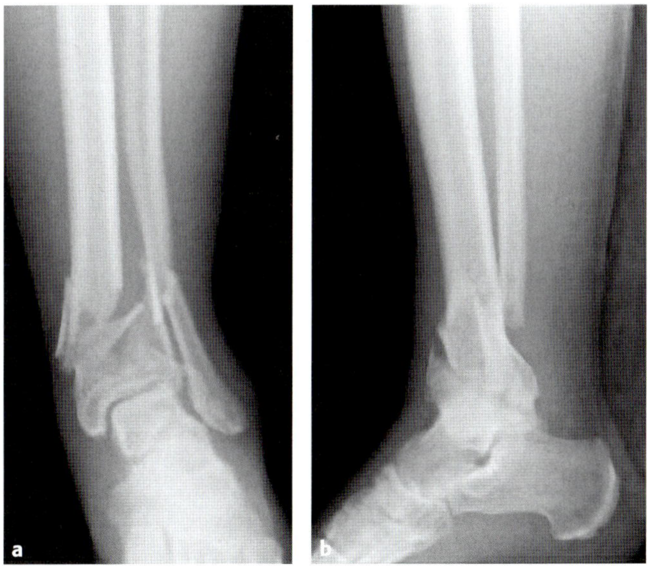

Fig 2.9-1a–b Postinjury x-rays of the left ankle after a fall from 3.6 m, prior to splint placement.
a AP view.
b Lateral view.

2 Preoperative planning

Indications for surgery

Initial indications for staged treatment of this pilon fracture included a displaced, articular tibial pilon fracture with an associated fibular fracture in a 37-year-old patient with significant soft-tissue injury.

Indication for return to the operating room (OR) immediately in the postoperative period included the development of suspected acute foot compartment syndrome (FCS) with progressive neurological changes.

Indications for the salvage surgeries included the development of a symptomatic nonunion with concern for infection.

Acute management

Stage 1: Closed manipulative reduction of the ankle and spanning external fixator placement

The fibular fracture can be addressed at the same time or at the time of definitive management of the pilon fracture. The fibular fracture can be fixed with a plate and screw construct, intramedullary screw or rod (if the fracture pattern is amenable), or left to heal without internal fixation. In this case, a plate and screw construct was used.

Fibular malreduction and improper surgical approach can impede later tibial plafond reconstruction. Ideally, fibular fixation should be performed by the same surgeon who will ultimately perform the tibial fixation.

Stage 2: Pilon fracture open reduction and fixation

Pilon fractures can be accessed via direct lateral, anterolateral, anteromedial, posterolateral, or posteromedial exposures depending on the fracture pattern.

A posteromedial incision is ideally suited to address tendon entrapment in the fracture plane between the Volkmann and medial malleolar fragment. It is also useful for direct visualization and reduction of those fracture fragments. However, the posteromedial soft tissue was compromised in this case, so plans were made to use the anterolateral approach for reduction and stabilization of the entire joint (**Fig 2.9-2**). Two separate 5 mm incisions were planned to reduce and fix the medial column with a modified point-to-point reduction (Weber) clamp and two compression screws.

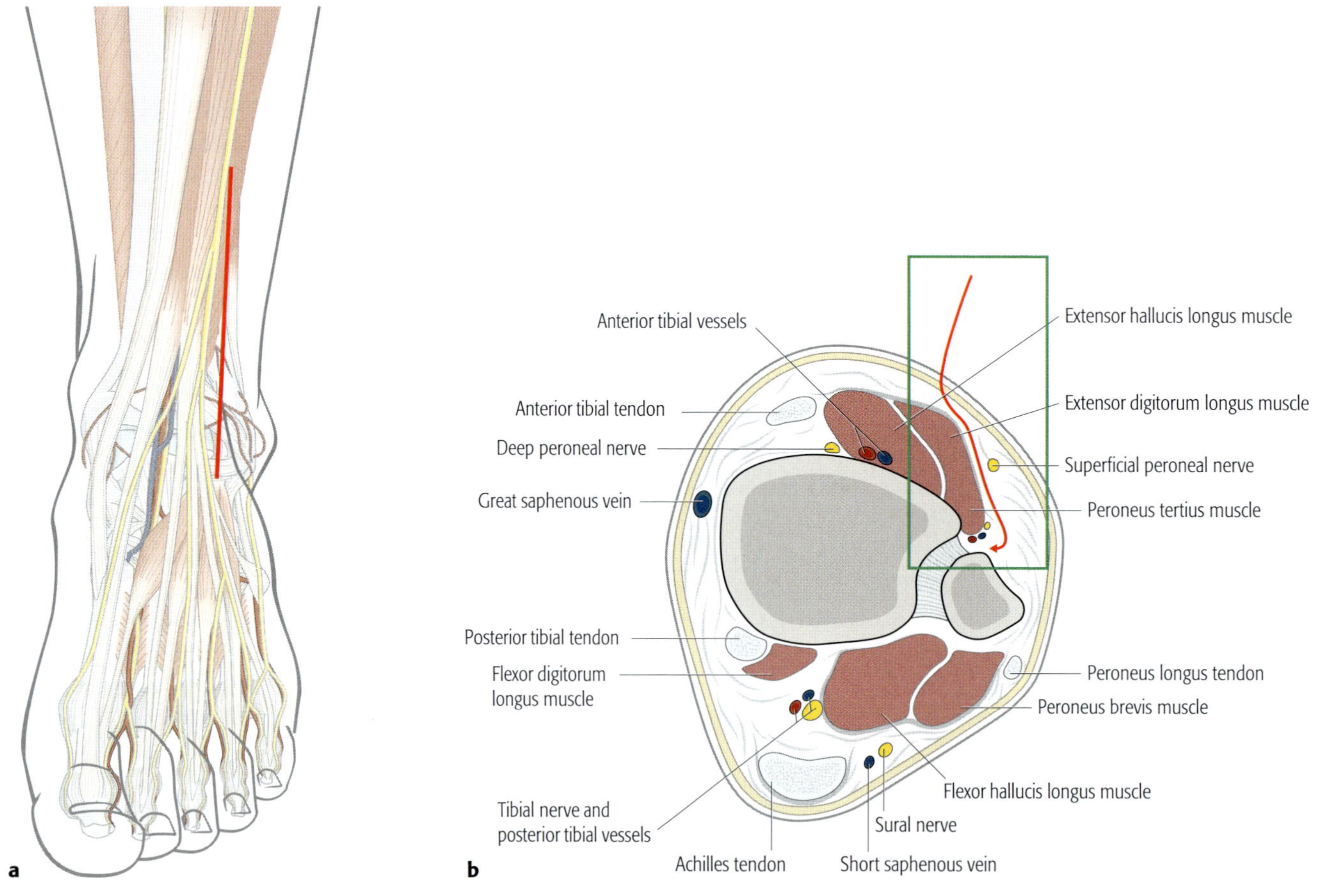

Fig 2.9-2a–b Anterolateral approach to the tibia. Landmarks for skin incision (red line, arrow) and interval (green box).

Salvage treatment

Salvage of a septic pilon nonunion is complex. Septic nonunion management follows a typical algorithm:

1. Debride all infected and necrotic bone. Osteomyelitis in infected pilon nonunions is typically localized rather than diffuse. This debridement can be accomplished with different instruments, but the high-speed precision burr with coolant allows for more precise bone removal back to viable bleeding bone.
2. Multiple sets of tissue samples are taken and sent for aerobic, anaerobic, acid fast bacilli, and fungi cultures.
3. Fill the defect created from debridement. Either antibiotic beads or an antibiotic spacer may be used.
4. Reduction and stabilization during the intravenous antibiotic stage. This can be accomplished with different techniques, but the ring fixator affords the advantage of multiplanar stability with avoidance of metal in the zone of infection.
5. Exchange of the spacer for bone graft. Different types of graft can be used, but autograft has clear advantages. Smaller defects can be filled with local graft harvest from the proximal tibia, distal femur, or calcaneus. Larger defects require harvesting bone graft from the iliac crest or an intramedullary canal.
6. Determine stabilization during the graft incorporation stage. The ring fixator can be continued or a plate can be placed with or without removal of the fixator.

Preoperative planning for salvage treatment includes ensuring that all equipment that may be needed is easily available in the OR.

3 Operating room setup

Patient positioning	• Supine on a radiolucent table
Anesthesia options	• General anesthesia is recommended • Alternatively, spinal or regional anesthesia can be used. • First-generation cephalosporin is administered for prophylaxis within 30 minutes of surgery.
C-arm location	• Entering from the medial aspect of the ankle • C-arm monitor placed at the head of the table
Tourniquet	• Can be applied, and inflated if needed

The setup is the same for all stages of surgery.

For illustrations and overview of anesthetic considerations, see chapter 1.

Equipment list

- Large external fixator or universal distractor
- Clamps, dental scalers, small (Freer) elevator
- K-wires
- Small plates of various shapes and sizes
- Precontoured distal tibial plates (variable angle locking)
- 3.5 mm (or 2.7 mm) cancellous screws
- 3.5 mm (or 2.7 mm) cortex screws
- For salvage treatment of the tibial malunion:
- High-speed precision burr
- Reamer-irrigator-aspirator (RIA) system
- Ring fixator

4 Surgical procedure

In this case, it would have been ideal to use a 2-incision approach for definitive fixation of the pilon fracture. A posteromedial incision would have made for easier reduction and posterior tibial tendon (PTT) removal from the fracture site; however, the soft-tissue injury did not allow for safe exposure. Regardless of which surgical approach is used in pilon fracture management, a general understanding of the six distinct angiosomes that feed the foot and ankle is helpful to limit soft-tissue complications (**Fig 2.9-3**).

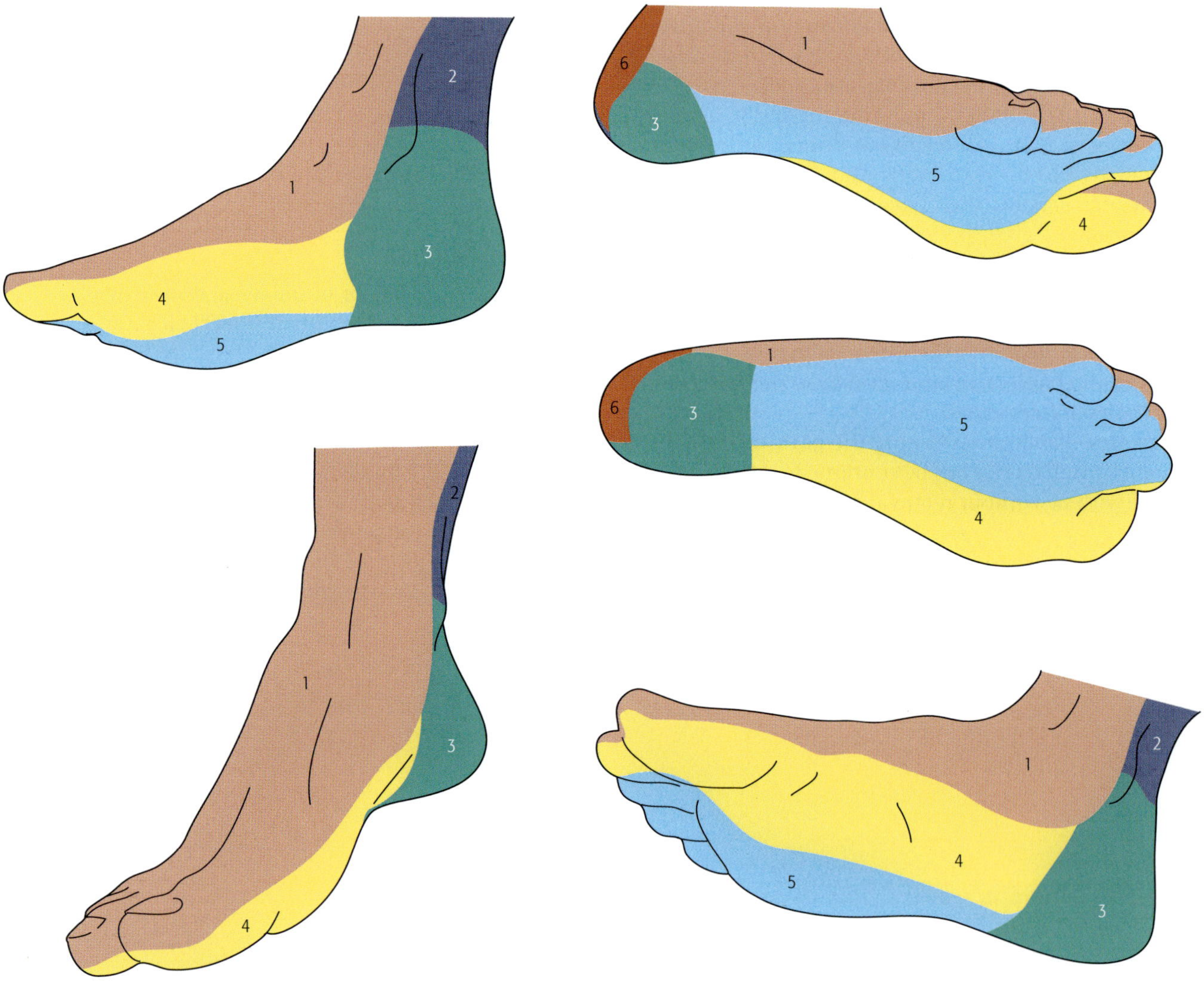

Fig 2.9-3 The foot and ankle is divided into six angiosomes. Three derive from the posterior tibial artery (PTA), one from the anterior tibial artery (ATA), and two from the peroneal artery (PA). (Adapted from LeBus, 2008.)

1. Dorsalis pedis artery (ATA)
2. Calcaneal branch (PTA) supplying medial ankle
3. Calcaneal branch (PTA) supplying plantar heel
4. Medial plantar branch (PTA)
5. Lateral plantar branch (PTA)
6. Lateral calcaneal artery (PA) plantar heel and lateral ankle

Stage 1: Closed manipulative reduction of the ankle and spanning external fixator placement

The patient is taken for external fixator placement on day 1 following the initial injury. The external fixator is applied providing relative stability. The fibular fracture was a simple fracture pattern and could be anatomically reduced, providing further stability to the soft-tissue envelope. To reduce the fibula a posterolateral incision is made, centered between the posterior border of the fibula and Achilles tendon centered at the fracture site. The peroneal musculature is mobilized. Length is achieved through traction on the transcalcaneal pin. Alternatively, a smaller ratcheting distractor can be used. Once the fracture surfaces are inter-digitated into anatomical position, there is a large amount of intrinsic stability of the fracture and a 6-hole, one-fourth tubular plate 2.7 is used for stabilization of the fibular fracture. Although a one-fourth tubular plate is used in this case, a one-third tubular plate is more commonly used for fibular fixation.

Postoperatively, the patient developed swelling with severe fracture blisters, ecchymosis along the posteromedial ankle, increasing pain, and progressive neurological deficits (**Fig 2.9-4**). It was unclear what was causing the progressive neurological deficit with possible causes including acute FCS, entrapment and stretching of the tibial nerve in the fracture line exiting posteromedially, or progression of a traumatic nerve injury. An urgent computed tomographic (CT) scan was then performed for preoperative planning and evaluation of the posteromedial structures (**Fig 2.9-5**). The CT revealed PTT entrapment within the fracture gap between the posteromedial and the medial malleolar fragment, but no tibial nerve entrapment.

In cases where FCS is a concern, an intracompartmental pressure monitor is used to measure foot compartment pressures. In this case the pressures ranged from 30–65 mm Hg, with a baseline diastolic blood pressure of approximately 80–85 mm Hg. A clinical diagnosis of FCS was made, so the patient was taken back to the OR for fasciotomies of the foot and revision of the external fixator to relax distraction.

Foot fasciotomies

The patient is returned to the OR for fasciotomies of the left foot. This is accomplished with incisions in the first and second web space and between the third and fourth web space extending onto the dorsal aspect of the foot to release the dorsal and plantar interosseous compartments. Once the compartments are released the foot is noted to be significantly softer. An incision is made along the medial aspect of the foot in order to allow for access to the plantar and calcaneal compartments, in addition to the abductor compartment. For treatment of FCS, see chapter 6.8.

The patient had significant improvement in pain and swelling following completion of fasciotomies; however, the decreased sensation throughout the foot was still present after the procedure.

Stage 2: Open reduction and internal fixation of the pilon

The patient is taken for definitive management when the swelling has reduced and soft tissues have recovered.

According to the preoperative plan an anterolateral approach is made along the line of the fourth metatarsal and centered at the ankle joint. Dissection is carried down through skin and subcutaneous tissue at the level of the intermediate dorsal cutaneous branch of the superficial peroneal nerve (SPN), which is protected and retracted medially. The anterior compartment fascia is opened including the extensor retinaculum, and the anterior compartment musculature is mobilized from lateral to medial.

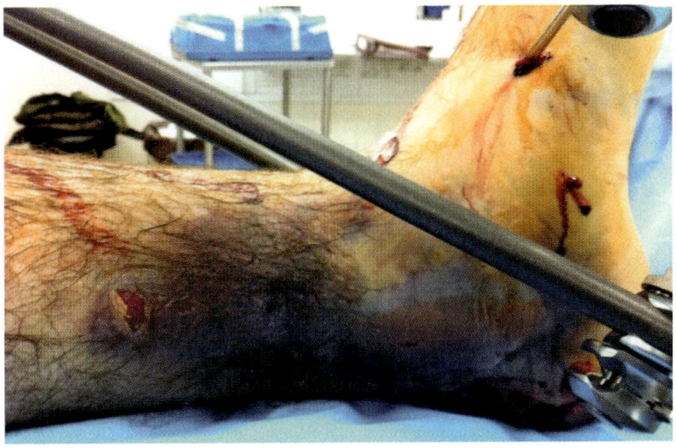

Fig 2.9-4 Compromised medial ankle soft tissue due to ecchymosis, fracture blisters, and skin tearing proximally.

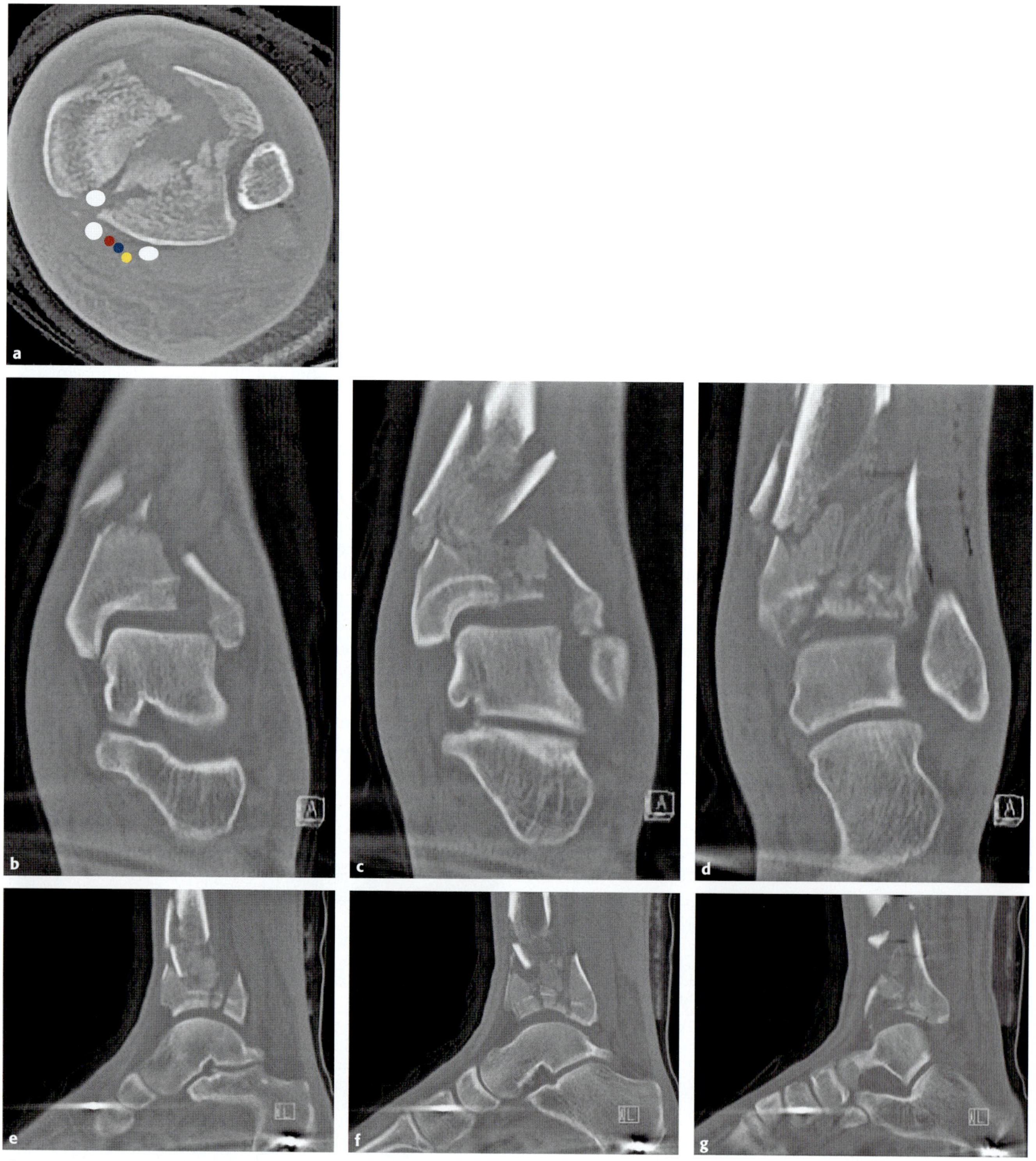

Fig 2.9-5a–g Preoperative CT images.

a Axial cut reveal entrapment of the posterior tibial tendon within the fracture plane between the medial malleolar and Volkmann fragment. A common articular fracture pattern is noted with a Chaput fragment (anterolateral), a medial malleolar fragment, and a Volkmann fragment (posterolateral). Central comminution is also visible.

b–g Coronal (**b–d**) and sagittal (**e–g**) views showing significant metaphyseal comminution along the medial and lateral column of the tibia, with complete dissociation of the articular surface from the diaphysis.

Based on the CT images, the articular surface consisted of a Chaput, medial malleolar, and Volkmann fragment, as well as a significant amount of osteochondral impaction at the central portion of the joint. Through the anterolateral surgical approach, the goal is to move from a C-type to an A-type fracture by combining segments, followed by reducing the reconstructed articular component to the shaft. The PTT (incarcerated between the Volkmann and medial malleolar fragment) is first moved out of the fracture site by pushing with a small (Freer) elevator. The reduction between these two fragments is often challenging and may be accomplished using threaded wires followed by provisional stabilization with K-wires (**Fig 2.9-6**).

Next, the central impaction noted on the CT imaging is addressed and osteochondral fragments are reduced back into appropriate position using an osteotome. Multiple wires are used to hold the fragments in the appropriate position (**Fig 2.9-6c**). The anterolateral Chaput fragment is then reduced to the remainder of the articular surface, followed by reducing the posterolateral extension of the Volkmann fragment to the shaft. The anterior distal tibial angle and lateral distal tibia angle are compared to x-ray images of the contralateral uninjured ankle to ensure appropriate anatomical reduction. A reconstruction plate 2.0 is cut to the desired length, placed along the subchondral rim, and used to hold the articular surface in position and allow for wire removal (**Fig 2.9-6d-g**). This eases the process of sliding the precontoured anterolateral plate into place.

A nonlocking 12-hole anterolateral distal tibia plate is slid in submuscular fashion beneath the anterior compartment and fixed with screws. Next, a percutaneous clamp is placed along the medial column from the medial malleolus to a drill hole in the tibial shaft in order to improve reduction of the medial column without dissecting the damaged medial soft tissue. This allows placement of two 3.5 mm screws to stabilize the medial column (**Fig 2.9-6h-j**). Then the ankle is taken through a range of motion to assess stability. If stability is present, a layered closure including the extensor retinaculum and anterior compartment fascia is completed. Skin closure is done using the Allgöwer modification of the Donati technique. This is a vertical tension relieving suture technique. A well-padded, 3-sided, below-knee splint is applied postoperatively and remains in place for the first 2 weeks, without being taken off to inspect the incisions.

At the 2-week orthopedic follow-up visit, the incision appeared to be healing without complication and the sutures were removed. One week later, the patient developed drainage from a small area along his incision. He presented to his primary care doctor for a short course of oral antibiotics. It was unclear whether this represented a superficial suture abscess or a deep infection. At his 6-week return visit with the orthopedic surgeon, his incisions looked sealed and pristine.

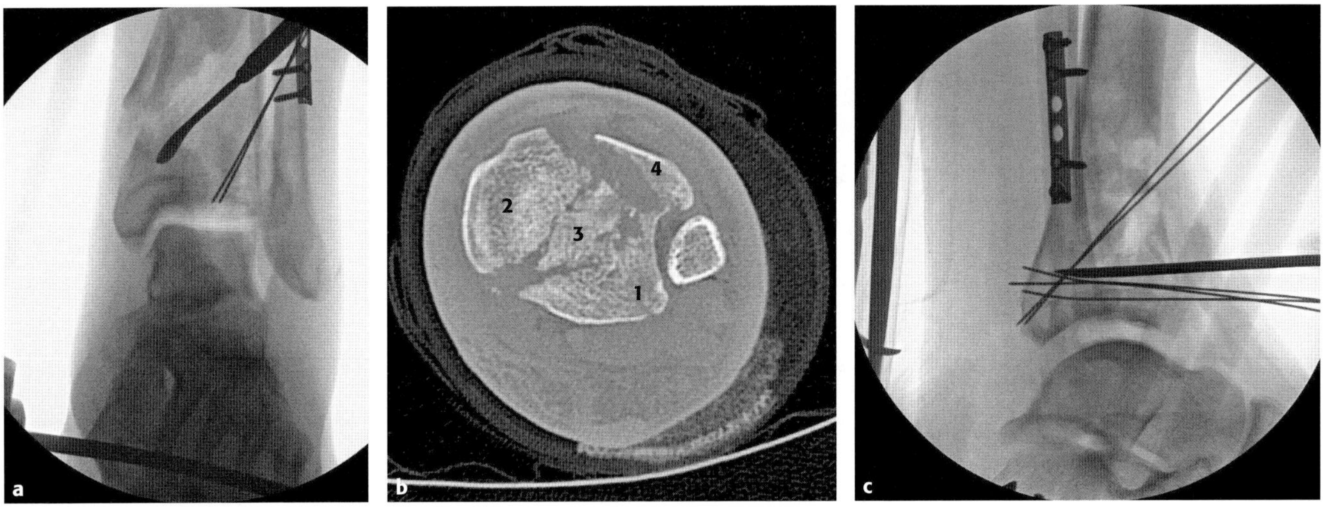

Fig 2.9-6a–j Open reduction internal fixation of pilon fracture.
a–b A small (Freer) elevator was used to push the PTT out from its incarcerated position within the fracture fragments. This was especially difficult with the anterolateral approach. The PTT was pushed out while rotating the posterior malleolar segment (1) and the medial malleolar segment (2).
c Demonstrating reduction of osteochondral fragmentation (3) to the medial articular block, Chaput fragment (4).

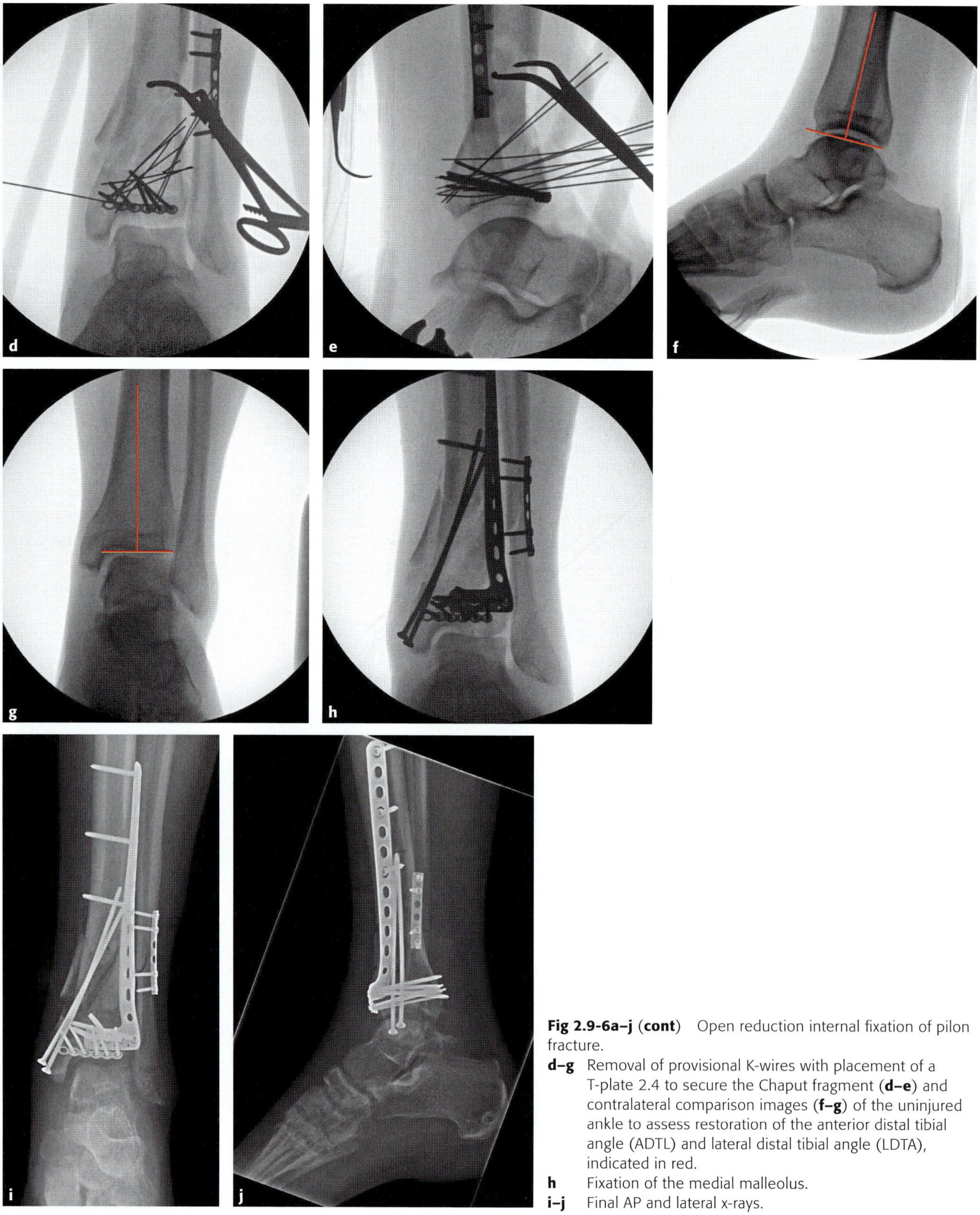

Fig 2.9-6a–j (cont) Open reduction internal fixation of pilon fracture.

d–g Removal of provisional K-wires with placement of a T-plate 2.4 to secure the Chaput fragment (**d–e**) and contralateral comparison images (**f–g**) of the uninjured ankle to assess restoration of the anterior distal tibial angle (ADTL) and lateral distal tibial angle (LDTA), indicated in red.

h Fixation of the medial malleolus.

i–j Final AP and lateral x-rays.

At his 3-month orthopedic visit, there was radiographic concern for a nonunion due to atrophy at the fracture edges and lack of healing at any fracture site (**Fig 2.9-7**). Clinically, he was having pain with weight bearing (WB) but no signs of infection. His surgical incisions were well healed and his posteromedial soft tissue was recovering. His white blood cell count, C-reactive protein, and erythrocyte sedimentation rate were all normal. The decision was made to proceed with a staged reconstruction because of concern for an indolent infection.

Preoperative antibiotics are withheld until deep cultures can be taken and then antibiotics are given as per protocol.

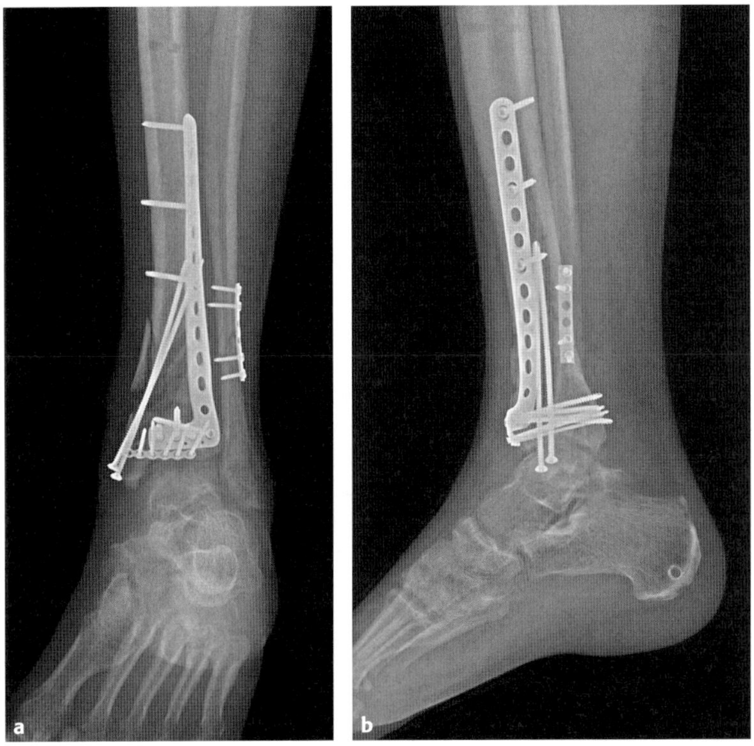

Fig 2.9-7a–b X-rays of the left ankle at 3 months postoperatively demonstrating atrophy at the fracture edges raising concerns for atrophic bone segments and a lack of healing at the fracture site.
a AP view.
b Lateral view.

Salvage treatment of nonunion

The anterolateral surgical exposure is used. All implants are removed and a high-speed precision burr is used under irrigation coolant to debride bone back to bleeding surfaces. The posterior cortex was partially healed, but there was obvious concern for secondary displacement in the absence of further stabilization. Multiple sets of cultures are taken. Antibiotic-laden cement is used as a defect filler and to increase the local concentration of antibiotics in the area. The intraoperative cultures revealed infection with methicillin-sensitive Staphylococcus aureus. The ankle was deemed to be too unstable to treat in a cast and the decision was made to use a ring fixator to maintain stability and alignment during a 6-week period of culture-specific treatment with intravenous antibiotics. A foot plate is included and the ankle joint is spanned (**Fig 2.9-8**).

The staged bone grafting is performed 6–8 weeks after the ring fixator and cement spacer are applied.

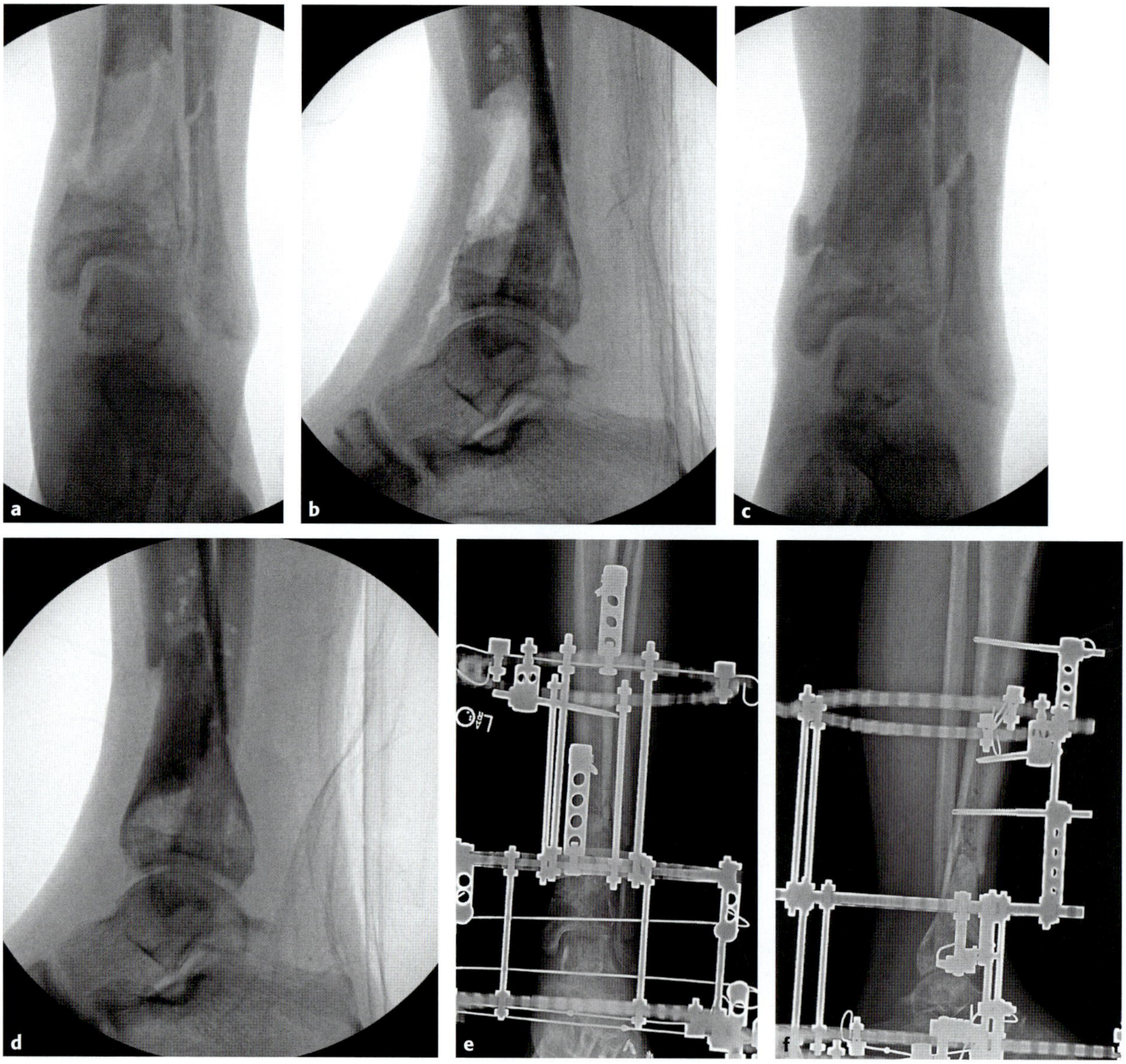

Fig 2.9-8a–f Intraoperative and postoperative images showing debridement, cement spacer placement, and ring fixator application.
a–b AP and lateral x-rays of the ankle after debridement and hardware removal with residual bony void.
c–d Repeat AP and lateral x-rays of the ankle following antibiotic cement spacer placement using a Masquelet technique.
e–f X-ray and clinical images after circular frame placement.

Staged bone grafting

At 6–8 weeks, the patient did not exhibit any signs of infection—his inflammatory laboratory results remained normal. In light of the large amount of bone required for the defect and his lack of infectious signs when he was diagnosed with the nonunion (normal laboratory results, healed incisions, normal vital signs, limited swelling), it was decided that two separate procedures were indicated during the same hospitalization: single stage spacer removal, and then bone graft harvest.

The first procedure was the exchange of his antibiotic spacer and multiple biopsies for culture. The ring fixator remains on the leg and is disinfected and draped into the surgical field after extensive scrubbing. The anterolateral incision is once again opened. The antibiotic cement is removed piecemeal and tissue biopsies for new cultures are taken. A new cement spacer is placed.

For the second step of the procedure, the patient returns to the OR only when the cultures come back negative. This patient was returned to the OR after 72 hours for spacer removal and massive grafting using the RIA system with a filter for bone harvest (**Fig 2.9-9**). The ring fixator was left in place for another 2 months.

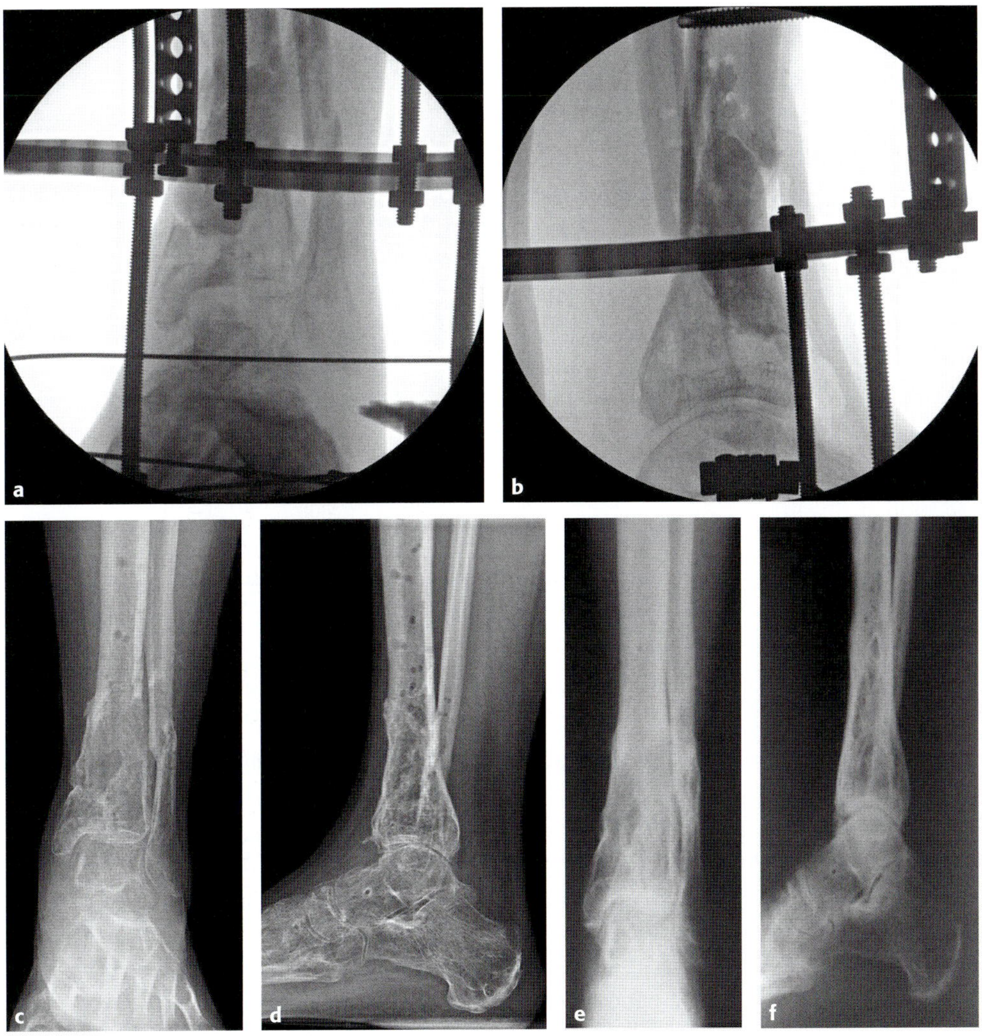

Fig 2.9-9a–f Postoperative images after bone grafting and frame removal.
a–b Cement spacer removal and bone graft placement using RIA bone graft harvesting.
c–f The 1-year (**c–d**) and 2-year (**e–f**) follow-up after grafting and frame removal.

5 Complications

- Injury to the intermediate cutaneous branch of the SPN in the anterolateral approach and lateral approach to the fibula
- Acute compartment syndrome requiring fasciotomy and subsequent skin grafting
- Loss of fixation
- Malunion/nonunion
- Infection
- Posttraumatic arthritis of the ankle and adjacent joints
- Arthrofibrosis with loss of motion

6 Alternative techniques

Amputation is indicated when the patient has comorbidities that do not allow reconstruction or when the infection does not heal.

7 Postoperative management and rehabilitation

Acute pilon management

Postoperatively, the ankle is immobilized in a well-padded below-knee splint and the lower leg is elevated. The patient is advised to maintain nonweight-bearing status and assigned the appropriate walking aids. At the 2-week follow-up the splint is removed and the incisions are evaluated with suture removal if ready. If there is still a moderate amount of swelling, the patient can be brought back a week later for re-evaluation for possible suture removal at that time. The sutures should not be removed too soon as this may cause the wound to split.

Physical therapy is prescribed at this visit and the patient is encouraged to begin active and passive range-of-motion exercises as well as toe contracture prevention measures. The patient is seen at 6 weeks, 12 weeks, and 6 months. Transition to weight bearing as tolerated begins at week 12.

Implant removal

Implant removal is generally not planned unless required. For this patient, removal was done because of the development of a septic nonunion.

Septic nonunion salvage

Ring fixator treatment has the potential for substantial toe stiffness and contractures. Rehabilitation includes toe contracture prevention and weight bearing, once the incisions have sealed and swelling is controlled. After the fixator has been removed, aggressive therapy and manual manipulation will allow for an improvement in motion and function.

The patient's original injury healed, but subsequently he developed posttraumatic arthritis and stiffness of the ankle (**Fig 2.9-10**).

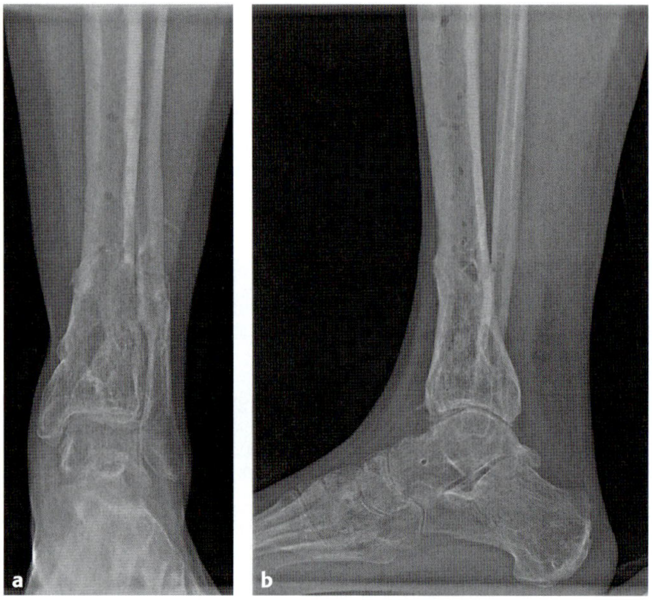

Fig 2.9-10a–b X-rays taken 1 year after bone grafting showing a healed pilon and distal fibular fracture with the development of posttraumatic arthritis.
a AP view.
b Lateral view.

8 Recommended reading

Attinger CE, Evans KK, Bulan E, et al. Angiosomes of the foot and ankle and clinical implications for limb salvage: reconstruction, incisions, and revascularization. *Plast Reconstr Surg.* 2006 Jun;117(7 Suppl):261s–293s.
Dunbar RP, Taitsman LA, Sangeorzan BJ, et al. Technique tip: use of "pie crusting" of the dorsal skin in severe foot injury. *Foot Ankle Int.* 2007 Jul;28(7):851–853.
Eastman JG, Firoozabadi R, Benirschke SK, et al. Entrapped posteromedial structures in pilon fractures. *J Orthop Trauma.* 2014 Sep;28(9):528–533.
LeBus GF, Collinge C. Vascular abnormalities as assessed with CT angiography in high-energy tibial plafond fractures. *J Orthop Trauma.* 2008 Jan;22(1):16–22.
Taylor GI, Pan WR. Angiosomes of the leg: anatomic study and clinical implications. *Plast Reconstr Surg.* 1998 Sep;102(3):599-616; discussion 617–598.

2.10 Free flap coverage

Marschall Berkes, John W Munz

1 Case description

A 46-year-old man was involved in a high-speed motor vehicle collision. He was driving and restrained with a seatbelt. He presented with an open right AO/OTA 43C3.2 (complete, multifragmentary articular epiphyseal and metaphyseal, distal tibial fracture) pilon fracture with a 5 x 5 cm open wound over the anteromedial aspect of the distal tibia (**Fig 2.10-1** and **Fig 2.10-2**). His neurovascular status was intact. The patient had a medical history of elevated cholesterol. Social history revealed no use of tobacco products, and occasional use of alcohol. He was independent in all activities prior to this injury.

Initial treatment consisted of urgent irrigation and debridement (I&D) of the wound.

Bone fragments without attached soft tissue were removed. Gross particulate matter was found impacted into the proximal fracture fragment and was removed with a dental scaler and small curette. Near circumferential periosteal stripping involving the distal third of the tibia was noted at the time of the I&D.

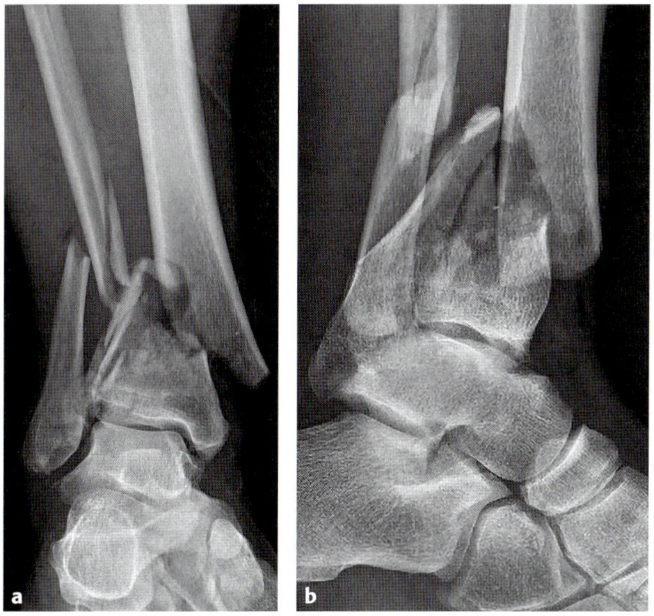

Fig 2.10-1a–b Injury x-rays demonstrating the AO/OTA 43C3.2 open pilon and fibular fracture.
a AP view.
b Lateral view.

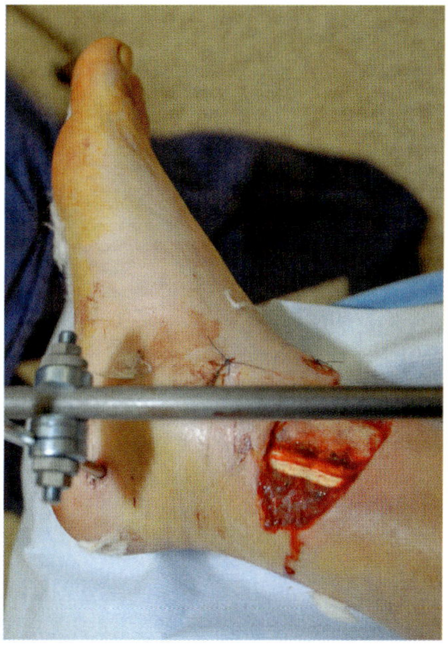

Fig 2.10-2 Open anteromedial wound following initial debridement and external fixation.

Next, closed reduction and application of ankle-spanning external fixation was performed and a wound vacuum-assisted closure (VAC) device was applied (**Fig 2.10-3**).

The soft tissues were amenable to limited articular reduction and fixation 4 days later, with plans for subsequent soft-tissue coverage by the plastic surgeon within 72 hours of definitive fixation.

2 Preoperative planning

Indications for surgery

Surgical indications include this fracture being an open, displaced, complete articular plafond fracture. Open reduction and internal fixation (ORIF) for this fracture allows for bone and ankle stability.

Open reduction and internal fixation restores articular congruity to maximize ankle range-of-motion (ROM) function and allow for subsequent soft-tissue healing by creating a stable environment. Fracture repair also restores the long axis alignment of the leg.

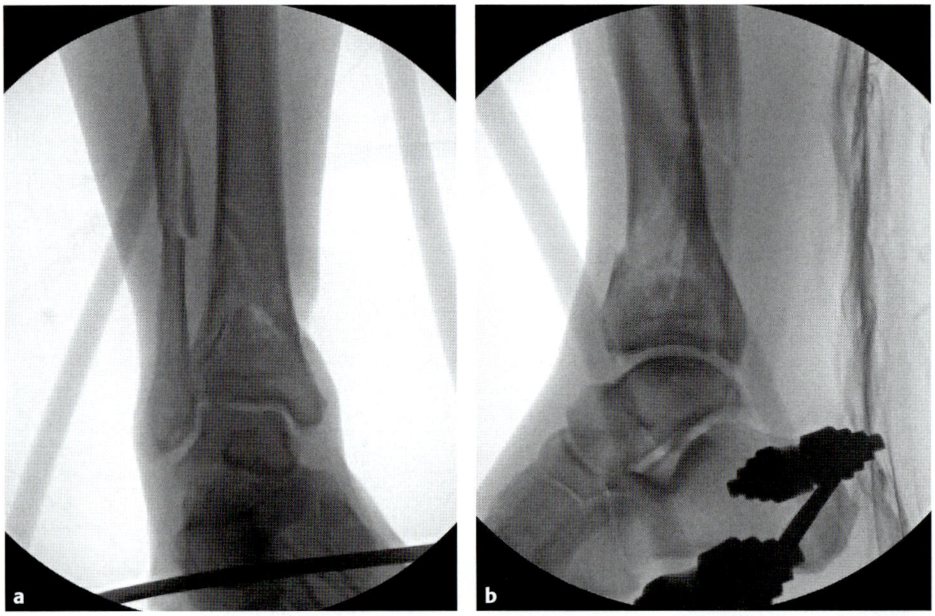

Fig 2.10-3a–b C-arm images following the initial closed manipulative reduction and ankle-spanning external fixator with restoration of gross alignment and length.
a AP view.
b Lateral view.

Considerations for surgery

In this case, the fracture involved three main articular fragments with anterolateral comminution of the joint and metaphysis. This can be better appreciated on the preoperative computed tomographic (CT) scan (**Fig 2.10-4–Fig 2.10-7**). Given the magnitude of the soft-tissue injury, a limited articular fixation strategy was adopted to limit the risk of infection imposed by surface implants and further soft-tissue dissection. This was accomplished with percutaneous mini incisions. A direct lateral approach was selected to stabilize the fibula and provide an anatomically reduced lateral buttress.

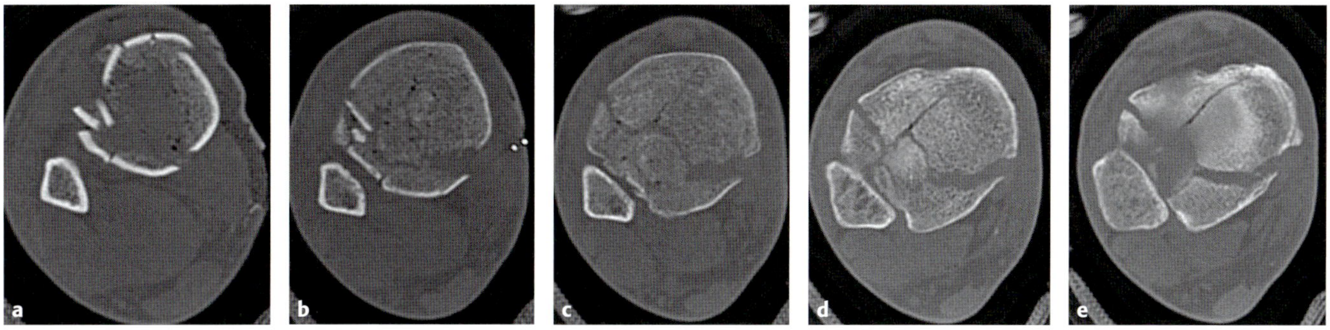

Fig 2.10-4a–e Axial CT scan images of the distal tibia and fibula demonstrating the fracture planes exiting the ankle joint.

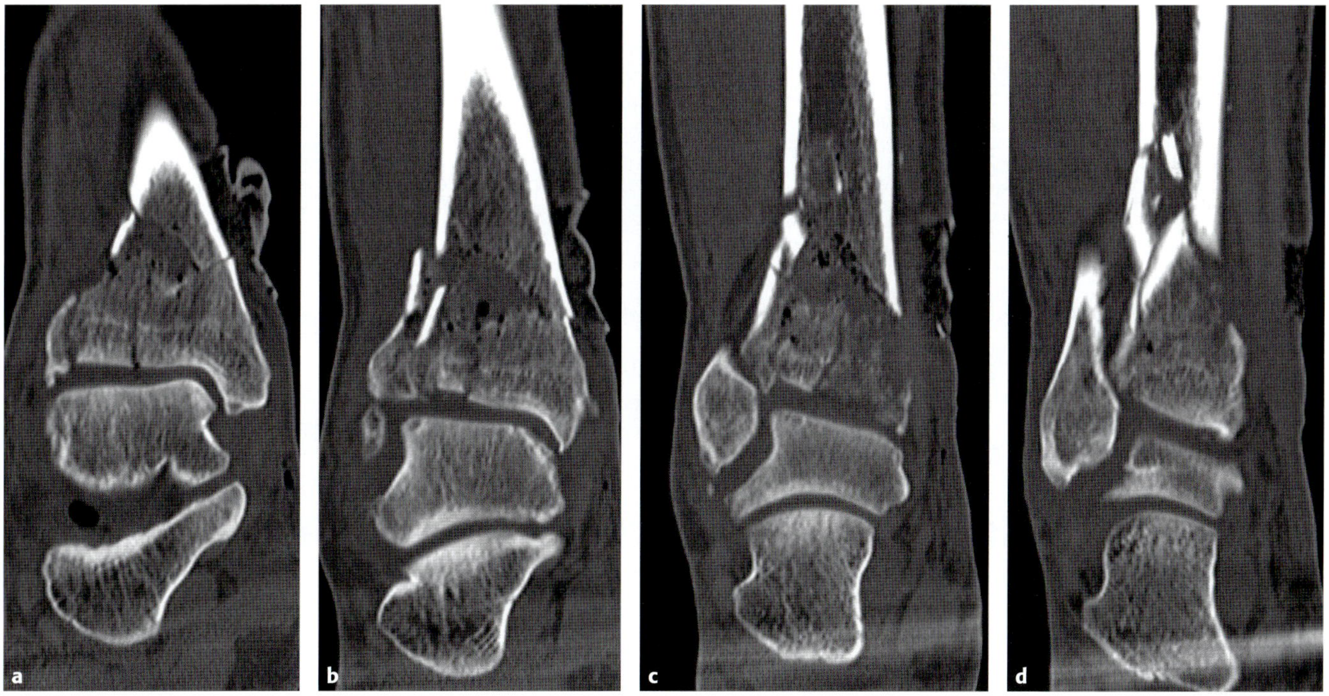

Fig 2.10-5a–d Coronal CT scan images of the distal tibia and fibula demonstrating the fracture planes exiting the ankle joint and metaphyseal comminution.

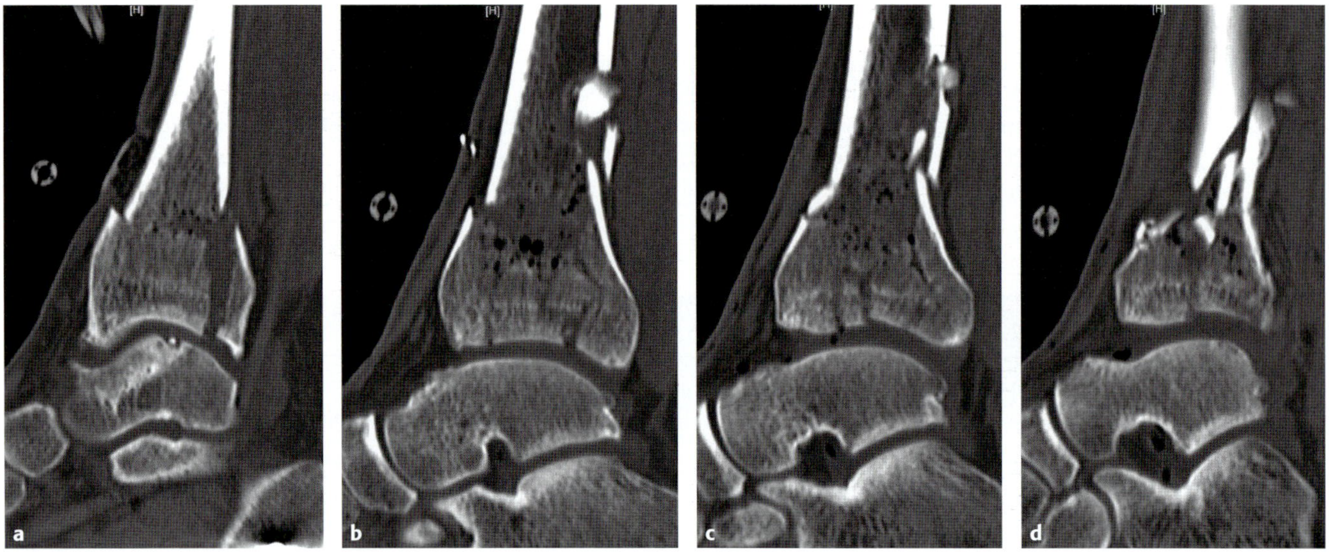

Fig 2.10-6a–d Sagittal CT scan images of the distal tibia and fibula demonstrating the articular and metaphyseal fracture comminution.

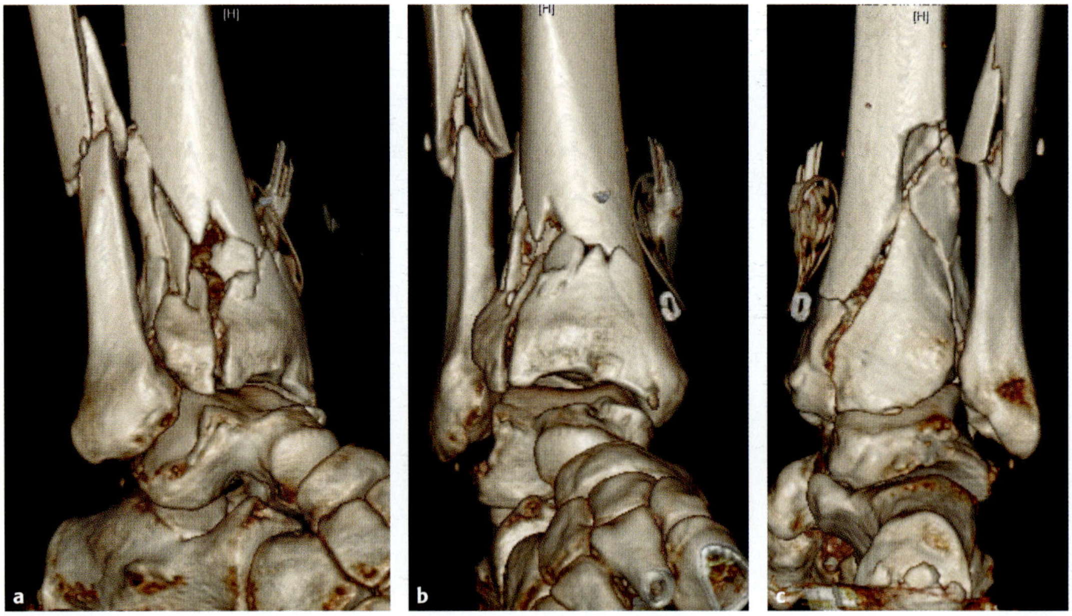

Fig 2.10-7a–c 3D CT reconstruction images demonstrating the overall fibula and pilon fracture morphology.

3 Operating room setup

Patient positioning	• Supine on a radiolucent table with a bump under the ipsilateral hip
Anesthesia options	• General endotracheal anesthesia • Antibiotics as per surgeon preference and guidelines
C-arm location	• C-arm from the side of the table, monitor towards the head of the operative table
Tourniquet	• Applied to the ipsilateral upper thigh
Tips	• The external fixator can be prepared into the sterile field if needed to maintain stability or alignment. • Alternatively, it can be removed, sterilized, and replaced as a device to assist reduction.

For illustrations and overview of anesthetic considerations, see chapter 1.

Equipment

- Small fragment set
- Mini fragment set
- Point-to-point reduction (Weber) clamps (various sizes)
- Wound VAC device

4 Surgical procedure

The procedure begins with a repeated I&D of the open wound and fracture surface after removing the external fixator bars. Inspection for any residual contamination of the wound is performed, and if identified, it is removed. New gloves and drapes are then applied. The articular surface reduction is next with care to avoid excessive dissection. The medial joint surface is then reduced. A point-to-point reduction (Weber) clamp is applied from the medial side, using the medial wound to safely pass the posterior reduction tip. The anterior tine is placed percutaneously with a mini incision. The posterior fragment and dominant anteromedial fragments are compressed with the reduction device to gain an acceptable joint reduction and compression (**Fig 2.10-8**). A single 2.7 mm lag screw is then placed through a percutaneous mini incision, which is appropriately located with the assistance of C-arm images taken in both AP and lateral planes.

Fixation of the fibula is then performed using a lateral approach, taking care to avoid injury to the superficial peroneal nerve as it crosses the fibula. The fracture surfaces are identified and cleaned of hematoma and interposing soft tissue with a pituitary rongeur and curette. The wedge fragment of the fibula is reduced to the proximal fibula using point-to-point reduction (Weber) clamps and fixed with two 2.0 mm lag screws. Next, the proximal and distal fragments of the fibula are reduced with point-to-point reduction (Weber) clamps and secured with a single 2.0 mm lag screw (**Fig 2.10-9**). A 10-hole one-third tubular plate is then placed in neutralization mode to finalize the fibular fixation.

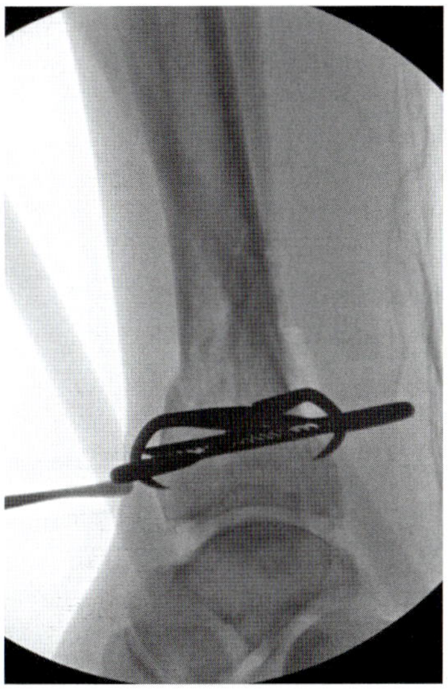

Fig 2.10-8 Lateral C-arm view demonstrating clamp placement and joint reduction prior to lag screw placement.

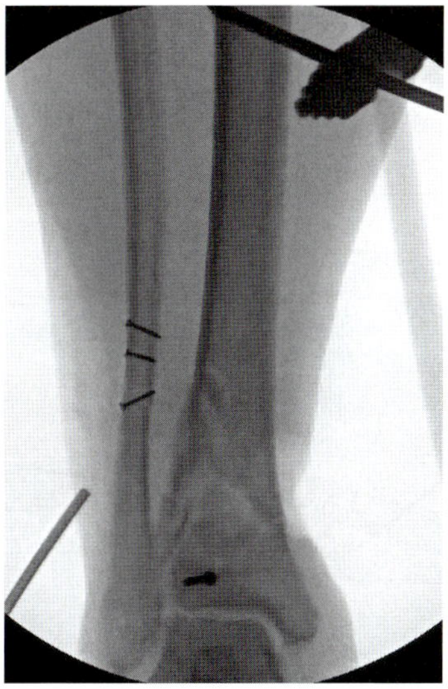

Fig 2.10-9 AP C-arm view demonstrating reduction and lag screw fixation of the fibula fracture as well as overall ankle alignment and lag screw fixation of the pilon fracture.

An additional anterior to posterior 2.7 mm lag screw is placed in subchondral bone parallel to the first screw using a percutaneous mini incision. This screw supplemented the fixation of the anteromedial fragment to the posterior articular fragment.

The medial malleolus component is then addressed. Using the open medial wound, the medial malleolus component is reduced with a point-to-point reduction (Weber) clamp. A single 3.5 mm screw placed from the intact anterolateral tibia is then inserted to maintain the reduction (**Fig 2.10-10**).

The lateral wound is closed in layers. Mini incisions are closed with horizontal mattress nylon sutures. The medial wound is dressed with a wound VAC device. The external fixator construct is reassembled to provide additional stability and maintain the articular reduction. The final intraoperative x-rays are seen in **Fig 2.10-11**.

In this case, the plastic surgeon provided definitive coverage 2 days later. This consisted of a latissimus dorsi free flap, with an end-to-side anastomosis with the posterior tibial artery and split-thickness skin graft (**Fig 2.10-12**). Coordination for early wound coverage is a key component of the fracture repair and is necessary for successful management of these severe injuries.

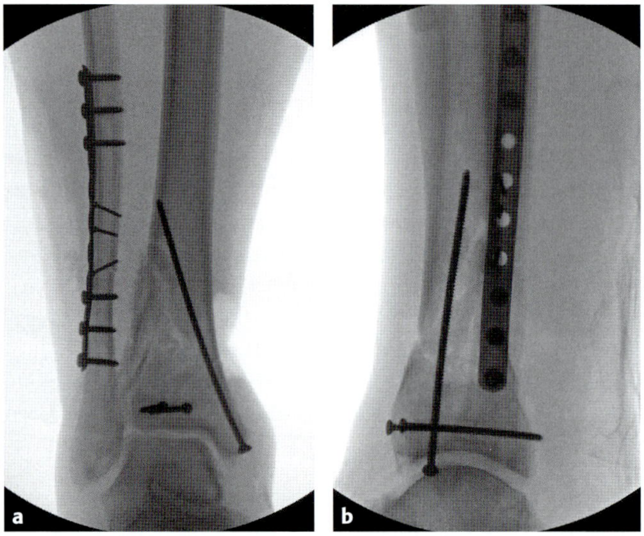

Fig 2.10-10a–b C-arm images showing the final intraoperative construct consisting of fibular fixation, limited articular reduction and screw fixation of the pilon and maintenance of the external fixator as supplemental fixation.
a AP view.
b Lateral view.

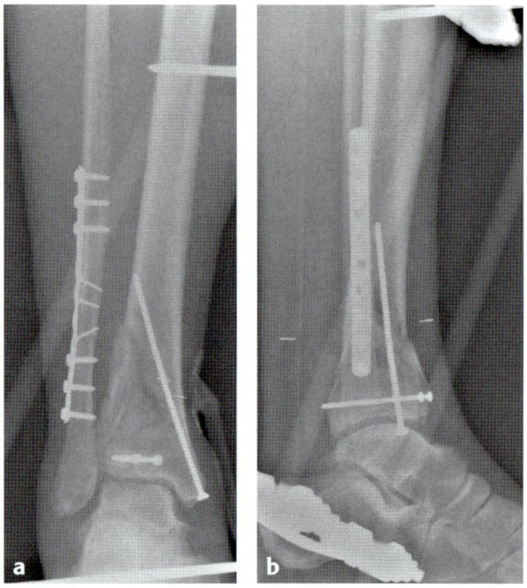

Fig 2.10-11a–b Immediate postoperative x-rays again reveal the final construct prior to soft-tissue coverage.
a AP view.
b Lateral view.

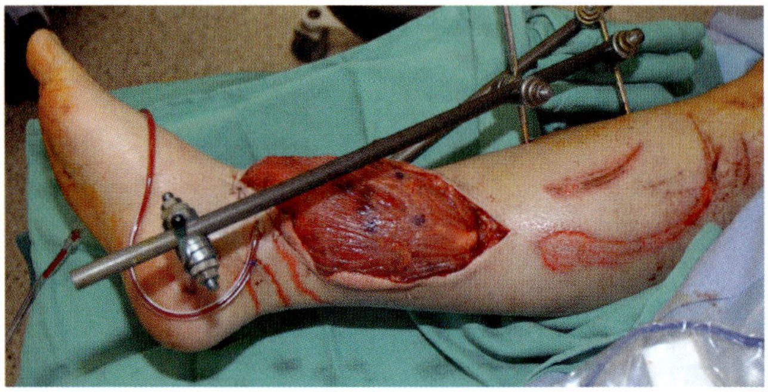

Fig 2.10-12 Immediately following latissimus free-flap coverage of the soft-tissue defect prior to skin graft.

5 Pitfalls and complications

Pitfalls

Bone viability

Significant stripping of the metaphyseal bone may lead to devascularized and necrotic bone. If retained, it may both serve as a nidus of infection, and also impede bone healing. The bone ends should be debrided to ensure visible bleeding ("paprika sign"). Even if this requires significant bone resection with resultant critical-sized defects, this is preferable to retention of dead bone.

Finally, the strategy of limited articular reduction relies on the external fixator to remain in place until some bone healing has occurred. External fixator pin-site infection is likely. Also, the flexible internal fixation is at risk of failing particularly with any weight bearing (WB).

Complications

- Infection is a serious risk when limb salvage is attempted in a Gustilo-Anderson grade III B open pilon fractures (**Fig 2.10-13**). Despite the use of limited articular reduction, infection can occur and may prove disastrous to limb salvage.
- External fixator pin-site infection is likely. Pin-site care should be meticulously performed.
- Nonunion or delayed union, which may require secondary interventions
- Failure of fixation and malunion
- The strategy of limited articular reduction relies on the external fixator to remain in place until some bone healing has occurred. The flexible internal fixation is at risk of failing, particularly with any WB, and thus supervised rehabilitation is essential.
- Posttraumatic arthritis
- Failure of soft-tissue coverage

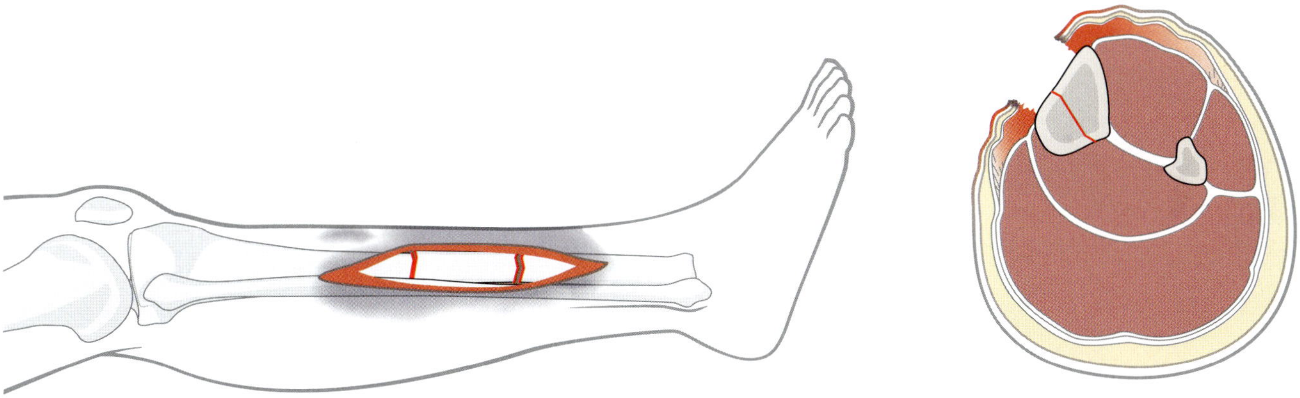

Fig 2.10-13 Gustilo-Anderson grade III open fracture.

6 Alternative techniques

Internal fixation with plates and screws

Rigid internal fixation with plates and screws is certainly preferable from a stability standpoint. This could be undertaken through an anteromedial approach incorporating the wound. However, in a wound of this magnitude with significant soft-tissue stripping, the strategy of limited articular reduction and fixation with a minimized surgical footprint and external fixator augmentation has helped to prevent disastrous infectious complications.

Small-wire external fixation

Small-wire fixation is an alternative option for these injuries. Limitations of this technique include inability to anatomically restore the articular surface and difficulty in wound management around the external fixator. Additionally, the external fixator is often poorly tolerated by the patient.

Surgical fixation and long-term wound care

This method of treatment results in an unacceptably high infection rate and is discouraged for these injuries.

7 Postoperative management and rehabilitation

In this case, the wounds healed uneventfully (**Fig 2.10-14**). The patient was maintained in an external fixator for 8 weeks, at which point it was removed and a short-leg cast placed. Two weeks later, he was transitioned into a fracture boot and range of motion (ROM) initiated. Weight bearing was initiated at 4 months postoperatively. At 6 months postoperatively, persistent pain with weight bearing was reported and a CT scan revealed posterolateral healing but lack of bridging bone elsewhere (**Fig 2.10-15–Fig 2.10-19**). Thus, the patient was indicated for flap elevation, iliac crest bone graft of the distal tibial metaphysis, and additional medial plating with return of the flap. Intraoperative C-arm images and immediate postoperative x-rays are seen in **Fig 2.10-20** and **Fig 2.10-21**. This was done in conjunction with the plastic surgeon.

The patient was not allowed to bear weight for 6 weeks following the bone graft, at which time WB was initiated in a fracture boot. Six months after the bone graft, the fracture was healed.

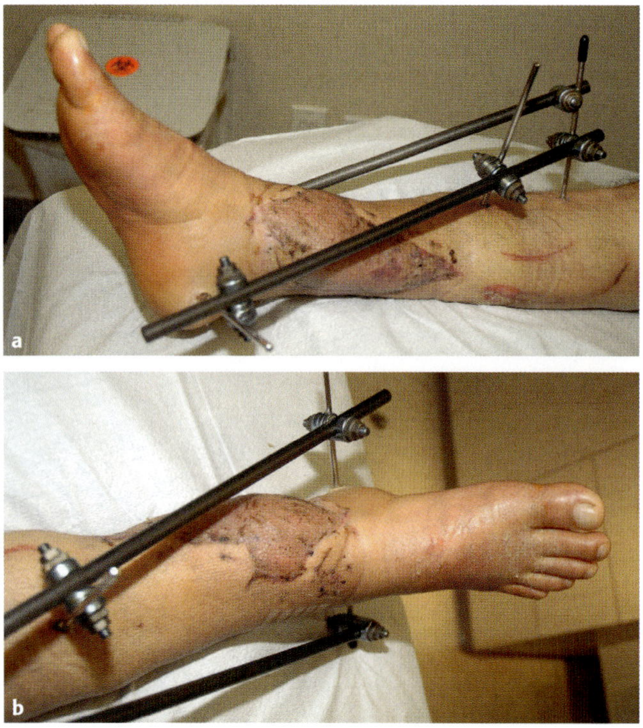

Fig 2.10-14 A healthy flap and skin graft incorporation prior to the second stage surgical intervention.

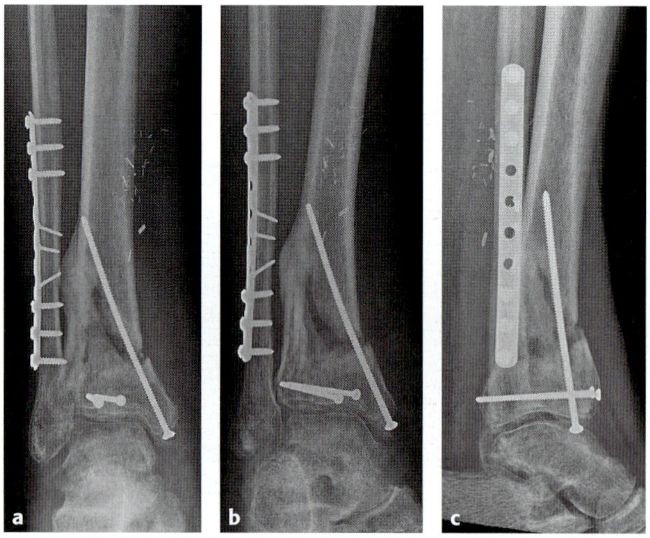

Fig 2.10-15a–c X-rays at 6 months postoperative show partial healing (lateral cortex) of the metaphyseal component of the tibial fracture and complete healing of the joint and fibular fractures. A bone void is seen in the majority of the tibial metaphysis.

- **a** AP view.
- **a** Mortise view.
- **c** Lateral view.

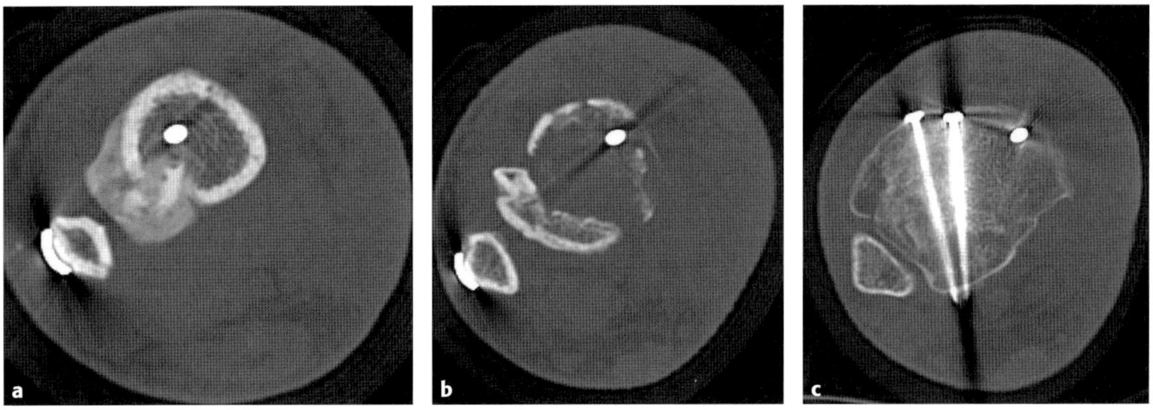

Fig 2.10-16a–c Axial CT scan images again demonstrate healing of the lateral tibial metaphysis, a large central and medial tibial metaphyseal void, and a healed fracture of the plafond.

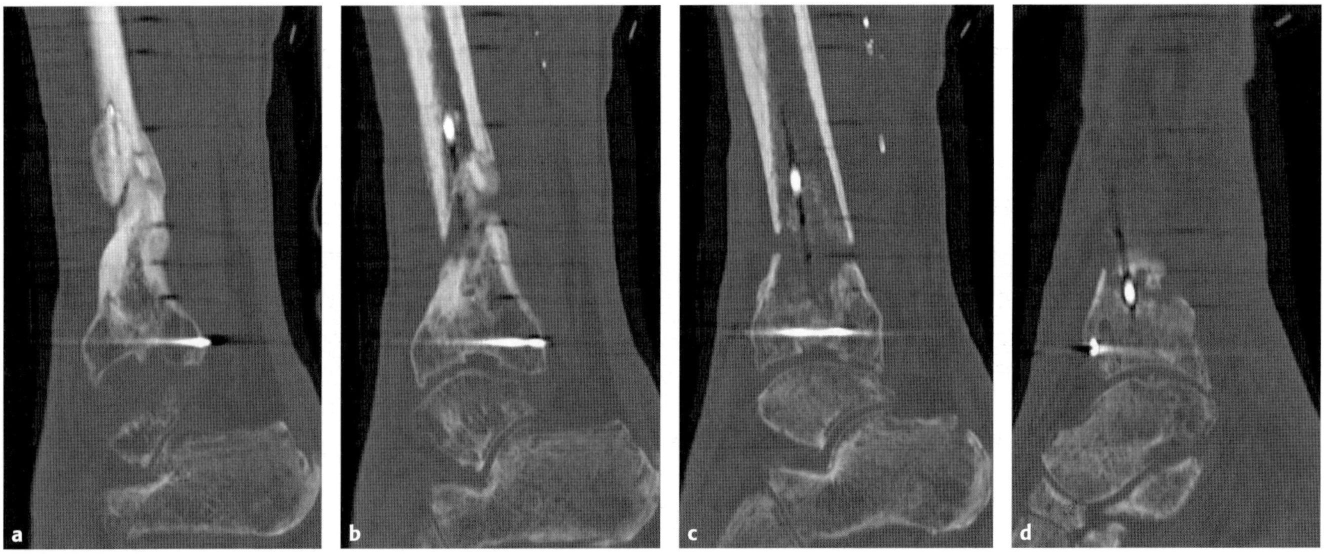

Fig 2.10-17a–d Sagittal CT scan images demonstrating the healed lateral tibial metaphysis, healed plafond with residual malreduction, and central and medial distal tibial metaphyseal bone void.

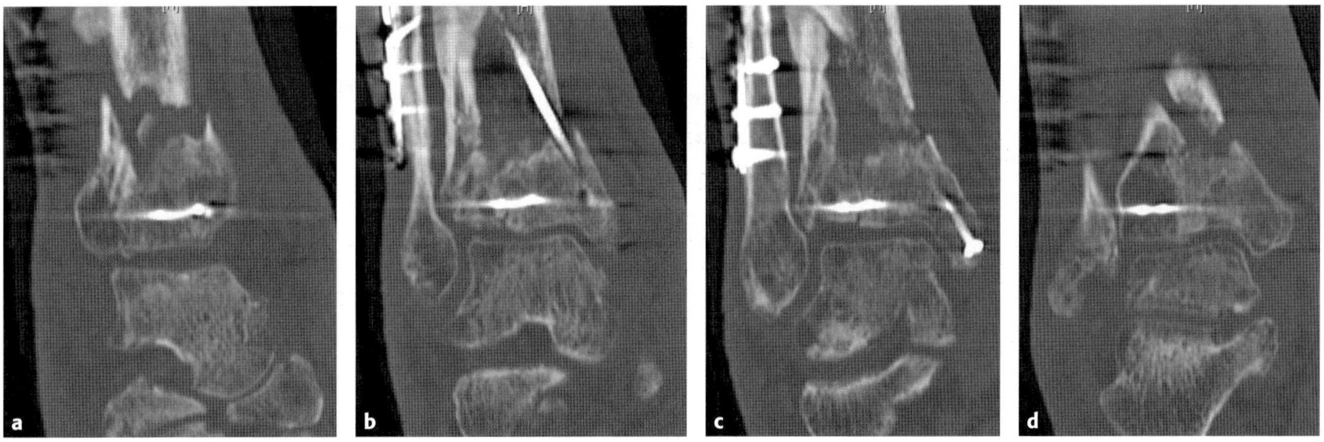

Fig 2.10-18a–d Coronal CT images at 6 months postoperative.

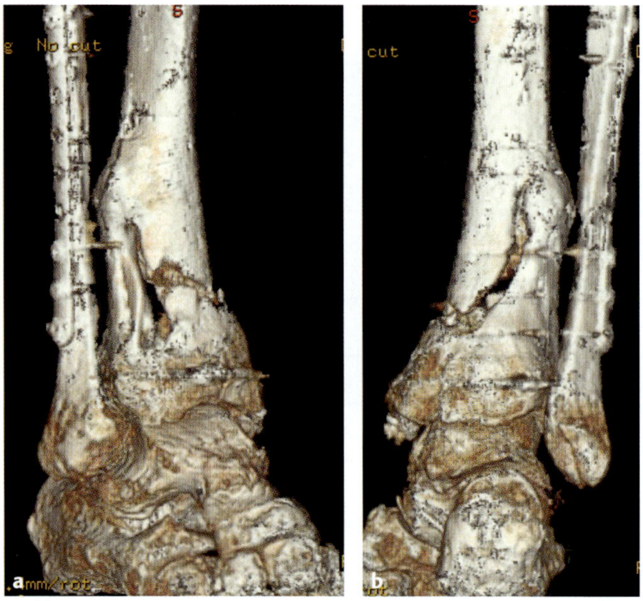

Fig 2.10-19a–b 3D CT reconstructions at 6 months postoperatively.

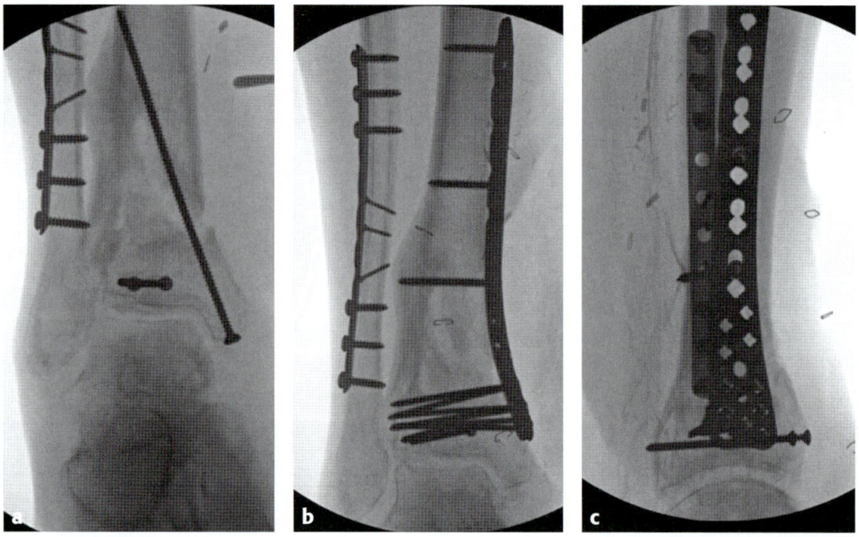

Fig 2.10-20a–c C-arm images prior to and at the completion of the flap elevation, bone grafting, and medial plating.

a AP view.
b Mortise view
c Lateral view.

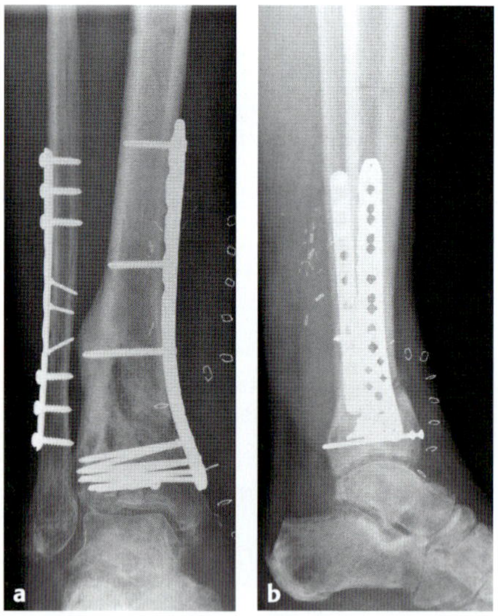

Fig 2.10-21a–b Immediate postoperative x-rays which demonstrate overall alignment following bone grafting, plate fixation.

a AP view.
b Lateral view.

At the 4-year follow-up, the patient demonstrated good function and used antiinflammatory medication on an occasional basis. There was decreased ankle ROM, as might be expected. X-rays demonstrated a healed fracture and posttraumatic ankle arthritis (**Fig 2.10-22** and **Fig 2.10-23**).

Implant removal

Implant removal is only performed if the patient is symptomatic. Hardware may also need to be removed if the patient develops severe posttraumatic arthritis and surgical management is necessary.

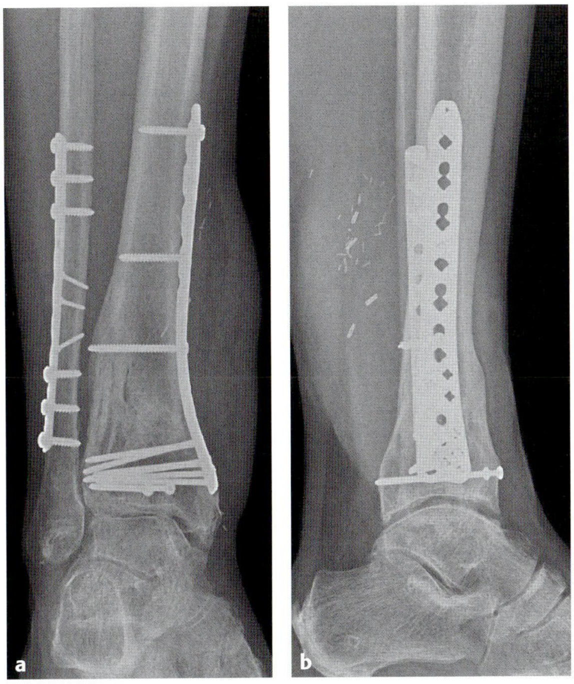

Fig 2.10-22a–b Final x-rays at 4 years after the injury reveal complete bony union and the final result.
a AP view.
b Lateral view.

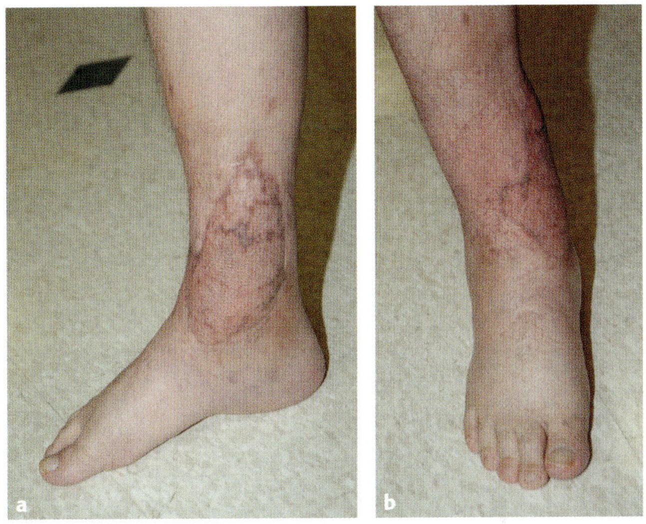

Fig 2.10-23a–b The leg at final follow-up.

8 Recommended reading

Blauth M, Bastian L, Krettek C, et al. Surgical options for the treatment of severe tibial pilon fractures: a study of three techniques. *J Orthop Trauma.* 2001 Mar–Apr;15(3):153–160.
Boraiah S, Kemp TJ, Erwteman A, et al. Outcome following open reduction and internal fixation of open pilon fractures. *J Bone Joint Surg Am.* 2010 Feb;92(2):346–352.
Gardner MJ, Mehta S, Barei DP, et al. Treatment protocol for open AO/OTA type C3 pilon fractures with segmental bone loss. *J Orthop Trauma.* 2008 Aug;22(7):451–457.
Godina M. Early microsurgical reconstruction of complex trauma of the extremities. *Plast Reconstr Surg.* 1986 Sep;78(3):285–292.
Gustilo RB, Anderson JT. Prevention of infection in the treatment of one thousand and twenty-five open fractures of long bones: retrospective and prospective analyses. *J Bone Joint Surg Am.* 1976 Jun;58(4):453–458.
Gustilo RB, Mendoza RM, Williams DN. Problems in the management of type III (severe) open fractures: a new classification of type III open fractures. *J Trauma.* 1984 Aug;24(8):742–746.
Pollak AN, McCarthy ML, Bess RS, et al. Outcomes after treatment of high-energy tibial plafond fractures. *J Bone Joint Surg Am.* 2003 Oct;85-a(10):1893–1900.
Sirkin M, Sanders R, DiPasquale T, et al. A staged protocol for soft tissue management in the treatment of complex pilon fractures. *J Orthop Trauma.* 1999 Feb;13(2):78–84.

3

Malleoli

Malleoli

3 Malleolar fractures

Stefan Rammelt

1 Introduction

Ankle fractures represent the most frequent intraarticular fractures to a weight-bearing joint. Their incidence has been calculated with 100 to 187 per every 100,000 people per year in recent studies from Europe and the United States, respectively. Due to the complex anatomy, ankle fractures cover a wide range of bony and ligamentous injuries. Isolated malleolar fractures account for two-thirds of ankle fractures, bimalleolar fractures account for nearly 25%, and trimalleolar fractures account for 5–10% of ankle fractures. The distal tibiofibular syndesmosis is injured in 20–45% of all operatively treated ankle fractures. Proper management therefore requires a thorough understanding of the fracture mechanism and a precise determination of the amount of bony and ligamentous injury, especially with regard to stability of the fracture.

This chapter pertains to malleolar fractures which typically result from rotational, abduction, and adduction forces. Fractures of the weight-bearing portion of the distal tibia are addressed in chapter 2. However, several malleolar fractures may exhibit partial impaction of the tibial plafond. They have been termed "partial pilon" fractures. These include medial impaction in supination-adduction (SA) fractures, lateral impaction in pronation-abduction (PA) fractures, and posterior impaction with fractures of the posterior tibial rim, also termed "posterior malleolus". The distinction between a "partial" and "true" pilon is sometimes difficult and rather a matter of convention.

The long-term outcome after bimalleolar and trimalleolar fractures is a matter of concern. Several long-term studies have shown that one-third of the patients display clinical signs and up to 97% display radiographic signs of posttraumatic osteoarthritis 10–21 years after the injury. In an epidemiological study, Salzman et al estimated that up to 78% of the cases of end-stage arthritis (with patients presenting for ankle fusion or total ankle replacement) are of traumatic origin. Improper reduction and fixation may be a major factor contributing to less favorable results and several clinical and biomechanical studies suggest that even minor step-offs and incongruities, axial malalignment, and residual ligamentous instability lead to considerable redistribution of intraarticular pressure and therefore predispose to the evolution of posttraumatic arthritis. Other factors, such as primary damage to the articular cartilage or the blood supply to the distal tibia and comorbidities (eg, diabetes and osteoporosis) are also reported to have a negative impact on outcome.

2 Anatomy and pathomechanics

Anatomy

The ankle joint is an irregular 3-part joint formed by the articular facets of the distal tibia and fibula, connected via the syndesmotic complex, the talar dome, the medial and lateral collateral ligaments, and the anterior and posterior joint capsule (**Fig 3-1**). The shape of the talar dome is asymmetric, resembling part of a cone rather than a cylinder. It is broader anteriorly than posteriorly and has a steeper slope laterally than medially. The retromalleolar groove of the distal fibula holds the peroneal tendons and may be shallow or absent in a substantial percentage of patients. The medial malleolus consists of a larger anterior and smaller posterior colliculus separated by an intracollicular groove. The posterior tibial tendon is in direct contact with the posterior colliculus.

The axis of the ankle joint runs from the tip of the lateral malleolus to the tip of the medial malleolus and thus ascends 8° in the frontal plane and 6° in the transverse plain. The lateral slope of the talar dome is perpendicular to the axis, while the medial side is inclined by 6°, which leads to a "pseudorotation" of the talus during movement in the ankle mortise. The irregular shape of the talus also results in a 3D movement of the fibula with respect to the tibia during tibiotalar movement. The movements of the ankle joint are also closely coupled with that of the subtalar and midtarsal joints (the "lower ankle joint"). Plantar flexion at the ankle is coupled with supination at the subtalar joint and adduction at the midtarsal (Chopart) joint; dorsal extension of the foot at the ankle joint is accompanied by pronation at the subtalar joint and abduction at the mid-tarsal joint.

Bony congruence itself results in a considerable inherent stability at the ankle joint. The medial and lateral collateral ligaments as well as the tibiofibular syndesmosis provide dynamic support (**Fig 3-1**). In addition, the ankle is stabilized by the extrinsic foot muscles from the leg that span the ankle joint.

Pathomechanics

Most malleolar fractures and fracture dislocations result from a rotational or twisting force of the foot against the tibia, such as in a misstep or fall. Only about 10% of malleolar fractures are produced by high-energy trauma like motor vehicle accidents. A direct force against the medial or lateral malleolus is less frequent. An increasing number of irregular osteoporotic fracture patterns from low-energy trauma is seen in developed countries.

The sequence of ligamentous and bony injuries has been extensively studied in a landmark series of biomechanical and clinical investigations by the Danish surgeon Lauge-Hansen. His classification consists of two components: the position of the foot at the time of injury (pronation or supination) and the direction of the deforming force (adduction, abduction, or external rotation). With the foot in pronation, the broader anterior part of the talus wedges in between the distal tibia and fibula, putting increased strain on the distal tibiofibular syndesmosis. Therefore, pronation type injuries are more likely to be accompanied with syndesmotic disruption. Although several recent biomechanical studies failed to reproduce the injury patterns as predicted by Lauge-Hansen, the use of this classification forces the surgeon to consider the pathomechanism of ankle fractures and the full range of possible bony and ligamentous injuries.

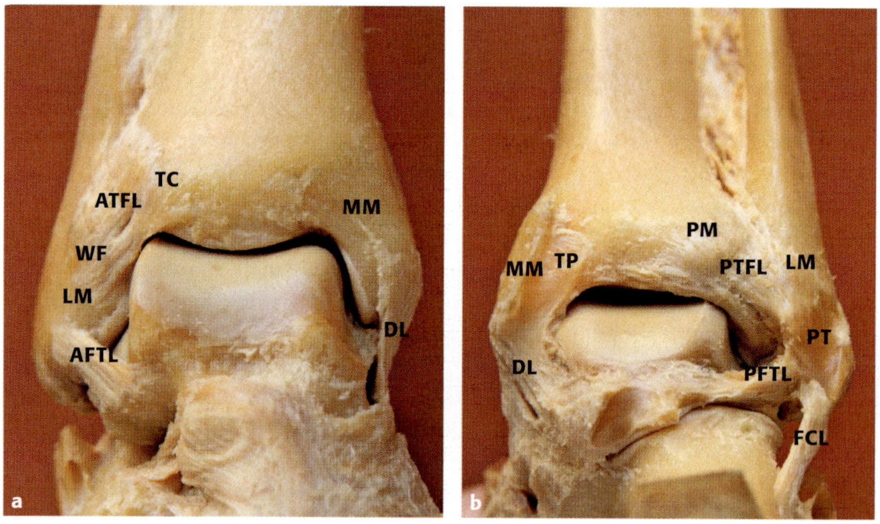

Fig 3-1a–b Anatomy of the ankle joint.

a The ankle joint is formed by the medial (MM) and lateral malleolus (LM), containing the talar dome. The distal tibia and fibula are held together by the tibiofibular syndesmosis. From the front, the anterior tibiofibular ligament (ATFL) with 2–3 strands is seen. It attaches to the anterior tubercles of the distal tibia and fibula. The anterior tubercle of the distal tibia is also called "tubercule de Chaput" (TC), an osseous avulsion from the anterior tubercle of the fibula is called "Wagestaffe fragment" (WF). The collateral ligaments seen from the front are the anterior fibulotalar ligament (AFTL) laterally and the superficial tibiotalar, tibiocalcanear, and tibionavicular portion of the deltoid ligament (DL) medially.

b From the back, the posterior tibial tubercle or posterior malleolus (PM) to which the strong posterior tibiofibular ligament (PTFL) attaches is seen. An osseous avulsion of the posterior syndesmosis from the tibia or fracture of the posterior malleolus is often called "Volkmann fragment" or "Volkmann triangle" (which is historically incorrect), disrupts the posterior contributions to syndesmotic stability. The medial malleolus (MM) has a groove for the posterior tibial tendon (TP), the lateral malleolus (LM) for the peroneal tendons (PT). The collateral ligaments seen from the back are the posterior fibulotalar ligament (PFTL) and fibulocalcaneal ligament (FCL) laterally, and the tibiocalcaneal and deep tibiotalar portion of the deltoid ligament (DL) medially. Notice the proximity of the ankle and subtalar joints.

(Specimen prepared and photographed by Jan Bartoníček, MD, at the Anatomical Institute of the Charles University, Prague, Czech Republic.)

In SA injuries the lateral strain produces a lateral ligament rupture, bony avulsion, or transverse infrasyndesmal fibular fracture (stage 1). Continued adduction produces a perpendicular fracture of the medial malleolus (stage 2). Frequently this fracture mechanism also produces an impression of the medial tibial plafond which may be regarded as either a stage 3 or a partial pilon fracture (**Fig 3-2**; see chapter 3.3).

Pronation-abduction injuries are produced by the reverse mechanism. The medial strain results in a deltoid ligament rupture, bony avulsion, or horizontal fracture of the medial malleolus (stage 1). Continued abduction produces a rupture or bony avulsion of the anterior and posterior syndesmosis (stage 2). With continued force, the fibula is fractured by an indirect, bending force that produces irregular fracture patterns at the level of the syndesmosis (stage 3) (**Fig 3-3**; see chapter 3.7).

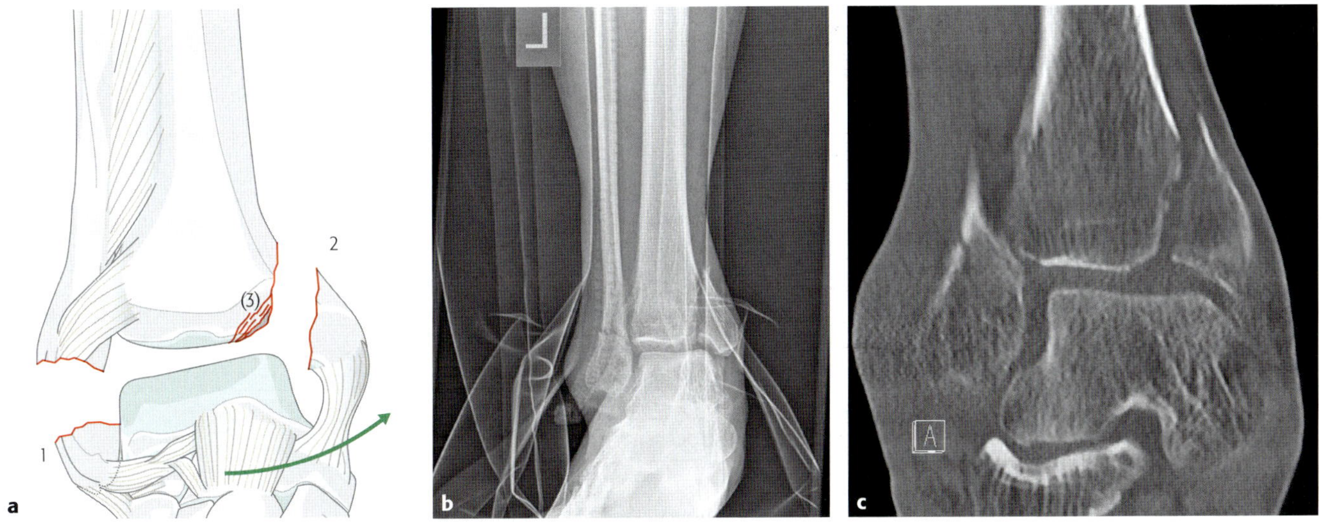

Fig 3-2a–c Supination-adduction (SA) injury.
a Lauge-Hansen stages 1, 2, and (3)
b Plain x-ray with the patient's leg in a pneumatic splint.
c Coronal CT imaging of a SA 2 injury with additional medial plafond impaction, which may be considered stage 3.

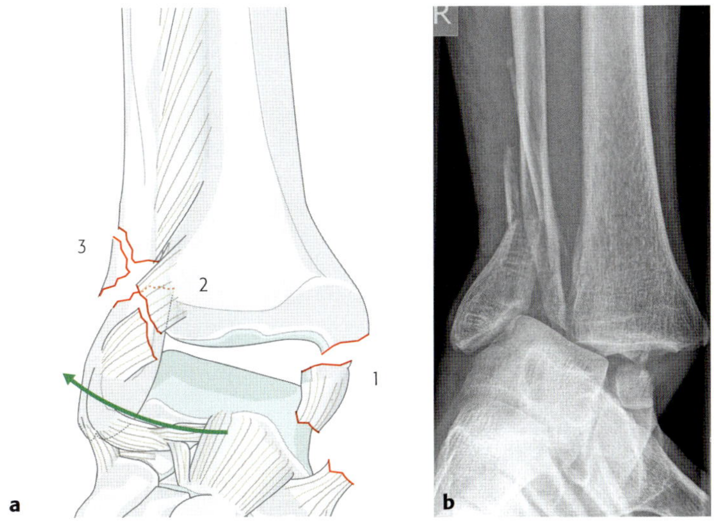

Fig 3-3a–b Pronation-abduction (PA) injury.
a Lauge-Hansen stages 1, 2, and 3.
b Plain x-ray with the foot still in abduction in relation to the lower leg.

Supination-external rotation (SER) injuries start laterally with a rupture or bony avulsion of the anterior syndesmosis (stage 1). A bony avulsion at the tibia is referred to as Tubercúle de Tillaux-Chaput (Tillaux-Chaput avulsion fracture, first described by Cooper). An avulsion fracture at the fibula is termed Wagstaffe fragment. External rotation of the foot (or internal rotation of the tibia with the foot fixed) then produces the typical spiral fracture of the distal fibula at the level of the syndesmosis (stage 2) (see chapter 3.1). Continued rotation results in a rupture of the posterior syndesmosis or fracture of the posterior tibia, also referred to as a "posterior Volkmann triangle" that was first described by Earle (stage 3). With continuing force, finally a transverse or oblique fracture of the medial malleolus or rupture of the deltoid ligament follows (stage 4) (**Fig 3-4**; see chapter 3.2).

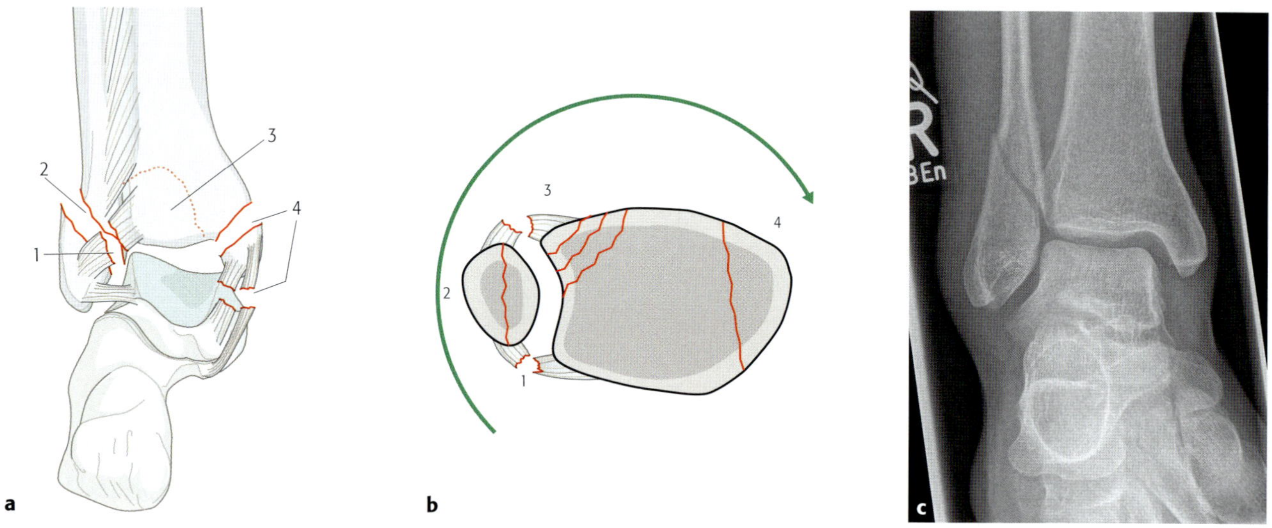

Fig 3-4a–c Supination-external rotation (SER) injury.
a–b The Lauge Hansen stages (1, 2, 3, and 4) in the coronal (**a**) and axial (**b**) plane.
c Plain x-ray of a SER 4 fracture with obvious widening of the MCS due to deltoid ligament rupture.

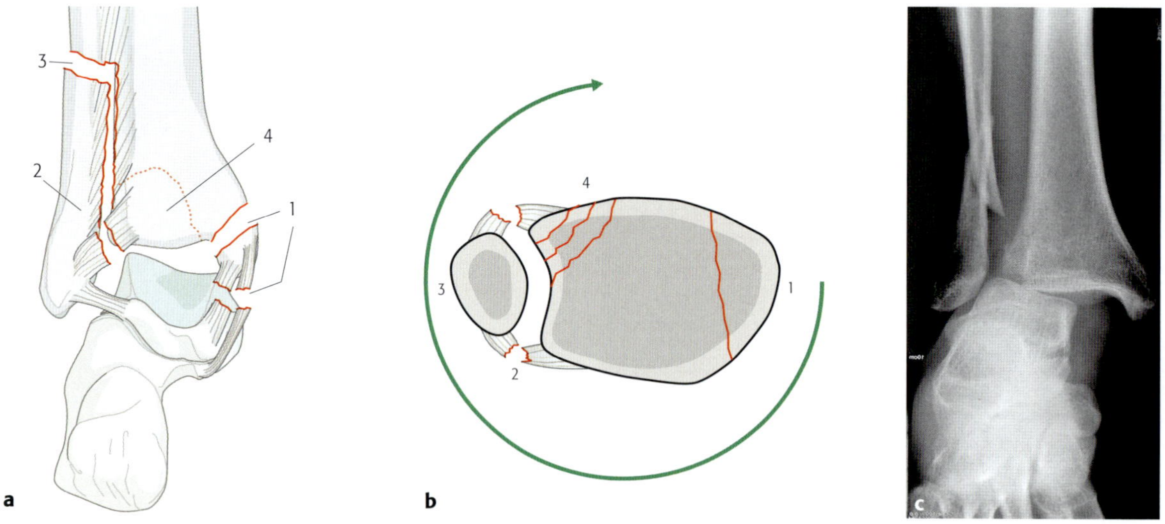

Fig 3-5a–c Pronation-external rotation (PER) injury.
a–b The Lauge Hansen stages (1, 2, 3, and 4) in the coronal (**a**) and axial (**b**) plane.
c Plain x-ray of a PER 4 fracture with obvious widening of the MCS and TCS due to syndesmotic disruption.

Pronation-external rotation (PER) injuries follow a similar sequence as SER fractures with the medial malleolus or deltoid ligament being injured first (stage 1). External rotation then produces a rupture or avulsion of the anterior syndesmosis (stage 2), a disruption of the interosseous ligament, a suprasyndesmotic fibular fracture (stage 3) (see chapter 3.4), and finally rupture of the posterior syndesmosis or posterior malleolar fracture (stage 4) (**Fig 3-5**). A special form of a PER injury is the Maisonneuve fracture consisting of a medial malleolar fracture or deltoid ligament rupture (stage 1), disruption of the anterior and interosseous syndesmotic ligaments (stage 2), and a high diaphyseal or subcapital fibular fracture (stage 3), and sometimes even a dislocation of the fibular head because of a rupture of the proximal tibiofibular syndesmosis (**Fig 3-6**). However, studies using magnetic resonance imaging have shown that the interosseous membrane is not always ruptured up to the level of the fibular fracture. On computed tomographic (CT) examination, 80% of Maisonneuve fractures also display a posterior malleolar fracture (stage 4). Consequently, any seemingly "isolated" medial or posterior malleolar fracture should always raise the suspicion of a Maisonneuve-type injury and lead to assessment of the proximal fibula and syndesmotic stability (see chapter 3.5). Rarely, a high fibular fracture is caused by a direct lateral impact.

Although this sequence of injuries appears plausible in most malleolar fractures, the Lauge-Hansen system should be used cautiously. Lauge-Hansen himself could not assign one of the stages of his classification to about 5% of all malleolar fractures in his clinical series. In more recent studies, 5–53% of fractures revealed bony or ligamentous injury patterns that were not compatible with the Lauge-Hansen stages. Several studies failed to show a clear correlation of the height of the fibular fracture and syndesmotic injury. Furthermore, it appears from both clinical and human anatomical studies, that a substantial number of injuries appearing radiographically as supination injuries may have actually been produced by an abduction force with the foot in dorsiflexion or pronation.

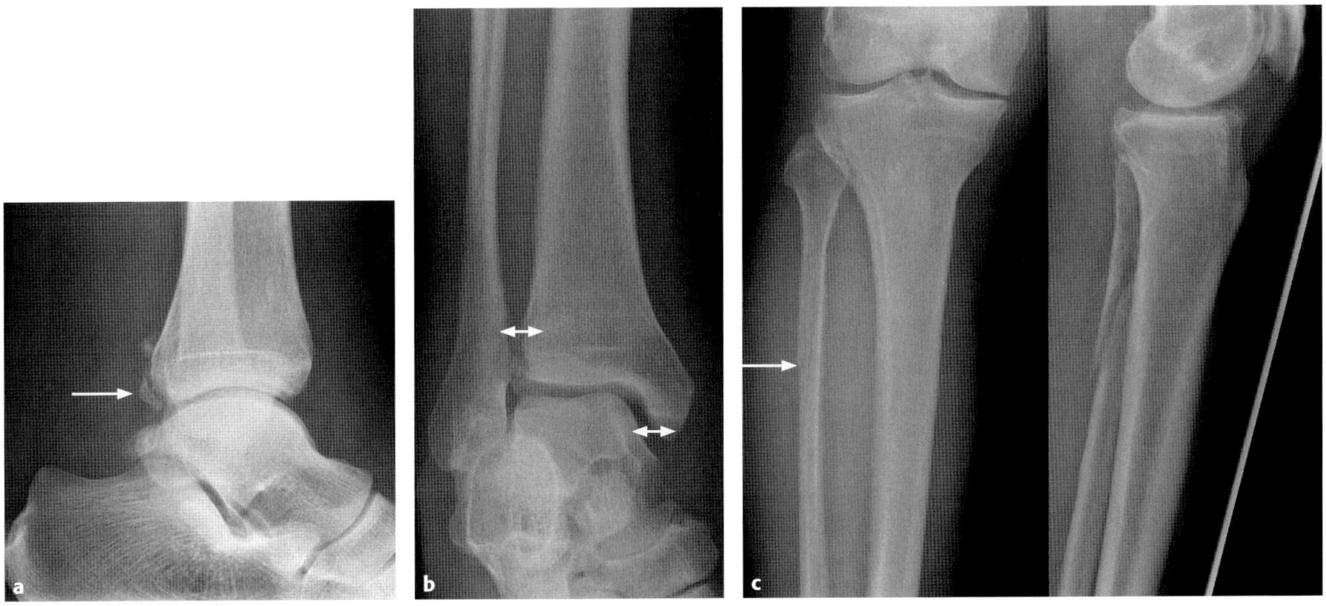

Fig 3-6a–c Maisonneuve fracture with syndesmotic disruption and high fibular fracture.
a The lateral ankle view shows a small avulsion of the posterior syndesmosis (arrow).
b In the AP view, not centered on the ankle joint, there is suspect widening of the MCS and TCS (double arrows) indicating syndesmotic instability.
c X-rays of the lower leg and knee reveal a high fibular fracture (arrow).

3 Fracture classification

The Danis-Weber classification is most frequently used for describing malleolar fractures:

Type A Infrasyndesmal fibular fracture with the syndesmosis intact

Type B Transsyndesmal fibular fracture with questionable syndesmotic instability

Type C Suprasyndesmal fibular fracture with obligatory syndesmotic disruption

This classification is easy to apply in daily practice but only considers the height of the fibular fracture with respect to the syndesmosis (**Fig 3-7**). Because the medial, anterior, and posterior structures are not considered, with exception of type C fractures, no assessment can be made with respect to the stability of the fracture and thus the indication to surgery.

The AO/OTA classification (see appendix) is based on the Danis-Weber classification with respect to the level of the fibular fracture. It adds two hierarchical levels (numbers) that refer to the medial structures and both anterior and posterior bony avulsions of the syndesmosis resulting in a total of 27 subgroups. The malleolar segment is assigned number 44.

The genetic Lauge-Hansen classification of malleolar fractures as described above is valuable for assessing the amount of bony and ligamentous injury. However, with 13 subgroups it is rather complex for daily use and has only a moderate intraobserver agreement. Because the injury pattern is not always compatible with the Lauge-Hansen subgroups, the treating surgeon is encouraged to describe all bony and ligamentous components of the injury as seen on plain x-rays and, for an increasing number of fractures, also CT scans.

A simple description which is frequently used, distinguishes between isolated (see chapter 3.1), bimalleolar (see chapters 3.2–3.4), and trimalleolar fractures, the latter representing a fracture of the medial and lateral malleolus and the posterior rim of the tibia (see chapters 3.6 and 3.7). Consequently, with an additional fracture of the anterior tibial or fibular rim, one could speak of a quadrimalleolar fracture (see chapter 3.9). Typical patterns of fractures and fracture dislocations are often described with eponyms, like the Maisonneuve fracture (see chapter 3.5) and Bosworth fracture dislocation (see chapter 3.8).

Fractures of the medial malleolus have been classified by Pankovich and Shivaram into six types. This classification was later modified by Boszczyk et al into four main types which are weakly correlated to the patient-reported fracture mechanism:

Type A Avulsion fracture or deltoid ligament rupture

Type B Fracture of the anterior colliculus

Type C Fracture of the posterior colliculus

Type D Supracollicular fracture

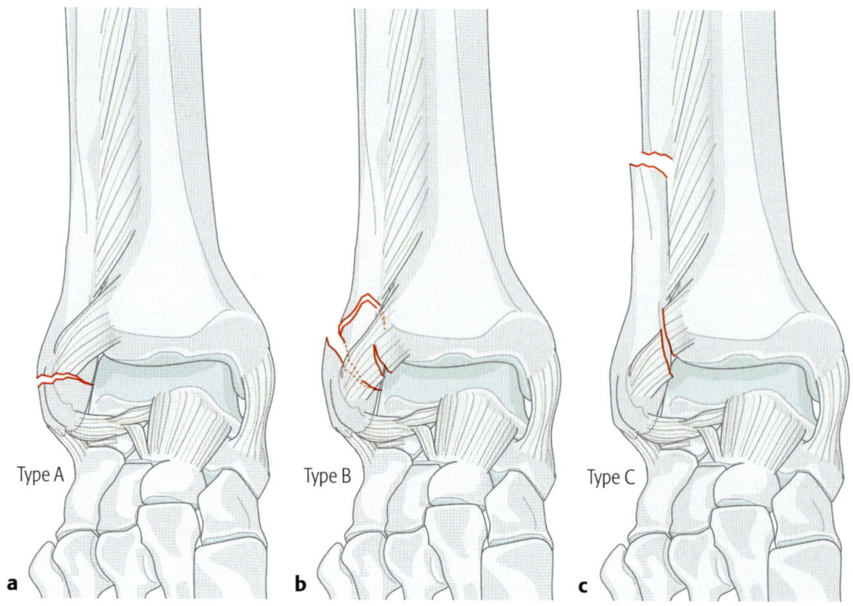

Fig 3-7a–c Danis-Weber classification of malleolar fractures with respect to the height of the fibular fracture in relation to the syndesmosis.

According to Herscovici et al, medial malleolar fractures can be classified according to the orientation (obliquity) of the main fracture line.

Fractures of the posterior malleolus can be classified with respect to involvement of the tibial incisura and require CT imaging. Bartoníček et al distinguish four types (**Fig 3-8**):

Type 1 Extraincisural fragment
Type 2 Posterolateral fragment
Type 3 Posteromedial, 2-part fragment with medial extension
Type 4 Large, posterolateral triangular fragment

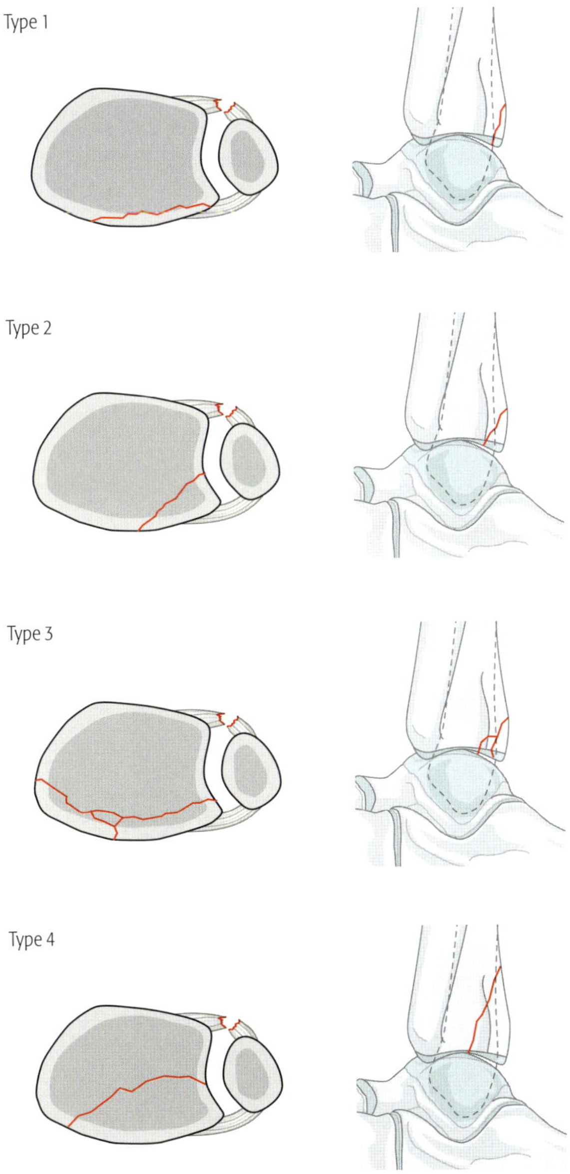

Fig 3-8 Bartoníček et al classification of posterior malleolar fractures with respect to incisura involvement, medial extension, and fragment size.

4 Assessment

Clinical assessment

Clinical examination of the affected foot and ankle focusses on visible deformities and dislocations, open wounds, local skin conditions, and peripheral neurovascular supply. Patients typically present with a local perimalleolar swelling and hematoma (ecchymosis) and pain on palpation over the malleoli. The fibula should be palpated along its entire length to exclude a Maisonneuve fracture. Ankle range of motion is painful and usually restricted. Weight bearing on the affected foot and ankle is impaired or impossible in most cases. Visible dislocations with marked bony prominence and local pressure to the skin—typically over the medial malleolus—require urgent reduction to avoid further damage to the soft tissues (**Fig 3-9**). Massive swelling with loss of skin wrinkling and blister formation must raise the suspicion of a compartment syndrome.

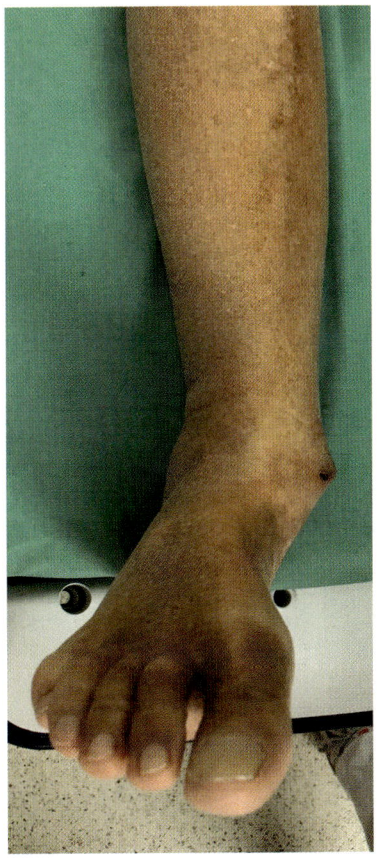

Fig 3-9 Clinical aspect of an acute malleolar fracture dislocation (PA stage 3, same patient as in **Fig 3-3**). Note the valgus deformity and the protrusion of the proximal medial malleolar fragment that will rapidly lead to a full thickness skin necrosis if not reduced promptly.

Imaging

Standard x-rays for suspected malleolar fractures include an exact lateral view and an AP view (mortise view) with 15° of internal rotation of the leg (**Fig 3-10**). A true AP view allows a more precise assessment of the medial malleolus. The following landmarks are important for both preoperative and postoperative assessment of joint congruity on the mortise view:

- A fibulotibial distance 1 cm above the joint line (Chaput ligne claire) or tibiofibular clear space (TCS) of more than 5 mm raises the suspicion of an unstable syndesmosis.
- The medial clear space (MCS) should not exceed 4 mm and not be broader than the superior joint space, ie, the trilateral intervals of the ankle joint should be equal and parallel.
- The medial spike of the fibula ("Weber-Nase", "Weber nose") should indicate the level of the tibial subchondral bone (Shenton line of the ankle).
- The contour of the lateral process of the talus continues as an unbroken curve to the peroneal recess in the distal fibula (Weber ball, "Weber Kreis", "dime sign").

Preoperative computed tomographic CT imaging should be obtained for the following fracture patterns that cannot be reliably assessed by conventional x-rays (**Fig 3-11**):

- Malleolar fractures with an unstable syndesmosis (particularly with bony avulsions)
- Malleolar fractures involving the posterior malleolus
- Suspected impaction of the tibial plafond
- Spiral fractures of the distal tibial shaft
- Transitional ankle fractures in adolescents
- Irregular fracture patterns (eg, in osteoporotic bone)

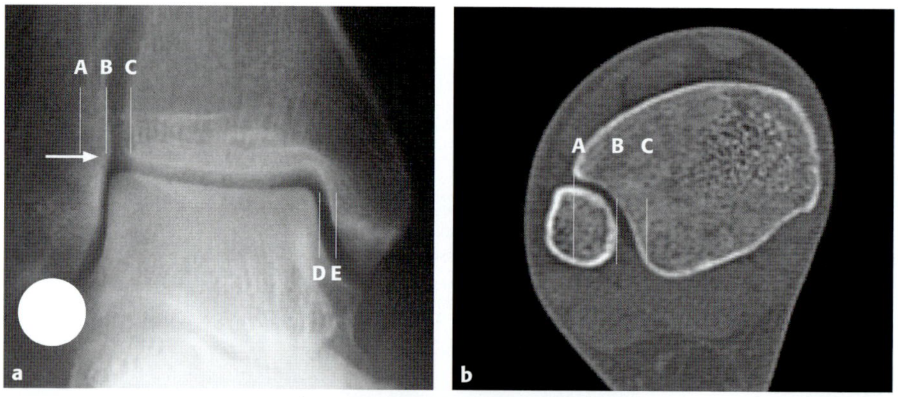

Fig 3-10a–b Radiographic landmarks for a congruent ankle joint are:
AB: Tibiofibular overlap
BC: TCS (ligne claire)
DE: MCS
Weber ball ("dime sign", see circle) and Weber nose (arrow) at the distal fibula.

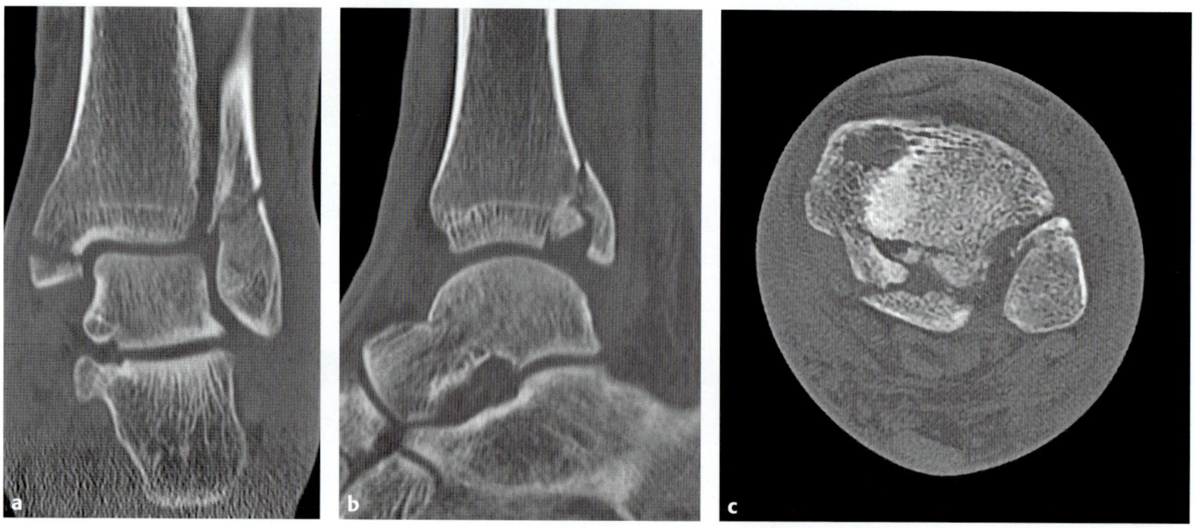

Fig 3-11a–c The CT scans after closed reduction and external fixation reveals a multifragmentary posterior malleolar fracture with extension (type 3 according to Bartoníček et al), partial impaction of the tibial plafond and a rotated intercalary fragment. Therefore, the decision was to approach the posterior malleolar fracture from posterolateral. (Same patient as in **Figs 3-13**, **3-14**, and **3-15**.)

Magnetic resonance imaging has a limited role and is most useful in soft-tissue injury patterns and suspected cartilage injury or complex injuries to the ligaments and tendons. For the latter, ultrasound examination is a valuable tool for an experienced examiner.

5 Nonoperative treatment

Stable and nondisplaced malleolar fractures can be treated nonoperatively. These include isolated fibular fractures without additional syndesmotic or medial ligamentous instability and isolated medial malleolar fractures without syndesmotic or lateral instability. With any medial or posterior malleolar fracture, a ligamentous syndesmotic injury and a high fibular fracture (Maisonneuve) must be ruled out.

In case of an isolated, nondisplaced or minimally (< 2 mm) displaced lateral malleolar fracture, relevant injury to the tibiofibular syndesmosis and/or deltoid ligament must be ruled out. Static instability is detected on the mortise view with a TCS of > 5 mm, a MCS of > 4 mm or widening of more than 1 mm compared to the superior joint space. Dynamic mortise instability can be detected with stress x-rays as clinical signs of medial ligament injury, such as pain, swelling, and ecchymosis, are nonspecific. Stability can be tested with either manual lateral shift of the foot, external rotation (about 4 kp) of the foot with the lower leg fixed (**Fig 3-12**), or passive lateral overhanging of the affected foot with the leg being placed on a pad ("gravity stress test").

Because of the intrinsic stability of the joint surfaces, not all lateral malleolar fractures with positive stress testing will result in significant instability during axial loading while standing and walking. Therefore, weight-bearing x-rays may be more adequate to detect relevant ankle instability under physiological conditions.

Fractures that are stable under stress x-rays or axial loading can be treated with either a stable orthosis or a special walker/boot that puts the foot in neutral and limits supination and weight bearing as tolerated. With severe soft-tissue swelling, a leg cast is applied initially for 3–5 days. In the case of a poorly compliant patient, the splint may be overwrapped for better stability and may be kept in place until the fracture shows evidence of healing on x-rays. The orthosis or boot is worn until bony union is demonstrated with follow-up x-rays, usually at 6 weeks. Physical therapy starts with isometric exercises within the boot and is supplemented with isotonic exercises after 2 weeks.

In cases of contraindication to open reduction and internal fixation (ORIF), closed reduction aims at axial realignment of the ankle and relieving the strain on the soft tissues. Closed reduction usually is carried out with longitudinal traction and reversal of the suspected fracture mechanism. Retention is achieved either with ankle-spanning external fixation or a split below-knee cast that may be converted into a circular cast after soft-tissue swelling has subsided. Secondary ORIF may be carried out after improvement of the patient's overall condition or soft-tissue consolidation.

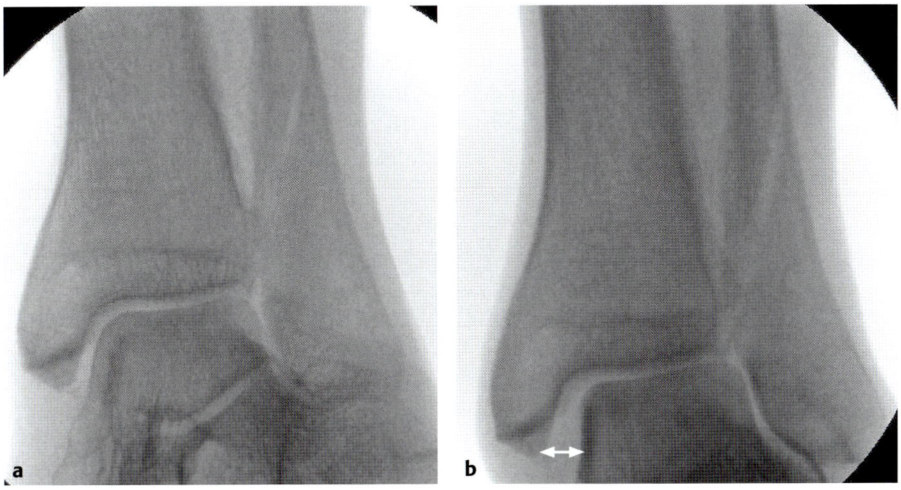

Fig 3-12a–b Dynamic instability of the ankle mortise is detected with external rotation of the foot against the fixed lower leg. Widening of the MCS (double arrow) demonstrates deltoid ligament rupture and therefore indicates a SER 4 injury warranting surgical treatment. Alternatively, weight-bearing x-rays can be obtained to detect mortise instability.

a Unstressed x-ray.

b Stress x-ray.

6 Operative treatment

Indications for surgery

Isolated malleolar fractures that are displaced more than 2 mm or unstable on plain imaging or stress testing/weight bearing (**Fig 3-12**) and all bimalleolar and trimalleolar fractures should be treated operatively. According to biomechanical and clinical studies, any fibular displacement of 2 mm or more compared to the uninjured side carries the risk of posttraumatic arthritis. In addition, fibular malrotation of more than 5° led to a significant load alteration in a human anatomical experiment by Thordarson et al while in a clinical study by Vasarhelyi et al malrotation of more than 15° was associated with less favorable outcome.

Contraindications for surgery include a critical overall condition of the patient (eg, polytraumatized or critically ill patients), and a poor local soft-tissue status like contaminated wounds, chronic ulcers, or infected soft tissues. In patients with complicated diabetes mellitus, perioperative control of serum glucose levels is advised. Advanced peripheral vascular disease may warrant a vascular intervention.

Patient positioning

For most unimalleolar and bimalleolar fractures requiring lateral and/or medial approaches, the patient is placed supine on a radiolucent table with the injured leg elevated. A bump is placed under the ipsilatetal hip to have the foot in neutral position. This enables the surgeon to access both the medial and lateral side and allows adequate visualization in the lateral C-arm projections.

For direct access to the posterior tibia the patient is placed prone on a radiolucent table with the leg draped free. The ability to rotate the limb internally and externally and to bend the knee is essential to allow all necessary incisions. A roll is placed under the fractured ankle to allow adequate lateral C-arm projections. In addition to posterolateral or posteromedial approaches, the standard lateral and medial approaches can be performed as well.

Considerations for surgery

Grossly displaced fracture dislocations should be reduced as soon as possible under sufficient analgesia to avoid further soft-tissue damage (**Fig 3-9**). After closed reduction using longitudinal traction and reversal of the fracture mechanism, the ankle is immobilized with a radiolucent pneumatic or vacuum splint.

Open and closed fractures with significant soft-tissue damage like subcutaneous delamination, compartment syndrome, soft-tissue incarceration, and impeding skin necrosis represent surgical emergencies. Open wounds are debrided after copious lavage. The decision on the timing of definite surgery depends on the individual fracture pattern, wound contamination, location, and extent of soft-tissue damage. For optimal immobilization and soft-tissue monitoring, a tibiometatarsal external fixator is applied. Definite wound closure is achieved during planned revisions ("second look") either by direct suture, skin graft, or local or free flaps.

Closed malleolar fractures are best addressed early (within 8–12 hours) after the injury. Soft-tissue swelling alone is no contraindication to early internal fixation because soft-tissue swelling will diminish after evacuation of the hematoma and stable fracture fixation. In cases of delayed patient presentation or contaminated soft-tissues, definite internal fixation should be carried out after soft tissue consolidation. Highly unstable fractures, especially pronation fracture dislocations should be treated initially with closed reduction and external fixation (**Fig 3-13**) until definite internal fixation because they tend to redislocate with immobilization in a cast only. A CT imaging, if warranted, is performed after closed reduction and external fixation (**Fig 3-11**).

Surgical approaches

Lateral approach

The distal fibular fracture can be addressed through a standard lateral approach. The incision lies centrally over the palpable distal fibula at the level of the fracture. Care is taken not to injure the branches of the superficial peroneal nerve anteriorly and the peroneal tendons posteriorly. The lateral joint compartment is routinely explored for loose fragments or capsular impingement and the lateral talar dome inspected for cartilage damage and osteochondral fragments. Displaced or unstable infrasyndesotic (Weber A) fractures are fixed with either an intramedullary screw or tension band wiring. For larger fragments, a plate can be used (see chapter 3.3). With small, osteoporotic, and multiple fragments, several minifragment screws or a hook plate can be used.

The classic spiral fracture in transsyndesmotic (Weber B, SER) injuries is fixed with one or two compression screws and a lateral neutralization plate (see chapter 3.1). Alternatively, a posterior antiglide plate provides more stability (see chapter 3.6). The plate should end at least 1 cm above the tip of the fibula in order to avoid irritation of the peroneal tendons. Irregular and highly unstable fibular fractures may warrant the use of a bridging plate, preferably an interlocking plate (see chapter 3.9). After fixation of all bony injuries, syndesmotic stability is tested with a hook that pulls the fibula laterally and posteriorly (see chapters 3.1–3.9). Alternatively, external rotation of the foot against the distal tibia or insertion of a lamina spreader between the distal tibia and fibula can be performed. In cases with TCS widening of ≥ 2 mm, the fibula is reduced into the tibial notch with a curved point-to-point reduction (Weber) clamp under direct vision and palpation of the anterior tibial and fibular rim. A tibiofibular syndesmotic screw (alternatively a flexible implant eg, suture button) is introduced 1–4 cm above the joint at an angle of about 30° anteriorly which corresponds to the axis of the clamp between the tip of the lateral and medial malleolus (see chapter 3.6).

Suprasyndesmotic (Weber C) fractures are fixed with a lateral plate (see chapter 3.4). Care must be taken to respect the individual physiological torsion of the fibula to avoid malrotation through a rigid and straight plate. After fixation of all bony injuries, the distal fibula is reduced into the tibial notch and a syndesmosis screw or dynamic implant is used for syndesmotic stabilization.

High fibular fractures in Maisonneuve injuries do not need internal fixation. However, they must be reduced anatomically in order to reestablish correct fibular length and rotation. The anterior syndesmosis is explored via a small anterolateral approach over the syndesmotic region and cleared from intervening ligaments or debris. The distal fibula is reduced into the tibial incisura and two syndesmotic screws (alternatively flexible implants) are inserted (see chapter 3.5). While fibular length can be easily checked with conventional C-arm images, anteroposterior translation and particularly malrotation of the distal fibular is hard to detect with 2D imaging. A postoperative CT scan or intraoperative 3D imaging is advocated after syndesmotic stabilization to ensure exact placement of the distal fibula into the tibial notch. Malreduction should be corrected as soon as possible after detection.

Several biomechanical studies failed to show a mechanical advantage of stainless steel over titanium screws, 4.5 mm over 3.5 mm screws, and quadricortical over tricortical screws. Bioabsorbable screws from polylactic acid and endobutton suture appear to provide equivalent stability. Thus, the quality of reduction and not the type of fixation is of clinical importance in syndesmotic stabilization.

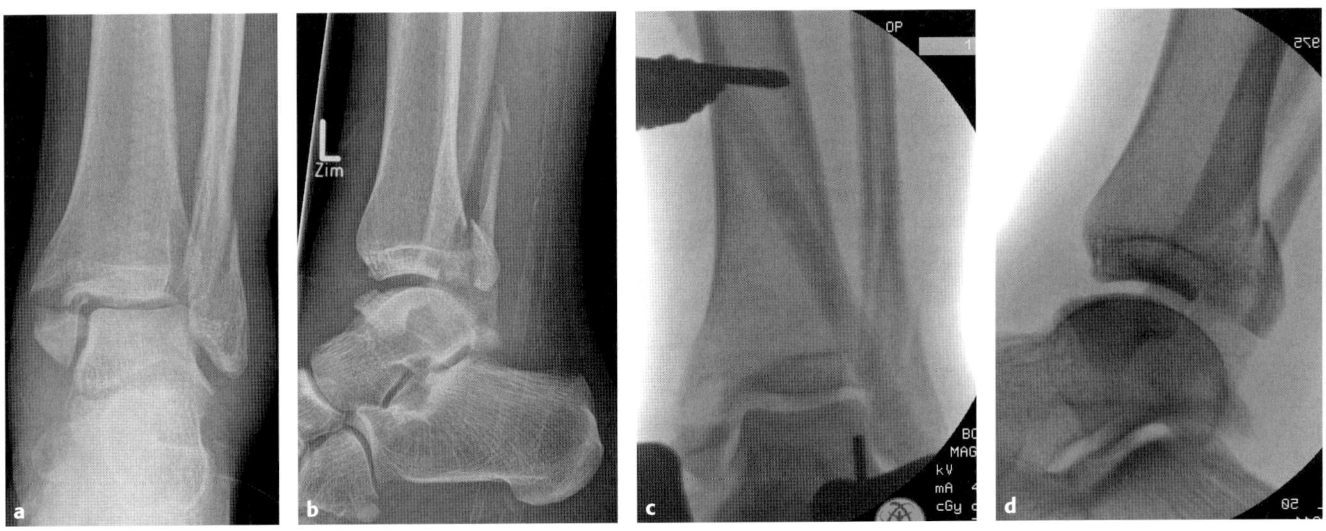

Fig 3-13a–d Temporary external fixation. (Same patient as in **Figs 3-11**, **3-14**, and **3-15**.)

a–b Closed reduction and temporary external fixation is warranted in grossly unstable fractures and fracture dislocations that are not amenable to immediate internal fixation.

c–d The external fixator is left in place until soft tissue consolidation and definite internal fixation.

Medial approach

The medial malleolus is approached via a direct epimalleolar medial incision that is slightly curved anteriorly in its distal end. The fracture is freed from intervening periosteum and small fragments. The medial joint compartment is cleared of debris and the talar dome is explored for chondral injuries. The medial aspect of the tibial plafond is inspected for impaction, especially in Weber A (SA 2) injuries with a vertical malleolar fracture (see chapter 3.3). Anatomical reduction is controlled at the exposed medial joint angle. Fixation of the medial malleous is achieved with either compression screws (see chapter 3.2), K-wires with olives (see chapter 3.6), or tension band wiring depending on bone quality and fragment size. Implants should be placed into the anterior colliculus or the intracollicular groove to avoid damage to the posterior tibial tendon which curves around the posterior colliculus.

In SA 2 injuries, the vertical fracture of the medial malleolus warrants a horizontal screw placement if the fragment is large enough. Alternatively, a medial buttress plate can be used (see chapter 3.3). Any articular impaction of the medial tibial plafond must be lifted and supported by local cancellous bone graft from the tibial metaphysis. Suture of the ruptured deltoid ligament complex is not necessary.

Posterior approaches

Despite recent advances in understanding the pathoanatomy of posterior malleolar fractures, there is still controversy as to when and how to fix a posterior tibial fragment. There is no support in the literature for traditional recommendation to fix any fragment containing more than 25% (or 33%) of the joint surface. Rather, the dislocation of the posterior fragment and the presence of an intercalary fragment and/or joint impaction are criteria for ORIF (**Fig 3-14**). Additionally, fixation of any posterior fragment with incisura involvement reestablishes the integrity of the tibial incisura and physiological tension of the tibiofibular syndesmosis which attaches to it. Anatomical reduction and fixation of the posterior fragment may obviate the need for a syndesmotic screw and appears to be associated with a lower rate of malreduction of the syndesmosis on postoperative CT scans (see chapter 3.9).

The incision for the posterolateral approach lies parallel to the Achilles tendon. The sural nerve is identified within the subcutaneous tissue in the proximal part of the incision and gently retracted medially together with the lesser saphenous vein. The superficial and deep fasciae are incised longitudinally and the flexor hallucis longus muscle and tendon are retracted medially to protect the posterior tibial neurovas-

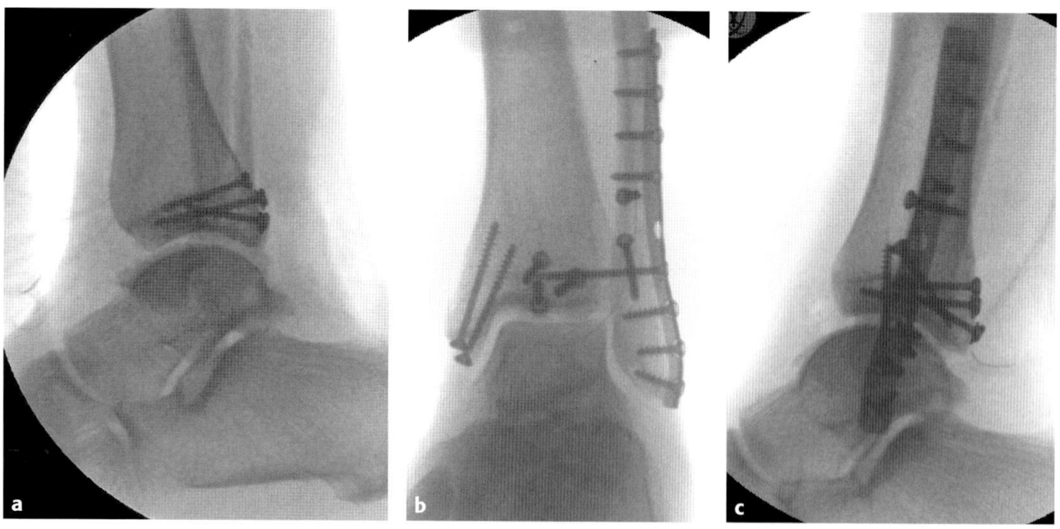

Fig 3-14a–c Trimalleolar fracture fixation with the patient in a prone position. (Same patient as in **Figs 3-11**, **3-13**, and **3-15**.)
a The multifragmentary posterior malleolar fracture is fixed with screws via a posterolateral approach.
b–c The distal fibular fracture is fixed with a lateral plate via a lateral approach and the medial malleolus is fixed with two lag screws via a medial approach.

cular bundle. The fractured posterior tibial fragment is hinged on the posterior syndesmosis and cleared of debris. Larger intercalary fragments are reduced and fixed to the anterior tibia (see chapter 3.7), smaller fragments are discarded. The posterior fragment is reduced and fixed with lag screws or a dorsal antiglide plate (see chapters 3.6–3.9).

In selected cases, single, large fragments (Bartoníček type 4) can be visualized and reduced through the oblique fibular fracture, which lies in the same plane via a lateral approach and fixed indirectly with anterior to posterior screws. A small anterior approach is used for screw insertion respecting the extensor tendons and anterior neurovascular bundle. However, biomechanical studies have shown that posterior plating provides a more stable fixation than anterior screws. Reduction of the posterior fragment before fixing the fibula will control joint reduction in the lateral view (**Fig 3-14**). Alternatively, reducing the fibula prior to fixation of the posterior malleolar component may restore length and aid in reduction of the posterior malleolar fracture, as the posterior malleolar fragment shortens with the fibula because it is attached to the intact the posterior inferior tibiofibular ligament.

As the exact position of the distal fibula in the incisura and fibular rotation cannot be determined reliably on plain x-rays, postoperative CT (alternatively intraoperative 3D) imaging is useful after fixation of an unstable syndesmosis and complex injuries with partial tibial plafond impaction (**Fig 3-15**). Because of the considerable interindividual variation of the incisura morphology, bilateral imaging is advantageous.

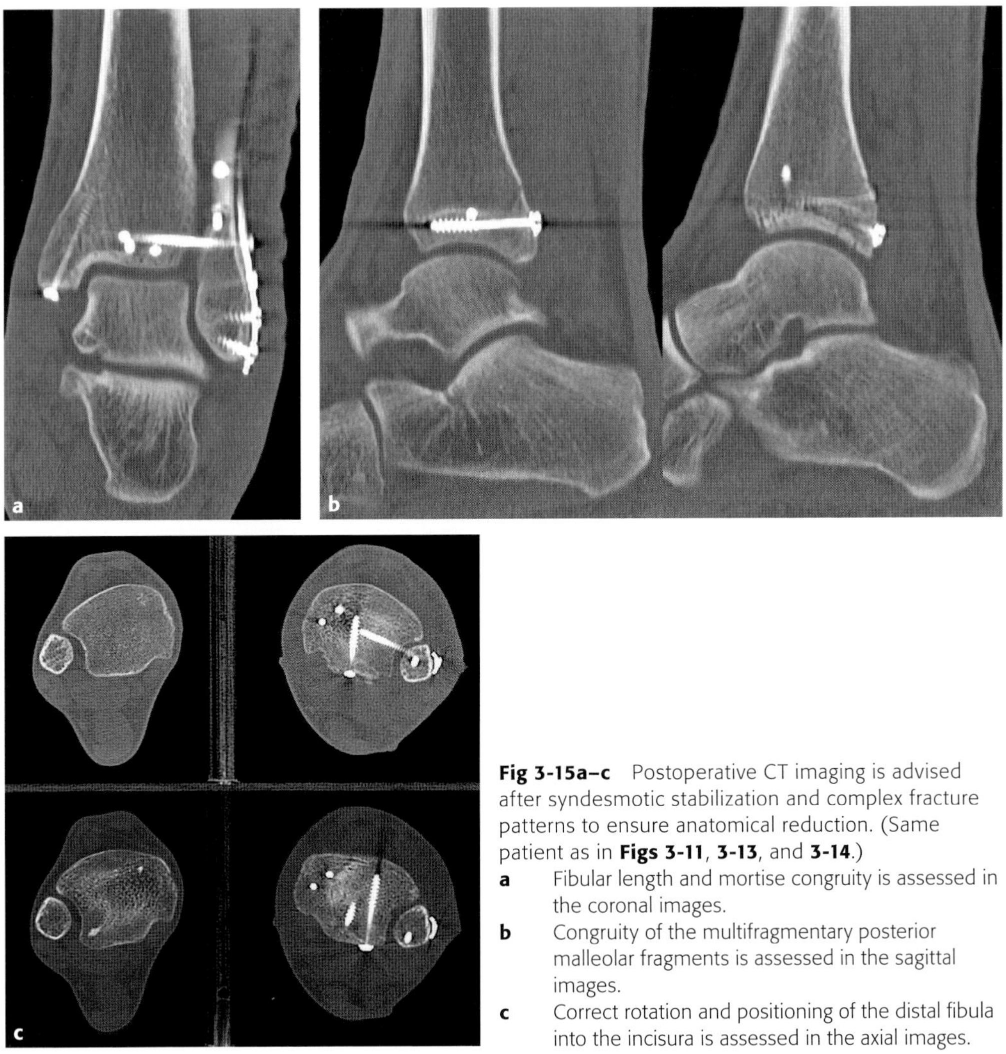

Fig 3-15a–c Postoperative CT imaging is advised after syndesmotic stabilization and complex fracture patterns to ensure anatomical reduction. (Same patient as in **Figs 3-11**, **3-13**, and **3-14**.)

- **a** Fibular length and mortise congruity is assessed in the coronal images.
- **b** Congruity of the multifragmentary posterior malleolar fragments is assessed in the sagittal images.
- **c** Correct rotation and positioning of the distal fibula into the incisura is assessed in the axial images.

7 Postoperative care

In the early postoperative period, the operative ankle is immobilized in a splint or cast. If there has been extensive associated soft-tissue injury, including open fractures, an external fixator is applied until soft-tissue consolidation. At that time a removable boot is applied and patients are restricted to partial weight bearing (15–20 kg) pending adequate compliance and ability to walk on crutches. The boot is removed for range-of-motion exercises. Trimalleolar, osteoporotic, and comminuted fractures should be protected in a leg cast with partial weight bearing or complete offloading.

Gradual transition to full weight bearing is initiated after radiographic evidence of bone healing, typically 6 weeks after surgery. This period may last considerably longer in the presence of comorbidities, most notably in patients with diabetes or other neuropathy. It appears from published literature, that removal of a syndesmotic screw is not needed unless symptomatic. Patients should be counseled about the possibility of screw loosening or breakage.

Isolated fibular or medial malleolar fractures can be treated in a removable boot with full weight bearing as tolerated after internal fixation.

8 Complications and outcomes

Complications

The rate of short-term complications after ankle fractures is low. In a database of more than 57,000 patients from California, wound infections were seen in 1.44% and amputation in 0.16%. Open fractures, increased age, and medical comorbidities are associated with a higher risk of postoperative complications. Patients with diabetes have significantly higher infection rates of up to 50% particularly with poor blood glucose control and diabetic neuropathy.

Nonunions are rare after stable internal fixation and may be due to improper stabilization or poor bone quality. Solid malunions are associated with pain, functional disability, and sometimes a visible deformity. They represent a greater risk for posttraumatic arthritis and can be treated successfully with corrective osteotomies if no symptomatic arthritis is present. Chronic syndesmotic instability may be treated with fibular reduction and flexible implants, a split peroneus longus ligamentoplasty that reconstructs all three syndesmotic ligaments, or tibiofibular fusion. In cases of progressive posttraumatic arthritis, corrective fusion or total ankle replacement with correction of the deformity is indicated.

Outcomes

Numerous clinical studies with substantial numbers of patients have shown that the most important prognostic factor in malleolar fractures that may be influenced by the treating surgeon is anatomical reduction of the malleoli, irrespective of the type of fracture. Precise positioning of the distal fibula into the tibial incisura is of utmost importance in ankle fractures with syndesmotic instability. Exact reduction of posterior malleolar fragments not only restores articular congruity but also the shape of the fibular incisura and stability of the syndesmosis. Anatomical reduction and stable internal fixation of these posterior fragments is therefore of prognostic relevance even in smaller fragments, so long as there is displacement and involvement of the incisura. However, initial cartilage damage may cause posttraumatic arthritic and less favorable results even with perfect reduction.

The prognosis clearly worsens with the number of injured bony and ligamentous structures around the ankle. Bimalleolar fractures are associated with poorer 1-year outcomes than fibular fractures with deltoid ligament rupture and the presence of a posterior fragment further worsens the prognosis.

Prospective randomized studies and several nonrandomized comparative studies showed significantly better outcome with ORIF than with closed reduction and cast immobilization for unstable and displaced ankle fractures. Stable isolated lateral and medial malleolar fractures have good to excellent outcomes with nonoperative treatment when accompanying bone and ligament injuries could be ruled out.

In the absence of severe systemic comorbidities, the results after ORIF of malleolar fractures in patients older and younger than 60 years are nearly identical while nonoperative treatment leads to significantly inferior outcomes. Therefore, the general indications for surgery in elderly patients should not differ from that in younger patients. If relevant comorbidities are present, above all diabetes with neuropathy, severe osteoporosis, dementia, and peripheral vascular disease, the treatment regimen must be adapted accordingly as outlined above.

9 Recommended reading

Bartoníček J, Rammelt S, Kašper Š, et al. Pathoanatomy of Maisonneuve fracture based on radiologic and CT examination. *Arch Orthop Trauma Surg.* 2019 Apr;139(4):497–506.
Bartoníček J, Rammelt S, Kostlivý K, et al. Anatomy and classification of the posterior tibial fragment in ankle fractures. *Arch Orthop Trauma Surg.* 2015 Apr;135(4): 505–516.
Bartoníček J, Rammelt S, Kostlivý K. Bosworth fracture: A report of two atypical cases and literature review of 108 cases. *FussSprungg.* 2017 June 15(2):126–137.
Baumbach SF, Herterich V, Damblemont A, et al. Open reduction and internal fixation of the posterior malleolus fragment frequently restores syndesmotic stability. *Injury.* 2019 Feb;50(2):564–570.
Berkes MB, Little MT, Lazaro LE, et al. Articular congruity is associated with short-term clinical outcomes of operatively treated SER IV ankle fractures. *J Bone Joint Surg Am.* 2013 Oct 2;95(19):1769–1775.
Boszczyk A, Fudalej M, Kwapisz S, et al. X-ray features to predict ankle fracture mechanism. *Forensic Sci Int.* 2018 Oct;291:185–192.
Boszczyk A, Fudalej M, Kwapisz S, et al. Ankle fracture — correlation of Lauge-Hansen classification and patient reported fracture mechanism. *Forensic Sci Int.* 2018 Jan;282:94–100.
Broos PL, Bisschop AP. Operative treatment of ankle fractures in adults: correlation between types of fracture and final results. *Injury.* 1991 Sep;22(5):403–406.
Davidovitch RI, Walsh M, Spitzer A, et al. Functional outcome after operatively treated ankle fractures in the elderly. *Foot Ankle Int.* 2009 Aug;30(8):728–733.
Dingemans SA, Rammelt S, White TO, et al. Should syndesmotic screws be removed after surgical fixation of unstable ankle fractures? A systematic review. *Bone Joint J.* 2016 Nov;98-b(11):1497–1504.
Donken CC, Verhofstad MH, Edwards MJ, et al. Twenty-one-year follow-up of supination-external rotation type II-IV (OTA type B) ankle fractures: a retrospective cohort study. *J Orthop Trauma.* 2012 Aug;26(8):e108–114.
Drijfhout van Hooff CC, Verhage SM, Hoogendoorn JM. Influence of fragment size and postoperative joint congruency on long-term outcome of posterior malleolar fractures. *Foot Ankle Int.* 2015 Jun;36(6):673–678.
Egol KA, Amirtharajah M, Tejwani NC, et al. Ankle stress test for predicting the need for surgical fixation of isolated fibular fractures. *J Bone Joint Surg Am.* 2004 Nov;86(11):2393–2398.
Egol KA, Koval KJ, Zuckerman JD. *Handbook of Fractures.* 4th ed. Philadelphia: Lippincott Williams & Wilkins; 2010.
Futamura K, Baba T, Mogami A, et al. Malreduction of syndesmosis injury associated with malleolar ankle fracture can be avoided using Weber's three indexes in the mortise view. *Injury.* 2017 Apr;48(4):954–959.
Gardner MJ, Demetrakopoulos D, Briggs SM, et al. The ability of the Lauge-Hansen classification to predict ligament injury and mechanism in ankle fractures: an MRI study. *J Orthop Trauma.* 2006 Apr;20(4):267–272.
Haraguchi N, Armiger RS. A new interpretation of the mechanism of ankle fracture. *J Bone Joint Surg Am.* 2009 Apr;91(4):821–829.
Hartwich K, Lorente Gomez A, Pyrc J, et al. Biomechanical analysis of stability of posterior antiglide plating in osteoporotic pronation abduction ankle fracture model with posterior tibial fragment. *Foot Ankle Int.* 2017 Jan;38(1):58–65.
Heim D, Niederhauser K, Simbrey N. The Volkmann dogma: a retrospective, long-term, single-center study. *Eur J Trauma Emerg Surg.* 2010 Dec;36(6):515–519.
Heim U, Pfeiffer KM. *Internal Fixation of Small Fractures: Techniques Recommended by the AO-ASIF Group.* 3rd ed. Berlin Heidelberg New York: Springer; 1988.
Herscovici D Jr, Scaduto JM, Infante A. Conservative treatment of isolated fractures of the medial malleolus. *J Bone Joint Surg Br.* 2007 Jan;89(1):89–93.
Lauge-Hansen N. Fractures of the ankle. II. Combined experimental-surgical and experimental-roentgenologic investigations. *Arch Surg.* 1950 May;60(5):957–985.
Lindsjö U. Operative treatment of ankle fractures. *Acta Orthop Scand Suppl.* 1981;189:1–131.
Makwana NK, Bhowal B, Harper WM, et al. Conservative versus operative treatment for displaced ankle fractures in patients over 55 years of age. A prospective, randomised study. *J Bone Joint Surg Br.* 2001 May;83(4):525–529.
McConnell T, Tornetta P 3rd. Marginal plafond impaction in association with supination-adduction ankle fractures: a report of eight cases. *J Orthop Trauma.* 2001 Aug;15(6):447–449.
Miller AN, Carroll EA, Parker RJ, et al. Posterior malleolar stabilization of syndesmotic injuries is equivalent to screw fixation. *Clin Orthop Relat Res.* 2010 Apr;468(4):1129–1135.
Mont MA, Sedlin ED, Weiner LS, et al. Postoperative radiographs as predictors of clinical outcome in unstable ankle fractures. *J Orthop Trauma.* 1992;6(3):352–357.
Ovaska MT, Makinen TJ, Madanat R, et al. A comprehensive analysis of patients with malreduced ankle fractures undergoing re-operation. *Int Orthop.* 2014 Jan;38(1):83–88.
Pankovich AM, Shivaram MS. Anatomical basis of variability in injuries of the medial malleolus and the deltoid ligament. II. Clinical studies. *Acta Orthop Scand.* 1979 Apr;50(2):225–236.
Pelton K, Thordarson DB, Barnwell J. Open versus closed treatment of the fibula in Maissoneuve injuries. *Foot Ankle Int.* 2010 Jul;31(7):604–608.
Rammelt S, Boszczyk A. Computed tomography in the diagnosis and treatment of ankle fractures: a critical analysis review. *JBJS Rev.* 2018 Dec;6(12):e7.
Rammelt S, Obruba P. An update on the evaluation and treatment of syndesmotic injuries. *Eur J Trauma Emerg Surg.* 2015 Dec;41(6):601–614.
Rammelt S, Zwipp H. Ankle fractures. In: Bentley G, ed. *European Instructional Course Lectures, Volume 12.* Berlin Heidelberg New York: Springer; 2012:205–219.
Rammelt S. Management of ankle fractures in the elderly. *EFORT Open Rev.* 2016 May;1(5):239–246.
Sagi HC, Shah AR, Sanders RW. The functional consequence of syndesmotic joint malreduction at a minimum 2-year follow-up. *J Orthop Trauma.* 2012 Jul;26(7):439–443.
Saltzman CL, Salamon ML, Blanchard GM, et al. Epidemiology of ankle arthritis: report of a consecutive series of 639 patients from a tertiary orthopaedic center. *Iowa Orthop J.* 2005;25:44–46.
Schock HJ, Pinzur M, Manion L, et al. The use of gravity or manual-stress radiographs in the assessment of supination-external rotation fractures of the ankle. *J Bone Joint Surg Br.* 2007 Aug;89(8):1055–1059.
SooHoo NF, Krenek L, Eagan MJ, et al. Complication rates following open reduction and internal fixation of ankle fractures. *J Bone Joint Surg Am.* 2009 May;91(5):1042–1049.
Stufkens SA, van den Bekerom MP, Kerkhoffs GM, et al. Long-term outcome after 1822 operatively treated ankle fractures: a systematic review of the literature. *Injury.* 2011 Feb;42(2):119–127.
Tejwani NC, McLaurin TM, Walsh M, et al. Are outcomes of bimalleolar fractures poorer than those of lateral malleolar fractures with medial ligamentous injury? *J Bone Joint Surg Am.* 2007 Jul;89(7):1438–1441.
Thordarson DB, Motamed S, Hedman T, et al. The effect of fibular malreduction on contact pressures in an ankle fracture malunion model. *J Bone Joint Surg Am.* 1997 Dec;79(12):1809–1815.

Tochigi Y, Rudert MJ, Saltzman CL, et al. Contribution of articular surface geometry to ankle stabilization. *J Bone Joint Surg Am.* 2006 Dec;88(12):2704–2713.

Vasarhelyi A, Lubitz J, Gierer P, et al. Detection of fibular torsional deformities after surgery for ankle fractures with a novel CT method. *Foot Ankle Int.* 2006 Dec;27(12):1115–1121.

Verhage SM, Krijnen P, Schipper IB, et al. Persistent postoperative step-off of the posterior malleolus leads to higher incidence of post-traumatic osteoarthritis in trimalleolar fractures. *Arch Orthop Trauma Surg.* 2019 Mar;139(3):323–329.

Weber BG, Colton C. Malleolar fractures. In: Müller M, Allgöwer M, Schneider R, et al, eds. *Manual of internal fixation: Techniques Recommended by the AO-ASIF Group.* Berlin: Springer; 1991:595–612.

Weber BG. Lengthening osteotomy of the fibula to correct a widened mortice of the ankle after fracture. *Int Orthop.* 1981;4(4):289–293.

Weber M. Trimalleolar fractures with impaction of the posteromedial tibial plafond: implications for talar stability. *Foot Ankle Int.* 2004 Oct;25(10):716–727.

Weber M, Burmeister H, Flueckiger G, et al. The use of weightbearing radiographs to assess the stability of supination-external rotation fractures of the ankle. *Arch Orthop Trauma Surg.* 2010 May;130(5):693–698.

Weening B, Bhandari M. Predictors of functional outcome following transsyndesmotic screw fixation of ankle fractures. *J Orthop Trauma.* 2005 Feb;19(2):102–108.

3.1 Distal fibular transsyndesmotic fracture (Weber B)

Lubomír Kopp, Petr Obruba

1 Case description

A 32-year-old man slipped on wet grass and twisted his right ankle. The next day, he presented to the emergency department with ongoing pain in the right lower extremity. X-rays of the ankle revealed a fracture of the lateral malleolus (AO/OTA 44B1.1, Danis/Weber B, supination-external rotation stage 2 fracture according to Lauge-Hansen) (**Fig 3.1-1**). The patient had no comorbidities. Despite the delay of 1 day in diagnosis and treatment, his ankle was not swollen and his foot was neurovascularly intact (**Fig 3.1-2**).

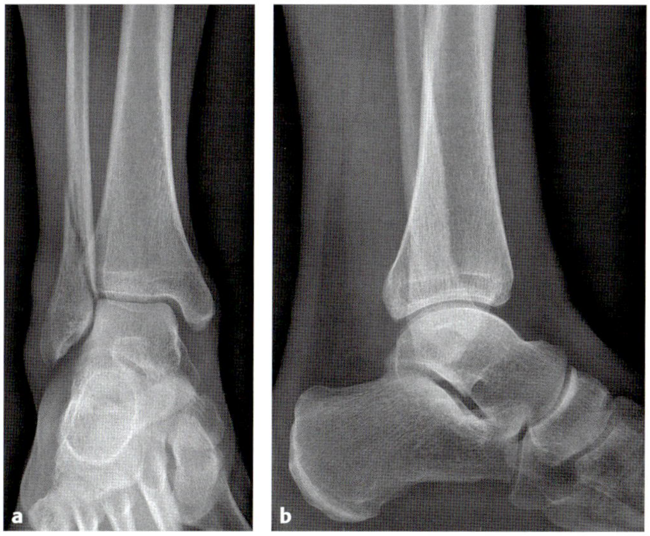

Fig 3.1-1a–b Diagnostic x-rays after injury showing a simple oblique fibular fracture with displacement of more than 2 mm. Note the widening of the medial clear space.
a AP view.
b Lateral view.

2 Preoperative planning

Indications for surgery

Due to a displaced AO/OTA 44B1 fracture with gentle swelling of the soft tissues the indication for early open reduction and internal fixation (ORIF) was seen. In general, longitudinal or lateral displacement of more than 2 mm is an indication for surgery. According to the fracture type, the syndesmosis was expected to be stable after fibular fixation. Critical assessment of syndesmotic stability is essential in all operatively treated ankle fractures, as it may occur with any ankle fracture pattern.

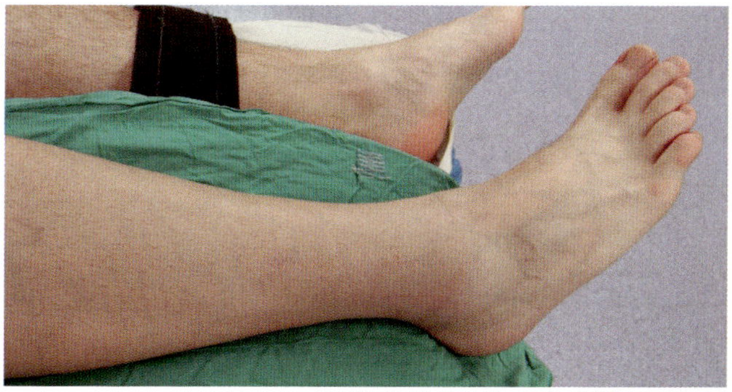

Fig 3.1-2 Clinical image showing mild edema around the lateral malleolus.

Considerations for surgery

The simple oblique fibular fracture is typically fixed with an interfragmentary lag screw and a neutralization plate from a lateral approach (**Fig 3.1-3**).

Deltoid and syndesmotic ligament stability should be tested under C-arm control after completion of the fibula osteosynthesis. Stability of the deltoid and syndesmosis are essential contributors to reestablishing normal ankle mortise.

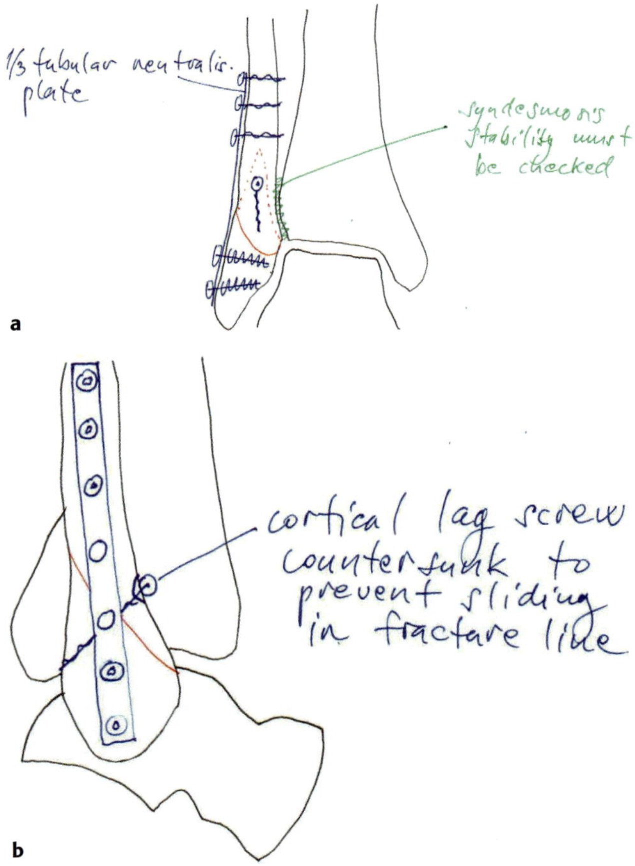

Fig 3.1-3a–b Preoperative plan. The simple oblique fibular fracture is fixed with an interfragmentary lag screw and neutralization plate from a lateral approach. The syndesmosis is then tested for stability with the C-arm.

3 Operating room setup

Patient positioning	• Supine with a bump under the ipsilateral hip
Anesthesia options	• General, regional, or spinal
C-arm location	• Positioned on contralateral side of the patient with monitor near the patient's shoulder and the C-arm positioned at a 90° angle to the operative table.
Tourniquet	• Usually not necessary in simple fracture patterns
Tips	• Elevate the operative extremity on a radiolucent ramp or a stack of blankets to allow easier instrumentation and prevent the other limb from interfering with lateral C-arm imaging.

For illustrations and overview of anesthetic considerations, see chapter 1.

Equipment

- 3.5 mm (2.7 or 2.4 mm) cortex screws
- 4.0 mm cancellous screws
- One-third tubular plate
- Point-to-point reduction (Weber) clamps

4 Surgical procedure

For ORIF of simple oblique fibular fractures, a lateral approach is typically used. After fibular fracture fixation, stability of the syndesmosis is tested with the C-arm.

The longitudinal lateral incision is placed centrally over the distal fibula (**Fig 3.1-4**). Attention must be paid to gentle manipulation of the soft tissues. The oblique fracture line is identified, cleared of hematoma (**Fig 3.1-5**), and reduced with forceps. Correct length and rotation of the distal fragment must be restored (**Fig 3.1-6**). A cortex lag screw is then placed anteroposteriorly and craniocaudally perpendicular to the fracture line on the anterior side. With good bone quality, the screw head is countersunk to prevent dislocation of the screw head and the fracture line during tightening (**Fig 3.1-7**).

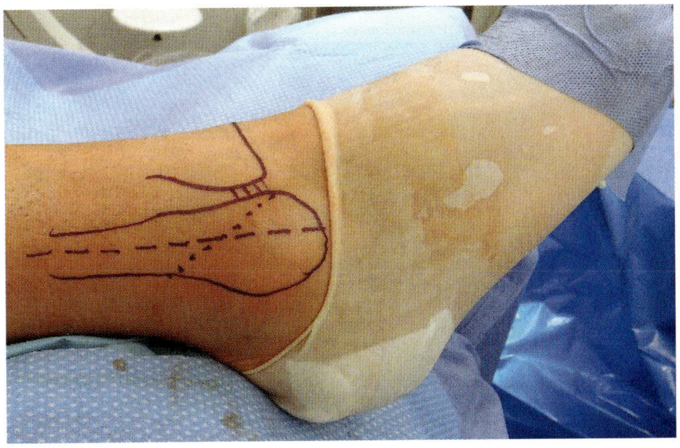

Fig 3.1-4 The standard lateral approach for fibular fixation.

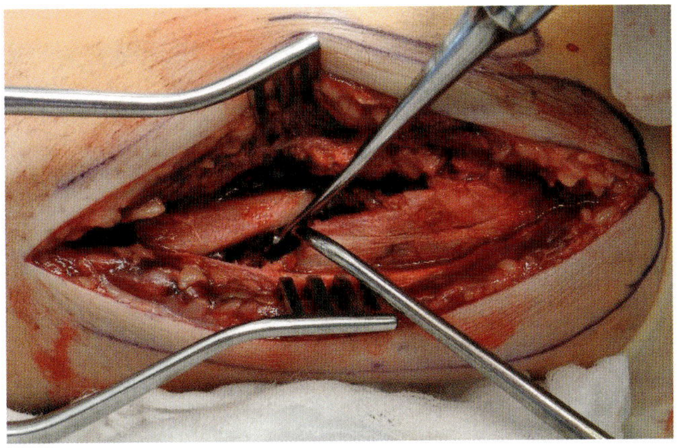

Fig 3.1-5 The oblique fracture line is identified, cleared of hematoma, and irrigated. The distal fragment is gently held away with a bone hook.

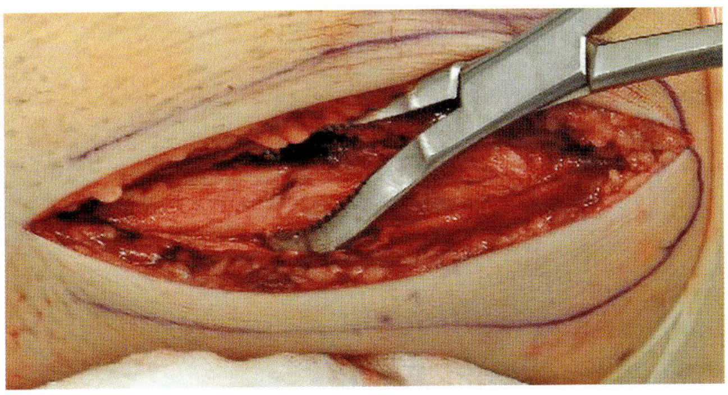

Fig 3.1-6 The fracture is reduced with a forceps. Correct length and rotation of the distal fragment must be achieved.

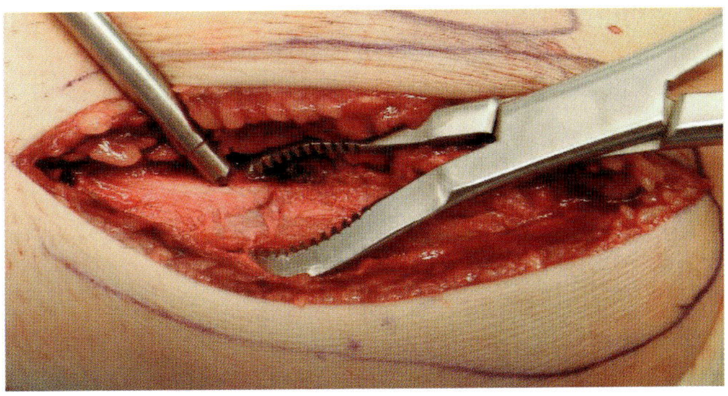

Fig 3.1-7 Countersinking of the lag screw prevents the screw head and fracture line from dislocation during tightening.

The position of the screw is checked with the C-arm (**Fig 3.1-8**).

For neutralization, a one-third tubular plate is slightly bent at the fibular tip to imitate the contour of distal fibula. Undercontouring in the central part maximizes the pressure on the distal fibular fragment during tightening, which further pushes the distal fibula back into proper alignment (**Fig 3.1-9**).

A minimum of two fully threaded screws are placed into the distal fragment and preferably three cortex screws proximally. Self-tapping screws may be used in patients with hard cortical bone but this is rarely required (**Fig 3.1-10**).

Completion of fibular fixation is followed by inspection of tibiofibular ligaments. If a bony syndesmotic avulsion from the anterior tibia or fibula (a Tillaux-Chaput or Wagstaffe fragment) is present, it should be reduced and reattached with 2.7 or 3.5 mm screws, pins, or suture anchors to restore stability of the syndesmosis and integrity of the tibial incisura. Syndesmotic stability is checked using the C-arm with a lamina spreader or a hook inserted at the anteromedial rim of the distal fibula that is pulled dorsolaterally (**Fig 3.1-11**).

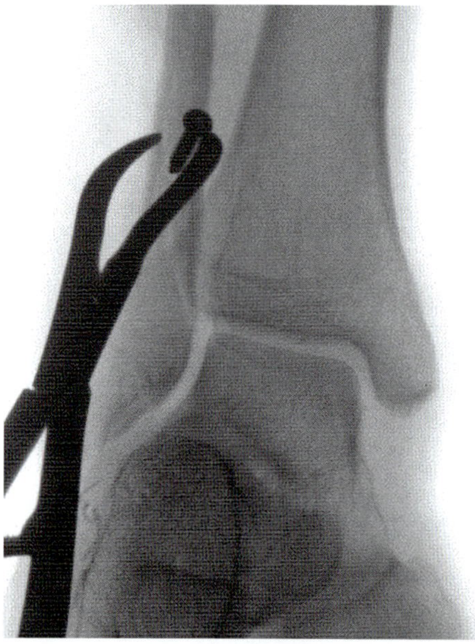

Fig 3.1-8 The cortex lag screw is placed anteroposteriorly and perpendicularly to the fracture line. The position of screw and the talus in the ankle mortise is checked using the C-arm.

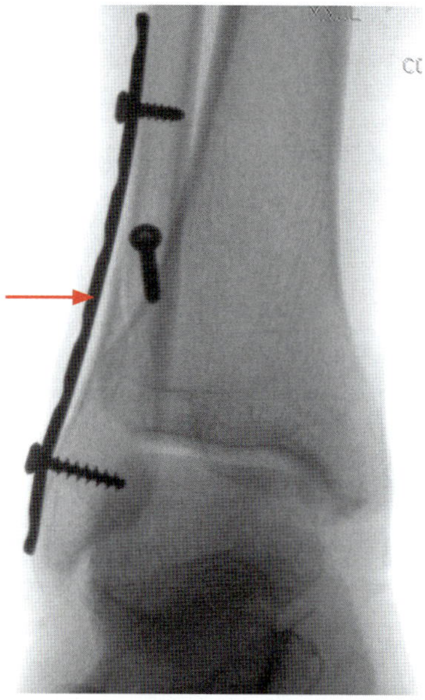

Fig 3.1-9 The plate is undercontoured to allow for maximal compression of the distal fragment. Before screw tightening, the plate is therefore slightly detached from the bone surface (red arrow).

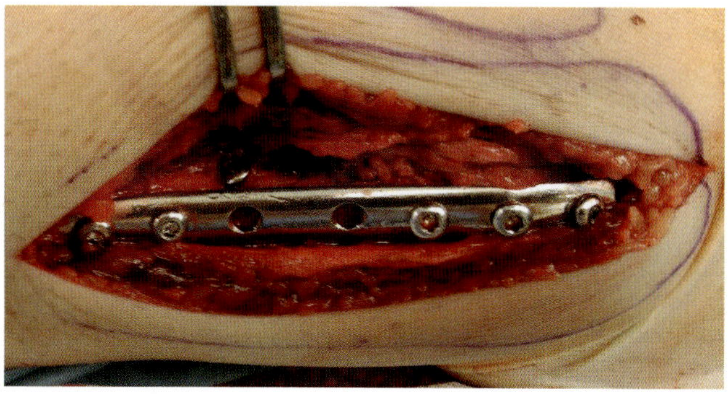

Fig 3.1-10 Completed osteosynthesis using a lag screw combined with a lateral neutralization plate. The plate is fixed distally with three fully threaded cancellous screws and proximally with three cortex screws.

Alternatively, the foot is externally rotated with the lower leg fixed. However, care must be always taken while testing the syndesmosis as over-strenuous stressing may cause failure and pull out of the hardware construct in cases of altered bone density. If the syndesmosis is unstable, it must be reduced into the tibial incisura under C-arm control and direct visualization and fixed to the distal tibia with syndesmotic screws or flexible implant.

The medial side is only opened if perfect mortise reduction is not possible. The deltoid ligament may be interposed between the talus and malleolus in the medial gutter, preventing correct talus position within the mortise. Otherwise, opening the medial side is not indicated as there is no need to directly repair the medial ligaments if the ankle mortise is congruent after a successful osteosynthesis.

Standard x-rays in AP, mortise, and lateral views are obtained after internal fixation (**Fig 3.1-12**).

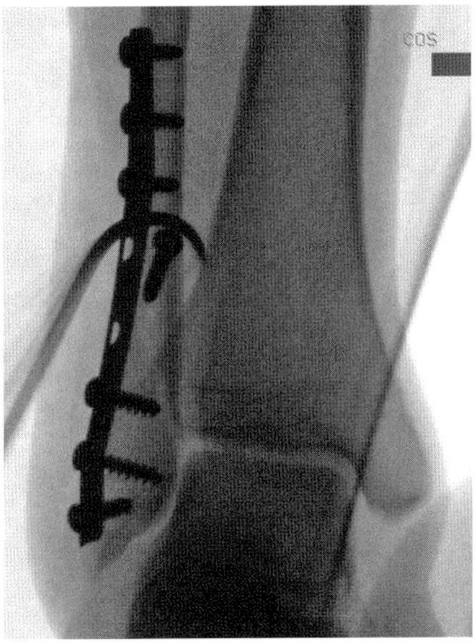

Fig 3.1-11 Hook test for syndesmosis stability under C-arm control (mortise view). The fibula is pulled laterally and dorsally.

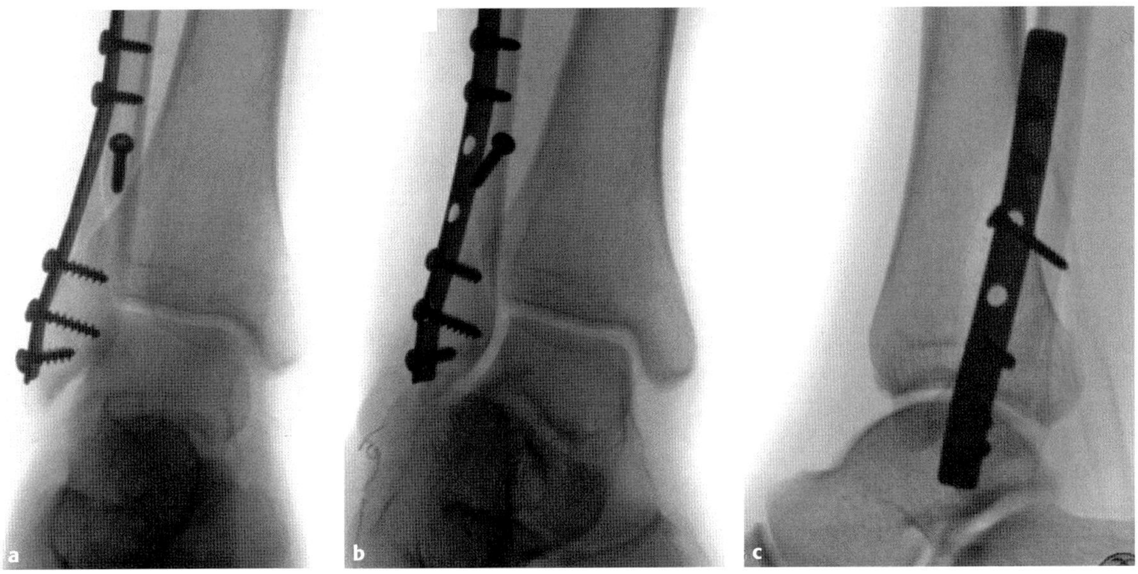

Fig 3.1-12a–c C-arm images taken directly after surgery showing anatomical fracture reduction and correct position of the implants.

a AP view.
b Mortise view.
c Lateral view.

5 Pitfalls and complications

Pitfalls

Malreduction of the distal fibular fragment regarding length and rotation

Small comminution zones on the lateral or anterior side of the distal fibular fragment can cause malreduction. Reduction can best be assessed after removing the periosteum from the posterior aspect along the fracture line at a length of about 1 mm. Here, the distal fragment continues in a spike-like shape proximally and fits precisely into the groove of the proximal fragment (**Fig 3.1-13**).

The anterior aspect of the distal tibia and fibula with the insertion of the anterior tibiofibular (syndesmotic) ligament should be inspected for bony avulsions, as these fragments can prevent proper reduction and lead to syndesmotic instability. The lateral aspect of the joint should be inspected for loose fragments and osteochondral fractures of the talar dome.

In cases of more severe comminution, x-rays of the contralateral ankle can provide a guide to correct anatomy. The fibula must be brought out to length and malrotation has to be corrected. This can be done by using distraction devices to obtain correct length and rotation. Alternatively, correct length can be achieved by securing the plate to the distal fragment and pushing the plate with its attached bony fragment distally using a lamina spreader and a push screw inserted into the fibula proximal to the plate. Rotation must be corrected before distraction is carried out. Care must be taken, especially in osteoporotic bone, to not push the hardware out from within the bone. This is a common problem in locking constructs which are especially useful in soft bone. Any defects should be bone grafted.

Intraarticular insertion of the distal screws

Drilling of the opposite cortex of distal fragment could lead to wrong screw length measurement. A slightly posterior direction of the drill bit is preferred. The depth gauge should be inserted close to the opposite cortex and 2 mm should be subtracted from the measured length (**Fig 3.1-14**). This ensures that a screw of a correct length can be inserted.

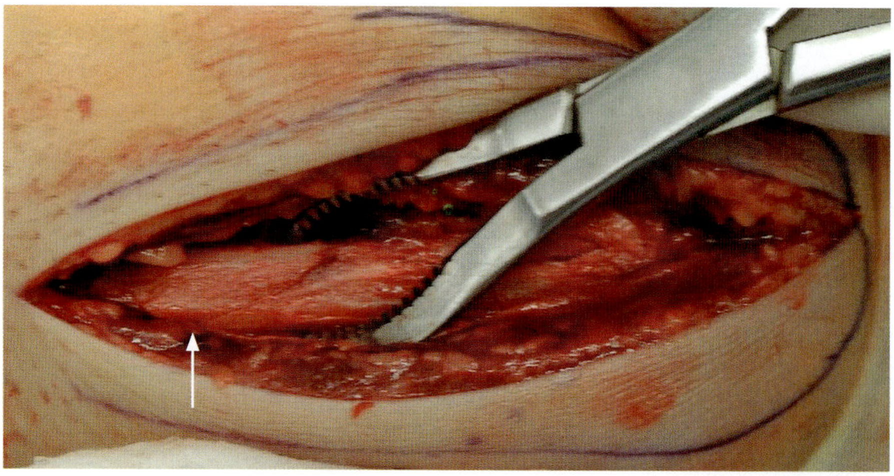

Fig 3.1-13 Anatomical reduction can be assessed best on the dorsal aspect of the fracture line, where distal fragment continues proximally in a spike-like shape (white arrow).

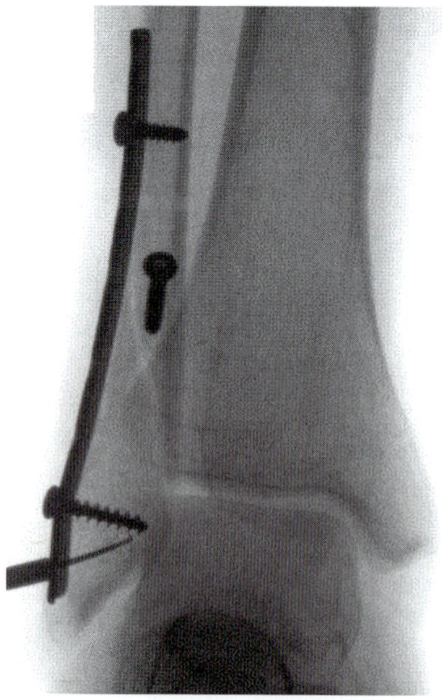

Fig 3.1-14 A slightly posterior direction of drilling is preferred in the distal fragment. The depth gauge should be inserted close to the opposite cortex and 2 mm subtracted from the length measurement.

Overlooking syndesmotic instability

As syndesmotic disruption may be present with AO/OTA 44B1.1 malleolar fractures with syndesmotic instability should be ruled out intraoperatively after fibular fixation. Failure to address syndesmotic bony avulsions can result in both instability and incongruity.

Complications

- Injury to the superficial peroneal nerve—may be prevented by careful dissection in the proximal aspect of the incision
- Loss of fixation (**Fig 3.1-15**)
- Malunion of the distal fibula (mainly malrotation but also shortening, rarely valgus) leading to ankle arthritis (see pitfalls topic for prevention)
- Chronic instability of the syndesmosis resulting in talus dislocation and arthritis (see pitfalls topic for prevention)

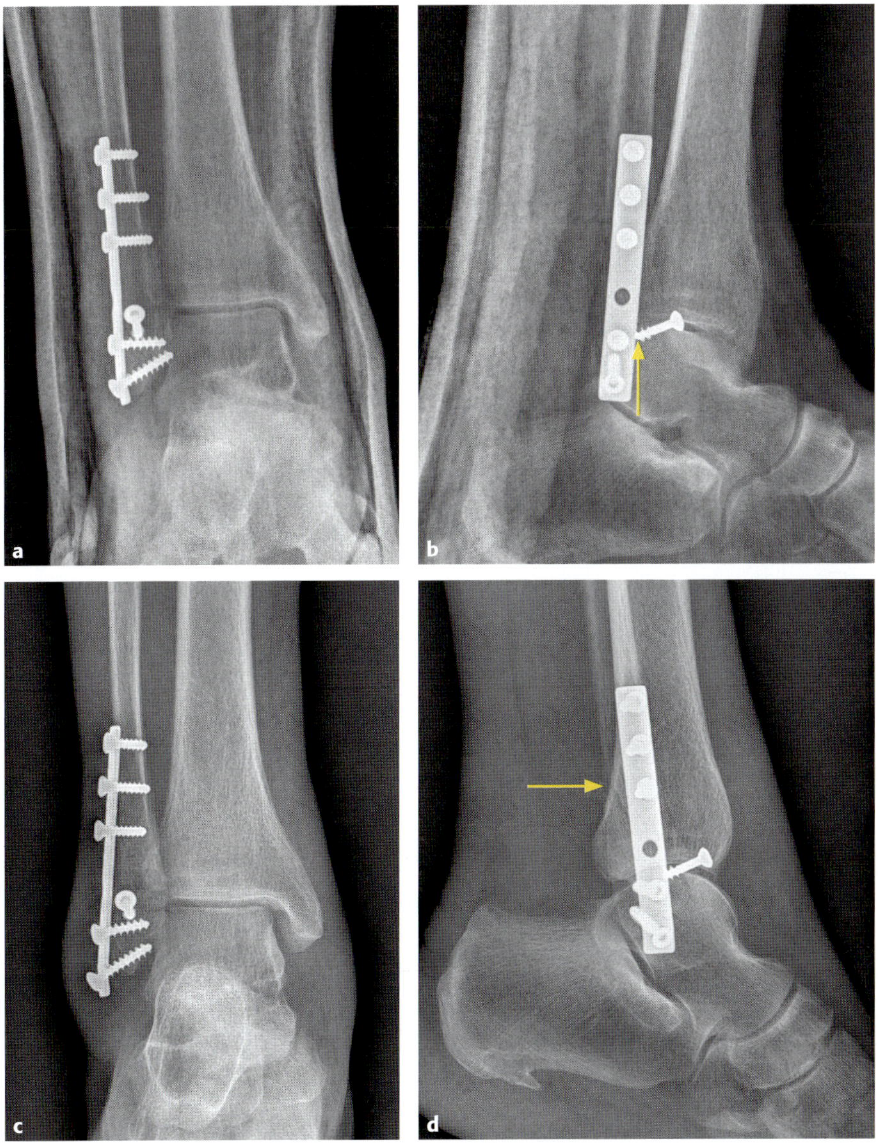

Fig 3.1-15a–d Example from a different case showing loss of fixation as a result of insufficient fixation.

a–b A Weber type B fracture is treated with lag screw and neutralization plate. The lag screw is too short to produce compression (yellow arrow in **b**). The distal screws in the plate are too long. The plate is not contoured properly at the distal end.

c–d Loss of fixation as a result of a lag screw insufficiency. Proximal dislocation of the distal fragment (yellow arrow in **d**) with loosening of the implants distally.

6 Alternative techniques

Longer oblique fracture lines can be stabilized using two or three lag screws without neutralization plate (**Fig 3.1-16**). The patient must be compliant with the postoperative treatment protocol, where weight bearing is restricted for about 6 weeks.

Short oblique or transverse fibular fractures can be fixed with tension band plate applied from the lateral or posterior side.

A one-third tubular antiglide plate may be placed posteriorly with lag screw inserted through plate. Precontouring of the plate is not needed. The plate will fit on the flat surface of the posterolateral fibula. This technique is often used in trimalleolar or pilon fractures reduced from posterolateral approach (**Fig 3.1-17**).

Screws through the distal end of the plate may be placed in bicortical fashion as they exit the fibula anteriorly. However, screw heads might cause irritation to the peroneal tendons if placed within 1 cm to the fibular tip.

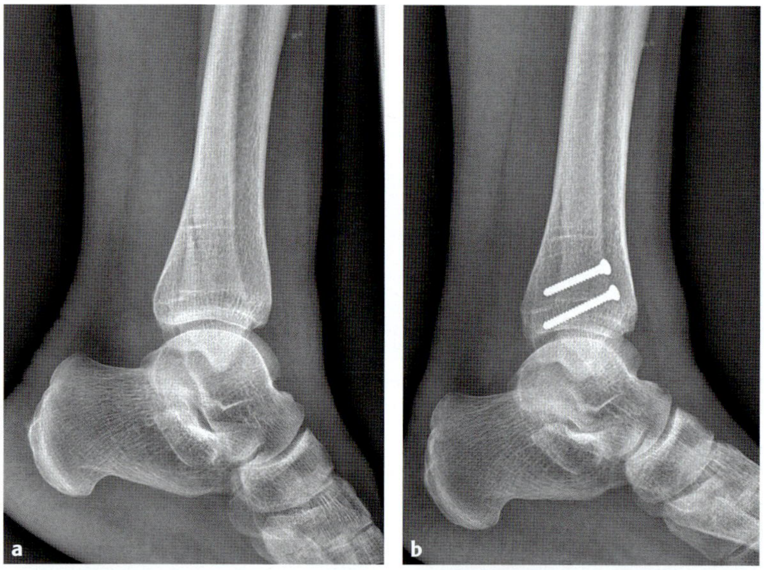

Fig 3.1-16a–b Example from a different case showing two lag screws used for fixation of an oblique distal fibular fracture. Good bone quality is needed to attempt this technique.

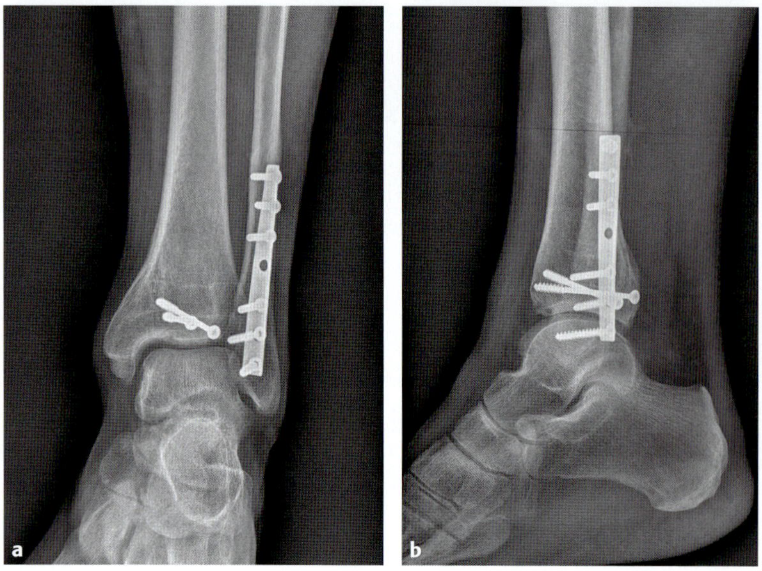

Fig 3.1-17a–b Example from a different case showing an antiglide plate is placed posteriorly with the lag screw inserted through plate in the treatment of a trimalleolar fracture via a posterolateral approach. The plate must stop at least 1 cm proximal to the fibular tip to avoid peroneal tendon irritation.

7 Postoperative management and rehabilitation

For this patient, postoperative passive range-of-motion (ROM) training was initiated after suction drainage removal. X-rays of his ankle joint in three planes after mobilization with partial weight bearing did not reveal any loss of reduction (**Fig 3.1-18**).

After 6 weeks a rehabilitation protocol consisting of ROM exercises and muscle training was initiated. Weight bearing was gradually increased over the next 4 weeks. The patient achieved full bony union 10 weeks after surgery with a final ROM comparable to the uninjured side.

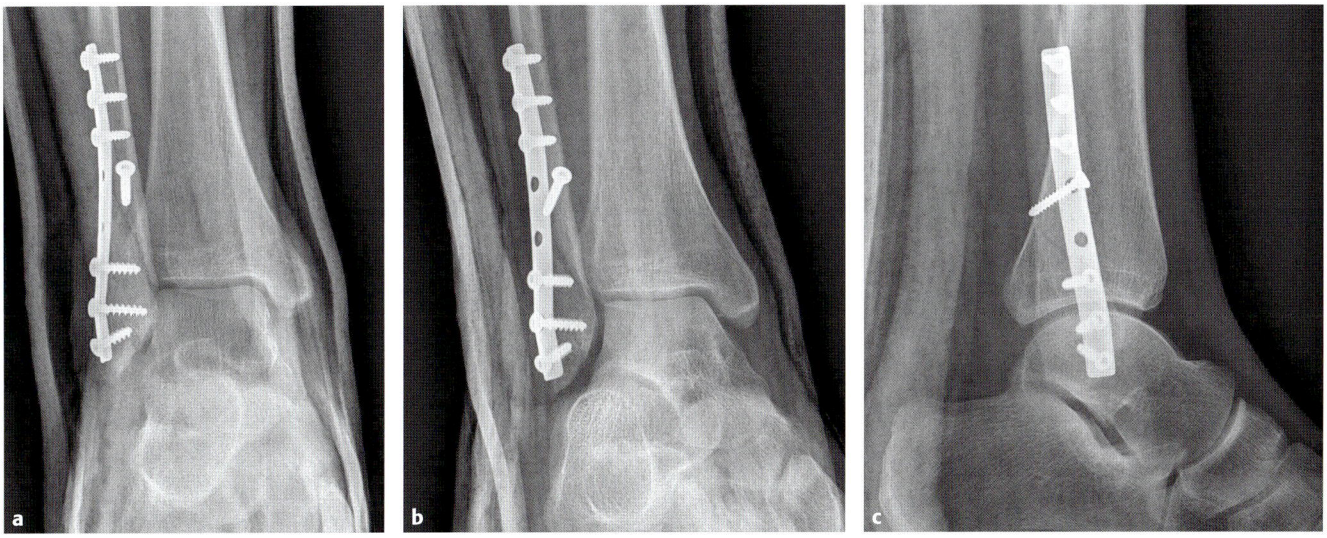

Fig 3.1-18a–c X-rays in three planes after removal of the suction drain.
a AP view.
b Mortise view.
c Lateral view.

8 Recommended reading

Heim D, Schmidlin V, Ziviello O. Do type B malleolar fractures need a positioning screw? *Injury.* 2002 Oct;33(8):729–734.
Jenkinson RJ, Sanders DW, Macleod MD, et al. Intraoperative diagnosis of syndesmosis injuries in external rotation ankle fractures. *J Orthop Trauma.* 2005 Oct;19(9):604–609.
Kortekangas T, Flinkkila T, Niinimaki J, et al. Effect of syndesmosis injury in SER IV (Weber B)-type ankle fractures on function and incidence of osteoarthritis. *Foot Ankle Int.* 2015 Feb;36(2):180–187.
McKenna PB, O'Shea K, Burke T. Less is more: lag screw only fixation of lateral malleolar fractures. *Int Orthop.* 2007 Aug;31(4):497–502.
Michelson JD. Ankle fractures resulting from rotational injuries. *J Am Acad Orthop Surg.* 2003 Nov-Dec;11(6):403–412.
Nortunen S, Lepojarvi S, Savola O, et al. Stability assessment of the ankle mortise in supination-external rotation-type ankle fractures: lack of additional diagnostic value of MRI. *J Bone Joint Surg Am.* 2014 Nov 19;96(22):1855–1862.
Rammelt S, Zwipp H. Ankle fractures. In: Bentley G, ed. *European Instructional Course Lectures, Volume 12.* Berlin Heidelberg New York: Springer; 2012:205–219.
Spering C, Lesche V, Dresing K. Osteosynthesis of Weber B ankle fractures using the one-third tubular plate and refixation of the syndesmosis. *Oper Orthop Traumatol.* 2015 Aug;27(4):317–333.

3.2 Bimalleolar transsyndesmotic fracture (Weber B) with transverse medial malleolar fracture

Lubomír Kopp, Petr Obruba

1 Case description

A 52-year-old man twisted his left ankle when walking on rough terrain. The resulting severe dislocation was reduced immediately by a paramedic at the scene and immobilized in a vacuum splint. Intravenous analgesia was administered, and he was transferred to hospital. Diagnostic x-rays of the ankle revealed a bimalleolar fracture dislocation (AO/OTA type 44 B3.2, Danis/Weber type B, supination-external rotation stage 4 fracture according to Lauge-Hansen) (**Fig 3.2-1**).

There were no comorbidities. Initial reduction alleviated pressure on the soft tissues. The injury was closed and was neurovascularly intact after reduction (**Fig 3.2-2**).

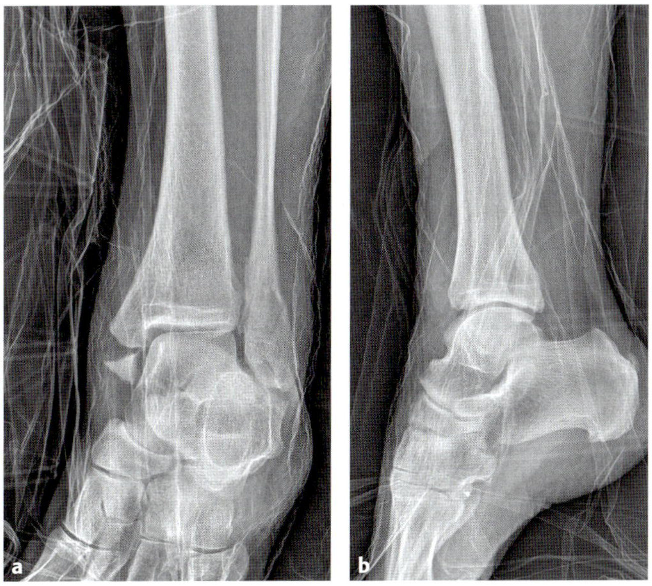

Fig 3.2-1a–b Diagnostic x-rays of the left ankle after gross reduction and immobilization in a vacuum splint after the injury.
a Mortise view.
b Lateral view.

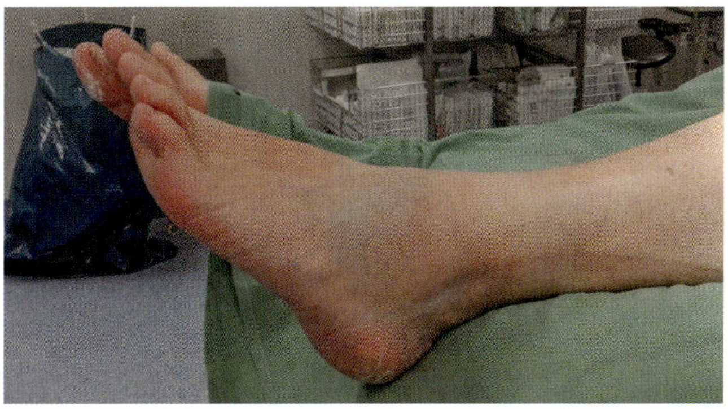

Fig 3.2-2 Correct initial reduction protected the soft tissues from further damage and enabled early surgery.

Computed tomographic (CT) scanning with 2D and 3D reconstructions was performed to exclude fracture of the posterior malleolus, which could require different incisions as part of the treatment strategy (**Fig 3.2-3**).

2 Preoperative planning

Indications for surgery

Surgery is indicated as this is an unstable (AO/OTA 44B3.2) bimalleolar fracture dislocation with gentle swelling of soft tissues allowed for early open reduction and internal fixation (ORIF). According to the injury mechanism and fracture type, the syndesmosis is usually stable after fixation of the distal fibula. However, it should be stress tested to assure no instability is present.

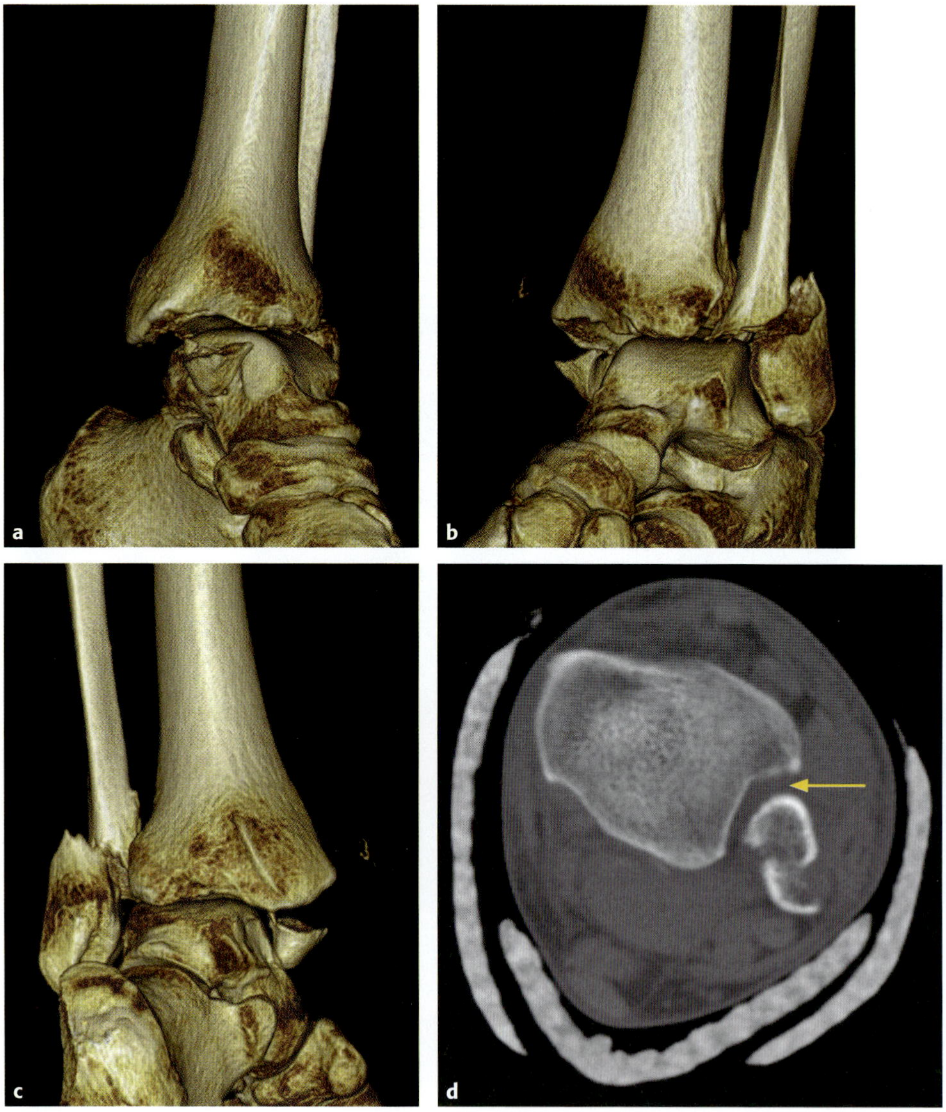

Fig 3.2-3a–d Computed tomographic images.

a–c 3D reconstructions of the CT scans reveal characteristic supination-external rotation injury. Bony avulsions of the syndesmosis and a fracture of the posterior tibial rim (posterior malleolar fracture) is ruled out.

d Axial CT scan shows a correct position of the distal fibular fragment with respect to the distal tibia at the level of the syndesmosis as a sign of intact anterior and interosseous tibiofibular ligaments (yellow arrow).

The short, simple oblique fibular fracture should be fixed with a lag screw and neutralization plate or a posterior antiglide plate.

The fracture of the medial malleolus should be fixed via an axial medial approach with screws or tension band wiring, depending on fragment size (**Fig 3.2-4**). A combination of a compression screw and a K-wire does not provide uniform compression and rigid fixation across the fracture plane.

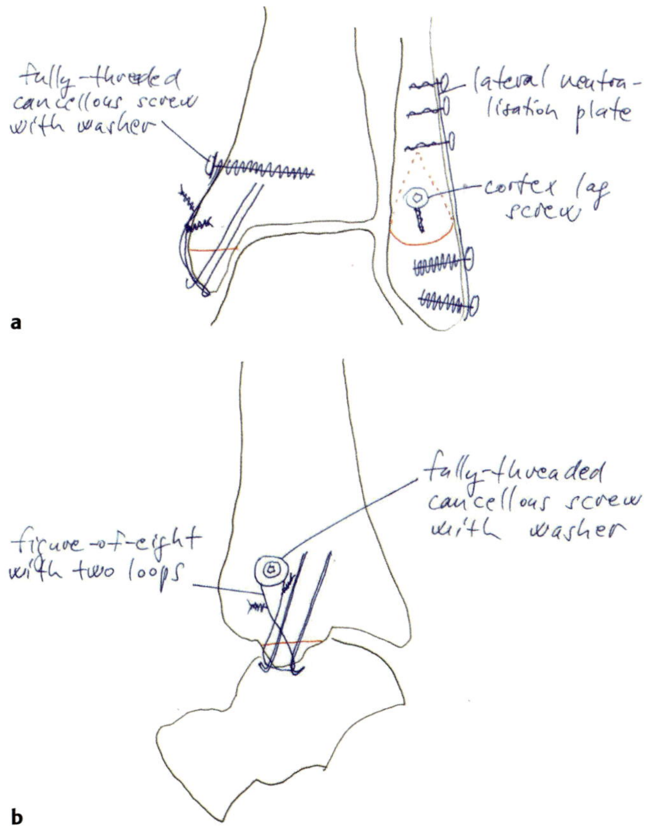

Fig 3.2-4a–b Preoperative plan.

a The short simple oblique fibular fracture is fixed first via a lateral approach using a lag screw and a neutralization plate.

b The fracture of the medial malleolus is fixed via a medial approach with tension band wiring.

3 Operating room setup

Patient positioning	• Supine on a radiolucent table with the injured leg placed on a foam block and draped above the ankle. This enables the surgeon to access both the medial and lateral side.
Anesthesia options	• Regional or general anesthesia (or a combination of both)
C-arm location	• C-arm is placed on the patient's uninjured side with the screen positioned near the head of patient.
Tourniquet	• Used at surgeon's discretion

For illustrations and overview of anesthetic considerations, see chapter 1.

Equipment

- 1.6–2.0 mm K-wires, tension band wire
- 3.5 mm (2.7 or 2.4 mm) fully threaded cortex screws
- 4.0 mm cancellous screws, washers
- One-third tubular plate (can be locking which might be helpful in soft bone)
- Bone hook or lamina spreader

4 Surgical procedure

For ORIF of bimalleolar fractures, lateral and medial approaches are needed. The type B fibular fracture should be reduced first followed by direct inspection of the anterior tibiofibular ligament and anterolateral aspect of the ankle joint.

Fibular fixation

The longitudinal lateral incision is placed slightly anteriorly to enable direct visualization of the anterior tibiofibular ligament (**Fig 3.2-5**). The superficial peroneal nerve is identified and protected (**Fig 3.2-6**). Alternatively, the incision may be placed more posterior, allowing the nerve to remain safely in the anterior soft tissues, bearing in mind that the course of the nerve may be variable. The incision should be long enough to avoid tension on the soft tissues. Carefully placed small retractors allow for visualization of reduction. The oblique fracture line is identified and cleared of hematoma and interposed periosteum and then reduced with a point-to-point reduction clamps. Attention must be paid to correct length and rotation of the distal fragment. A cortex lag screw is then placed in an anteroposterior direction nearly perpendicular to the fracture line and firmly tightened, taking care to not break the anterior cortex. A neutralization plate is contoured in its distal part to follow the shape of the distal fibula. No bending in the central part is necessary (**Fig 3.2-7**). When tightening such a plate to the fibular diaphysis, this undercontouring will compress the distal fragment medially against the externally rotated talus and thus help with reduction and enhance the stability of fixation. The plate is secured with a minimum of two screws distally and preferably three screws proximally. Although most screws are self-tapping, a tap may be used in patients with hard cortical bone but this is rarely necessary.

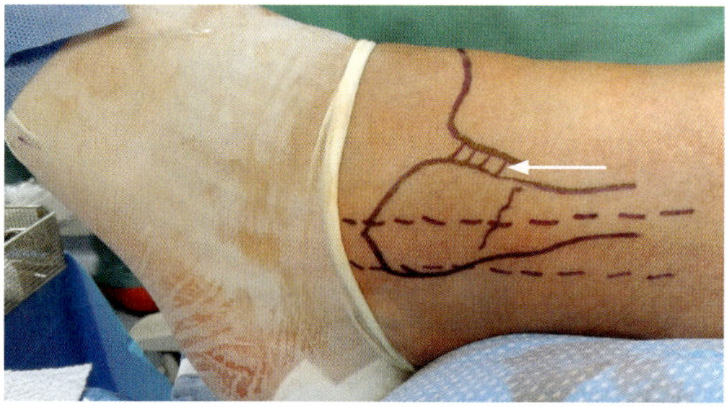

Fig 3.2-5 Lateral approach to the fibula, through a slightly ventral incision is used to enable direct visual control of anterior tibiofibular ligament (white arrow).

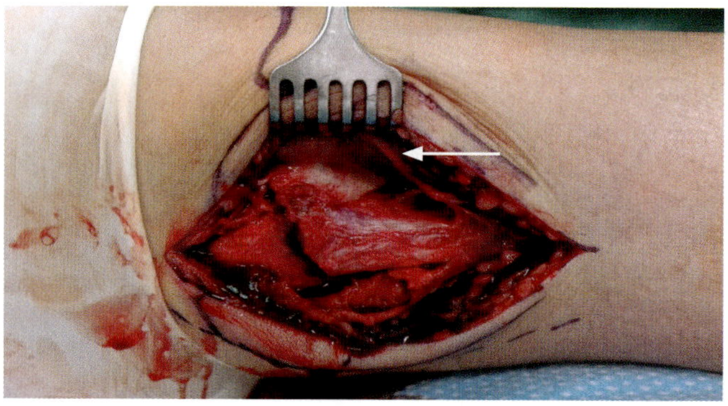

Fig 3.2-6 The superficial peroneal nerve (white arrow) should be protected.

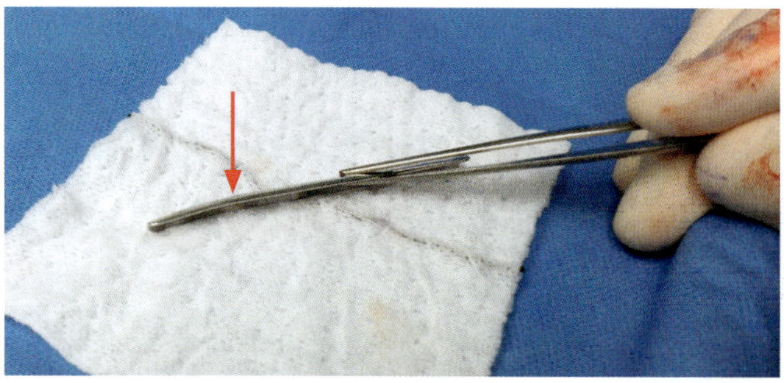

Fig 3.2-7 The neutralization plate is slightly contoured in its distal part (red arrow) to imitate the shape of the distal fibula. Preloading of the central part compresses the distal fragment medially.

Completion of fibular osteosynthesis is followed by inspection of the syndesmosis for any intervening anterior and interosseous tibiofibular ligament and the presence of a Tillaux-Chaput or Wagstaffe fragment at the anterior tubercle of the tibia or fibula, respectively. A stress test of syndesmosis stability under the C-arm is essential. Testing can be accomplished with a bone hook or lamina spreader. It is necessary to position the ankle in the mortise view to allow for exact visualization of distal fibular mobility (**Fig 3.2-8**). The fibula is then pulled laterally and posteriorly, and the ligamentous stability of the syndesmosis is assessed with the C-arm and visually. Any observed instability must be addressed with syndesmosis stabilization (see chapter 3.4).

Medial malleolar fixation

The medial malleolar fracture is reduced via an axial incision starting along the medial malleolus then curving slightly anterior toward the medial utility line (**Fig 3.2-9**). The fracture line and the underlying joint area are inspected and any talar impact lesions are noted. The gutter and superior joint facets are cleared of any fracture debris and fragments that could otherwise prevent anatomical reduction (**Fig 3.2-10**). The posterior margin of the fracture is inspected for any soft-tissue interposition.

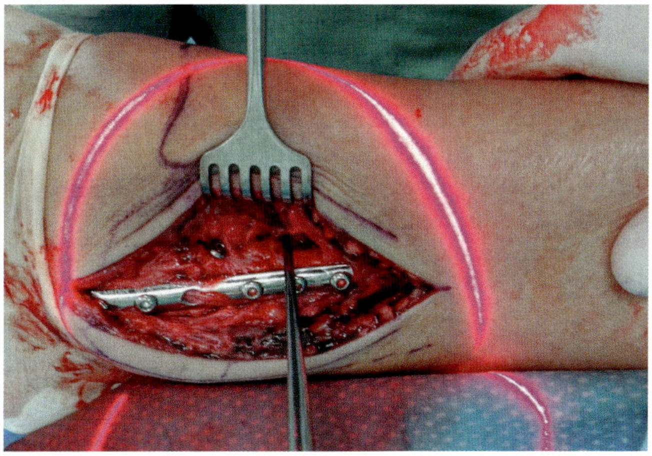

Fig 3.2-8 Hook test of syndesmotic stability. The fibula is pulled laterally and posteriorly and the ligamentous stability of the syndesmosis is assessed using the C-arm and visually. A laser pointer helps in aiming the C-arm, thus reducing the amount of radiation.

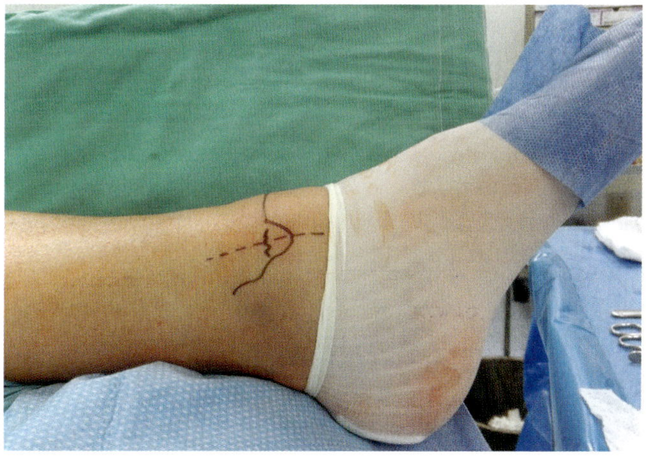

Fig 3.2-9 Longitudinal medial approach. The greater saphenous vein should be protected.

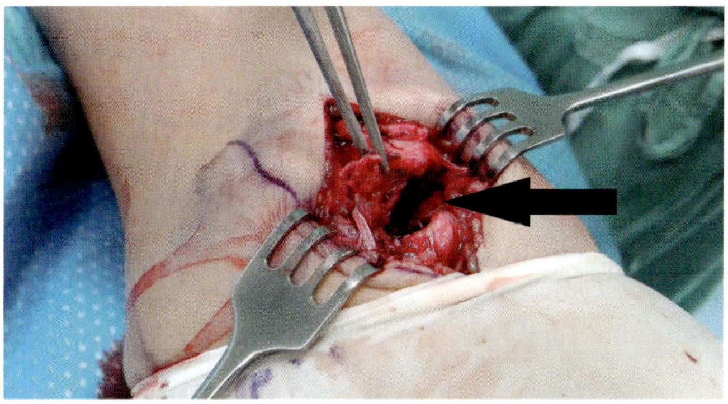

Fig 3.2-10 Longitudinal medial approach. The fracture line is cleared of periosteum and small fragments, which could otherwise intervene with reduction (black arrow). The joint surface is visualized in the anterior part of the approach, the flexor tendons are protected behind the medial malleolus.

Reduction is usually achieved with a pointed clamps or manually with a dental scaler, and joint congruity is controlled visually at the anterior/superior margin, along the shoulder of the medial malleolus. The fracture fragment may be small and fixation can be performed with 2.7 mm screws or tension band wiring. If tension band technique is used, the wires should be advanced to the intact opposite cortex to achieve stable fixation. Two parallel K-wires are inserted into the reduced medial malleolus perpendicularly to the fracture line. A unicortical cancellous screw with washer is inserted approximately 2 cm above the fracture line and parallel to the joint surface. A figure-of-eight with two loops is formed from wire. Both loops must be tightened at the same time and in the same direction to prevent unequal distribution of compression forces, leading to loss of reduction (**Fig 3.2-11**). Use of the parallel 2.0 mm wire guide facilitates placement of parallel wires while also helping to maintain reduction.

If lag screw technique is used, the fracture is reduced and provisionally fixed with K-wires. The reduction is checked on AP and lateral C-arm views and the wires are replaced with screws. The wires are removed one at a time. The near fracture fragment track is then overdrilled using a 2.7 mm drill and a 40–50 mm screw is carefully inserted but not overtightened. Once the first screw is in place, the second wire is removed, the track overdrilled with the 2.7 mm drill, and a second 2.7 mm screw is inserted, again taking care not to overtighten across the fracture as this may displace the fragments. Washers are rarely if ever needed, as the two screw heads adequately hold the fragment. If the fragment is extremely small or comminuted, smaller diameter screws including 2.4 mm screws can be used. Alternatively, small wires can be used to reduce the fracture, then bent at the ends, inserted to the cortex, and left in place.

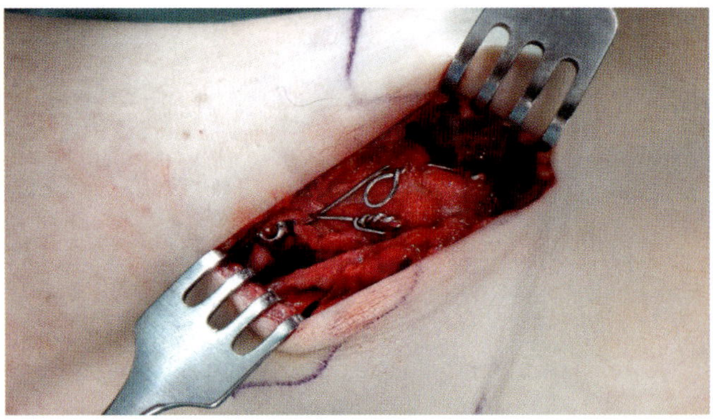

Fig 3.2-11 Tension band wiring. A figure-of-eight with two loops is formed from wire and fixed proximally with a cancellous screw with washer.

Precise C-arm images in all three planes (AP, mortise, and lateral) are made after completion of internal fixation (**Fig 3.2-12**). If in doubt, especially concerning rotation of distal fibular fragment and position of the medial malleolus, an intraoperative 3D C-arm imaging can be performed if available. As the rotation of distal fibula varies according to patients' bone anatomy, the specificity of this examination is not high and cannot be recommended in general if the other side is not examined, too.

5 Pitfalls and complications

Pitfalls

Inadequate reduction of distal fibular fragment in means of length, axis, and rotation

Inserting a lag screw nearly perpendicular to a short oblique fracture line can bring the dorsal part of screw head into contact with the proximal fragment during tightening, causing deviation of the screw and loss of reduction. In shorter oblique fractures lag screw fixation may not be possible and reduction should be maintained in anatomical fashion using reduction clamps until all implants have been inserted. Alternatively, the plate may be placed posterior to provide an antiglide effect on these short oblique fractures.

Tightening of an eccentrically positioned, laterally placed fibular neutralization plate can generate torque forces on the distal fragment caused by uneven pressure distribution and leading to rotational malposition of the distal fragment. The plate must be always centered on the long axis of the fibula when placed laterally.

Malreduction of the distal fibula (shortening, malrotation, anteroposterior translation) can be avoided in simple, oblique fractures with adequate visual control of the fracture line and intraoperative imaging of the proper fibular length using Weber radiographic indices (**Fig 3.2-13**):

- Trilateral intervals of the ankle joint should be equal and parallel.
- The medial spike of the fibula ("Weber nose") should indicate the level of the tibial subchondral bone (Shenton line of the ankle).
- The contour of the lateral part of the articular surface of the talus continues as an unbroken curve to the peroneal recess in the distal fibula (Weber ball ["dime sign"]).

Inadequate medial malleolar fixation in patients with osteoporosis

Monocortically inserted screws could be pulled out in osteoporotic bone. Bicortical screw insertion enhances the stability but if two parallel screws are used loss of reduction is extremely rare, provided that they are long enough to enter the metaphyseal bone.

In smaller medial fragments with osteoporotic bone the tightening of screws or tension band could cause comminution, compression, or medial dislocation of the fragment (**Fig 3.2-14**). In such cases, screws or tension band should be tightened gently. In some cases, smaller diameter screws may be necessary.

Any implant should be placed in the anterior two thirds of the medial malleolus to avoid irritation of the tibialis posterior tendon.

Complications

- Injury to the superficial peroneal nerve
- Injury to the greater saphenous vein
- Missed ligamentous instability of the syndesmosis resulting in chronic syndesmotic instability with lateral talar shift and posttraumatic arthritis
- Malunion resulting in posttraumatic arthritis
- Nonunion of the medial or lateral malleolus (mostly after inadequate fixation)

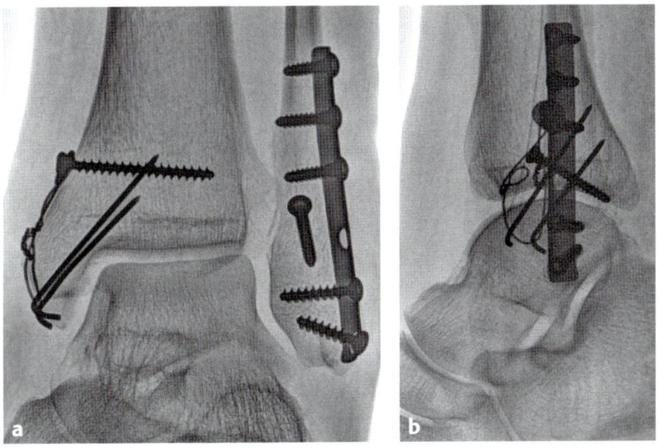

Fig 3.2-12a–b C-arm images taken directly after surgery showing anatomical fracture reduction and correct position of implants. The fibula is fixed with a lag screw and neutralization plate, and the medial malleolus with tension band wiring. K-wires are inserted perpendicularly to the fracture line and parallel to each other to enable axial compression when tensioning the wire.

a Mortise view.

b Lateral view.

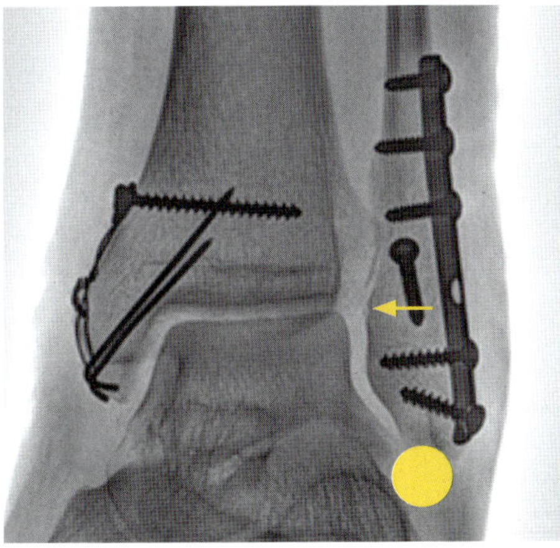

Fig 3.2-13 Radiographic indices include the fibular spike ("Weber nose", see arrow) and circle from the distal fibula to the lateral talar process (Weber ball ["dime sign"]) see circle).

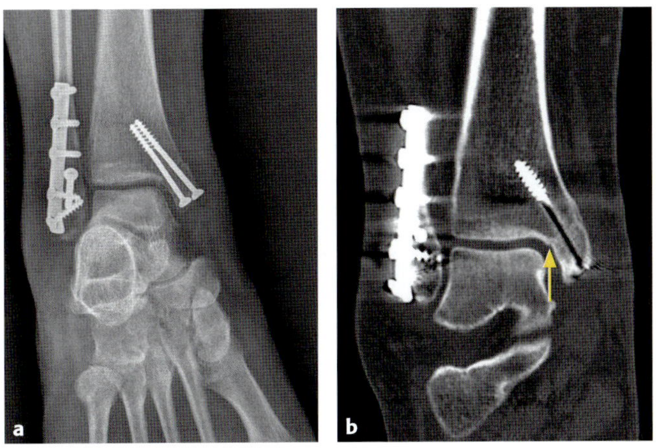

Fig 3.2-14a–b Example from a different case showing dislocation of the medial malleolus during screw tightening.

a In patients with osteoporosis, excessive load exerted by lag screws can cause compression of medial cortex and medial dislocation of fragment.

b The 2D CT reconstruction in coronal plane confirms medial dislocation of fragment (yellow arrow). Lag screws or tension band should be tightened gently in patients with osteoporosis.

6 Alternative techniques

A large medial malleolar fragment can be fixed with two 4.0, 3.5, or 2.7 mm lag screws introduced in a parallel fashion. The length of the required approach is shorter (**Fig 3.2-15**). Larger screws can irritate soft tissues (**Fig 3.2-16**).

A tension band plate can be used for fibular fracture fixation in cases of a short oblique fibular fracture line, where a lag screw cannot be used (**Fig 3.2-17**). In patients with osteoporosis, a locking plate can increase stability of fixation (**Fig 3.2-18**).

Alternatively, for fibular fixation a one-third tubular plate may be placed posterior on the fibula in antiglide fashion. This position allows bicortical fixation using cortex screws distally.

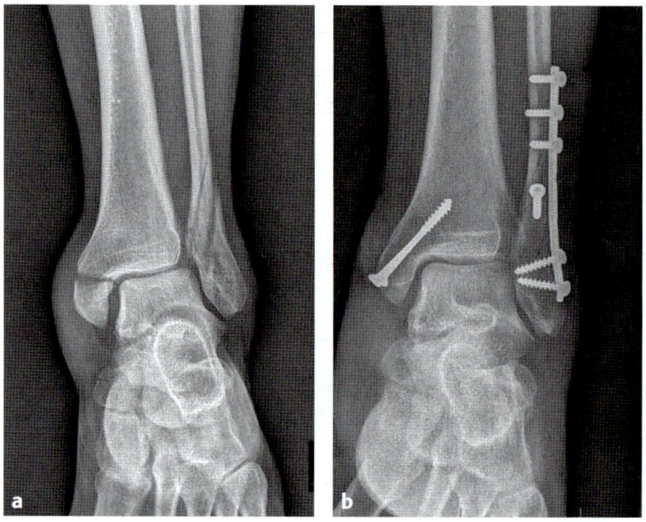

Fig 3.2-15a–b Example from a different case showing a medial malleolus fixed with 4.0 mm lag screws. The length of the required approach is smaller than for a tension band wire cerclage.

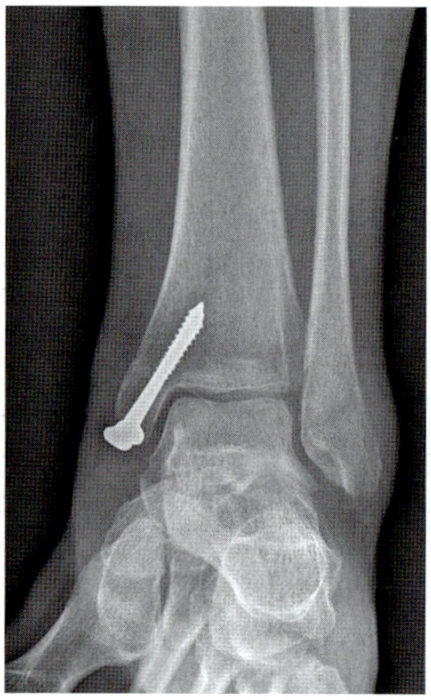

Fig 3.2-16 Example from a different case showing the large screw heads of these "malleolar" screws which can easily irritate the soft tissues and break smaller fragments. These screws offer no advantage over smaller sized screws and should probably not be used.

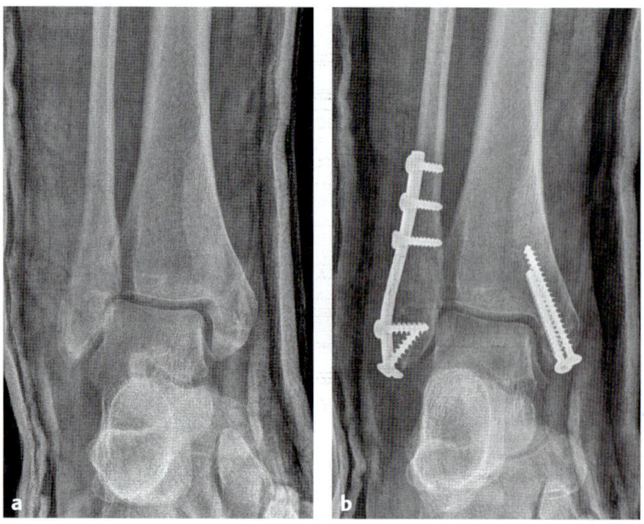

Fig 3.2-17a–b Example from a different case showing a tension band plate used for fixation of a very short oblique or transverse fibular fracture.

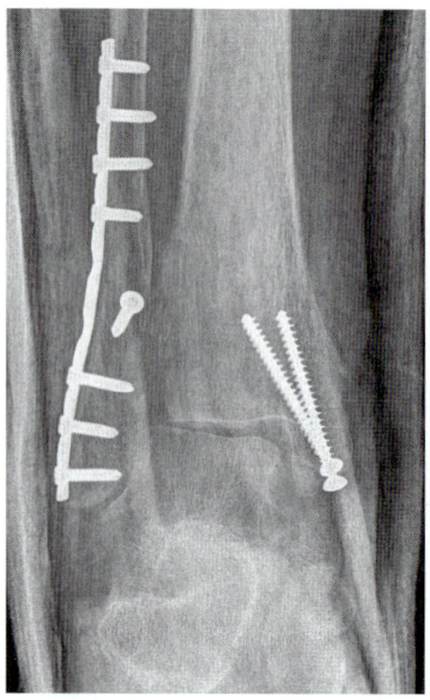

Fig 3.2-18 Example from a different case showing locking plate used as a neutralization plate in a patient with severe osteoporosis to increase stability of fixation.

7 Postoperative management and rehabilitation

For this patient the ankle joint was immobilized postoperatively in a short lower leg cast and cryotherapy was applied. Standard x-rays of the ankle joint in three planes were performed (**Fig 3.2-19**).

In case of any doubt CT scan is recommended to detect fragment malreduction or material malposition. Both ankles should be scanned to assess correct length and rotation of distal fibular fragment on the injured side compared with the uninjured ankle when there is concern for malreduction.

For this patient, active and passive range-of-motion training were initiated on postoperative day 2 and the patient was restricted to partial weight bearing (up to 20 kg) for the next 6 weeks. Upon radiographic bony union, weight bearing was gradually increased over the next 4 weeks.

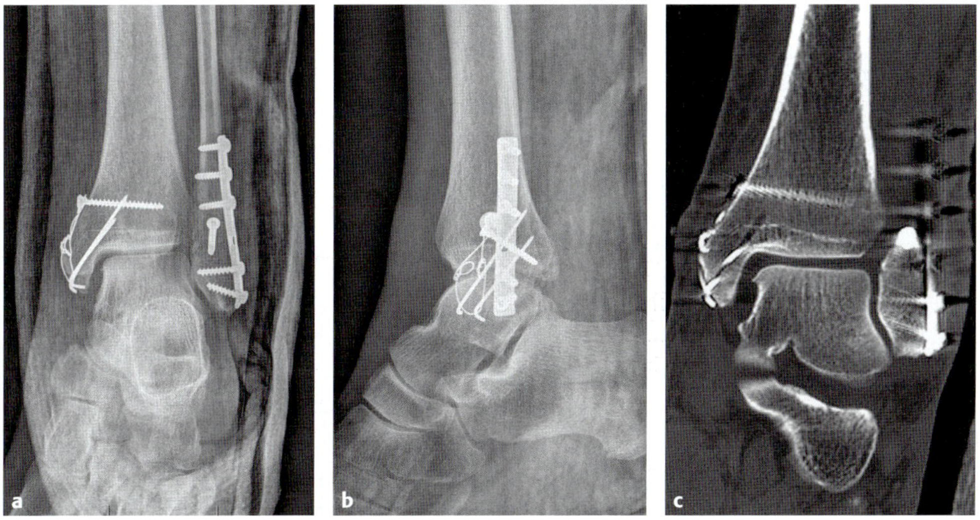

Fig 3.2-19a–c X-ray and CT images after removal of the suction drain.
a–b AP and lateral view in lower leg cast.
c The 2D CT in coronal plane confirms anatomical reduction of the medial and lateral malleolus.

The patient achieved full bony union 10 weeks after surgery (**Fig 3.2-20**) with a final range of motion comparable with the uninjured side.

Implant removal

Ideally implants are maintained for at least a year after fixation. Prominent implants on the medial and lateral malleolus are removed only after achieving full bony union and clinical findings consistent with hardware irritation.

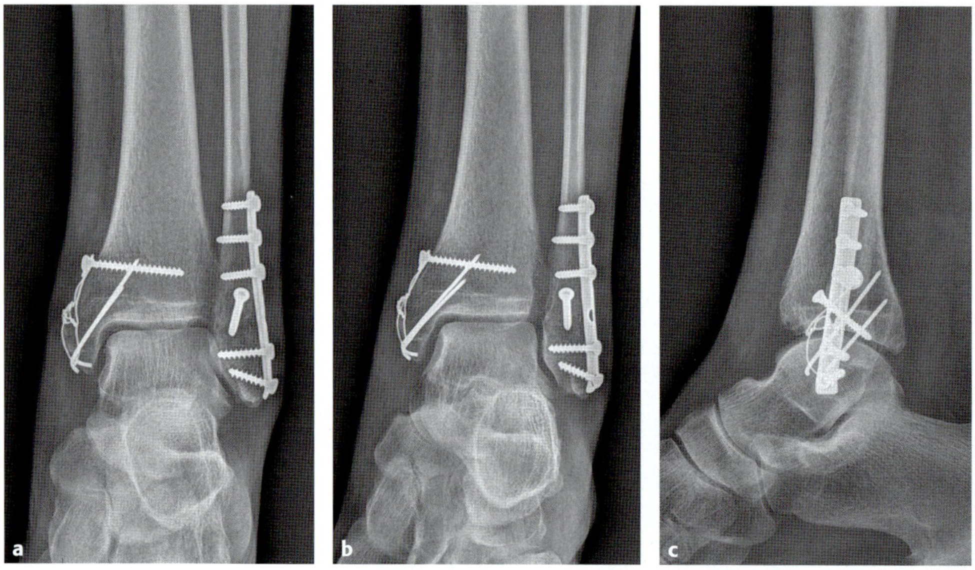

Fig 3.2-20a–c X-rays 10 weeks after surgery showing full bony union and correct position of the talus within the mortise.
- **a** AP view.
- **b** Mortise view.
- **c** Lateral view.

8 Recommended reading

Barnes H, Cannada LK, Watson JT. A clinical evaluation of alternative fixation techniques for medial malleolus fractures. *Injury*. 2014 Sep;45(9):1365–1367.

Heim D, Schmidlin V, Ziviello O. Do type B malleolar fractures need a positioning screw? *Injury*. 2002 Oct;33(8):729–734.

Kwon JY, Gitajn IL, Walton P, et al. A cadaver study revisiting the original methodology of Lauge-Hansen and a commentary on modern usage. *J Bone Joint Surg Am*. 2015 Apr 1;97(7):604–609.

Lauge-Hansen N. Fractures of the ankle: II. Combined experimental-surgical and experimental-roentgenologic investigations. *Arch Surg*. 1950 May;60(5):957–985.

McKenna PB, O'Shea K, Burke T. Less is more: lag screw only fixation of lateral malleolar fractures. *Int Orthop*. 2007 Aug;31(4):497–502.

Michelson JD. Ankle fractures resulting from rotational injuries. *J Am Acad Orthop Surg*. 2003 Nov–Dec;11(6):403–412.

Mohammed AA, Abbas KA, Mawlood AS. A comparative study in fixation methods of medial malleolus fractures between tension bands wiring and screw fixation. *Springerplus*. 2016;5:530.

Rammelt S, Boszczyk A. Computed tomography in the diagnosis and treatment of ankle fractures: a critical analysis review. *JBJS Rev*. 2018 Dec;6(12):e7.

SooHoo NF, Krenek L, Eagan MJ, et al. Complication rates following open reduction and internal fixation of ankle fractures. *J Bone Joint Surg Am*. 2009 May;91(5):1042–1049.

Tan EW, Sirisreetreerux N, Paez AG, et al. Early weightbearing after operatively treated ankle fractures: a biomechanical analysis. *Foot Ankle Int*. 2016 Jun;37(6):652–658.

Verhage SM, Schipper IB, Hoogendoorn JM. Long-term functional and radiographic outcomes in 243 operated ankle fractures. *J Foot Ankle Res*. 2015 Aug 25;8:45.

Wang X, Zhang C, Yin JW, et al. Treatment of medial malleolus or pure deltoid ligament injury in patients with supination-external rotation type IV ankle fractures. *Orthop Surg*. 2017 Feb;9(1):42–48.

Weber BG, Colton C. Malleolar fractures. In: Müller M, Allgöwer M, Schneider R, et al, eds. *Manual of Internal Fixation*. Berlin: Springer; 1991:595–612.

3.3 Distal fibular infrasyndesmotic fracture (Weber A) with medial malleolar vertical fracture and joint impaction

Lubomír Kopp, Petr Obruba

1 Case description

A 46-year-old man severely twisted his left ankle when he fell from a scaffold. The primary injury pattern was described as supination which resulted in ankle dislocation. The injury was self-reduced. He was immediately brought to hospital. The ankle was immobilized in vacuum splint, and intravenous analgesics were administered. Diagnostic x-rays of the ankle revealed a transverse fracture of the distal fibula below the syndesmosis, a suspected fracture of the medial malleolus, and a fracture of the anterior tibial rim (**Fig 3.3-1**).

Computed tomographic (CT) scans with 2D and 3D reconstructions revealed a AO/OTA 44A2.3 fracture (Danis/Weber type A, supination-abduction stage 2 according to Lauge-Hansen) with a vertical medial malleolar fracture, impacted articular segment, avulsion fracture of the anterior tibial rim, and horizontal infrasydesmotic fibular fracture (**Fig 3.3-2**). The patient had no comorbidities.

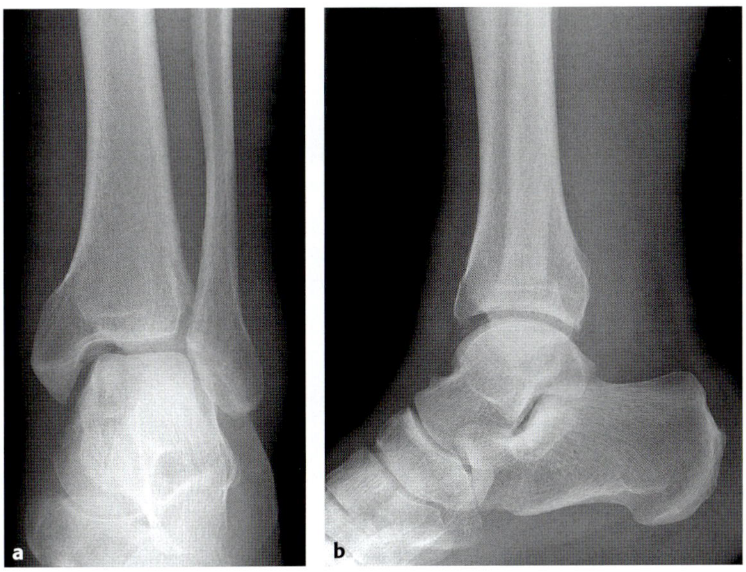

Fig 3.3-1a–b Diagnostic x-rays of the injury with a suspected fracture of the medial malleolus and anterior tibial rim.

a AP view.
b Lateral view.

2 Preoperative planning

Indications for surgery

An unstable AO/OTA 44A2.3 fracture with minimal swelling of the soft tissues may be considered for early open reduction and internal fixation (ORIF). According to the fracture type, the syndesmosis is not expected to be injured. Bimalleolar injuries are unstable, consequently surgery is indicated.

Articular impaction of the medial plafond is another indication for surgical treatment of this injury.

Treatment options

The simple transverse fibular fracture should be provisionally fixed first to regain proper anatomical alignment, which results in an anatomical position of the talus and enables

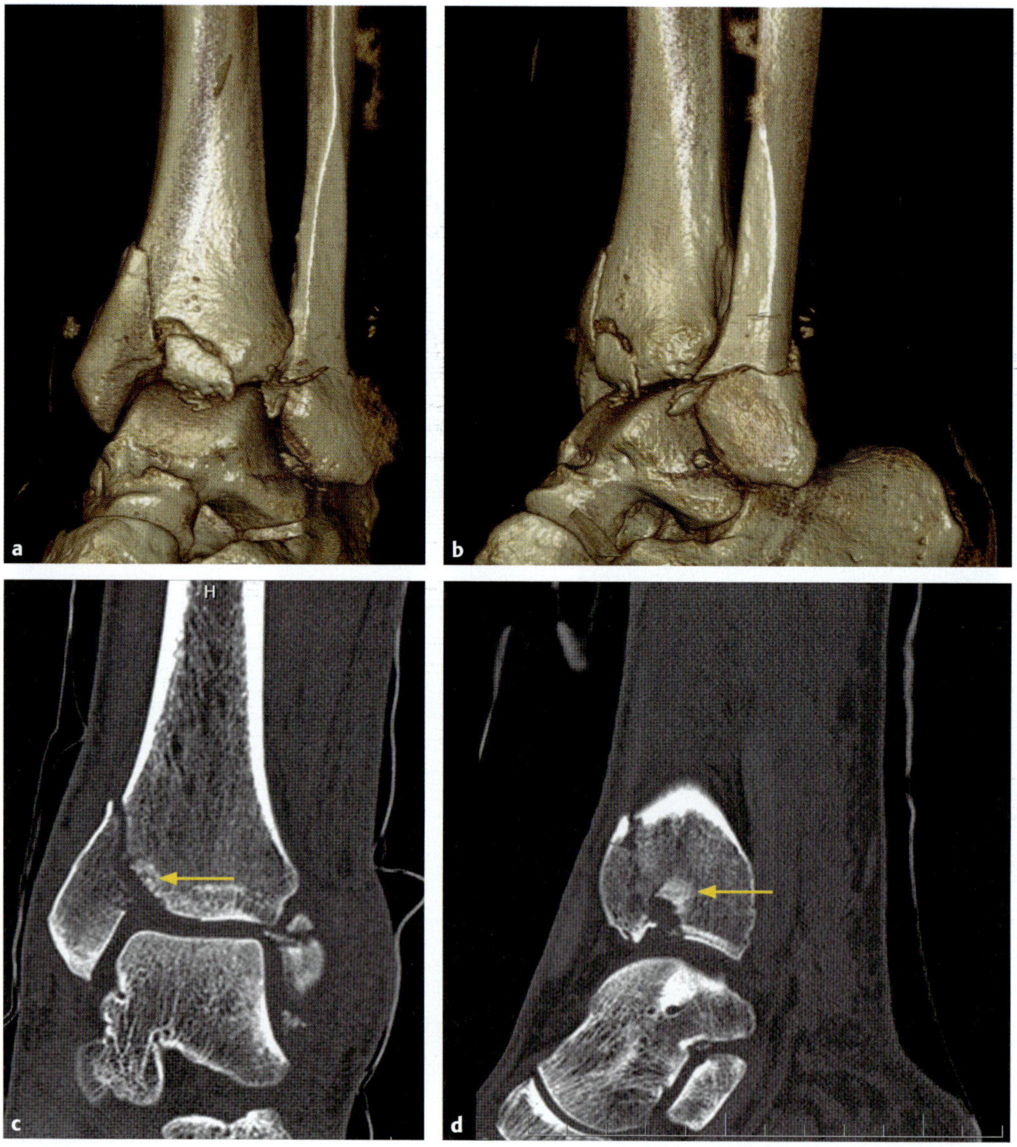

Fig 3.3-2a–d Computed tomographic images.

a–b The 3D CT reconstructions reveal a vertical medial malleolar fracture, an avulsion fracture of the anterior tibial rim and a nearly horizontal infrasyndesmotic fibular fracture.

c–d The 2D CT reconstructions in the coronal (**c**) and sagittal plane (**d**) demonstrate a medially impacted articular segment (yellow arrows).

precise reconstruction of the comminuted medial side. The fibular fracture can then be fixed with a tension band plate, plating, or an axial screw through a lateral approach (**Fig 3.3-3**). Because of small comminution on the far fibular cortex, a plate is the preferred option for treatment. It can be applied along the anterior aspect of the fibula to gain a bony buttress against the plate.

The vertical medial malleolar fracture with the impacted joint segment can be fixed from an anteromedial approach with screws and a neutralization plate after disimpacting the joint surface (**Fig 3.3-4**).

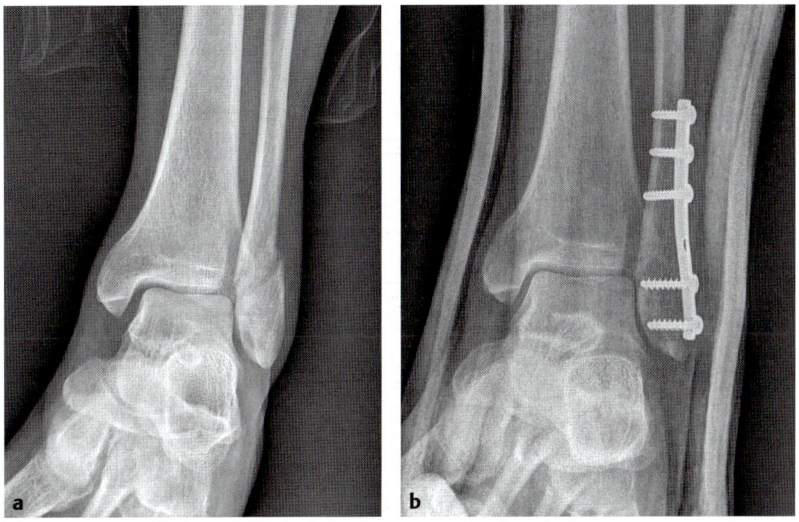

Fig 3.3-3a–b Example from a different case showing tension band plating of a short oblique fibular fracture. The far fibular cortex is intact and able to withstand compression forces. Therefore, the plate can be applied from the lateral side.

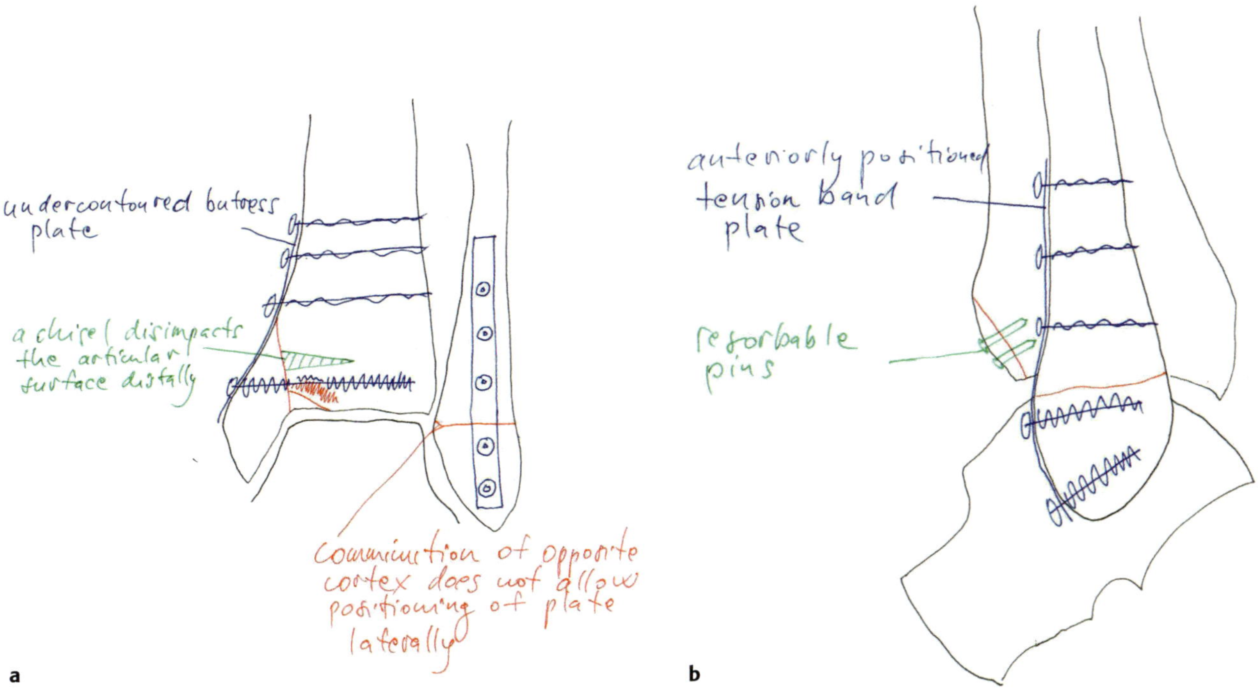

Fig 3.3-4a–b Preoperative plan.

- **a** The simple transverse fibular fracture is fixed first with a tension band plate placed anteriorly from a lateral approach. The vertical medial malleolar fracture with impacted joint segment should be fixed from an anteromedial approach with lag screws and buttress plate.
- **b** The small avulsion of the anterior tibial rim will be fixed with resorbable pins or small screws. A tension band plate will be fixed proximally with a cortex screw followed by the first distal screw inserted eccentrically to achieve compression.

3 Operating room setup

Patient positioning	• Supine on a radiolucent table with the injured leg elevated. This enables the surgeon to access both the medial and lateral side and allows adequate visualization in the lateral C-arm projections.
Anesthesia options	• Regional or general anesthesia (or a combination of both)
C-arm location	• Positioned on the injured or uninjured side of the patient, depending on complexity of the medial malleolar fracture and joint impaction, with the screen positioned near the head of patient.
Tourniquet	• May speed up fracture cleaning and reduction but is not necessary

For illustrations and overview of anesthetic considerations, see chapter 1.

Equipment

- K-wires 1.6–1.8 mm
- 3.5 mm (2.7 or 2.4 mm) cortex screws
- 4.0 mm cancellous screws
- Resorbable pins
- One-third tubular plate or variable angle locking distal fibula plate 2.7 if bone quality is poor but is locking fixation rarely necessary
- Chisel or sharp elevator

4 Surgical procedure

For ORIF, lateral and anteromedial approaches are needed. The simple transverse fibular fracture is fixed first, followed by reconstruction of the vertical medial malleolar fracture and joint impaction.

Fixation of the simple transverse fibular fracture
The longitudinal lateral incision is placed slightly anteriorly so that the plate can be placed on the anterior aspect of the fibula (**Fig 3.3-5**). The superficial peroneal nerve is identified and protected. Tension band plating can be used in patients with good bone quality and a large infrasyndesmotic fragment. A minimum of two screws must be securely inserted through the plate into the distal and proximal fibular fragments. The plate is contoured to perfectly fit the shape of the underlying bone. The fracture line is cleared of hematoma and fragments reduced with pointed forceps. The plate is positioned and fixed proximally with a cortex screw (**Fig 3.3-6**). The first distal screw is inserted eccentrically to achieve compression. Drilling is performed through the most distal hole of the plate and a cancellous screw is inserted. The remaining cancellous and cortex screws are inserted distal and proximal to the fracture, respectively, always perpendicular to the plate.

Plate position and screw length are checked using the C-arm and the fracture line is inspected visually to exclude distal fragment malrotation.

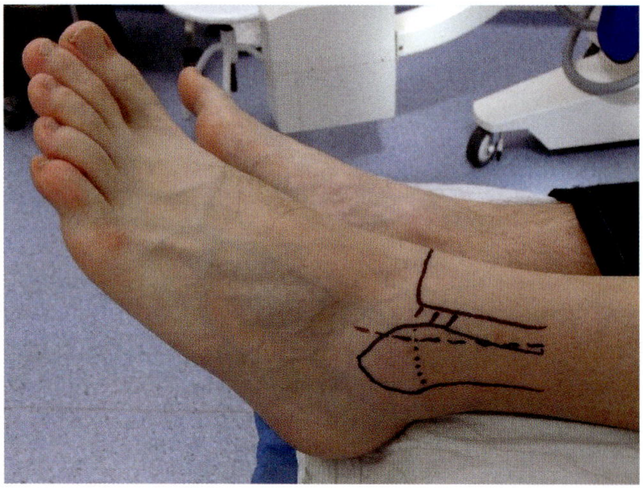

Fig 3.3-5 Lateral approach to the fibula. A slightly anterior incision is used to facilitate positioning of the plate.

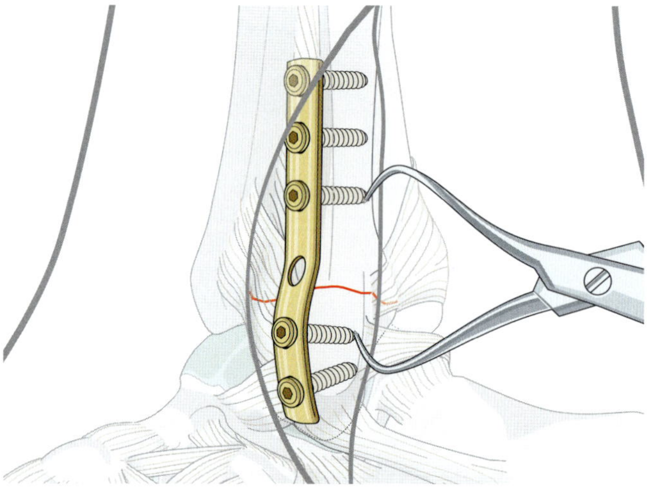

Fig 3.3-6 Tension band plate for a transverse fibular fracture. The plate is contoured precisely and tensioned by tightening with the first screw proximally to the fracture.

Testing the syndesmosis for stability is generally not necessary after fixation of an infrasyndesmotic injury. It may be considered in rare cases of an irregular fracture pattern.

Reconstruction of the vertical medial malleolar fracture and joint impaction

The vertical fracture of medial malleolus is approached via a longer axial anteromedial incision (**Fig 3.3-7**). The greater saphenous vein is identified and protected. The fracture is opened anteromedially, the malleolar fragment is gently retracted distally; and the impacted articular segment is identified and evaluated for size and vitality. If the cartilage adheres to subchondral bone and the impaction site is not comminuted, then it is reduced and fixed. A chisel or sharp elevator is placed into the cancellous metaphyseal bone proximal to the joint impaction from medial to lateral side and the articular surface is elevated distally (**Fig 3.3-8**). The resulting metaphyseal defect can usually be filled with bone graft, eg, from the distal tibial metaphysis. The malleolar fragment is then reduced and held with a pointed forceps or K-wires.

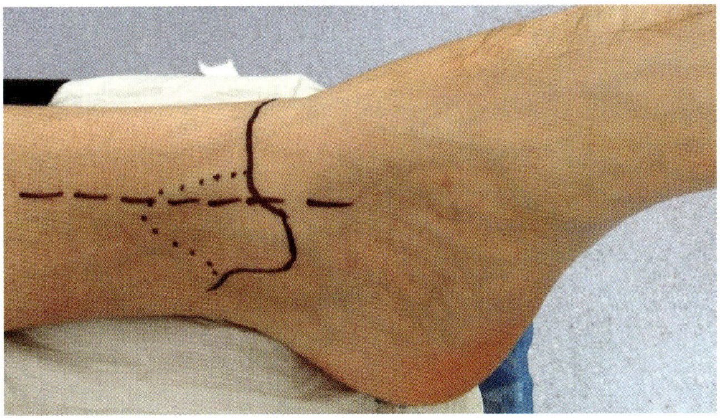

Fig 3.3-7 Anteromedial approach to the medial malleolus. The fracture line can be easily accessed, the medial malleolar fragment held aside, and the impacted articular segment elevated.

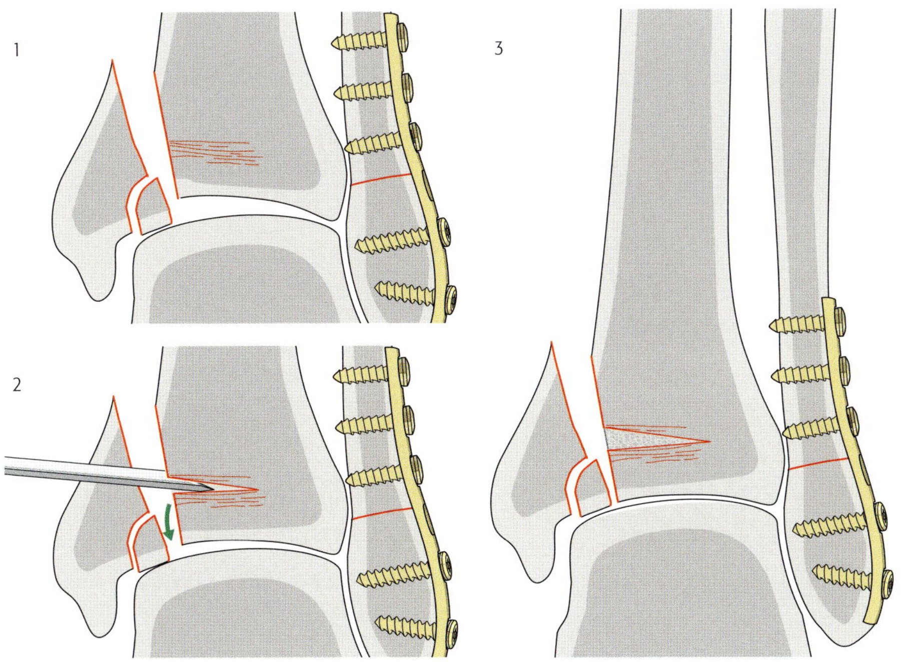

Fig 3.3-8a–c Reduction of the impacted articular segment. A chisel is placed into the cancellous metaphyseal bone proximal to the joint impaction and the articular surface is elevated distally.

Reduction is assessed visually from the anterior aspect of the ankle joint and with the C-arm. A small distractor can be placed from the tibia to the talar neck to improve visualization and assist with reduction. A screw is inserted across the fracture line from the tip of the medial malleolus into the distal tibial metaphysis. A medial buttress plate is applied with additional screws placed through the plate, above and below the fracture line.

A one-third tubular plate is slightly contoured at the distal end to conform to the shape of the medial malleolus and avoid protrusion of the implant (**Fig 3.3-9**). Bending at the central part is not necessary. The plate is fixed with a cortex screw just above the fracture line. Tightening of the central screw maximizes the pressure on the distal fragment (**Fig 3.3-10**). Two additional cortex screws fix the plate proximally, followed by two screws inserted through the distal plate holes. The avulsion of the anterior tibial rim is too

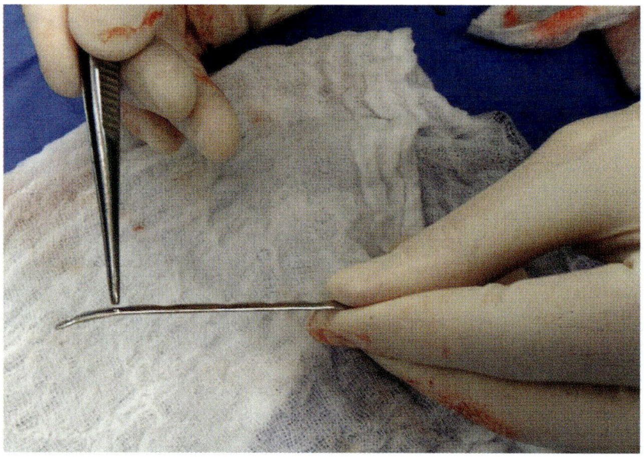

Fig 3.3-9 Contouring of the one-third tubular plate at the distal end to imitate the shape of medial malleolus. No bending of the central part is necessary.

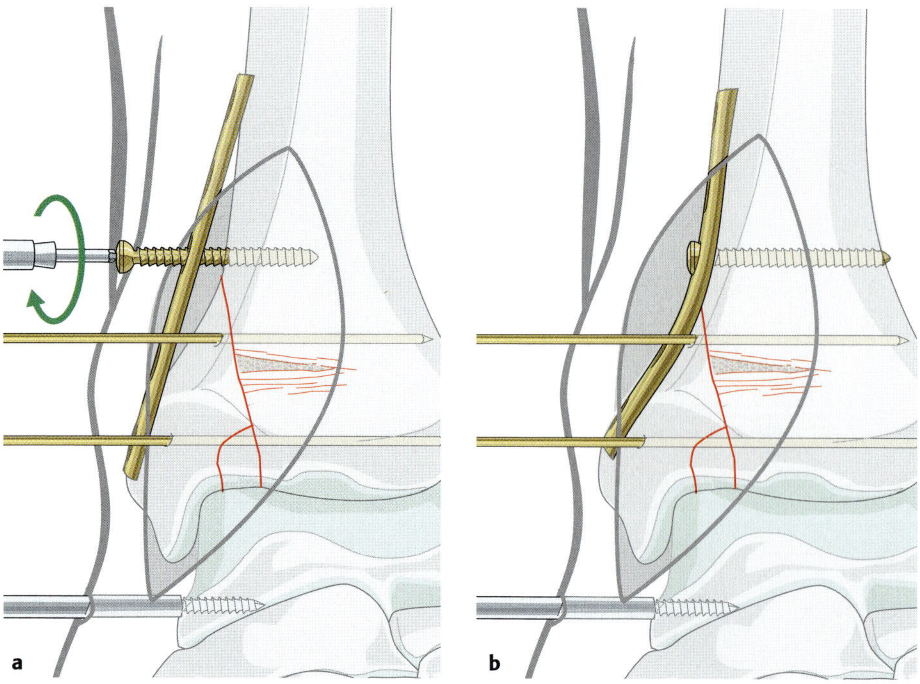

Fig 3.3-10a–b The under-contoured plate maximizes the pressure on the distal fragment when tightening the proximal screw.

small for screw fixation (**Fig 3.3-11**) and is therefore fixed with resorbable pins.

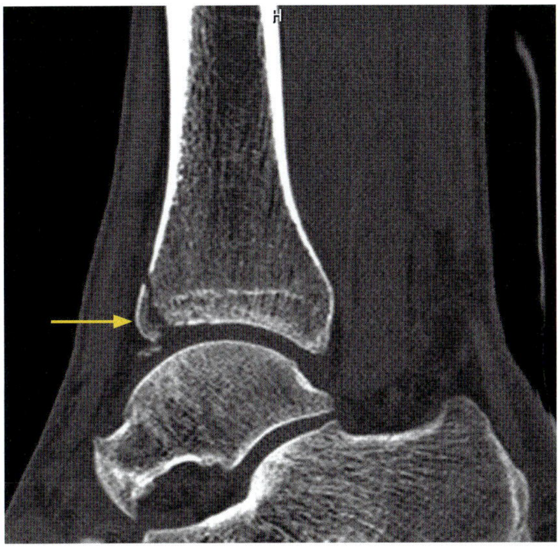

Fig 3.3-11 The anterior rim avulsion fragment is too small for screw fixation (yellow arrow). Therefore, use resorbable pins for fixation.

Precise C-arm imaging is carried out after completion of internal fixation (**Fig 3.3-12**). If there are concerns about the correct reduction of impacted central articular segment, perioperative 3D imaging or postoperative CT imaging can be performed if available.

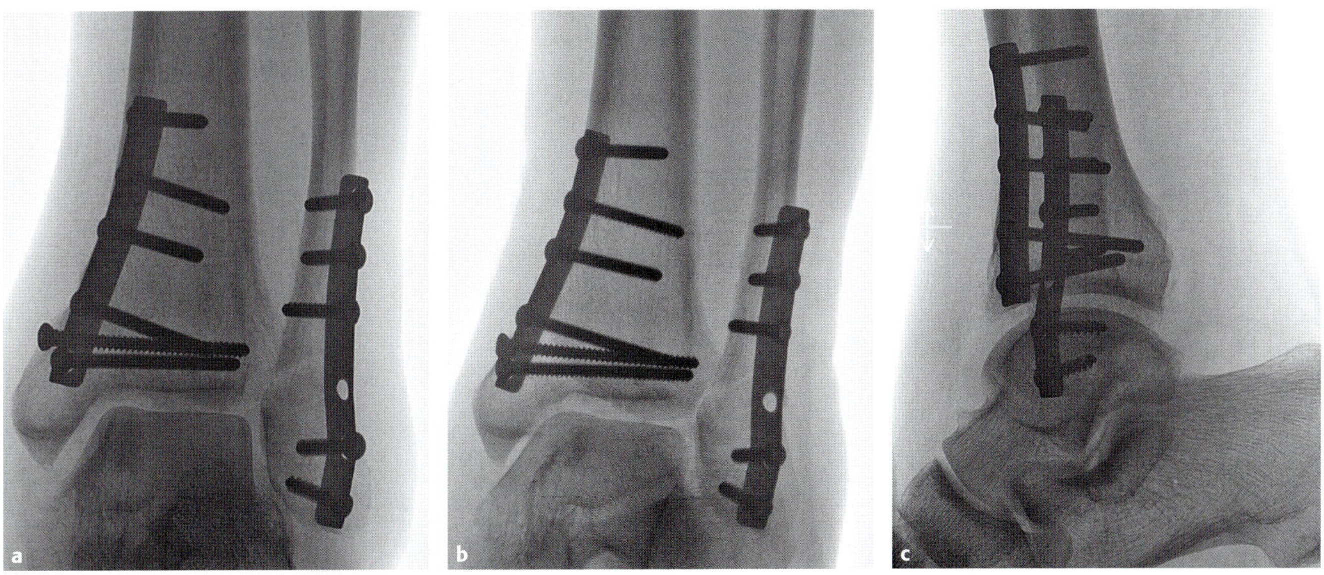

Fig 3.3-12a–c C-arm images taken after surgery showing fracture reduction and correct position of the implants. The fibula is fixed with a tension band plate and the medial malleolus with lag screws and a buttress plate.

a AP view.

b Mortise view.

c Lateral view.

5 Pitfalls and complications

Pitfalls

Wrong technique in tension band plating and wiring of the fibular fracture

When using a plate as a tension band, it must be contoured precisely to allow for the pressure to be exerted on the opposite cortex. This cortex must be intact. If any comminution is present, the plate position must be changed (**Fig 3.3-13**).

The distal screw tips should not penetrate the posterior cortex, in order to avoid damage to the peroneal tendons behind the fibula.

When using a tension band wiring, the tip of the screw or K-wire can irritate the syndesmosis which potentially leads to ossification (**Fig 3.3-14**). Thus, appropriate length of implants must be ensured.

Inadequate timing in the treatment of high-energy fractures

High-energy trauma causes more complex vertical fracture patterns at the medial malleolus and more severe injuries to the soft tissues. Primary ORIF is associated with higher incidence of wound-healing complications and infection. A staged treatment protocol is advisable with primary external fixation and definitive internal fixation after soft-tissue recovery. Smaller plates and screws can be used to achieve compression between comminuted fragments (**Fig 3.3-15**).

Failure to recognize plafond impaction

Fixation of the malleoli without elevation and bone grafting of the articular impaction leads to varus stress on the talus and early degenerative changes within the ankle joint. In the presence of a stage 2 supination-adduction fracture with vertical medial malleolar fracture, the indication to perform a preoperative CT scan should be made generously as medial plafond impaction frequently occurs with this fracture type.

Complications

- Injury to the greater saphenous vein
- Irritation of the peroneal tendons with a dorsally placed fibular plate or protruding screw/wire tips
- Chondral defects on the talus and tibial plafond with resulting posttraumatic arthritis
- Malunion with resulting varus deformity and arthritis
- Nonunion of the medial or lateral malleolus

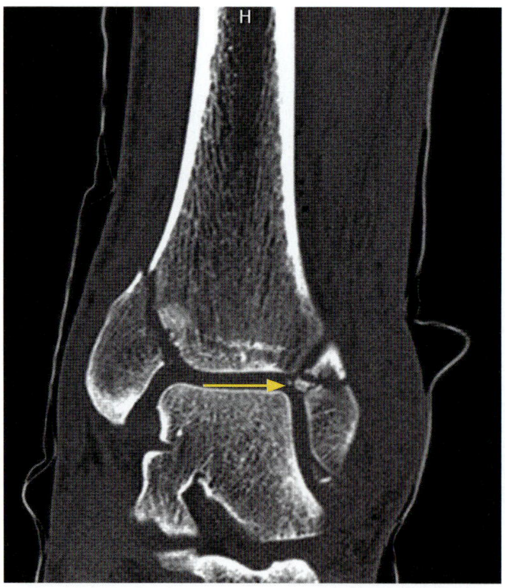

Fig 3.3-13 Example from a different case of a transverse fibular fracture. Comminution of the opposite cortex (yellow arrow) prevents positioning of a tension band plate from the lateral side.

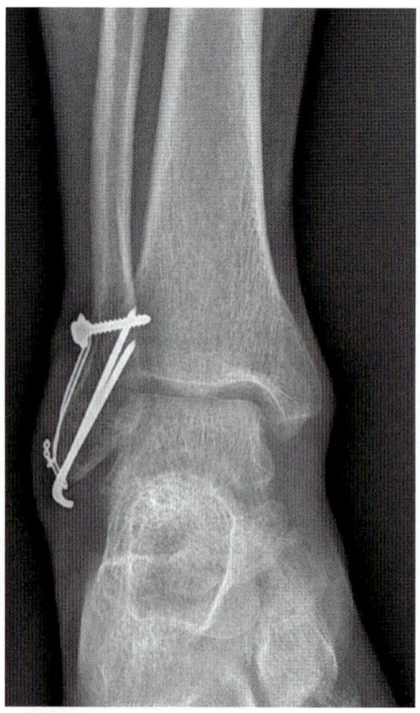

Fig 3.3-14 Example from a different case showing tension band wiring of a low transverse fibular fracture. The tip of the proximal screw potentially irritates the syndesmosis.

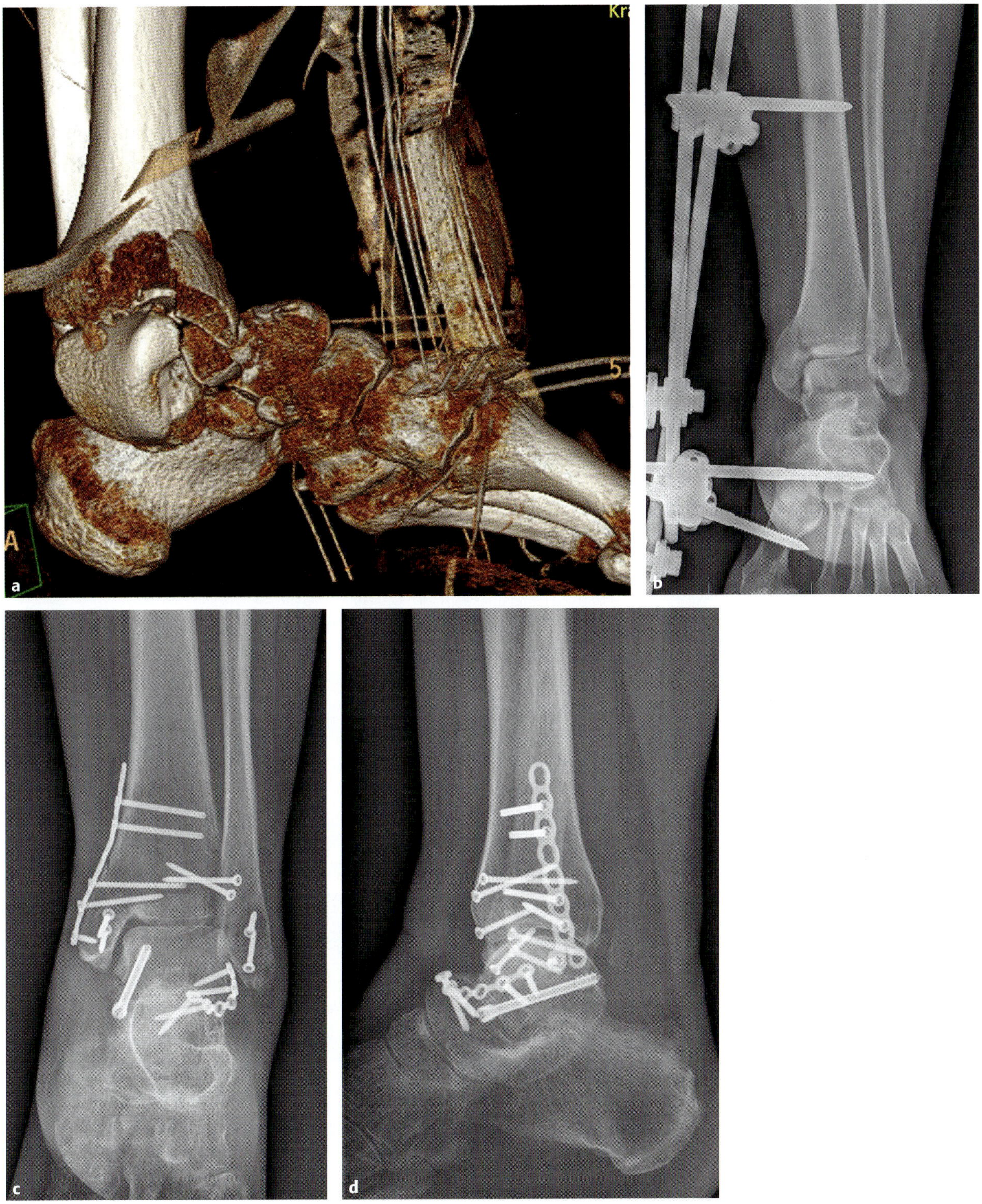

Fig 3.3-15a–d Example from a different case showing a high-energy trauma with injury to soft tissues and complex fracture pattern at the medial malleolus and talus.

a Talar neck fracture dislocation with vertical comminution of the medial malleolus.

b Staged treatment with an ankle-spanning external fixator as a first line treatment.

c–d The 2.4 and 2.7 plates and screws can be used for fixation of small fragments.

6 Alternative techniques

A low transverse fibular fracture, which cannot accommodate two screws in the small distal fragment, can be fixed using tension band wiring (**Fig 3.3-16**), a hook plate, or a single screw placed through the tip of the medial malleolus in a vertical direction. Intramedullary screw fixation is reserved for fracture patterns that are length stable and essentially transverse.

With open physeal plates, screws must be inserted parallel to the physeal growth plate.

The buttress plate for fixation of the medial malleolar fracture can be positioned more anteriorly to accommodate more complex fracture patterns (**Fig 3.3-17**).

7 Postoperative management and rehabilitation

Postoperatively the ankle was immobilized in a lower leg cast and elevated. Because of the articular compression and small anterior tibial rim fragment, range-of-motion (ROM) exercises were delayed for 10 days. Four weeks after surgery the lower leg cast was removed, and an ankle orthosis applied. The patient was restricted to partial weight bearing (approximately 20 kg) for the next 2 weeks and rehabilitation started, consisting of ROM exercises, muscle strengthening and gait training. Weight bearing was gradually increased after radiographic evidence of bony consolidation. This patient achieved full bony union at 4 months after surgery (**Fig 3.3-18**) with a final ROM that was comparable with the uninjured side (**Fig 3.3-19**). X-rays at a 3-year follow-up reveal osteophyte formation at the anterior tibial rim as a radiographic sign of mild posttraumatic arthritis (**Fig 3.3-20**). Osteophytes can be removed with arthroscopic assistance.

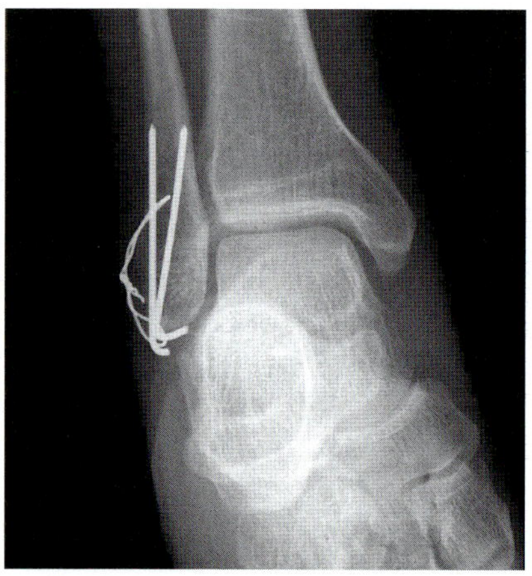

Fig 3.3-16 Example from a different case showing tension band wiring of a transverse fibular fracture with a small distal fragment.

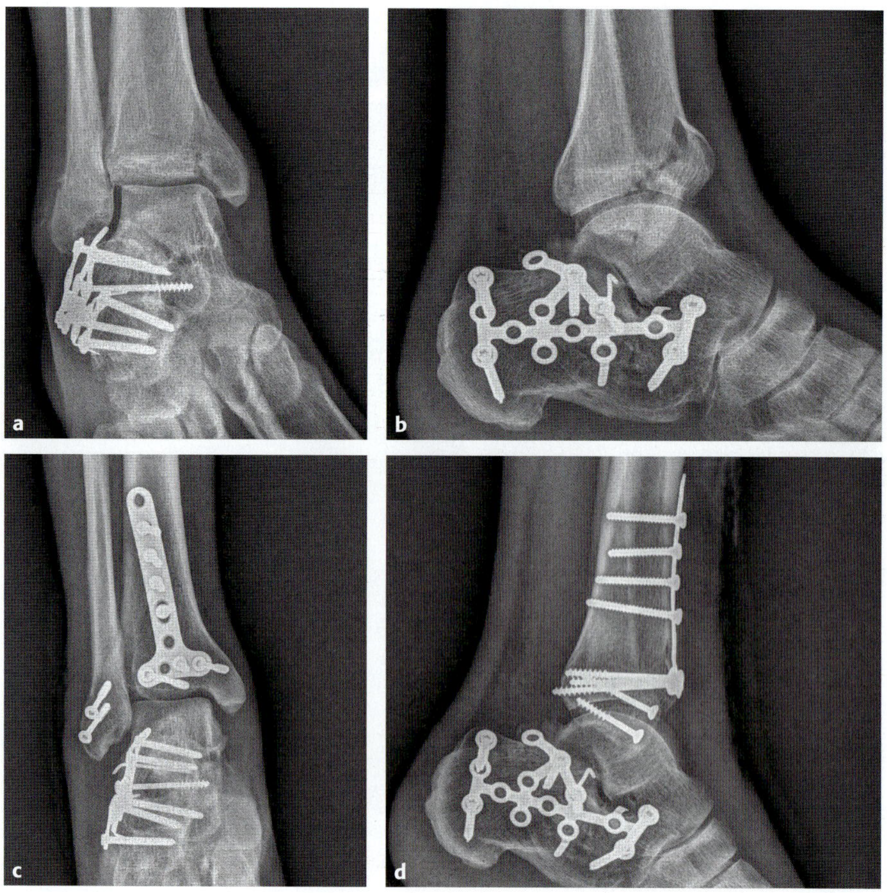

Fig 3.3-17a–d Example from a different case showing buttress plating in case of a more complex fracture pattern (with additional calcaneal fracture).
a–b AP and lateral x-rays showing a vertical fracture of the medial malleolus with an anterior extension.
c–d Anterior position of the buttress plate (perpendicular to the main fracture lines).

Implant removal

Prominent plates and screws on medial and lateral side are removed using the same incisions 9–12 months after surgery, after full bony union has been documented. Implant removal can be combined with arthrolysis in case of restricted ROM because of adhesions and scar formation.

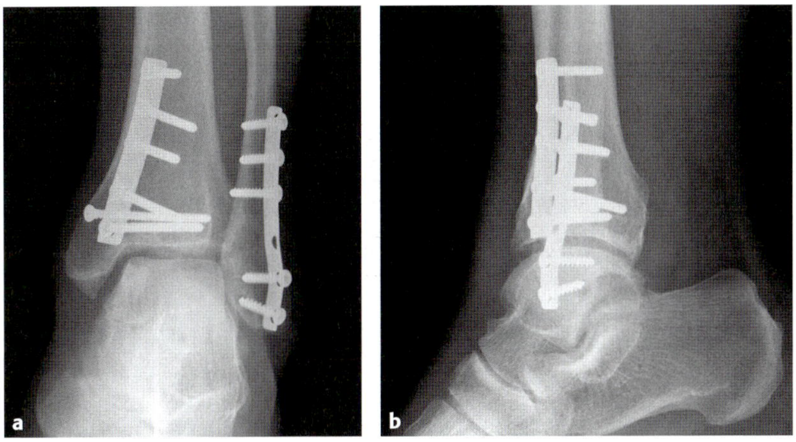

Fig 3.3-18a–b Control x-rays 4 months after surgery. Full bony union is achieved.

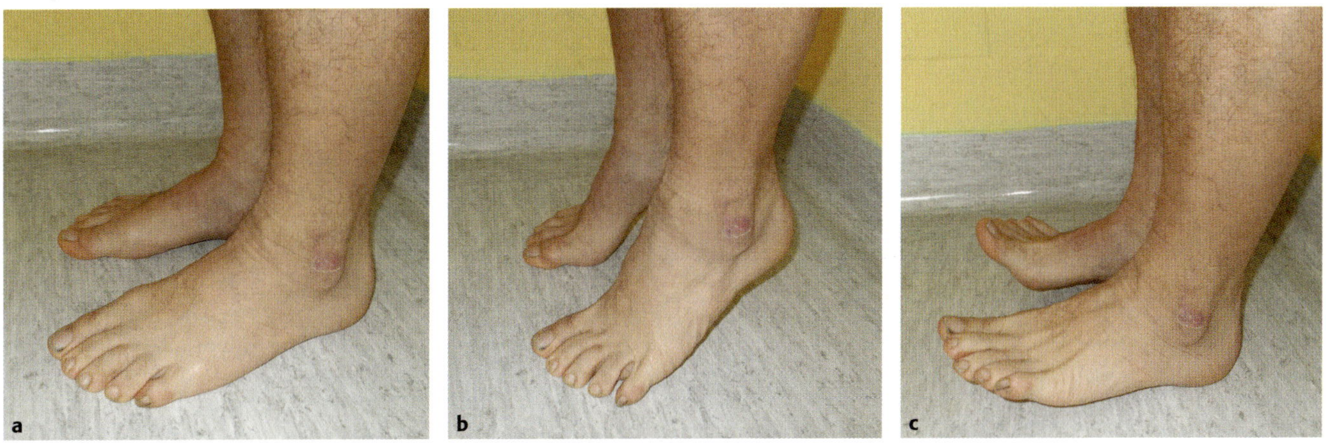

Fig 3.3-19a–c Range of motion at the 3-year follow-up.

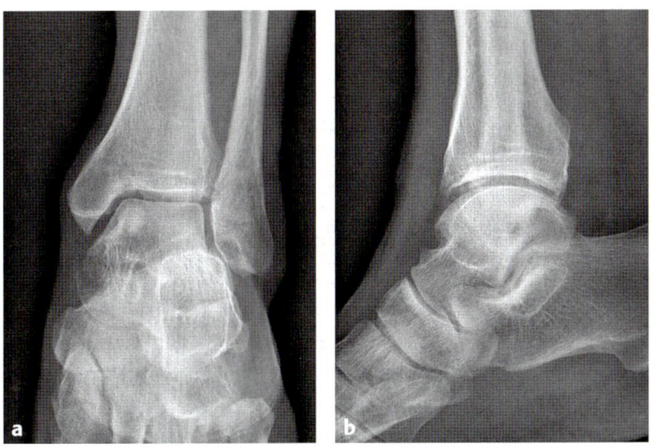

Fig 3.3-20a–b Follow-up x-rays 3 years after surgery reveal osteophyte formation at the anterior tibial rim (the site of the former avulsion fracture) as a radiographic sign of mild posttraumatice ankle arthritis.

a Mortise view.

b Lateral view.

8 Recommended reading

Barnes H, Cannada LK, Watson JT. A clinical evaluation of alternative fixation techniques for medial malleolus fractures. *Injury.* 2014 Sep;45(9):1365–1367.

Davidovitch RI, Egol KA. The medial malleolus osteoligamentous complex and its role in ankle fractures. *Bull NYU Hosp Jt Dis.* 2009;67(4):318–324.

Ebraheim NA, Ludwig T, Weston JT, et al. Comparison of surgical techniques of 111 medial malleolar fractures classified by fracture geometry. *Foot Ankle Int.* 2014 May;35(5):471–477.

Futamura K, Baba T, Mogami A, et al. Malreduction of syndesmosis injury associated with malleolar ankle fracture can be avoided using Weber's three indexes in the mortise view. *Injury.* 2017 Apr;48(4):954–959.

Lauge-Hansen N. Fractures of the ankle. II. Combined experimental-surgical and experimental-roentgenologic investigations. *Arch Surg.* 1950 May;60(5):957–985.

Lübbeke A, Salvo D, Stern R, et al. Risk factors for post-traumatic osteoarthritis of the ankle: an eighteen-year follow-up study. *Int Orthop.* 2012 Jul;36(7):1403–1410.

McConnell T, Tornetta P 3rd. Marginal plafond impaction in association with supination-adduction ankle fractures: a report of eight cases. *J Orthop Trauma.* 2001 Aug;15(6):447–449.

Parada SA, Krieg JC, Benirschke SK, et al. Bicortical fixation of medial malleolar fractures. *Am J Orthop (Belle Mead NJ).* 2013 Feb;42(2):90–92.

Rammelt S, Zwipp H. Ankle fractures. In: Bentley G, ed. *European Instructional Course Lectures, Volume 12.* Berlin Heidelberg New York: Springer; 2012:205–219.

Rammelt S, Boszczyk A. Computed tomography in the diagnosis and treatment of ankle fractures: a critical analysis review. *JBJS Rev.* 2018 Dec;6(12):e7.

Weber BG, Colton C. Malleolar fractures. In: Müller M, Allgöwer M, Schneider R, et al, eds. *Manual of Internal Fixation.* Berlin: Springer; 1991:595–612.

Zhenhua F, Waizy H, Ming X, et al. Lateral malleolus hook plate for comminuted Weber A and B fractures: a retrospective study. *Indian J Orthop.* 2013 Jul;47(4):364–369.

3.4 Bimalleolar fracture with syndesmotic disruption

Michaël Houben, Martijn Poeze

1 Case description

A 35-year-old woman tripped, sustaining a pronation injury of her left ankle. Directly after the incident the ankle was painful on both the medial and lateral side and she was unable to walk. The patient's only related medical history was a medial meniscus lesion of her left knee.

Upon arrival at the emergency department the left ankle was severely swollen and hematoma was visible around the medial and lateral malleoli.

Physical examination revealed that the malleoli were painful to palpation. Movement of the ankle joint was limited in all directions, as a result of swelling and pain. There was no indication of neurovascular injury of the ankle or foot.

X-rays of the ankle in AP and lateral views revealed a bimalleolar ankle fracture with lateral displacement of the talus (**Fig 3.4-1**). There was a horizontal medial malleolar fracture and an AO/OTA 44C2.2 (Weber type C) fibular shaft fracture, pronation-external rotation (Lauge-Hansen) injury. The fracture was considered unstable, requiring surgery for stabilization of the ankle.

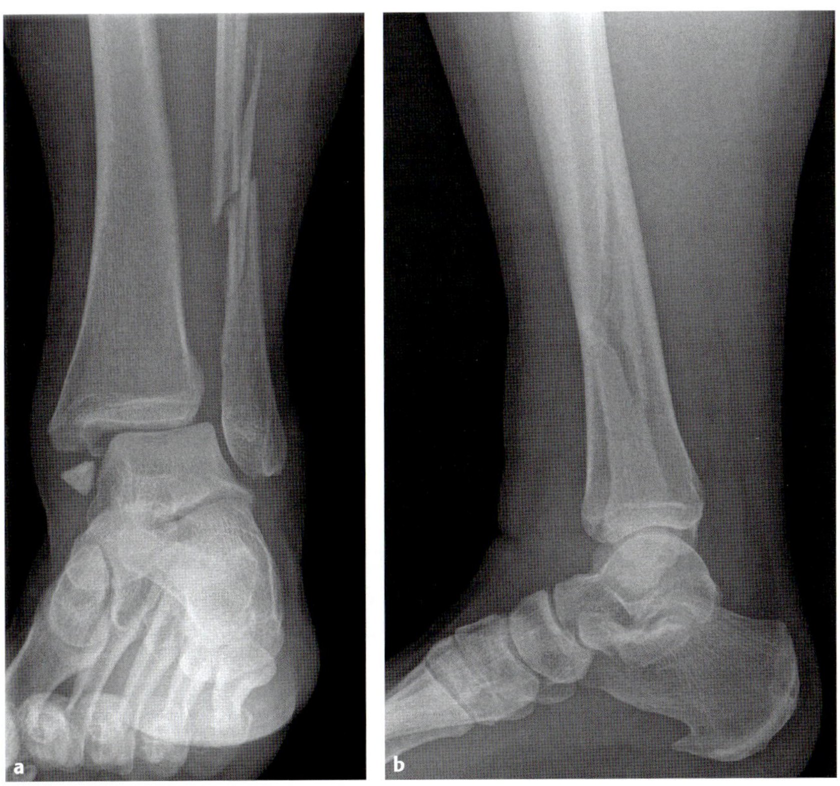

Fig 3.4-1a–b Typical x-rays of a pronation-external rotation injury obtained directly after arrival in the emergency department.

a AP view.

b Lateral view.

After closed reduction and padded splint placement, repeated x-rays were performed (**Fig 3.4-2**). Surgery was postponed for 7 days secondary to allow the severe soft-tissue swelling to adequately subside. Two days before surgery the skin was checked to assess the swelling and soft-tissue condition. Surgery was approved, as the skin demonstrated the "wrinkle sign" indicating soft-tissue recovery (**Fig 3.4-3**).

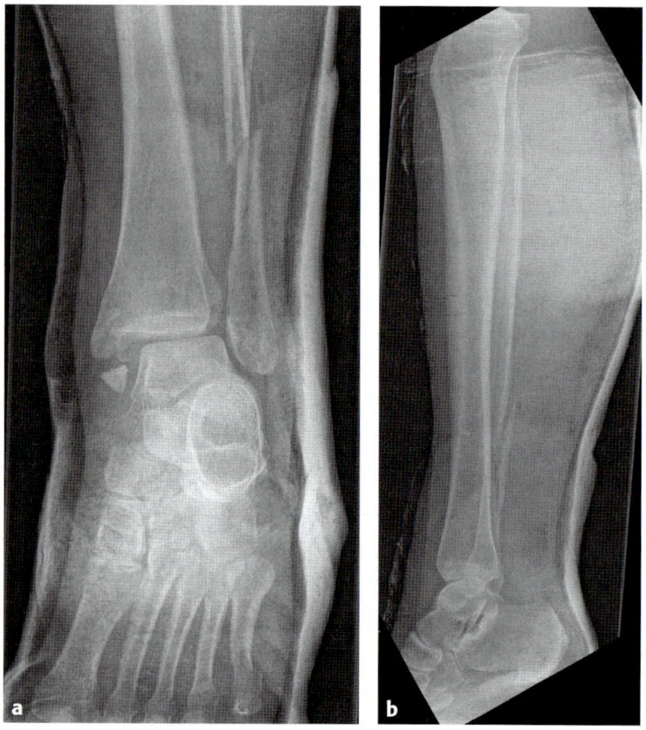

Fig 3.4-2a–b Lower leg x-rays after closed reduction and plaster cast immobilization.
a AP view.
b Lateral view.

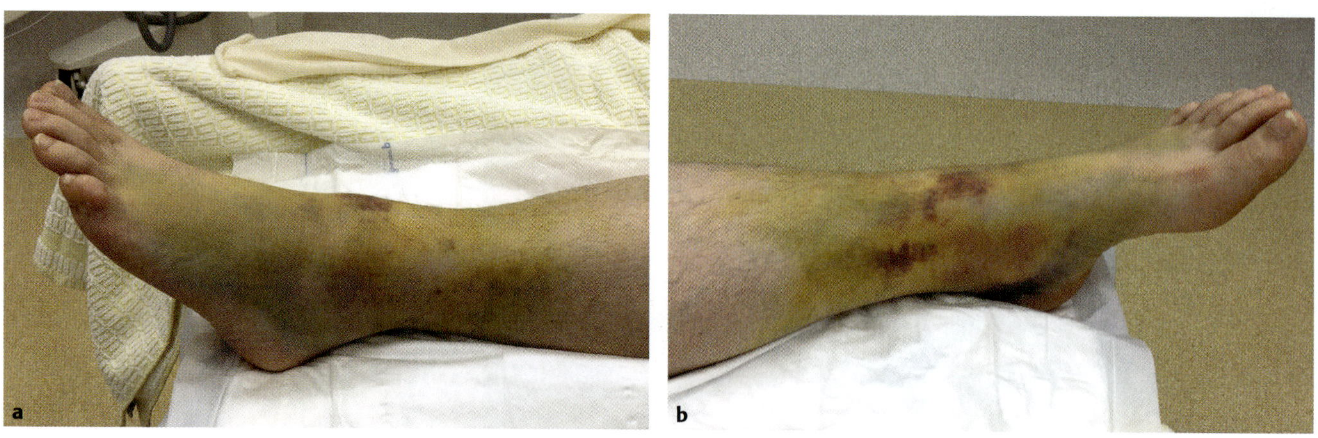

Fig 3.4-3a–b Left ankle 8 days after trauma demonstrating wrinkling of the skin.

2 Preoperative planning

The approaches used in this case were:

- Straight lateral approach of the distal fibula (**Fig 3.4-4a**)
- Straight medial approach for the medial malleolus fragment (**Fig 3.4-4b**).

The position of the lateral fracture was determined by C-arm to reduce the size of the incision. A posterolateral approach is not useful with a high-fibular fracture.

A lateral metaphyseal plate can be used for fixation of the fibula. K-wires or screws can be used for stabilization of the medial malleolus, depending on the size of the medial fragment.

Equipment

- K-wires
- 2.5 mm and 3.5 mm drill with guide sleeve and electric drill
- Various retractors
- Point-to-point reduction (Weber) clamp
- Silicon vessel loop (optional)
- 2-0 synthetic braided absorbable suture, 2-0 and 3-0 synthetic nonabsorbable nylon suture, 3-0 absorbable synthetic suture
- Plaster and cast
- Metaphyseal plates
- Interfragmentary (lag) screws
- Various screws as per surgeon preference, fragment size, and individual bone quality

3 Operating room setup

Patient positioning	• Supine on a radiolucent table with a sandbag under the ipsilateral buttock and with the knee slightly flexed, creating more visibility for the lateral approach. • The position of the surgeon is typically at the lateral side for the direct lateral approach. • For complex reconstruction of the ankle, the surgeon may also take position at the plantar aspect of the foot.
Anesthesia options	• General anesthesia, regional anesthesia, or spinal anesthesia as per surgeon preference and patient comorbidities
C-arm location	• Positioned on contralateral side over the patient with the monitor in front of the surgeon. • Ipsilateral or contralateral at the cranial side
Tourniquet	• Temporary tourniquet (only applied when visualization is hampered by bleeding)

For illustrations and overview of anesthetic considerations, see chapter 1.

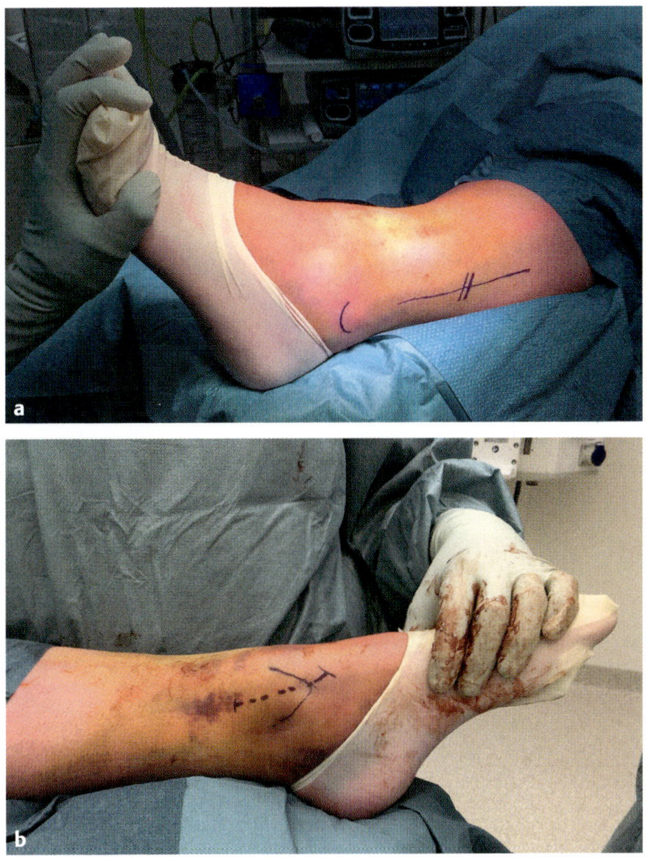

Fig 3.4-4a–b Preoperative plan for the positioning of the lateral incision (**a**) and the medial incision (**b**).

4 Surgical procedure

Lateral approach

First, the lateral approach is used to reestablish enough length and rotation of the fibula.

The lateral incision is made with special attention to the superficial peroneal nerve in the proximal end of the skin incision (**Fig 3.4-5**). Visibility is created using blunt retractors. Dissection is carried down to the fracture. Hematoma and debris are cleared aiding in reduction (**Fig 3.4-6a**).

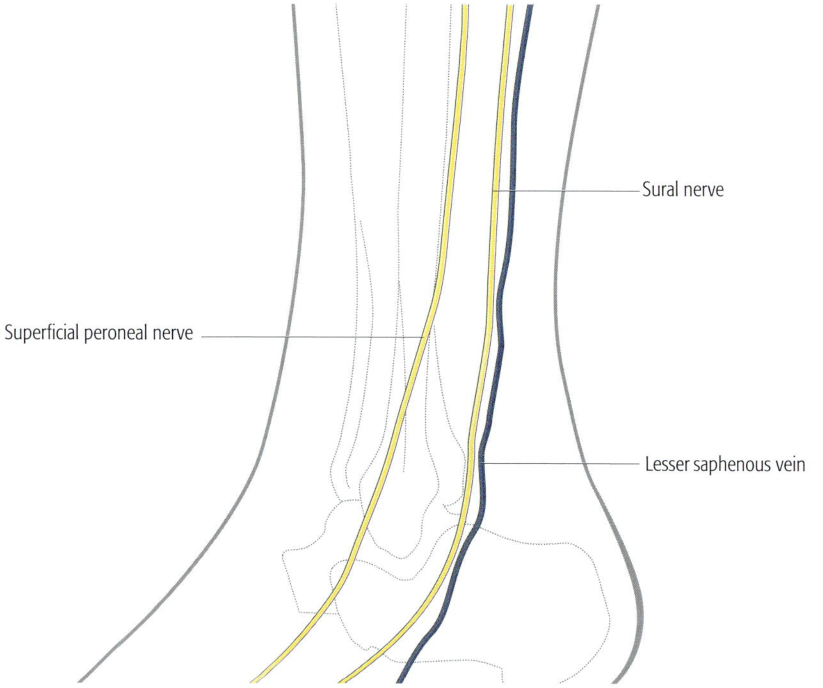

Fig 3.4-5 Lateral incision with special attention to the superficial peroneal nerve anterior to the incision and the sural nerve and lesser saphenous vein posterior to the incision.

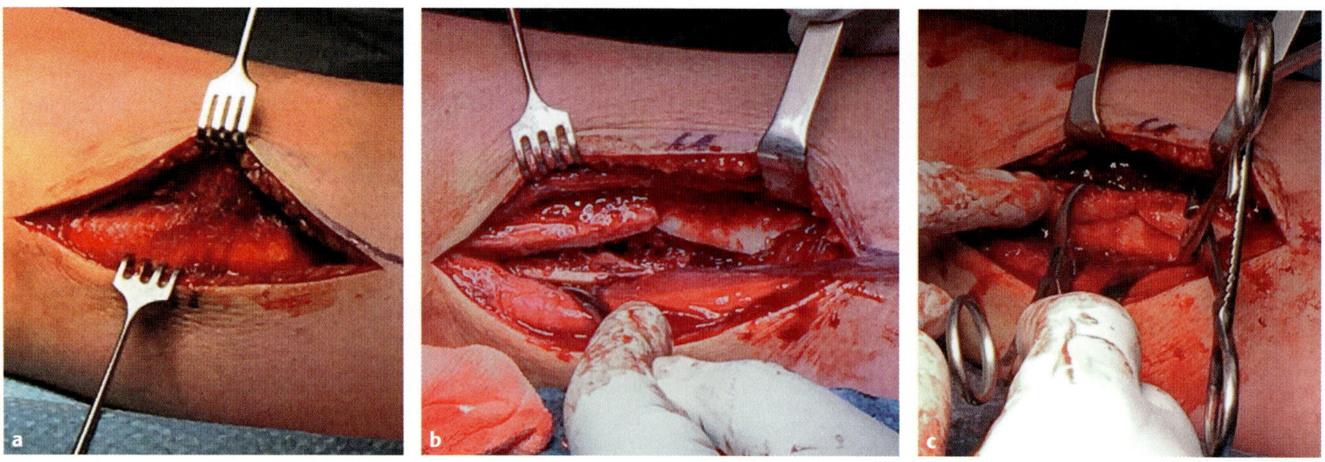

Fig 3.4-6a–c Steps in the fibular fracture fixation.
- **a** Lateral skin incision to access a Weber C fracture.
- **b** Reduction of the three fragments using blunt (Hohmann) retractors.
- **c** Reduction of the fibular fracture fragments with two point-to-point reduction (Weber) clamps with full closure of the fracture gap.

Anatomical reduction of the fibular fragments is achieved using a point-to-point reduction (Weber) clamp (**Fig 3.4-6b–c**). By restoring the length and rotation of the fibula, the position of the tibial fragments will be easier to restore. The use of an interfragmentary (lag) screw across the fracture site helps to achieve absolute stabilization. Hereafter a metaphyseal neutralization plate can be placed over the fragments. It is fixed with six cortex screws or interlocking screws, if the quality of the bone requires a more rigid fixation (**Fig 3.4-7a**). The anatomical reduction should be checked using C-arm (**Fig 3.4-7b**). Reduction should be congruent according to the Weber criteria in a mortise view x-ray (10° internal rotation of the fifth metatarsal), ie, Shenton line of the ankle, a line from the lateral part of the articular surface of the tibia to that of the distal fibula, and a circle drawn between the distal fibula and the talus, the Weber ball ("dime sign") (**Fig 3.4-8**).

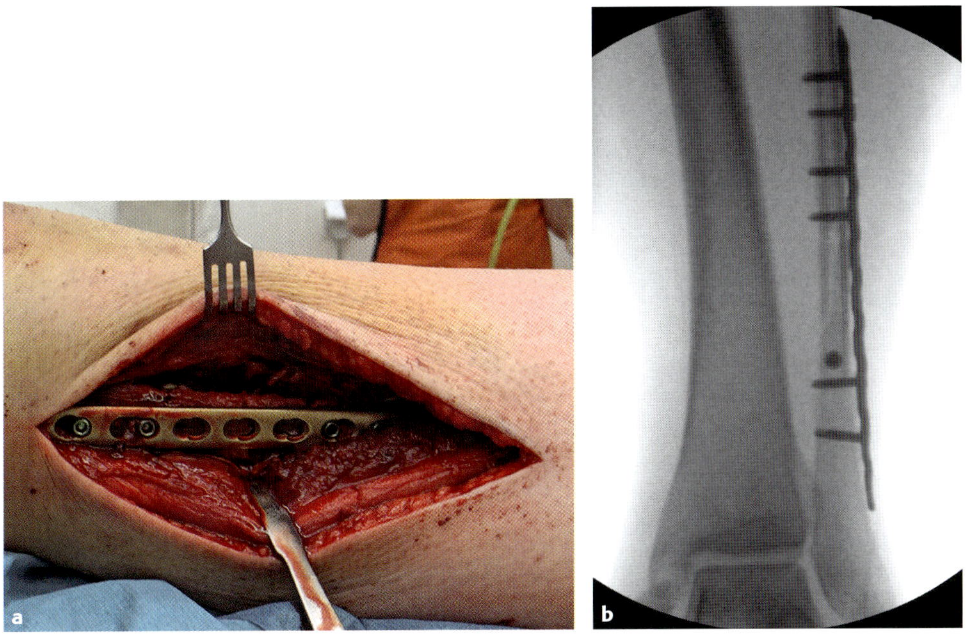

Fig 3.4-7a–b Results of lateral fixation.
a Metaphyseal plate fixation of the distal fibula for neutralization of the interfragmentary lag screw.
b Metaphyseal plate screw fixation on the distal fibula and the use of a single interfragmentary lag screw.

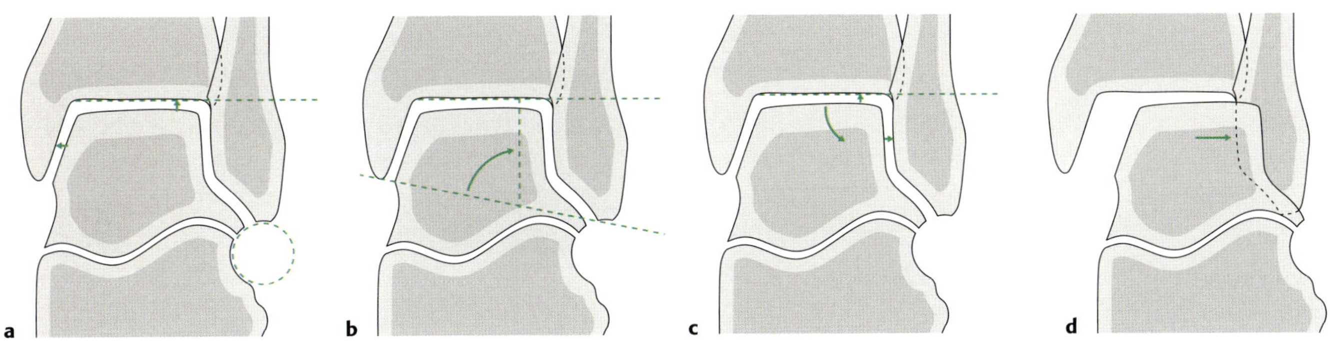

Fig 3.4-8a–d Radiographic criteria for evaluating the congruity of the articular surface in the mortise view.
a Medial clear space of ≤ 4 mm and no larger than the superior clear space (arrows), tibiofibular clear space of ≤ 5 mm, Weber ball ("dime sign") (dotted circle).
b Talocrural angle of 83° ± 4°.
c Talar tilt of ≤ 2 mm.
d No talar displacement.

Medial approach

After fixing the lateral malleolus, the medial malleolus should be corrected to its anatomical position. Surgical dissection is done by a 10 cm longitudinal incision with its center over the tip of the medial malleolus, distally curving the incision onto the medial aspect of the midfoot. Alternatively, an incision tangentially to the previous option can be used to provide better access to the anterior border of the ankle joint (see the dotted line in **Fig 3.4-9a–b**). Retract the skin, the greater saphenous vein and the saphenous nerve (using vessel loop) anterior to the medial malleolus.

A small longitudinal incision is made in the anteromedial ankle joint capsule and directly posterior to the medial malleolus in the flexor retinaculum over the tibialis posterior tendon (**Fig 3.4-9c**).

Under direct vision the medial malleolus is reduced and fixed by using a point-to-point reduction (Weber) clamp (**Fig 3.4-9d–e**). Different options exist for definite fixation: large fragments are preferably stabilized with two screws (**Fig 3.4-9f–g**). Smaller fragments can be fixed by using two fracture fixation system wires or K-wires. In case of severe comminution, miniplate fixation can be used (**Fig 3.4-9h**).

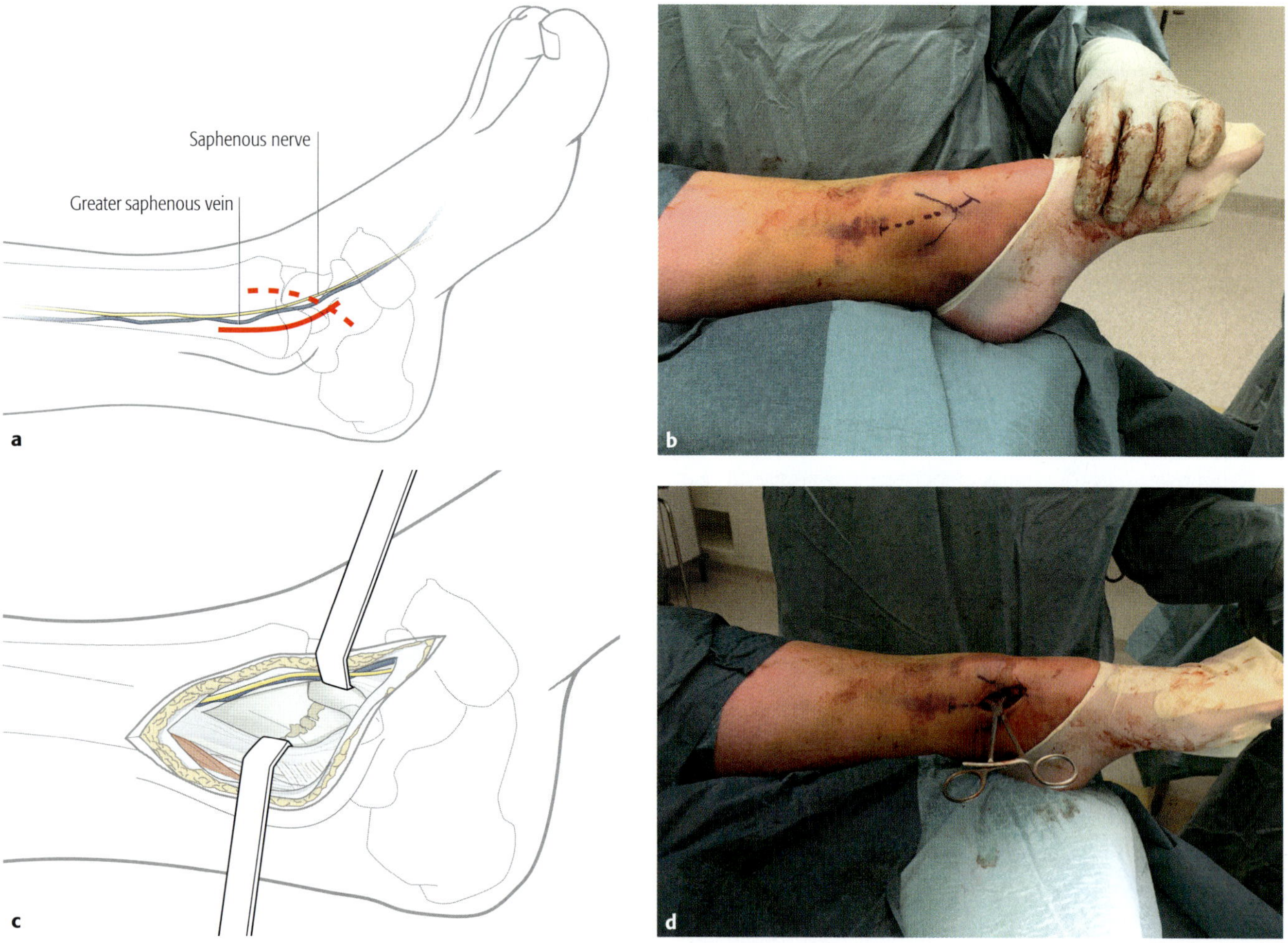

Fig 3.4-9a–g Steps in medial malleolar fracture fixation.
- **a** Greater saphenous vein and the saphenous nerve anterior of the medial malleolus and incision.
- **b** A longitudinal incision centered over the tip of the medial malleolus.
- **c** Incision in anteromedial ankle joint capsule and flexor retinaculum over the tibialis posterior tendon.
- **d** Reduction clamp to temporarily hold the medial malleolar fragment before fixation with two screws.

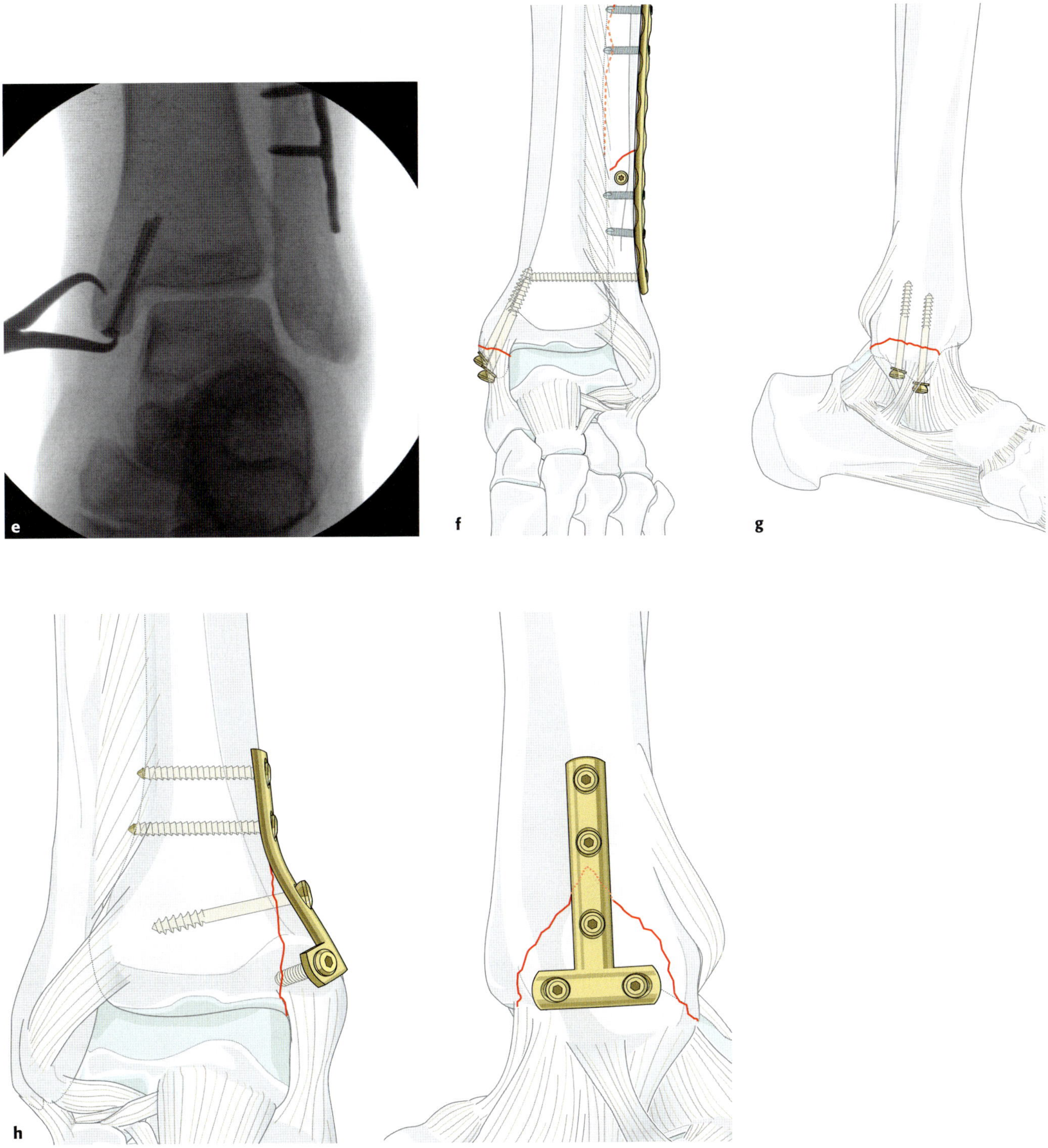

Fig 3.4-9a–h (cont) Steps in medial malleolar fracture fixation.
e Intraoperative C-arm image of the medial malleolar and fibular fixation.
f–g Medial malleolar and fibular fixation.
h Fixation with a 3-hole miniplate.

After the fixation of the medial malleolus, stabilization of the syndesmosis should be performed. A pronation-external rotation injury with a high (Weber C) fibular fracture has a syndesmosis injury in all cases that must be addressed. In the absence of a frank diastasis between the distal tibia and fibula after malleolar fracture fixation, syndesmotic stability should be tested with one of the many syndesmosis stress tests. A pointed reduction clamp is placed along the axis of the ankle joint (ideally from the tip of the medial malleolus to the tip of the lateral malleolus of the fracture and bone quality allow this position) (**Fig 3.4-10a**). Care is taken to reduce the distal fibula into the tibial incisura. Direct visualization of the anterior syndesmosis is recommended to avoid anteroposterior malreduction of the distal fibula. Anatomical reduction of the ankle mortise is checked again using the Weber criteria (**Fig 3.4-8**).

An additional tricortical or quadricortical screw is placed through the lateral incision, alternatively a fiber wire or suture-button is used for securing the syndesmotic articulation (**Fig 3.4-10b–c**). Wound closure is performed without tension as per surgeon preference.

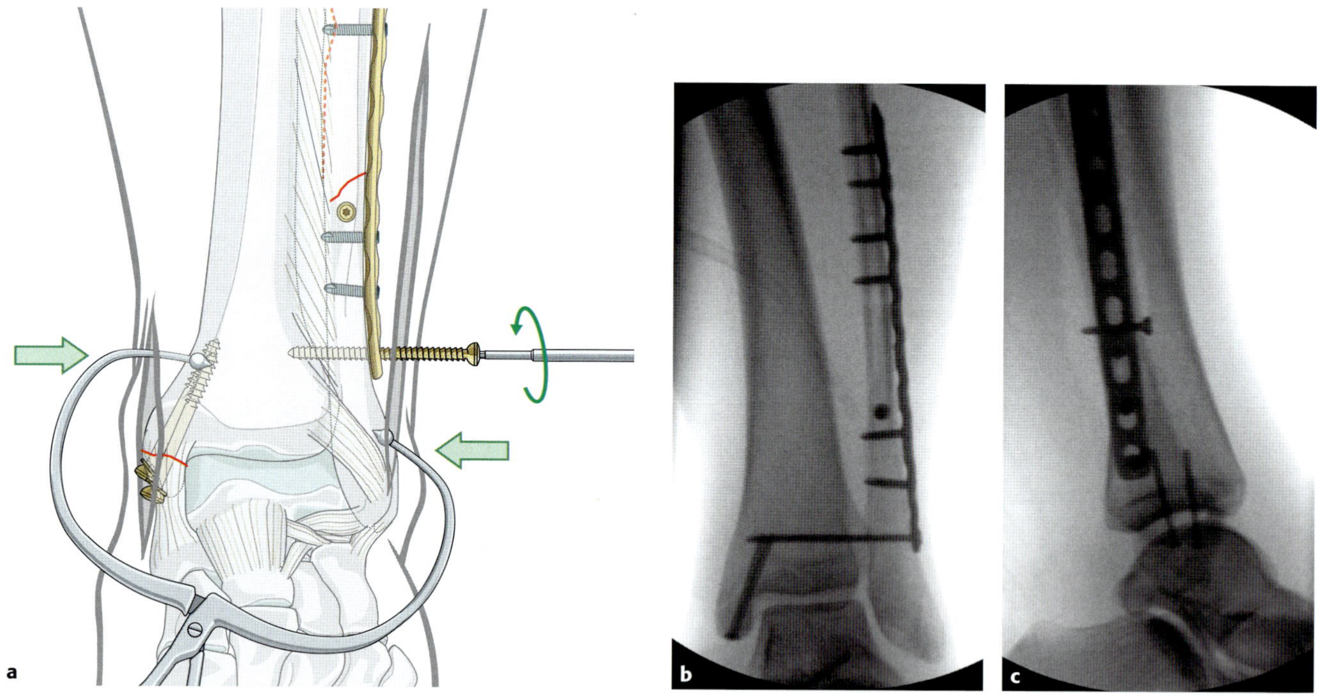

Fig 3.4-10a–c Positioning the syndesmotic screw.
a Syndesmotic screw placement aided by using a reduction clamp.
b Syndesmotic screw for securing the syndesmosis between the fibula and tibia in a correct position (mortise view).
c Syndesmotic screw, medial fixation and metaphyseal plate fixation (lateral view).

5 Pitfalls and complications

Pitfalls

Malpositioned screws

During medial malleolar fixation there is the risk of putting a screw through the cartilage of the talocrural joint (intraarticular screw at the medial superior corner) or interference of the screws with the posterior tibial tendon. Hardware malposition can be prevented by direct inspection into the joint and C-arm imaging in AP and lateral views (**Fig 3.4-11**). The safe zone for screw placement is the anterior colliculus. The risk zones for posterior tibial tendon abutment or injury lie in the intercollicular groove (high risk) and screws placed in the posterior colliculus inevitably result in abutment of the posterior tibial tendon.

Malreduction of the fibula

A (multifragmentary) fibular fracture must be brought out to length and rotation to prevent malreduction of the ankle joint. By starting with the lateral incision, it is possible to create anatomical reduction of the mortise of the ankle joint.

Malreduction of the syndesmosis

Syndesmotic instability will potentially result in prolonged pain and discomfort during rehabilitation and is the most common cause of chronic ankle dysfunction.

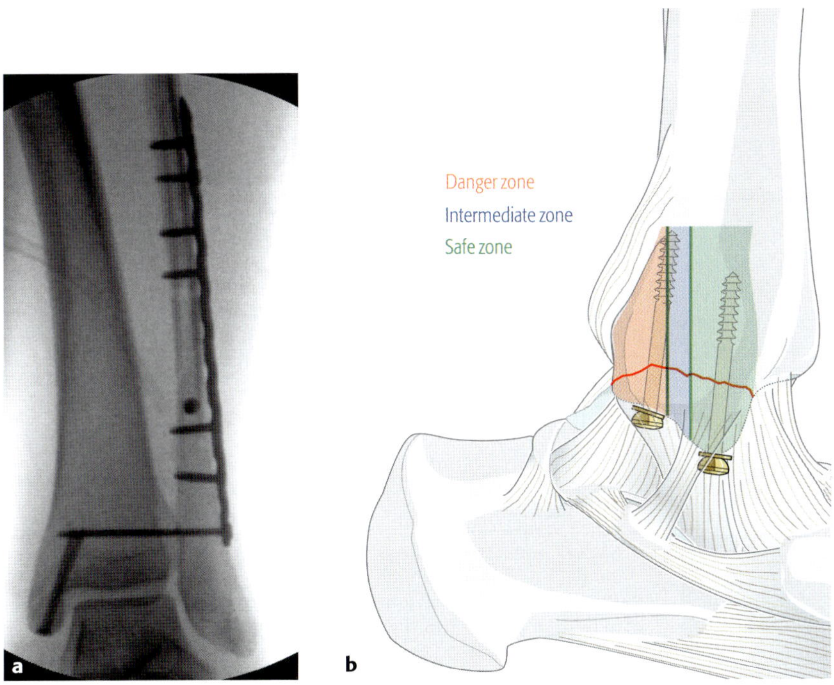

Fig 3.4-11a–b Pitfall for medial malleolus fixation.
a C-arm images from adequate AP position.
b If the posterior screw is too far posterior, it will result in irritating the posterior tibial tendon (circle).

Malposition of screws and inadequate fixation of the syndesmosis

A malposition of screws and inadequate fixation of the syndesmosis can be detected using intraoperative 3D C-arm imaging or postoperative CT scanning (**Fig 3.4-12**). Therefore, a low threshold should be applied for performing intraoperative or postoperative 3D imaging, but only if the surgeon is willing to return the patient to the OR for correction of position.

Complications

- Injury to the superficial peroneal nerve (lateral approach)
- Injury to the posterior tibial neurovascular bundle, if dissecting medially beyond the FHL tendon
- Irritation of the posterior tibial tendon with posterior screw placement in the medial malleolus
- Inadequate reduction and/or fixation of the syndesmosis
- Loss of fixation
- Malunion
- Nonunion
- Posttraumatic arthritis

6 Alternative techniques

Higher fibular fractures are treated as detailed in chapter 3.5. Fractures including a posterior tibial fragment are treated as trimalleolar fractures as detailed in chapter 3.6, by using the posterolateral approach.

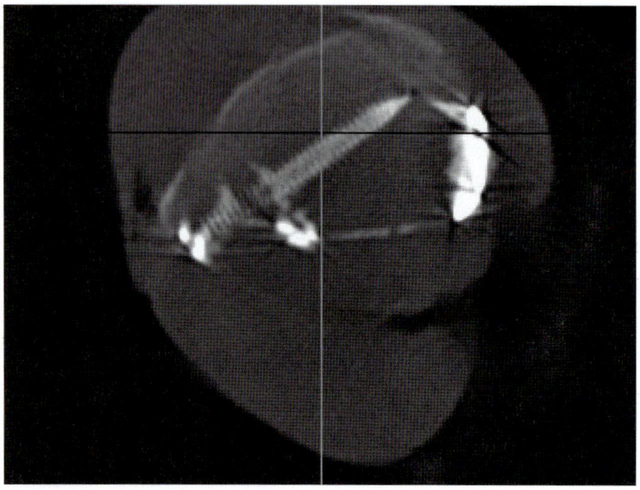

Fig 3.4-12 Anatomical reduction of the syndesmosis can be confirmed by intraoperative 3D imaging.

7 Postoperative management and rehabilitation

Postoperative immobilization in a splint for 2 weeks and elevation for reducing the swelling is enough to heal the skin. Early progressive weight bearing is recommended when tolerated by the reduction. The patient can mobilize on crutches with weight bearing limited by the pain.

Follow-up visits are recommended at 2, 6, 12, and 26 weeks postoperatively until bony consolidation is confirmed radiographically. Postoperative control x-rays are recommended at the 6, 12, and 26 weeks follow-up.

Implant removal

Implant removal is not generally recommended, as there is no evidence for improved functional outcome unless protruding hardware with soft-tissue irritation or objective functional limitations are found. Current evidence suggests retaining syndesmosis screws, unless complaints or limitations in absence of screw breakage with pain.

8 Recommended reading

Abu-Laban RB, Rose N. Ankle and foot. Emergency Medicine. June 2015. Available at: https://clinicalgate.com/ankle-and-foot-3/. Accessed March 11, 2018.

Del Buono A, Florio A, Boccanera MS, et al. Syndesmosis injuries of the ankle. *Curr Rev Musculoskelet Med.* 2013 Dec;6(4):313–319.

Dingemans SA, Rammelt S, White TO, et al. Should syndesmotic screws be removed after surgical fixation of unstable ankle fractures? A systematic review. *Bone Joint J.* 2016 Nov;98-b(11):1497–1504.

Femino JE, Gruber BF, Karunakar MA. Safe zone for the placement of medial malleolar screws. *J Bone Joint Surg Am.* 2007 Jan;89(1):133–138.

Graves M. Ankle Fracture Update, OTA Resident Core Curriculum Lecture Series, Updated November 2010. University of Mississippi Medical Center. Available at: https://slideplayer.com/slide/4329303/. Accessed March 11, 2018.

Rammelt S, Obruba P. An update on the evaluation and treatment of syndesmotic injuries. *Eur J Trauma Emerg Surg.* 2015 Dec;41(6):601–614.

3.5 High fibular fracture with syndesmotic disruption (Maisonneuve)

Michaël Houben, Martijn Poeze

1 Case description

A 25-year-old man fell while riding his scooter bike. He immediately had pain localized to the right ankle but was able to bear weight. Once at home, he applied ice and elevated his foot to reduce the swelling. The next morning, he noted that there was progressive edema and pain along the medial aspect of the ankle. He consulted a physician.

X-rays of the right ankle revealed a displaced ankle joint—most notably there was medial clear space widening (**Fig 3.5-1a–b**).

The patient had no history of ankle injuries and no comorbidities. Physical examination revealed significant edema of the medial aspect of the ankle and superficial lacerations. The areas of the deltoid ligament and proximal fibula were painful on palpation. He was next seen in the emergency department, where x-rays of the entire length of the tibia and fibula revealed a high fibular fracture and a posterior malleolar fracture (AO/OTA 44C3.3) (**Fig 3.5-1c**).

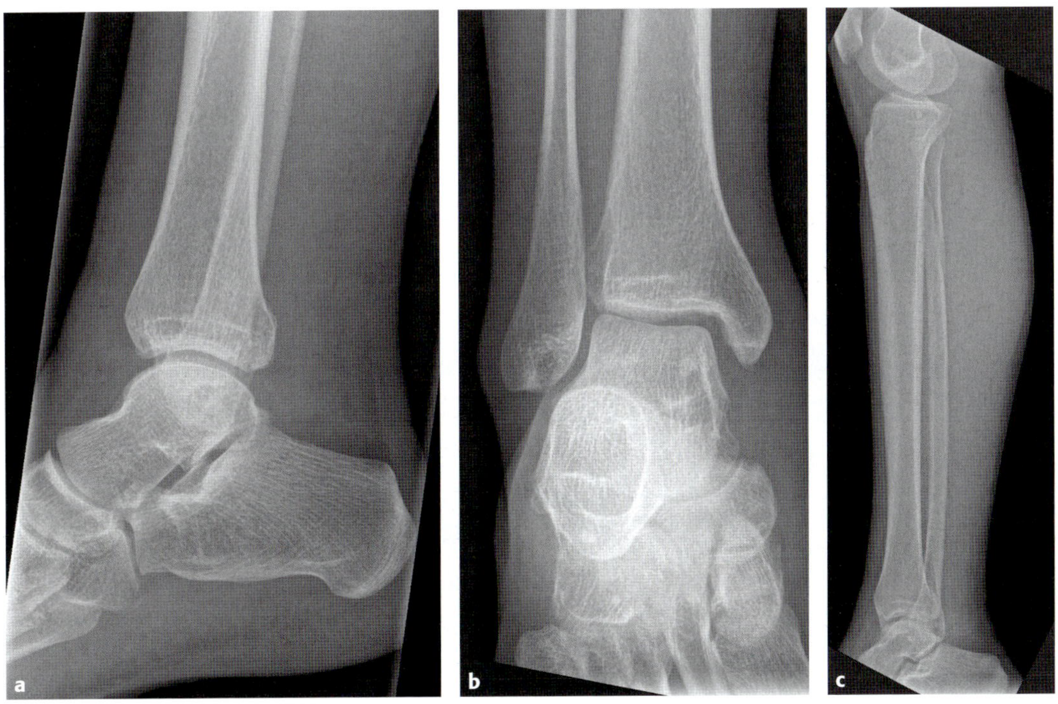

Fig 3.5-1a–c Preoperative x-rays.
a Lateral view of the ankle with small nondisplaced posterior malleolus fracture.
b AP view of the ankle showing talar tilt and widened tibiofibular clear space with loss of overlap.
c Lateral view of the leg showing a high fibular fracture and a nondisplaced posterior tibial fracture.

A computed tomographic (CT) scan was obtained for surgical preoperative planning—specifically the CT was used to determine the size and configuration of the posterior fragment to determine if it required open reduction and internal fixation (ORIF) (**Fig 3.5-2**).

2 Preoperative planning

The combination of the incongruent ankle joint with the high fibular fracture plus the posterior malleolar fragment are pathognomonic of a syndesmosis injury.

For this patient, fixation of the posterior fragment was not required due to the small size of the fragment (here, less than the amount needed for stability of the posterior malleolus) and because there was no displacement of the fibular notch (incisura). The high fibular fracture itself did not require fixation, although attention should be focused on restoring length and rotation of the fibula and thus the syndesmotic articulation in the incisura requires accurate reduction and stabilization.

3 Operating room setup

Patient positioning	• Supine on a radiolucent table with a sandbag under the ipsilateral buttock, the knee slightly flexed, the foot in neutral position
Anesthesia options	• General anesthesia, alternatively spinal anesthesia
C-arm location	• The C-arm is positioned on the foot end of the table, with the screen positioned for optimal viewing by the surgeon.
Tourniquet	• Temporary tourniquet (placed at the top of the thigh but only inflated if visualization is hampered by bleeding).

For illustrations and overview of anesthetic considerations, see chapter 1.

Equipment

- K-wires
- Drills with appropriate size sleeves
- Retractors as per surgeon preference
- Point-to-point reduction (Weber) clamp
- Periarticular reduction clamp
- Screws as per surgeon preference, fragment size, and individual bone quality
- Washers if needed for soft bone

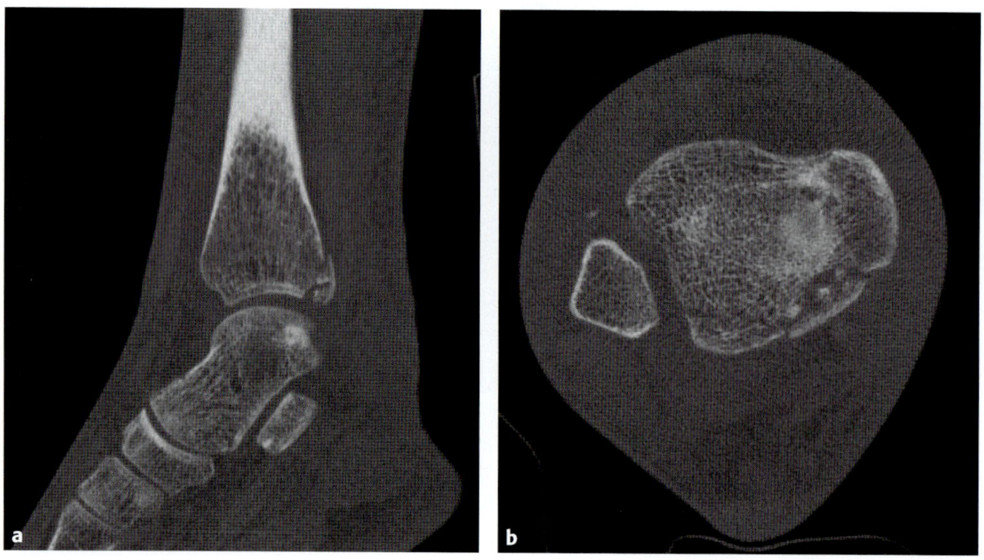

Fig 3.5-2a–b Preoperative CT scan.
a Sagittal cuts showing a small posterior malleollar fragment.
b Axial cuts showing small posterior fragment and syndesmotic incongruity but no displacement at the incisura.

4 Surgical procedure

A skin incision is made in line with the distal fibula. Sharp dissection is carried out to reach the periosteum and then continued anteriorly. The syndesmosis is visualized, and the syndesmotic space is cleared of any intervening tissue which hampers reduction of the fibula into the incisura.

A point-to-point reduction (Weber) clamp is applied to the distal fibula for traction to restore length and rotation. The syndesmotic incisura is usually reduced with traction and internal rotation. When perfect alignment and congruency of the tibiofibular joint is achieved, a 2.0 mm K-wire can be used to temporarily hold the reduction. The wire is inserted distal to the planned fixation screw. The screw should be placed approximately 1–2 cm above the plafond (**Fig 3.5-3a**).

Alternatively, a large periarticular reduction clamp can be used to restore the position of the distal fibula in the incisura, taking care not to displace the distal fibula by positioning the clamp off axis. Ideally, the clamp is placed from the tip of the lateral malleolus to the tip of the medial malleolus, thus lying exactly in the axis of the ankle joint. Direct visual inspection and palpation of the distal tibiofibular joint through the incision, or intraoperative C-arm imaging should be used to confirm reduction of the syndesmotic articulation, ie, the correct positioning of the distal fibula into the tibial incisura.

Reduction should be congruent according to the Weber criteria (**Fig 3.5-3b**). This must be assessed in a mortise view x-ray, with 10° internal rotation of the leg and the fifth metatarsal directly in line with the center of the calcaneum. Three characteristics should be comparable to the contralateral uninjured side:

1. The Shenton line of the ankle—a continuous line from the lateral part of the articular surface of the tibia to that of the distal fibula without any interruptions.
2. The Weber ball ("dime sign")—if the reduction is adequate the tip of the fibula and the lateral process of the talus can be connected by a circle (**Fig 3.5-3b**).
3. The medial and lateral joint space should equal the superior joint space.

With the ankle held in neutral position, a 2.5 mm hole is drilled through the fibula and tibia with an angle of 30° from posterior to anterior and parallel to the tibial plafond (**Fig 3.5-3c**). The length of the screw is measured with the depth gauge and the 3.5 or 4.0 mm cortex screw is inserted through three or four cortices of the fibula and tibia (**Fig 3.5-3d**).

Generally, a second screw is placed approximately 1.5–2 cm proximal to the first (**Fig 3.5-3e**) and the K-wire is removed (**Fig 3.5-3f–g**).

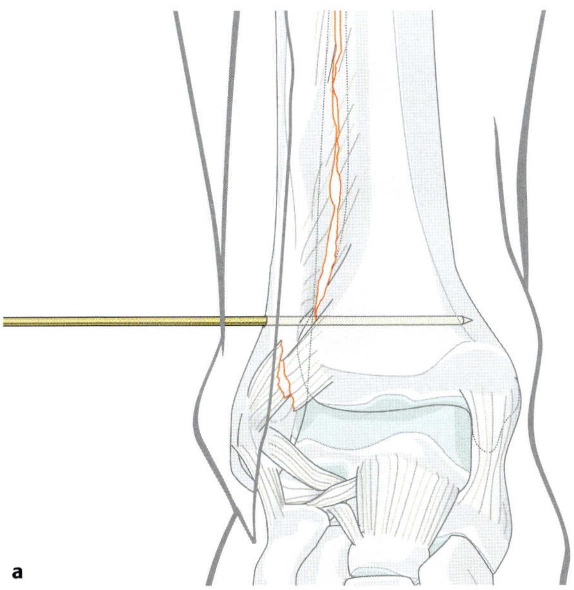

a

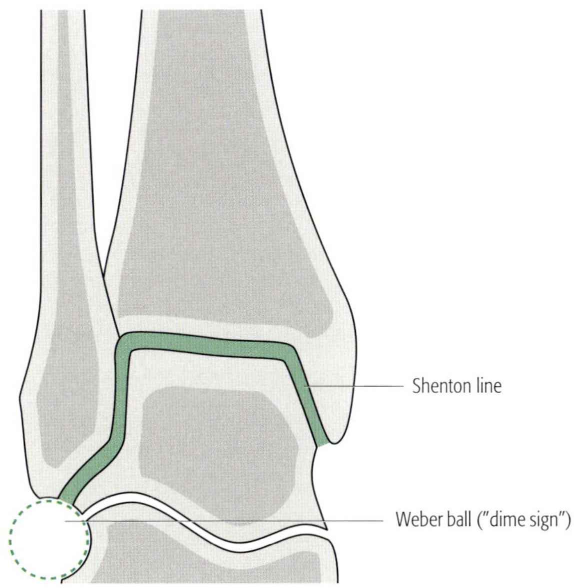

b

Fig 3.5-3a–g Syndesmotic fixation with two syndesmotic screws.
a Temporary fixation of the reduced fibula with a K-wire.
b Shenton line—the green continuous line from the lateral part of the articular surface of the tibia to that of the distal fibula. The Weber ball ("dime sign")—if the reduction is adequate the tip of the fibula and the lateral process of the talus can be connected by a circle.

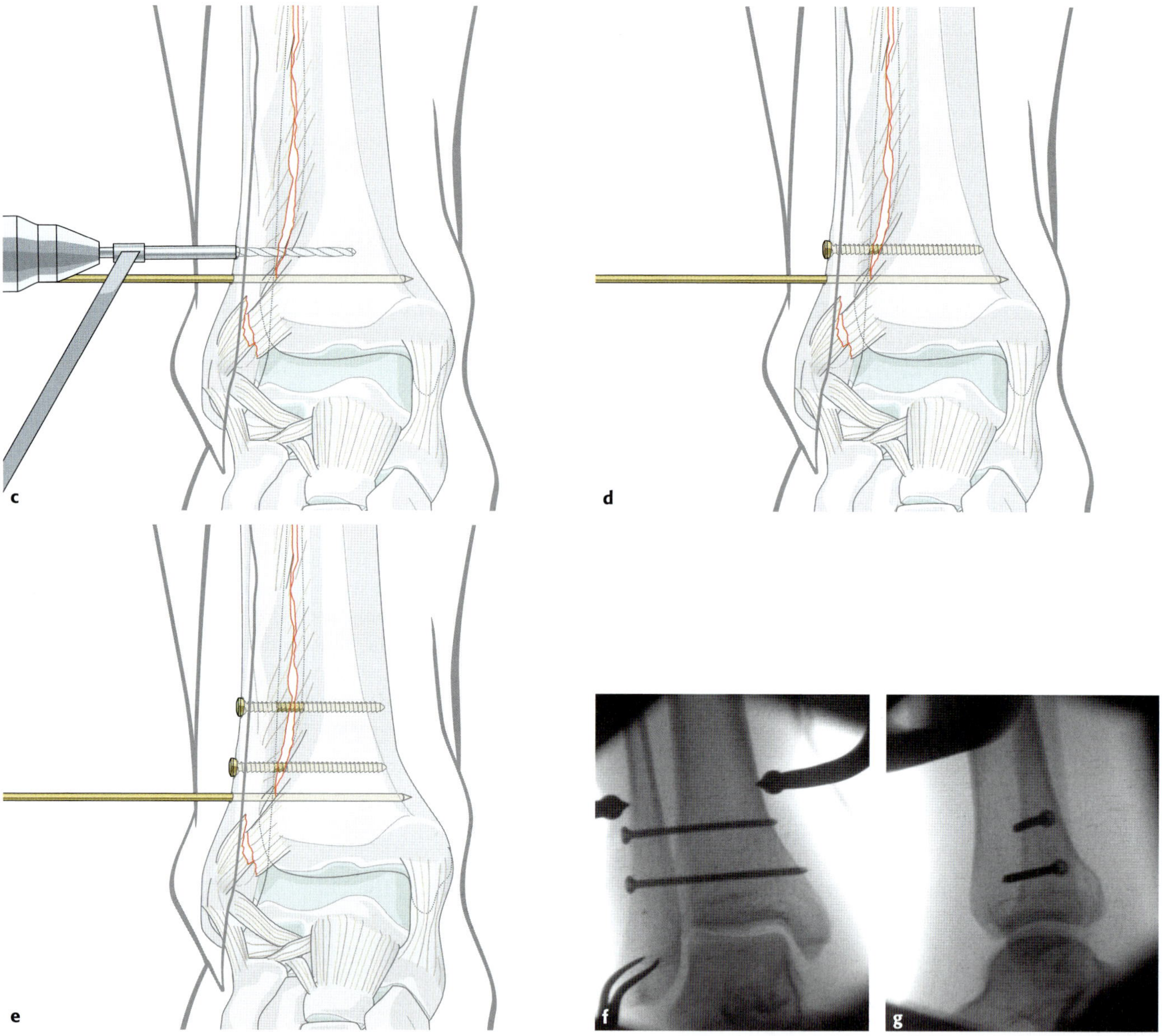

Fig 3.5-3a–g (cont) Syndesmotic fixation with two syndesmotic screws.

- **c** A 2.5 mm hole is drilled through the fibula and tibia.
- **d** A 3.5 mm cortex screw is inserted through the three or four cortices of the fibula and tibia.
- **e** A second screw can be placed in the same manner.
- **f** The AP C-arm image with a reduction clamp over the syndesmotic articulation showing the oblique screw placement from posterolateral to anteromedial.
- **g** Lateral C-arm image with a reduction clamp over the syndesmotic articulation showing the oblique screw placement from posterolateral to anteromedial.

The surgeon may choose to use a small one-third tubular plate along the posterolateral fibula through which two screws are placed. This helps spread the forces out and prevent fibular fracture, either at time of insertion or when walking commences.

Postoperative x-rays should be taken to confirm the congruence of the fibulotalar joint and the reduction in the syndesmosis (**Fig 3.5-4**).

If no intraoperative 3D imaging was made, a postoperative CT scan of both ankles is advised to ensure correct position of the distal fibula within the tibial incisura. If postoperative CT imaging shows an imperfect reduction, the surgeon must be prepared to discuss this with the patient with the goal of returning the patient to the operating room for revision ORIF.

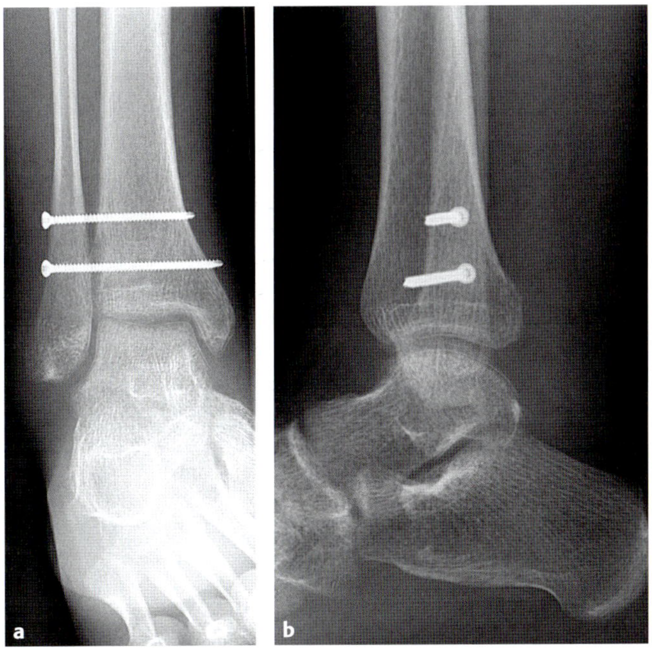

Fig 3.5-4a–b Postoperative x-rays showing fixation with two screws and a reduced syndesmosis.
a Good reduction and stable fixation of the syndesmosis (AP view).
b Note that the posterior fracture is also in an acceptable position (lateral view).

5 Pitfalls and complications

Pitfalls

Inadequate reduction of the syndesmotic articulation resulting in an incongruent talucrural joint

This can be caused by:

- Inadequate reduction of the length, anteroposterior position, and rotation of the distal fibula (particularly the latter two are hard to evaluate with 2D imaging).
- Malpositioning of the syndesmotic screws forcing the fibula into malposition.

Malreduction

The risk of malreduction can be minimized by correct axial clamp placement, which is aided by direct visual assessment and palpation of the alignment of the distal tibia and fibula; this is supplemented by obtaining adequate C-arm images in the mortise and lateral views using Weber indices. Secondary displacement by insertion of the screw can be avoided using K-wires to temporarily secure the reduction

Incongruity and loss of integrity

Failure to reduce and fix a displaced posterior tibial fragment may result in incongruity and loss of integrity of the tibial incisura leading to malpositioning of the distal fibula. Although the exact size of the fragment that needs fixation is debated, lateral incongruency of the ankle joint indicates a clinically relevant injury to the posterior malleolus. Failure to reduce and stabilize these fragments can result in persistent syndesmotic instability. However, a proper reduction of the distal fibula usually allows the posterior malleolus to move distally together with the fibula to which it is attached via the posterior syndesmosis and thus is more easily reduced.

Complications

- Superficial peroneal nerve damage (lateral approach)
- Failure of healing of the syndesmotic ligaments leading to chronic instability

6 Alternative techniques

Fixation of displaced posterior tibial fragments is discussed in chapters 3.6–3.9.

Fixation of the syndesmotic articulation can be achieved by the use a flexible implant (fiber wire or suture button fixation). The screws can be inserted through a 2-hole one-third tubular plate to reduce strain on the fibula.

7 Postoperative management and rehabilitation

The patient is placed into a 3-sided ("AO") splint for the first 2 weeks. After inspection of the skin and removal of the sutures, a circular plaster or removable boot is applied for an additional 4–6 weeks. The patient is restricted to non-weight-bearing on the operated ankle for 6–8 weeks postoperatively.

Implant removal

Some surgeons prefer to remove the syndesmotic screws at 8 weeks before weight bearing is started. The need for syndesmotic screw removal is unclear and it has been shown that screw breakage after full weight bearing may lead to improved functional results. Flexible implants are only removed when symptomatic.

8 Recommended reading

Bartoníček J, Rammelt S, Kašper Š, et al. Pathoanatomy of Maisonneuve fracture based on radiologic and CT examination. *Arch Orthop Trauma Surg.* 2019 Apr;139(4):497–506.
Dingemans SA, Rammelt S, White TO, et al. Should syndesmotic screws be removed after surgical fixation of unstable ankle fractures? A systematic review. *Bone Joint J.* 2016 Nov;98-b(11):1497–1504.
Miller AN, Barei DP, Iaquinto JM, et al. Iatrogenic syndesmosis malreduction via clamp and screw placement. *J Orthop Trauma.* 2013 Feb;27(2):100–106.
Mittal, A. Ankle fractures. Available at: https://www.slideshare.net/mittal87/ankle-fractures-final. Accessed March 22, 2019.
Peek AC, Fitzgerald CE, Charalambides C. Syndesmosis screws: how many, what diameter, where and should they be removed? A literature review. *Injury.* 2014 Aug;45(8):1262–1267
Pelton K, Thordarson DB, Barnwell J. Open versus closed treatment of the fibula in Maisonneuve injuries. *Foot Ankle Int.* 2010 Jul;31(7):604–608.
Phisitkul P, Ebinger T, Goetz J, et al. Forceps reduction of the syndesmosis in rotational ankle fractures: a cadaveric study. *J Bone Joint Surg Am.* 2012 Dec 19;94(24):2256–2261.
Rammelt S, Zwipp H, Grass R. Injuries to the distal tibiofibular syndesmosis: an evidence-based approach to acute and chronic lesions. *Foot Ankle Clin.* 2008 Dec;13(4):611–633.
Walley KC, Hofmann KJ, Velasco BT, et al. Removal of hardware after syndesmotic screw fixation: a systematic literature review. *Foot Ankle Spec.* 2017 Jun;10(3):252–257.
Wang C, Ma X, Wang X, et al. Internal fixation of distal tibiofibular syndesmotic injuries: a systematic review with meta-analysis. *Int Orthop.* 2013 Sep;37(9):1755–1763.

3.6 Trimalleolar fracture with syndesmotic disruption

Michaël Houben, Martijn Poeze

1 Case description

A healthy 69-year-old woman lost her balance while getting onto her bicycle, landing directly on her right foot before falling to the ground. She immediately felt severe pain in her ankle. There was an associated severe displacement of her ankle and she was unable to move her foot. An attempt at immediate reduction of the ankle was performed.

On arrival at the emergency department, physical examination revealed massive swelling of her right lower leg. The area was painful on palpation. AP and lateral x-rays of the ankle and leg revealed a trimalleolar transsyndesmotic fracture (AO/OTA 44B3.2) (**Fig 3.6-1**). AP and lateral x-rays of the whole lower leg were taken to rule out any other fractures of the adjacent joints. After adequate reduction of the ankle, a splint was used to temporarily stabilize the ankle.

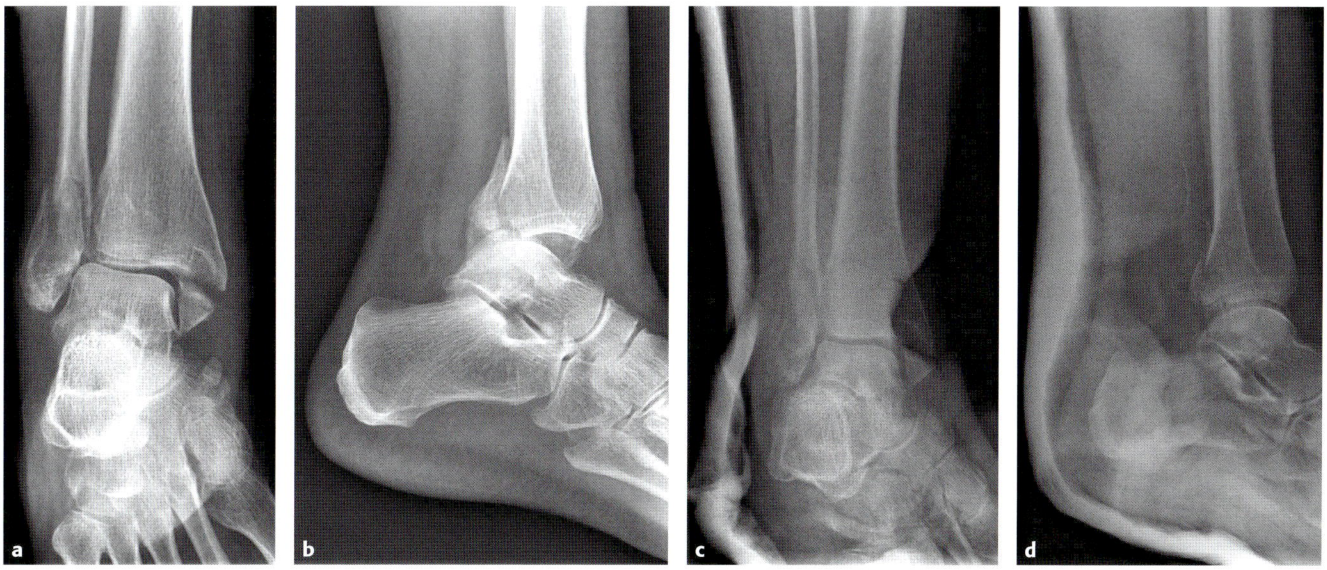

Fig 3.6-1a–d X-rays at presentation.
a AP x-ray with a decrease in talocrucal joint space and obvious medial and lateral malleolar fractures (AO/OTA 44B3.2).
b Lateral x-ray revealing a posteriorly dislocated ankle mortise.
c–d Postreduction AP and lateral x-rays views showing adequately reduced ankle joint in a plaster cast.

Computed tomographic (CT) imaging obtained for preoperative planning of the surgical approach revealed a large posterior malleolus (Volkmann) fragment and type Weber B fibular fracture (**Fig 3.6-2**). A mechanically significant posterior malleolar fracture (at least 30%) with posterosuperior displacement and intraarticular comminution, Haraguchi type 2/Bartoníček and Rammelt type 4 was present.

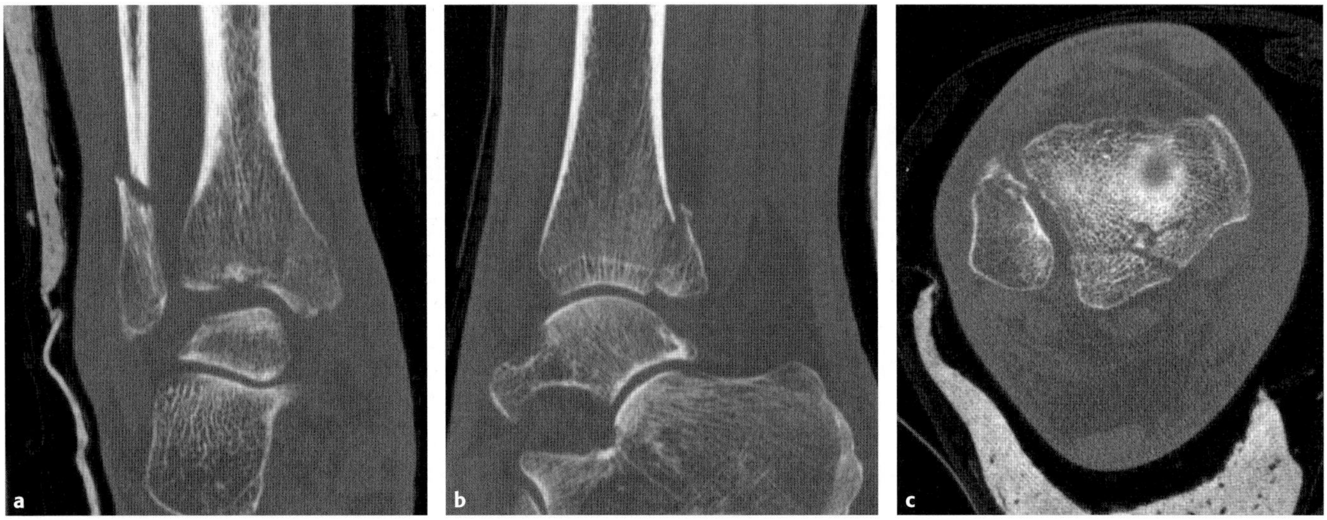

Fig 3.6-2a–c Preoperative CT scan demonstrating the Haraguchi type 2 posterior malleolar fracture.
a Coronal view.
b Sagittal view.
c Axial view.

2 Preoperative planning

Indications for surgery

The indication for surgery was instability of the ankle joint.

Considerations for surgery

A posterolateral approach is most suitable for accessing the posterior fragment when necessary (**Fig 3.6-3**).

For adequate reduction of the medial malleolar fragment a standard medial incision can be used, although a posteromedial approach may be an alternative approach. Open reduction and internal fixation with buttress plates and screws is performed. Perioperative manual stress testing of the syndesmosis is helpful in detecting syndesmosis residual instability after stabilizing the other fracture components. In the case of persistent syndesmotic instability, one or two screws (across three or four cortices), or a suture button implant can be inserted.

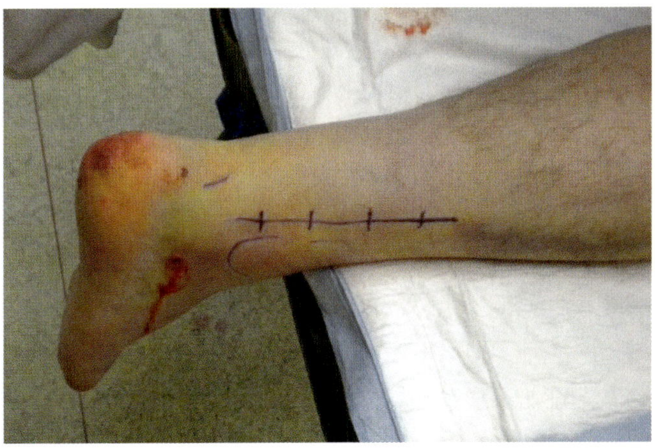

Fig 3.6-3 Preoperative positioning and marking of the posterolateral incision.

3 Operating room setup

Patient positioning	• Prone for the best visibility on the posterolateral approach and posterior malleolar fragment. A small pillow can be put below the distal tibia for foot manipulation
Anesthesia options	• General anesthesia, alternatively regional anesthesia
C-arm location	• C-arm is positioned lateral to the patient's leg and foot
Tourniquet	• Temporary tourniquet (only applied when visualization is hampered by bleeding)

For illustrations and overview of anesthetic considerations, see chapter 1.

Equipment

- K-wires
- 2.5 mm, 3.5 mm, and 4.0 mm drills with soft-tissue protection sleeves
- Drill
- Assorted retractors
- Point-to-point reduction (Weber) clamp
- Silicon vessel loop (optional)
- One-third tubular plates
- T-buttress plates
- Screws
- Washers
- Threaded K-wires

4 Surgical procedure

Fixation of the fibular fracture

The posterolateral approach uses a 10 cm vertical incision midway between the fibula and Achilles tendon (**Fig 3.6-4a**). The skin is retracted. Special care is taken to identify and to protect the sural nerve. Surgical dissection is performed through the fascia cruris to the interval between the flexor hallucis longus (FHL) and peroneus brevis muscles (**Fig 3.6-4b**). Deep retractors (Hohmann) can then be placed to facilitate visualization. Care must be taken to avoid trauma to the skin edges. The peroneal retinaculum is retracted laterally and anteriorly, and a longitudinal incision is made along the origin (lateral fibers) of the FHL. Now the FHL is retracted medially to expose the periosteum of the posterior tibia and fibula, while protecting the neurovascular bundle medially.

The fibular fracture is reduced manually by using the retractors for leverage and fixed temporarily with K-wires. Then, the posterior malleolar fragment is visualized. The posterior fragment is brought to the level of the ankle joint surface and first fixed with K-wires (**Fig 3.6-4c–d**). Fixation by an antiglide buttress plate provides compression on the posterior fragment as well as resistance to superior displacement. Use of a partially threaded or fully threaded lag screw ensures that the distal part of the posterior fragment will be compressed. Care must be taken to not over compress the distal screws or deformity of the plafond may occur.

Definitive fixation is achieved by using cortex and interlocking screws in the proximal fragment through the plate (**Fig 3.6-4e**). Distal fixation is done under compression. Intraoperative imaging with the C-arm is used to verify the reduction and confirm that screws are not penetrating the articular surface (**Fig 3.6-4f**). Fixation of the distal fibula is achieved with a posterolateral antiglide plate using the same interval between FHL and peroneus brevis muscles. The distal end of the fibular plate should be placed a minimum of 1 cm above the tip of the fibula to avoid peroneal tendon irritation.

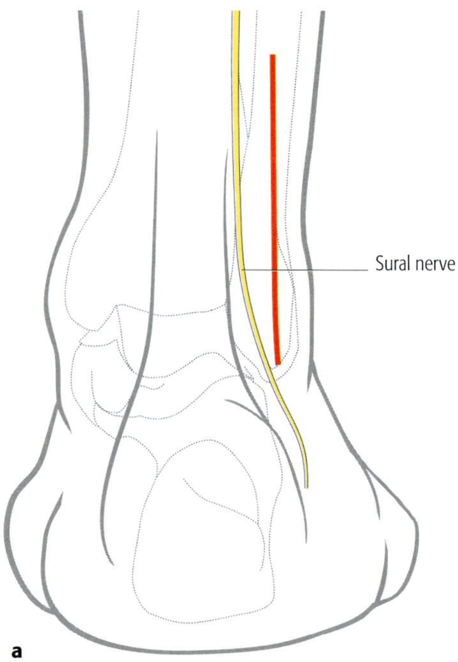

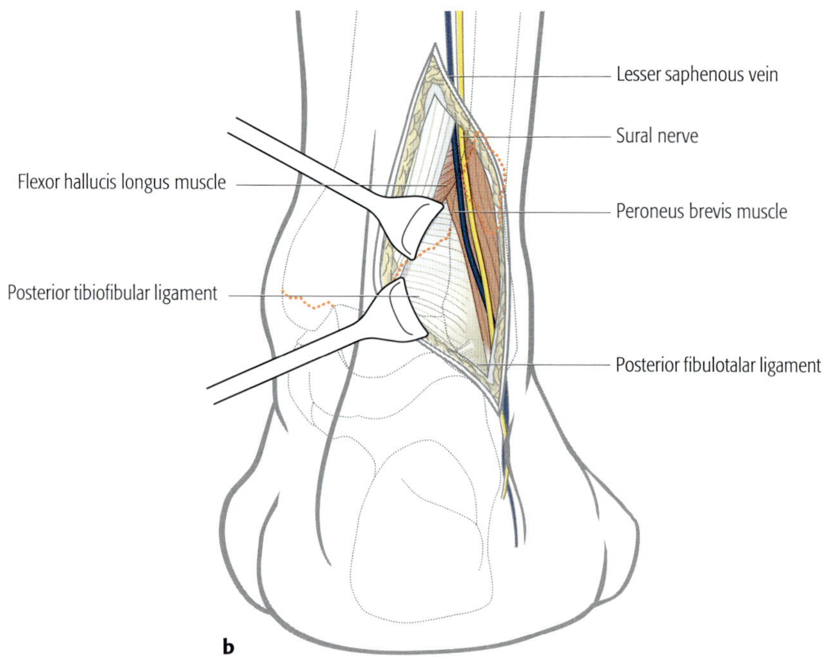

Fig 3.6-4a–f Fixation of the posterior fragment.
a Posterolateral approach, with identification of the sural nerve.
b Deeper dissection with the neurovascular bundle protected to the medial side.

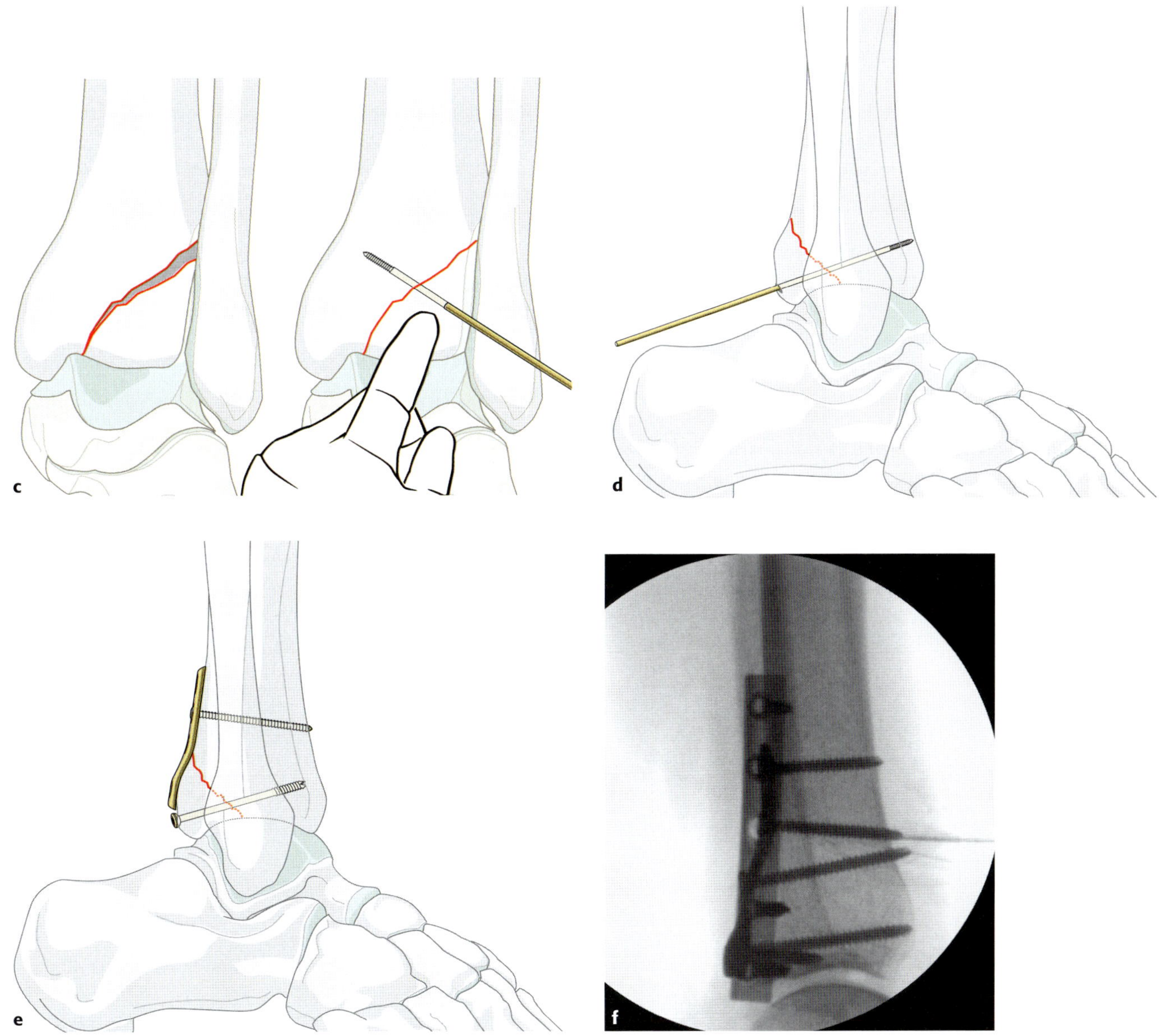

Fig 3.6-4a–f (cont) Fixation of the posterior fragment.

- **c** Volkmann fragment manipulation.
- **d** Temporary K-wire fixation.
- **e** After anatomical reduction, fixation is performed by using a compression screw through the plate for a fixation under compression, then a partially threaded cannulated screw is inserted to keep the fragment from moving cranially.
- **f** Intraoperative imaging of the posterior fragment fixation and fibular fixation.

Fixation of the malleolar fracture

Next, a longitudinal incision centered over the tip of the medial malleolus is made. The incision is curved distally toward the navicular tuberosity (**Fig 3.6-5a**). After retracting the skin, the greater saphenous vein and the saphenous nerve are identified anterior to the medial malleolus and protected using a vessel loop or are retracted anteriorly. A small longitudinal incision is made in the anteromedial ankle joint capsule, directly posterior to the medial malleolus in the flexor retinaculum, just above the tibialis posterior tendon (**Fig 3.6-5b**). Under direct vision, the medial malleolus is fixed using two fracture fixation system wires. Alternatively, screws can be used when dealing with a larger fragment (**Fig 3.6-5c–d**).

There are several different methods to test syndesmosis stability after fracture fixation:

- Using lateral and posterior translation stress
- Via external rotation of the foot with the tibia fixed
- Using a reduction clamp or lamina spreader between the distal tibia and fibula

Testing should be done gently so as not to disrupt the fractures which were just fixed. If testing results in significant tibiofibular displacement, indicating syndesmotic instability, a tibiofibular cortex screw is added through the posterolateral incision to secure the incisura (**Fig 3.6-5e–f**). In most cases, however, fixation of a large posterior fragment will also stabilize the syndesmosis.

5 Pitfalls and complications

Pitfalls

Difficulty in maintaining reduction and fixation

In case of multifragmentary posterior malleolar fracture, reduction and fixation can be difficult to maintain. Possible failure of fixation can result in serious consequences for the patient. Buttress plating is essential for adequate stabilization, especially in elderly patients with osteoporotic bone.

Injury to the posterior tibial tendon and neurovascular structures

The posterior tibial tendon is in danger when making the medial incision and placing implants into the posterior part of the medial malleolus. Care must be taken not to injure the neurovascular structures anterior and posterior to the medial malleolus.

Intraarticular fragmentation

Intraarticular fragmentation is a serious pitfall. Depending on the amount of comminution, location, and size of the intraarticular fragment a deliberate decision should be made whether to fix or remove the fragments to avoid loose intraarticular bodies.

Complications

- Injury to the sural nerve (posterolateral approach)
- Injury to the superficial peroneal nerve (lateral approach)
- Injury to the posterior tibial neurovascular bundle, if preparing medially beyond the FHL tendon
- Irritation of the posterior tibial tendon with posterior implant placement in the medial malleolus
- Inadequate fixation of the syndesmosis
- Loss of fixation
- Malunion
- Nonunion
- Posttraumatic arthritis

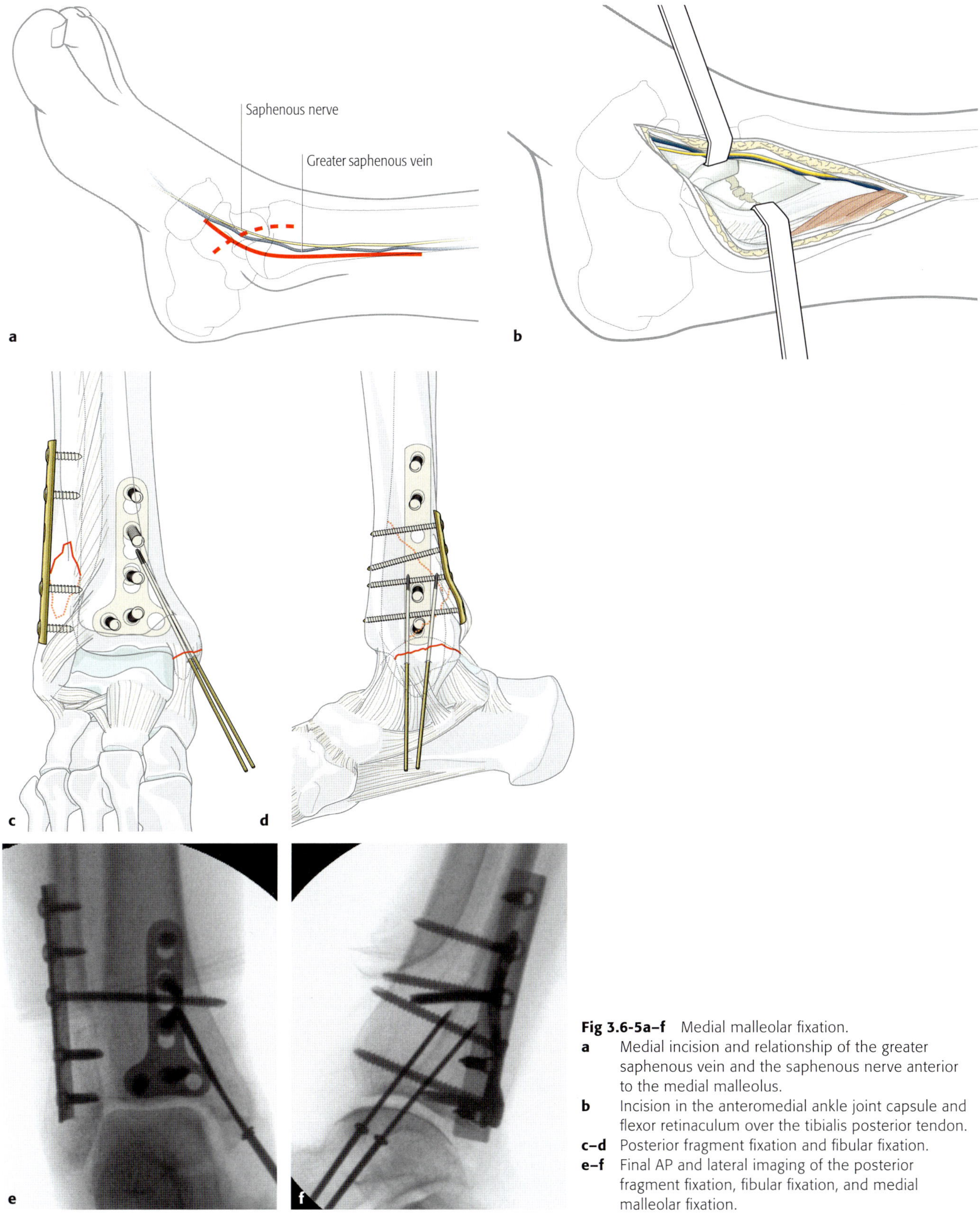

Fig 3.6-5a–f Medial malleolar fixation.

a Medial incision and relationship of the greater saphenous vein and the saphenous nerve anterior to the medial malleolus.

b Incision in the anteromedial ankle joint capsule and flexor retinaculum over the tibialis posterior tendon.

c–d Posterior fragment fixation and fibular fixation.

e–f Final AP and lateral imaging of the posterior fragment fixation, fibular fixation, and medial malleolar fixation.

6 Alternative techniques

A single large posterior fragment can be visualized through the fibular fracture using a lateral approach and reduced indirectly and fixed with two anterior to posterior screws.

With multifragmentary posterior fractures, adequate visualization and direct fixation of the posterior fragment is advisable using the posterolateral approach (see chapter 3.9).

For a medial malleolar fracture a direct posteromedial approach can be used for reduction and fixation (**Fig 3.6-6**).

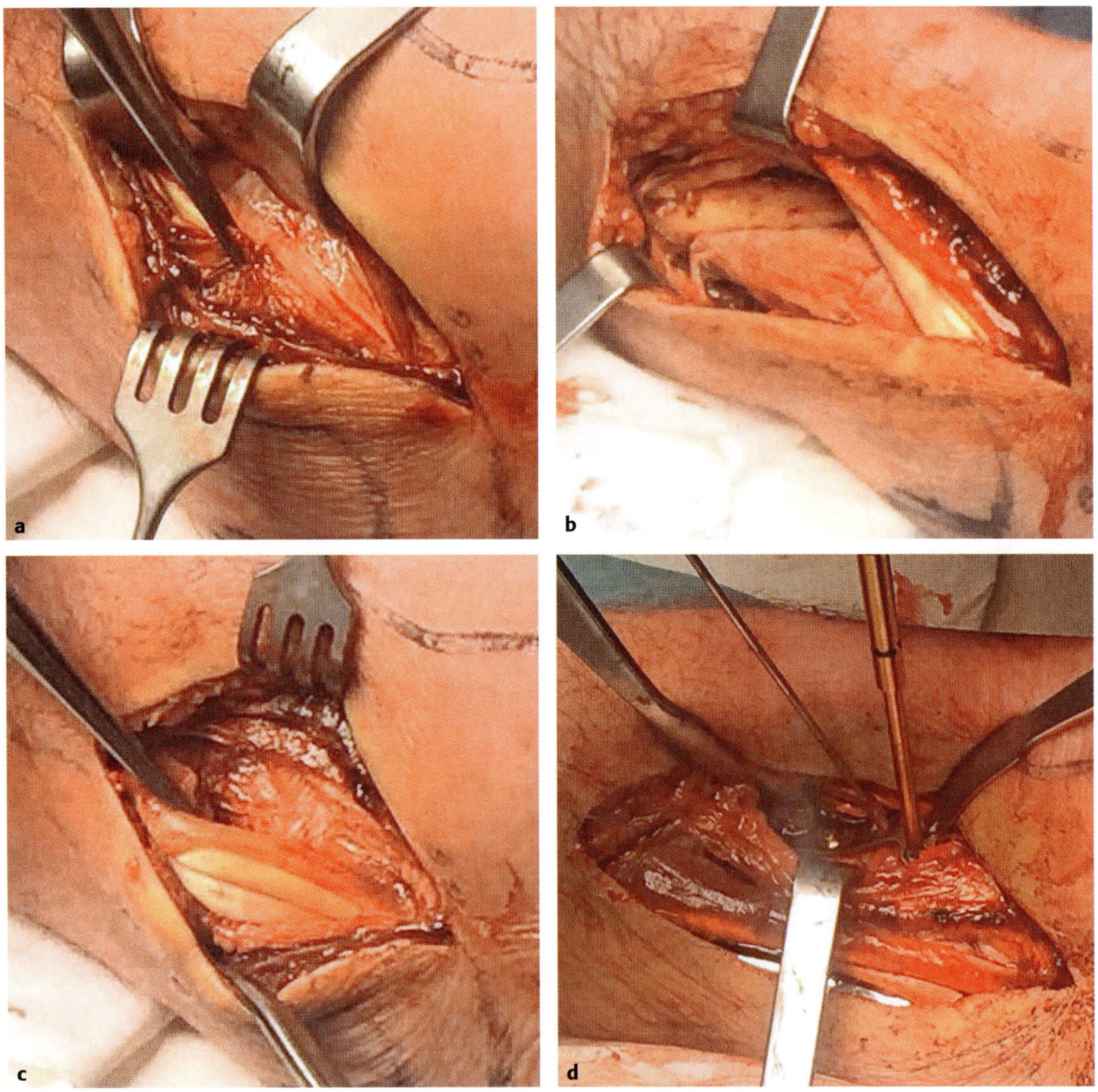

Fig 3.6-6a–d Example from a different case showing the posteromedial approach opening of the fascia of the posterior tibial tendon (**a**), lifting of the posterior tibial and flexor digitorum tendons (**b**), window between posterior tibial, flexor digitorum tendons and neurovascular bundle (**c**), and plate fixation lateral from neurovascular bundle and testing for syndesmotic instability (**d**).

7 Postoperative management and rehabilitation

Postoperative immobilization in a splint for 2 weeks and elevation for reducing the swelling provides enough time for the skin to heal. Early progressive weight bearing is recommended when tolerated by reduction and fixation. Subsequently, the patient can mobilize weight bearing depending on the pain.

Follow-up is recommended at 2, 6, 12, and 26 weeks postoperatively until consolidation; with x-rays taken at the 6-, 12- , and 26-week follow-up (**Fig 3.6-7**).

Implant removal

Implants are not routinely removed. They are removed only in cases where they are prominent or bothersome. Syndesmotic fixation screws may also remain in situ as there is no evidence of better functional outcome when no objective limitations are found. Current evidence suggests retaining syndesmotic screws, unless there are complaints or limitations in absence of screw breakage with pain. Suture button implants are only removed if they become symptomatic, which reportedly occurs in about 17% of patients.

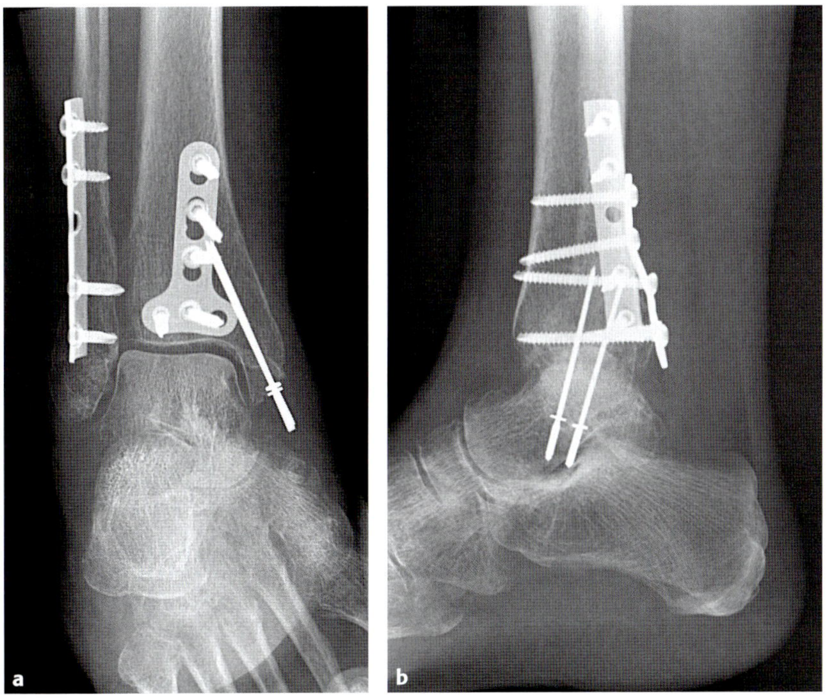

Fig 3.6-7a–b Postoperative imaging at 3 months. The syndesmotic fixation screw was removed due to functional limitations.
a AP view.
b Lateral view.

Recommended reading

Bartoníček J, Rammelt S, Tuček M. Posterior malleolar fractures: changing concepts and recent developments. *Foot Ankle Clin.* 2017 Mar;22(1):125–145.

Degroot H, Al-Omari AA, El Ghazaly SA. Outcomes of suture button repair of the distal tibiofibular syndesmosis. *Foot Ankle Int.* 2011 Mar;32(3):250–256.

Dingemans SA, Rammelt S, White TO, et al. Should syndesmotic screws be removed after surgical fixation of unstable ankle fractures? A systematic review. *Bone Joint J.* 2016 Nov;98-b(11):1497–1504.

Hoppenfeld S, de Boer P, Buckley R. *Surgical Exposures in Orthopaedics: The Anatomic Approach.* 5th ed. Philadelphia: Lippincott Williams & Wilkins; 2016.

Peek AC, Fitzgerald CE, Charalambides C. Syndesmosis screws: how many, what diameter, where and should they be removed? A literature review. *Injury.* 2014 Aug;45(8):1262–1267.

Sman AD, Hiller CE, Refshauge KM. Diagnostic accuracy of clinical tests for diagnosis of ankle syndesmosis injury: a systematic review. *Br J Sports Med.* 2013 Jul;47(10):620–628.

Verhage SM, Boot F, Schipper IB, et al. Open reduction and internal fixation of posterior malleolar fractures using the posterolateral approach. *Bone Joint J.* 2016 Jun;98-b(6):812–817.

Walley KC, Hofmann KJ, Velasco BT, et al. Removal of hardware after syndesmotic screw fixation: a systematic literature review. *Foot Ankle Spec.* 2017 Jun;10(3):252–257.

Wiesel SW, ed. *Operative Techniques in Orthopaedic Surgery* (4 Volume Set). 1st ed. Philadelphia: Wolters Kluwer; 2015.

3.7 Trimalleolar ankle fracture with impaction of the posterior tibial rim

Stefan Rammelt

1 Case description

A 55-year-old woman heavily twisted her left ankle on a curb when falling off her bicycle. She immediately experienced a sharp pain at the ankle and noted an obvious displacement of her foot. The ankle was grossly reduced on site by an emergency physician after administration of intravenous anesthetics and immobilized with a vacuum splint. Upon arrival in the hospital, x-rays of the ankle and whole lower leg revealed a trimalleolar fracture dislocation (AO/OTA type 44B3.3, pronation abduction stage 3 according to Lauge-Hansen). A high fibular fracture or dislocation of the fibular head was ruled out (**Fig 3.7-1**).

Computed tomographic (CT) scanning was performed for thorough fracture assessment, particularly of the posterior tibial rim (**Fig 3.7-2**).

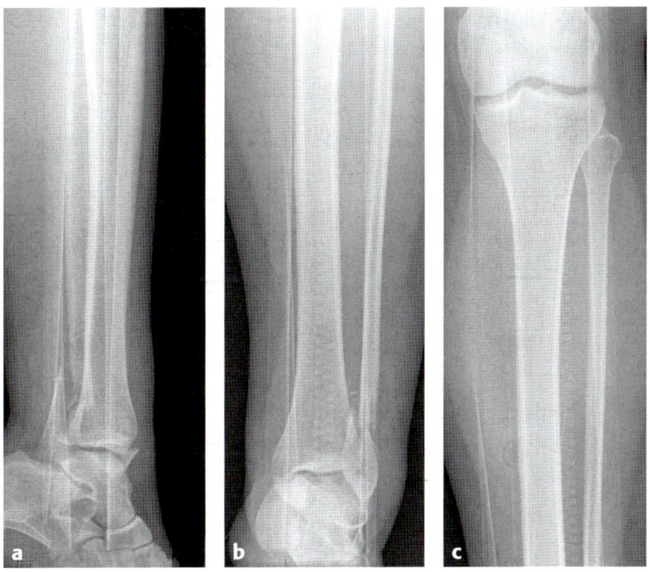

Fig 3.7-1a–c Postinjury images.

a–b X-rays of the ankle after gross reduction of the dislocation and immobilization with a vacuum splint.

c A high fibular fracture is ruled out with x-rays of the whole lower leg including the knee.

2 Preoperative planning

Indication for surgery was obvious with a trimalleolar fracture dislocation in an otherwise healthy patient. The fibular fracture is typically fixed with a plate. Options include a lateral neutralization plate or a posterior antiglide plate. In this case, the multifragmentary fibular fracture was fixed with a bridge plate.

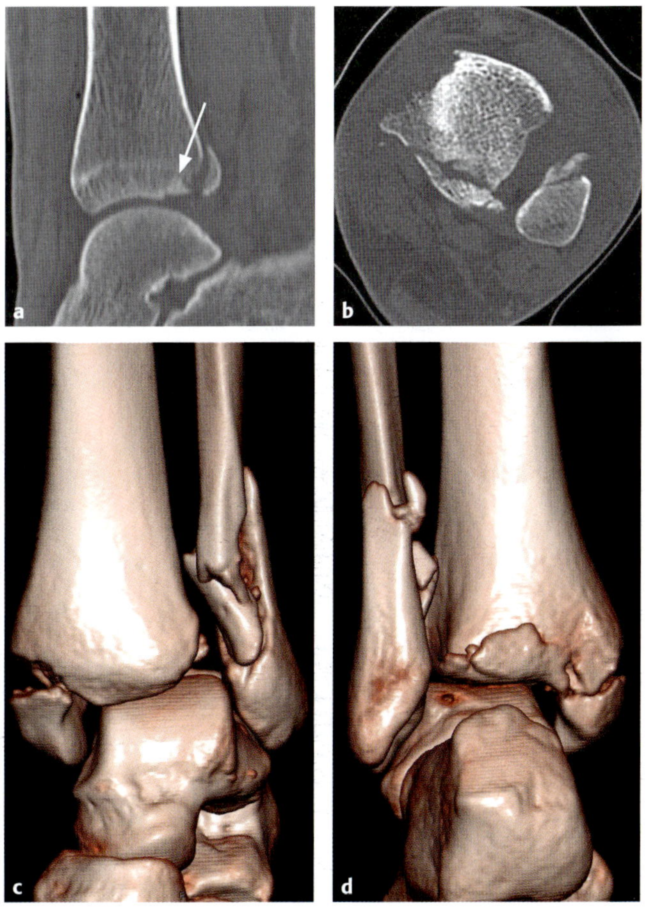

Fig 3.7-2a–d Computed tomographic images.

a–b The CT scans revealed a posterolateral fracture of the distal tibial rim with a depressed intercalary fragment (white arrow, Bartoncíček type II) in addition to the multifragmentary fibular fracture and the medial malleolar fracture.

c–d 3D reconstructions of the CT scans.

The oblique medial malleolar fracture can be accessed via a medial approach and fixed with compression screws, a tension band wire, or, in case of comminution, a small medial plate.

The posterior tibial fragment should be fixed directly from posterior to allow proper reduction of the displaced posterior rim and the impacted, intercalary fragment (**Fig 3.7-3**).

3 Operating room setup

Patient positioning	• Prone on a radiolucent table with the upper foot draped free
Anesthesia options	• General anesthesia • Alternatively, spinal or regional anesthesia may be used.
C-arm location	• Placed at the foot of the operative table with the monitor facing toward the head of the operative table.
Tourniquet	• Used at surgeon's discretion

For illustrations and overview of anesthetic considerations, see chapter 1.

Equipment

- K-wires, resorbable pins
- One-third tubular plate (with poor bone quality rather use an interlocking plate)
- 3.5 mm (or 2.7 mm) cancellous screws
- 3.5 mm (or 2.7 mm) cortex screws
- Smooth and sharp elevators

Size of system, instruments, and implants may vary according to the anatomy of the patient.

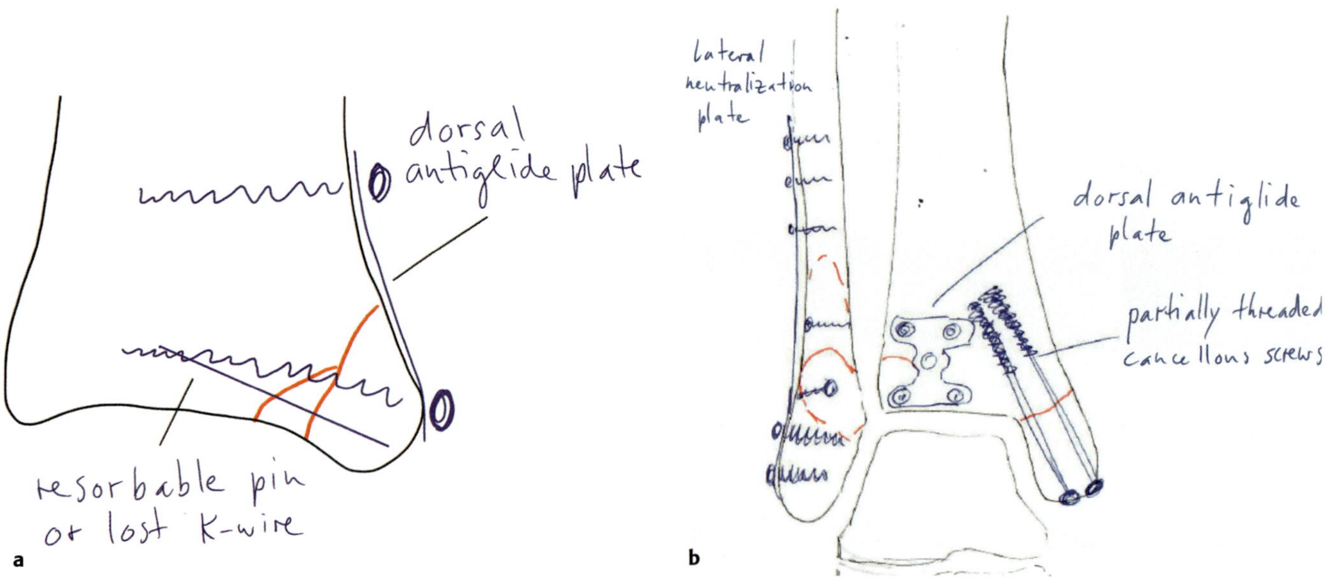

Fig 3.7-3a–b Preoperative plan.
a The posterior malleolus is fixed directly from posterior with a small antiglide plate. The intercalary fragment is assessed for stability and carticlage cover and eventually fixed with a resorbable pin or K-wire.
b The larger fibular fragments is fixed with interfragmentary (lag) screws, then a lateral neutralization plate is applied via a lateral approach. The medial malleolus is stabilized with cancellous lag screws via a slightly curved medial approach.

4 Surgical procedure

For internal fixation according to the preoperative plan, three approaches are needed: posterolateral, lateral, and medial.

Reduction and fixation of the posterior tibial fragments—posterolateral approach

Reduction of the posterior tibial fragments should be performed first to allow adequate visualization in the lateral C-arm projections. The incision for the posterolateral approach lies parallel to the Achilles tendon (**Fig 3.7-4**). The sural nerve is identified within the subcutaneous tissue in the proximal part of the incision and gently retracted medially. The superficial and deep fasciae are incised longitudinally and the flexor hallucis longus (FHL) muscle belly and tendon are retracted medially so that the posterior tibial neurovascular bundle is protected. The fractured posterior tibial fragment is identified and cleared of hematoma and debris and held away laterally. The posterior tibiofibular ligament is used as a hinge and left intact.

The intercalary fragments are then identified and evaluated for bone quality and cartilage cover. If the cartilage is intact and a stable fragment with a diameter of 5 mm or more is present, this fragment is reduced to the intact anterior portion of the tibial plafond and fixed temporarily with a K-wire.

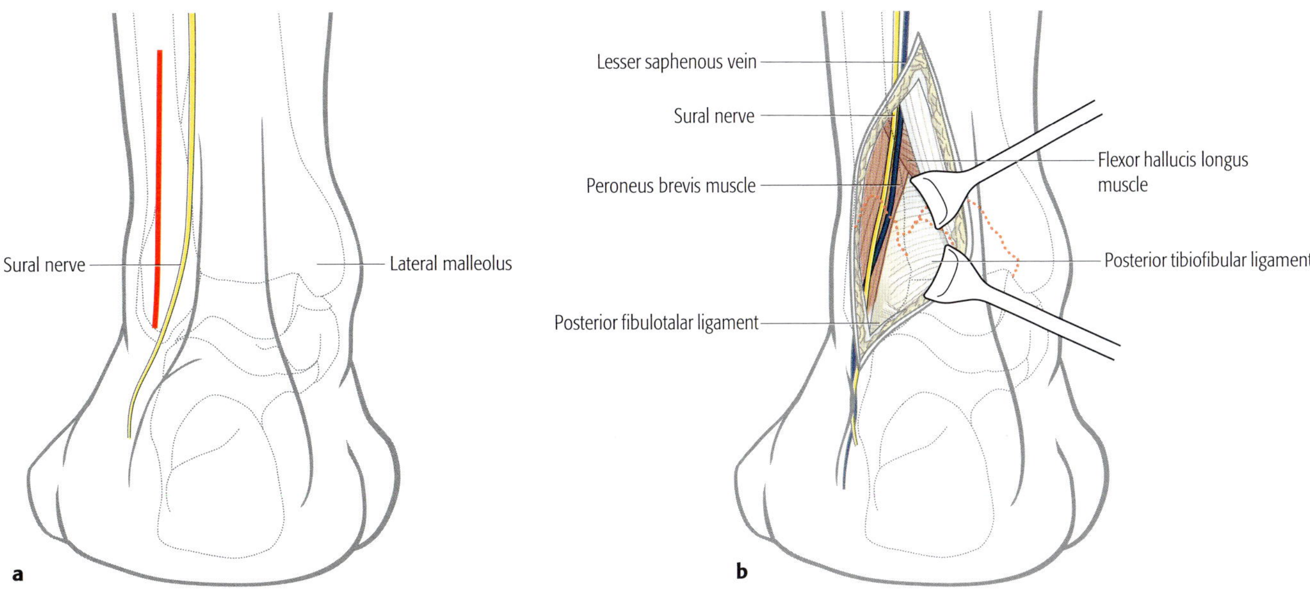

Fig 3.7-4a–b Posteolateral approach to the posterior tibia (and fibula).
a Landmarks for the skin incision (red line).
b Intraoperative exposure of the posterior tibial fragment which is attached to the posterior tibiofibular ligament.

Definite fixation of this fragment can be achieved with either a resorbable pin or a K-wire that is cut flush with the intercalary fragment and acts as a lost or buried K-wire. The posterolateral rim with the posterior syndesmosis attached is then brought back and realigned with the posterior tibial plafond. Anatomical reduction of the tibial joint surface is controlled with a lateral C-arm view. Definite fixation is achieved with screws (and washers in the case of shallow fragments) or a posterior antiglide plate depending on the size of the fragment and the bone quality (**Fig 3.7-5**). Fixation of the posterior fragment stabilizes the posterior syndesmosis and recreates the tibial incisura which eases fibular reduction.

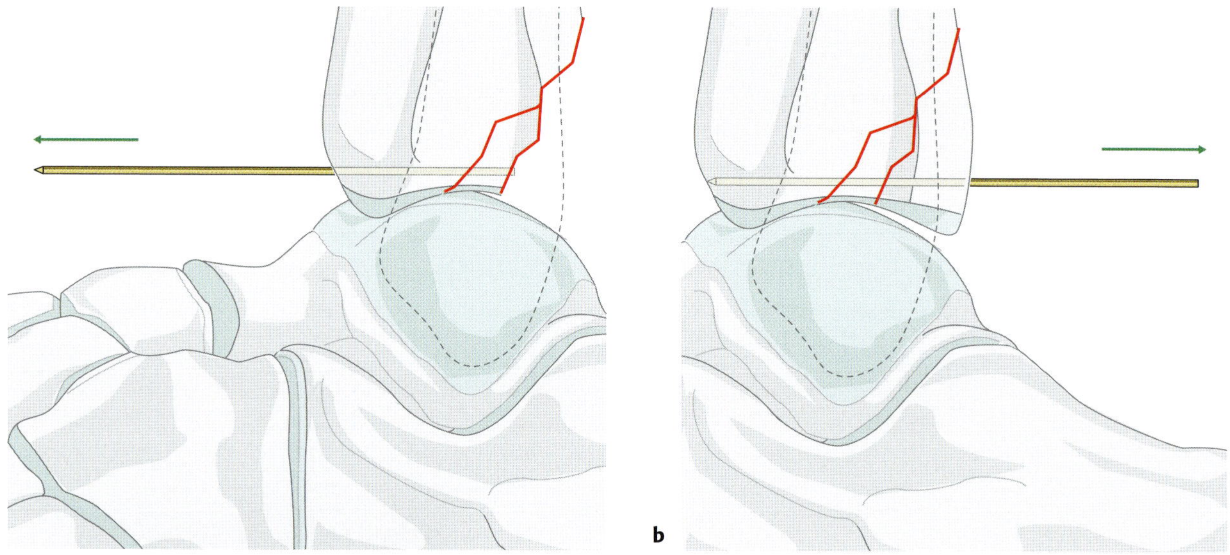

a b

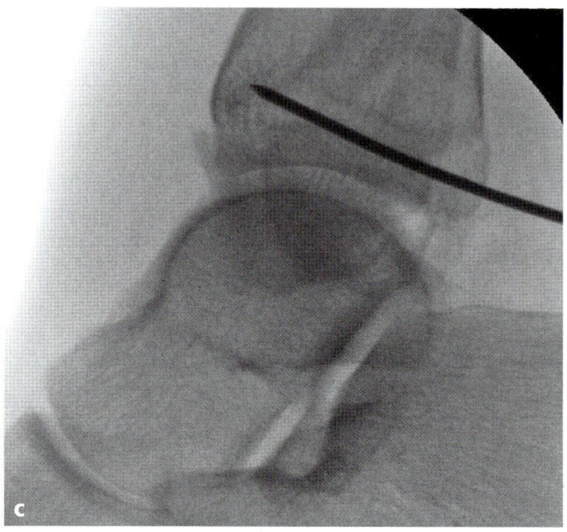

c

Fig 3.7-5a–f Sequence of reduction and fixation of the posterior tibial rim.
a–b Reduction of the intercalary fragment and temporary fixation with a K-wire. The space between the peroneal muscles and FHL is used for reduction and fixation of the posteior tibial rim. The talar dome serves as a template.
c Intraoperative x-ray.

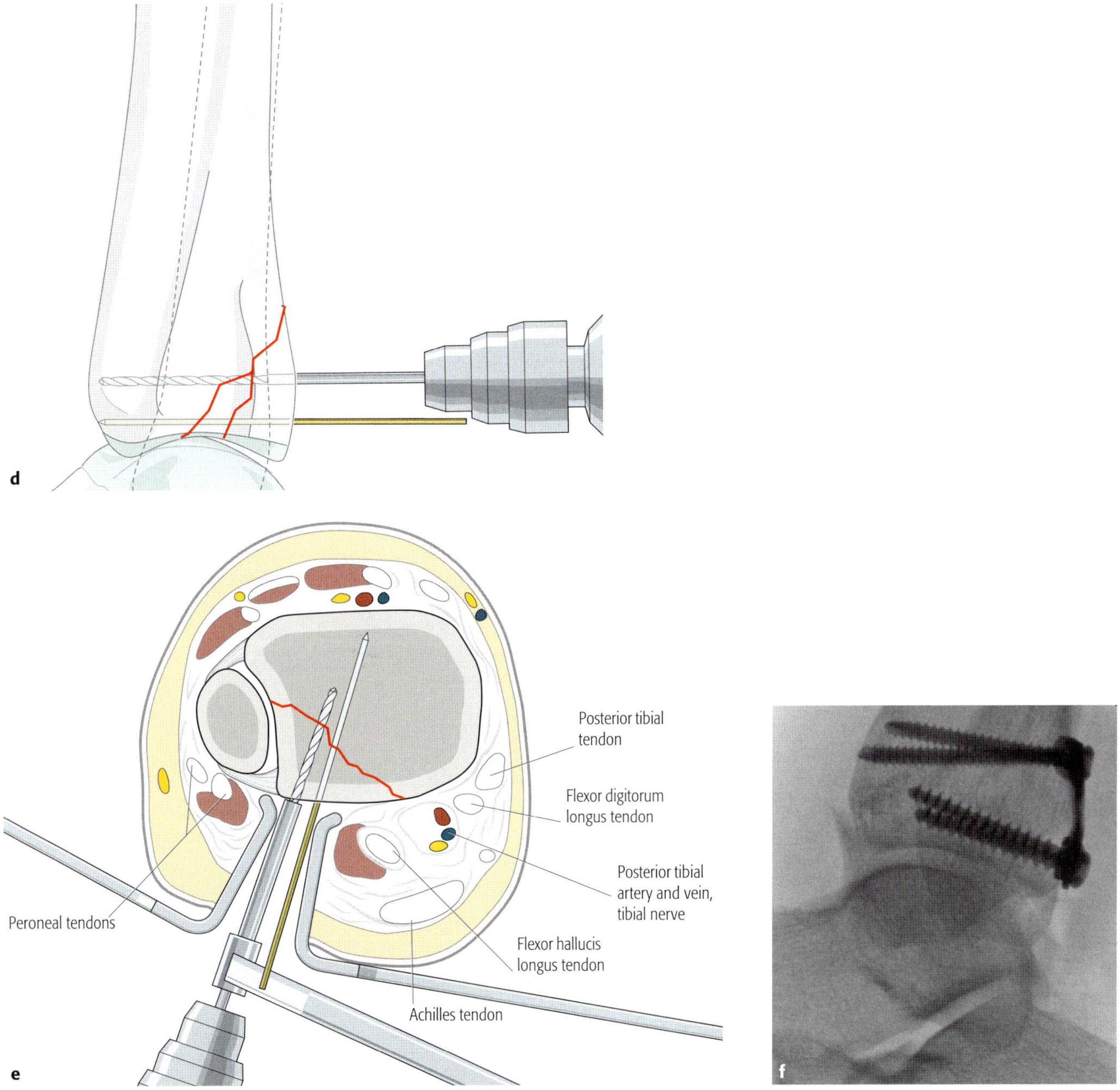

Fig 3.7-5a–f (cont) Sequence of reduction and fixation of the posterior tibial rim.

d–e The K-wire is brought out anteriorly until it is flush with the intercalary bone fragment. The posterior fragment is then reduced and the K-wire brought back posteriorly.

f Fixation with a posterior antiglide plate and C-arm control of the anatomical joint reduction.

Reduction and fixation of the multifragmentary fibular fracture—lateral approach

The multifragmentary fibular fracture is reduced via a standard lateral approach with the patient still in the prone position (**Fig 3.7-6**).

Two interfragmentary screws are used to fix the main fragments. A lateral bridge plate is then applied and fixed with three cortex screws proximally and one cortical and one cancellous screw distally.

The medial malleolar fracture is reduced via a standard medial approach (**Fig 3.7-7**). The fragments are cleared of hematoma and debris. The medial malleolus is then reduced to the distal tibia under direct vision of the medial aspect of the ankle joint. Screw fixation is carried out with 3.5 mm cancellous compression screws. Anatomical reduction is checked with the C-arm (**Fig 3.7-8**).

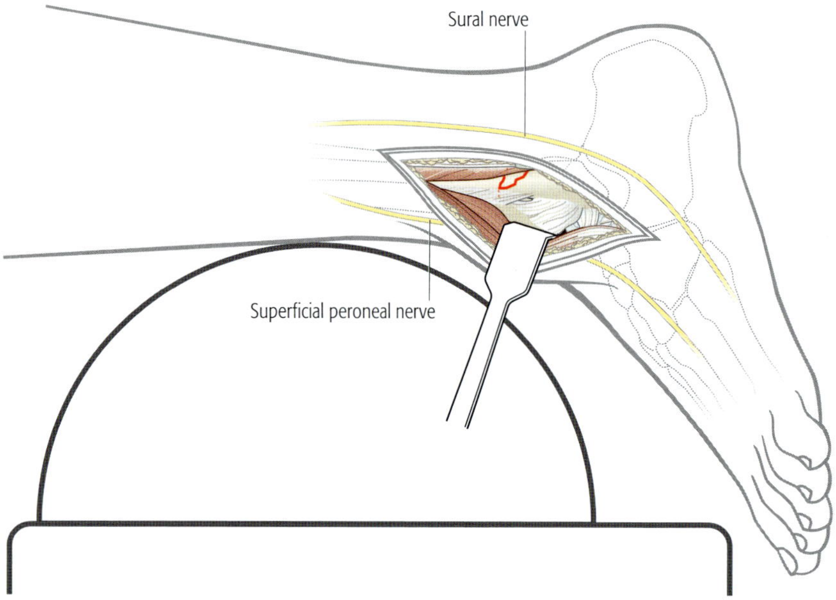

Fig 3.7-6 Lateral approach to the distal fibula with the patient in the prone position.

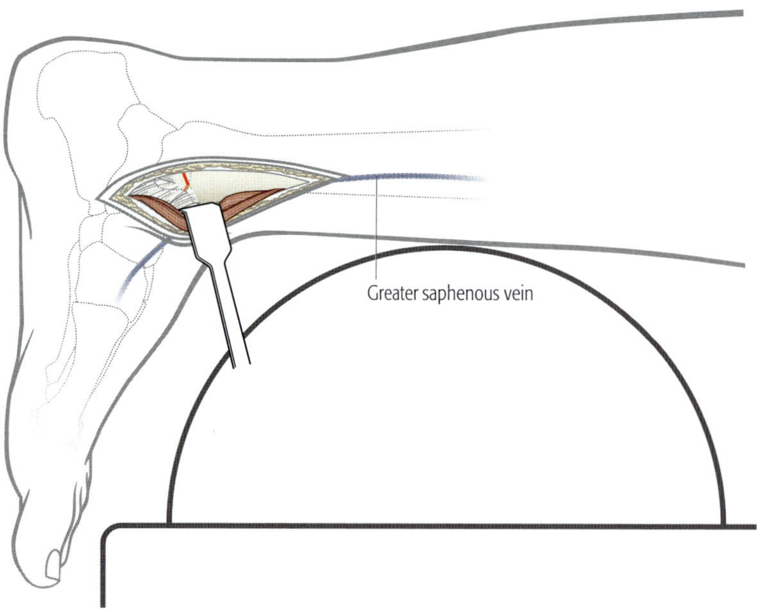

Fig 3.7-7 Medial approach to the medial malleolus with the patient in the prone position.

Reduction and fixation of the posterior tibial fragment—medial approach

Reduction and stable fixation of the posterior tibial fragment with the attached posterior tibiofibular ligament increases syndesmotic stability by providing a bone-to-bone fixation. Typically, after stable fixation of the posterior malleolus and the distal fibula the syndesmotic complex is stable and no additional fixation with either a syndesmostic screw or flexible implant (suture button) is needed.

Syndesmotic stability is tested intraoperatively with external rotation or the hook test (**Fig 3.7-9**). The fibula is pulled laterally and posteriorly to detect syndesmotic instability. With rupture of the anterior and interosseous syndesmotic ligaments, syndesmotic instability may persist despite fixation of the posterior malleolus. In these cases, an additional syndesmotic fixation with a syndesmotic screw or flexible implant is indicated (see chapter 3.6).

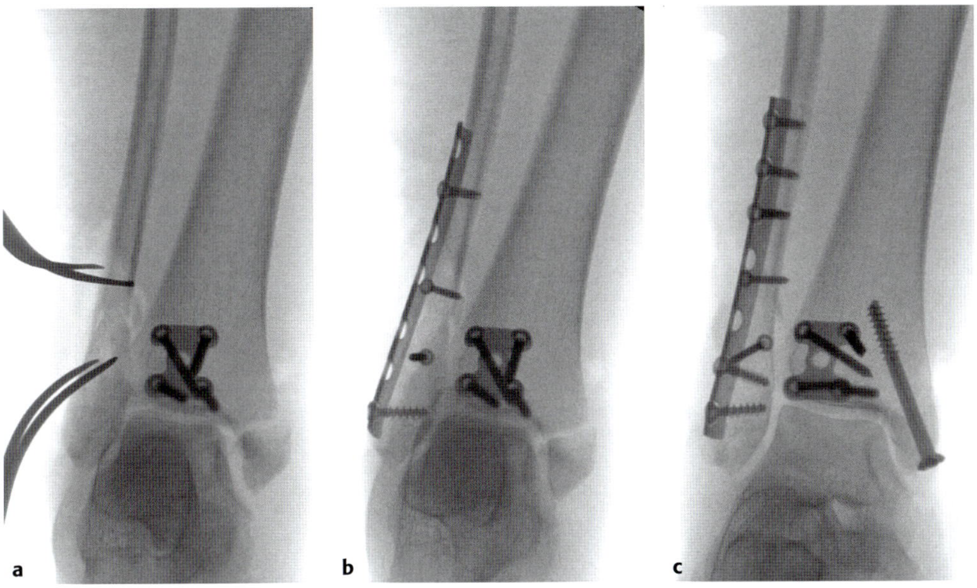

Fig 3.7-8a–c Intraoperative C-arm images of fixation of the medial and lateral malleolus.
a Reduction of the main fragments of the fibula with pointed reduction clamps.
b Fibular fixation with two interfragmentary screws and a lateral neutralization plate.
c Medial malleolar fixation with two screws.

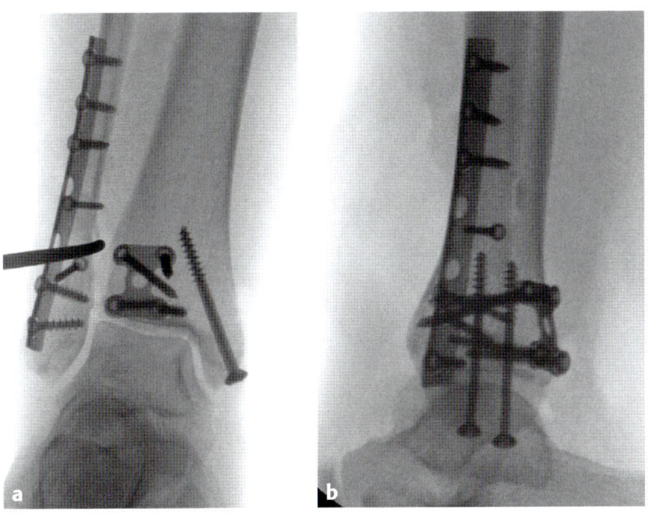

Fig 3.7-9a–b C-arm images taken directly after internal fixation.
a Syndesmotic stability is restored by fixation of the posterior malleolus and the distal fibular fracture as demonstrated by the classic hook test. Therefore, no additional fixation of the tibiofibular syndesmosis with a screw is needed.
b Lateral view after internal fixation.

5 Pitfalls and complications

Pitfalls

Inadequate reduction and fixation of the posterior tibial fragment

The posterior tibial fragment can be fixed indirectly from the front with anteroposterior screws. Biomechanically this provides less stability than a posterior antiglide plate. It should therefore only be attempted with large posterior fragments to allow adequate purchase of the screws and interfragmentary compression. Indirect reduction also carries the risk of inadequate reduction (**Fig 3.7-10**) and cannot be achieved in case of intercalary fragments, as in the present case.

Inadequate C-arm projections with the patient in a prone position

Fixation of malleolar fractures with the patient in a prone position is carried out less frequently than with the patient supine. Care has to be taken to achieve the exact mortise and lateral C-arm projections to allow control of reduction.

With complex fracture patterns, 3D C-arm imaging is beneficial, if available. In case of doubt, postoperative CT scanning of both ankles is recommended.

Irreducible intercalary fragments

Small intercalary fragments (ie, less than 5 mm in diameter) and fragments that do not carry a cartilage cover should be removed rather than attempting fixation. These fragments do not contribute to joint congruity and may impede anatomical reduction or even displace into the joint as loose bodies.

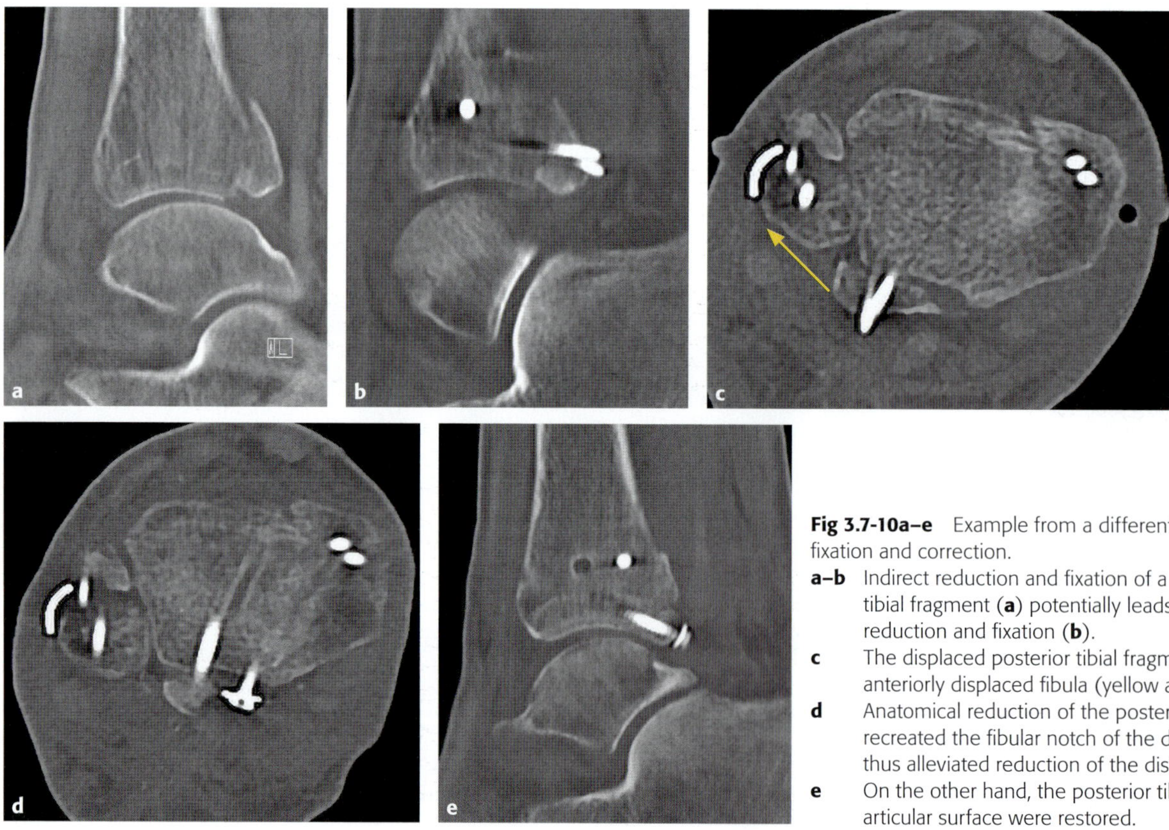

Fig 3.7-10a–e Example from a different case showing fixation and correction.
- **a–b** Indirect reduction and fixation of a posterior tibial fragment (**a**) potentially leads to improper reduction and fixation (**b**).
- **c** The displaced posterior tibial fragment follows the anteriorly displaced fibula (yellow arrow).
- **d** Anatomical reduction of the posterior malleolus recreated the fibular notch of the distal tibia and thus alleviated reduction of the distal fibula.
- **e** On the other hand, the posterior tibial rim and articular surface were restored.

Complications

- Injury to the sural nerve (posterolateral approach), superficial peroneal nerve (lateral approach)
- Injury to the posterior tibial neurovascular bundle, if dissecting medially beyond the FHL tendon
- Irritation of the posterior tibial tendon with posterior screw placement in the medial malleolus
- Loss of fixation
- Malunion
- Nonunion
- Posttraumatic arthritis

6 Alternative techniques

Screws (2.7–3.5 mm) and washers can be used to fix smaller fragments (**Fig 3.7-11**).

Interlocking plates can be used in osteoporotic bone and a posterior antiglide plate may be used for fibular fracture fixation to increase stability (**Fig 3.7-12**).

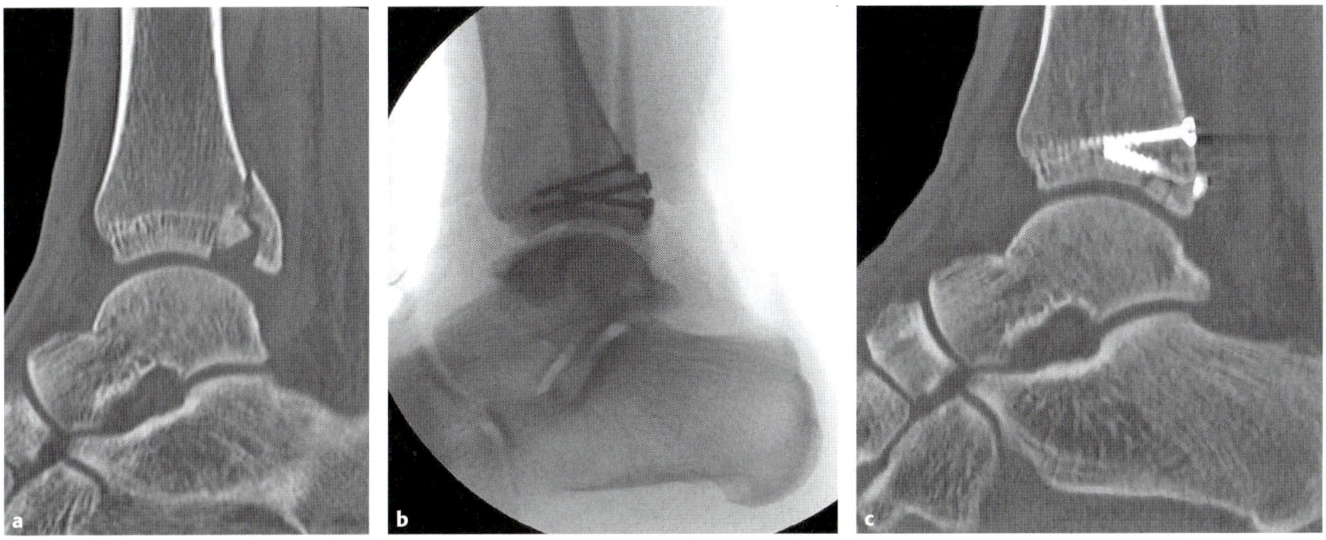

Fig 3.7-11a–c Example from a different case showing fixation of a multifragmented posterior malleolus with three 3.5 mm cortex screws.

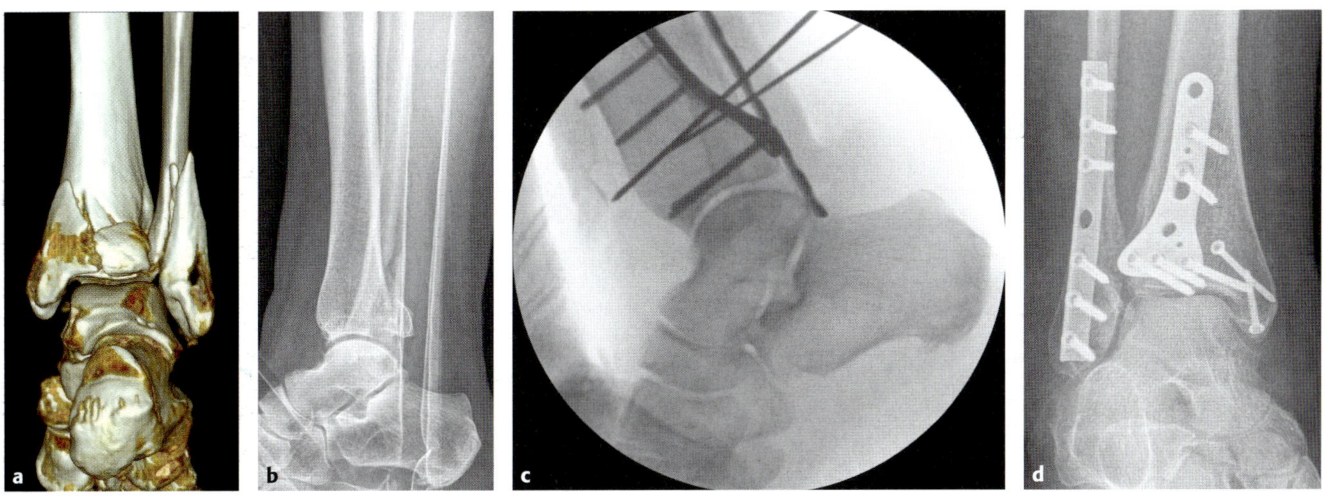

Fig 3.7-12a–d Example from a different case showing fixation of the posterior malleolus in a trimalleolar fracture with an interlocking plate in a patient with osteoporosis. The fibula is fixed with a posterior plate via the same posterolateral approach.

7 Postoperative management and rehabilitation

Postoperatively, the foot is immobilized in a splint or below knee cast and the lower leg is elevated. Any applied suction drain is removed on day 1 or day 2 postsurgery. Active and passive range-of-motion exercises are initiated on postoperative day 1 including continuous passive motion if available. A rigid boot or foot orthosis is applied, and the patient is restricted to partial weight bearing (up to 20 kg) on the injured leg for 6 weeks. Standard postoperative x-rays are taken to confirm anatomical reduction. In case of doubt or after fixation of an unstable syndesmosis, a postoperative CT scan of both ankles is recommended to detect relevant side-to-side differences that could warrant revision and repeated reduction. Weight bearing is gradually increased after 6 weeks if x-rays demonstrate bone union. An active rehabilitation protocol is then initiated including range-of-motion exercises, muscular balancing, and gait training (**Fig 3.7-13**).

Implant removal

Removal of plates or screws on the posterior aspect of the distal tibia is generally not necessary. Prominent implants on the medial and lateral malleolus are typically removed using the same approaches after 1 year.

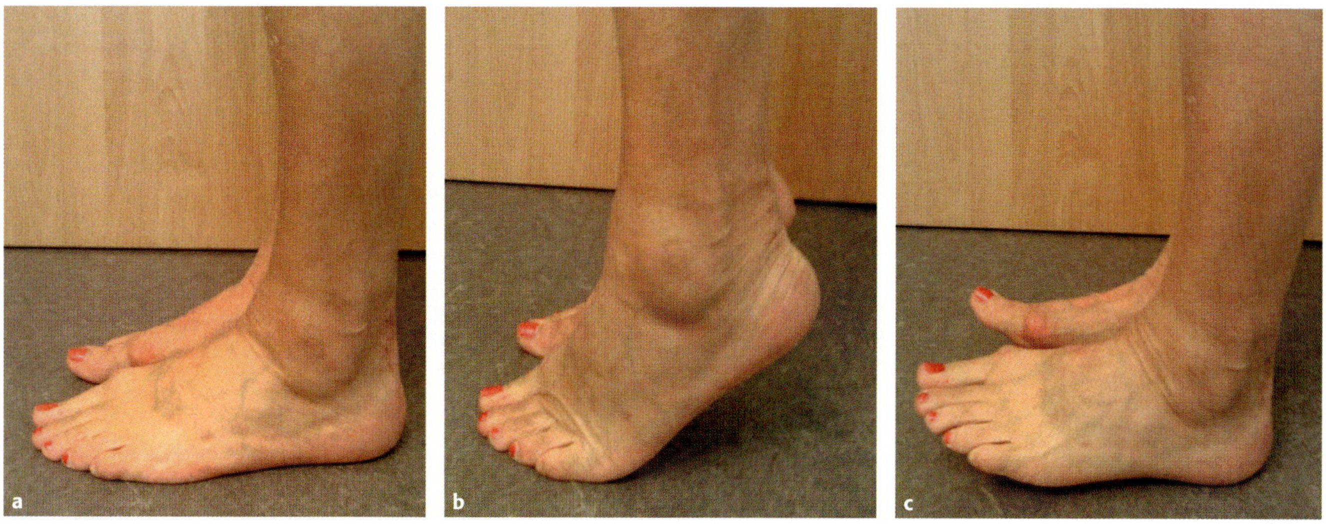

Fig 3.7-13 Range of motion and uneventful scars at 3-year follow-up.

8 Recommended reading

Bartoníček J, Rammelt S, Kostlivý K, et al. Anatomy and classification of the posterior tibial fragment in ankle fractures. *Arch Orthop Trauma Surg*. 2015 Apr;135(4):505–516.
Bartoníček J, Rammelt S, Tuček M. Posterior malleolar fractures: changing concepts and recent developments. *FootAnkle Clin*. 2017 Mar;22(1):125–145.
Gardner MJ, Brodsky A, Briggs SM, et al. Fixation of posterior malleolar fractures provides greater syndesmotic stability. *Clin Orthop Relat Res*. 2006 Jun;447:165–171.
Heim U. Trimalleoar fractures: late results after fixation of the posterior fragment. *Orthopedics*. 1989 Aug;12(8):1053–1059.
Rammelt S, Zwipp H, Mittlmeier T. Operative treatment of pronation fracture-dislocations of the ankle. *Oper Orthop Traumatol*. 2013 Jun;25(3):273–291.
Rammelt S, Zwipp H. Ankle Fractures. In: Bentley G, ed. *European Instructional Course Lectures, Volume 12*. Berlin Heidelberg New York: Springer; 2012:205 -219.
Shi HF, Xiong J, Chen YX, et al. Comparison of the direct and indirect reduction techniques during the surgical management of posterior malleolar fractures. *BMC Musculoskelet Disord*. 2017 Mar 14;18(1):109.
Verhage SM, Boot F, Schipper IB, et al. Open reduction and internal fixation of posterior malleolar fractures using the posterolateral approach. *Bone Joint J*. 2016 Jun;98-B(6):812–817.
Weber M. Trimalleolar fractures with impaction of the posteromedial tibial plafond: Implications for talar stability. *Foot and Ankle Int*. 2004 Oct;25(10):716–727.

3.8 Locked fracture-dislocation of the fibula (Bosworth) with impaction of the posterior tibial rim

Jan Bartoníček, Stefan Rammelt

1 Case description

A 35-year-old woman slipped while walking and twisted her right ankle. She immediately experienced severe pain at the ankle and noted a clear displacement of her foot. The ankle was immobilized in a vacuum splint by paramedics on site. On arrival in the hospital, a marked swelling around the ankle and external rotation of the right foot of nearly 90° in relation to the lower leg were noted.

X-rays of the ankle and lower leg revealed a fracture dislocation with the fibula locked behind the distal tibia (AO/OTA 44B3.1, Bosworth fracture) (**Fig 3.8-1**).

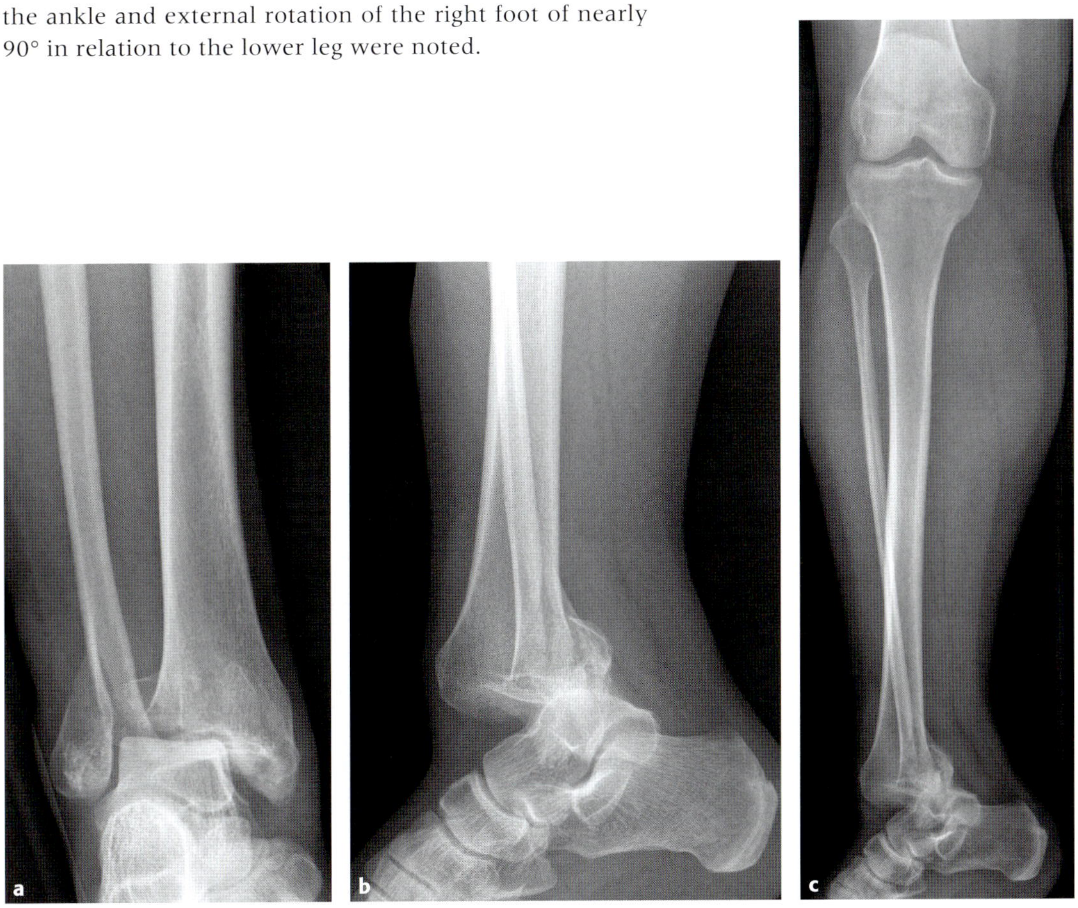

Fig 3.8-1a–c X-rays of the right ankle on admission, and immobilization with a vacuum splint.

a AP view.

b Lateral view.

c The AP x-ray of the leg shows rotational malalignment ("AP knee and lateral foot sign").

Closed reduction was attempted under intravenous analgesia. The position of the foot was somewhat improved but the ankle remained displaced. X-rays taken after reduction of the gross dislocation revealed residual tibiofibular subluxation with the typical overlapping of the distal tibia and fibula in the AP view (**Fig 3.8-2**). Computed tomographic (CT) imaging at this stage revealed incomplete reduction with the fibula still locked behind the tibia and additional fragmentation of the posterolateral tibial rim (**Fig 3.8-3**).

Bosworth fracture-dislocations are believed to result from forced external rotation of the foot. The common feature is a posterior dislocation of the intact or fractured fibula and its extraincisural entrapment behind the posterior tibial tubercle, or intraincisural entrapment into a gap between the distal tibia and the avulsed posterior tibial fragment, as in the present case (**Fig 3.8-4**).

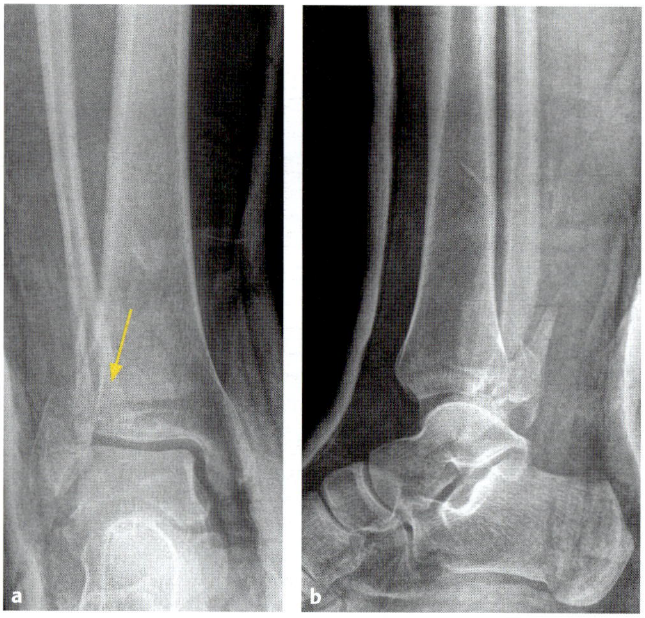

Fig 3.8-2a–b X-rays after reduction of the gross dislocation showing residual tibiofibular dislocation with the typical overlapping of the distal tibia and fibula in the AP view (**a**) (yellow arrow) and an irregular contour of the distal tibial rim ("posterior malleolus") in the lateral view (**b**).

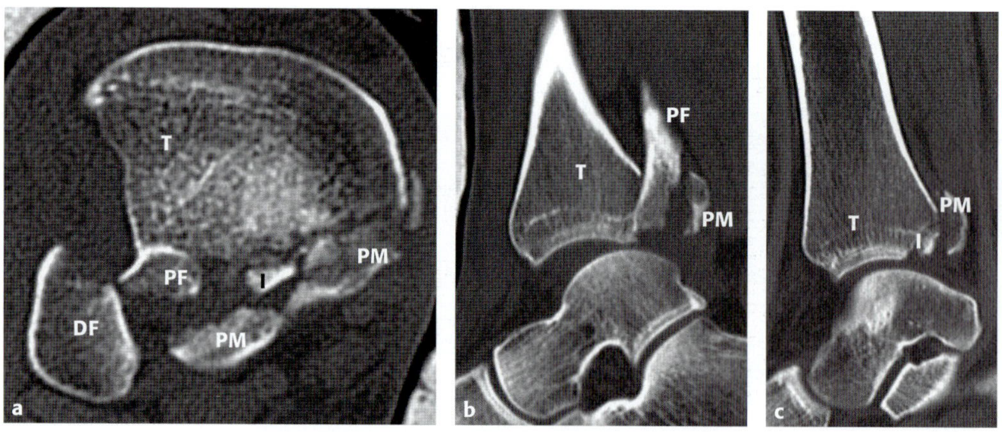

Fig 3.8-3a–c Computed tomographic scans.

- **a** The CT scans revealed a persistent dislocation of the distal fibular fragment (DF) behind the distal tibia (T) and an additional posterior malleolar fracture (PM) extending into the medial malleolus (Bartoníček and Rammelt type 3) with a rotated intercalary fragment (I) making indirect reduction impossible.
- **b** The proximal fibular fragment (PF) is trapped in the posterior tibial fracture behind the distal tibia (T) and the posterior malleolar fragment (PM).
- **c** The intercalary fragment (I) is tilted and impacted.

2 Preoperative planning

Indications for surgery

The indication for early surgery was the unstable trimalleolar fracture with persistent locked dislocation of the distal fibula behind the tibia and the resulting strain on the vulnerable soft tissues in an otherwise healthy 35-year-old patient. If excessive swelling of the soft tissues prevents the surgeon from early definitive fixation, the procedure is staged. After open reduction is completed and an ankle-spanning external fixator is placed, definitive internal fixation is delayed until the soft-tissue swelling has improved.

Treatment options

The simple oblique fibular fracture resulting from a rotational force is fixed with an interfragmentary compression screw and a plate. Options include a lateral neutralization plate or a posterior antiglide plate. In this case, a lateral plate was used.

The posterior tibial fracture is fixed directly via a posterolateral approach. An antiglide plate allows proper reduction of the displaced posterior rim and the rotated, intercalary fragment (**Fig 3.8-5**).

The extension of the posterior malleolar fracture into the medial malleolus can be accessed via a posterolateral approach, or via an additional posteromedial approach. The fragment is fixed directly to the distal tibia with a posteroanterior compression screw.

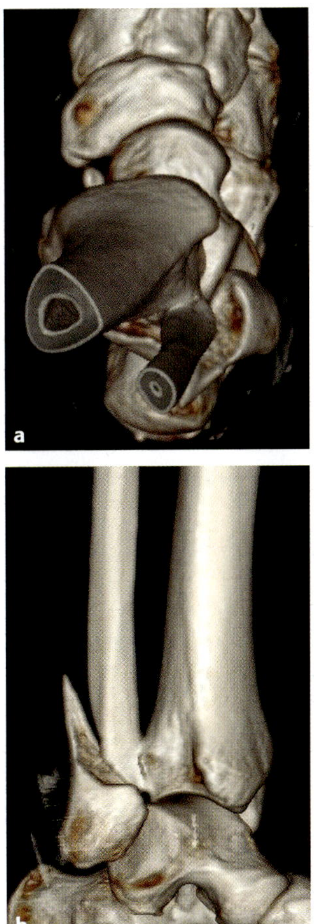

Fig 3.8-4a–b The 3D CT reconstructions show the displacement of the fibula behind the tibia and the empty incisura.

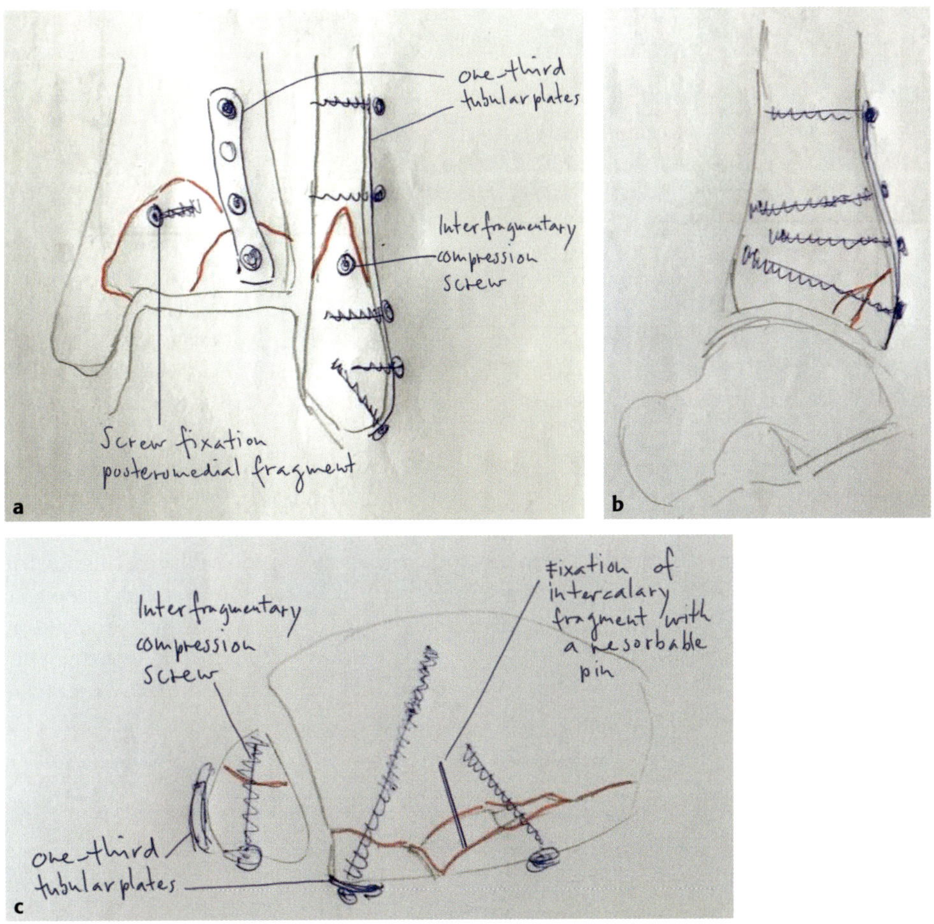

Fig 3.8-5a–c Preoperative plan.

3 Operating room setup

Patient positioning	• Prone on a radiolucent table for direct fixation of the posterior malleolus. A lateral approach to the fibula can be used without repositioning the patient. • The ability to rotate the limb internally and externally as well as to bend the knee is essential to allow all necessary incisions.
Anesthesia options	• General anesthesia due to the patient being in the prone position. • Alternatively, spinal or regional anesthesia can be used
C-arm location	• The C-arm is positioned on the foot end of the table. • The screen for the C-arm is placed more toward the head end of the operative table, so that the surgeon can have a free view while performing the reduction
Tourniquet	• Well-padded at the thigh and inflated before incision. • Released after joint reduction
Tips	• A bump may be placed under the anterior aspect of the contralateral hip if the limb is in too much external rotation allowing for greater ease in obtaining true mortise and lateral images. • Occasionally titling the C-arm toward the patient's head slightly will result in a better AP and mortise image

For illustrations and overview of anesthetic considerations, see chapter 1.

Equipment

- K-wires, resorbable pins
- Plate (usually one-third tubular, but in the case of poor bone quality a locking plate can be used)
- 3.5 mm (2.7 mm) cancellous and cortex screws
- Smooth and sharp elevators

Size of implants and instruments may vary according to anatomy, bone quality, and fracture fragment size.

4 Surgical procedure

Posterolateral approach

Reduction of the posterior tibial fragments should be performed first to allow adequate visualization in the lateral C-arm projections. The incision for the posterolateral approach lies parallel to the Achilles tendon (**Fig 3.8-6**). The sural nerve is identified within the subcutaneous tissue in the proximal part of the incision and gently retracted medially. The superficial and deep fasciae are incised longitudinally and the flexor hallucis longus (FHL) muscle belly and tendon are retracted medially. Thus, the FHL protects the posterior tibial neurovascular bundle. The fractured posterior tibial fragment is identified and cleared of hematoma and retracted laterally. The posterior tibiofibular ligament is used as a hinge and left intact.

The intercalary fragment is then identified and evaluated for bone quality and cartilage cover. If the latter is intact and the fracture fragment is 5 mm or more in size, the fragment is reduced to the intact anterior portion of the tibial plafond and fixed temporarily with a K-wire. Definite fixation of this fragment can be achieved with either a resorbable pin or a K-wire that is cut flush with the intercalary fragment and acts as a lost or buried K-wire. The posterolateral rim with the posterior syndesmosis attached is then reduced and realigned with the posterior tibial plafond. Anatomical reduction of the tibial joint surface is evaluated on the lateral C-arm view.

For this patient definitive fixation was achieved with a posterior one-third tubular antiglide plate because of the relatively small and brittle posterior malleolar fragment.

The medial malleolar fracture is a medial extension of the posterior malleolar fracture, which is fixed directly with a compression screw via the same approach (**Fig 3.8-7**). Alternatively, a separate posteromedial approach can be used. Fixation of the posterior fragments helps to stabilize the syndesmotic complex through bone-to-bone fixation of the posterior tibiofibular ligament and recreates the tibial incisura which helps with fine reduction of the fibula.

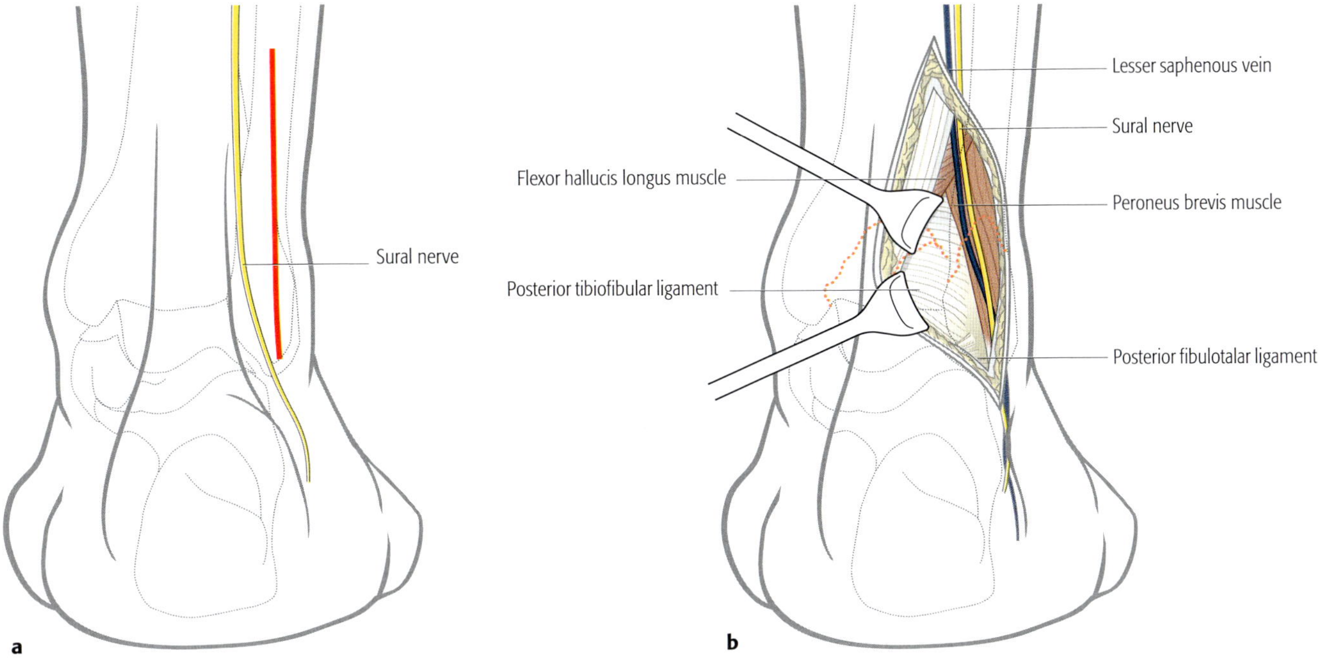

Fig 3.8-6a–b Posterolateral approach to the posterior tibia (and fibula).

a The surgical incision is in the interval between the Achilles and the peroneal tendons. Care must be taken to identify and to protect the sural nerve.

b Deep dissection requires retracting the FHL medially. The posterior tibiofibular (syndemotic) ligament is intact but the syndesmosis is unstable due to the posterior malposition of the distal fibula.

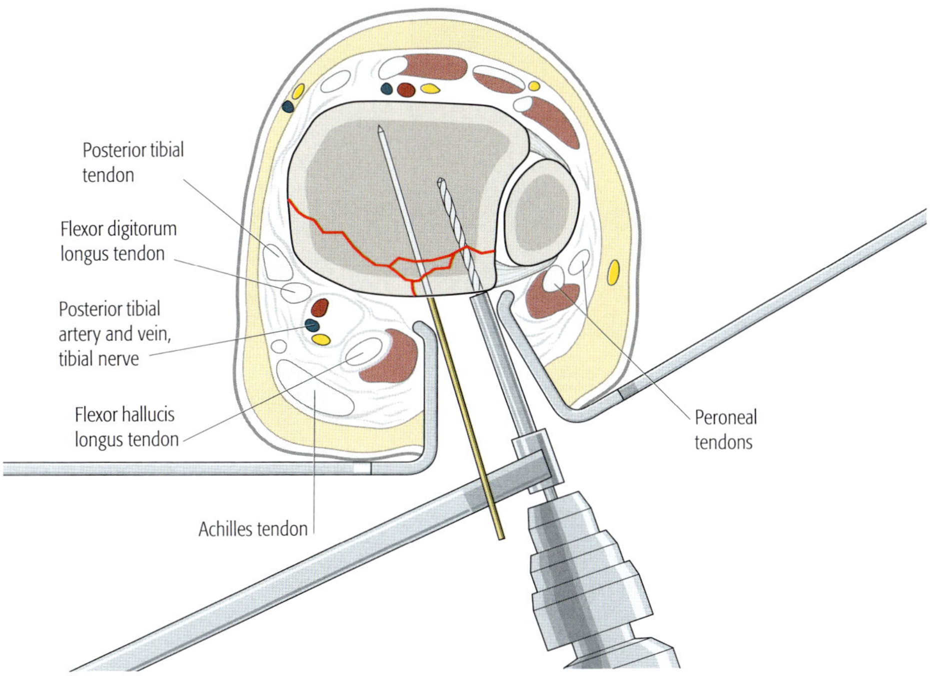

Fig 3.8-7 Reduction and fixation of the posterior tibial fragments. The interval between the peroneal muscles and FHL is used for reduction and fixation of the posterior tibial fragments. The intercalary fragment is reduced and fixed temporarily with a K-wire (see chapter 3.9). The medial extension of the posterior malleolar fracture is fixed directly with a compression screw via the same approach.

Lateral approach

The distal fibular fracture is reduced via a standard lateral approach with the patient still in the prone position (**Fig 3.8-8**). The fragments are cleared of hematoma and small debris.

The oblique fracture is reduced anatomically with a point-to-point reduction (Weber) clamp. The posterior rim of the fibula serves as a template for the reduction. An interfragmentary compression screw is used to fix the main fragments. A lateral one-third tubular plate is then applied as a neutralization plate and fixed with 3.5 mm cortex screws proximally and distally.

Although fixation of the posterior malleolus typically restores syndesmotic stability, in this particular case a fibulotibial (syndesmotic) screw was applied to protect the relatively small and brittle posterior tibial fragments.

Anatomical reduction is checked with the C-arm and with postoperative x-rays (**Fig 3.8-9**).

Routine postoperative CT scanning for syndesmotic stabilization is often used to ensure proper reduction of the distal fibula into the tibial incisura and to exclude fibular malrotation and/or anteroposterior translation (**Fig 3.8-10**). Postoperative CT imaging is also advised for impacted posterior malleolar fractures, as in the present case.

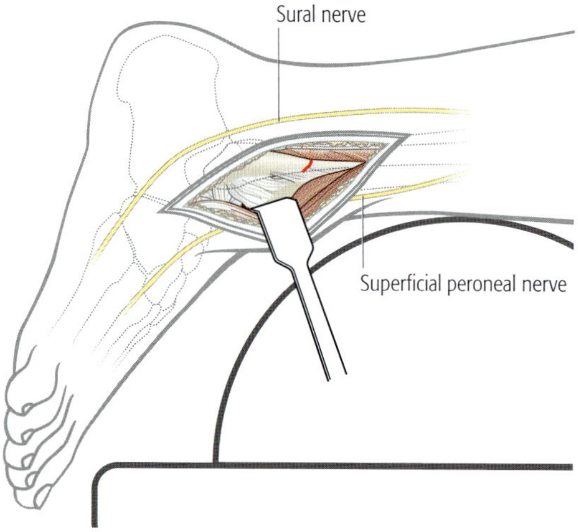

Fig 3.8-8 Lateral approach to the distal fibula with the patient prone.

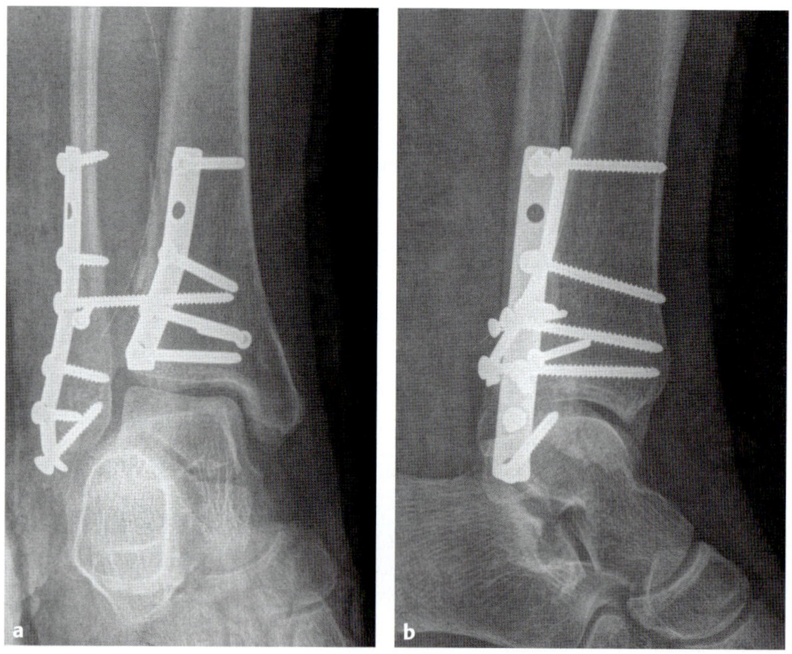

Fig 3.8-9 Postoperative x-rays.
a Mortise view.
b Lateral view.

5 Pitfalls and complications

Pitfalls

Failed closed reduction

Bosworth fracture-dislocations are especially difficult to reduce in a closed manner, as the fibula is locked behind the tibia. In this patient the fibula was even trapped in the posterior malleolar fracture, rendering closed reduction impossible. Repeated unsuccessful attempts at closed reduction put additional strain on the soft tissues and may be painful. Therefore, multiple attempts of closed reduction should be avoided, and open reduction should be performed if closed reduction cannot be achieved.

Inadequate reduction and fixation of the posterior tibial fragment

Indirect reduction of a small posterior tibial fragment carries the risk of inadequate reduction and is impossible with displaced intercalary fragments, as in the present case. Indirect fixation with an anteroposterior screw only provides adequate stability where there are large triangular posterolateral fragments without comminution (Bartoníček and Rammelt type 4).

Inadequate C-arm projections with the patient in a prone position

Fixation of malleolar fractures with the patient in a prone position is carried out less frequently than with the patient supine. Care must be taken to achieve the exact mortise and lateral C-arm projections to allow evaluation of the reduction. The limb is often considerably externally rotated when in the prone position. Placing a bump or blanket roll under the contralateral hip will improve alignment of the limb and improve the ability to obtain true lateral and mortise images during the procedure. Occasionally titling the C-arm toward the patient's head slightly will result in a better AP and mortise image. The bump placed anterior to the ankle results in the operative limb being slightly off plane.

With complex fracture patterns 3D imaging is beneficial, if available. Postoperative CT scanning of both ankles is recommended for further evaluation (**Fig 3.8-10**).

Irreducible intercalary fragments

Small intercalary fragments (< 5 mm in diameter) and fragments that do not carry a cartilage cover should be removed rather than attempting fixation. These fragments do not contribute to joint congruity and may impede anatomical reduction or even displace into the joint as loose bodies.

Complications

- Injury to the sural nerve (posterolateral approach), superficial peroneal nerve (lateral approach)
- Injury to the posterior tibial neurovascular bundle (if working medially beyond the FHL tendon)
- Irritation of the posterior tibial tendon with posterior screw placement in the medial malleolus
- Loss of fixation
- Malunion
- Nonunion
- Posttraumatic arthritis

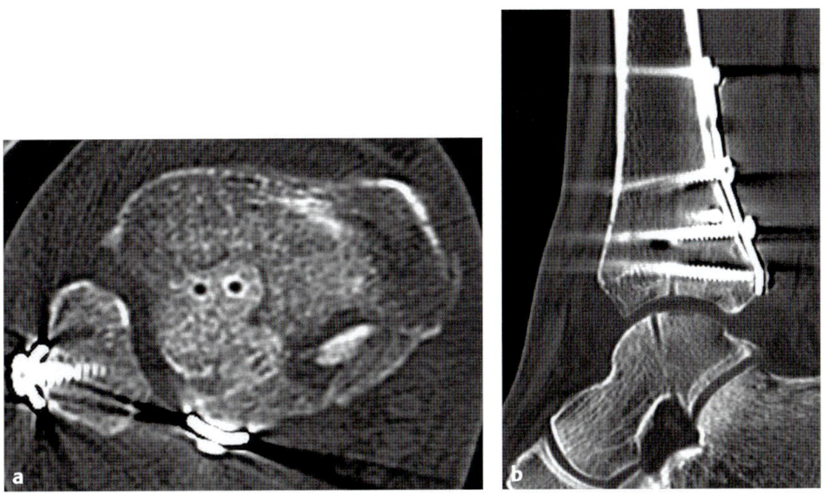

Fig 3.8-10a–b Postoperative CT (cross-section and sagittal) scan confirming exact reduction of the distal fibula into the tibial incisura.

6 Alternative techniques

Different types of Bosworth fracture-dislocations need different approaches.

Smaller posterolateral fragments may be also fixed with 2.7–3.5 mm screws. The size and quality of the fragments dictates the size of the implants.
Interlocking plates may be used in osteoporotic bone.

7 Postoperative management and rehabilitation

Postoperatively, the foot is immobilized in a splint or below knee cast and the lower leg is elevated. Active and passive range-of-motion exercises are initiated on the postoperative day 1 including continuous passive motion if available. A rigid boot or foot orthosis is applied, and the patient is restricted to partial weight bearing (up to 20 kg) on the injured leg for 6 weeks. In case of doubt, or after fixation of an unstable syndesmosis, a postoperative CT scan of both ankles is recommended to detect relevant side-to-side differences that warrant revision and repeat reduction. At 6 weeks any temporary fixation including the syndesmotic screw can be removed, if x-rays demonstrate bony union (**Fig 3.8-11**).

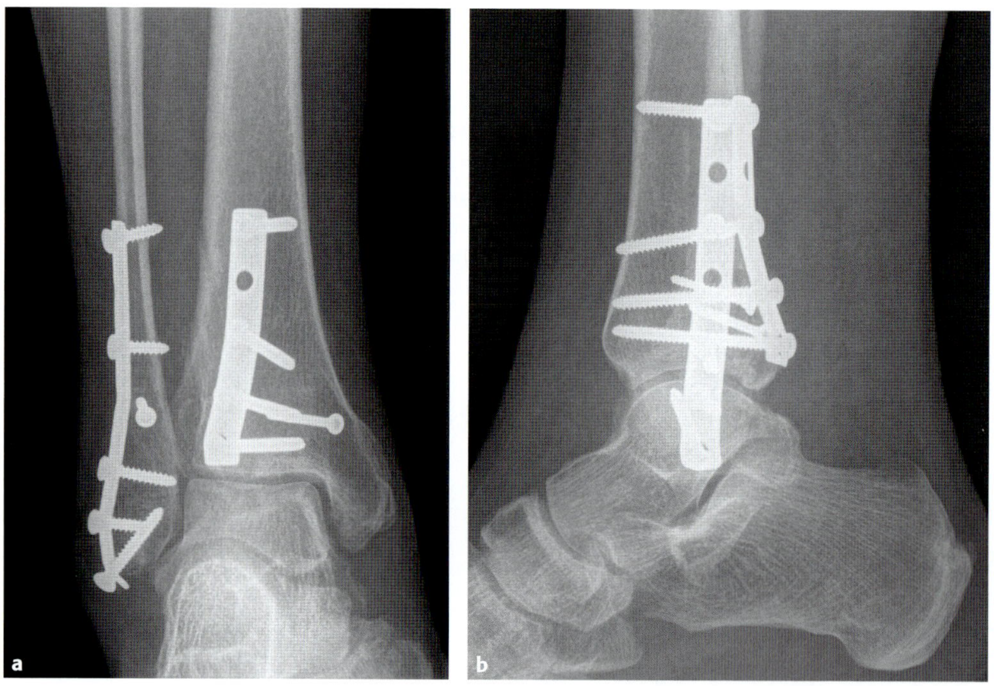

Fig 3.8-11a–b X-rays taken after bony healing and removal of the syndesmotic screw 8 weeks after surgery.
a Mortise view.
b Lateral view.

Weight bearing is then gradually increased over the next 2 weeks until full weight bearing is achieved. An active rehabilitation protocol is initiated including range-of-motion exercises, muscular balancing, proprioceptive, and gait training (**Fig 3.8-12**).

Implant removal

Removal of plates or screws on the posterior aspect of the distal tibia is generally not necessary. Prominent and symptomatic implants on the medial and lateral malleolus are typically removed using the same approaches after 1 year. Removal of syndesmotic fixation is controversial and there is no current consensus on timing and the overall necessity to remove syndesmotic screws.

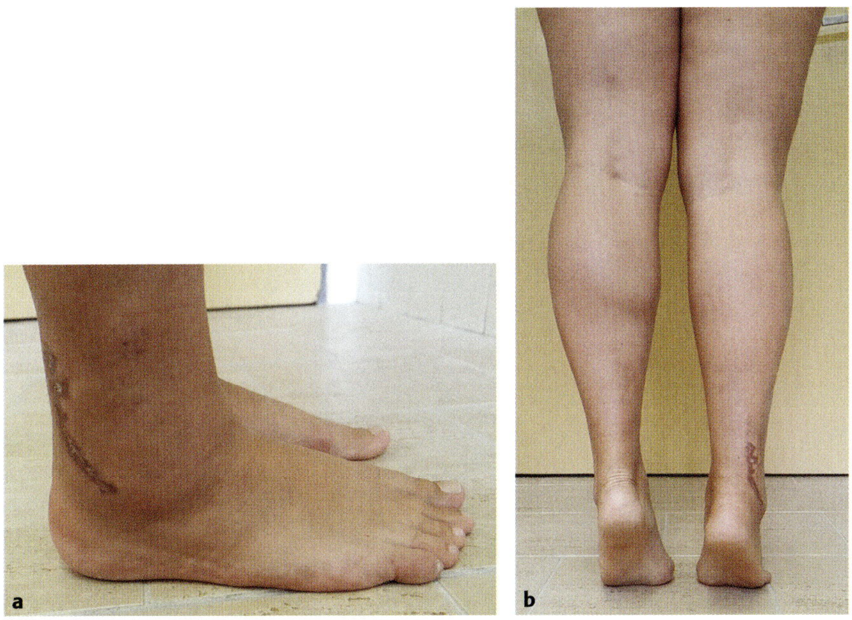

Fig 3.8-12a–b Clinical appearance and ability to stand tiptoe at 1-year follow-up.

8 Recommended reading

Bartoníček J, Frič V, Svatoš F, et al. Bosworth-type fibular entrapment injuries of the ankle: the Bosworth lesion. A report of 6 cases and literature review. *J Orthop Trauma.* 2007 Nov–Dec;21(10):710–717.

Bartoníček J, Rammelt S, Kostlivý K, et al. Anatomy and classification of the posterior tibial fragment in ankle fractures. *Arch Orthop Trauma Surg.* 2015 Apr;135(4):505–516.

Bartoníček J, Rammelt S, Kostlivý K. Bosworth fracture: a report of two atypical cases and literature review of 108 cases. *Fuß Sprunggelenk.* 2017 June;15(2):126–137. German.

Bosworth DM. Fracture-dislocation of the ankle with fixed displacement of the fibula behind the tibia. *J Bone Joint Surg Am.* 1947 Jan;29(1):130–135.

Delasotta LA, Hansen RH 3rd, Sands AK. Surgical management of the posterior fibula fracture dislocation: case report. *Foot Ankle Int.* 2013 Oct;34(10):1443–1446.

Rammelt S, Zwipp H, Mittlmeier T. [Operative treatment of pronation fracture-dislocations of the ankle]. *Oper Orthop Traumatol.* 2013 Jun;25(3):273–291. German.

Woods RS. Irreducible dislocation of the ankle-joint. *Br J Surg.* 1942;29:(115)359–360.

3.9 Osteoporotic trimalleolar fracture with additional fracture of the anterior tibial rim (Chaput)

Stefan Rammelt

1 Case description

A 66-year-old man was the restrained driver of a car involved in a head-on collision. An outward displacement of his foot was observed, but there were no other obvious injuries. The foot and ankle were immobilized in a plastic splint on site by an emergency physician. He was transported to the hospital by ambulance.

On arrival at the hospital, the man was awake and fully oriented. The right ankle was highly unstable. The skin was stretched and compromised over the medial side but no open wound was visible. There was a marked swelling over the whole right foot and ankle and also a submalleolar hematoma. No acute neurovascular deficits were noted but there was a slight global decreased sensation over both feet indicative of preexisting neuropathy. Medical history revealed comorbidities including terminal/chronic renal failure, and chronic venous insufficiency with chronic edema of both lower legs and feet.

X-rays of the right ankle revealed a trimalleolar fracture dislocation (AO/OTA 44B3.3). Gross reduction was attempted after administration of intravenous anesthetics. The foot was immobilized in a pneumatic splint. Repeat x-rays revealed continued lateral subluxation of the talus (**Fig 3.9-1**). A high fibular fracture or dislocation of the fibular head was ruled out during the physical examination and x-rays of the whole lower leg including the knee.

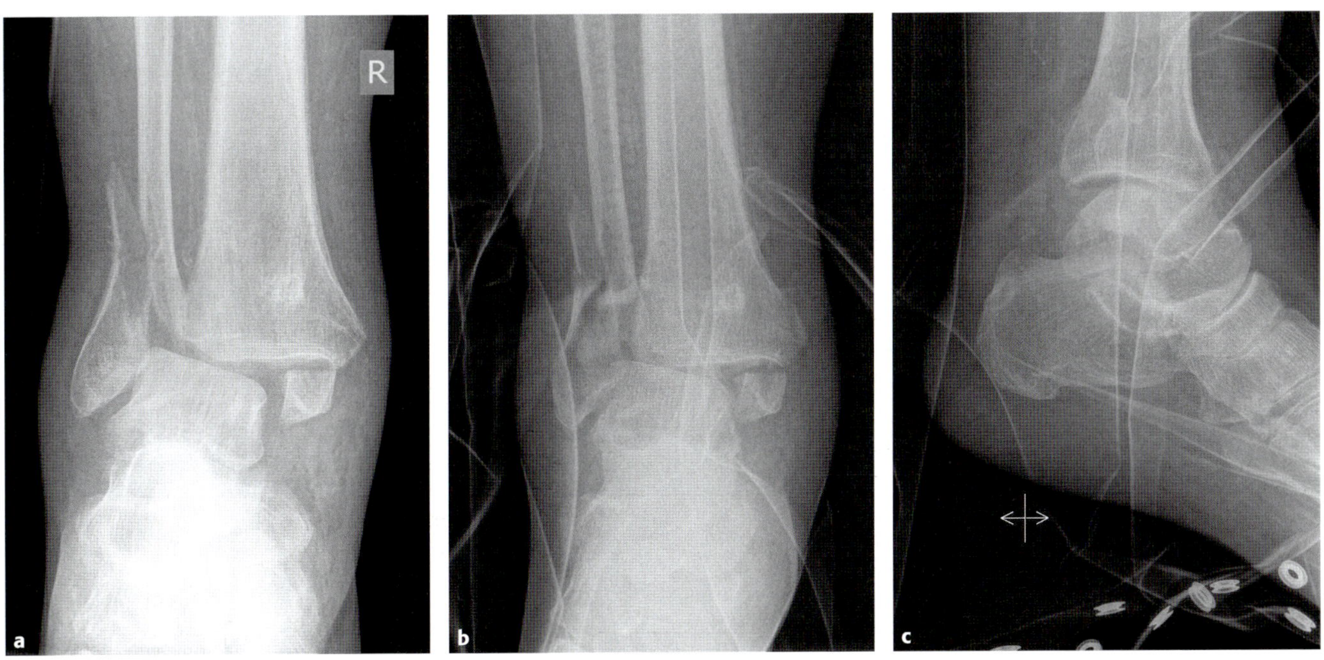

Fig 3.9-1a–c X-ray in AP view on admission showing fracture dislocation of the right ankle (**a**). After attempted reduction of the dislocation and immobilization in a pneumatic splint, there is still lateral subluxation of the talus. Therefore, the indication to external fixation is made (**b–c**).

As a result of a highly unstable fracture pattern with threatening possible soft-tissue breakdown at the medial aspect of the ankle, the patient was taken to the operating room for immediate closed reduction and ankle spanning external fixation (**Fig 3.9-2**).

After closed reduction and external fixation, computed tomographic (CT) imaging was performed for thorough fracture assessment before definitive internal fixation. The images revealed a "quadrimalleolar" fracture pattern, ie, a fracture of lateral, medial, posterior malleoli, and Chaput tubercle (**Fig 3.9-3**).

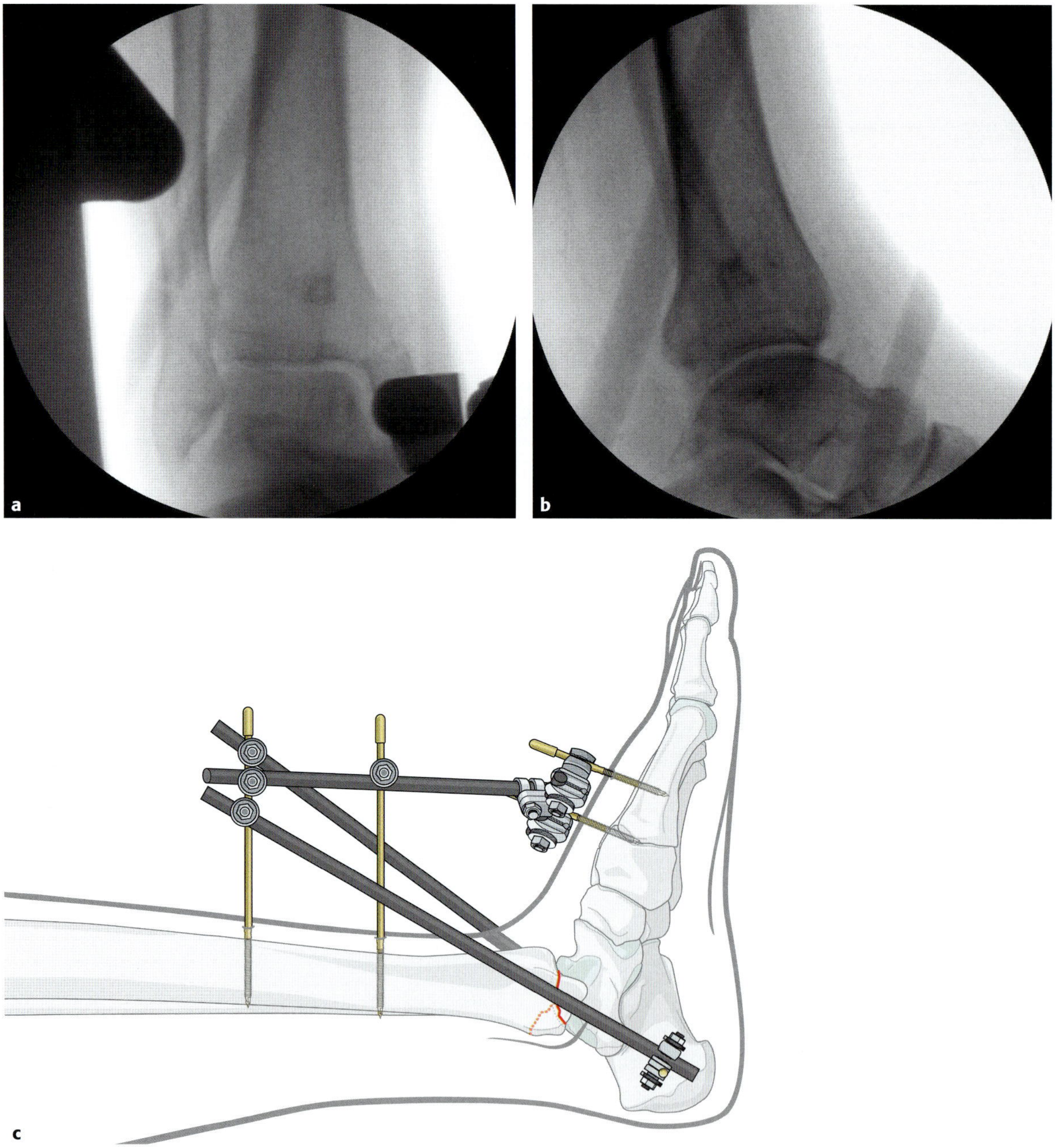

Fig 3.9-2a–c For this patient, closed reduction and external fixation was performed under spinal anesthesia (**a–b**). Because of the highly unstable fracture pattern and relatively poor bone quality, an additional transcalcaneal pin is used to enhance stability of the tibiometatarsal external fixator (**c**).

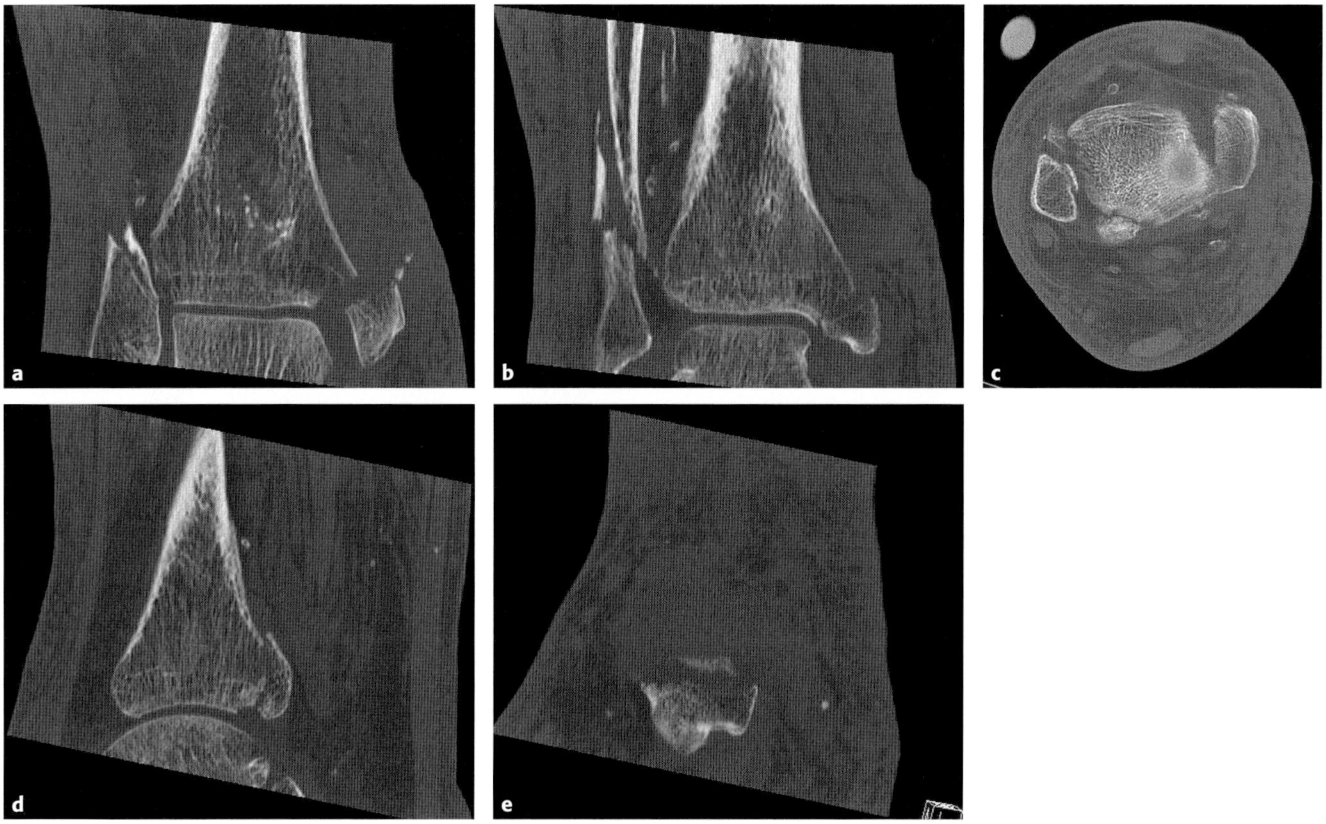

Fig 3.9-3a–e Computed tomographic scanning revealing a multifragmentary transsyndesmotic fracture of the distal fibula (Weber type B) (**a–b**), a posterolateral fracture of the distal tibial rim with a depressed intercalary fragment (Bartonícek and Rammelt type 2) (**c**), an additional fracture of the anterior tibial (Tillaux-Chaput) tubercle (**d**), and a medial malleolar fracture (**e**). Thus, all four malleoli are fractured and displaced ("quadrimalleolar").

2 Preoperative planning

Indications for surgery

The indication for surgery in the present case is obvious, as there is a highly unstable fracture dislocation. In addition to the trimalleolar fracture pattern, the anterior tibial tubercle (tubercule of Tillaux-Chaput) was fractured, resulting in a "quadrimalleolar" fracture. The patient had comorbidities including a mild polyneuropathy and end-stage chronic renal failure resulting in osteoporosis. Osteodensitometry revealed moderate to severe osteoporosis (T-score-1.5).

Treatment options

The fibular fracture is fixed with a locking plate because of fragmentation and poor bone quality. The plate acts as a bridge plate.

The oblique supracollicular medial malleolar fracture (ie, large medial malleolar fragment containing the anterior and posterior colliculus) can be accessed via a small medial approach and fixed with two compression screws, tension band wire, or, if there is comminution, a small medial plate.

The posterolateral tibial fragment is fixed directly from posterolateral. This allows proper reduction of the displaced posterior rim and the impacted intercalary fragment. The poor bone quality dictates that it be fixed with a posterior antiglide plate.

The anterolateral tibial fragment (tubercle) is fixed with a screw. A washer is added because of the poor bone quality (**Fig 3.9-4**).

Anatomical reduction of both the anterior and posterior tibial fragments recreates the tibial incisura. This reconstructs the anatomy of the incisura and restores syndesmotic stability by providing bone-to-bone fixation of the anterior and posterior tibiofibular ligaments.

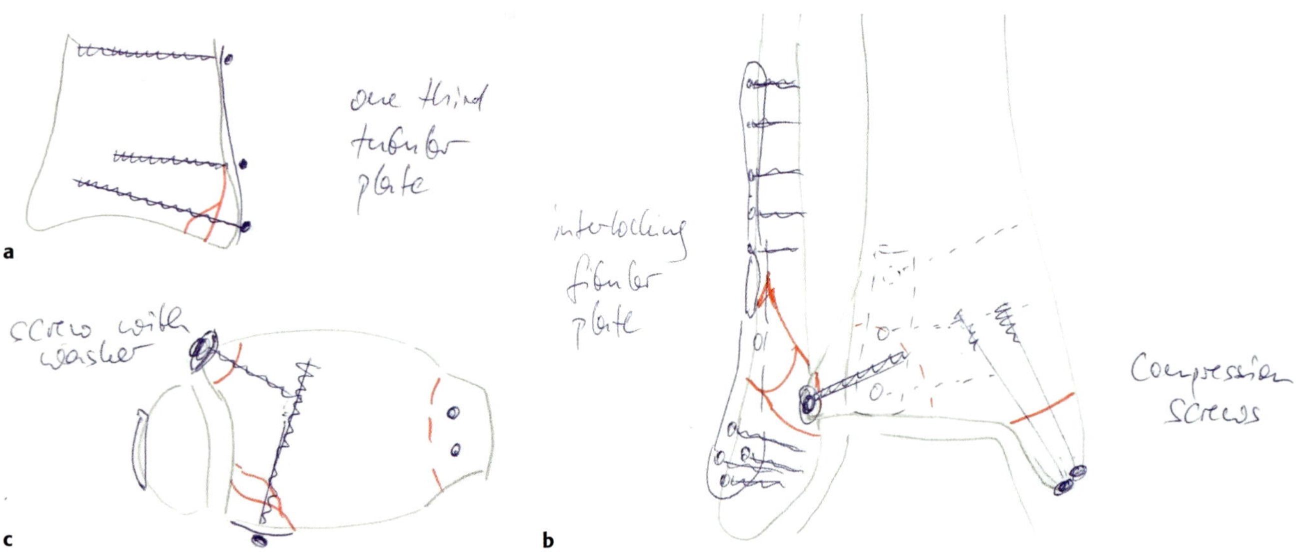

Fig 3.9-4a–c Preoperative plan.

a The posterior malleolus is fixed directly from posterior with a small antiglide plate. The intercalary fragment is assessed for stability and cartilage cover and eventually fixed with a resorbable pin or K-wire.

b The multifragmentary distal fibular fracture is bridged with a lateral interlocking plate via a lateral approach. The medial malleolus is stabilized with lag screws via a small, curved medial approach.

c The anterolateral tibial fragment (tubercle) is fixed with a screw and washer.

3 Operating room setup

Patient positioning	• Prone on a radiolucent table with the leg draped free • The ability to rotate the limb internally and externally as well as bend the knee is essential to allow all necessary incisions.
Anesthesia options	• General anesthesia due to the patient being in the prone position • Alternatively, spinal or regional anesthesia may be used.
C-arm location	• The C-arm is positioned on the foot end of the table. • The screen for the C-arm is placed more toward the head end of the table, so that the surgeon can have a free view while performing the reduction.
Tourniquet	• Well padded at the thigh and inflated before incision, deflated after reduction
Tips	• A bump may be placed under the anterior aspect of the contralateral hip if the limb is in too much external rotation allowing for greater ease in obtaining true mortise and lateral images. • Occasionally titling the C-arm toward the patient's head slightly will result in a better AP and mortise image.

For illustrations and overview of anesthetic considerations, see chapter 1.

Equipment

- K-wires, resorbable pins
- Small fragment one-third tubular and interlocking plates (for osteoporotic bone)
- 3.5 mm (2.7 mm) screws
- Smooth and sharp elevators
- Curved point-to-point reduction (Weber) clamp for reduction of the distal fibula into the incisura (if needed)

Size of implants and instruments may vary according to anatomy, bone quality, and fracture fragment size.

4 Surgical procedure

For internal fixation according to the preoperative plan, three approaches are needed:

- Posterolateral approach for the posterior tibial fragments
- Lateral approach for the fibular fracture
- Medial approach for the medial malleolar fracture

Posterolateral approach for the posterior tibial fragments

Reduction of the posterior tibial fragments should be performed first to allow adequate visualization in the lateral C-arm projections. The incision for the posterolateral approach lies parallel to the Achilles tendon (**Fig 3.9-5**). The sural nerve is identified within the subcutaneous tissue in the proximal part of the incision and gently retracted medially. The superficial and deep fasciae are incised longitudinally and the flexor hallucis longus (FHL) muscle belly and tendon are retracted medially, thereby protecting the posterior tibial neurovascular bundle. The fractured posterior tibial fragment is identified and retracted laterally which allows for removal of fracture hematoma. The posterior tibiofibular ligament is used as a hinge and left intact.
The intercalary fragments are then identified and evaluated for bone quality and cartilage cover. If the fragments are intact and the fracture fragment is 5 mm or more in size, the fragment is reduced to the intact anterior portion of the tibial plafond and fixed temporarily with a K-wire (**Fig 3.9-6a**).

Definite fixation of this fragment can be achieved with either a resorbable pin or a K-wire that is cut flush with the intercalary fragment and acts as a lost or buried K-wire. The posterolateral rim with the posterior syndesmosis attached is then brought back and realigned with the posterior tibial plafond. Once this is accomplished, the articular surface cannot be assessed by direct inspection. Anatomical reduction of the tibial joint surface is therefore performed using C-arm imaging in the lateral view. Definitive fixation is achieved with a posterior antiglide plate secondary to the osteoporotic bone quality (**Fig 3.9-6b**).

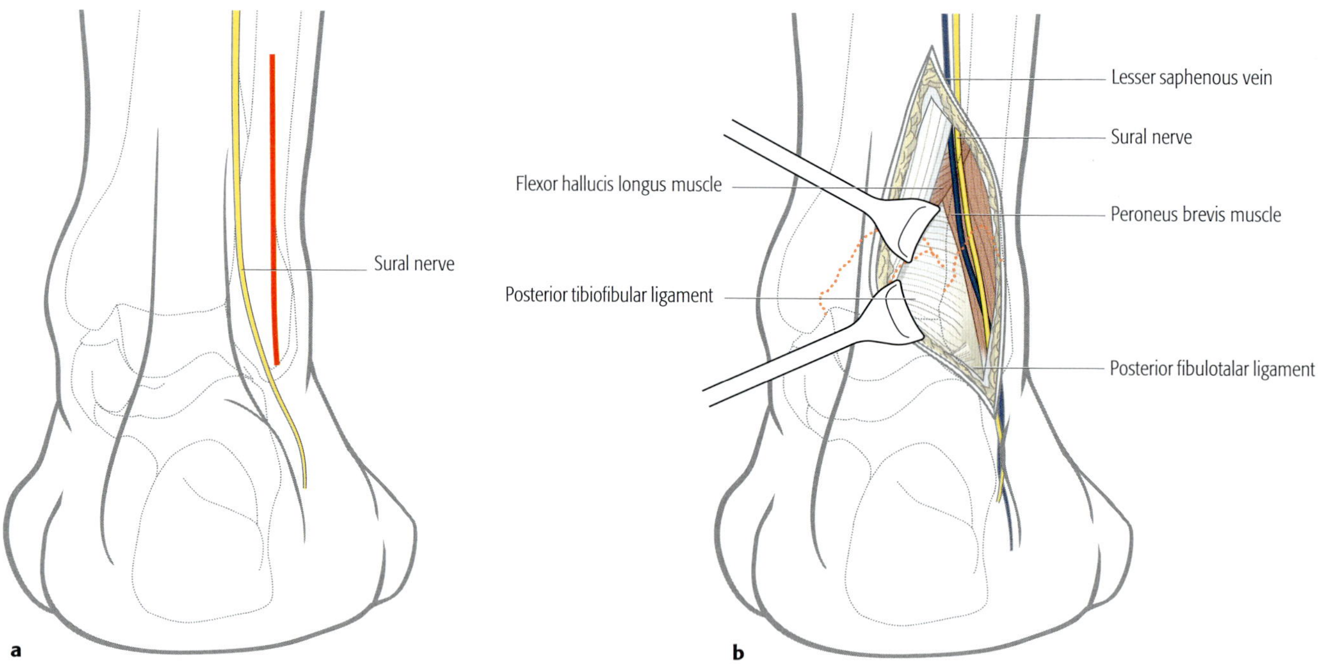

Fig 3.9-5a–b Posterolateral approach.
a Landmarks of the posterolateral approach to the ankle. The incision lies in the interval between the Achilles and the peroneal tendons. Care must be taken to identify and protect the sural nerve in the proximal end of the incision.
b Deep dissection requires cutting the superficial and deep crural fascia and retracting the FHL medially. The posterior tibiofibular (syndesmotic) ligament is attached to the posterolateral tibial fragment and the distal fibular fragment.

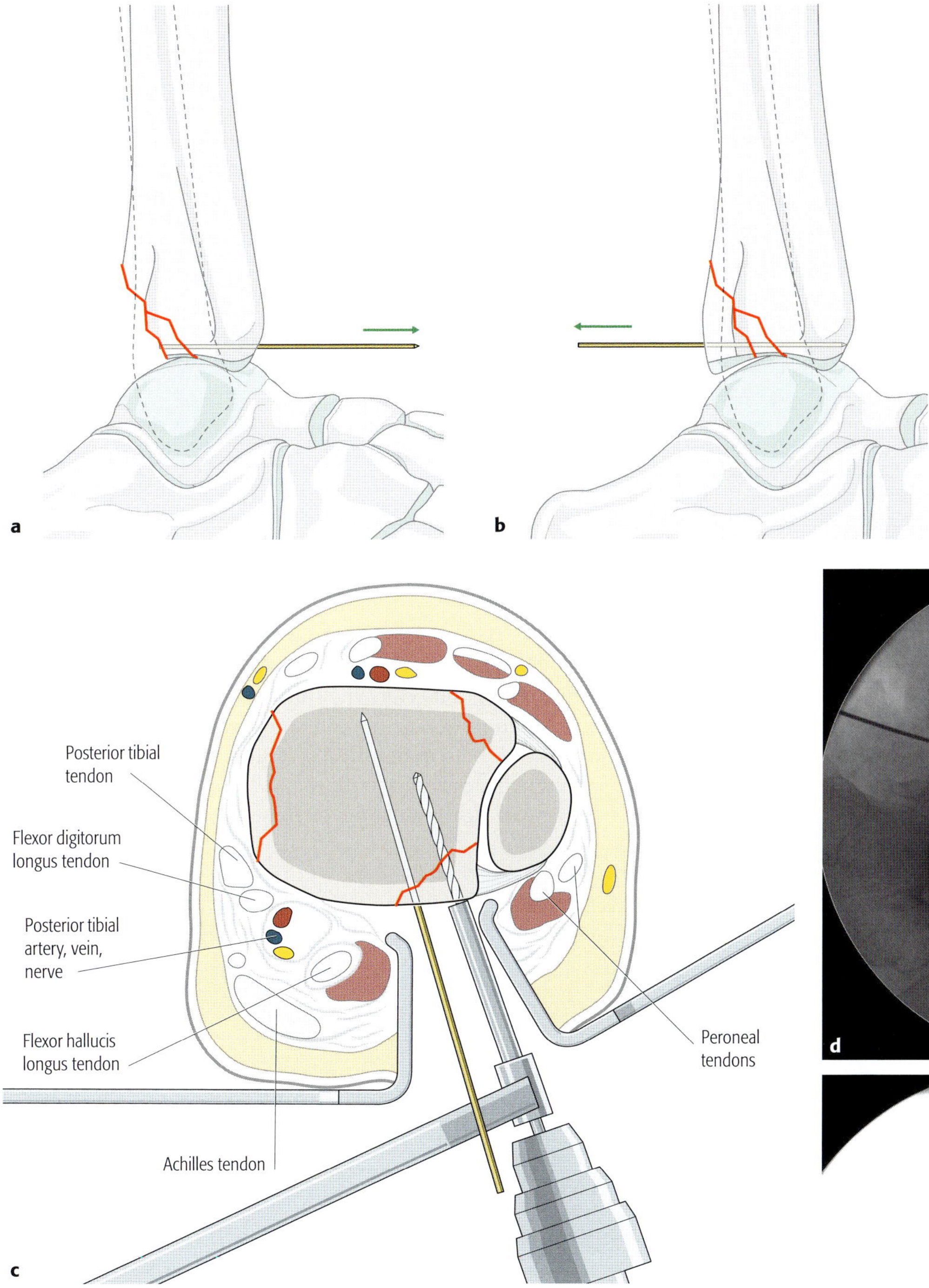

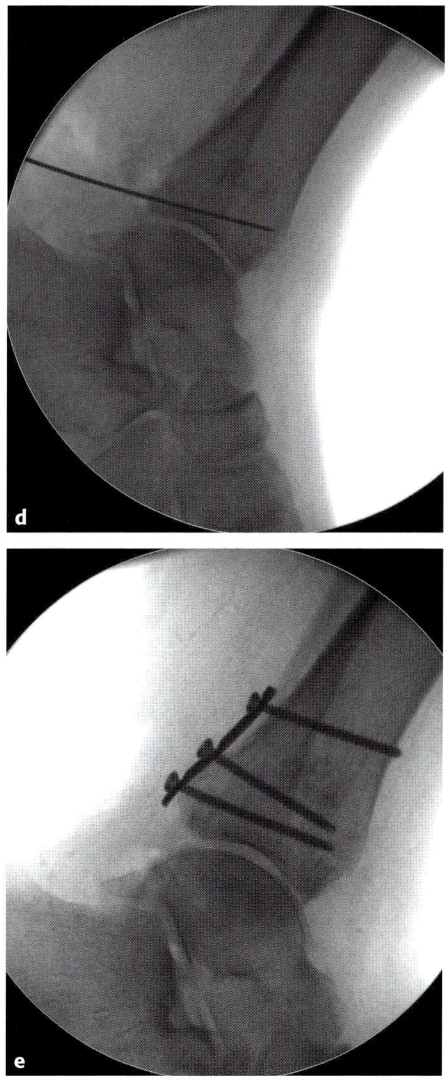

Fig 3.9-6a–e Reduction of the posterior tibial fragments.

a–b For reduction of the intercalary posterior tibial fragment, the talar dome serves as a template. The K-wire is brought out anteriorly until it is flush with the intercalary bone fragment. The posterior fragment is then reduced, and the K-wire brought back posteriorly.

c The K-wire is brought out anteriorly until it is flush with the intercalary bone fragment. The posterior fragment is then reduced and the K-wire brought back posteriorly.

d Temporary fixation with a K-wire.

e Definite fixation of the posterolateral fragment with a one-third tubular antiglide plate. Anatomical reduction of the joint surface is controlled with a lateral C-arm view.

Lateral approach for the fibular fracture

The comminuted fibular fracture is reduced next via a standard lateral approach with the patient still in the prone position (**Fig 3.9-7).** The leg may be rotated internally as needed for fracture manipulation.

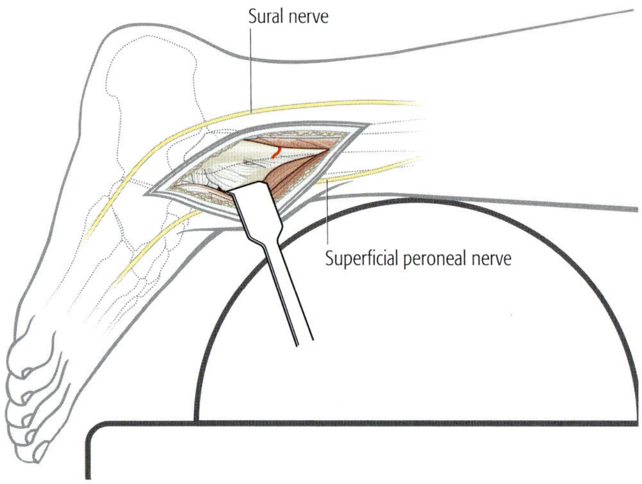

Fig 3.9-7 Lateral approach to the distal fibula with the patient in prone position. The anterior tibial tubercle (Tillaux-Chaput fragment) can be accessed via the distal anterior part of the incision.

The fibular fracture is fixed with a locking plate because of the poor bone quality. The plate is first fixed to the distal fibular fragment with locking screws. A screw is then placed proximal to the plate. A lamina spreader is inserted between the independent proximal screw and the proximal end of the plate. The lamina spreader is opened, gently pushing the plate and distal fragment to achieve appropriate length and alignment (**Fig 3.9-8**). Alternatively, a linear distractor can be used. Some plate systems have an olive wire push-pull device which may also be used to achieve proper fibular length. The key is to achieve appropriate fibular length allowing anatomical reconstruction.

Next, the proximal screws are placed. The first screw is introduced in a nonlocking fashion to compress the plate to the bone. The other screws are placed as locking screws. The fracture zone with comminution is bridged by the plate and no screws are placed into this region.

The anterior tibial tubercle (Tillaux-Chaput fragment) is accessed via the distal anterior part of the lateral incision. The knee may be bent 90° by an assistant to ease access to the anterior tibial rim. The fracture is cleared of debris and entrapped fibers of the anterior syndesmosis. Large fragments are fixed anatomically to the tibia with a screw and washer, if needed. Small and shallow fragments may be fixed with suture anchors or transosseous sutures.

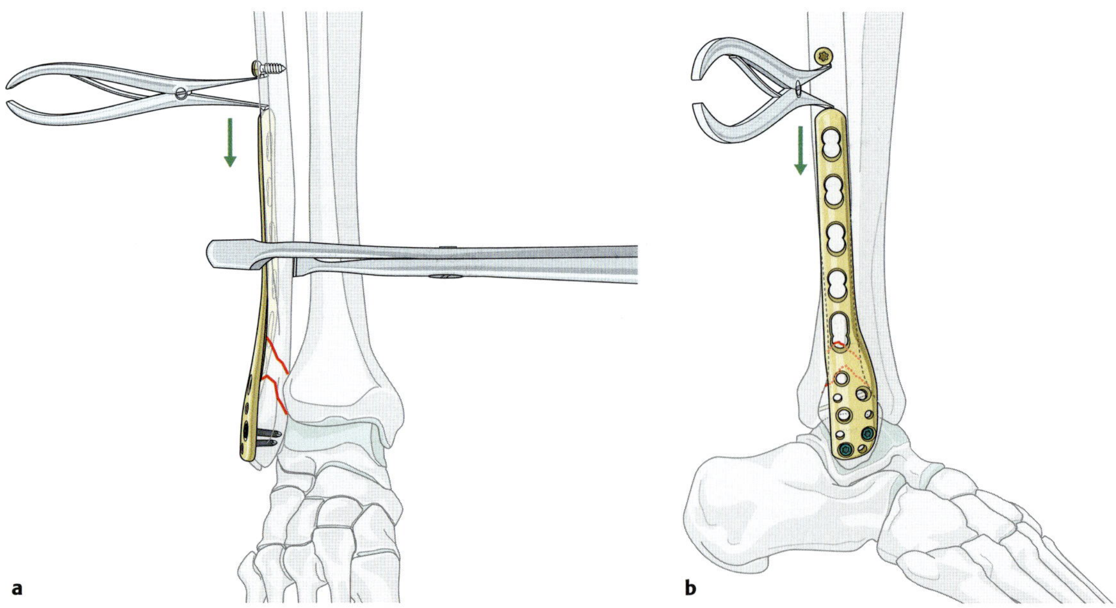

Fig 3.9-8a–b Technique of indirect fibular reduction with the plate fixed at the distal fragment in patients with osteoporotic bone. Direct manipulation of the distal fragment with a point-to-point reduction clamps carries the risk of further fragmentation. The same is true for interfragmentary compression screws in cases of multiple fragmentation of the distal fibula.

Medial approach for the medial malleolar fracture

The medial malleolar fracture is reduced via a standard medial approach, with the patient in prone position (**Fig 3.9-9**). The leg is turned slightly externally, a position that it assumes almost naturally.

The fragments are cleared of debris and hematoma. The medial malleolus is then reduced to the distal tibia under direct vision on the medial aspect of the ankle joint. Screw fixation is carried out and the anatomical reduction is checked with the C-arm (**Fig 3.9-10**).

Reduction and stable fixation of the anterior and posterior tibial fragments with the attached respective tibiofibular ligaments restores syndesmotic stability by providing a bone-to-bone fixation. This leads to stabilization of the syndesmotic complex. No additional fixation with either a syndesmotic screw or flexible implant (suture button) is required. Syndesmotic stability is tested intraoperatively with external rotation or the hook test (**Fig 3.9-11**). When using the hook test, the fibula is pulled laterally and posteriorly to detect syndesmotic instability.

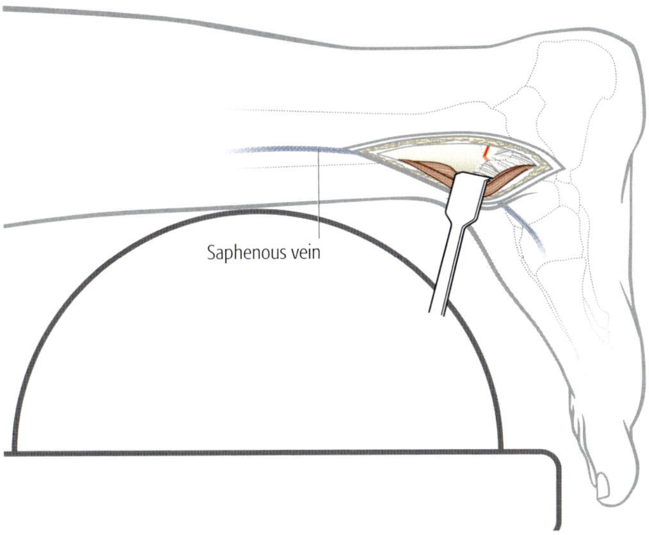

Fig 3.9-9 Medial approach to the medial malleolus with the patient in the prone position.

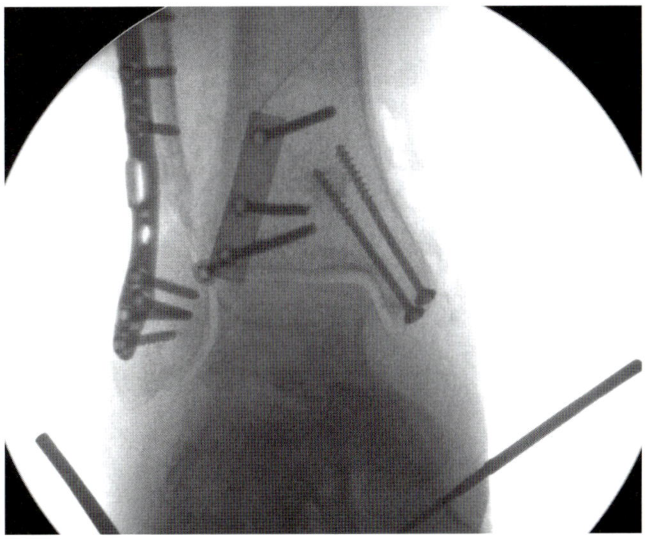

Fig 3.9-10 Reduction and fixation of: the distal fibula with a lateral interlocking neutralization plate; the medial malleolus with two screws; the anterior tibial with a screw and washer; the posterior tibial with an antiglide plate, result in a congruent ankle mortise and a well-centered talus below the distal tibia.

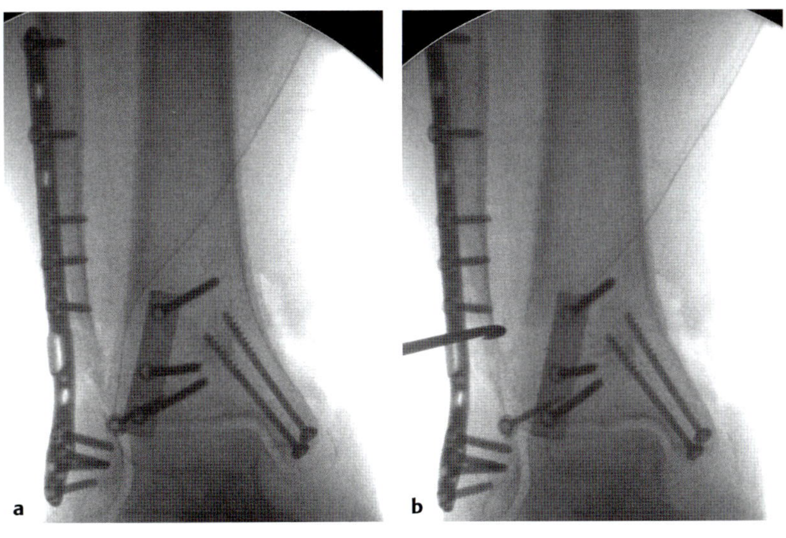

Fig 3.9-11a–b Syndesmotic stability is restored by fixation of the anterior and posterior tibial fragments carrying the respective tibiofibular ligaments and the distal fibular fracture as demonstrated by the classic hook test. Therefore, no additional fixation of the tibiofibular syndesmosis is needed.

5 Pitfalls and complications

Pitfalls

Inadequate reduction and fixation of the posterior tibial fragment

Attempts to fix a small posterior tibial fragment indirectly from the front with anteroposterior screws will result in a less stable fixation than with a posterior antiglide plate. Indirect reduction from the front also carries the risk of inadequate reduction and cannot be achieved in case of intercalary fragments, as in the present case.

Inadequate C-arm projections with the patient in a prone position

Fixation of malleolar fractures with the patient in a prone position is still carried out less frequently than with the patient supine. Care must be taken to achieve the exact mortise and lateral C-arm projections to allow visualization of reduction. The leg must be draped in such a manner that internal and external rotation or bending of the knee can be achieved easily. The limb is often externally rotated when in the prone position. Placing a bump or blanket roll under the contralateral hip will improve alignment of the limb and improve the ability to obtain true lateral and mortise images during the procedure. Occasionally, slightly tilting the C-arm toward the patient's head will result in better AP and mortise images. The bump placed anterior to the ankle results in the operative limb being slightly off plane (**Fig 3.9-5**).

The posterior approach and reduction should be performed before the lateral open reduction and internal fixation (ORIF). If lateral ORIF is performed first, the plate may obscure the C-arm views of the posterior area and impede ORIF of the posterior fracture.

With complex fracture patterns, 3D imaging is beneficial. In case of doubt or with complex fracture patterns, as in the present case, postoperative CT scanning of both ankles is recommended (**Fig 3.9-12**).

Irreducible intercalary fragments

Small intercalary fragments (< 5 mm in diameter) and fragments that do not carry a cartilage cover should be removed rather than attempting fixation. These fragments do not contribute to joint congruity and may impede anatomical reduction or even displace into the joint as loose bodies.

Complications

- Injury to the sural nerve (posterolateral approach), or superficial peroneal nerve (lateral approach)
- Injury to the posterior tibial neurovascular bundle (if dissecting medially beyond the FHL tendon)
- Irritation of the posterior tibial tendon with posterior screw placement in the medial malleolus
- Loss of fixation
- Malunion
- Nonunion
- Posttraumatic arthritis

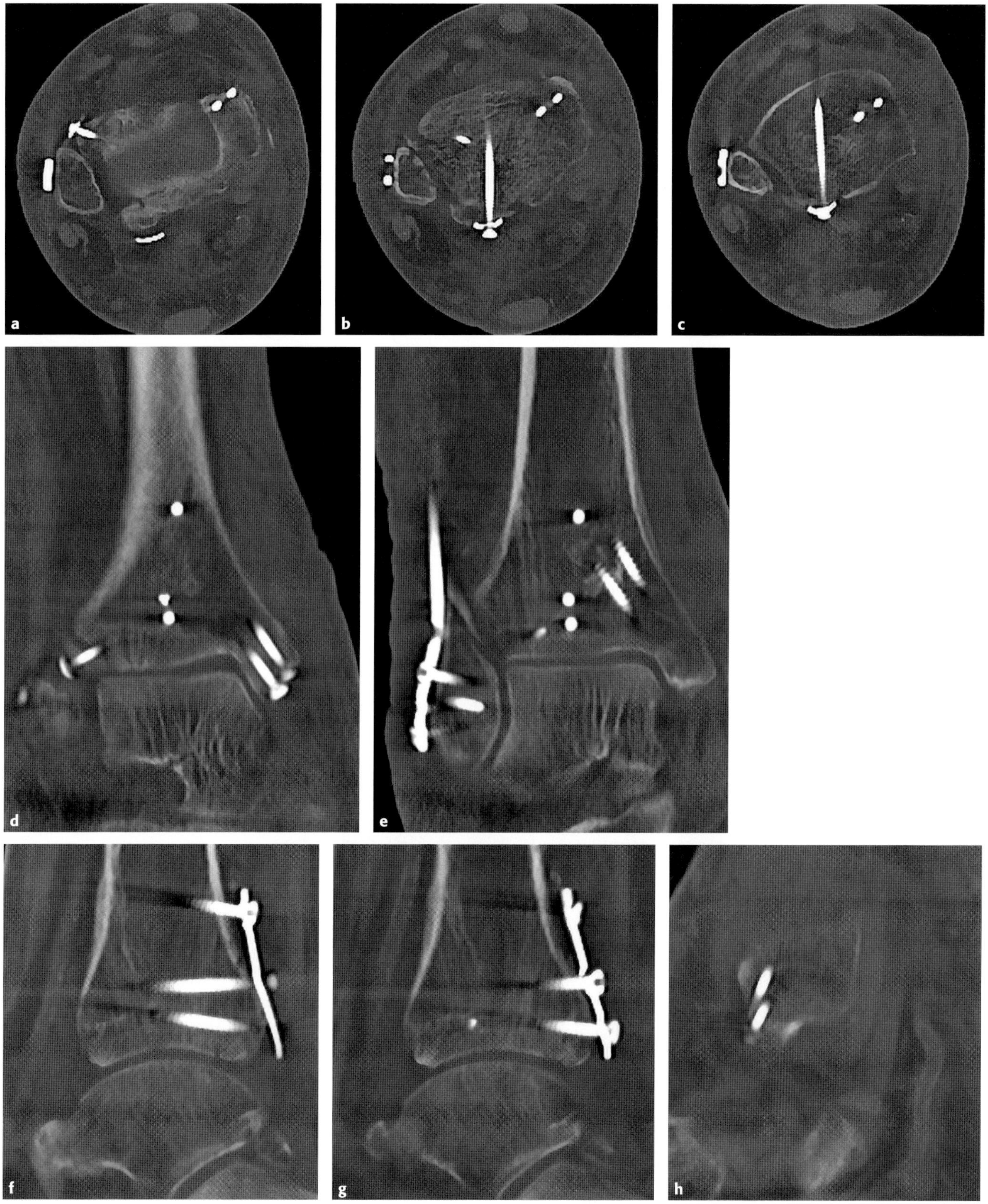

Fig 3.9-12a–h Postoperative CT scans revealing anatomical restoration of all four malleoli: the medial and lateral malleolus, anterior and posterior tibial fragments including the depressed intercalary posterior fragment, resulting in a congruent joint surface and ankle mortise.

6 Alternative techniques

Osteoporotic ankle fractures are increasing in frequency. Numerous fixation techniques have been described including:

- Dorsal antiglide plate (instead of a lateral neutralization plate) or a hook plate to the distal fibula
- Additional intramedullary fixation of the distal fibula with fanned K-wires
- Intramedullary fixation of the distal fibula with a nail
- Locking plates on the medial and posterior malleolus, which can enhance stability.
- The use of several syndesmotic screws through a fibular plate (tibia pro fibula ,ie, the distal tibia serves as an additional stabilization for the distal fibula)
- Cement augmentation of screws
- Tibiotalocalcaneal fusion with a retrograde nail or external fixation is a treatment option for patients with dementia, bedridden patients, and for patients with Charcot neuroosteoarthropathy
- Bicortical medial malleolar screw placement

With extremely soft bone, a combination of the above-mentioned measures may be warranted. Treatment strategies should be tailored to the patient according to the fracture pattern, comorbidities, patient compliance, and individual bone quality.

7 Postoperative management and rehabilitation

Postoperatively, the foot is typically immobilized in a splint or below-knee cast and the lower leg is elevated. Any applied suction drain is removed on day 1 or 2 after surgery.

For this patient, because of the high degree of instability at first presentation and the poor bone quality with preexisting polyneuropathy, external fixation was kept in place for 6 weeks after definite surgery to protect internal fixation (**Fig 3.9-13**). After removal of the external fixator, the patient was allowed only partial weight bearing (up to 20 kg) for another 6 weeks in an ankle-spanning walker boot.

Weight bearing is gradually increased after radiographic union is seen. An active rehabilitation protocol is then initiated including range-of-motion exercises, muscular balancing, and gait training (**Fig 3.9-14**).

Implant removal

Removal of plates or screws on the posterior aspect of the distal tibia is generally not necessary. Prominent implants on the medial and lateral malleolus are typically removed using the same approaches after 1 year, when x-rays show bony healing.

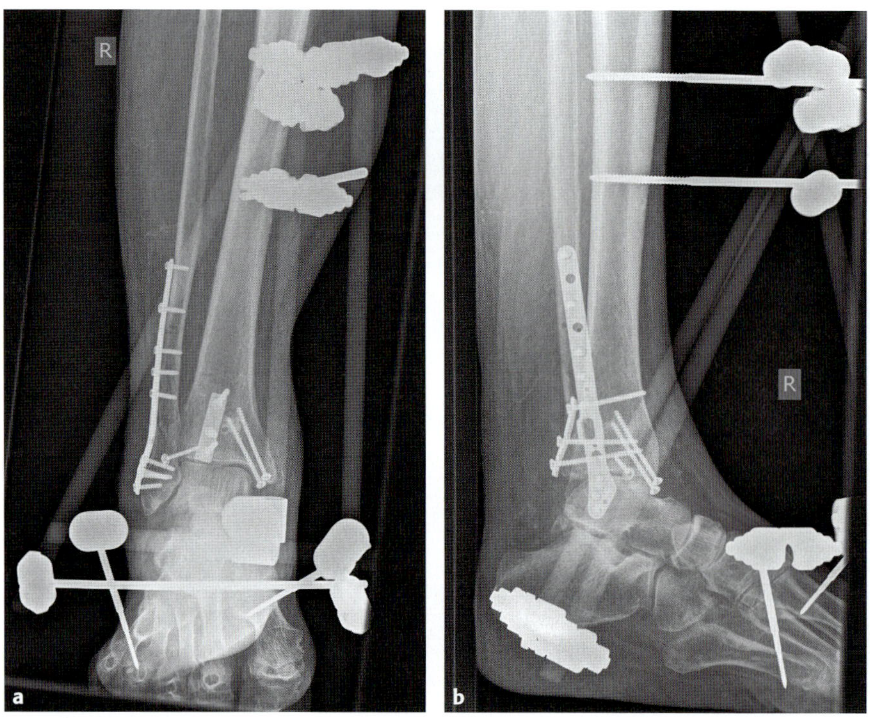

Fig 3.9-13a–b X-rays taken 1 week after surgery with the external fixator still in place.
a AP view.
b Lateral view.

Treatment of comorbidities

Treatment of osteoporosis and relevant comorbidities is essential to obtain adequate wound and fracture healing. This includes antiresorptive agents, vitamin D3 supplementation, tight control of blood glucose serum levels in patients with diabetes, and professional foot care for patients with neuropathy. Bone mineral density is controlled in patients with suspicious findings. In many instances, the orthopedic surgeon treating an osteoporotic fracture will be the first to diagnose that condition. It is their obligation to initiate further diagnosis and treatment, often via referral to the patient's primary care physician or metabolic bone consultant.

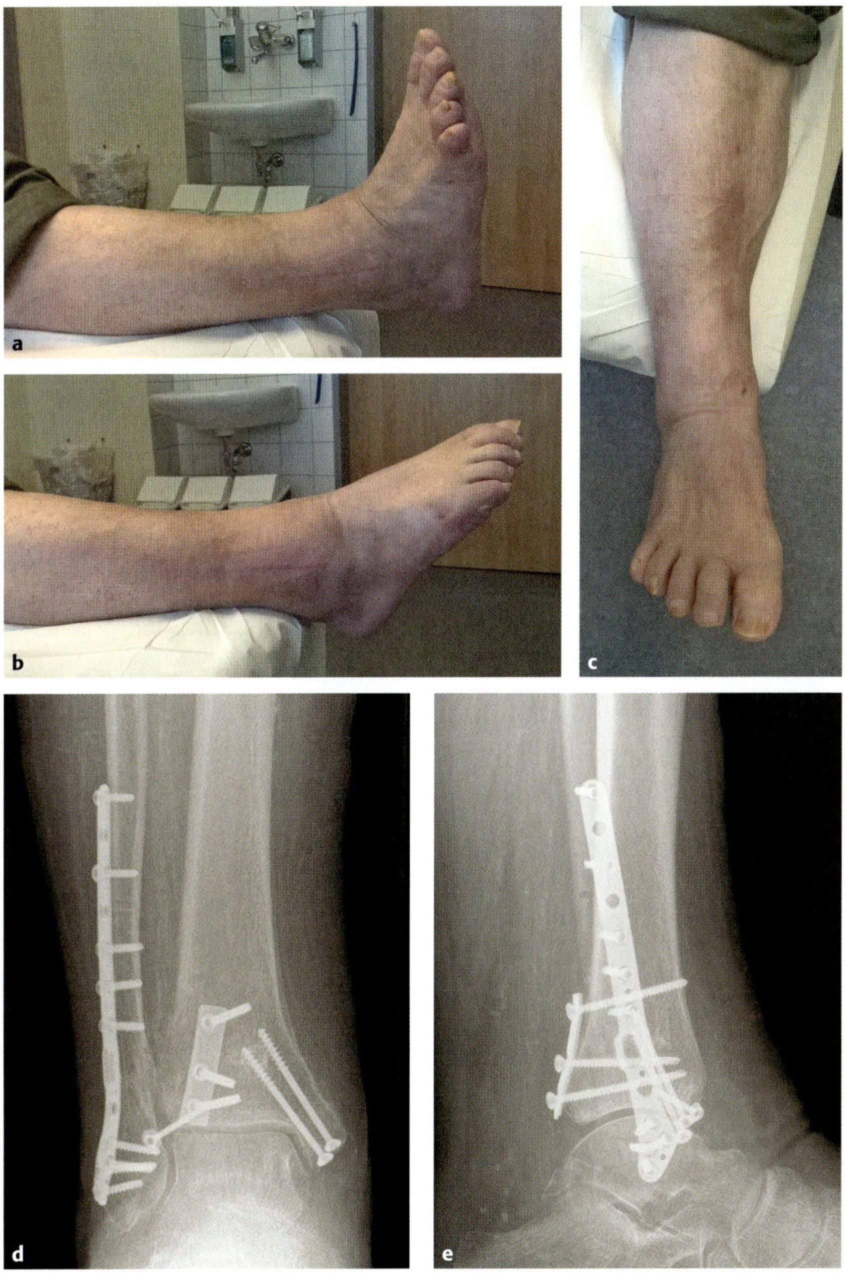

Fig 3.9-14a–e Follow-up at 3 months after surgery.
a–c Soft-tissue status and range of motion.
d–e Standing x-rays demonstrating good alignment and bone healing. At this point the patient is allowed full weight bearing.

8 Recommended reading

Anand N, Klenerman L. Ankle fractures in the elderly: MUA versus ORIF. *Injury.* 1993 Feb;24(2):116–120.
Bartoníček J, Rammelt S, Kostlivý K, et al. Anatomy and classification of the posterior tibial fragment in ankle fractures. *Arch Orthop Trauma Surg.* 2015 Apr;135(4):505–516.
Court-Brown CM, Biant LC, Clement ND, et al. Open fractures in the elderly. The importance of skin ageing. *Injury.* 2015 Feb;46(2):189–194.
Davidovitch RI, Walsh M, Spitzer A, et al. Functional outcome after operatively treated ankle fractures in the elderly. *Foot Ankle Int.* 2009 Aug;30(8):728–733.
Koval KJ, Petraco DM, Kummer FJ, et al. A new technique for complex fibula fracture fixation in the elderly: a clinical and biomechanical evaluation. *J Orthop Trauma.* 1997 Jan;11(1):28–33.
Makwana NK, Bhowal B, Harper WM, et al. Conservative versus operative treatment for displaced ankle fractures in patients over 55 years of age. A prospective, randomised study. *J Bone Joint Surg Br.* 2001 May;83(4):525–529.
Panchbhavi VK, Mody MG, Mason WT. Combination of hook plate and tibial pro-fibular screw fixation of osteoporotic fractures: a clinical evaluation of operative strategy. *Foot Ankle Int.* 2005 Jul;26(7):510–515.
Rammelt S. Management of ankle fractures in the elderly. *EFORT Open Rev.* 2016 May;1(5):239–246.
Rammelt S, Zwipp H. Ankle fractures. In: Bentley G, ed. *European Instructional Course Lectures,* Volume 12. Berlin Heidelberg New York: Springer; 2012:205–219.
Rammelt S, Zwipp H, Mittlmeier T. [Operative treatment of pronation fracture-dislocations of the ankle]. *Oper Orthop Traumatol.* 2013 Jun;25(3):273–291. German

4 Calcaneus

Calcaneus

4 Calcaneal fractures

Michael Swords

1 Introduction

Calcaneal fractures are rare but represent approximately 60% of tarsal bone fractures. The anatomy of the hindfoot is complex, increasing the difficulty of management. Unlike most traumatic orthopedic injuries there is much debate on the ideal treatment of these injuries. Treatment may be non-operative in certain fractures. Operative treatment should be chosen based on the specific fracture pattern and patient.

2 Anatomy and pathomechanics

The calcaneus is an oddly shaped bone with three articular facets on the superior surface articulating with the undersurface of the talus to form the subtalar joint. The posterior facet is the largest of the articular facets and sits on the calcaneal body. The middle facet is the superior surface of the sustentaculum tali. The anterior facet is located on the anterior process and is sometimes an independent articular surface and at other times is an extension (in the shape of an 8) of the middle facet. The distal articular surface of the calcaneus articulates with the cuboid and is essential in maintaining lateral column length and function (**Fig 4-1**).

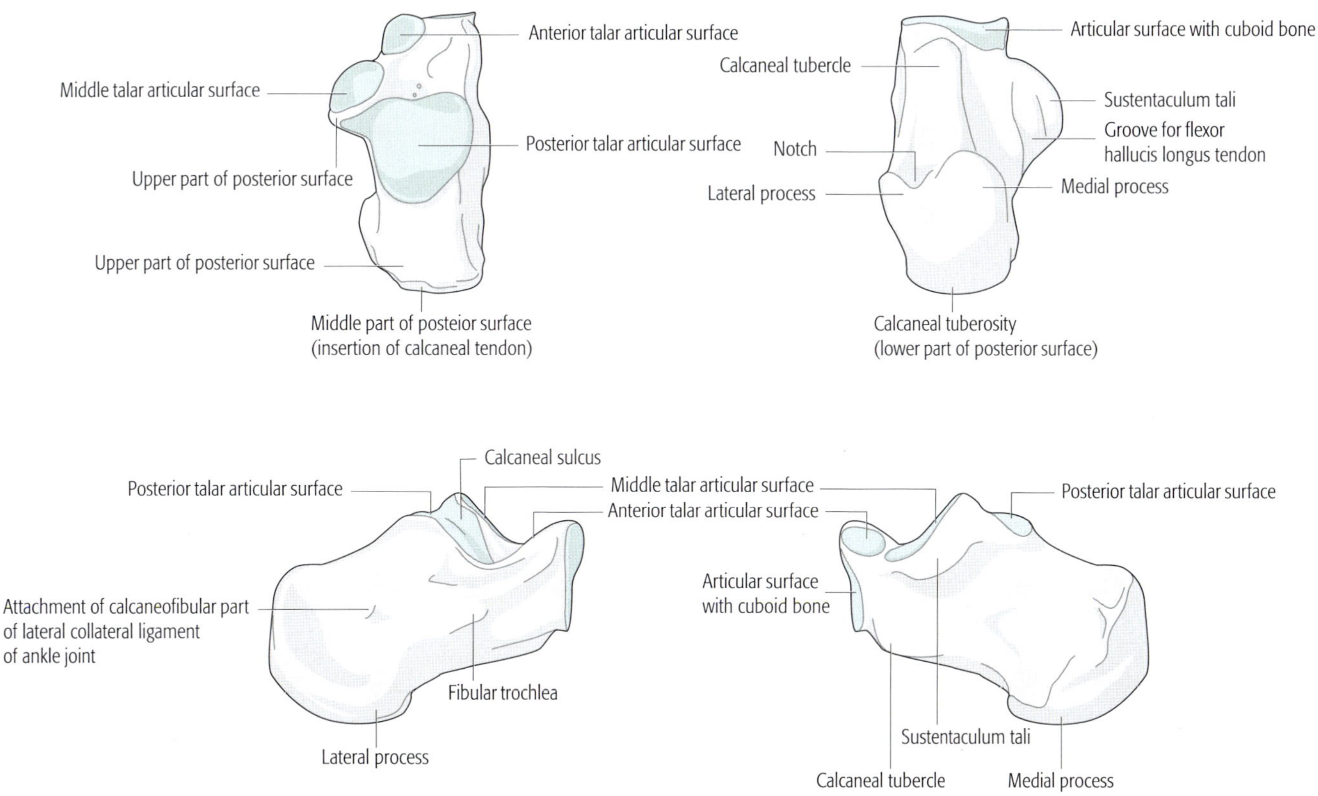

Fig 4-1 The calcaneus has three articular facets. The posterior facet is the largest while the anterior and middle facets sit on the anterior process. The middle facet is located on the superior surface of the sustentaculum.

The Achilles tendon attaches to the posterior of the tuber. The peroneal tendons run diagonally along the lateral aspect of the calcaneus and are held in position by the superior peroneal retinaculum behind the fibula, and the inferior peroneal retinaculum which attaches to the peroneal tubercle on the lateral wall of the calcaneus. The flexor hallucis longus runs along the medial aspect of the posterior facet and then under the sustentaculum tali.

The glabrous plantar skin is uniquely structured for shock absorption and to dissipate shear forces. The skin and soft tissue covering the remainder of the calcaneus is thin and vulnerable both to traumatic injury and to development of chronic wounds which can occur as a result of posttraumatic deformity.

Knowledge of the vascular supply to the soft tissues on the lateral side of the calcaneus is important. Surgical treatment in most cases requires incisions to be made on the lateral side of the foot. Much of the lateral side of the calcaneus receives arterial supply from the lateral calcaneal artery. The plantar heel pad obtains arterial supply from the medial calcaneal branches of the posterior tibial artery. The posterior heel takes arterial supply from the perforating branches of the peroneal artery and branches of the posterior tibial artery (**Fig 4-2**). The sural nerve runs along the lateral side of the foot and is at risk at the proximal and distal ends of the lateral extensile approach.

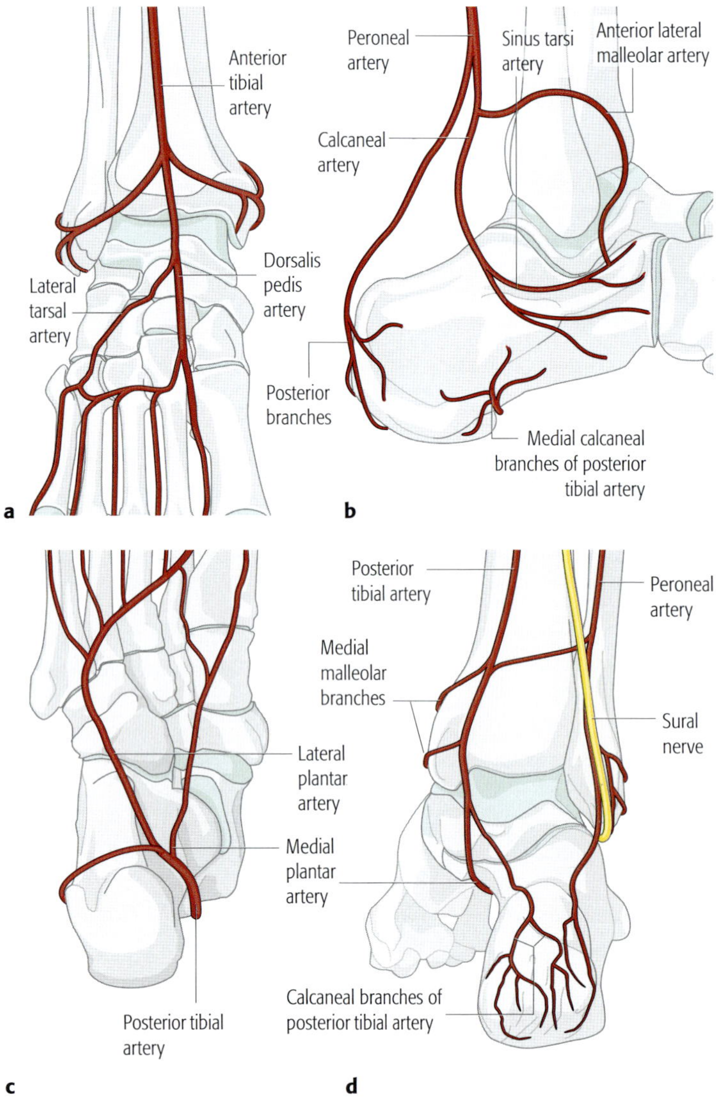

Fig 4-2a–b Blood supply to the calcaneus from anterior (**a**), lateral (**b**), inferior (**c**), and posterior (**d**). The lateral calcaneal artery is one of the perforating branches of the peroneal artery and is the dominant blood supply to the lateral extensile flap. The heel pad receives most of its vascular supply from branches of the posterior tibial artery (**b**), which is vulnerable to injury with significant fracture displacement along the medial wall.

Fractures are typically the result of an axial load, most commonly from a fall from height or a motor vehicle injury. The lateral process of the talus impacts on the calcaneus creating the primary fracture line at the critical angle. A secondary fracture line exits superiorly resulting in a joint depression fracture or posteriorly resulting in a tongue-type fracture.

Fractures of the sustentaculum occur as a result of varus force, either in isolation or in combination with other fractures to the calcaneus or hindfoot.

Beak fractures occur more commonly in individuals with altered bone density or neuropathy and are often the result of lower-energy mechanisms.

3 Fracture classification

Fracture classification for calcaneal fractures includes both x-ray and computed tomography (CT) based classification systems. The most common radiographic classification system is the Essex-Lopresti classification (**Fig 4-3**). This system divides calcaneal fractures initially into extraarticular and intraarticular fractures. The intraarticular fractures are further subdivided into either joint depression or tongue type fractures.

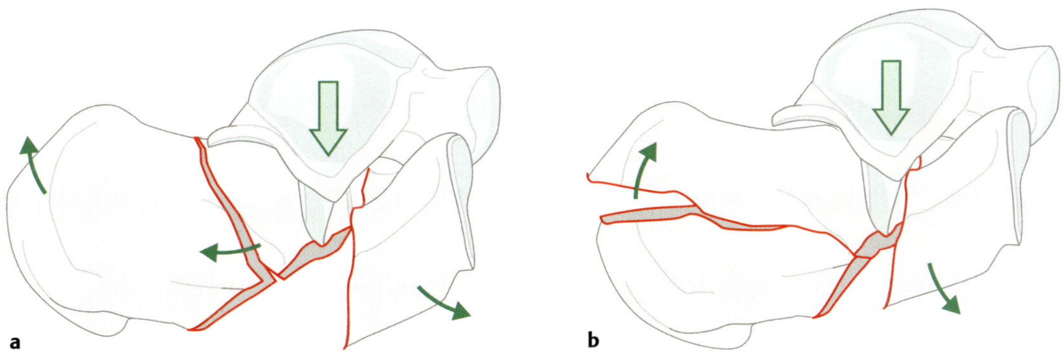

a b

Fig 4-3a–b Example of an Essex-Lopresti classification. In both fracture patterns impaction creates the primary fracture line at the critical angle.

a In joint depression-type fractures the secondary fracture line exits superiorly isolating the posterior facet fragment.

b In tongue-type fractures the secondary fracture line exits posteriorly and the posterior superior aspect of the calcaneus is part of the articular fragment with the posterior facet.

The AO/OTA Fracture and Dislocation Classification incorporates both the Essex-Lopresti and Sanders classifications. It is comprehensive and includes all but rare fracture variants (see appendix for the detailed AO/OTA calcaneal classification). It follows this pattern:

- Extraarticular fractures are divided into two groups: fractures that are avulsion or extraarticular tongue or tuberosity fractures (82A1) or extraarticular body fractures (82A2).
- Intraarticular tongue-type fractures include fractures where the intraarticular fracture fragment includes the Achilles tendon attachment. These may be simple fractures (82B1) or multifragmentary (82B2).
- The joint depression fractures (82C) include intraarticular fractures where the intraarticular fracture does not include the Achilles tendon attachment at posterior superior calcaneus. The joint depression portion of the classification generally follows the Sanders classification (**Fig 4-4**). Joint depression fractures with two articular fragments (82C1) are equivalent to Sanders 2, fractures with three articular fragments (82C2) are equivalent to Sanders 3, while multifragmentary fractures (82C3) are equivalent to Sanders 4.

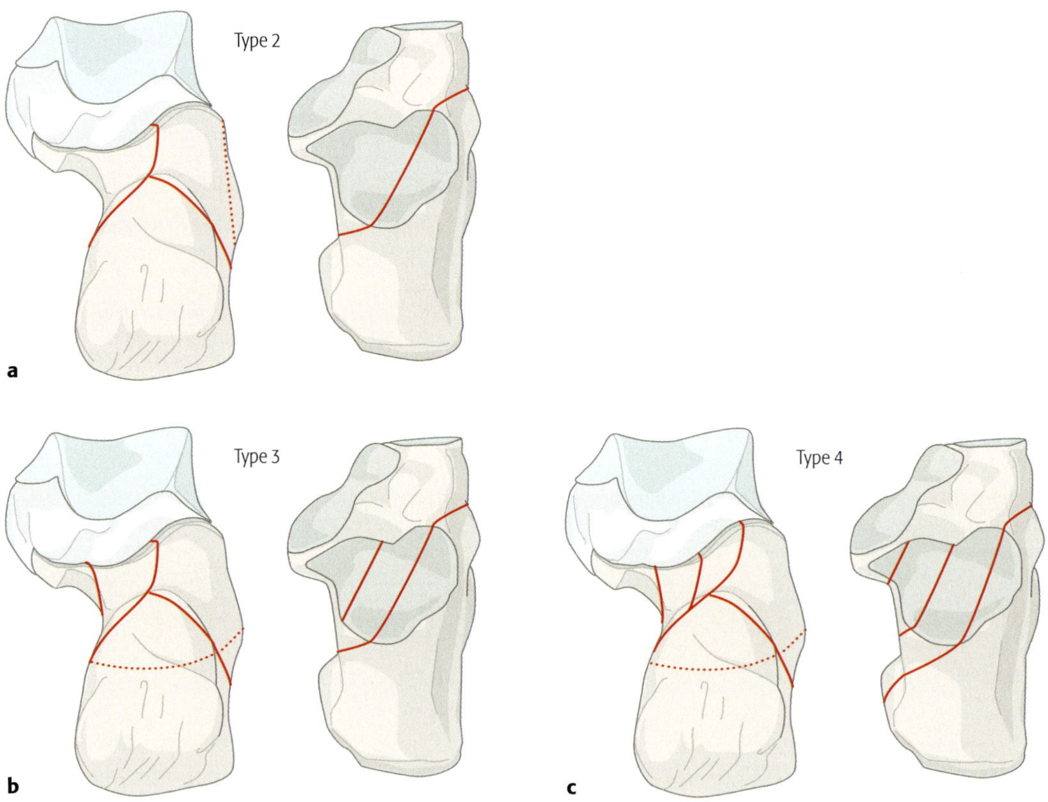

Fig 4-4a–c The Sanders classification is based on the CT coronal projection of the posterior facet. The prognosis worsens due to increasing articular comminution and the difficulty of the surgical reconstruction increases with increasing Sanders classification. In Sanders 2 (**a**), the posterior facet is divided in two fragments. These fractures are easier to reduce and have a better prognosis than Sanders 3 (**b**), or Sanders 4 (**c**) fractures which are much more challenging to reduce and have a more guarded prognosis.

4 Preoperative assessment

Clinical assessment

The initial evaluation of calcaneal fractures should be thorough. Examination of sensation should include assessment of the sural nerve distribution. Additionally, the plantar sensation provided by the medial and lateral plantar nerves should be examined and recorded. Occasionally, the tibial nerve may be stretched from the fracture displacement of the tuberosity. The lateral plantar nerve is more commonly affected as it travels the longest distance so is the most vulnerable to stretch neuropraxia.

The soft tissues must be examined. Most calcaneal fractures are the result of high-energy injuries, such as a fall from height or a motor vehicle accident. These injuries result in significant soft-tissue swelling that may increase over time. The soft tissues should be monitored over time and surgical fixation, if indicated by the fracture, should only be considered when the swelling has resolved enough to allow safe closure of the wound. This is often when the swelling has resolved to the point the skin will wrinkle when tested (**Fig 4-5**). Surgical treatment is usually performed between days 7 and 21 postinjury.

The posterior portion of the hindfoot should be examined. In tuberosity or beak fractures skin may be blanched or ischemic resulting in the early development of catastrophic wound complications unless intervention is made emergently (**Fig 4-6**). Gardner reported that tongue-type fractures additionally are associated with a 10–20% risk of posterior soft-tissue complications. This complication is best avoided by using appropriate padding when splinting and preventing pressure on the posterior calcaneus when elevating is necessary.

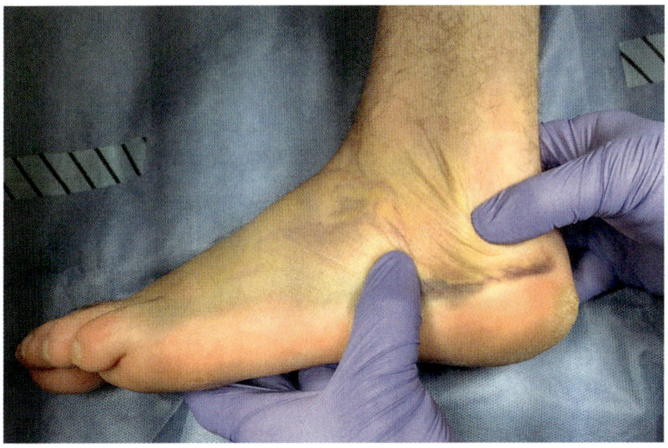

Fig 4-5 Surgical management using an extensile lateral approach should only be considered when the swelling has resolved enough that it will allow safe closure of the wound. This is often when the swelling has resolved to the point the skin will wrinkle when tested (wrinkle sign). This generally occurs 7–21 days postinjury.

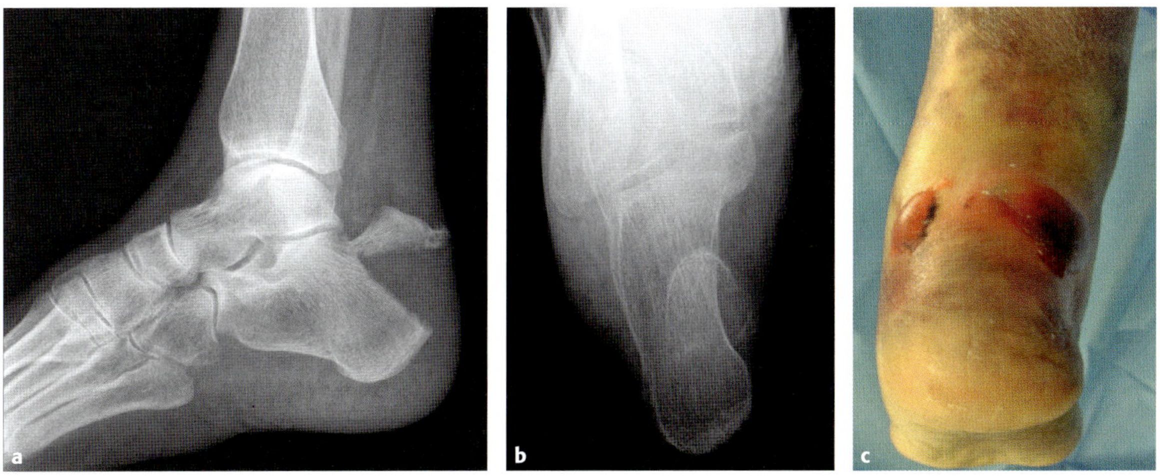

Fig 4-6a–c Lateral (**a**) and axial (**b**) x-rays demonstrating an avulsion (beak) fracture with marked displacement. The displaced fragment causes injury to the posterior soft tissues and must be addressed in a timely manner to avoid pressure necrosis from developing (**c**).

Lateral displacement of the tuberosity results in a medial fracture spike that may traumatize the medial soft tissues. Close examination of the medial hindfoot is important as fracture blisters and wounds from open fractures are more commonly found on the medial side. Open fractures should be treated with surgical debridement. Early provisional reduction in cases with severe displacement should be considered.

Imaging

Initial imaging for calcaneal fractures includes lateral, axial, and Brodén views. Böhler angle demonstrates the severity of joint injury and displacement (depression) and is measured on the lateral x-ray (**Fig 4-7**). The axial view shows joint displacement as well as increase in width and varus/valgus malalignment. Brodén views are special views to assess the congruency of the subtalar joint surface taken at 30°, 50°, and 70° off the horizontal plane. In certain situations, contralateral imaging may be helpful. Additional foot or ankle x-rays may be needed based on the individual injury being evaluated.

Intraarticular fractures are best examined with a CT scan including sagittal, axial, and semicoronal (perpendicular to the posterior facet) planes (**Fig 4-8**). This will allow full assessment of the fracture pattern and aid in surgical planning.

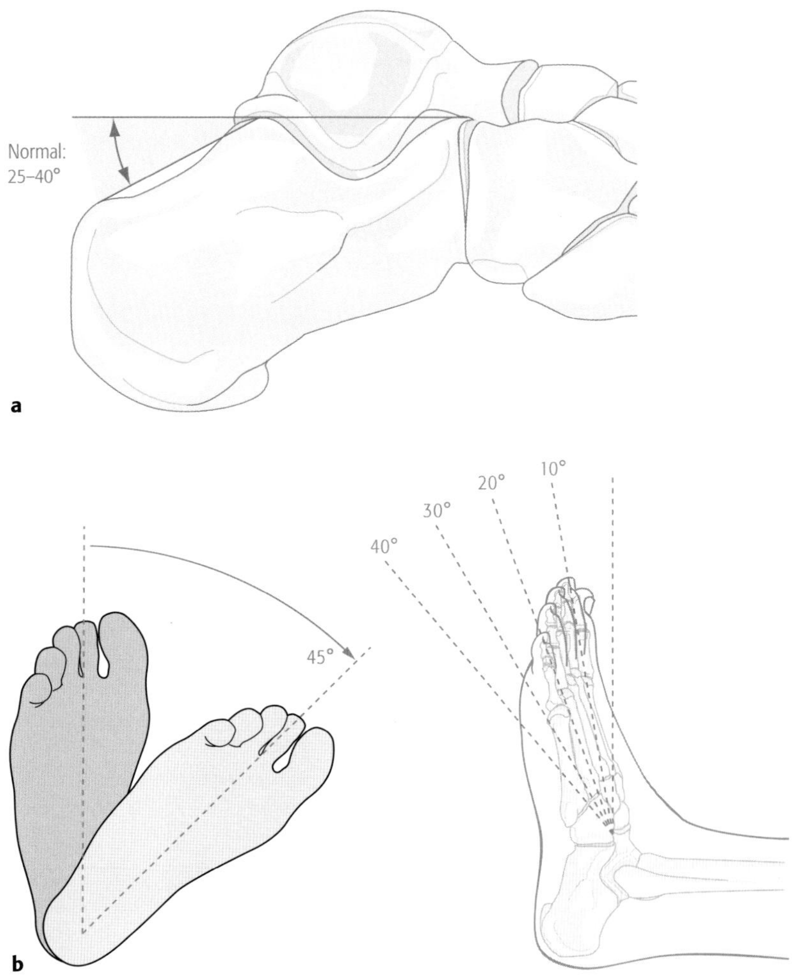

Fig 4-7a–b Böhler angle.
a Böhler angle is measured on the lateral x-ray. A normal Böhler angle is between 25° and 40°.
b Brodén views are special views to assess the congruence of the subtalar joint and are taken at 45° with the ankle tilted 10–40° off the horizontal plane.

5 Nonoperative treatment

Systemic diseases, such as dense neuropathy, peripheral vascular disease, poorly controlled diabetes, or noncompliance from substance abuse, may be contraindications for surgical treatment.

Nonoperative treatment is reserved for fracture patterns with minimal displacement. Extraarticular fractures with minimal alteration of the overall shape and alignment of the calcaneus may be treated without surgery. Gross alteration of the shape of the calcaneus may interfere with shoe wear or cause problems with weight bearing if excessive. Fractures resulting in varus or valgus less than 10° may be considered for nonoperative treatment.

Select intraarticular fractures may also be treated nonoperatively. Fractures with intraarticular involvement with less than 2 mm of articular step off and less than 3 mm of gap may be considered for nonoperative treatment if there is also minimal loss of Böhler angle.

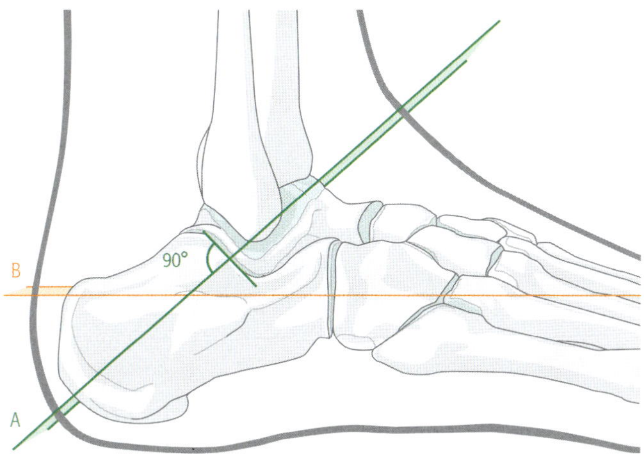

Fig 4-8 For best CT imaging careful foot position is mandatory. The planes of reconstruction are (A) perpendicular to the posterior facet and (B) parallel to the sole of the foot.

6 Operative treatment

Emergent operative treatment is indicated for open fractures, fractures with an associated dislocation, and fractures with soft tissues at risk of breakdown due to gross fracture fragment displacement or malalignment, such as beak fractures. Impending compartment syndrome is also an indication for surgical treatment.

Operative treatment is also generally indicated for fractures that result in gross alteration of the shape of the calcaneus that may interfere with either shoe wear or result in plantar deformity leading to painful callosities or ulceration over time.

Extraarticular fractures that result in more than 10° of varus or valgus alignment should be treated operatively. Excessive shortening, lengthening, or broadening of the calcaneus should also be considered for operative treatment. Many of these extraarticular fractures are amenable to small incision techniques, and in many cases, screw fixation.

Displaced intraarticular calcaneal fractures with an articular step off more than 2 mm or an articular gap of more than 3 mm should also be considered for operative treatment. Fractures with severe loss of Böhler angle should also be treated operatively to increase the likelihood of a good functional result.

Patient positioning

The patient is positioned in the lateral position with the operative leg up on a table that is radiolucent distally. A bean bag may be used to secure the patient to the table. The down leg, which is just anterior to operative leg, is padded with pillows to prevent pressure injury to the peroneal nerve. A foam-positioning ramp is placed under the operative leg with the ramp wedged into the beanbag. Alternatively, pillows or blankets can be used to elevate the operative limb to avoid interference with C-arm imaging. A tourniquet is placed on the upper thigh and a nonsterile U-drape placed circumferentially just distal to the tourniquet (**Fig 4-9**).

The knee of the operative leg is slightly flexed to position the foot in the corner of the end of the table. The surgeon sits directly behind the heel of the operative foot.

C-arm positioning

The C-arm is positioned oblique to the foot of table with the monitor in front of the patient (**Fig 4-10**). This position allows for necessary imaging throughout the case with limited movement of the C-arm base needed (**Fig 4-11**).

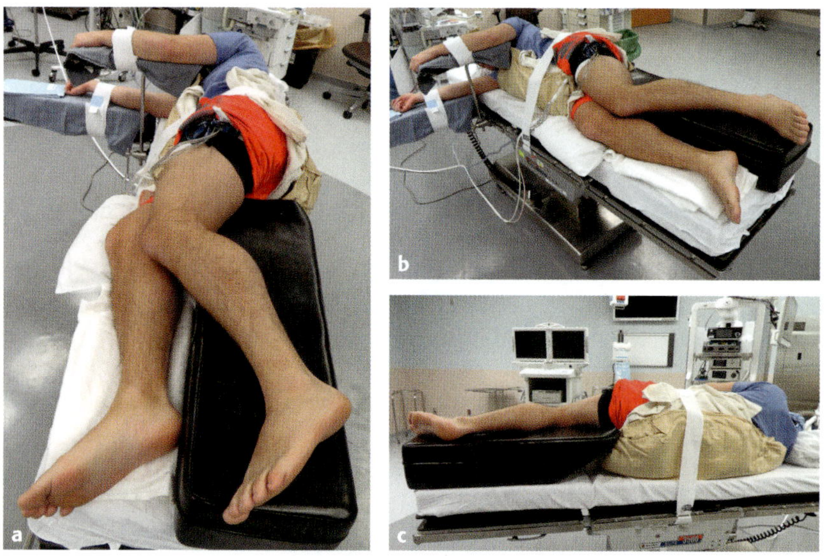

Fig 4-9a–c The patient is positioned lateral with operative leg elevated allowing easy access for a lateral approach to the calcaneus.

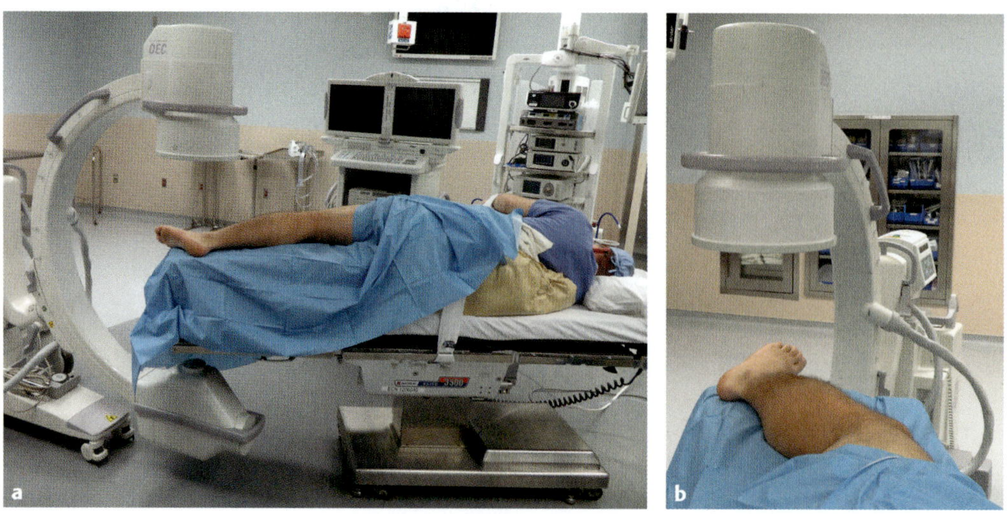

Fig 4-10a–b The C-arm is positioned at the foot of the operative table obliquely with the monitor in front of the patient.

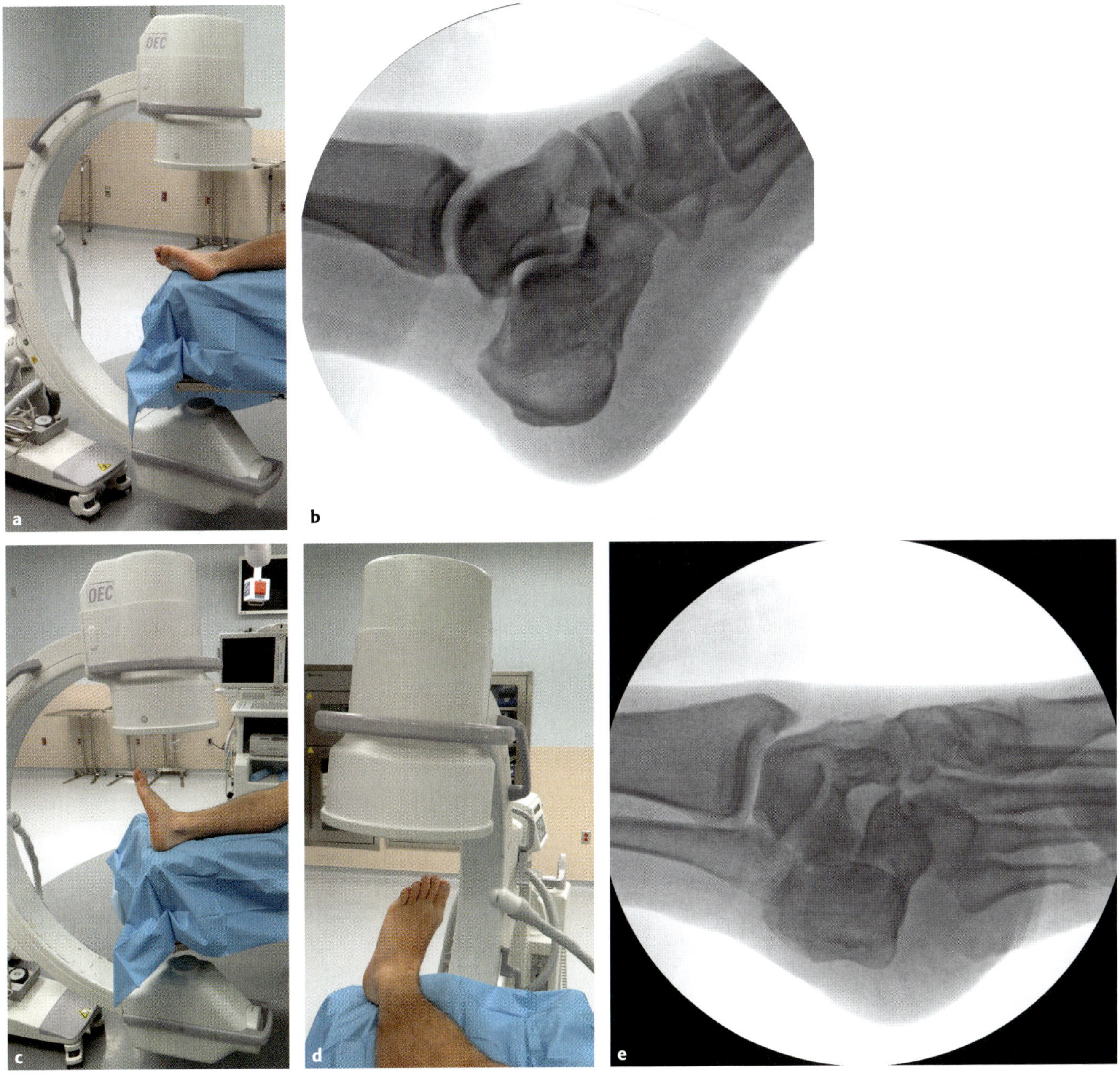

Fig 4-11a–j Obtaining the necessary images throughout the case is accomplished as shown.

a–b Lateral x-ray position and image: the C-arm shoots straight down at the lateral aspect of the foot. Care is taken during patient positioning to make sure the patient is truly lateral in position.

c–e Brodén view x-ray position and image: this image is achieved by extending the knee and necessary rotation is introduced by controlling the degree of rotation of the leg. Alternatively, the C-arm may be canted to achieve the necessary views.

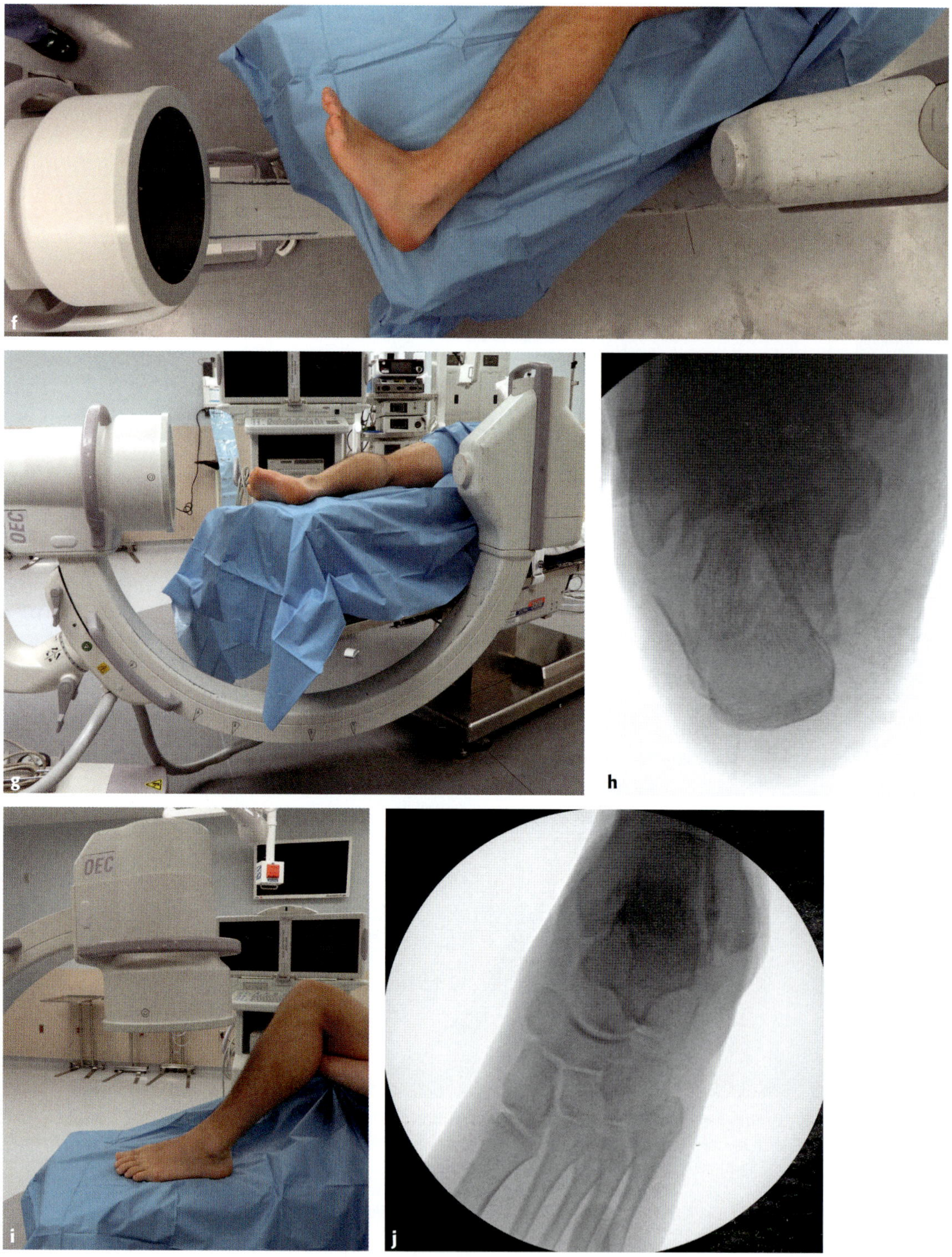

Fig 4-11a–j (cont) Obtaining the necessary images throughout the case is accomplished as shown.

f–h Harris view x-ray position and image: the knee is bent, and the ankle is dorsiflexed. The C-arm is rotated to a lateral position.

i–j AP hindfoot x-ray position: the hip is externally rotated, and the plantar surface of the foot placed on the table by flexing the knee. The C-arm shoots straight down at the foot.

Surgical approaches

Lateral extensile approach

Fractures with significant displacement and multiple intraarticular fracture lines can be treated with the lateral extensile approach. This approach allows for full visualization of the anterior process, lateral wall, and posterior facet. Surgery should be delayed until the soft-tissue swelling has resolved. Careful soft-tissue handling and closure techniques are necessary to reduce the risk of wound-healing complications. Soft-tissue flaps should be full thickness. Appropriate placement is essential as this approach is between two angiosomes. Apical wound necrosis, infection, and stiffness may occur even if meticulous surgical techniques are followed but are less likely to occur with an experienced surgeon.

See chapter 4.7 for further details on treatment of calcaneal fractures using a lateral extensile approach.

Sinus tarsi approach

This is a small lateral approach at the level of the angle of Gissane. The peroneal tendons are mobilized and retracted plantar. This approach is gaining popularity due to lower reported wound complications. This approach allows for direct visualization and reduction of the articular surface. The extraarticular components are reduced percutaneously. Fixation may be achieved using screws, a plate slid in thorough the incision, or a locking nail. Independent screws are often used to supplement fixation. This approach is associated with reduced soft-tissue complication rates while still allowing for direct articular reduction.

See chapter 4.5 for further details on treatment of calcaneal fractures using a sinus tarsi approach.

Percutaneous approach

Extraarticular and simple articular patterns may be amenable to reduction and screw insertion with small incisions. Soft-tissue complications are lowest with these techniques. More complex fractures are at increased risk of malreduction using percutaneous techniques. An arthroscope may be used at the surgeon's discretion to evaluate the articular reduction.

See chapter 4.4 for further details on treatment of calcaneal fractures using small incision or percutaneous approaches.

Dislocation approach

This approach is beneficial for calcaneal fractures, where the calcaneus dislocates laterally and abuts the distal end of the fibula. The incision runs from the fibula and follows along the lateral side of the calcaneus just above the peroneal tendons. This incision allows reduction of the lateral articular fragment from below the fibula, fixation of the fracture and repair of the peroneal tendon subluxation often seen with this fracture dislocation pattern.

See chapter 4.7 for further details on treatment of calcaneal fracture dislocations using a dislocation approach.

Sustentaculum approach

This incision is typically 3 cm in length directly over the palpable sustentaculum. It is most frequently used for isolated sustentaculum fractures but on a rare occasion may be needed in combination with a lateral approach in more complex fracture patterns. The posterior tibialis and flexor digitorum are retracted superiorly allowing access to the medial wall of the calcaneus and direct reduction of the medial facet.

See chapter 4.3 for further details on treatment of sustentaculum calcaneal fractures using this approach.

7 Postoperative care

The patient is instructed to elevate the extremity to prevent wound complications associated with postoperative swelling. Range of motion is encouraged as soon as the wound is stable to improve subtalar motion. A better functional outcome and gait are associated with improved range of motion.

Sutures are removed when the wound is healed. X-rays are taken periodically to assess for union. Weight bearing is allowed once the fracture is healed.

8 Complications and outcomes

Complications

Surgical treatment of calcaneal fractures is technically difficult. There is a significant learning curve and improved results occur with surgeon experience. Clinical series including low-volume surgeons have higher complication rates than those reported in series by higher-volume surgeons.

Fractures treated at institutions with low fracture volume have increased complications and less favorable outcomes.

Complications of operative treatment include apical wound necrosis and other wound-healing complications, infection, failure to reduce the fracture appropriately, and potential need for hardware removal. Wound complications are higher with lateral extensile approaches. Sinus tarsi and percutaneous approaches are associated with lower wound complications but may not allow adequate reduction in more complex fracture patterns.

Outcomes

Worse outcomes are associated with severe fracture patterns, open and bilateral injuries, workers compensation, and failure to restore Böhler angle. Two randomized controlled trials (Agren 2013, Buckley 2002) reported residual articular step-off of the subtalar joint in 22–40% of the operatively treated fractures. Operative treatment coupled with malreduction combines the potential of complications of surgical treatment with those related to malreduction including decreased function and development of arthritis.

Improved outcomes are seen in operative cases where the Böhler angle is recreated, and the articular surface reduction is within 2 mm.

Sanders et al reported a long-term follow up (10–20 years) where 29% of patients required an arthrodesis procedure after surgical fixation. Arthrodesis ultimately was necessary in 47% of Sanders 3 fractures compared with 19% of Sanders 2 fractures. If arthrodesis is not necessary, functional results with mild pain, minimal alterations in activities of daily living or work, and essentially normal shoe wear can be expected from a properly performed open reduction and internal fixation.

Rammelt, in his recent long-term evaluation of a large series of operatively treated fractures found factors leading to improved function to include the absence of workers compensation, percutaneous fixation in less severe fractures, restoration of Böhler angle to within 5° of the unaffected side, and lower fracture severity as reflected in the Zwipp classification. Patients with better subtalar and ankle range of motion had less gait disturbance with dynamic pedobarography and improved functional scores.

Recommended reading

Agren PH, Mukka S, Tullberg T, et al. Factors affecting long-term treatment results of displaced intraarticular calcaneal fractures: a post hoc analysis of a prospective, randomized, controlled multicenter trial. *J Orthop Trauma.* 2014 Oct;28(10):564–568.

Agren PH, Wretenberg P, Sayed-Noor AS. Operative versus nonoperative treatment of displaced intraarticular calcaneal fractures: a prospective, randomized, controlled multicenter trial. *J Bone Joint Surg Am.* 2013 Aug 7;95(15):1351–1357.

Buckley R, Tough S, McCormack R, et al. Operative compared with nonoperative treatment of displaced intraarticular calcaneal fractures: a prospective, randomized, controlled multicenter trial. *J Bone Joint Surg Am.* 2002 Oct;84-a(10):1733–1744.

Crosby LA, Fitzgibbons T. Intraarticular calcaneal fractures. Results of closed treatment. *Clin Orthop Relat Res.* 1993 May(290):47–54.

Dürr C, Apinun J, Mittlmeier T, et al. Foot function after surgically treated intraarticular calcaneal fractures: correlation of clinical and pedobarographic results of 65 patients followed for 8 years. *J Orthop Trauma.* 2018 Dec;32(12):593–600.

Essex-Lopresti P. The mechanism, reduction technique, and results in fractures of the os calcis, 1951-52. *Br J Surg.* 1952 Mar;39(157):395–419.

Gardner MJ, Nork SE, Barei DP, et al. Secondary soft tissue compromise in tongue-type calcaneus fractures. *J Orthop Trauma.* 2008 Aug;22(7):439–445.

Griffin D, Parsons N, Shaw E, et al. Operative versus non-operative treatment for closed, displaced, intra-articular fractures of the calcaneus: randomised controlled trial. *Bmj.* 2014 Jul 24;349:g4483.

Poeze M, Verbruggen JP, Brink PR. The relationship between the outcome of operatively treated calcaneal fractures and institutional fracture load. A systematic review of the literature. *J Bone Joint Surg Am.* 2008 May;90(5):1013–1021.

Rammelt S, Zwipp H, Schneiders W, et al. Severity of injury predicts subsequent function in surgically treated displaced intraarticular calcaneal fractures. *Clin Orthop Relat Res.* 2013 Sep;471(9):2885–2898.

Sanders R, Fortin P, DiPasquale T, et al. Operative treatment in 120 displaced intraarticular calcaneal fractures. Results using a prognostic computed tomography scan classification. *Clin Orthop Relat Res.* 1993 May(290):87–95.

Sanders R, Vaupel ZM, Erdogan M, et al. Operative treatment of displaced intraarticular calcaneal fractures: long-term (10–20 Years) results in 108 fractures using a prognostic CT classification. *J Orthop Trauma.* 2014 Oct;28(10):551–563.

Sharr PJ, Mangupli MM, Winson IG, et al. Current management options for displaced intra-articular calcaneal fractures: non-operative, ORIF, minimally invasive reduction and fixation or primary ORIF and subtalar arthrodesis. A contemporary review. *Foot Ankle Surg.* 2016 Mar;22(1):1–8.

Thordarson DB, Krieger LE. Operative vs nonoperative treatment of intra-articular fractures of the calcaneus: a prospective randomized trial. *Foot Ankle Int.* 1996 Jan;17(1):2–9.

Zwipp H, Tscherne H, Thermann H, et al. Osteosynthesis of displaced intraarticular fractures of the calcaneus. Results in 123 cases. *Clin Orthop Relat Res.* 1993 May(290):76–86.

4.1 Extraarticular fracture (beak)

Michael Swords, Candice Brady

1 Case description

A 78-year-old woman was walking out her front door to get the mail. She tripped over the doorway and had immediate onset of pain in her left foot and inability to ambulate. The injury was closed. Comorbidities included only osteoporosis. The patient was independent in all activities of daily living and was otherwise healthy.

X-rays revealed an extraarticular posterior tuberosity avulsion or "beak" fracture AO/OTA 82A1 (**Fig 4.1-1**).

2 Preoperative planning

Indications for surgery

Prompt identification of the injury and the need for early surgical fixation are necessary for a successful recovery.

Surgical indications include a marked displacement of the tuber and loss of function of the Achilles with plantarflexion weakness. Additionally, surgical fixation is indicated to prevent soft-tissue breakdown posteriorly. Displacement of the fracture fragment may cause posterior soft-tissue breakdown as a result of pressure-related ischemia and necrosis. The patient should be counseled as to the high risk of complications from this injury, including soft-tissue breakdown, failure of fixation, and pain with shoe wear.

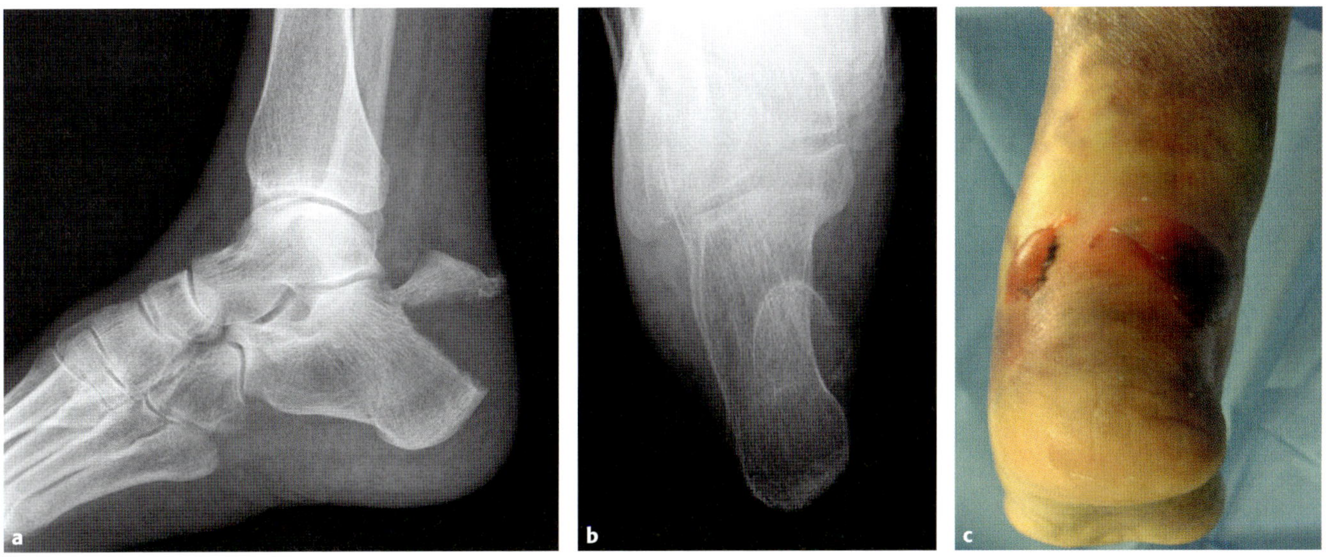

Fig 4.1-1a–c Preoperative images.
a–b Lateral (**a**) and axial (**b**) x-rays demonstrating an avulsion (beak) fracture with marked displacement.
c The displaced fragment causes injury to the posterior soft tissues and must be addressed in a timely manner to avoid pressure necrosis from developing.

Considerations for surgery

Surgical approaches include a direct posterior approach or use of the vertical limb of the lateral extensile approach. In open injuries the wound is typically transverse and treatment through the traumatic wound is required, with vertical and distal extension at the corners if needed.

Reduction is critical in restoring the anatomy and function of the hindfoot. The fractured tuberosity must be brought back down to the rest of the tuber to repair the plantar flexion mechanism of the foot. The tuber reduction must also be correct in rotation, as rotational malalignment will interfere with the heel contour of shoes, causing irritation. Occasionally, this fracture fragment will extend into the posterior facet but most commonly it is an extraarticular injury.

Procedures such as a tendo-Achilles lengthening or gastrocnemius recession may be necessary at the time of surgery. The contralateral limb should be evaluated for the presence of equinus contracture. If present, it may be assumed that the injured limb also has a contracture. Procedures may be necessary to treat preexisting equinus or alternatively help with contracture, which may have developed from the time of injury. Generally, the greater the displacement, the more likely the patient has concomitant equinus.

Surgical intervention for extraarticular beak fractures is difficult. This fracture pattern is most commonly seen in patients who may have altered bone density, diabetes, and neuropathy. If any of these risk factors are present, they must be considered during planning. Numerous techniques exist and share the goal of restoration of normal anatomy as well as counteracting the deforming forces. There is no single ideal way to provide stability to this injury pattern and all are at risk of failure.

The soft tissues posteriorly are often traumatized and usually not amenable to incisions. The vertical limb of the lateral extensile approach allows the incision to be placed in better soft tissues and works well for this injury.

3 Operating room setup

Patient positioning	• Lateral decubitus on a radiolucent table (injured side up)
Anesthesia options	• General or spinal anesthesia • Complete muscle relaxant is necessary to decrease the deforming force of the gastrocnemius soleus complex.
C-arm location	• Monitor placed on the opposite side of the operative table with the C-arm entering at an oblique angle from the foot of the bed.
Tourniquet	• Used at surgeon's discretion • Generally, improves visualization of anatomy
Tips	• Avoid positioning the patient with the knee extended. • Having the knee bent with the operative foot closest to the surgeon relaxes the gastrocnemius and may be beneficial at the time of reduction.

For illustrations and overview of anesthetic considerations, see chapter 1. For illustrations and overview of patient and C-arm positioning for calcaneal fracture treatment in the lateral decubitus position refer to chapter 3.

Equipment

- Point-to-point reduction (Weber) clamps
- K-wires
- Small locking plates
- Screws for lag screw placement (may be small or large fragment)
- Suture for augmentation if necessary
- C-arm
- Plaster for postoperative splinting

4 Surgical procedure

The contralateral limb should be thoroughly examined for any preexisting equinus. If present, it will be necessary to address the equinus to aid in reduction. This can be assessed by performing the Silfverskjöld test, which is used to determine if contracture is present in the Achilles or in the gastrocnemius. This test should be performed on the contralateral limb.

The fracture is approached using a small vertical incision on the lateral side of the foot. The incision is essentially the vertical limb of a standard extensile lateral approach (**Fig 4.1-2a**). After the incision is made, all fracture hematoma is removed using suction and careful use of a curette. Be careful when manipulating the fracture fragments, as these fractures occur in the soft cancellous bone of the calcaneal body. Bone loss, resulting in the loss of the ability to obtain an accurate fracture reduction read, is a risk if aggressive curettage is performed. When all hematoma is removed, a point-to-point reduction (Weber) clamp is placed over the superior ridge of the calcaneus. If the fragment is large, a small incision can be made posterior and a Schanz pin can be placed axially to act as a joystick in the fragment. Reduction is achieved by plantar flexion at the ankle while carefully closing the reduction clamp and manipulating the Schanz pin (**Fig 4.1-2b**). Assessment of reduction should be made at both the anterior and posterior aspects of the fracture to avoid rotational malalignment. The fracture is then held provisionally with multiple K-wires and additional reduction clamps, as necessary.

If using a small locking plate, place it onto the lateral aspect of the calcaneus. Drill sleeves and K-wires are placed through the plate into the proximal fragment. If using non-variable angle locking (VAL) plates, the K-wires must be placed through the plate before insertion of independent lag screws, as placement of lag screws may first block the trajectory needed for the locking screws in the proximal fragment. Lag screws are then inserted from the superior ridge of the calcaneus, making sure the length is appropriate to penetrate the plantar cortex (**Fig 4.1-2c**). If the fragment is large, additional screws may be directed from posterior into the anterior process. Locking screws are then inserted into the proximal limb of the plate (**Fig 4.1-2d**).

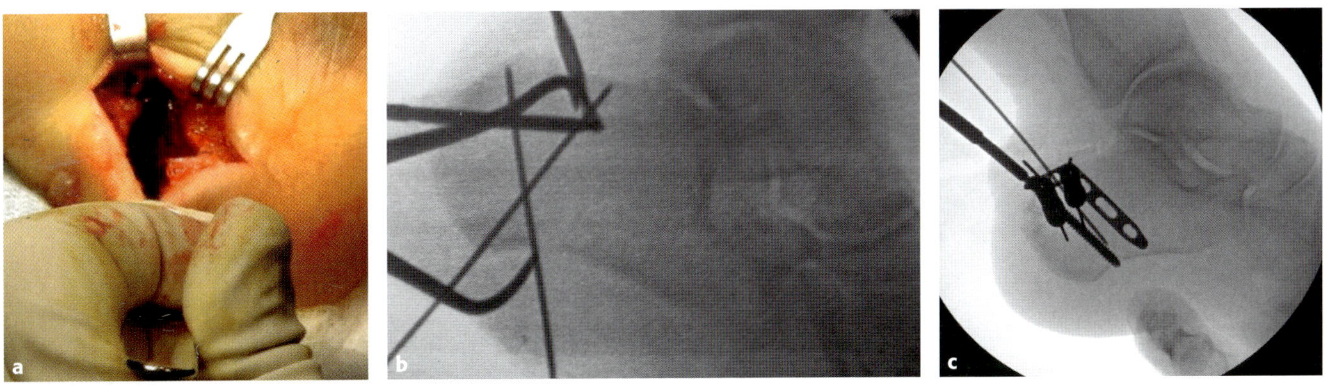

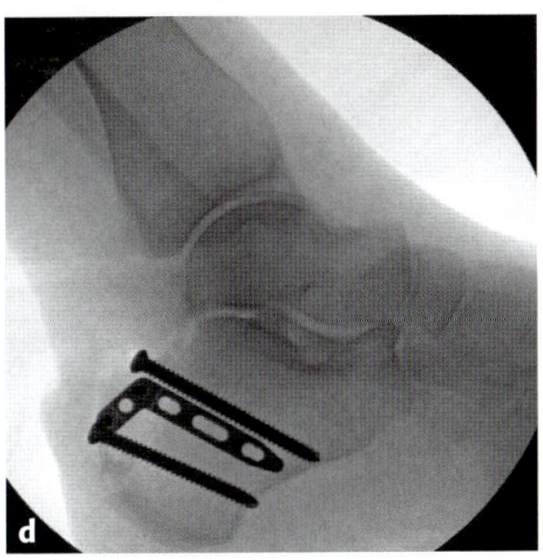

Fig 4.1-2a–g Surgical fixation with a locking plate and lag screws.
- **a** The fracture is approached using a small vertical incision on the lateral side of the foot. This falls in line with the vertical limb of a standard extensile lateral approach.
- **b** The fracture is reduced by inserting a Schanz screw into the fracture fragment and rotating this down while maximally plantar-flexing the foot to bring it up to the avulsed segment. Once reduced, a pointed reduction clamp and multiple K-wires are used to provide provisional fixation.
- **c** A small plate is inserted and slid under the soft tissues of lateral side of the hindfoot. Two wires are placed through the plate into the fracture fragment. The fragment is then compressed by inserting two lag screws through the avulsed fragment to the plantar cortex.
- **d** The proximal end of the plate is secured using two locking screws.

The plate is compressed either by using an external compression device or by standard compression plating techniques. A small incision is made using x-ray guidance to place the incision directly over the distal end of the plate. A standard screw is then inserted using compression plating techniques through the second to last screw hole. (**Fig 4.1-2e**). The last step is locking the most plantar and distal hole in the plate (**Fig 4.1-2f**). Finally, all provisional fixation is removed. The wound is closed (**Fig 4.1-2g**) and the ankle is splinted in slight plantar flexion to avoid pull of the gastrocnemius soleus complex.

5 Pitfalls and complications

Pitfalls

Failure to appropriately obtain and maintain reduction

The foot should be reduced to the displaced fragment as opposed to trying to pull the fragment down to the foot. Maximum plantar flexion may be necessary until fixation is complete.

The tuberosity fragment may be of poor bone density or comminuted. Often clamps or other reduction aids will further damage the displaced segment. Sutures can be placed in the distal portion of the Achilles tendon and used to aid in reduction by pulling the sutures distal, decreasing the pull on the displaced fragment.

Tendo-Achilles lengthening and/or gastrocnemius lengthening are often necessary at the time of fixation and should be part of the anticipated surgical plan.

Catastrophic loss of posterior soft tissues

Delay in surgical treatment may result in catastrophic loss of the posterior soft tissues including the Achilles attachment. These injuries must be recognized and treated with urgency. If surgery must be delayed, the foot should be splinted in plantar flexion.

Loss of bony insertion

If the fractured portion with the Achilles is small, or the bone density is excessively poor, sutures can be placed in the Achilles tendon to help reduce the fracture fragment by pulling the Achilles distally, reducing the risk of creating comminution of the fracture fragment. The sutures can be removed after use, or alternatively, placed through a transverse drill hole in the calcaneus to provide a secondary means of fixation. On rare occasions, small fragments may be removed, and the Achilles reattached to the calcaneus with suture anchors or pull-through sutures.

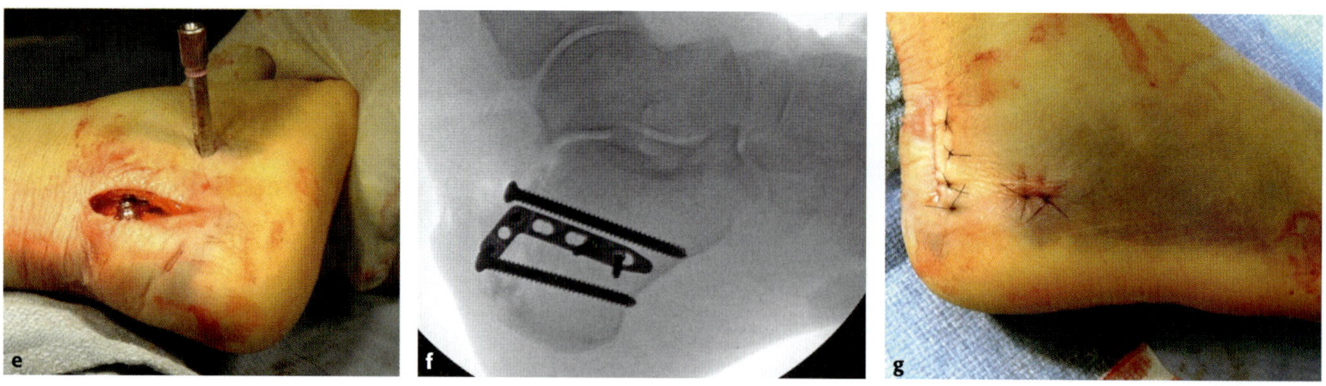

Fig 4.1-2a–g (cont) Surgical fixation with a locking plate and lag screws.
e A small incision is made with x-ray guidance.
f A standard screw is inserted using compression plating techniques through the second to last screw hole. The final locking screw is inserted in the most plantar and distal hole in the plate to complete the construct.
g Final wound closure.

Complications

Soft-tissue breakdown

Soft-tissue problems are present in most of these fractures. They range from bruising and blistering of the posterior skin to full thickness necrosis. Unlike many calcaneal fractures, this fracture pattern requires prompt attention. Surgery should be performed early to restore the normal bony morphology of the posterior aspect of the calcaneus to prevent soft-tissue breakdown. If splinting is necessary, the splint should be applied with the ankle in maximal plantar flexion to attempt to bring the foot up to the displaced fragment. Carefully advise the patient to avoid placing direct pressure on the posterior soft tissues of the heel. Pillows used to elevate the foot should be placed behind the calf to avoid pressure on the posterior aspect of the calcaneus (**Fig 4.1-3**).

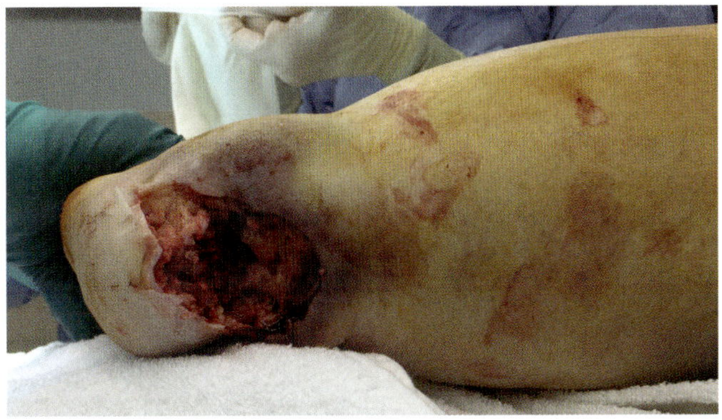

Fig 4.1-3 Example from a different case showing soft-tissue breakdown. The patient presented belatedly after inadequate initial treatment. Necrosis of the posterior soft tissues occurred. A large soft-tissue defect was present after debridement of non-viable tissue. The patient required a below-knee amputation.

Failure of fixation

This fracture pattern occurs most commonly in individuals with decreased bone density, diabetes, and neuropathy either individually or in some combination. Fixation is at risk in all patients. Equinus may be a preexisting factor and may need to be addressed at the time of fixation with gastrocnemious release (**Fig 4.1-4**).

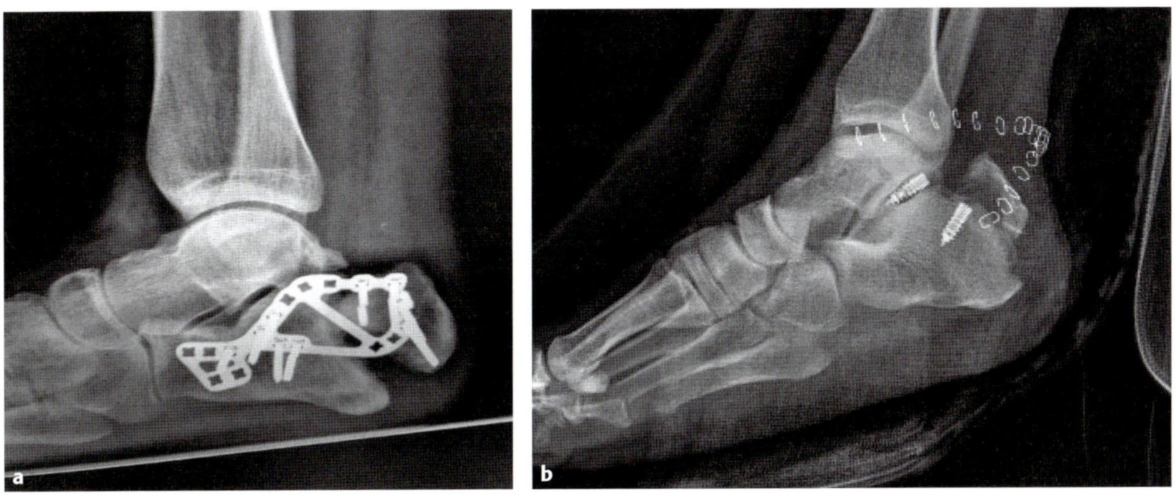

Fig 4.1-4a–b Example from a different case showing failure of fixation.

- **a** Failed fixation of a fracture treated with a lateral plate. Screws in the posterior superior portion of the plate have failed and there is loss of reduction.
- **b** Failed of fixation of a fracture with attempted fixation with suture anchors.

Malunion

Partial failure of hardware leads to displacement but not complete failure of fixation. This may lead to malunion of the tuber fragment but not failure of open reduction and internal fixation (**Fig 4.1-5**).

6 Alternative techniques

There is no consensus on the most successful fixation construct for these injuries. Treatment options include screws, locking plates, suture anchors, suturing through the distal Achilles and then through drill holes, lateral plates, posterior plates, and lateral extensile plates. All are options, but none are immune to failure (**Fig 4.1-6**).

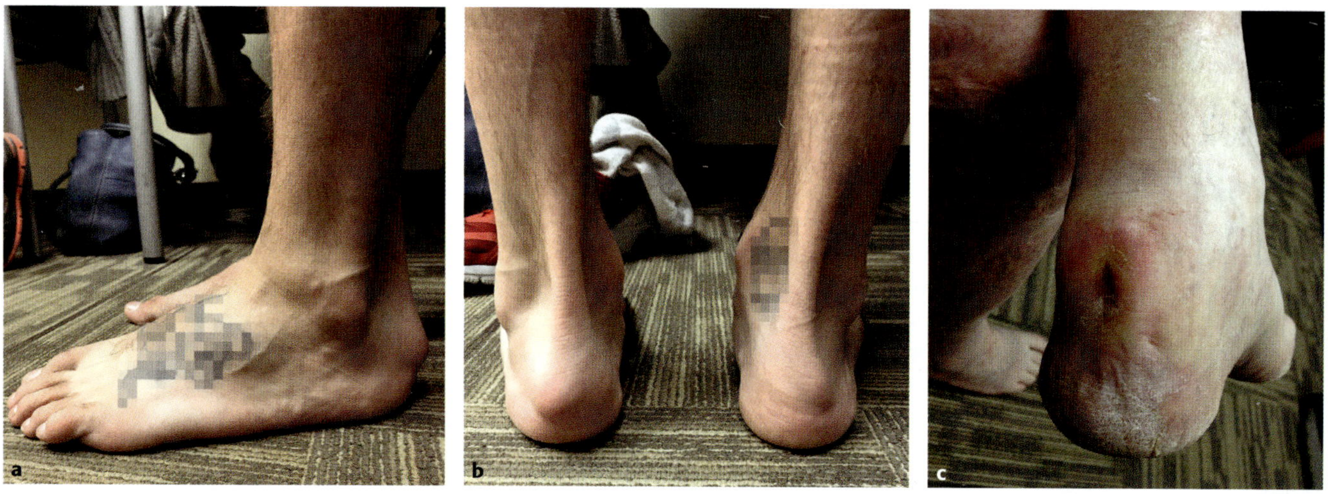

Fig 4.1-5a–c Example from a different case showing malunion of the posterior calcaneus.
a–b Malunion results in an abnormal shape to the contours of the hindfoot and will commonly interfere with shoe wear.
c A patient with a malunited avulsion fracture experiences chronic wound problems with shoe wear due to the underlying bony prominence.

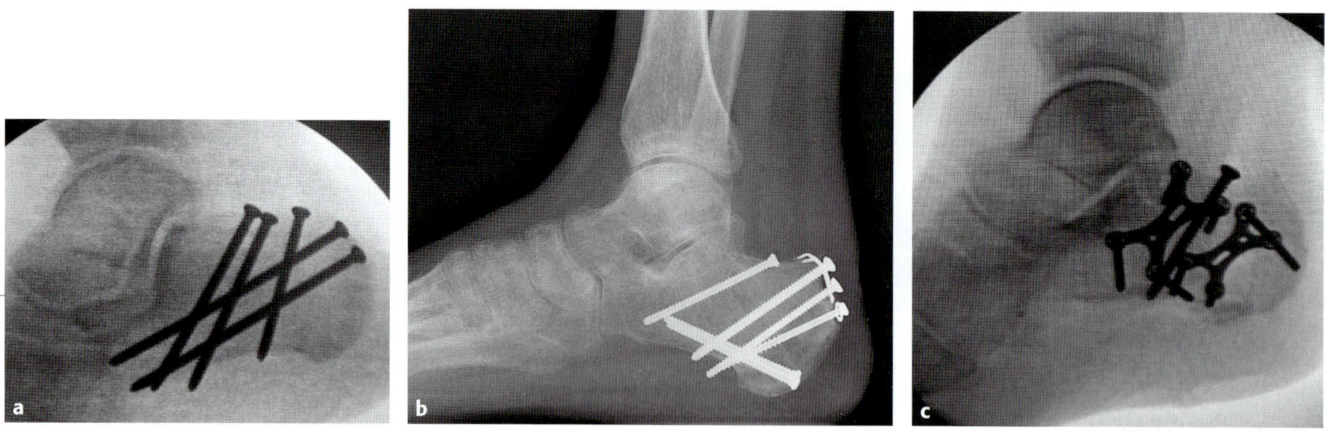

Fig 4.1-6a–c Example from a different cases showing alternative fixation options: fixation by screws only (**a**), screws and a posterior plate (**b**), and alternative combinations of locking plates and lag screws (**c**).

7 Postoperative management and rehabilitation

The patient is advised not to place pillows directly under the posterior aspect of the heel when elevating the limb, as doing so can further damage the traumatized tissues. Patients should be carefully informed and reminded that rehabilitation activities must be progressed slowly. Most patients with this fracture have decreased bone density and are at risk of fixation failure. Additionally, many have altered sensation and pain may not deter the patient from increasing activities and will not be a reliable indicator of complications developing.

The patient should be splinted in some degree of equinus to decrease tension on the fixation construct. The amount of equinus is dependent on stability of the construct and the quality of the bone. The patient is seen at 2 weeks postoperatively for suture removal and then advanced to a neutral position. In extreme cases, a heel wedge may be used and gradually diminished over time.

Range of motion of the ankle and subtalar joint typically are initiated 6–8 weeks postoperatively. The patient will maintain nonweight bearing until x-rays show union.

Implant removal

Implants are only removed if they cause irritation over time. This most often occurs with shoe wear. Patients with this fracture pattern often have sensitivity to the posterior aspect of the calcaneus with shoe wear. With appropriate reduction and implant placement the hardware is typically asymptomatic and patients with this fracture return to normal footwear (**Fig 4.1-7**).

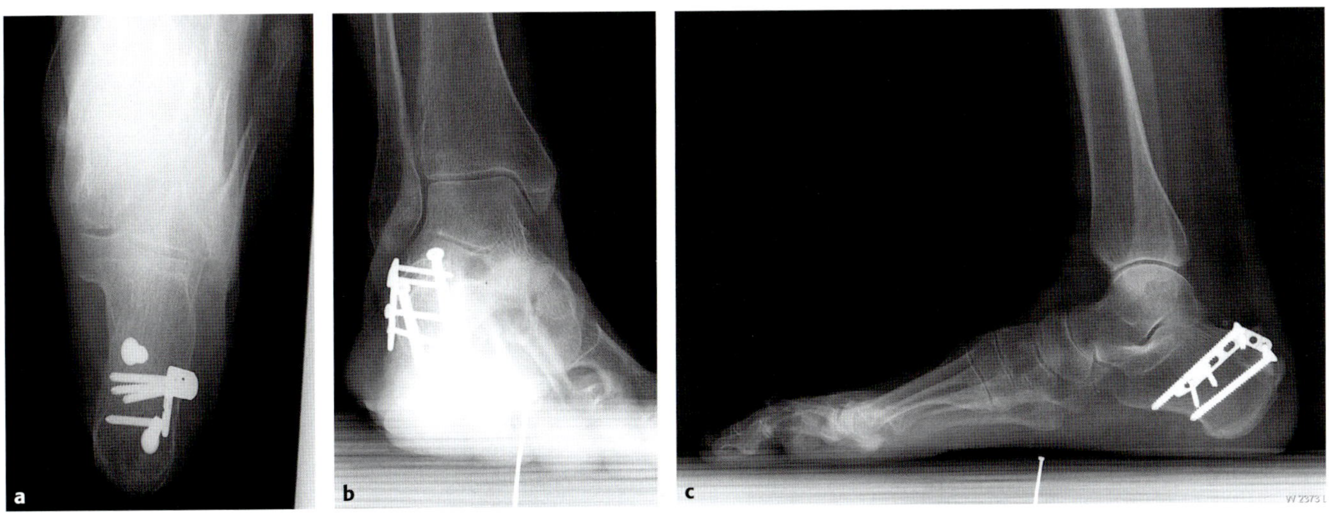

Fig 4.1-7a–c Final x-rays taken 3 years after injury demonstrate a well-aligned and healed fracture. The patient is asymptomatic and wears normal footwear.

8 Recommended reading

Beavis RC, Rourke K, Court-Brown C. Avulsion fracture of the calcaneal tuberosity: a case report and literature review. *Foot Ankle Int.* 2008 Aug;29(8):863–866.

Lee SM, Huh SW, Chung JW, et al. Avulsion fracture of the calcaneal tuberosity: classification and its characteristics. *Clin Orthop Surg.* 2012 Jun;4(2):134–138.

Swords MP, Penny P. Early fixation of calcaneus fractures. *Foot Ankle Clin.* 2017 Mar;22(1):93–104.

Foot Calcaneus

Section 1 Peripheral fractures

4.1 Extraarticular fracture (beak)

4.2 Medial tuberosity fracture

Stefan Rammelt

1 Case description

A 58-year-old construction worker fell from a scaffold and landed on his left heel. He immediately felt a dull pain over the heel and was unable to bear weight on the left foot. He was brought to the hospital by emergency services.

On physical examination, swelling was noted at the left hindfoot. No hematoma was seen. The heel was tender on palpation with the maximum pain at the plantar medial aspect, close to the insertion of the plantar aponeurosis into the calcaneus. No neurovascular deficits were noted. Lateral and axial x-rays of the left calcaneus were obtained (**Fig 4.2-1**).

A calcaneal fracture was diagnosed; consequently, a computed tomographic (CT) scan was performed (**Fig 4.2-2**) that confirmed an extraarticular, displaced fracture of the medial process of the calcaneal tuberosity with two main fragments. No extension of the fracture into the subtalar or calcaneocuboid joint was detected. The AO/OTA fracture classification is 82A1.

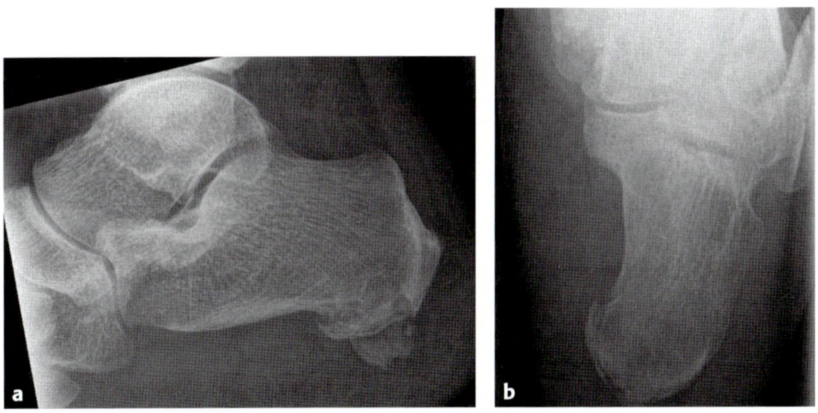

Fig 4.2-1a–b X-rays of the left calcaneus revealing a fracture of the medial process of the calcaneal tuberosity. The fragment is tilted and displaced in a plantar direction.
- **a** Lateral view.
- **b** Axial view.

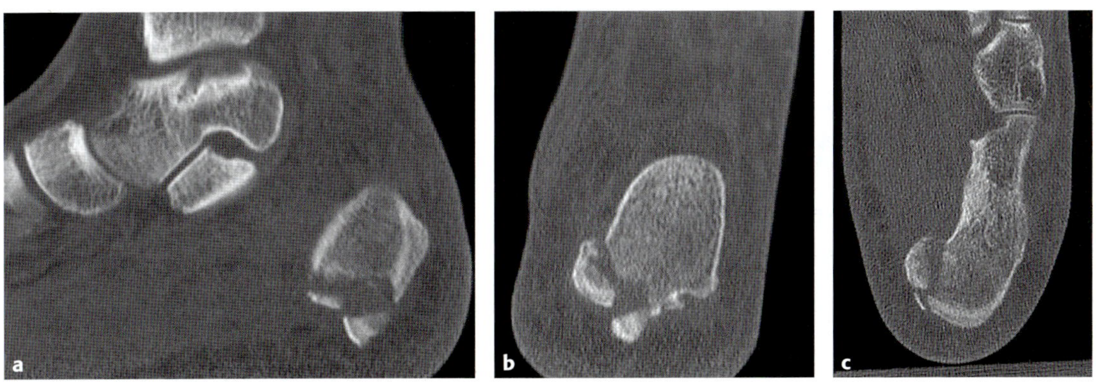

Fig 4.2-2a–c The CT scan showing a purely extraarticular, displaced fracture of the medial calcaneal tuberosity consisting of two main fragments.
- **a** Sagittal view.
- **b** Coronal view.
- **c** Axial view.

2 Preoperative planning

Indications for surgery

Extraarticular calcaneal fractures require surgery if there is a marked deformity in the heel that may result in mechanical axis deviation at the hindfoot or local soft-tissue compromise resulting in interference with shoe wear from displaced fragments.

Fractures of the medial process of the calcaneal tuberosity are uncommon. They possibly reflect a bony avulsion of the plantar aponeurosis. Alternatively, they may be produced by direct plantar impact (as in the case presented) or be part of a more complex injury. They must be differentiated from the rare presence of an accessory bone below the calcaneal tuberosity (os subcalcis). The latter has no trauma history, lies centrally below the tuberosity, and is oval without any bony connection to the calcaneus. The cortex surrounding such an ossicle is smooth and regular.

For the patient in the case presented here, indication for surgery was the presence of plantar displaced fragments. If malunion occurs, these fragments may produce local pressure on the highly specialized plantar skin of the heel resulting in painful callosities or even ulcerations. Owing to the large size of the two fragments, fixation with two screws was planned (**Fig 4.2-3**).

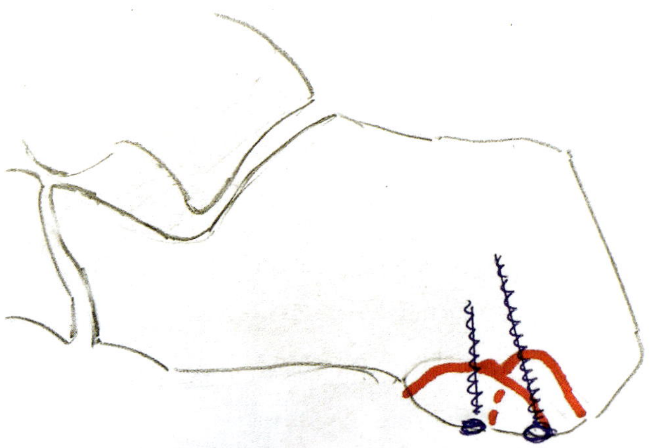

Fig 4.2-3 Preoperative plan. The two fragments are reduced and fixed with one screw each. The fragments partially overlap in both the sagittal and coronal plane (see **Fig 4.2-1** and **Fig 4.2-2**).

3 Operating room setup

Patient positioning	• Supine on a radiolucent table with the foot draped free
Anesthesia options	• General or regional
C-arm location	• Opposite side of the operative table, so the surgeon has a free view while performing reduction
Tourniquet	• Optional
Tips	• Foot is placed on a bump and slightly rotated externally, a position the limb assumes spontaneously on the operative table

For illustrations and overview of anesthetic considerations, see chapter 1.

Equipment

- Point-to-point reduction (Weber) clamps
- 2.7 mm (3.5 mm) cortex screws and drill bit
- K-wires (for provisional fixation)

Size of system, instruments, and implants may vary according to anatomy.

4 Surgical procedure

The medial process of the calcaneal tuberosity is accessed by a small medial approach (**Fig 4.2-4**). The skin incision has a length of 3–5 cm. It is placed parallel to the sole at the transition zone between the plantar and dorsal (glaborous) skin of the foot. If possible, avoid a plantar incision, as it may result in a painful scar and hyperkeratosis. Care should be taken to avoid injury to the terminal branches of the lateral plantar nerve that are running obliquely down the medial calcaneal wall. The fan-like insertion of the flexor retinaculum and the abductor hallucis muscle are gently detached from the displaced fragments of the medial tuberosity. Do not detach the plantar skin from the fragments.

The superior margin of the fracture is visualized, and the plantar fragments are reduced anatomically to the main tuberosity fragment starting with the fragment that is situated more laterally. The forefoot is held in maximal plantar flexion during reduction which eases reduction by relaxing the pull of the plantar aponeurosis. The fragments are fixed temporarily with 1.6 mm K-wires (**Fig 4.2-5a**). Definite internal fixation is achieved with screws placed from medial. The screw heads should be flush with the plantar-medial aspect of the fragments and should not protrude on the plantar aspect. Therefore, use of washers is discouraged. Anatomical reduction is ensured with intraoperative C-arm lateral and axial views (**Figs 4.2-5b–c**).

The incision is closed in layers. A suction drain is usually not required, but a compressive dressing is applied.

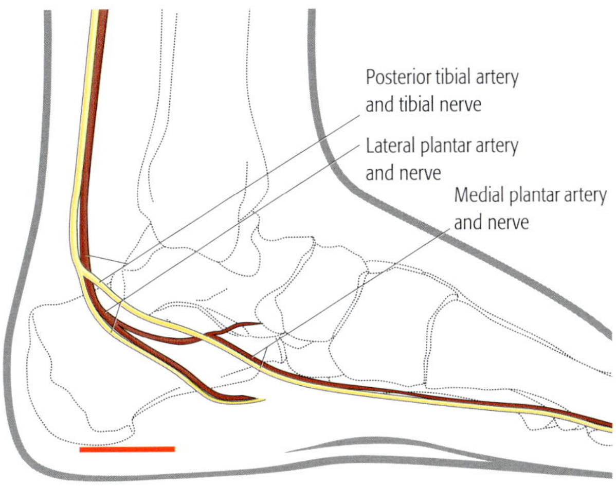

Fig 4.2-4 Medial approach to fractures of the medial process of the calcaneal tuberosity.

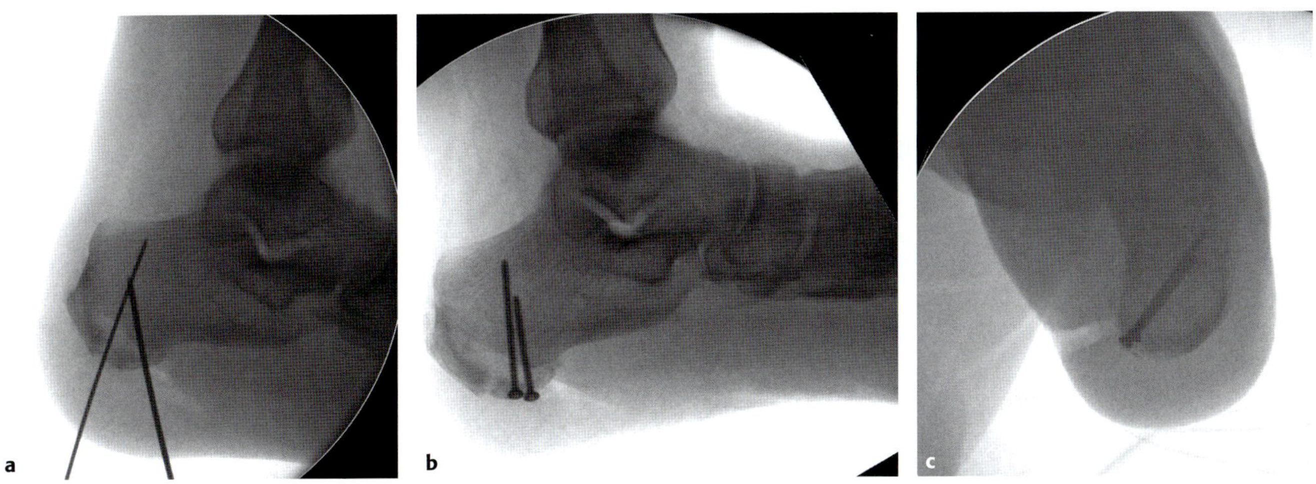

Fig 4.2-5a–c Anatomical reduction and temporary K-wire fixation of the two displaced fragments (**a**). After definite fixation with two 2.7 mm cortex screws, correct screw position and length is checked again with the standard lateral (**b**) and axial (**c**) C-arm projections.

5 Pitfalls and complications

Pitfalls

Inadequate reduction

Poor reduction is a potential complication when using a limited incision. Possible reasons include intervening ligament or bony debris, gross instability or further fragmentation of the fragment(s) while attempting reduction and fixation. In such cases, alternative fixation methods (resorbable pins, suture anchors, etc) may be used.

Nonoperative treatment of displaced fractures

Closed nonoperative treatment may lead to painful malunions with local pressure caused by fragments that are displaced plantarly or far medially. Malunion results in problems with shoe wear, painful callosities, or ulcerations.

Complications

- Injury to the terminal branches of the medial plantar nerve
- Injury to the plantar skin
- Loss of reduction/fixation
- Malunion
- Nonunion
- Hypertrophic scarring, keratosis

6 Alternative techniques

For smaller, displaced fragments or in case of further fragmentation upon reduction, alternative fixation methods include resorbable pins, suture anchors, and transosseous sutures. Small and brittle fragments, not amenable to fixation, may be resected. Open fractures extending into the calcaneal body may be treated with plate fixation. The position and size of the plate must be tailored to the individual fracture pathoanatomy. Displaced fragments interfering with reduction are removed.

Nonoperative treatment with partial weight bearing (WB) for 6 weeks and early range-of-motion (ROM) exercises is adequate for nondisplaced or minimally displaced fractures (**Fig 4.2-6**).

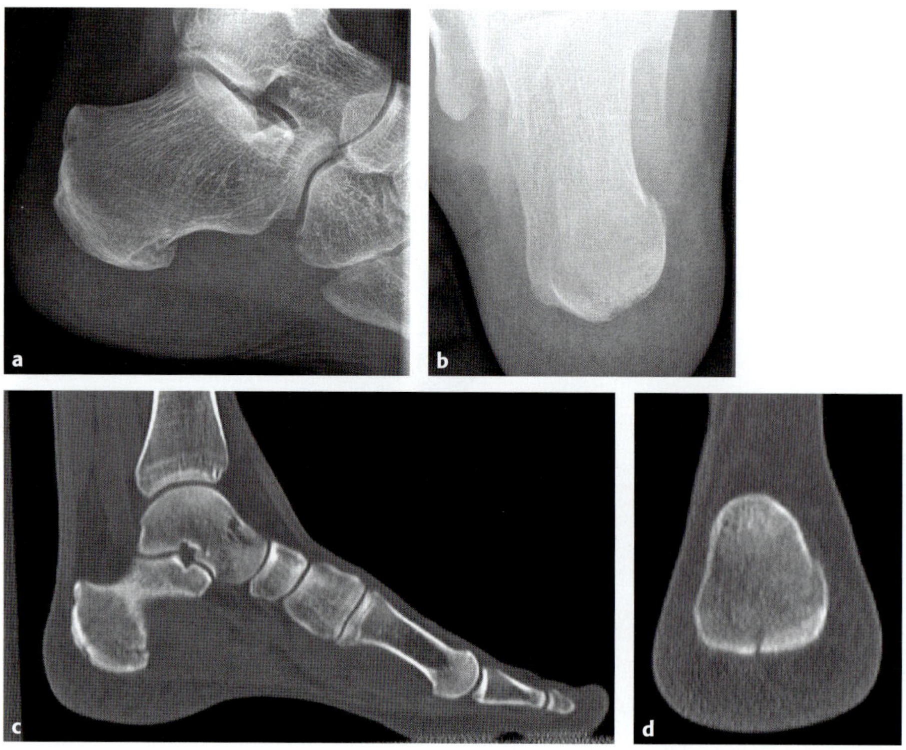

Fig 4.2-6a–d Example from a dfferent case of a minimally displaced medial tuberosity fracture treated nonoperatively with partial weight bearing (WB) and early motion. Lateral (**a**) and axial (**b**) x-rays and CT imaging (**c–d**).

7 Postoperative management and rehabilitation

Postoperatively the leg is elevated. In case of an isolated medial tuberosity fracture, no splint or cast is needed.

Active and passive ROM exercises of the ankle, subtalar, and mid-tarsal joints are initiated on postoperative day 1. The patient is mobilized in his own shoe as soon as the swelling has subsided and restricted to partial WB (up to 20 kg) on the injured leg for 6 weeks. At this point, standing lateral and axial x-rays are obtained. If images demonstrate bony union, WB is gradually increased over the next 1–2 weeks. The post-operative regimen should be adapted to the individual bone quality, comorbidities, and pattern of injury for more complex injury or multiple fractures (**Fig 4.2-7**).

Implant removal

Implant removal is indicated only when the screw heads are prominent and cause local skin irritation or problems with shoe wear.

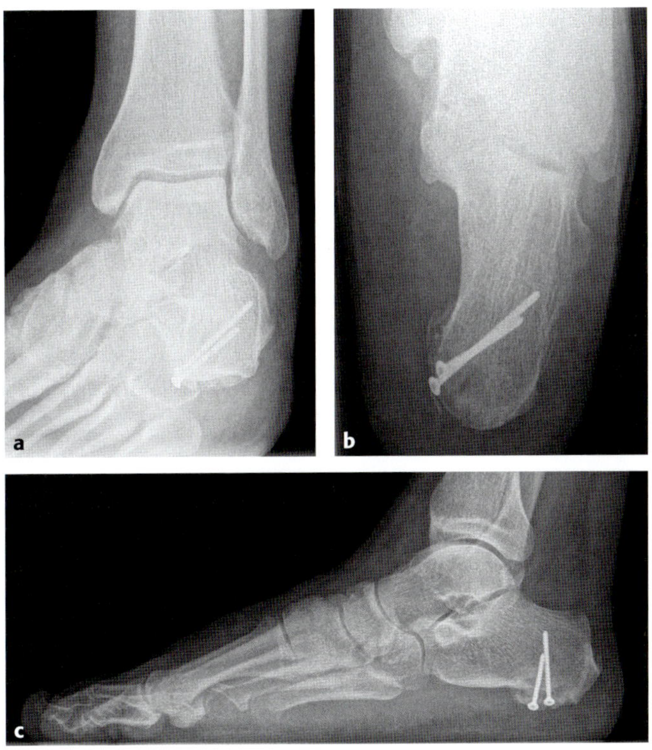

Fig 4.2-7a–c AP (**a**), axial (**b**), and standing lateral (**c**) x-rays at 6 weeks postoperatively confirming union in anatomical position.

8 Recommended reading

Li B, Wu G, Yang Y. Conservative versus surgical treatment for displaced fracture of the medial process of the calcaneal tuberosity. *J Orthop Surg (Hong Kong).* 2016 Aug;24(2):163–166.
Milliken RA. Os subcalcis. *Am J Surg.* 1937; 37:116–117.
Rammelt S, Zwipp H. Calcaneus fractures: facts, controversies and recent developments. *Injury.* 2004 May;35(5):443–461.
Sanders RW, Rammelt S. Fractures of the calcaneus. In: Coughlin MJ, Saltzman CR, Anderson JB, eds. *Mann's Surgery of the Foot & Ankle.* 9th ed. Philadelphia: Elsevier Saunders; 2013:2041–2100.
Squires B, Allen PE, Livingstone J, et al. Fractures of the tuberosity of the calcaneus. *J Bone Joint Surg Br.* 2001 Jan;83(1):55–61.
Zwipp H, Rammelt S. *Tscherne Unfallchirurgie: Fuß.* Berlin: Springer; 2014:434–435. German

4.3 Sustentacular fracture

Michael Swords

1 Case description

A 45-year-old man presented to the emergency department by ambulance after a motorcycle accident with a closed injury to his right hindfoot.

The patient initially had an obvious deformity, and was reduced and splinted by emergency personnel. He had no other associated injuries.

Foot x-rays demonstrated an irregularity of the sublatar joint suspicious for fracture (**Fig 4.3-1a–b**). The lateral process talar fracture and sustentacular fracture were well defined by a computed tomographic (CT) scan (**Fig 4.3-1c–g**).

2 Preoperative planning

Indications for surgery

- Loss of articular congruity of the medial facet, which is the superior surface of the sustentaculum tali.
- Subtalar stiffness as many of these injuries are associated with subtalar dislocations.

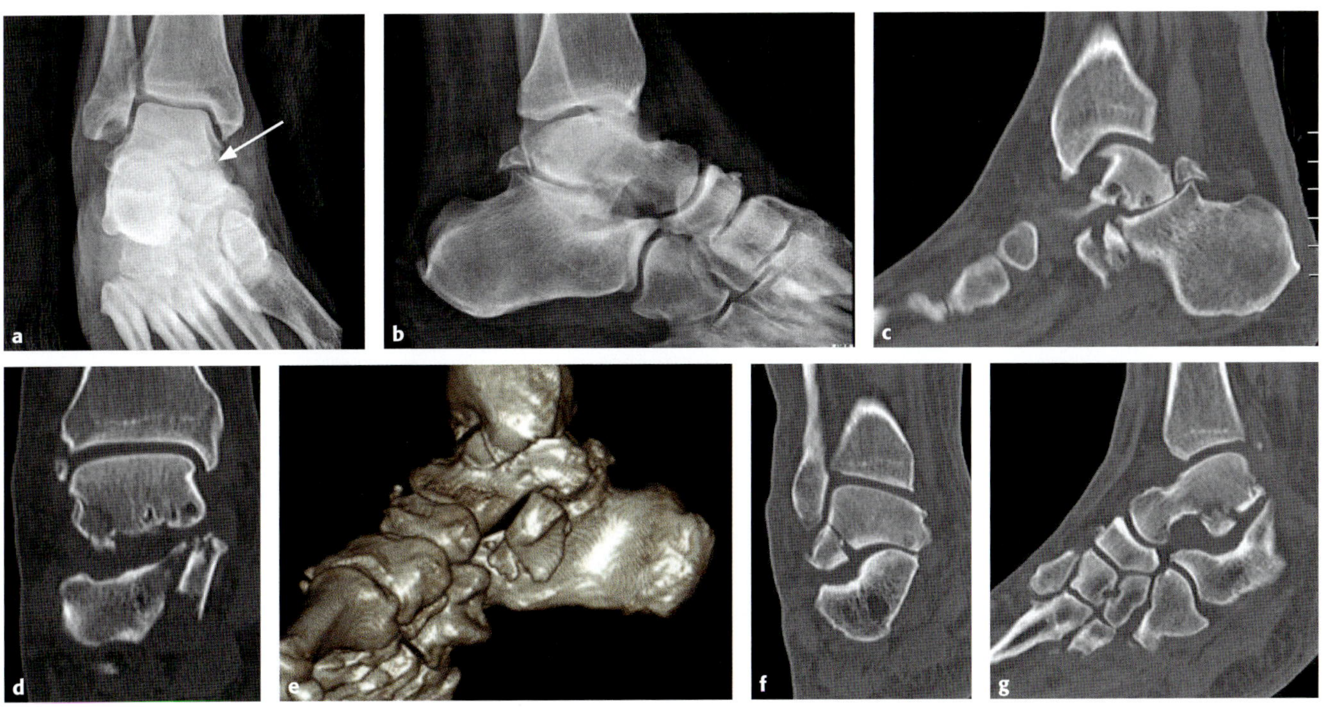

Fig 4.3-1a–g Fracture of the sustentaculum with associated lateral process fracture.
a–b AP and lateral x-rays from the initial presentation. Note the subtle irregularity of the lateral process of the talus (white arrow).
c–g The CT scans demonstrating a comminuted displaced sustentacular fracture (**c–e**) and an associated lateral process fracture (**f–g**).

If the depressed sustentaculum is not elevated up to the level of the medial talar facet, hindfoot varus will develop in addition to joint incongruity. Surgical timing and planning of surgical approaches must be well thought out, taking into consideration the treatment required for any other injuries present in the foot or ankle (**Fig 4.3-2–Fig 4.3-4**).

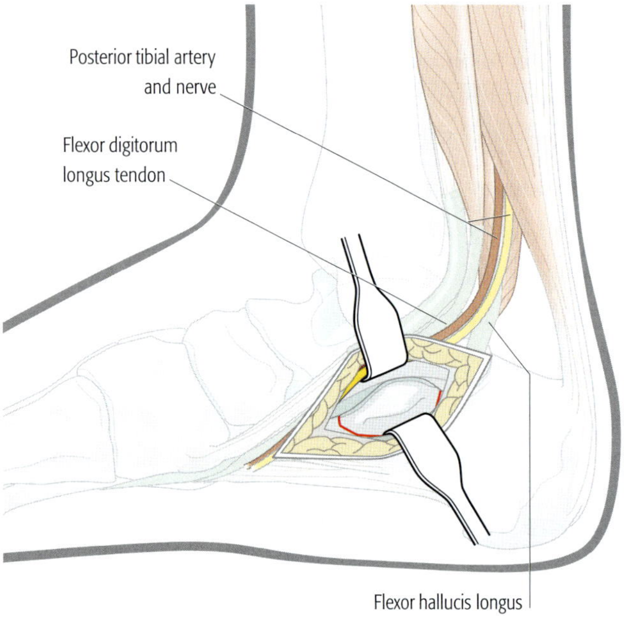

Fig 4.3-2 The surgical interval for fixation is between the flexor digitorum longus and extensor hallucis longus tendons.

3 Operating room setup

Patient positioning	• Supine
Anesthesia options	• General, spinal, or regional
C-arm location	• Placed on the lateral side of the injured extremity with the monitor facing toward the head of the patient
Tourniquet	• Used at surgeon's discretion • Generally improves visualization
Tips	• A bump can be placed under the ipsilateral hip to assist in positioning as needed. • Place the operative limb on an elevating ramp to aid in obtaining clear C-arm images and improve instrumentation of the foot

For illustrations and overview of anesthetic considerations, see chapter 1.

Equipment

- Headlight
- K-wires
- Elevators
- Small and minifragment screws
- Minifragment plates 2.0 and 2.4, available for comminuted injuries
- External fixator or distractor, if needed, to improve joint visualization

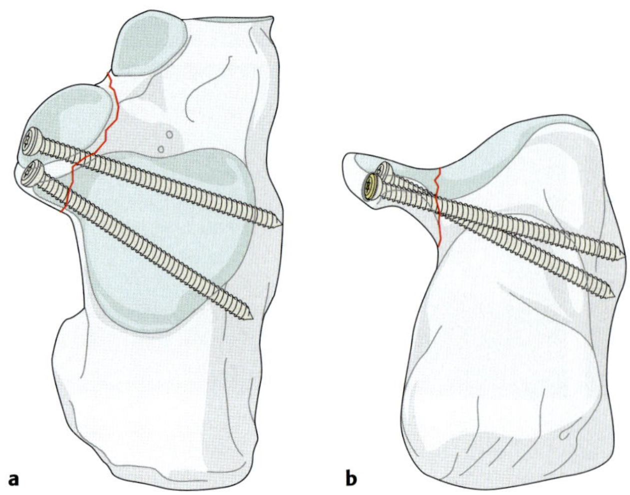

Fig 4.3-3 Simple fractures may be stabilized with 2.7 or 3.5 mm screws.

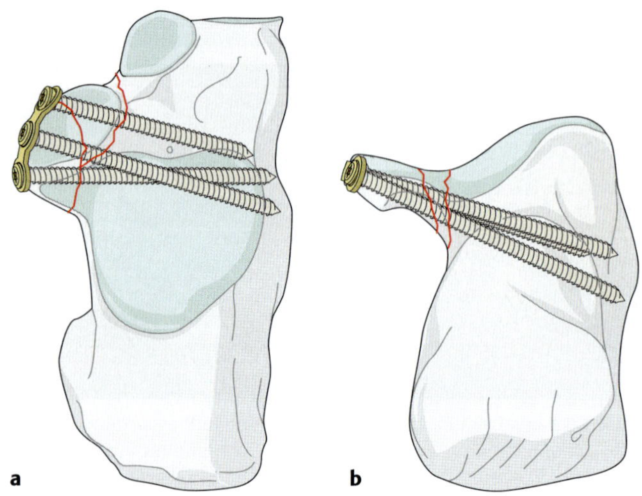

Fig 4.3-4a–b Comminuted injuries may be stabilized with minifragment plate fixation.

4 Surgical procedure

The described technique may be used in isolation or in addition to other procedures.

A marker is used to outline the distal medial malleolus and the navicular tuberosity. The posterior tibial tendon is palpated. A longitudinal incision is made below the posterior tibial tendon (**Fig 4.3-5**). Dissection continues to the flexor digitorum longus (FDL). Both tendons are released from their sheaths and retracted superiorly (**Fig 4.3-6**). This allows visualization of the fracture along the medial wall of the calcaneus. The joint capsule of the subtalar joint is usually traumatically open from the injury, but if it is still intact, it is incised. Sometimes the flexor retinaculum must be incised to adequately visualize the joint. Care should be taken to avoid injury to the tibiocalcaneal portion of the deltoid ligament which can result in medial ankle instability.

The articular injury can be seen by retracting the posterior tibialis and FDL tendons superiorly, or by using the interval between the two tendons. The flexor hallucis longus (FHL) is dissected out and retracted in a plantar direction. Dissection is carried down the medial wall to expose the fracture and ensure there are no entrapped structures such as the FHL tendon which may become entrapped in this fracture. A K-wire is then placed in the sustentacular fragment and the fracture is manipulated using this wire as a joystick. The fracture line is cleaned of hematoma and any osseus or cartilaginous debris, which may block reduction. Next, any small joint fragments that are displaced are reduced.

The fracture is reduced by lifting the fragment up, with the K-wire again used as a joystick to manipulate the fragment (**Fig 4.3-7**). The articular reduction is assessed by direct visualization of the joint surface and not indirectly by reducing the fracture as it exits the medial wall. K-wires are advanced across the fragment into the body of the calcaneus. In cases with a single large fragment, two wires are still necessary to prevent rotational deformity. In comminuted cases, multiple fragment-specific K-wires may be necessary.

A large point-to-point reduction (Weber) clamp may be used by placing one tip on the sustentaculum and the other tip through a small incision laterally onto the lateral wall taking care to avoid the peroneal tendons. This aids in reduction and provisional fixation (**Fig 4.3-8**). If comminution is present, caution must be used when applying the clamp to not over compress the fracture which creates a mismatch between the articular surface of the medial facet and the corresponding surface on the talus. If the fracture is one large piece, fixation may be performed using two screws. If comminution exists, evaluation of the reduction is made entirely by direct visualization of the joint surface and pal-

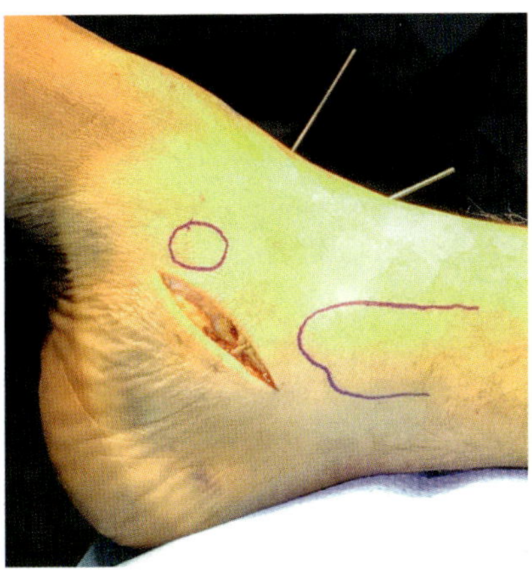

Fig 4.3-5 The incision is made on the medial side of the foot.

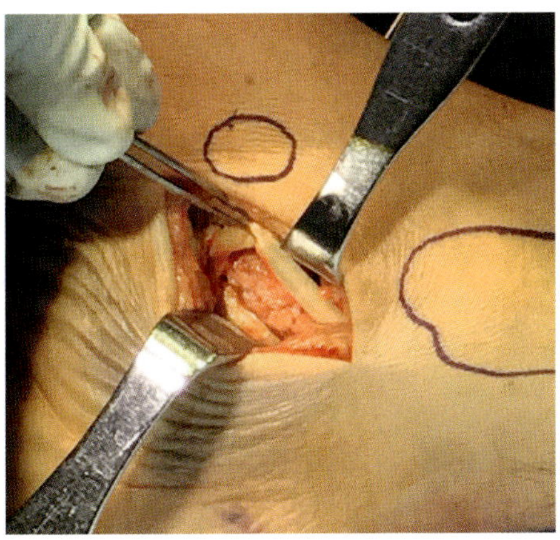

Fig 4.3-6 The FDL tendon is elevated.

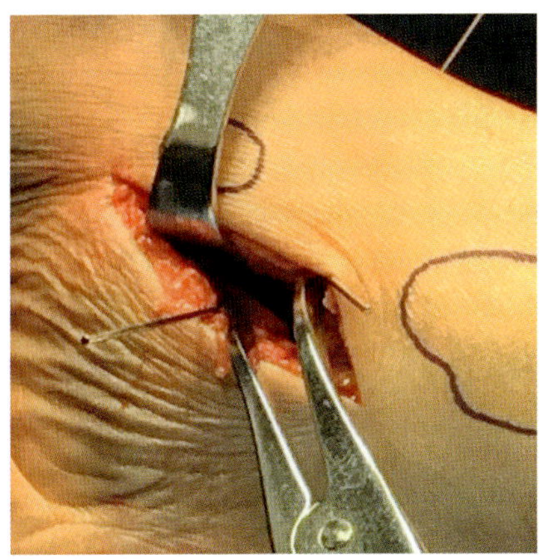

Fig 4.3-7 A lamina spreader is used to distract the subtalar joint and a temporary K-wire is inserted into the sustentacular fragment.

pation of the articular surface with a small (Freer) elevator (**Fig 4.3-9**). Multiple small K-wires are used for provisional fixation to prevent rotation (**Fig 4.3-10**). A minifragment plate is then slid over the K-wires (**Fig 4.3-11**). Wires are removed one at a time and replaced by screws (**Fig 4.3-12**).

The final construct is low profile and stable (**Fig 4.3-13**). The screws may be inserted in lag fashion if all bony elements are present or as positional non-lag screws if comminution is severe or there is bone loss. Final images are obtained at the conclusion of the case (**Fig 4.3-14**).

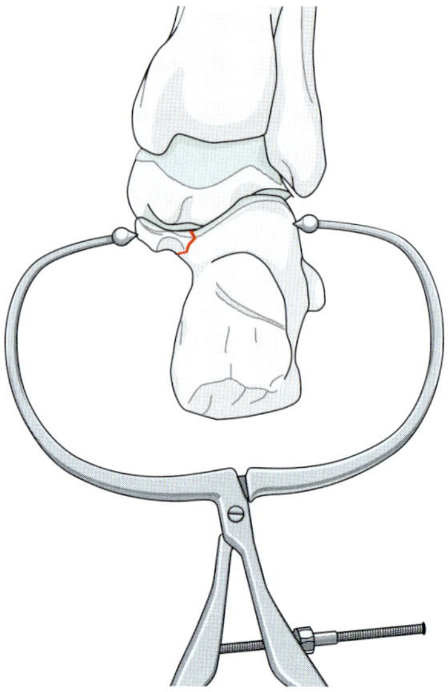

Fig 4.3-8 A large reduction clamp may be placed to aid in reduction.

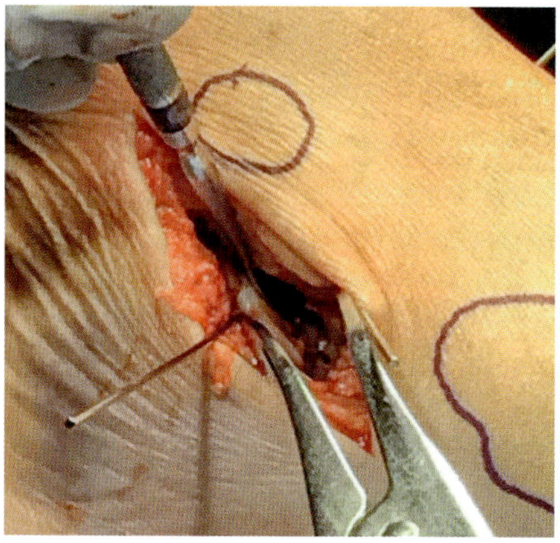

Fig 4.3-9 The reduction is completed and held with a provisional K-wire and a small (Freer) elevator is used to palpate the joint to assess for any residual malreduction.

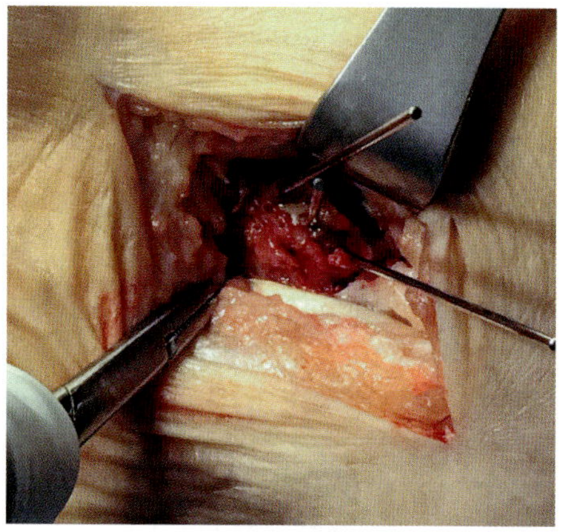

Fig 4.3-10 Multiple K-wires are used for provisional fixation to prevent fragment rotation.

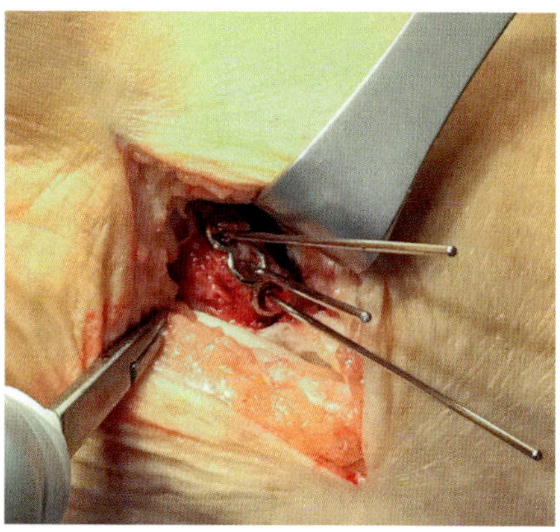

Fig 4.3-11 A small minifragment plate is then slid over the K-wires.

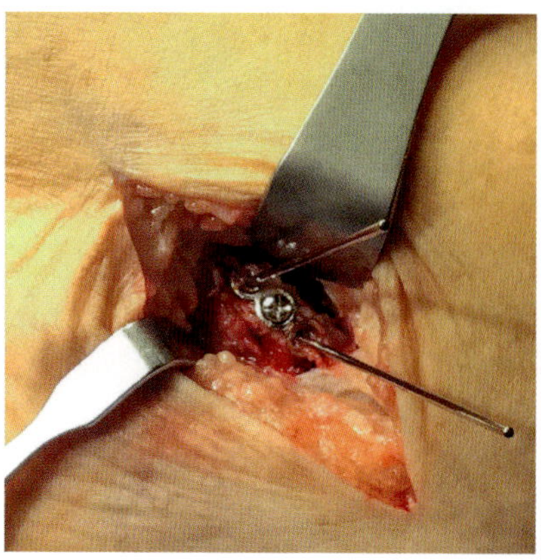

Fig 4.3-12 The K-wires are removed one at a time and exchanged for screws. The central wire has been removed and replaced with a 2.4 mm screw.

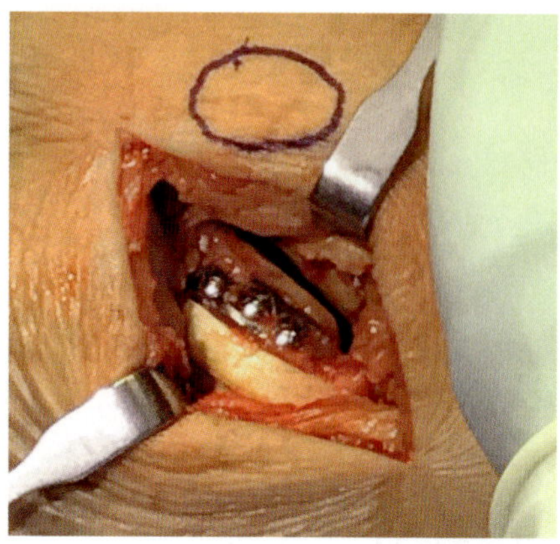

Fig 4.3-13 Final fixation with a 2.0 mm plate with minifragment screws.

5 Pitfalls and complications

Pitfalls

Inadequate visualization

Using a headlight greatly improves the ability to fully visualize the injury. Additionally, if further assistance is needed, a small distractor or external fixator may be placed from the medial face of the tibia to a medial calcaneal pin. Visualization of the now distracted medial facet may be improved by distraction.

Complications

- Wound dehiscence
- Stiffness in subtalar motion, intolerance to uneven surfaces, and potential development of subtalar arthritis over time. Stiffness is best avoided by initiation of early subtalar range-of-motion (ROM) exercises but will still occur in most patients.
- Posttraumatic arthritis:
  - Best prevented by anatomical reconstruction, but many patients will still develop arthritis due to the high-energy nature of this injury.
  - More common in individuals who also have an associated talar fracture.
  - If severe posttraumatic arthritis occurs, a subtalar arthrodesis is the salvage procedure (**Fig 4.3-15**).

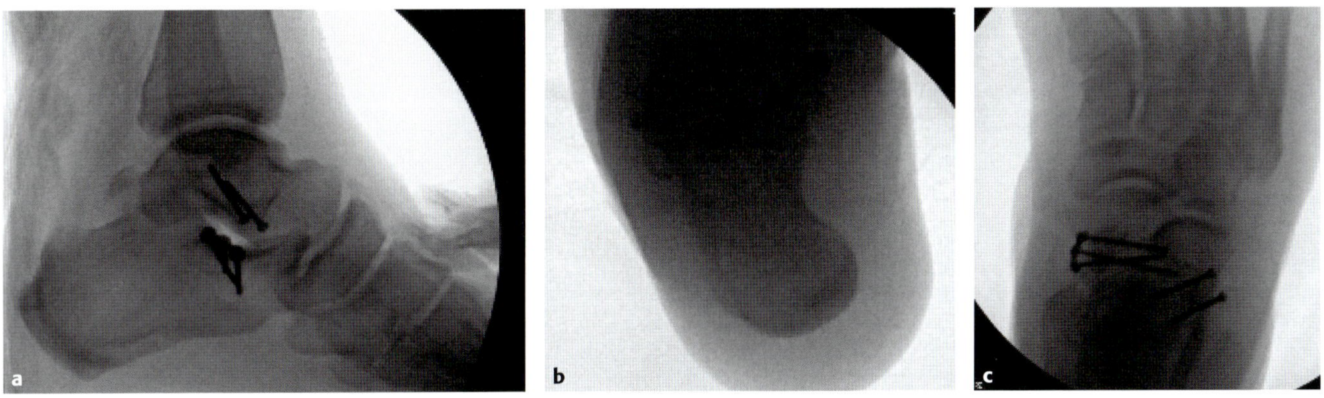

Fig 4.3-14a–c Hindfoot after fixation is completed.
a Lateral view.
b Axial view.
c AP view.

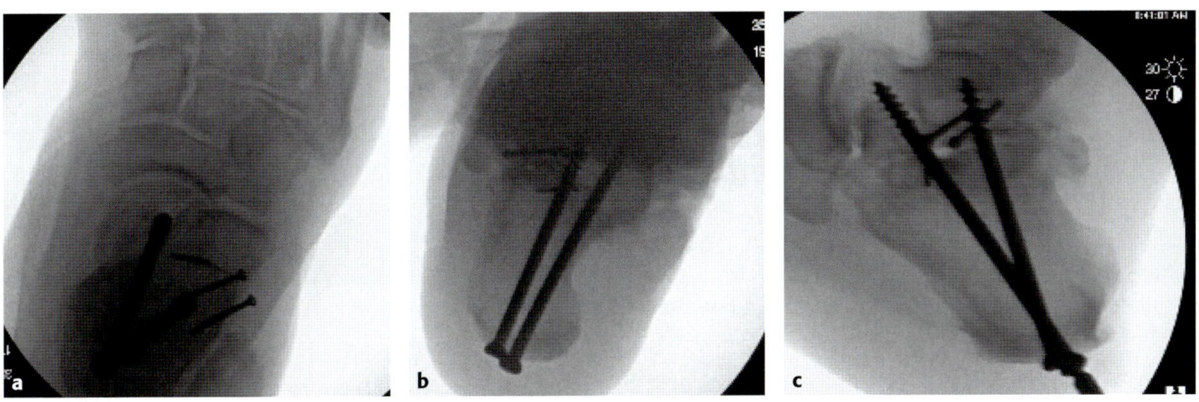

Fig 4.3-15a–c Example from a different case showing x-rays after arthrodesis for posttraumatic arthritis.
a AP view.
b Axial view.
c Lateral of subtalar arthrodesis performed due to development of posttraumatic subtalar arthritis after a sustentacular fracture.

- Irritation to the posterior tibial and/or FDL tendons may occur from hardware and may be improved by implant removal.
- Varus malalignment of the hindfoot may occur in missed or neglected fractures. If neurologic signs are present in the tarsal tunnel, nerve entrapment by displaced fragments must be considered.
- Injury to the neurovascular bundle or tendons may occur and is more common with percutaneous approaches.
- Entrapment of tendons may occur, particularly in missed fractures. Treatment for all subtalar dislocations should include a CT scan after reduction to assess for fractures, as there is a high association of fracture with subtalar dislocation. Late entrapment of the FHL with bony tunnel overgrowth is also possible.

6 Alternative techniques

Surgical excision with immediate aggressive ROM exercises may be performed for small peripheral fractures. Care must be taken to avoid excision of larger fragments that may result in the hindfoot falling into varus.

If an associated talar neck fracture is present, the sustentaculum may be fixed at the same time or in a staged fashion (**Fig 4.3-16**). Talar neck fractures are typically approached medially in the interval between the anterior tibialis and posterior tibialis. Occasionally both the talar neck fracture and sustentaculum fracture may be repaired by moving the incision slightly lower in this interval. If the talar neck fracture is not amenable to treatment with an altered approach, the talar neck fracture is treated through a traditionally

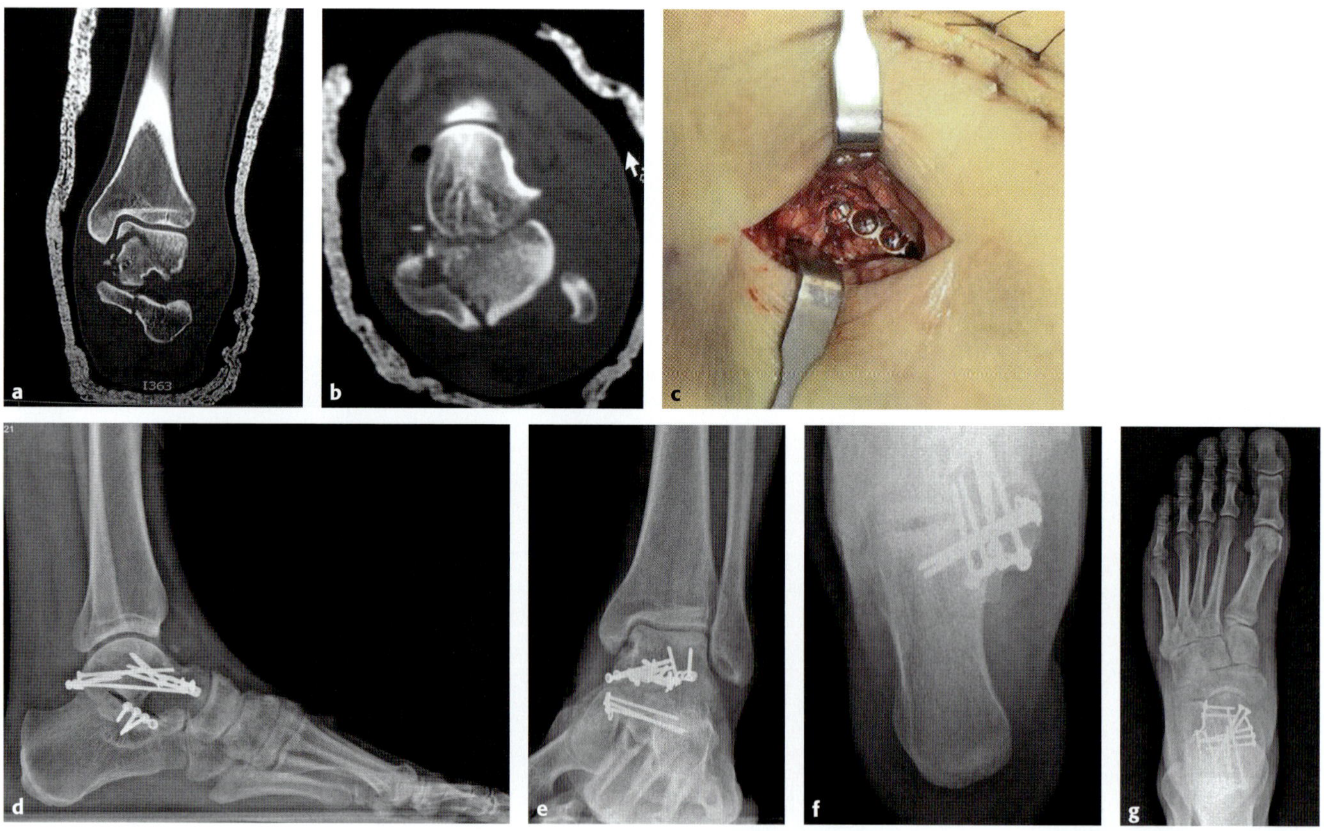

Fig 4.3-16a–g Example from a different case of a sustentaculum fracture with a comminuted fracture of the talar neck and posterior body with an associated sustentacular fracture from a fall from a ladder.
a–b Coronal and axial CT demonstrating a comminuted neck and body fracture with an associated sustentacular fracture.
c The patient was treated with three surgical procedures. The talar neck was treated at the first surgery by two incisions. The posterior talar body was repaired at the second surgery. The sustentaculum was repaired at the final operation by an independent incision.
d–g Final images of the hindfoot in lateral (**d**), mortise (**e**), axial (**f**), and AP (**g**) views after union was achieved.

placed medial incision at the index surgical event and the sustentaculum fracture is not addressed. When the skin and swelling have sufficiently recovered, the patient returns to the operating room and the sustentacular fracture is repaired through a separate incision.

Locking plate fixation may be necessary in osteoporotic patients.

Fracture dislocations of the calcaneus should not be considered sustentacular fractures even in cases of medial posterior facet fracture. Those injuries require management from a lateral approach. In that fracture pattern the posterior facet dislocates laterally and superiorly abutting the fibula. (For more details on appropriate treatment of fracture dislocation patterns, see chapter 4.7.)

7 Postoperative management and rehabilitation

Functional exercises

Range of motion of the subtalar, talonavicular, and tibiotalar joints is started at 2 days if the injury is isolated. In cases with associated injuries to the foot it may be necessary to refrain from motion for a longer period.

Follow-up

- 2 weeks: The patient is seen at 2 weeks for suture and splint removal. A removable fracture boot is placed. Range of motion exercises are reviewed and home exercises for ankle and subtalar and metatarsal phalangeal joints are initiated for most injuries. If the injury is part of a multiple fractures of the foot, then ROM may be held as dictated by the other injuries present.
- 6 weeks: The patient is seen for postoperative imaging. In isolated fractures if union is present, weight bearing (WB) may begin. If an external fixator was retained due to instability, then it is removed and ROM exercises are initiated. If an associated talar fracture was present, then nonweight bearing is continued until 12 weeks.
- 12 weeks: The patient is seen for postoperative imaging. Patients with isolated fractures are full WB and return-to-work issues are reviewed if the patient has a WB occupation. For more complex injuries, WB is typically initiated at 12 weeks.
- 6 months, 12 months: The patient is seen for continued follow-up at 6 months and 12 months; additional visits may be scheduled as deemed necessary. Risks of development of posttraumatic arthritis are reviewed and the patient is encouraged to avoid uneven surfaces. At each visit, ROM is assessed (**Fig 4.3-17**).

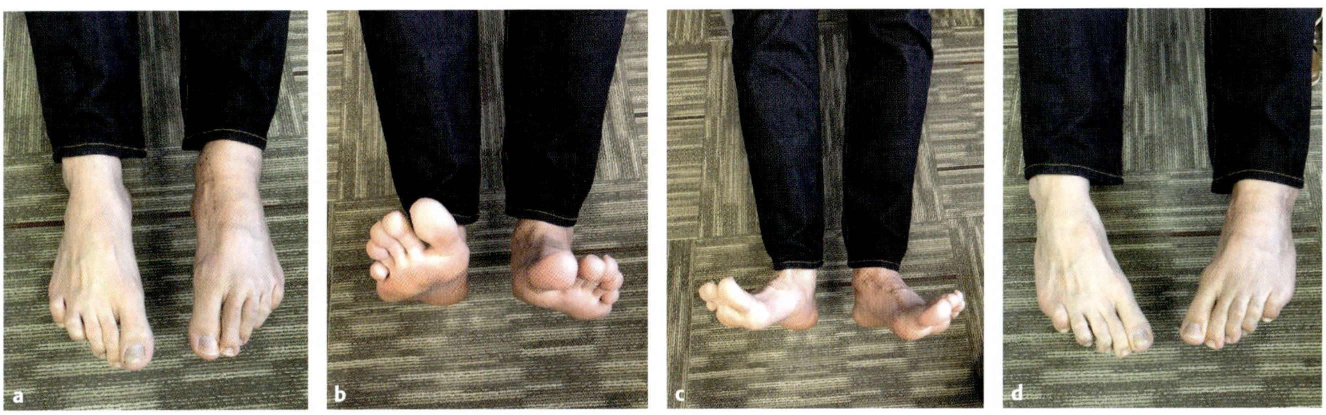

Fig 4.3-17a–d Final ROM after a combined talar and sustentacular fracture. (Patient from different case example, **Fig 4.3-16.**)
a Plantarflexion.
b Dorsiflexion.
c Eversion.
d Inversion.

Implant removal

The implants are not typically removed. They are only removed if they are symptomatic, which is unusual. They may need to be removed if severe posttraumatic arthritis develops and arthrodesis is required. Removal of the existing hardware may be required to allow for insertion of new hardware necessary for arthrodesis.

8 Recommended reading

Della Rocca GJ, Nork SE, Barei DP, et al. Fractures of the sustentaculum tali: injury characteristics and surgical technique for reduction. *Foot Ankle Int.* 2009 Nov;30(11):1037–1041.
Dürr C, Zwipp H, Rammelt S. Fractures of the sustentaculum tali. *Oper Orthop Traumatol.* 2013 Dec;25(6):569–578.

4.4 Simple articular fracture (Sanders 2)—minimally invasive screw fixation

Tim Schepers

1 Case description

A 23-year-old male window cleaner fell off a ladder from a height of 3 m and landed on his left foot. He was unable to bear weight on his left foot and was transferred to a local hospital. His medical history revealed him to be a smoker (20 cigarettes a day).

A complete physical examination revealed no injuries other than pain of both feet. There was no pain at the thoracolumbar spine. X-rays in multiple views of both feet and ankles were taken. The lateral and axial x-rays of the left foot showed a calcaneal fracture (Essex-Lopresti tongue-type calcaneal fracture) with Böhler angle measuring 13° (**Fig 4.4-1**).

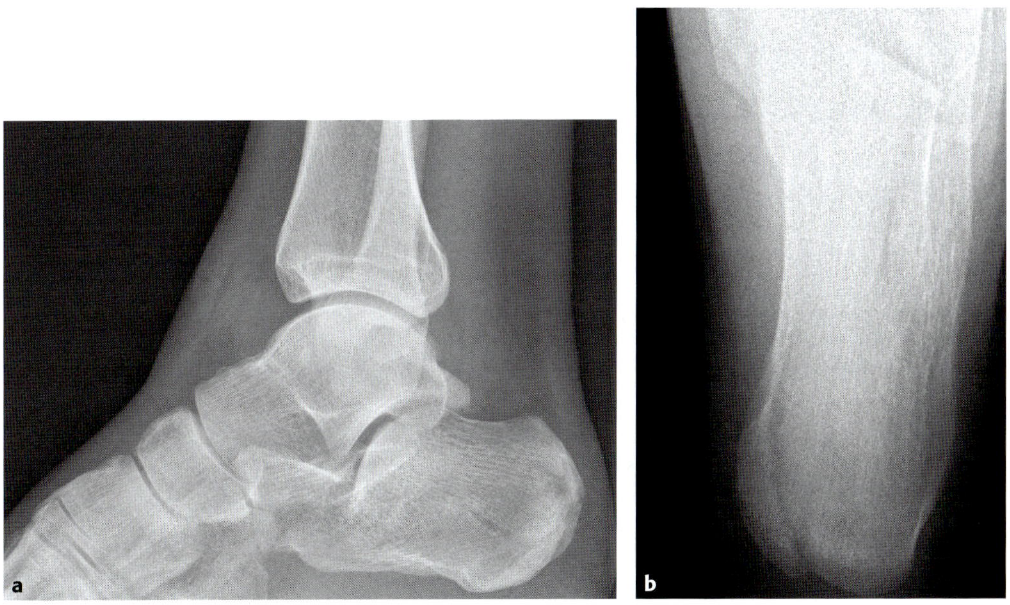

Fig 4.4-1a–b Postinjury images.
a Lateral x-ray of calcaneus showing tongue-type calcaneal fracture.
b Axial x-ray showing mild widening of calcaneus with neutral alignment.

In addition to plane x-rays, a computed tomographic (CT) scan was performed to assess the congruity of the posterior facet of the talocalcaneal/subtalar joint. The fracture was classified as an AO/OTA 82C1 (Sanders type 2C) (**Fig 4.4-2** and **Fig 4.4-3**). On postinjury day 5, the patient was transferred to another hospital which had more experience with treating displaced calcaneal fractures.

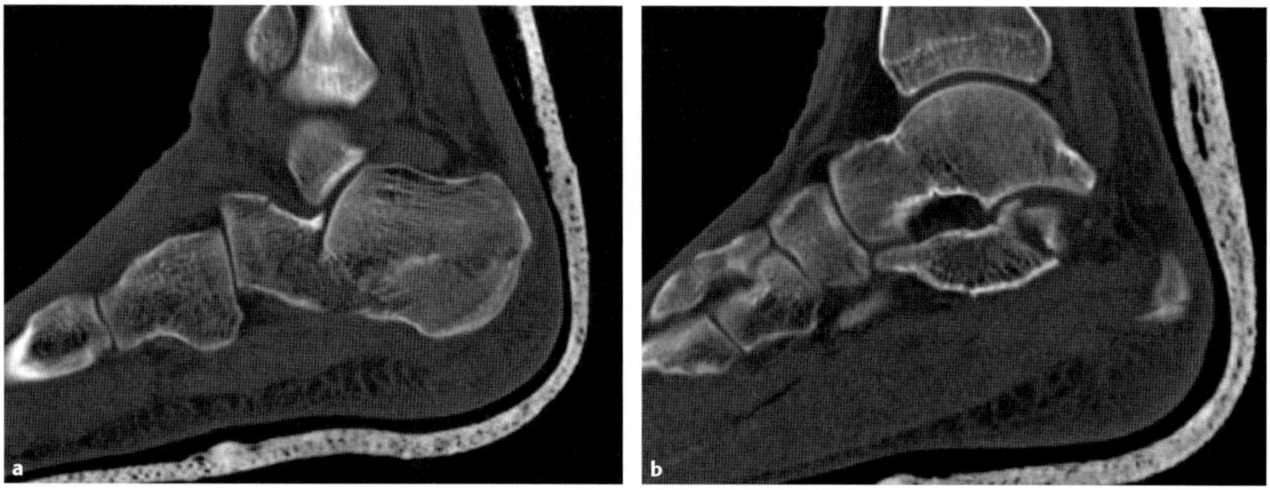

Fig 4.4-2a–b The CT images.
a Sagittal view of the lateral portion of the calcaneus at Gissane angle displaying depression of joint fragment.
b Sagittal view of the medial portion indicating step-off in posterior talocalcaneal joint.

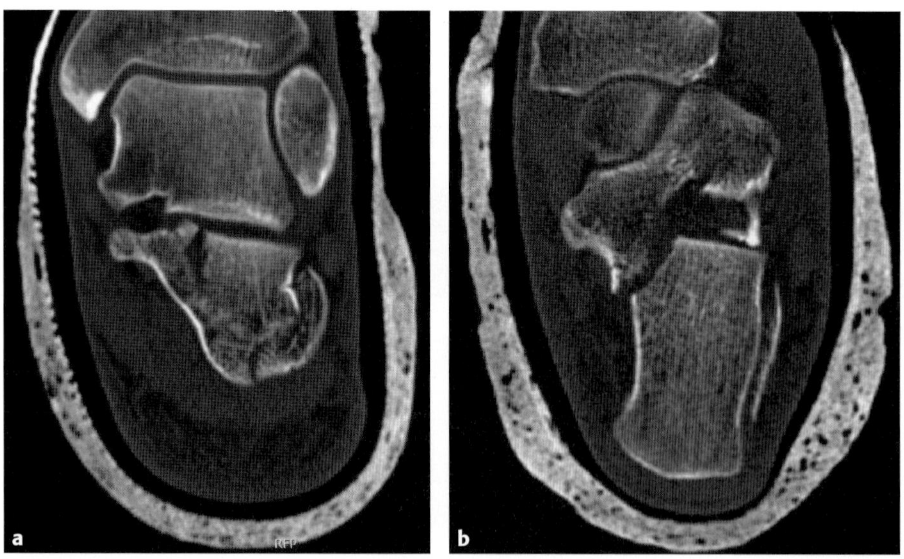

Fig 4.4-3a–b The CT images.
a Axial view revealing bulging of lateral wall and the fracture line through the most medial part of the posterior talocalcaneal joint.
b Sanders type 2C on semicoronal view.

2 Preoperative planning

Indications for surgery

The indication for surgery in less displaced intraarticular calcaneal fractures is still debatable. The reasons for and against surgical intervention were extensively discussed with the patient as part of the shared decision-making process.

A surgical approach was selected for the following reasons:

- Age of the patient
- Step-off at the level of the posterior facet
- Displaced Böhler angle, less than 15°

Considerations for surgery

Various options are available:

- Fully percutaneous with or without arthroscopic control
- A less invasive sinus tarsi approach
- Fully open extended lateral approach

For this patient, a percutaneous approach was chosen with screw-only fixation because of the less comminuted fracture pattern, the tongue-type configuration, and the patient's use of tobacco. A preoperative plan was made (**Fig 4.4-4**).

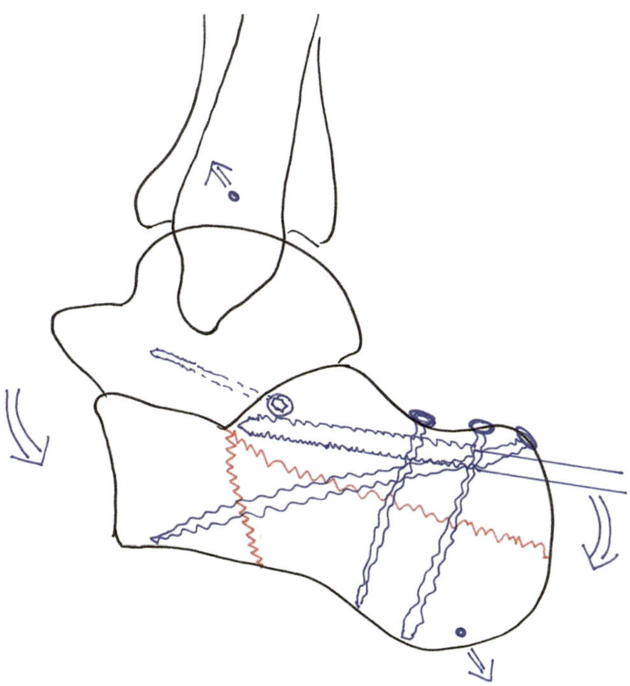

Fig 4.4-4 Preoperative planning sketch.

3 Operating room setup

Patient positioning	• Lateral decubitus (injured side up) with an elevating ramp or blankets under the operative limb
Anesthesia options	• General, spinal, or regional
C-arm location	• Monitor on the opposite side of the operative table with the C-arm entering at an oblique angle from the foot of the bed
Tourniquet	• Used at surgeon's discretion. • Improves ability to visualize both the joint and the reduction. • A tourniquet is necessary if arthroscopy is used
Tips	• Placing a small towel bump proximal to the malleoli improves the ability to instrument the foot and inverts the subtalar joint improving visualization (by open or arthroscopic techniques), if needed.

For illustrations and overview of anesthetic considerations, see chapter 1. For illustrations and overview of patient and C-arm positioning for calcaneal fracture treatment in the lateral decubitus position chapter 4.

Equipment

- K-wires in various lengths
- Small distraction device
- 3.0–5.0 mm Schanz pins
- 3.5 mm or 4.0 mm cancellous and cortex screws
- Periosteal elevator and small (Freer) or small spatula (Howard) elevator
- 2.7 mm, 30° arthroscope

4 Surgical procedure

After positioning the patient, skin markings are drawn indicating pertinent anatomical landmarks and the anticipated incisions (**Fig 4.4-5**). The procedure is performed guided by the C-arm from the start. The sinus tarsi approach is marked on the skin. If the necessary fracture reduction cannot be achieved by minimally invasive techniques, the case can be converted to a sinus tarsi approach. (See chapter 4.5 for the sinus tarsi approach and technique.)

Under C-arm guidance a 5.0 mm Schanz pin is inserted posteriorly into the tongue fragment. The tip of the pin is directed just underneath the posterior facet of the talocalcaneal subtalar joint, just underneath the strong subchondral cortex. To create space for reduction of the joint, a small distractor can be placed on the lateral side of the foot. One pin is placed inferiorly in the tuber and a second is placed in the talar neck, just anterior to the lateral process or distal fibula, allowing for subtalar distraction without interfering with hardware insertion (**Fig 4.4-6**). This also brings the tuber slightly inferiorly and posteriorly allowing the posterior cortex of the tongue fragment to reduce to the superior aspect of the tuber.

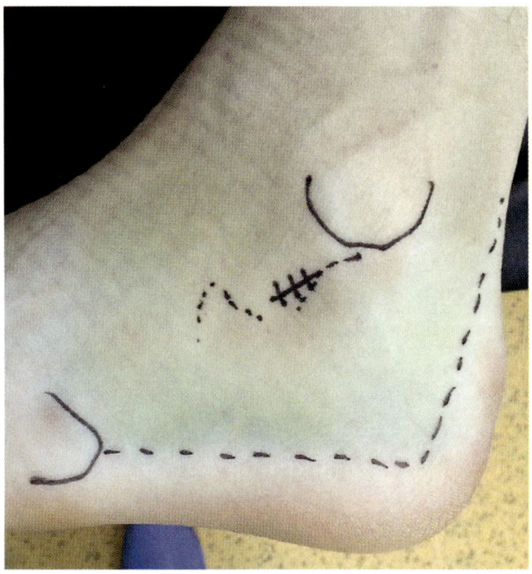

Fig 4.4-5 A sinus tarsi approach is outlined (extended lateral approach) for reference. An arthroscope can be introduced via small incision within the sinus tarsi approach.

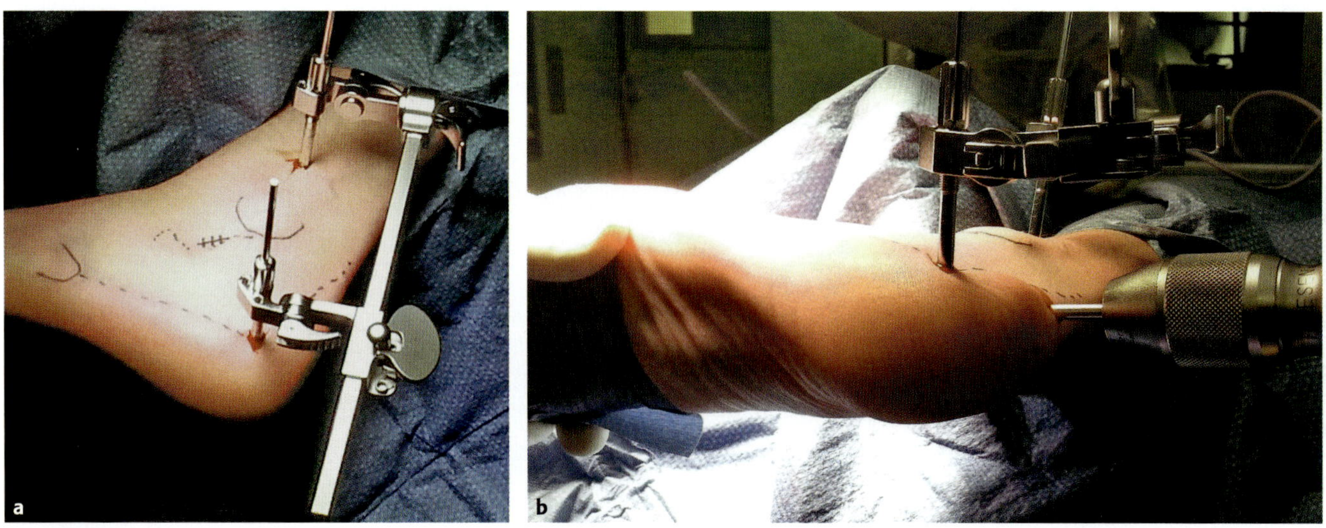

Fig 4.4-6a–b Intraoperative images.
a Placement of small distraction device with one pin in the calcaneal tuberosity and the second in the fibula.
b Insertion of Schanz pin.

The forefoot is then plantar flexed and the Schanz pin is pushed downward. The fragment, including the joint, is brought back up and derotated back into anatomical position. Sometimes the impaction or a delay in surgery prevents the tongue fragment from moving.

An additional small incision is then made just anterior and distal to the tip of the fibula (within the previously drawn sinus tarsi approach). Via this small incision, a periosteal elevator can be inserted over the lateral wall into the secondary fracture line, just underneath the deepest displacement of the joint fragment. Using a combined maneuver of lifting the periosteal elevator and pushing down on the Schanz pin, the fragment is brought back to the correct height. This incision can later be used to insert an arthroscope (anterolateral, sinus tarsi portal), if needed, to assess and confirm anatomical reduction of the posterior facet by direct visualization of the fracture line before insertion of hardware.

The reduction is checked in the lateral and Brodén views (**Fig 4.4-7a–b**). When reduction is achieved, temporary K-wires can be inserted (**Fig 4.4-7c**). A lateral-to-medial screw is inserted via small incisions into the sustentaculum tali (**Fig 4.4-7d**). This screw connects the two joint fragments. The tongue part of tuber is subsequently connected to the other half of the tuber. Finally, the entire tuber and joint are connected to the anterior process fragment with axially placed screws (**Fig 4.4-7e**). Care must be taken to engage the plantar cortex with the screws to avoid failure of fixation and late displacement of the tuber. Reduction may be evaluated with an intraoperative CT scan if available (**Fig 4.4-8**) or by a standard postoperative CT scan (**Fig 4.4-9**).

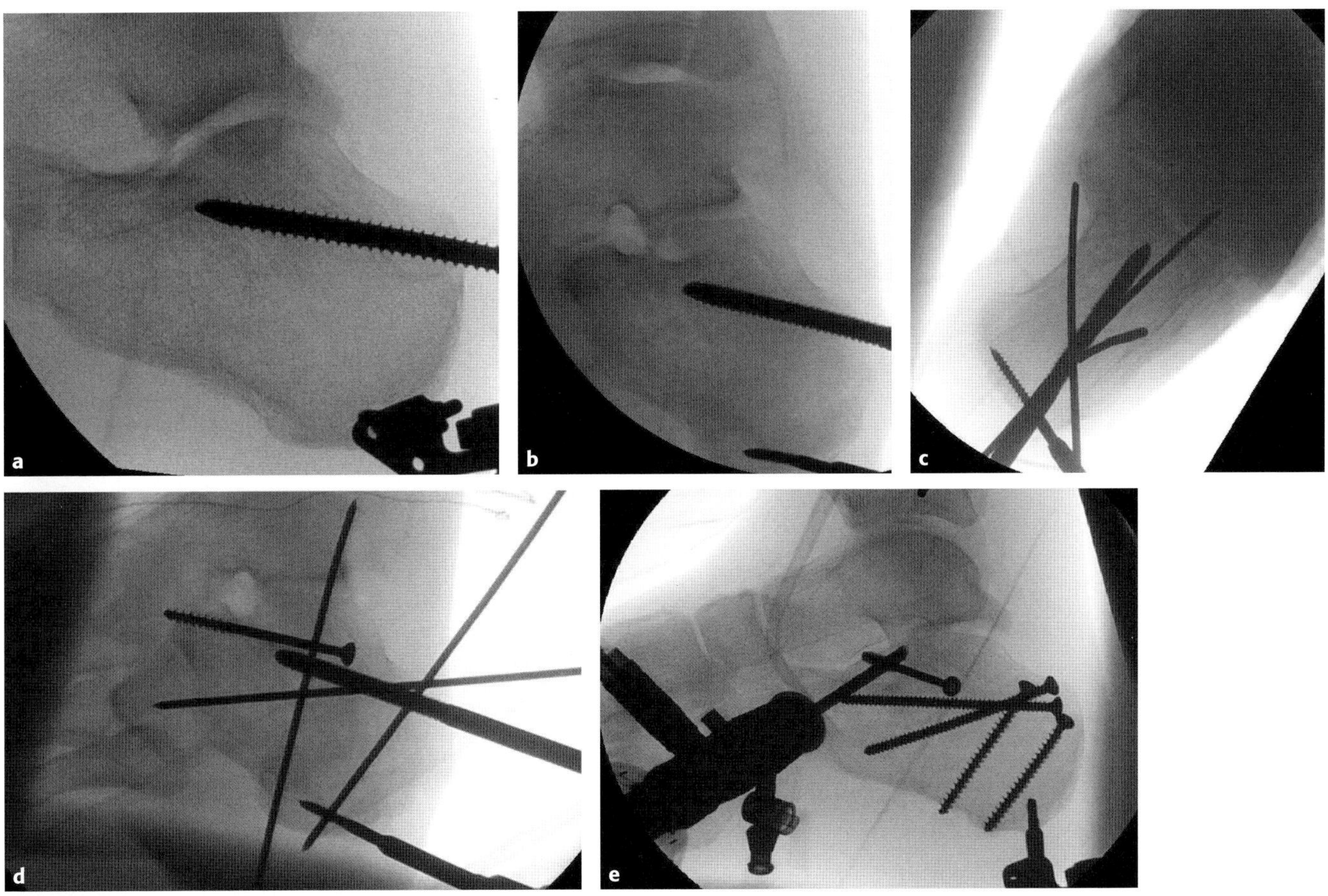

Fig 4.4-7a–e Intraoperative C-arm control.

a Insertion of a Schanz pin and application of the small distraction device, followed by leverage of posterior tongue fragment.
b By elevating the forefoot, a Brodén view is obtained showing reduction of talocalcaneal facet.
c The axial view is checked for axis, and temporary K-wires are inserted.
d A lateral-to-medial screw is inserted into the sustentaculum tali and checked in the Brodén view.
e The final reduction and stabilization achieved by the subarticular screw is checked using arthroscopy.

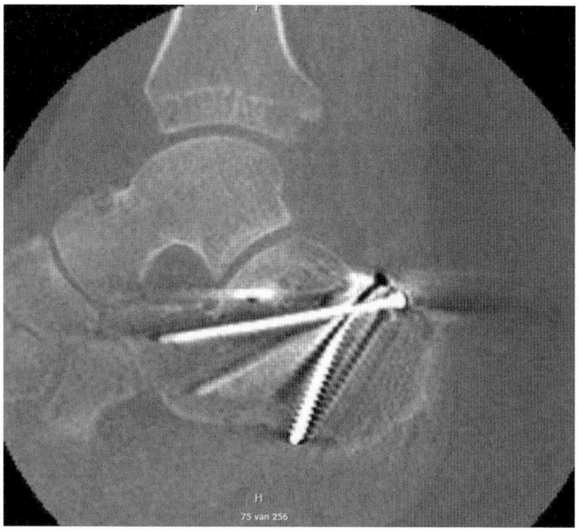

Fig 4.4-8 Intraoperative 3D scan to verify reduction and implant position.

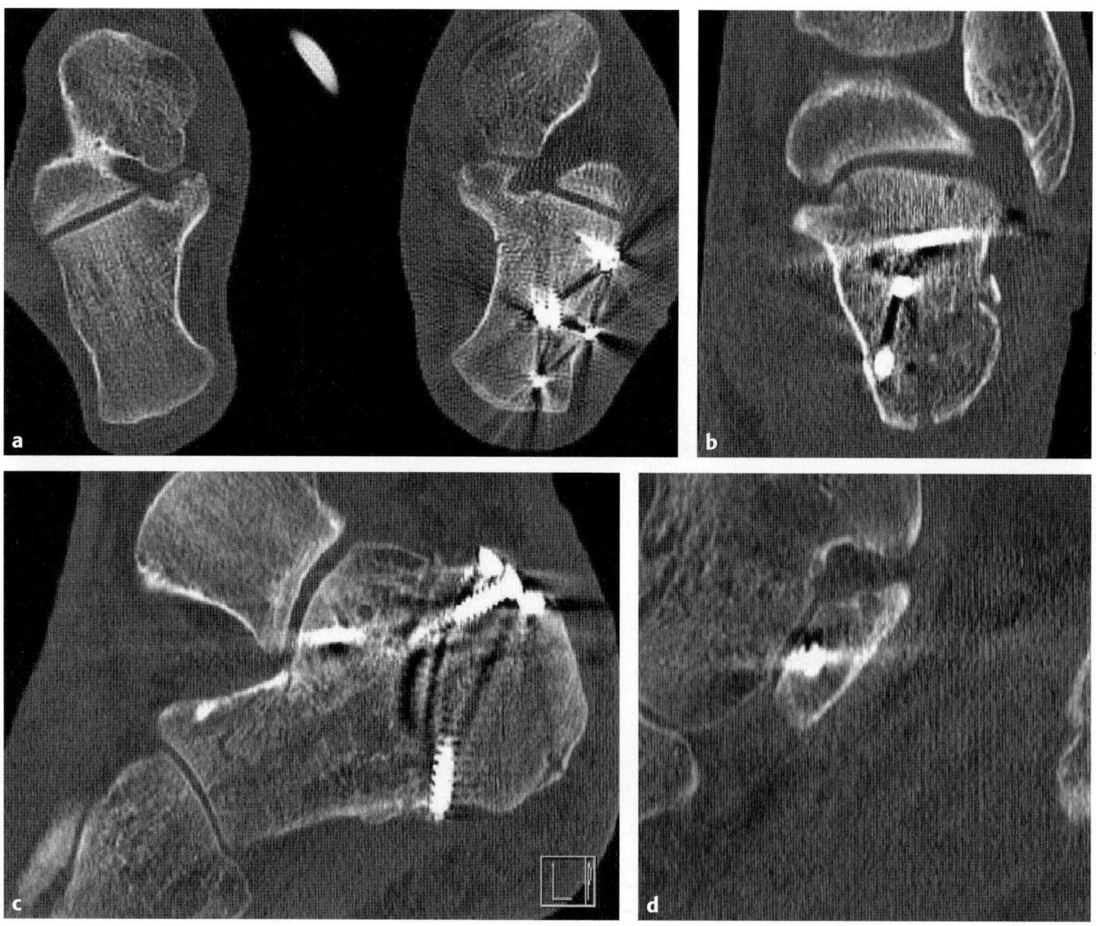

Fig 4.4-9a–d Postoperative CT scans showing adequate reduction.

5 Pitfalls and complications

Pitfalls

Possible conversion from minimally invasive to open technique

The patient should be counseled preoperatively that conversion to a more open technique might be necessary. An open technique is required when the fracture is too impacted, or if the delay between injury and surgery is too long, causing the fracture to be too stiff to manipulate percutaneously.

Preoperatively, the open incision can be drawn if the percutaneous technique is unsuccessful. If planning the sinus tarsi approach, a small incision can be made to insert a periosteal elevator. An additional Schanz pin can be inserted from posterior in the tongue fragment. If reduction cannot be achieved using the C-arm, the percutaneous procedure should be converted to an open procedure to ensure that correct reduction is achieved. The ability to clean out the fracture lines and mobilize fracture fragments is improved with the open surgical approaches (**Fig 4.4-10**).

Delay resulting in ischemia

A delay in severely depressed tongue-types can result into ischemia on the posterior aspect of the skin just above the tuber (see chapter 4.1). These type of injuries, with skin at risk, are orthopedic emergencies. Urgent reduction and (temporary 1.6 mm K-wire) fixation is warranted (**Fig 4.4-11**).

Alternatively, percutaneous screw or open reduction via a lateral approach should be performed. As the major deforming force displacing the posterior tuber is the Achilles, some form of calf or tendon release to correct the equinus is often necessary as part of the surgical procedure.

Complications

- Postoperative wound infection
- Sural nerve injury
- Screw malposition (eg, intraarticular or too long on medial side)
- Insufficient reduction of the posterior talocalcaneal joint
- Insufficient stabilization (loss of reduction)
- Intraarticular fragments
- Posttraumatic arthritis

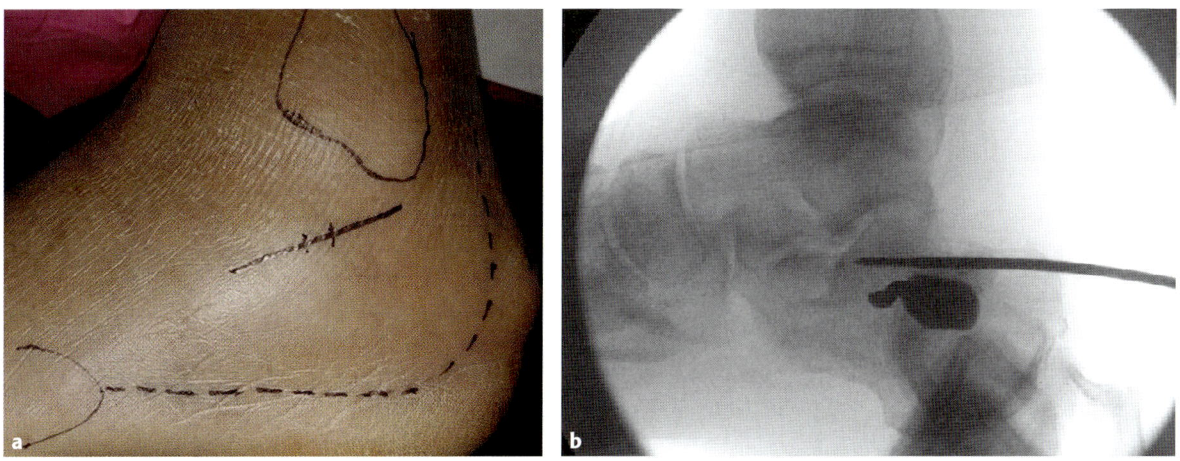

Fig 4.4-10a–b Is a less invasive approach possible? A surgical test (from a different case).
a Preoperative outlines of incisions on the skin. Within the sinus tarsi approach a small incision is made.
b Testing using a Schanz pin and periosteal elevator. If the tongue fragment can be reduced a less invasive approach is possible. In this case, the tongue fragment does not reduce. An open approach either by sinus tarsi or lateral extensile is required to clean out the fracture allowing for reduction.

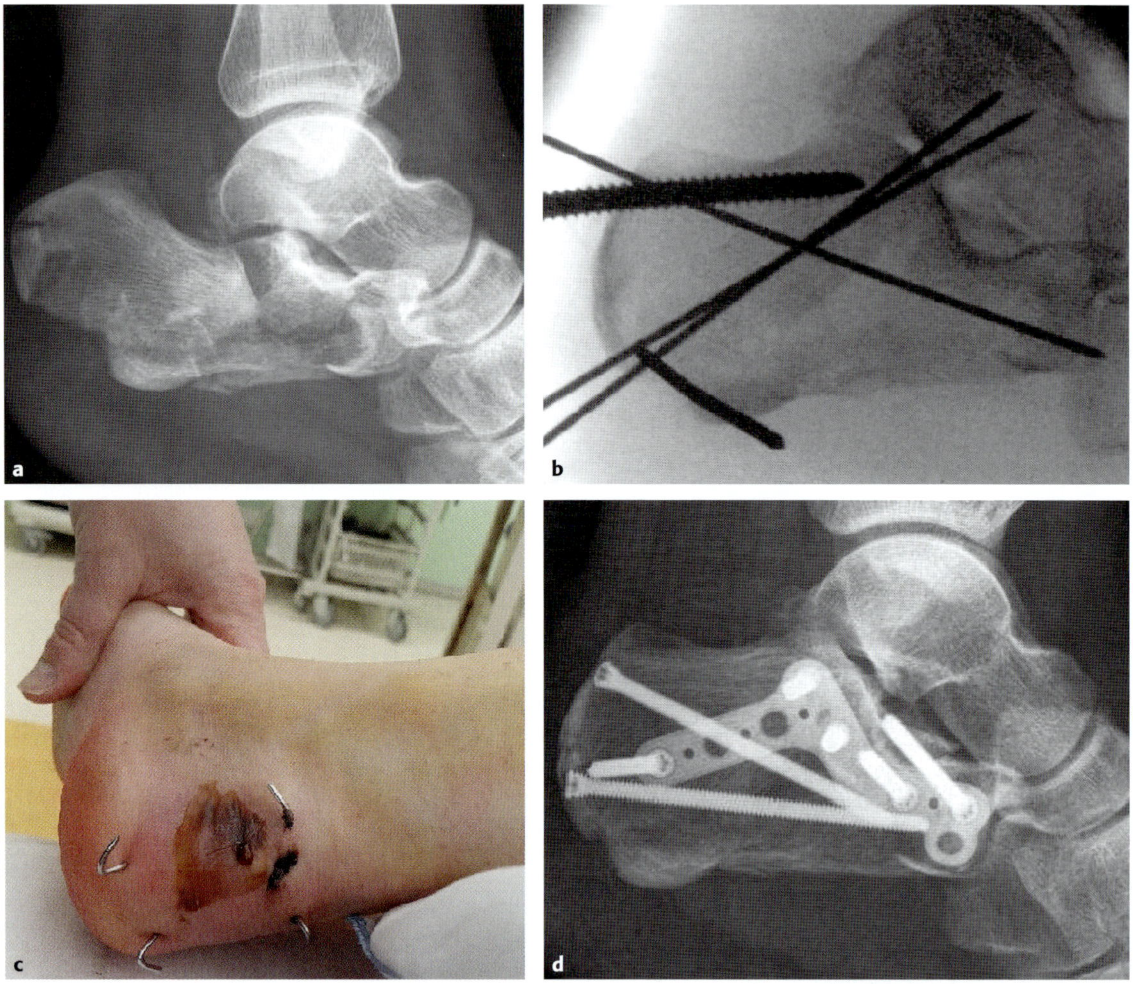

Fig 4.4-11a–d Example from a different case showing a severely depressed (with posterior displacement) tongue-type calcaneal fracture.

- **a** Postinjury images clearly demonstrating the posterior displacement of the tuber fragment and skin at risk on the conventional x-ray.
- **b** Temporary 1.6 mm K-wire fixation.
- **c** Preoperative clinical image at day 7 showing residual blister of posterior skin.
- **d** Postoperative image following definitive fixation via sinus tarsi approach.

6 Alternative techniques

The percutaneous techniques are the oldest surgical approach to the displaced intraarticular calcaneal fracture. Numerous modifications have been described with or without the use of distraction devices (ligamentotaxis).

The reduction can be fixed either with K-wires, percutaneous screws, external fixation (eg, Ilizarov frame), or using a calcaneal nail.

In some cases, the use of an injectable bone void filler can be beneficial and may allow for earlier weight bearing (WB) and lower the chance of loss of reduction.

The other surgical approaches most frequently used, besides the percutaneous technique, are:

- Sinus tarsi approach (chapter 4.5)
- Extended lateral approach (chapter 4.6)

7 Postoperative management and rehabilitation

Postoperatively the foot is placed in a bulky dressing.

The patient is discharged when the pain is controlled adequately and can safely ambulate with assist devices and while nonweight bearing on the operative extremity. Full range-of-motion (ROM) exercises can be started as soon as the wound is sealed.

The bandage is removed after 3 days, and the sutures at approximately 2 weeks. Patients are kept nonweight bearing for 8 weeks which is the time necessary for most fractures to heal when treated in this manner. Occasionally, in more severe fractures, WB will need to be delayed until union is present.

Rehabilitation should focus on full ROM exercises at the ankle and subtalar joints, muscle strength, proprioception, and gait. Formal physiotherapy following foot and ankle injuries is catered to the individual patient's needs.

The patient is followed up at 14–16 weeks to evaluate progress in WB return to activities. Return to work and other occupational concerns are also addressed during this follow-up (**Fig 4.4-12**).

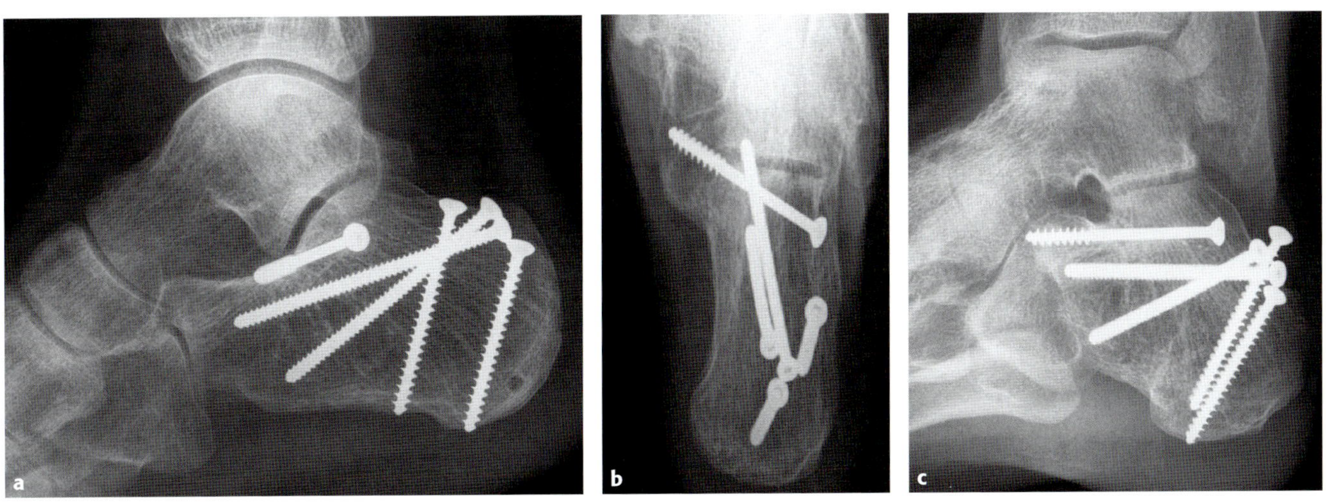

Fig 4.4-12a–c Follow-up x-rays at 6 months.
a Lateral view.
b Axial view.
c Brodén view.

Implant removal

Implant removal is performed in rare cases and only if specific symptoms of pain are reported over the hardware. However, this rarely occurs as no plates are used with this technique. Screws may sometimes be palpable and tender or irritating with shoe wear on the posterior aspect of the tuberosity. Peroneal tendon irritation with screw-only fixation is rare.

In this patient one of the posterolateral screws was removed after 16 months, as it was palpable and bothersome in shoes. The patient showed a full ROM of the ankle with near normal subtalar inversion and eversion compared with the contralateral side. He returned to work full time. No further follow-ups were necessary.

8 Recommended reading

Chen L, Zhang G, Hong J, et al. Comparison of percutaneous screw fixation and calcium sulfate cement grafting versus open treatment of displaced intraarticular calcaneal fractures. *Foot Ankle Int*. 2011 Oct;32(10):979–985.

Chhabra N, Sherman SC, Szatkowski JP. Tongue-type calcaneus fractures: a threat to skin. *Am J Emerg Med*. 2013 Jul;31(7):1151. e1153–1154.

Gardner MJ, Nork SE, Barei DP, et al. Secondary soft tissue compromise in tongue-type calcaneus fractures. *J Orthop Trauma*. 2008 Aug;22(7):439–445.

Ghorbanhoseini M, Kwon JY. Percutaneous method to determine optimal surgical approach for delayed treatment of calcaneus fracture. *Foot Ankle Int*. 2017 Jan;38(1):76–79.

Rammelt S, Gavlik JM, Barthel S, et al. The value of subtalar arthroscopy in the management of intra-articular calcaneus fractures. *Foot Ankle Int*. 2002 Oct;23(10):906–916.

Sangeorzan BJ, Benirschke S, Mills W. Technique of minimally invasive reduction and small fragment fixation of tongue-type calcaneus fractures. *Operative Tech Orthop*. 2004 Jan;14(1):36–40.

Schepers T, Backes M, Dingemans SA, et al. Similar anatomical reduction and lower complication rates with the sinus tarsi approach compared with the extended lateral approach in displaced intraarticular calcaneal fractures. *J Orthop Trauma*. 2017 Jun;31(6):293–298.

Schepers T, Patka P. Treatment of displaced intraarticular calcaneal fractures by ligamentotaxis: current concepts' review. *Arch Orthop Trauma Surg*. 2009 Dec;129(12):1677–1683.

Smerek JP, Kadakia A, Belkoff SM, et al. Percutaneous screw configuration versus perimeter plating of calcaneus fractures: a cadaver study. *Foot Ankle Int*. 2008 Sep;29(9):931–935.

Tantavisut S, Phisitkul P, Westerlind BO, et al. Percutaneous reduction and screw fixation of displaced intraarticular fractures of the calcaneus. *Foot Ankle Int*. 2017 Apr;38(4):367–374.

Tornetta P 3rd. Percutaneous treatment of calcaneal fractures. *Clin Orthop Relat Res*. 2000 Jun(375):91–96.

4.5 Displaced intraarticular fracture—sinus tarsi approach

Michael Swords, Candice Brady

1 Case description

A 56-year-old man fell approximately 1.5 meters off a ladder onto his left foot while working in construction. He experienced immediate pain on that heel. On arrival at the hospital, he underwent x-rays of the foot and ankle which demonstrated a left intraarticular, displaced, comminuted, joint depression fracture of the calcaneus (**Fig 4.5-1**). A thorough clinical examination ruled out additional injuries. There was no back pain. The injury was closed. The left leg was placed in a well-padded splint with the ankle and hindfoot in neutral position.

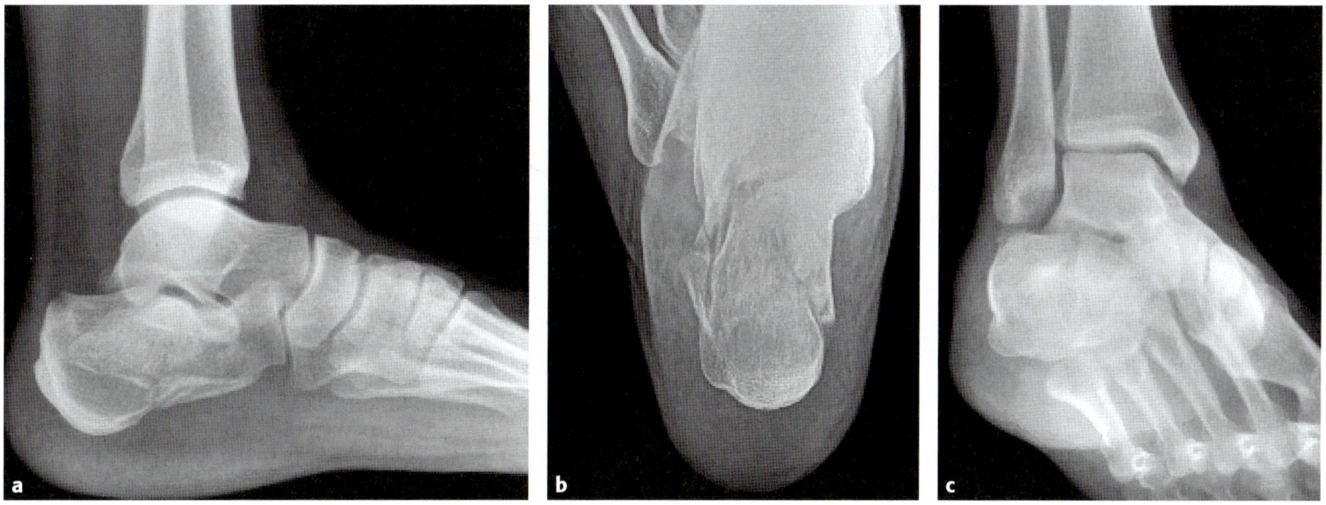

Fig 4.5-1a–c Postinjury x-rays of the calcaneus.
a Lateral view.
b Axial view.
c Brodén view.

A computed tomographic (CT) scan is necessary for full 3D understanding of the injury and operative planning. The CT revealed the fracture pattern and displacement to be an AO/OTA 82C2, Sanders 3AC (**Fig 4.5-2**). Given the amount of swelling, the patient was discharged home with strict orders to elevate the foot above the level of the heart and nonweight bearing (NWB). The following week he was examined up in the office for swelling and soft-tissue assessment.

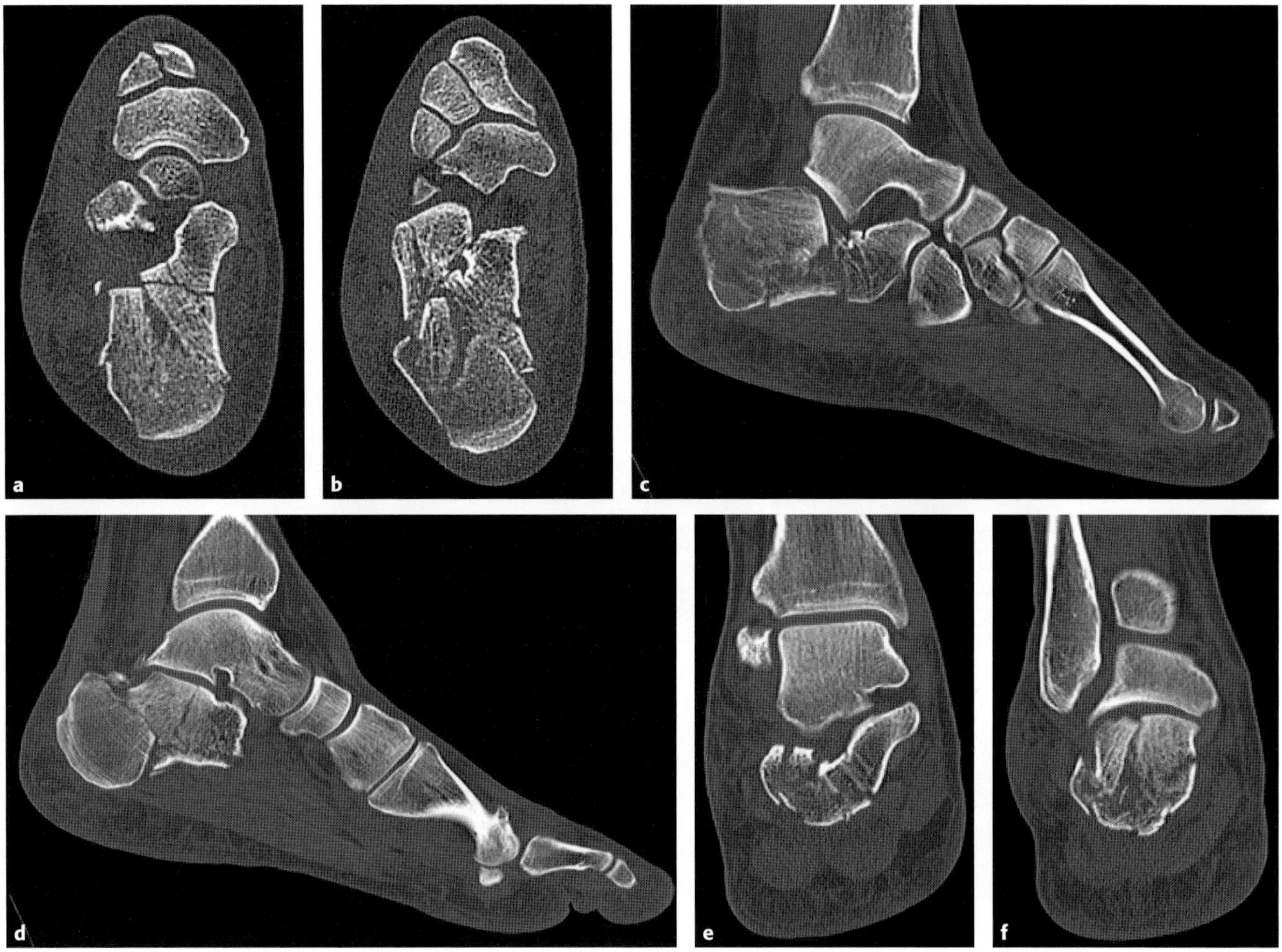

Fig 4.5-2a–f Computed tomographic scans.
a–b Axial view showing comminution of the articular surface and loss of articular congruity and widening of the calcaneal body.
c–d Lateral view showing comminution, intraarticular extension, and posterior facet joint depression.
e–f Coronal view showing comminution, intraarticular extension, and number of articular fragments at the widest portion of the posterior facet.

2 Preoperative planning

Indications for surgery

The indications for surgical treatment in this patient included gross displacement and incongruity of the articular surface. The tuberosity was in significant varus. There was a marked decrease in the Böhler angle and an increase in the angle of Gissane consistent with a significant loss of calcaneal height.

Treatment options

Options for approaches include:

- Lateral extensile (chapter 4.6)
- Sinus tarsi
- Percutaneous techniques (chapter 4.4)

For this patient, the sinus tarsi approach was chosen because it provides adequate visualization of the joint surface and causes limited soft-tissue disruption while still allowing restoration of overall calcaneal anatomy. A prerequisite for treating calcaneal fractures by a sinus tarsi approach is an in-depth understanding of the fracture patterns and reduction techniques necessary for successful fracture reduction. This approach should not compromise the quality of reduction.

A lateral plate can be used for maintaining the articular surface reduction. Several types of plates are available for calcaneal fractures. As the sinus tarsi approach is performed through a small incision, a smaller plate is typically used. A locking or a conventional T-plate 2.4 will maintain the articular surface of the posterior facet and attach it to the anterior process, maintaining the articular reduction. Variable angle (VA) anterolateral locking calcaneal plates 2.7 are also available and may be used in cases with more comminution or decreased bone density.

This patient was healthy, young, non-smoker, and with no diabetes, so a conventional plate (non-locking) was used. Unlike the lateral extensile plates, the smaller sinus tarsi plates do not provide fixation into the tuberosity. Fixation of the tuberosity and maintenance of alignment is achieved using independent screws, typically 3.5 or 4.0 mm, placed percutaneously into the tuberosity (**Fig 4.5-3**).

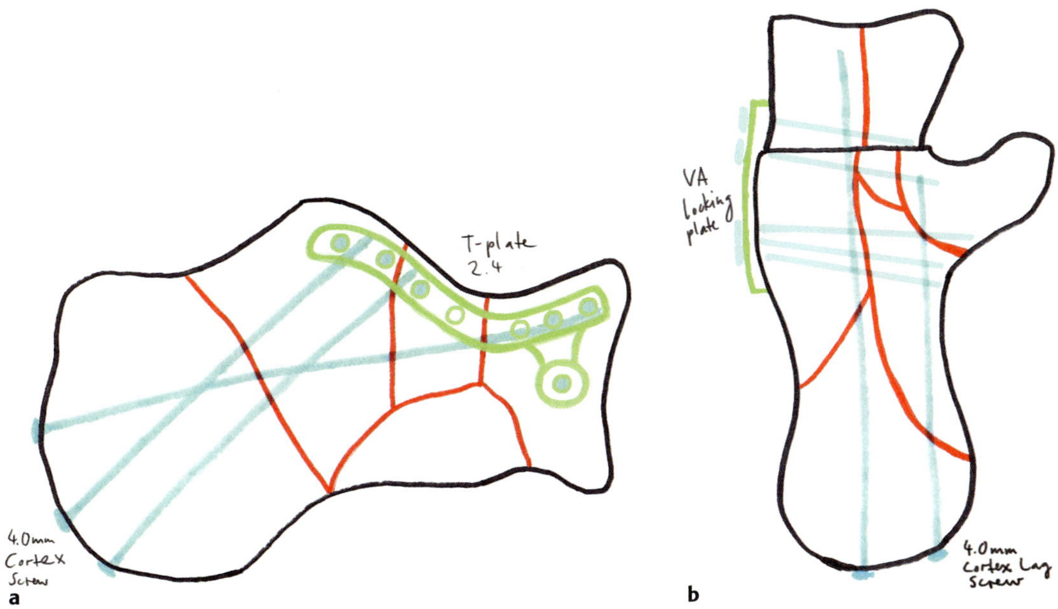

Fig 4.5-3a–b Preoperative plan. Through a sinus tarsi approach, a VA anterolateral locking plate 2.7 is used to maintain the posterior facet reduction, critical angle, and anterior process. Lag screws are inserted percutaneously to maintain the alignment of the medial wall reduction and tuberosity fixation.

3 Operating room setup

Patient positioning	• Lateral decubitus on a radiolucent operative table (injured side up)
Anesthesia options	• General, spinal, or regional
C-arm location	• Monitor on the opposite side of the table and the C-arm entering at an oblique angle from the foot of the bed
Tourniquet	• Used at the surgeon's discretion • Generally, improves fracture visualization
Tips	• Appropriate C-arm position allows all necessary images to be obtained without moving the limb. This is important as a large amount of the reduction and insertion of hardware is performed using the C-arm with the sinus tarsi approach.

For illustrations and overview of anesthetic considerations, see chapter 1. For illustrations and overview of patient and C-arm positioning for calcaneal fracture treatment in the lateral decubitus position refer to chapter 4.

Equipment

- Osteotome
- Small (Freer) elevator
- K-wires and olive wires
- Small plate (VA anterolateral locking plate 2.7, locking T-plate 2.4, or conventional T-plate)
- 2.7 mm fully threaded self-tapping cortex screws
- 4.0 mm fully threaded self-tapping cortex screws
- 4.0 mm Schanz pin
- Headlight for improved visualization

4 Surgical procedure

The skin is examined to ensure it wrinkles and no traumatic wounds or extensive fracture blisters are present where the sinus tarsi incision will be placed (**Fig 4.5-4**). A tourniquet may be used at surgeon's discretion. Joint visualization is often improved with tourniquet use.

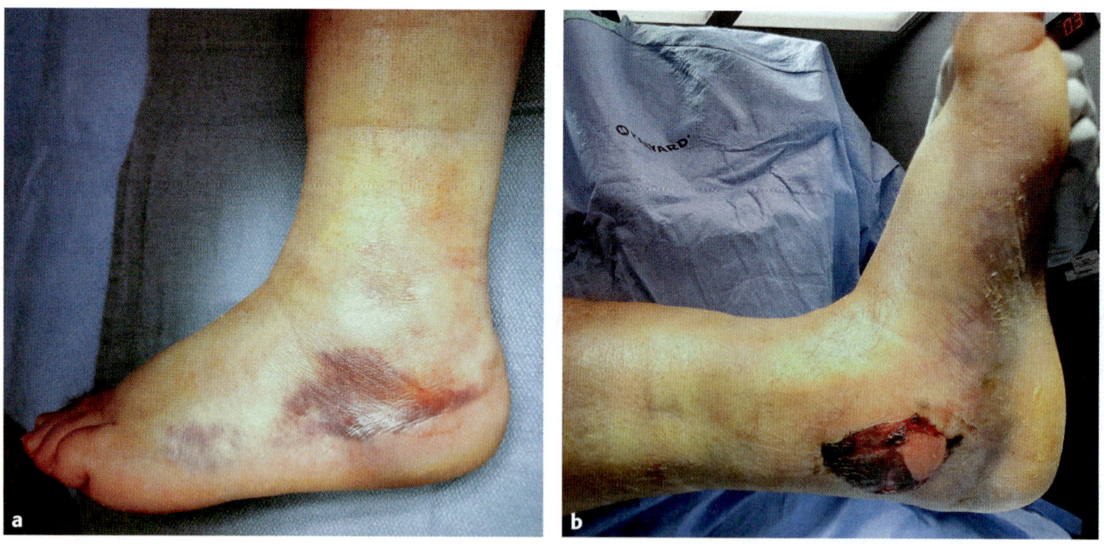

Fig 4.5-4a–b The skin at the beginning of the case showing appropriate swelling resolution with no traumatic skin issues laterally (**a**) and a large medial fracture blister (**b**).

An incision is made over the sinus tarsi just plantar to the tip of the fibula above the peroneal tendons and extended distally to the anterior process. This incision is along the superior aspect of the calcaneus, slightly lower than typically used to expose the subtalar joint for arthrodesis (**Fig 4.5-5**). Be aware that the sural nerve is plantar to the incision and the superficial peroneal nerve is dorsal. The peroneal tendons are identified and elevated off the lateral wall of the calcaneus.

Dissection is then carried down to the joint with a retractor protecting the peroneal tendons. The sinus tarsi soft tissue must be removed to allow visualization, and the lateral capsule of the subtalar joint incised if it is still intact. A small bump of towels can be placed proximal to the malleoli with the foot unsupported in inversion to help improve visualization. A small (Freer) elevator is inserted into the fracture line just below the posterior facet and used to disimpact the lateral fragment of the posterior facet. A small incision is made on the lateral aspect of the tuberosity and a 4.0 mm Schanz pin is inserted from lateral to medial (**Fig 4.5-6**).

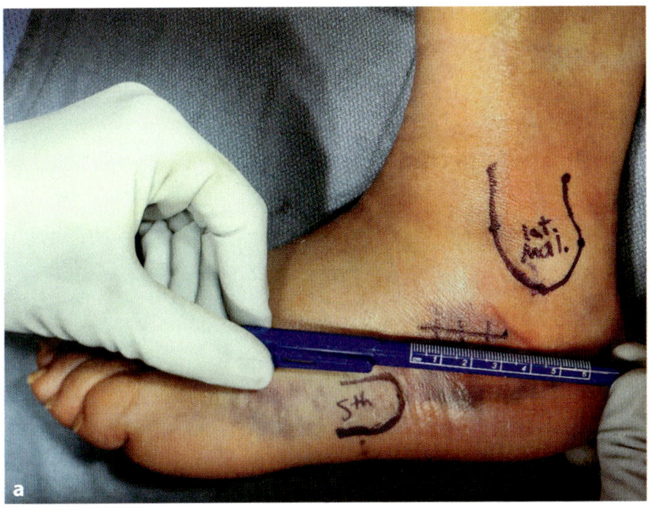

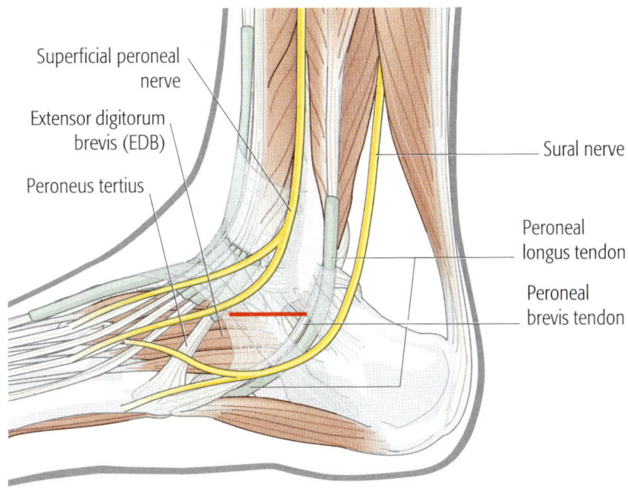

Fig 4.5-5a–b The sinus tarsi approach skin incision (**a**) with underlying anatomy (**b**).

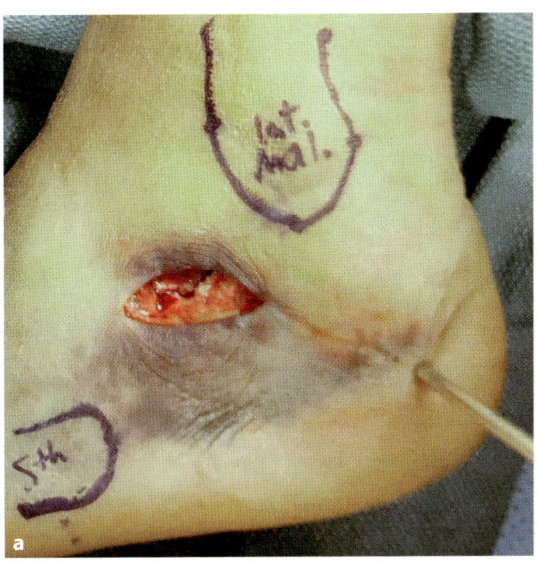

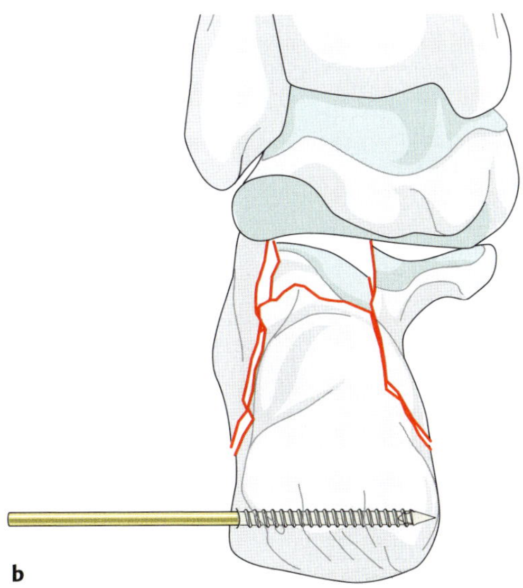

Fig 4.5-6a–b Bicortical placement of the Schanz pin in the tuberosity.

Two small K-wires are placed from the plantar medial tuberosity with one slightly superior to the other and inserted just inside the medial wall, angled dorsally up to the fracture line (**Fig 4.5-7**). An osteotome is then placed under the lateral posterior facet fragment and through the primary fracture line exiting out the medial wall (**Fig 4.5-8**).

A T-handle is placed on the Schanz pin. The medial wall is reduced by manipulating the medial joint surface with the osteotome to elevate and disimpact, combined with a Schanz pin to rotate and realign the tuberosity. This will restore the medial wall height and correct varus.

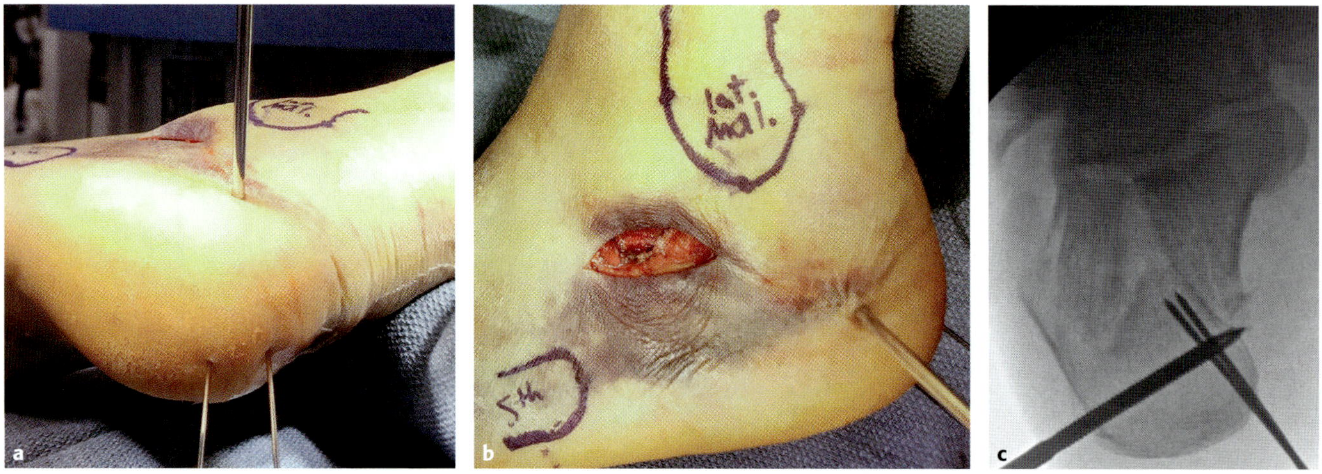

Fig 4.5-7a–c Intraoperative clinical images showing K-wire placement before tuberosity reduction. The wires are placed just inside the medial cortex and directed toward the posterior facet and are driven in just short of the fracture. Two wires are used to prevent rotation (**a–b**). Confirmation of appropriate K-wire position using the C-arm (**c**).

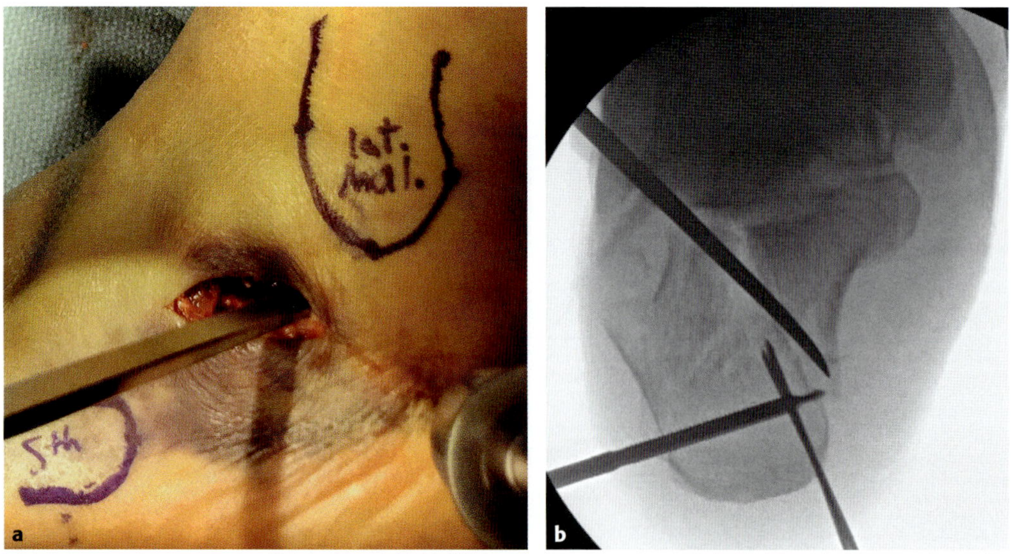

Fig 4.5-8a–b Osteotome placement through the primary fracture line and out the medial wall.

Once reduction is acceptable on the C-arm, an assistant advances the previously placed K-wires across the fracture while the surgeon holds the reduction (**Fig 4.5-9**). At the surgeon's discretion, a small distractor can be used to aid in reduction.

See chapter 4.4 for description on how to use a distractor as a reduction aid in calcaneal fracture fixation.

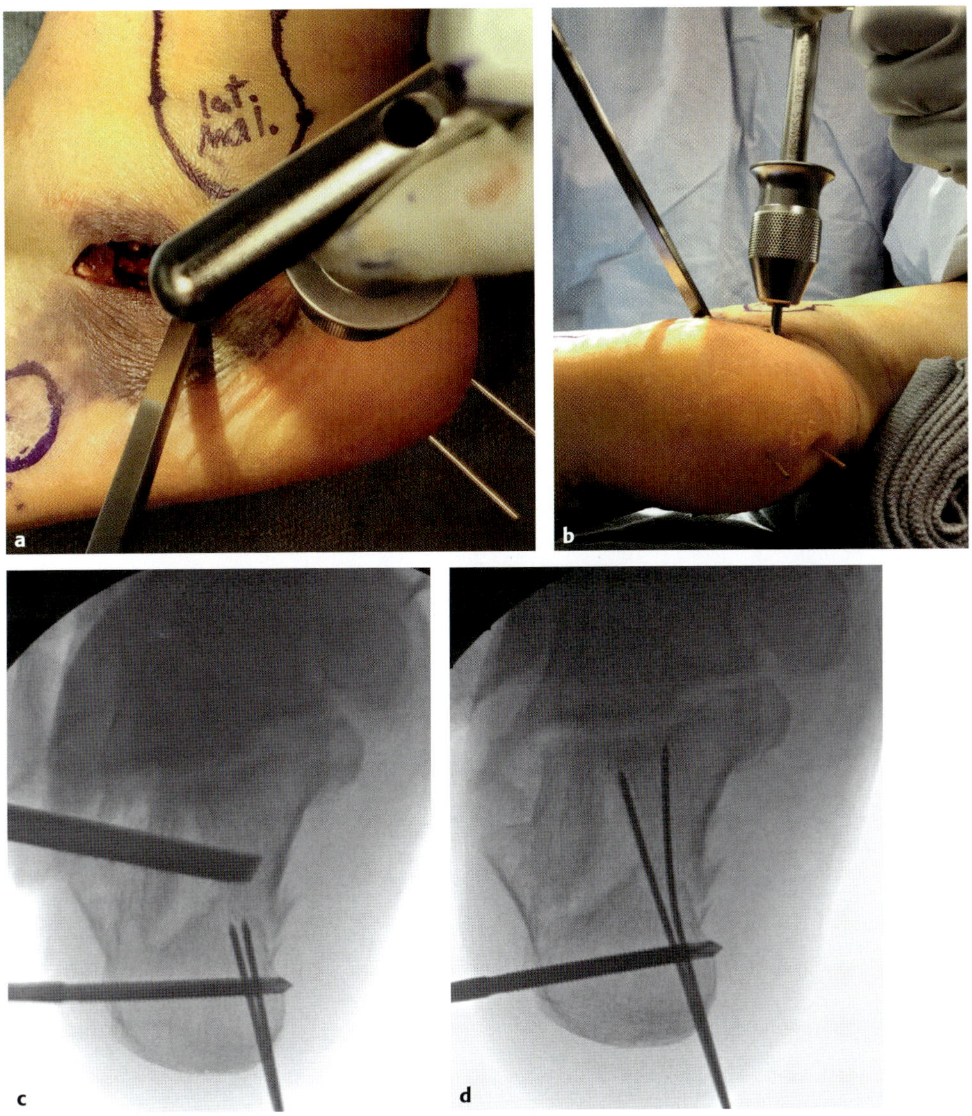

Fig 4.5-9a–d The osteotome is used to elevate the medial articular surface and the Schanz pin is used to align the tuber reducing the medial wall (**a–c**). The K-wires are then advanced across the fracture line (**d**).

Next, the articular surface of the posterior facet reduction can be accomplished by inserting a small K-wire into the lateral posterior facet fragment. This wire is placed just under the articular surface to avoid interfering with plate placement. A drill sleeve is placed over the K-wire and used as a joystick to maneuver the fragment into appropriate position. Often, more than one K-wire is needed. Once the fragment is in appropriate position, the K-wire is advanced to provisionally hold the reduction (**Fig 4.5-10**). Additional K-wires may be used, if necessary, to aid in reduction. A minimum of two provisional K-wires are required to maintain reduction and prevent rotation.

Next the anterior process and critical angle are reduced. Reduction is performed under direct visualization. The anterior process is typically elevated, and a dental instrument/scaler is used to reduce this down to the leading edge of the posterior facet at the critical angle. In this location the bone is dense and the fracture line will have an accurate reduction read. While the reduction is held in place, K-wires are brought through the skin into the anterior process and directed posterior into the calcaneal body for provisional fixation (**Fig 4.5-11**).

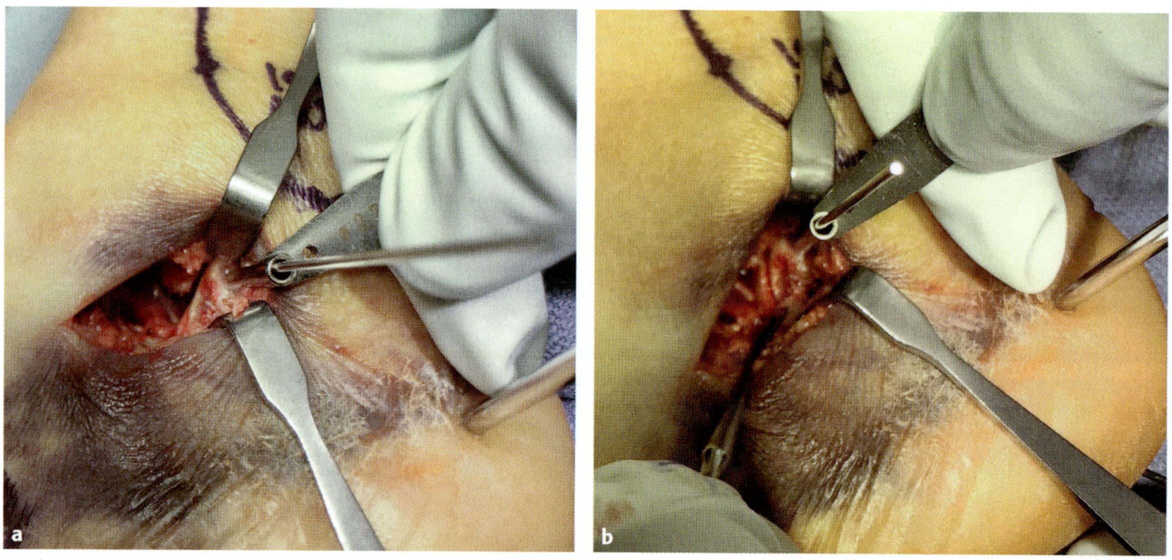

Fig 4.5-10a–b Reduction of the posterior facet.
a The posterior facet before reduction with a K-wire is positioned so that it will not interfere with plate placement. The drill guide is over the K-wire to use as a joystick to aid in reduction of the articular surface. Often more than one wire will be used.
b The posterior facet after reduction with the K-wire advanced to hold the reduction.

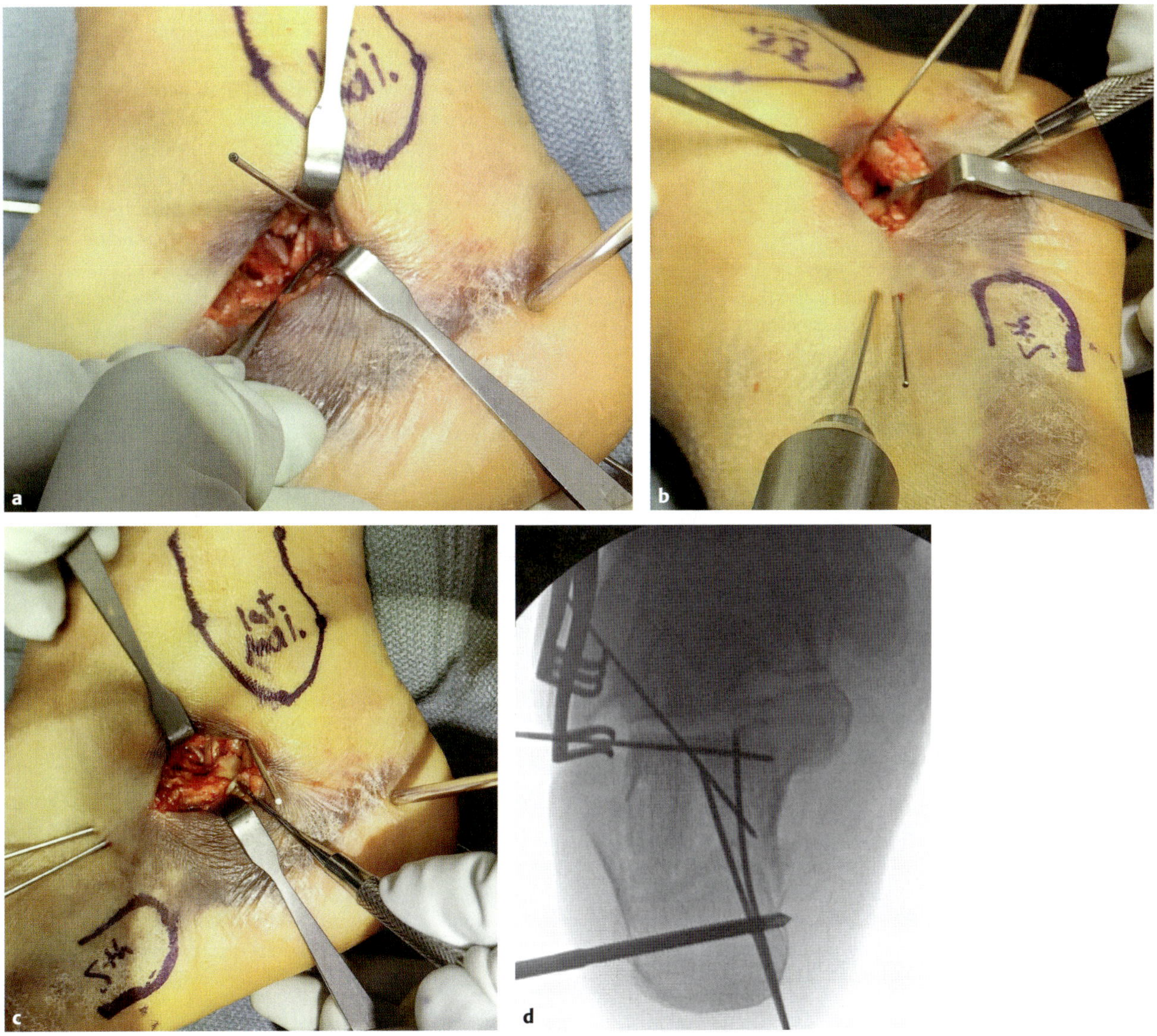

Fig 4.5-11a–d The critical angle and anterior process are before reduction (**a**). Two K-wires are inserted through the anterior process toward the calcaneal body to hold the reduction of the anterior process and critical angle (**b–d**).

Fixation of the posterior facet to the anterior process using a plate

A plate is inserted and placed on the lateral aspect of the calcaneus just plantar to the critical angle with holes in position to connect the posterior facet, critical angle, and anterior process. Care is taken to ensure the plate is not on the peroneal tendons and that the lateral wall fragment is contained under the plate.

A common error is to not release the peroneal tendons off the lateral wall of the calcaneus at the peroneal tubercle. The lateral cortical fragment, often referred as the lateral wall blow-out, is pulled away by the peroneal tendons. If the tendons are not released the plate may inadvertently be placed between the lateral cortical wall and the body of the calcaneus. After the plate is in the correct position, threaded ball-tipped compression wires can be used to hold the plate in place (**Fig 4.5-12**). Two 2.7 mm cortex lag screws are placed through the plate underneath the posterior facet to stabilize the articular surface. Two screws are placed into the anterior process and then the K-wires in the anterior process are removed.

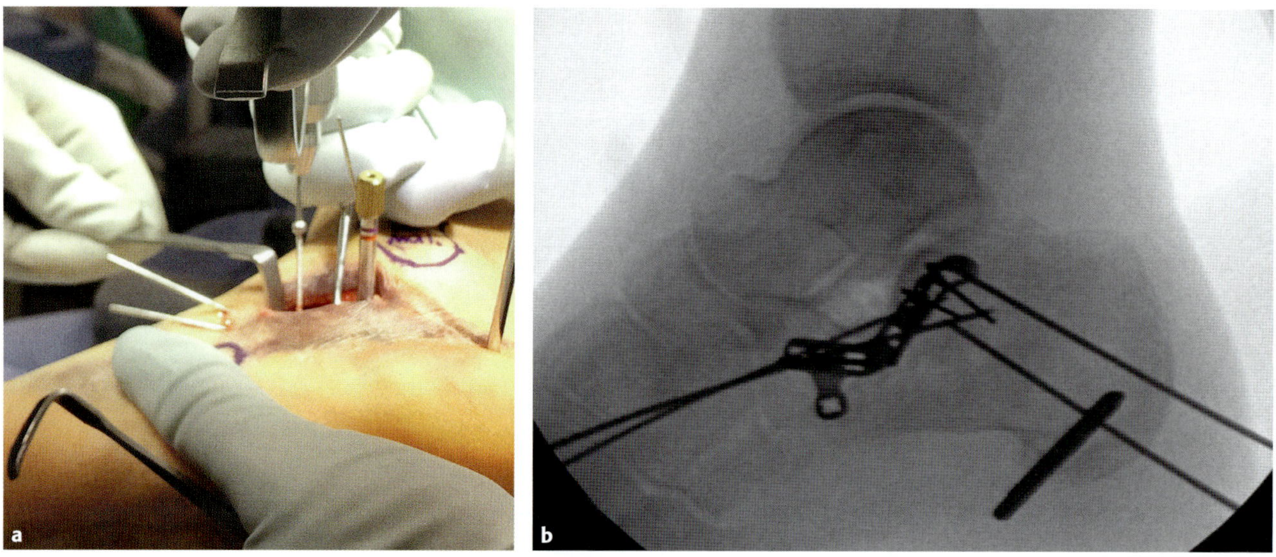

Fig 4.5-12a–b The plate is inserted onto the lateral of the calcaneus and holding in place with threaded ball-tipped compression wires (**a**). C-arm image showing the plate in correct position (**b**).

Fixation of the tuberosity to articular segment with screws

A small incision is made in the posterior tuberosity between the tuberosity K-wires holding the medial wall reduction. The Schanz pin is removed to avoid interfering with hardware insertion. A 4.0 mm cortex screw is inserted just inside the medial wall of the tuberosity in line with the K-wires to stabilize the calcaneal height and alignment. A second 4.0 mm screw is placed along the medial wall of the tuberosity directed toward the posterior facet (**Fig 4.5-13**). Both posterior tuberosity K-wires are removed. Two points of fixation are always necessary to prevent loss of reduction.

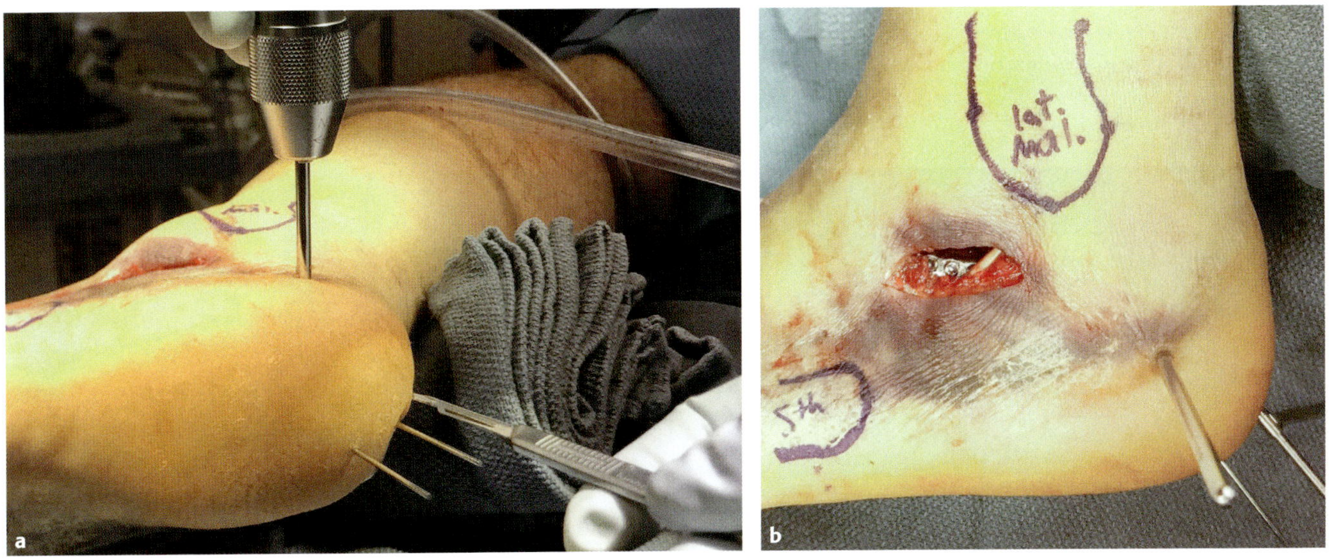

Fig 4.5-13a–b A small incision is made just superior to the K-wires used to maintain the medial wall reduction (**a**) and an appropriate length 4.0 mm cortex screw is drilled in line with the K-wire (**b**). A second screw will be placed between the two K-wires to complete fixation of the fracture line exiting the medial wall.

Fixation of the tuberosity to the anterior process with screws

Another small incision is made just medial to the previous two (centered medial to lateral). A small incision is then made centrally on the tuberosity and a 4.0 mm screw is drilled from the posterior tuberosity to the anterior process, measured and placed (**Fig 4.5-14**). Additional 4.0 mm cortex screws may be placed as needed based on the fracture pattern.

The joint is inspected under direct visualization, palpitation with a small (Freer) elevator and an C-arm to assess anatomical reduction (**Fig 4.5-15**). The wound is thoroughly irrigated. The tourniquet is deflated, and hemostasis is confirmed. Skin tension is relieved by placing a small towel bump distal to the malleoli everting the foot, assisting in wound closure (**Fig 4.5-16**). The sinus tarsi incision is closed with 2-0 braided absorbable for subcutaneous tissue and 3-0 nylon in a tension-relieving fashion for the skin. The small incisions are closed with simple sutures (**Fig 4.5-17**). A sterile dressing is applied consisting of adaptic, gauze, and nonadherent dressing with undercast roll padding. The patient is placed in a well-padded, posterior sugar-tong splint.

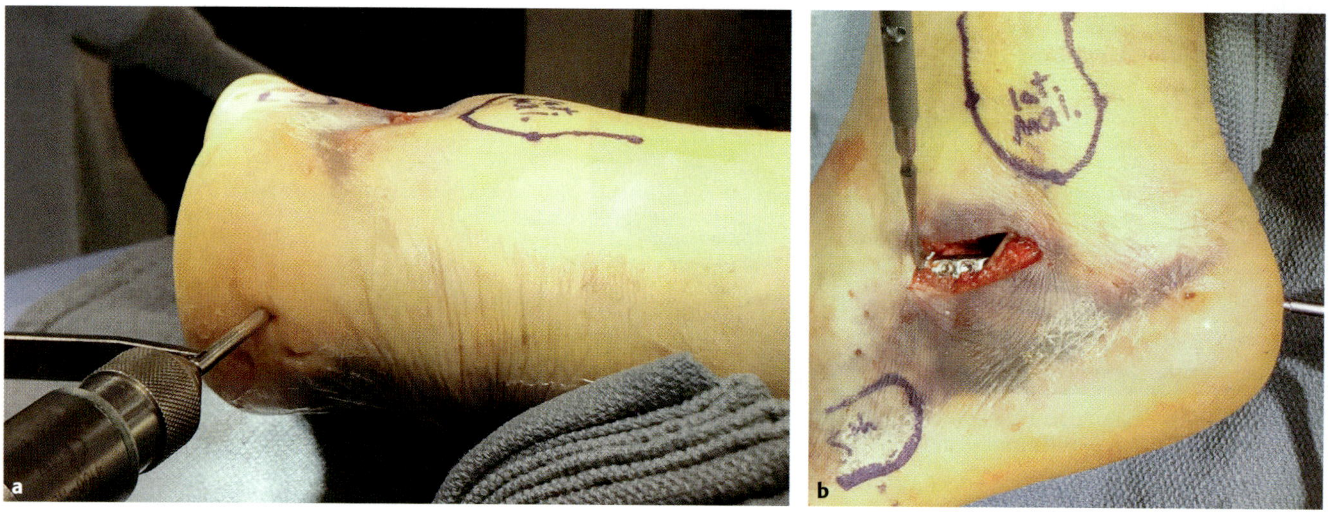

Fig 4.5-14a–b A final 4.0 mm cortex screw is drilled in starting just lateral to the previous two screws (**a**) and directed toward the anterior process. Ideally, the screw will be placed just inferior and distal to the plate as indicated by the small (Freer) elevator (**b**).

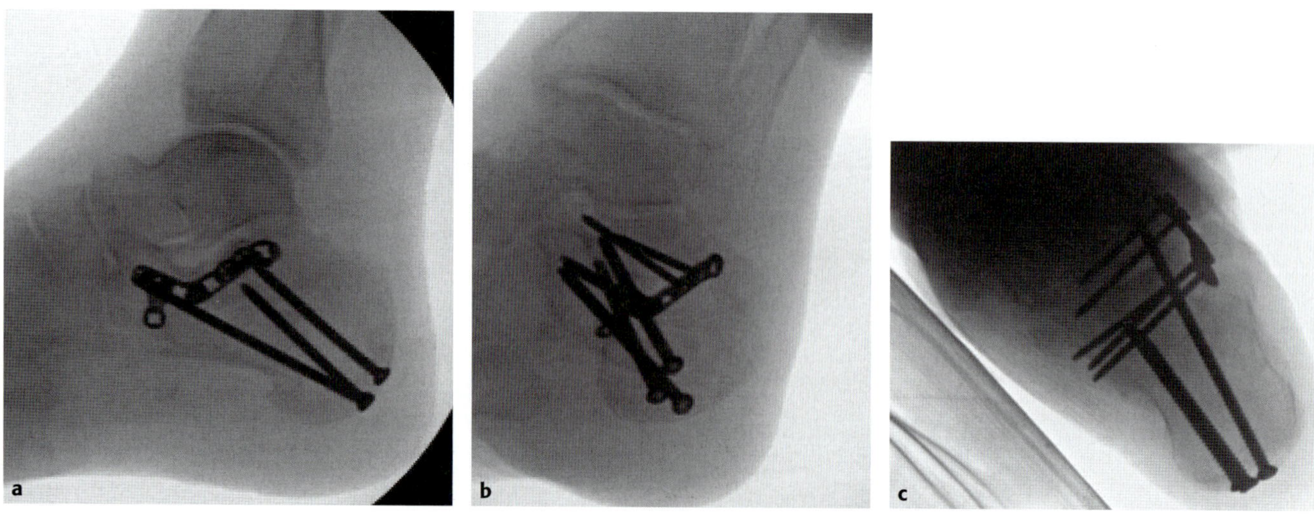

Fig 4.5-15a–c Final intraoperative images of the definitive fixation with anatomical reduction.
a Lateral view.
b Broden view.
c Axial view.

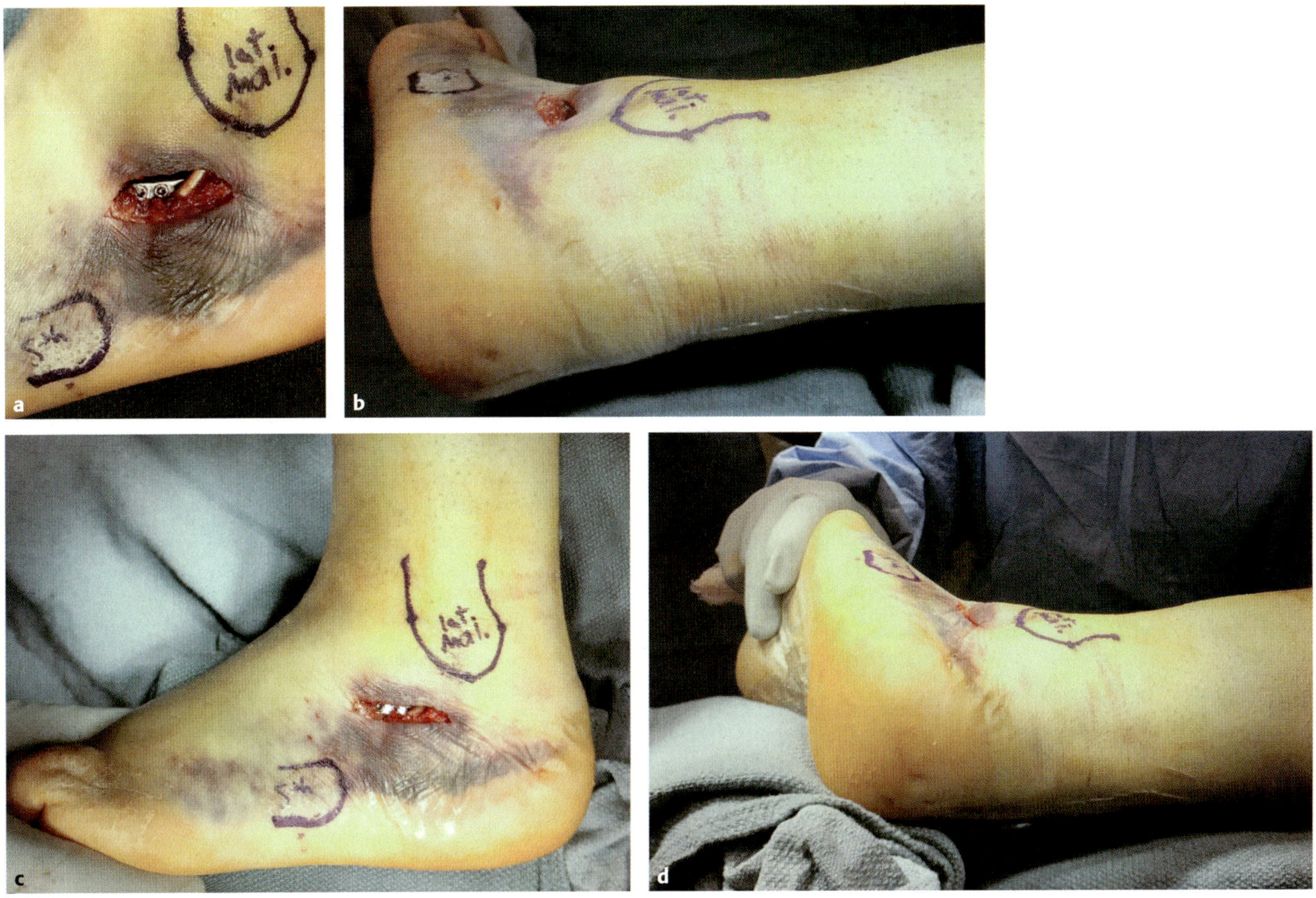

Fig 4.5-16a–d Final fixation and a small portion of the peroneal tendons are visible through the sinus tarsi incision (**a**). A towel bump is proximal to the malleoli improving visualization by allowing the subtalar joint to invert. The small incisions are used to insert the independent screws from the tuberosity (**b**). To decrease skin tension at the sinus tarsi incision the towel bump may be placed under the foot distal to the malleoli causing eversion aiding in wound closure with less tension (**c–d**).

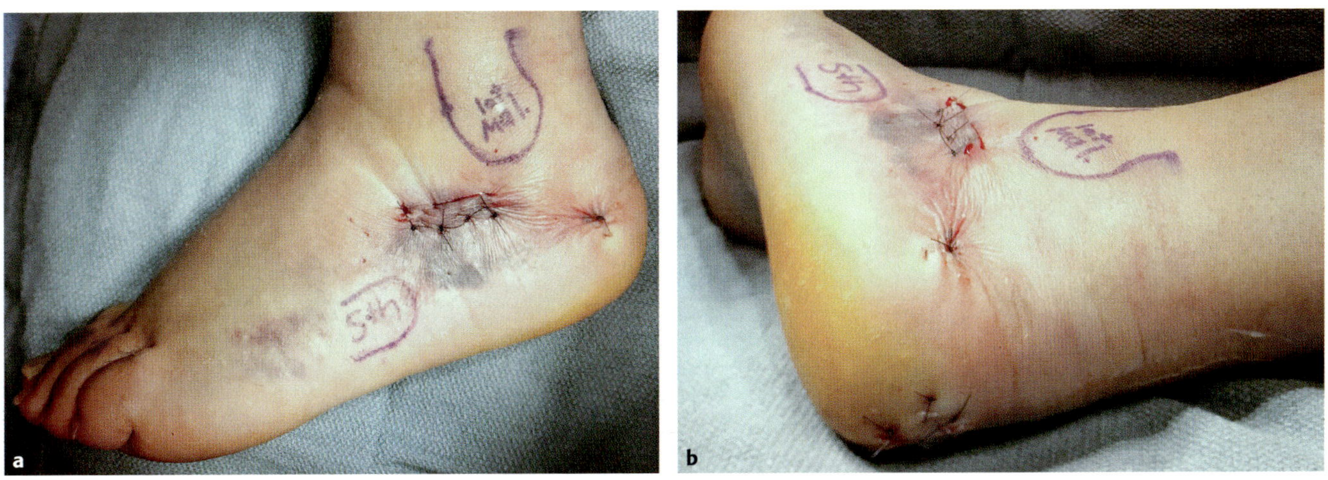

Fig 4.5-17a–b Closure of all incisions with 2-0 braided absorbable suture for subcutaneous tissue and 3-0 nylon suture for skin.

5 Pitfalls and complications

Pitfalls

Inadequate reduction of the posterior facet

The sinus tarsi approach allows for direct visualization of the posterior facet. However, in severely displaced injuries, anatomical landmarks are distorted which may result in the incision being placed too inferior or superior. A poorly placed incision makes it challenging to visualize the posterior facet but may be compensated by elongating the incision, thus creating a larger mobile window resulting in improved visualization.

Surgeon experience is essential. The surgeon must be familiar with the 3D geometry of the calcaneus, fracture patterns and reduction techniques required to reduce these difficult fractures. This knowledge increases the likelihood of successful reconstruction of the entire shape of the calcaneus. Surgeons unfamiliar with this technique are encouraged to begin with simpler fracture patterns.

Inadequate reduction and fixation of the varus malalignment

The varus malalignment is indirectly reduced. To verify correct reduction and placement of fixation, perfect intraoperative images must be obtained. If the C-arm is not set up correctly, or the person operating the C-arm is inexperienced, this can be difficult. It is important to take time at the beginning of the case to set up the C-arm properly and to discuss with the appropriate staff member how to obtain the necessary images, particularly the heel view of the calcaneus.

Irreducible fragments

Remove small intercalary fragments that cannot be stabilized with direct or indirect stabilization. These fragments can displace into the joint as a loose joint body.

Complications

- Wound-healing complications
- Injury or irritation of the peroneal tendons
- Irritation of the posterior heel with screw placement
- Loss of fixation
- Malunion
- Nonunion
- Subtalar posttraumatic arthritis

6 Alternative techniques

Alternative approaches include:

- Percutaneous techniques, see chapter 4.4 and chapter 4.6
- Lateral extensile approach, see chapter 4.6.

Plate options include plate 2.4, both locking (**Fig 4.5-18**) and nonlocking in addition to VA locking plates 2.7.

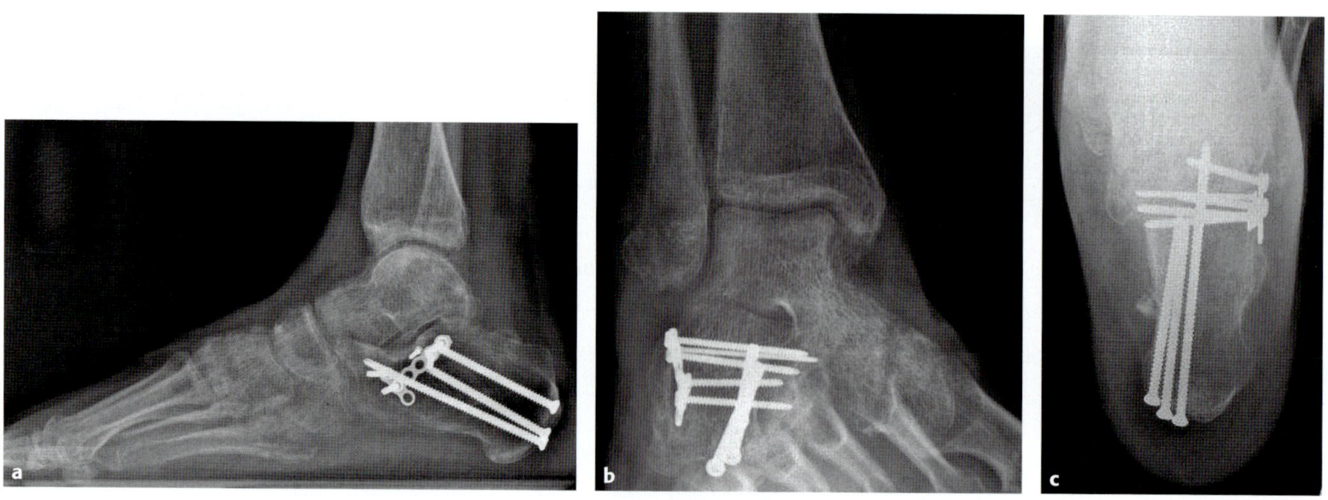

Fig 4.5-18a–c Example from a different case of a 77-year-old man treated with a locking plate 2.4.
a Lateral view.
b Brodén view.
c Axial view.

7 Postoperative management and rehabilitation

Postoperatively, the foot is immobilized in a bulky Jones splint without any pressure over the heel. The patient is administered antibiotics postoperatively for 24 hours. Patients are given instructions on NWB and elevation with specific counseling on the importance of maintaining these recommendations for wound healing.

The first follow-up is at 2 weeks postoperatively when the splint is removed, incisions inspected, and sutures removed. The foot is then placed in a posterior splint orthosis and the patient is instructed to maintain a NWB status. At this point, the patient can start active range-of-motion exercises.

At 6 weeks, the patient is seen in the outpatient office and an x-ray is taken (**Fig 4.5-19**). The images are scrutinized for anatomical reduction and healing. If the fracture is healed, the patient may increase weight bearing. Progression to full weight bearing typically occurs over of 2–4 weeks. If the fracture is not healed, the patient must maintain the NWB status and is reevaluated within another 2–4 weeks. If there are any concerns regarding healing, perform a CT scan.

Implant removal

Some patients experience hardware irritation. The implants causing the irritation may be removed. Hardware removal is typically not performed until at least 1 year after surgery. An arthrolysis of the subtalar joint is performed at the same time as hardware removal.

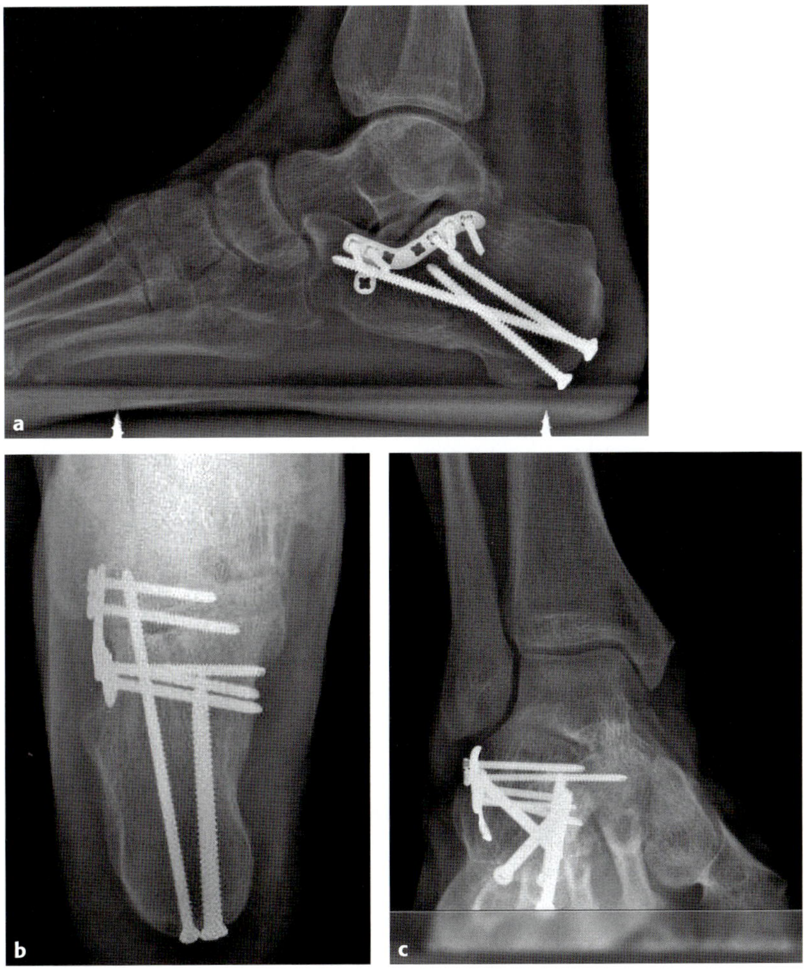

Fig 4.5-19a–c Postoperative x-rays at 6 weeks.
a Lateral view.
b Axial view
c Brodén view

8 Recommended reading

Basile A, Albo F, Via AG. Comparison between sinus tarsi approach and extensile lateral approach for treatment of closed displaced intraarticular calcaneal fractures: a multicenter prospective study. *J Foot Ankle Surg.* 2016 May–Jun;55(3):513–521.

Rammelt S, Sangeorzan BJ, Swords MP. Calcaneal fractures—should we or should we not operate? *Indian J Orthop.* 2018 May–Jun;52(3):220–230.

Schepers T, Backes M, Dingemans SA, et al. Similar anatomical reduction and lower complication rates with the sinus tarsi approach compared with the extended lateral approach in displaced intraarticular calcaneal fractures. *J Orthop Trauma.* 2017 Jun;31(6):293–298.

Swords M, Brady C, Popovich J. Wound complications in calcaneus fractures treated with the sinus tarsi approach: results in 164 consecutive fractures. *Foot Ankle Orthop.* 2017 Sept 1;2(3).

Swords MP, Rammelt S, Sands AK. Nonextensile techniques for treatment of calcaneus fractures. In: Pfeffer G, Easley M, Hintermann B, et al, eds. *Operative Techniques: Foot and Ankle Surgery.* 2nd Ed. New York: Elsevier; 2018:319–326.

Swords MP, Penny P. Early fixation of calcaneus fractures. *Foot Ankle Clin.* 2017 Mar;22(1):93–104.

Yao H, Liang T, Xu Y, et al. Sinus tarsi approach versus extensile lateral approach for displaced intraarticular calcaneal fracture: a meta-analysis of current evidence base. *J Orthop Surg Res.* 2017 Mar 14;12(1):43.

Yeo JH, Cho HJ, Lee KB. Comparison of two surgical approaches for displaced intra-articular calcaneal fractures: sinus tarsi versus extensile lateral approach. *BMC Musculoskelet Disord.* 2015 Mar 19;16:63.

4.6 Complex articular fracture (Sanders 3/4)—extensile approach

Tim Schepers

1 Case description

A 47-year-old healthy woman was involved in a head-on automobile crash. She was extracted from the vehicle by fire-fighters and brought to the hospital by ambulance where she underwent initial screening in the emergency department. She was hemodynamically stable and not in respiratory distress but had sustained multiple injuries which included a sternal fracture, a stable pelvis fracture, and a right foot-ankle injury. On the medial side of the ankle, there was a 3 cm laceration with protruding bone fragments.

The lateral and AP x-rays of the right foot and ankle showed a distal tibial fracture and a calcaneal fracture (Essex-Lopresti tongue-type calcaneal fracture) with a depressed Böhler angle of –28° (**Fig 4.6-1**).

The Gustilo-Anderson grade II open distal tibia fracture required an external fixator. As the definitive treatment was planned from lateral, it was decided to place the external fixator medially and to keep the calcaneal soft tissues clean (**Fig 4.6-2**).

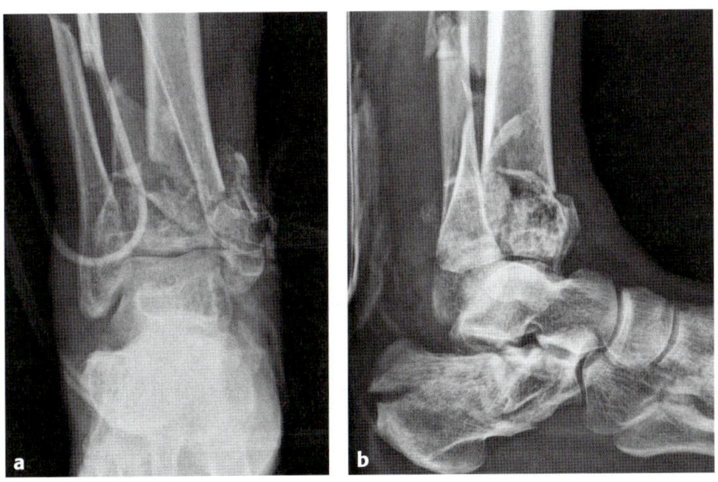

Fig 4.6-1a–b Postinjury images.
a AP x-ray of the ankle showing pilon fracture.
b Lateral x-ray of the ankle showing pilon and tongue-type calcaneal fracture.

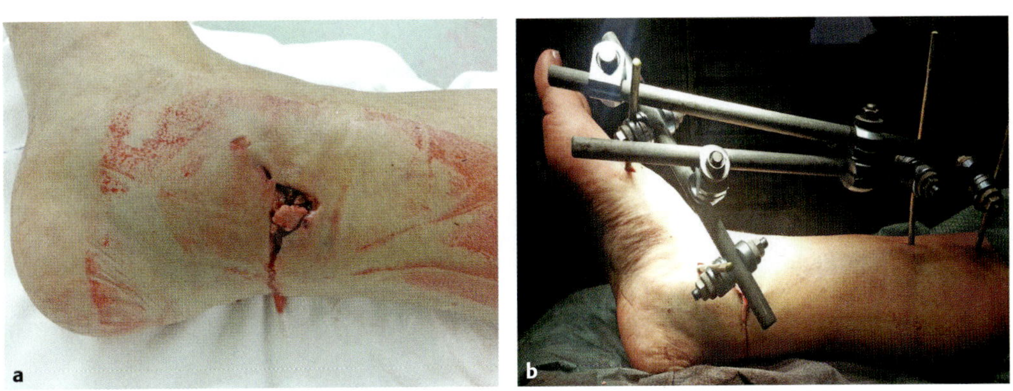

Fig 4.6-2a–b Soft tissues and external fixator placement.
a Soft-tissue injury on medial side of ankle.
b External fixator placement in the tibia, talar neck, and first metatarsal.

In addition to the conventional imaging, a computed tomographic (CT) scan was performed to assess the extent of the pilon and calcaneal fractures, as part of the preoperative plan. The fracture of the calcaneus was classified as a Sanders type 3BC injury (AO/OTA 82C2) (**Fig 4.6-3** and **Fig 4.6-4**). The management of the AO/OTA 43C3 pilon fracture is covered in chapter 2.3.

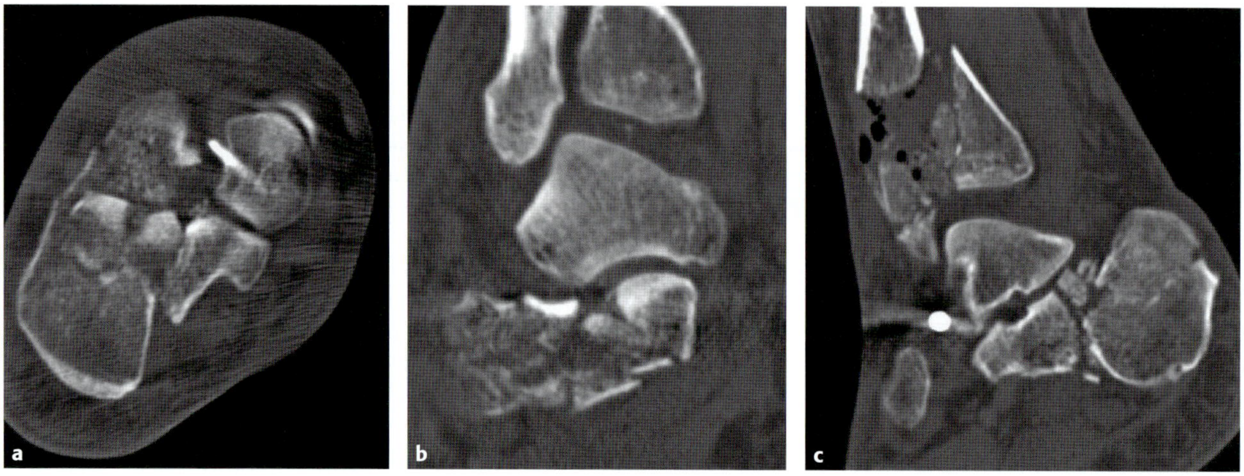

Fig 4.6-3a–c The CT images.
a Sanders type 3BC fracture on semicoronal view.
b Axial view showing comminuted fracture with bulging of lateral wall.
c Sagittal view of medial portion showing multifragmentary posterior talocalcaneal joint.

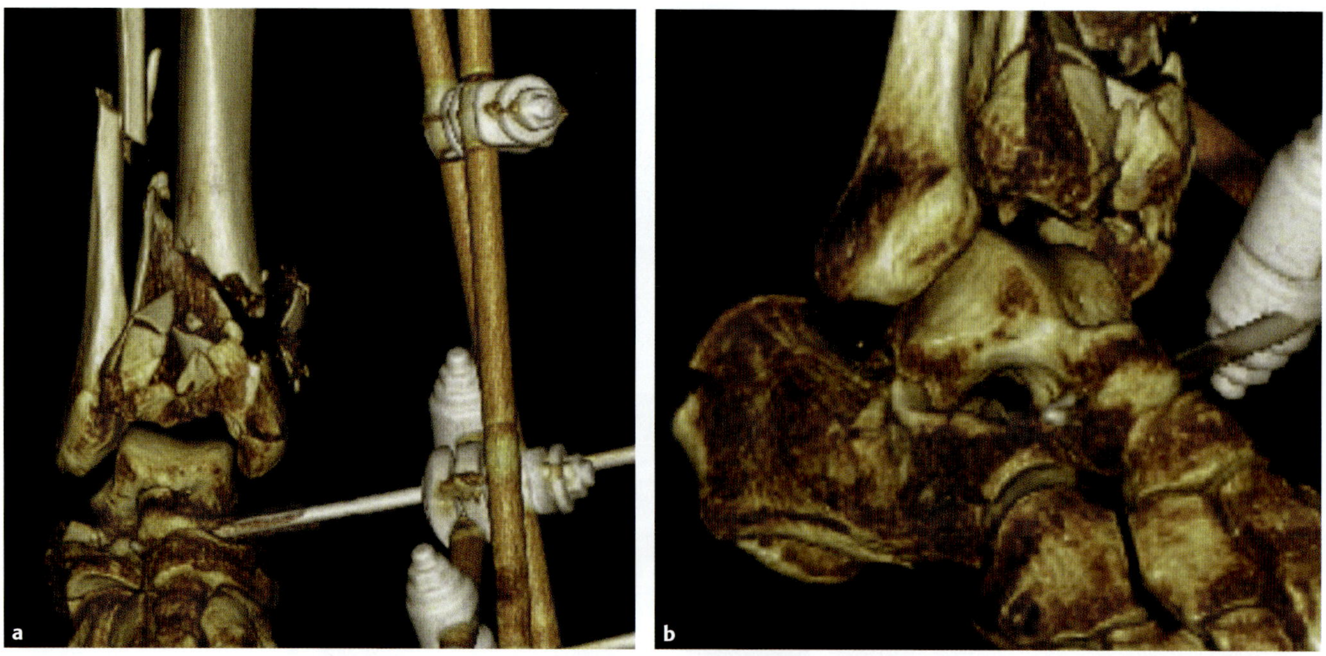

Fig 4.6-4a–b A 3D rendering of pilon and calcaneal fracture for preoperative planning.
a AP view of pilon fracture.
b Three-quarter projection showing calcaneal fracture.

2 Preoperative planning

Most surgeons agree that in comminuted fractures with severe displacement, surgery provides superior outcome over nonoperative management. Depending on the fracture anatomy, several approaches are available:

- Fully percutaneous with or without arthroscopic control
- Less invasive sinus tarsi approach
- Fully open extended lateral approach (ELA)

As the patient was a healthy nonsmoker, an ELA was scheduled for management. A preoperative plan was made (**Fig 4.6-5**).

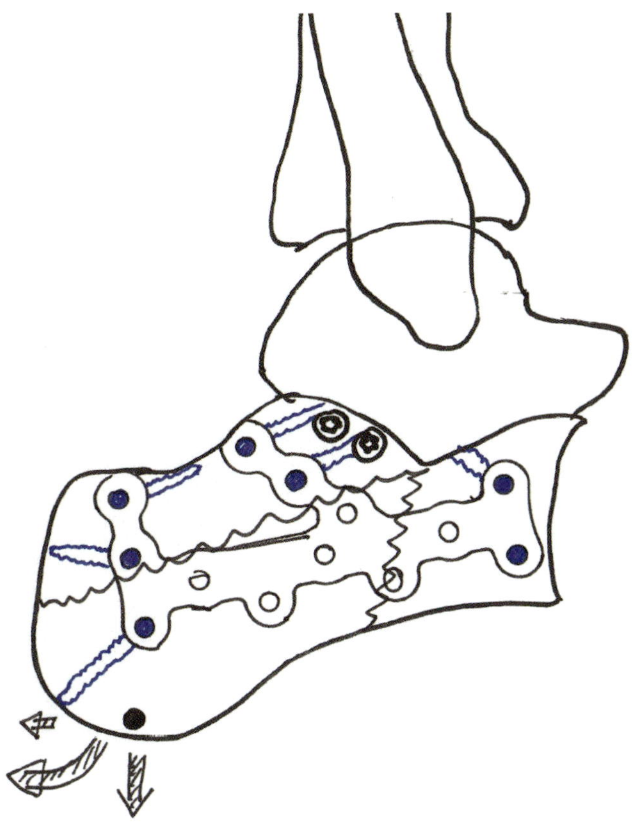

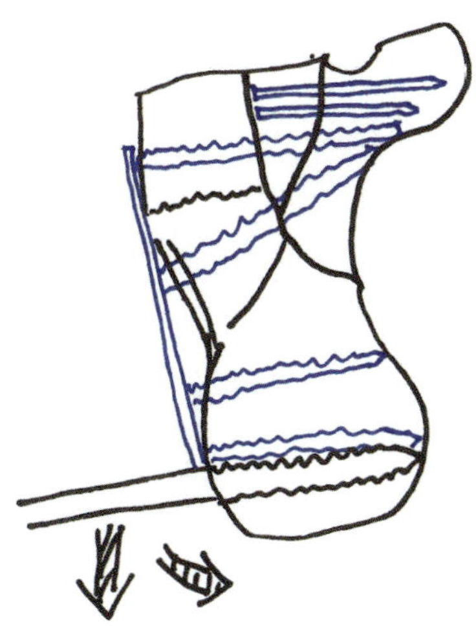

Fig 4.6-5 Preoperative plan.

3 Operating room setup

Patient positioning	• Lateral decubitus position on a radiolucent table (injured side up)
Anesthesia options	• General, spinal, or regional
C-arm location	• Monitor on the opposite side of the operative table with the C-arm entering at an oblique angle from the foot of the bed
Tourniquet	• At the surgeon's discretion • Generally, it improves fracture visualization
Tips	• A bean bag can be positioned just above the malleolus allowing for inversion of the subtalar joint (**Fig 4.6-6**). • Alternatively, if the leg is placed on an elevated ramp or blankets a small towel bump can be placed just proximal to the malleolus to allow for inversion of the subtalar joint improving visualization

For illustrations and overview of anesthetic considerations, see chapter 1. For illustrations and overview of patient and C-arm positioning for calcaneal fracture treatment in the lateral decubitus position refer to chapter 4.

Equipment

- K-wires in various lengths
- Small distraction device
- 3.0–5.0 Schanz pin
- 3.5 mm cancellous and cortex screws
- Periosteal elevator and small (Freer) or small spatula (Howard) elevator
- Calcaneal plate
- Power tools (drill, oscillating saw)

4 Surgical procedure

Adequate time between injury and definitive surgery allows for swelling to settle and soft-tissue recovery. This recovery is indicated by the return of soft-tissue wrinkles in the skin around the foot and ankle.

In most cases, a sharp 100–110° angled incision is used, with the vertical limb situated almost on the lateral edge of the Achilles tendon (**Fig. 4.6-6**). The straight horizontal limb of the incision is placed at the level at which the smooth skin of the lateral aspect transitions to the hyperkeratotic skin of the plantar aspect of the foot (glabrous junction) aimed slightly below the tip of the fifth metatarsal. A full-thickness flap containing the sural nerve, calcaneofibular ligament, and peroneal tendons is created, and is retracted superiorly using small hand-held retractors. Alternatively, the flap can be retracted by inserting temporary 2.0 mm K-wires into the fibula, talus and cuboid. The wires are then bent at 90° to facilitate operative exposure and retraction (commonly referred to as the no-touch technique). To prevent soft-tissue injury and wound edge necrosis the use of self-retaining retractors should be avoided. Either a Schanz pin is placed in the proximal plantar portion of the tuber to restore length or a small distractor is used, as in this case.

The lateral wall is opened, and the lateral joint fragment is either tilted outward in the case of a tongue-type fracture or temporarily removed and placed in saline on the back table, in a joint-depression type fracture. A Schanz pin can be inserted from posterior into the tongue fragment to manipulate it. The medial joint fragment (sustentaculum fragment) is pushed against the talus and the tuber is brought out to length and pushed medially back under the sustentaculum fragment to reestablish appropriate height and alignment. An osteotome or smooth elevator may be useful to realign the tuberosity beneath the sustentaculum thus restoring the medial wall (see chapter 4.5). Temporary K-wires are placed along the medial wall to stabilize the tuber and medial joint fragment.

The next step is to reduce and fix the central joint fragment. K-wires are used as joysticks and upon adequate reduction they are advanced. The axial view allows visualization of the medial wall assuring that the K-wires do not penetrate the area of the neurovascular bundle or flexor hallucis longus tendon. They are retracted a few millimeters and cut off, after which they are advanced again with a small bone-punch until they are flush with the level of the fragment. Alternatively, bioabsorbable pins may be used to stabilize the central fragment.

After reduction of the central fragment(s) the lateral joint fragment is placed back and reduced. The reduction is again held with temporary K-wires. The reduction can be checked using C-arm views and gentle manipulation of the hindfoot so as not to displace the reduced fragments. The next step is to reduce the anterior process restoring the angle of Gis-

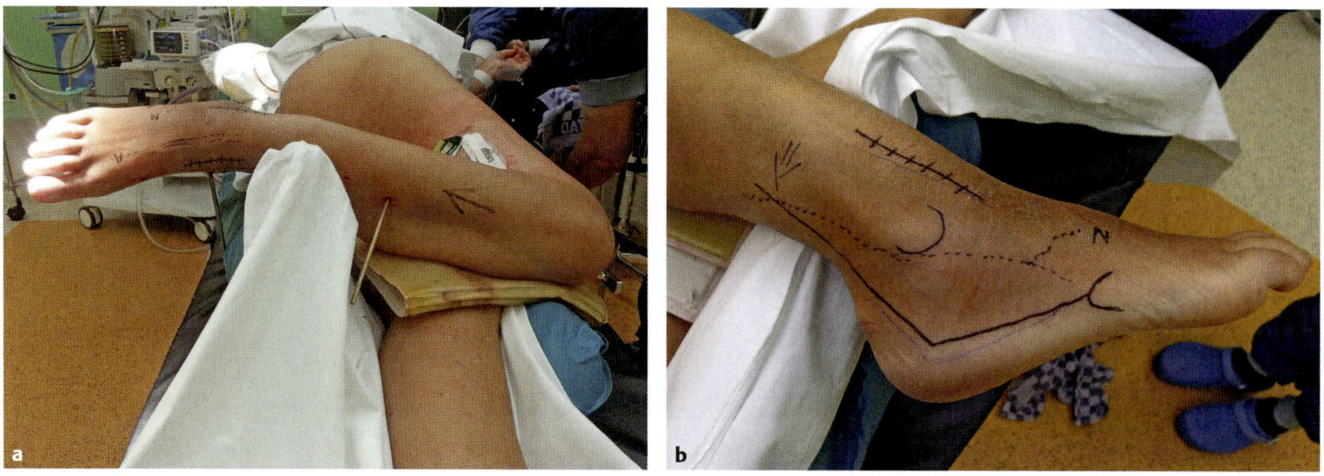

Fig 4.6-6a–b Patient positioning.
a The patient is positioned in a lateral decubitus position, with the injured leg flexed. The C-arm is on the opposite side. Adequate padding is provided.
b The extended lateral approach is drawn (with estimated course of the sural nerve for reference).

sane. This is sometimes a loose fragment which must be reduced separately. A smooth elevator can be inserted in the canalis tarsi to bring down the anterior process, until it lines up with the lateral subtalar joint fragment. A temporary K-wire is inserted from distal to posterior to stabilize the anterior process (**Fig 4.6-7**). A calcaneal plate is used with or without previous placement of one or two screws just beneath the subtalar joint surface (**Fig 4.6-8**). A closed suction drain is sometimes used as per surgeon preference. The skin is closed using interrupted subcuticular absorbable 2-0 sutures followed by nonabsorbable vertical tension relieving matrass sutures. A bulky dressing with a 3-sided ("AO") splint is applied.

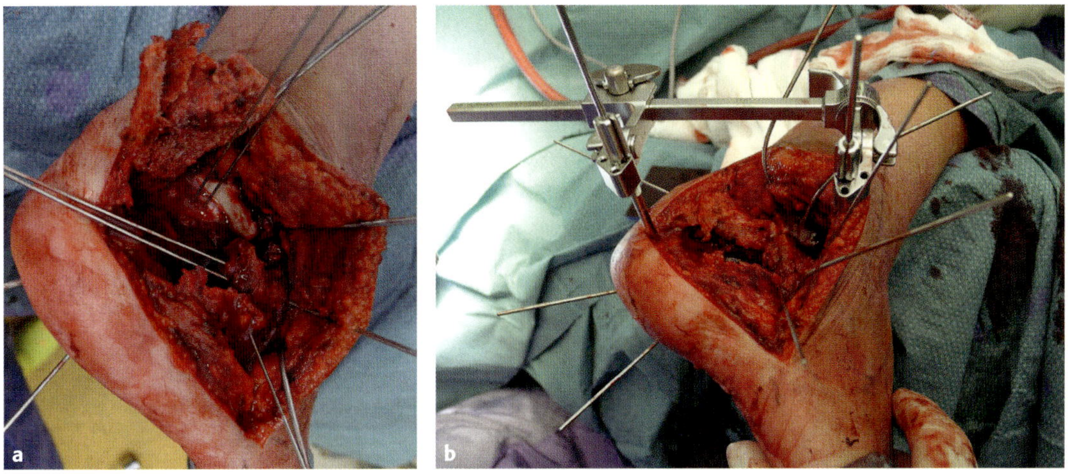

Fig 4.6-7a–b Intraoperative images.
a Extended lateral approach, with K-wires for flap retraction. Central fragment and anterior joint fragment reduced and held each with two K-wires.
b Placement of small distractor to facilitate reduction of height and length.

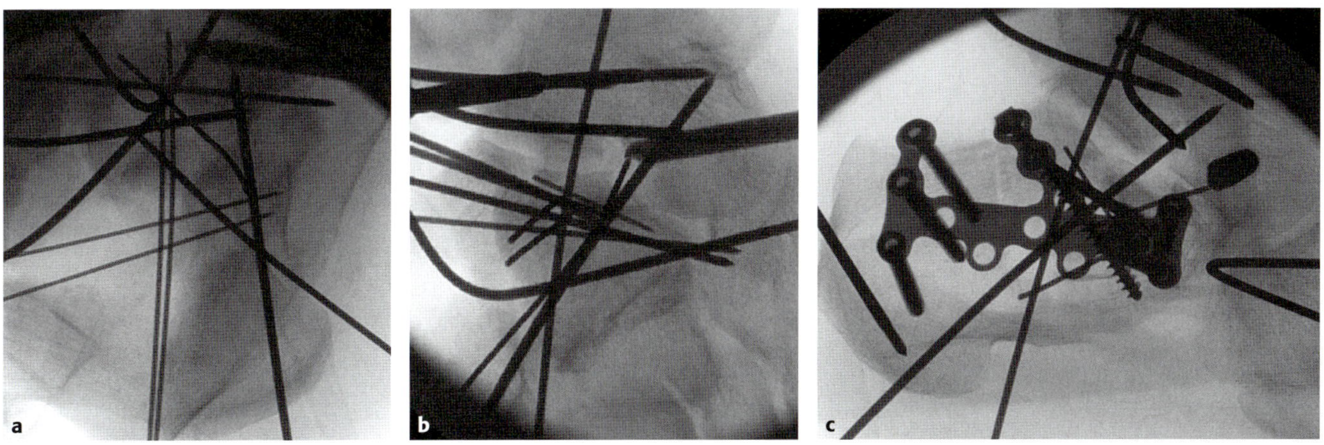

Fig 4.6-8a–c Intraoperative imaging control.
a Axial view to check alignment and medial cortex.
b Intraoperative Brodén view.
c Lateral view following plate fixation.

Once the wound is sealed, gentle range of motion (ROM) (inversion, eversion, dorsiflexion, plantarflexion, and complex circumduction) can be started. This usually happens at 3 days but may take longer in patients with soft-tissue problems or in tobacco users.

Postoperative CT scanning can be performed to assess quality of reduction at the surgeon's discretion (**Fig 4.6-9**).

5 Pitfalls and complications

Pitfalls

Postoperative wound complications

The patient should be counseled preoperatively about potential of postoperative wound complications. Postoperative wound complications affect outcome negatively in the extended lateral approach. Inadequate reduction and prolonged postoperative cast immobilization provide inferior outcome.

Timing of surgery

The timing of surgery should be carefully chosen. Operations too soon or too late increase postoperative complications.

Level of surgical experience

Significant experience is warranted to perform calcaneal surgery. Inexperience leads to a rise in complications.

Complications

- Postoperative wound infection including flap necrosis and osteomyelitis
- Sural nerve injury both at proximal and distal portion of incision
- Screw malposition (eg, intraarticular or too long on medial side)
- Insufficient reduction of the calcaneal shape and subtalar joint
- Insufficient stabilization (loss of reduction)
- Posttraumatic arthritis

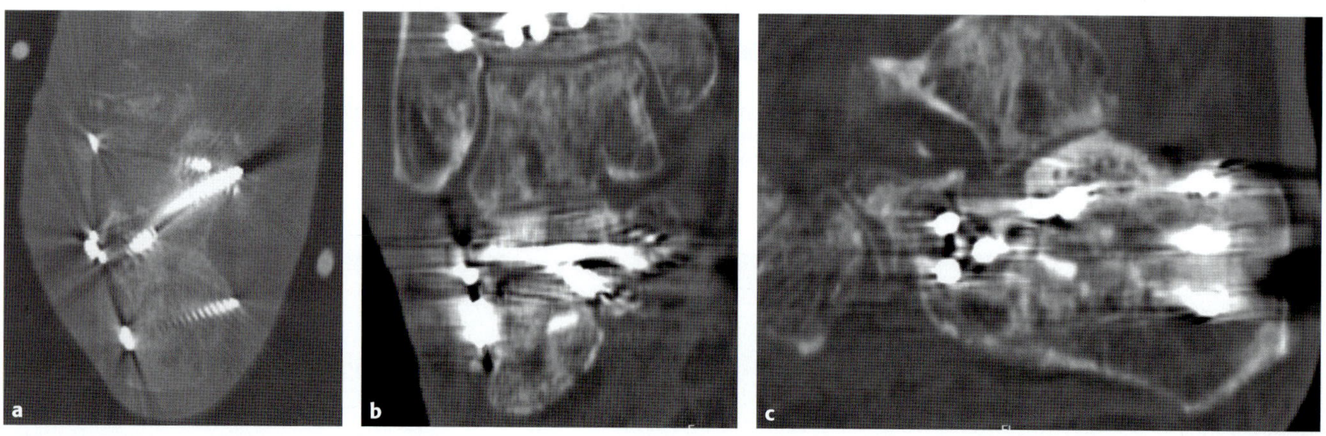

Fig 4.6-9a–c Postoperative CT scan at 3 months.
a Semicoronal view.
b Axial view.
c Sagittal view.

6 Alternative techniques

Other surgical approaches most frequently used are:

- Screws only approach approach (chapter 4.4)
- Sinus tarsi approach (chapter 4.5)

An alternative option to the "lost K-wire technique" is to advance the K-wires all the way through the medial skin where they are pulled out, until the end of the wire is flush at the level of the cancellous bone of the central fragment. After definitive screw fixation, remove the K-wires.

Occasionally, the tongue-type fractures are difficult to reduce. An osteotomy, as described by Sanders, can be used to convert a tongue-type into a joint-depression type, thereby facilitating an adequate reduction (**Fig 4.6-10**).

In cases with severe damage to the subtalar joint, eg, Sanders 4 fractures, fracture dislocations, and open calcaneal fractures, an option can be immediate primary arthrodesis. However, if the surgeon is confident that reduction and stabilization of the fracture is possible, avoid primary fusion as any small amount of subtalar motion is protective of the adjacent joints. Subtalar fusion inevitably leads to Chopart and ankle problems over time. Therefore, when surgeon skill and injury pattern allow, avoid fusion. Not all Sanders 4 fractures treated with surgical fixation will require late subtalar arthrodesis.

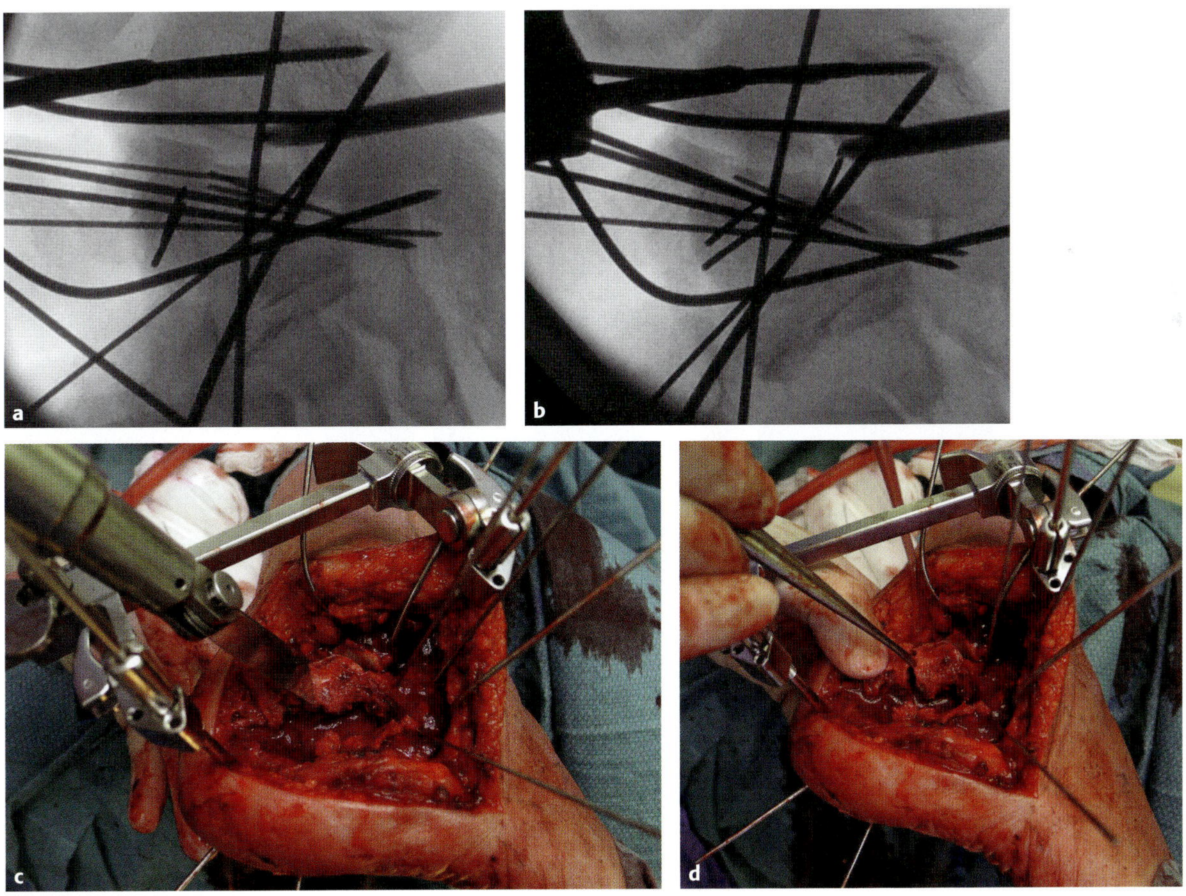

Fig 4.6-10a–d Sanders osteotomy to facilitate reduction.
a Attempted reduction with 3 mm residual step-off on the Brodén view.
b Reduction following osteotomy with less than 1 mm step-off.
c Intraoperative image of preparation of osteotomy.
d Intraoperative image following osteotomy.

7 Postoperative management and rehabilitation

Postoperatively the foot is put in a bulky dressing and a splint, the limb is elevated on a pillow with the heel free from pressure. If a drain was used, it is typically removed after 24–48 hours after surgery depending on the drainage amount.

Full ROM exercises can be started as soon as possible. The patient is routinely discharged when wound conditions and pain levels allow. In many centers these fractures are treated by ambulatory surgery. This requires absolute patient collaboration with the postoperative protocol.

The bandage is removed after 3 days, and sutures at approximately 2 weeks. Patients are kept nonweight bearing for 8–12 weeks.

Range of motion exercises by the patient are mandatory if a good postoperative functional outcome is to be achieved. Rehabilitation should focus on full ROM exercises, muscle strength, proprioception, and gait. Physiotherapy following foot and ankle injuries is started on an individual basis.

Follow-up is at 2 weeks (for suture removal and wound control), at 8 weeks (for conventional x-rays and subsequently start of weight bearing if x-rays show sufficient bone union). Additional visits are scheduled at 6 months and final check-up at 12 months for an isolated calcaneal fracture. This patient also had a type C open pilon fracture, so the final follow-up was scheduled at 24 months (**Fig 4.6-11**). The follow-up schedule is as per pattern of injury and surgeon preference.

The patient presented here had no postoperative wound complications. The calcaneus healed without incident. At the 2-year follow-up, the ankle had a pain-free ROM, but the subtalar joint was much stiffer with minimal inversion and eversion. She returned to work full time. The overall result was evaluated as good. No further check-ups were scheduled.

Implant removal

Implant removal is performed only in case of complaints. Plates can cause irritation of the peroneal tendons and screws can sometimes be palpable or cause irritation with shoewear.

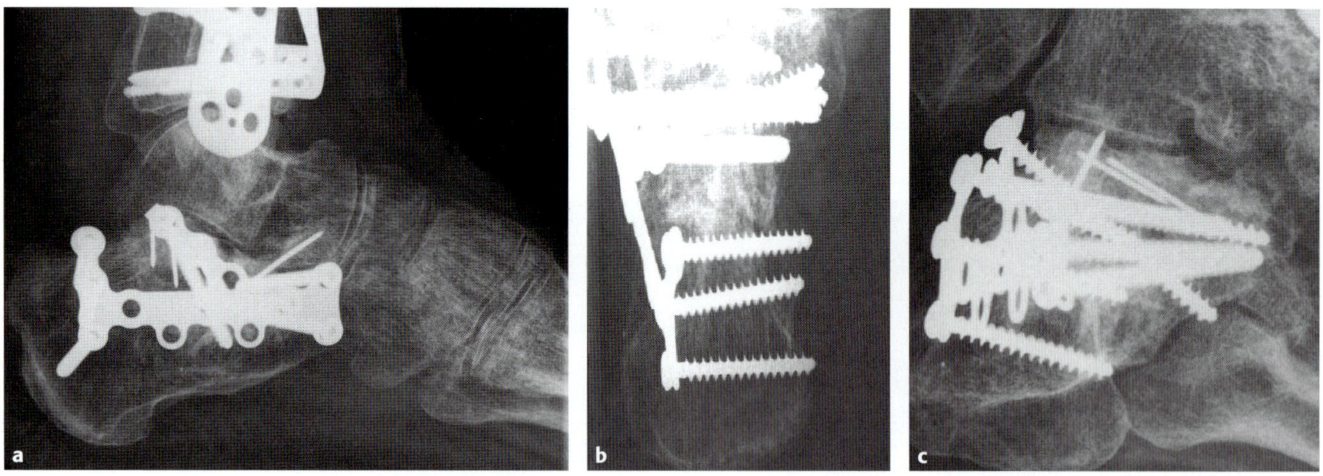

Fig 4.6-11a–c Follow-up x-rays at 24 months.
a Lateral view.
b Axial view.
c Brodén view.

8 Recommended reading

Backes M, Spierings KE, Dingemans SA, et al. Evaluation and quantification of geographical differences in wound complication rates following the extended lateral approach in displaced intra-articular calcaneal fractures: a systematic review of the literature. *Injury.* 2017 Oct;48(10):2329–2335.

Court-Brown CM, Schmied M, Schutte BG. Factors affecting infection after calcaneal fracture fixation. *Injury.* 2009 Dec;40(12):1313–1315.

Dingemans SA, de Ruiter KJ, Birnie MFN, et al. Comparable postoperative pain levels using 2 different nerve blocks in the operative treatment of displaced intraarticular calcaneal fractures. *Foot Ankle Int.* 2017 Dec;38(12):1352–1356.

Dingemans SA, Meijer ST, Backes M, et al. Outcome following osteosynthesis or primary arthrodesis of calcaneal fractures: a cross-sectional cohort study. *Injury.* 2017 Oct;48(10):2336–2341.

Freeman BJ, Duff S, Allen PE, et al. The extended lateral approach to the hindfoot. Anatomical basis and surgical implications. *J Bone Joint Surg Br.* 1998 Jan;80(1):139–142.

Rammelt S, Sangeorzan BJ, Swords MP. Calcaneal fractures—should we or should we not operate? *Indian J Orthop.* 2018 May–Jun;52(3):220–230.

Rammelt S, Zwipp H, Schneiders W, et al. Severity of injury predicts subsequent function in surgically treated displaced intraarticular calcaneal fractures. *Clin Orthop Relat Res.* 2013 Sep;471(9):2885–2898.

Sanders R, Fortin P, DiPasquale T, et al. Operative treatment in 120 displaced intraarticular calcaneal fractures. Results using a prognostic computed tomography scan classification. *Clin Orthop Relat Res.* 1993 May(290):87–95.

Schepers T, Den Hartog D, Vogels LM, et al. Extended lateral approach for intraarticular calcaneal fractures: an inverse relationship between surgeon experience and wound complications. *J Foot Ankle Surg.* 2013 Mar–Apr;52(2):167–171.

Zwipp H, Rammelt S, Barthel S. Calcaneal fractures: open reduction and internal fixation (ORIF). *Injury.* 2004 Sep;35 Suppl 2:Sb46–54.

4.7 Calcaneal fracture dislocation

Michael Swords, Stefan Rammelt

1 Case description

A 76-year-old woman fell down two steps when leaving her home. She presented to an emergency department and was diagnosed with a left ankle sprain. Subsequent imaging and evaluation demonstrated a calcaneal fracture dislocation. She had no medical problems or comorbidities (**Fig 4.7-1** and **Fig 4.7-2**).

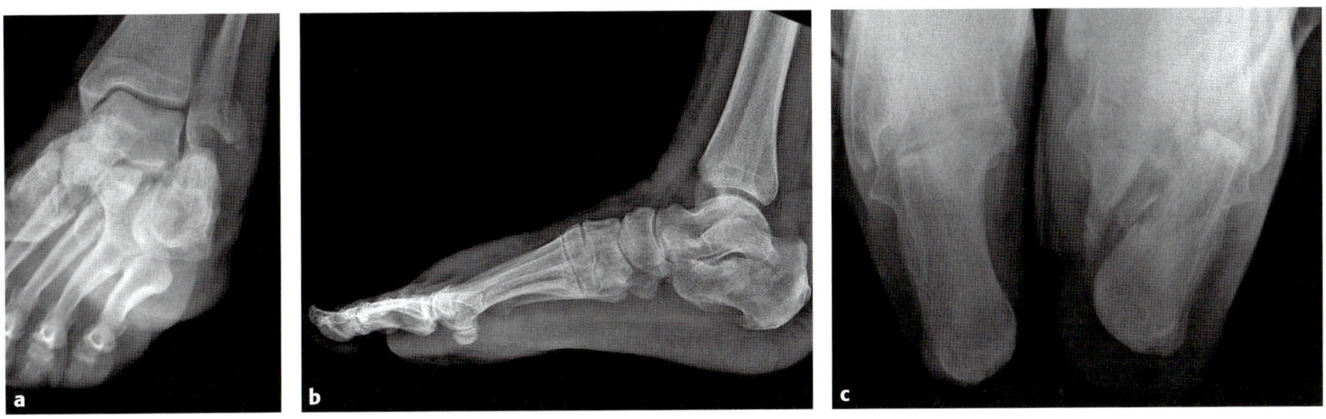

Fig 4.7-1a–c X-rays demonstrate a clear intraarticular fracture of the calcaneus with dislocation of the lateral portion of the calcaneus. Note the double contour in the lateral view and the comminution of the distal fibula from abutment of the calcaneus.

- **a** Mortise view.
- **b** Lateral view.
- **c** Axial view.

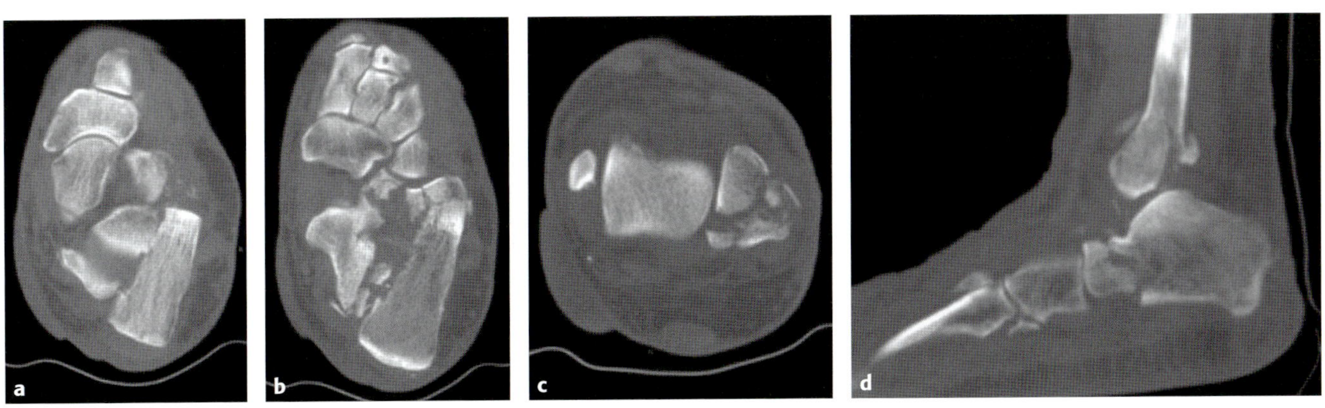

Fig 4.7-2a–d Preoperative CT scans.

- **a** Clear dislocation on the axial image.
- **b** There is comminution of the anterior process.
- **c** The most distal fibula is comminuted.
- **d** The entire lateral portion of the calcaneus is dislocated and has fractured the fibula. Anterior process comminution is visible.

2 Preoperative planning

Indications for surgery

Surgical fixation is necessary for calcaneal fracture dislocations. Goals of treatment include reduction of the dislocated tuberosity/body fragment that carries a substantial portion of the posterior facet, alignment of the articular surface of the posterior facet of the calcaneus, reduction and stabilization of the peroneal tendons back into the retrofibular groove, and fixation of the impaction injury of the distal fibula, if present.

If left untreated calcaneal fracture-dislocations lead to severe 3D foot deformities with chronic lateralization, shortening and varus deformity of the heel, painful calcaneofibular abutment, and dislocation of the peroneal tendons. In addition, loss of talar inclination from the dislocated portion of the posterior facet will result in tibiotalar impingement.

Considerations for surgery

The surgical approach is different for this fracture pattern compared with those typically used for treatment of intraarticular calcaneal fractures. The lateral extensile approach is not ideal for this injury. The dislocated lateral portion of the posterior facet makes access and visualization of the articular portion of the posterior facet challenging. Sinus tarsi approaches do not provide adequate access to the peroneal anatomy and the distal fibula, which may be necessary in treatment of calcaneal fracture dislocations.

The dislocation approach follows the course of the peroneal tendons starting at the tip of the fibula. This incision allows for reduction of the laterally dislocated joint fracture fragment from above. The posterior facet is easily visualized to ensure appropriate reduction. The incision can be extended proximally if repair of subluxed or dislocated peroneal tendons is necessary. If an associated distal fibular fracture is present, it can also be approached from the proximal extent of the incision. In this patient the fracture extended into the calcaneocuboid joint, so the approach was extended distally over the anterior calcaneal process.

Typically, there are two main fragments (sustentaculum and tuberosity/body of the calcaneus). Because the latter carries a substantial amount of the posterior facet, a Sanders 2B or 2C fracture results, with the lateral portion of the posterior facet dislocated. Calcaneal plates are seldom necessary for this pattern. If there is minimal comminution, the fracture can be stabilized with lag screws only. Generally, 3.5 mm screws are used. The fracture may extend into the anterior process of the calcaneus and calcaneocuboid joint. If there is significant comminution a small plate 2.4 or 2.7 may be necessary. In cases of decreased bone density, locked fixation with either plate 2.4 or 2.7 may be required.

3 Operating room setup

Patient positioning	• Lateral decubitis on a radiolucent table (injured side up)
Anesthesia options	• General, spinal, or regional
C-arm location	• Monitor on opposite side of the operative table with C-arm entering at an oblique angle from the foot of the bed
Tourniquet	• Used at surgeon's discretion • Generally it improves fracture visualization
Tips	• Early surgical treatment is recommended with this injury due to the increased difficulty in reducing the dislocation with delayed treatment.

For illustrations and overview of anesthetic considerations, see chapter 1. For illustrations and overview of patient and C-arm positioning for calcaneal fracture treatment in the lateral decubitus position refer to chapter 4.

Equipment

- Headlight
- K-wires
- Large point-to-point reduction (Weber) clamp
- Small fragment screws
- Nonabsorbable suture
- Minifragment plates
- Locking minifragment plates if decreased bone density is present
- Elevators
- Schanz pin

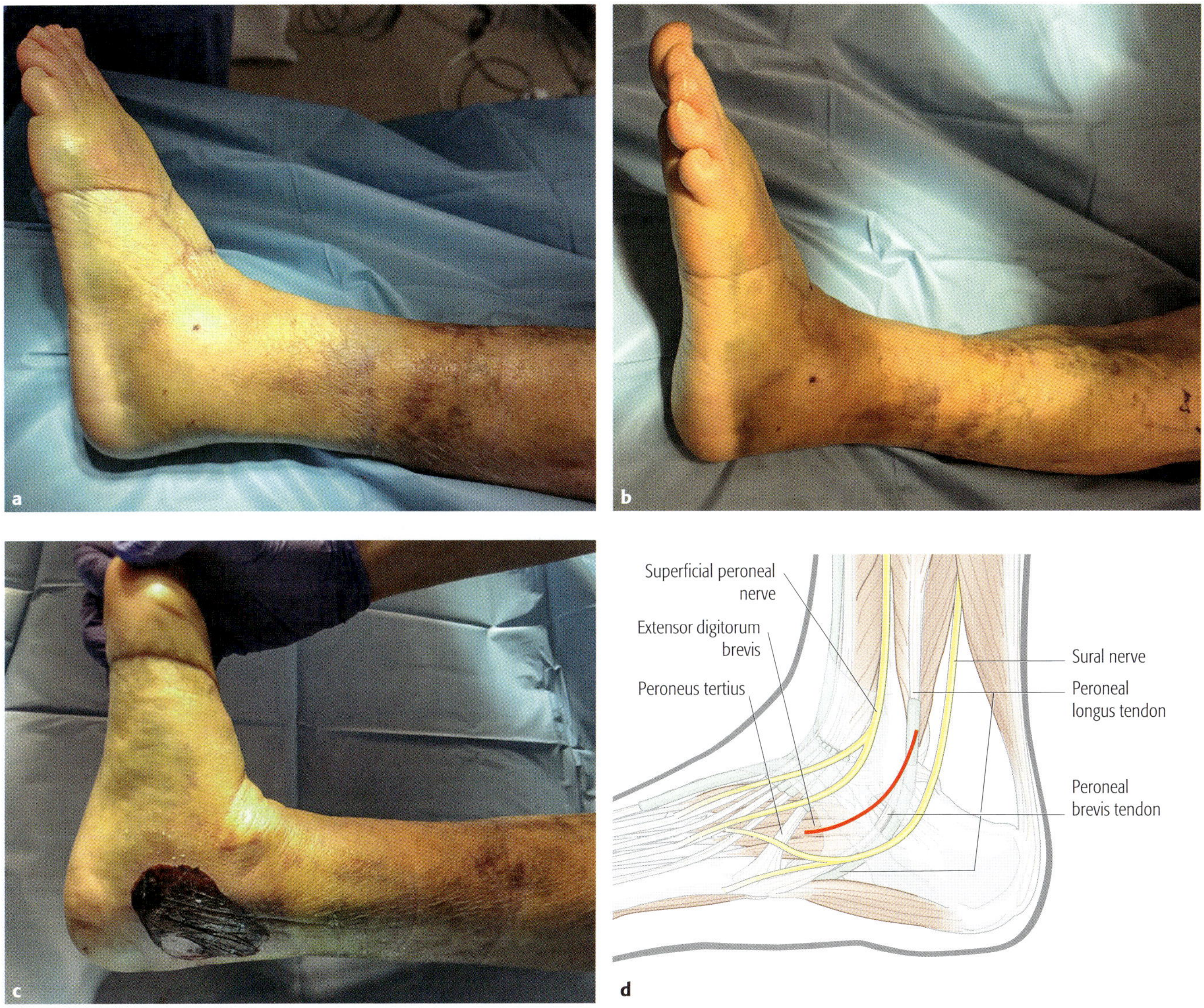

Fig 4.7-3a–d Preoperative images show appropriate resolution of swelling (**a–b**) and a resolving medial fracture blister (**c**). The incision follows along the course of the peroneals (**d**).

4 Surgical procedure

Once the skin swelling has decreased and the soft tissues have recovered after the injury, surgery can be considered. A slightly curved incision starting at the tip of the fibula is made just superior to the peroneal tendons along the lateral aspect of the hindfoot along the calcaneus (**Fig 4.7-3**). Be careful to avoid injury to the peroneal tendons, which are typically dislocated into the subcutaneous tissue. The tendons are identified and protected. Dissection continues down to the lateral aspect of the calcaneus. The articular surface of the dislocated lateral fragment is identified (**Fig 4.7-4**). The lateral fragment is then reduced back under the talus. A small osteotome is used to enter the fracture line through the posterior facet and the lateral portion of the joint is levered back under the talus (**Fig 4.7-5**). If the fracture is older and reduction is not easily achieved, a distractor can be used. A pin can be placed over the lateral fragment articular surface and into the talus. A second pin can be placed in the lateral calcaneus just below the articular surface. A small distractor or lamina spreader can be used to obtain the length necessary to aid in reducing the fragment.

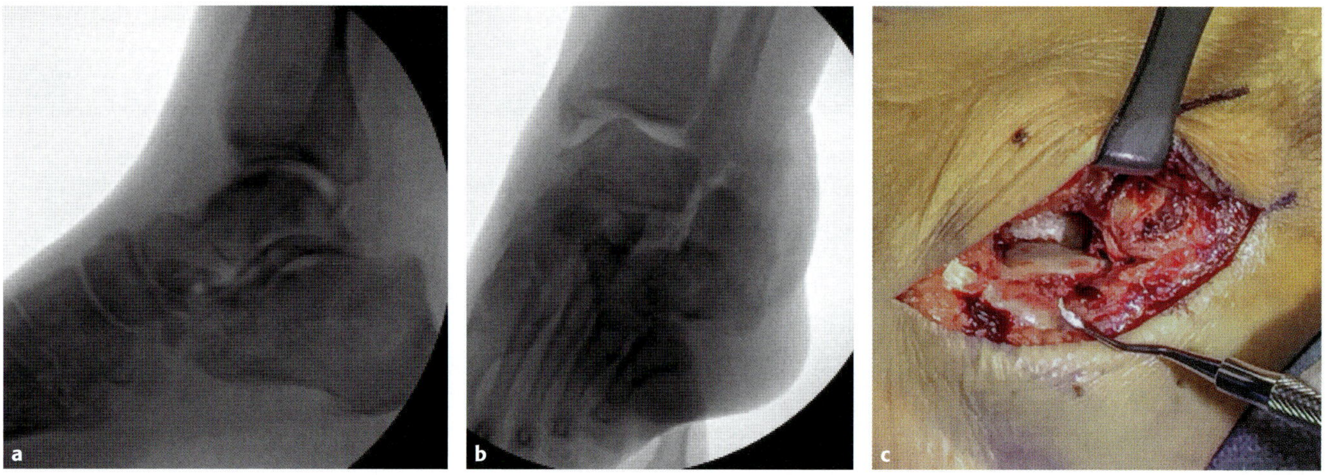

Fig 4.7-4a–c Intraoperative images and surgical approach demonstrating the dislocation.
a–b C-arm images in lateral and Brodén views clearly show the fracture dislocation pattern with subfibular abutment.
c The dislocation approach (Zwipp et al) was used and follows the course of the peroneals. The laterally dislocated portion of the calcaneus is clearly visible carrying the posterior fragment.

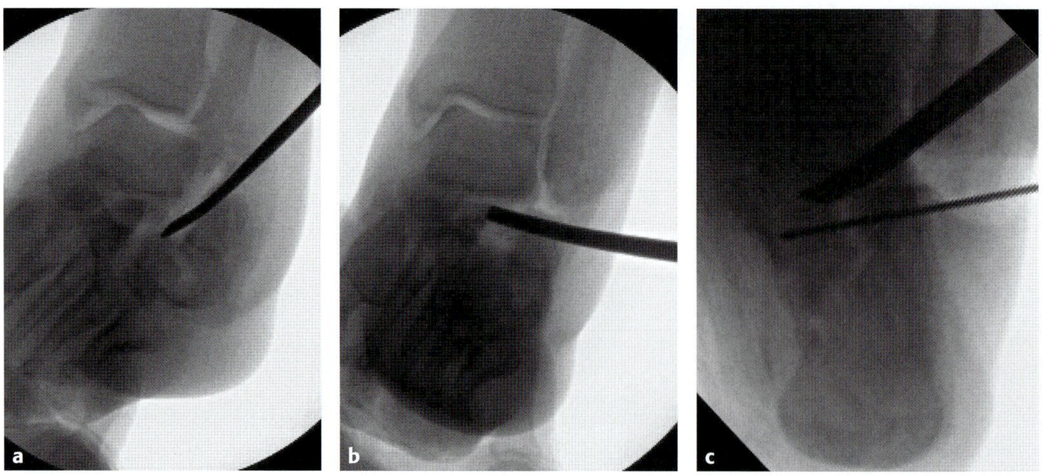

Fig 4.7-5a–c Reduction maneuver.
a The reduction is achieved by placing an osteotome or elevator carefully through over the dislocated lateral portion of the calcaneus. The instrument is then placed into the fracture line from superior as it exits the posterior facet.
b The instrument is then used as a lever to relocate the dislocated portion of the calcaneus back under the talus.
c Once reduced, stabilization is achieved with K-wires.

After the lateral fragment is no longer dislocated, the posterior facet of the calcaneus is reduced. The intraarticular fracture of the posterior facet is well visualized directly with a headlight if needed. Typically, this is fractured into two fragments. The articular surface is reduced under direct visualization and held with provisional K-wire fixation. If necessary, a small incision can be made medially over the sustentaculum and a large reduction clamp can be placed with one point on the sustentaculum medially and the other point on the lateral aspect of the calcaneus (**Fig 4.7-6**). This allows reduction and compression of the fracture line, which runs in the sagittal plane. K-wires are then inserted from lateral to medial to provide provisional fixation that is stable.

The reduction is then examined by direct visualization of the articular surface. Palpating the fracture line with a Freer elevator can also be used to assess the reduction. X-rays in lateral, axial, and Brodén views are also used to evaluate the reduction.

After reduction is confirmed to be anatomical, implants are selected. Hardware selection is based on both bone quality and comminution. If there is minimal comminution the fracture can be stabilized with lag screws only. Generally, 3.5 mm screws are used. If there is significant comminution a small plate 2.4 or 2.7 attached to the subchondral cortical bone may be necessary. In cases of decreased bone density locked fixation may be required, as in this patient. Any anterior process comminution must also be addressed.

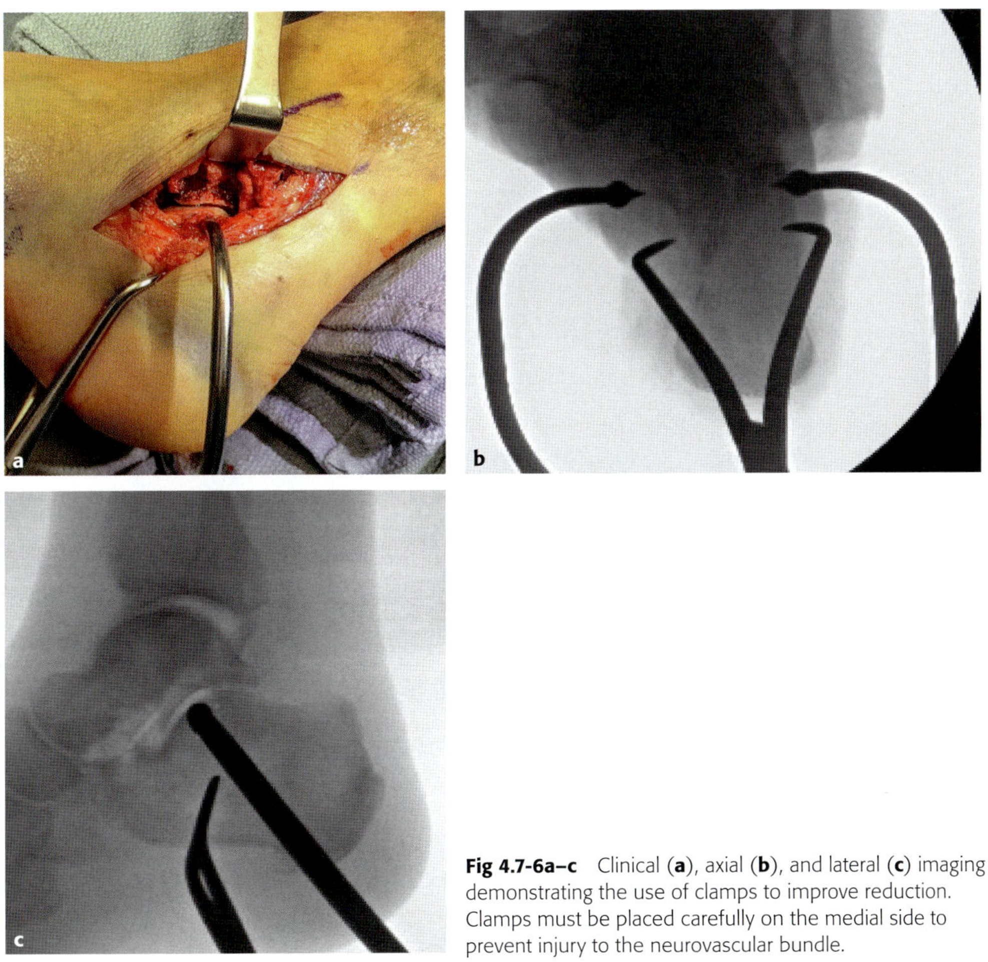

Fig 4.7-6a–c Clinical (**a**), axial (**b**), and lateral (**c**) imaging demonstrating the use of clamps to improve reduction. Clamps must be placed carefully on the medial side to prevent injury to the neurovascular bundle.

After fixation is complete, the peroneal tendons are examined to see if they are stable or if the peroneal retinaculum is torn. If the retinaculum is torn and/or the peroneals are unstable, the tendons are rerouted into the retrofibular groove and the superior peroneal retinaculum is repaired. Often, the injury pulls off a small portion of the posterior aspect of the fibula as an avulsion of the peroneal retinaculum. If it is a small fragment (less than 1 cm), the fracture fragment is excised before repair of the peroneal retinaculum. Larger fragments may be reduced and stabilized with a minifragment plate or two lag screws. Repair of this fragment will stabilize the peroneal tendons (**Fig 4.7-7**).

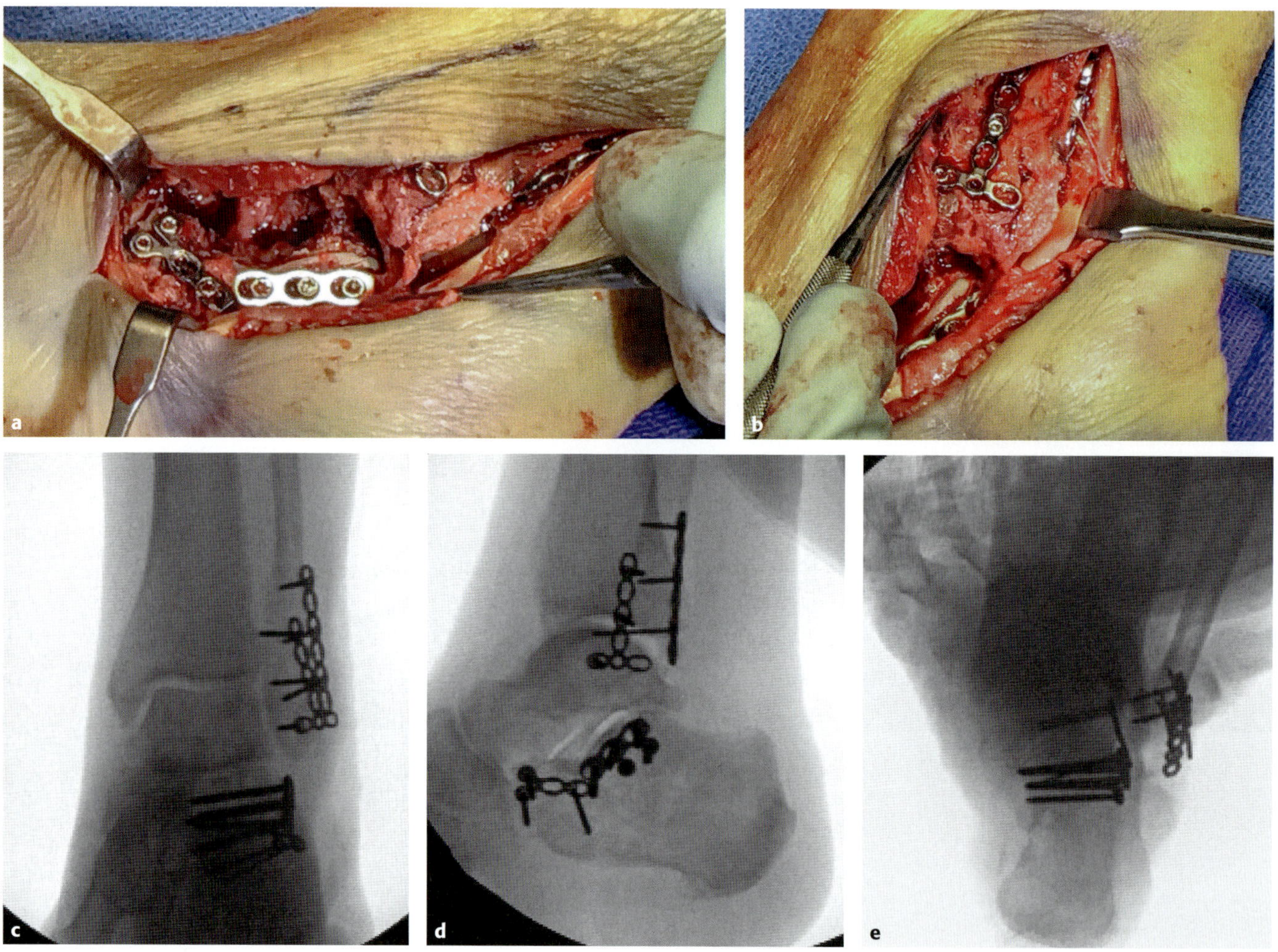

Fig 4.7-7a–e Final clinical images of the calcaneal fixation show a small locking plate and lag screws for the posterior facet and dislocation components of the injury. The anterior process is stabilized with a locking T-plate 2.4. The distal fibular fracture and the bony avulsion of the superior peroneal sheath are repaired using minifragment locked plates because of poor bone density (**a–b**). Final images in mortise (**c**), lateral (**d**), and axial (**e**) planes reveal anatomical reconstruction.

5 Pitfalls and complications

Pitfalls

Frequently, as for this patient, a calcaneal fracture is missed at the time of presentation because the x-rays do not show the characteristic features and the typical diagnosis then is that of an ankle sprain or infrasyndesmotic (Weber A) fibular fracture, when in fact, the fibula was fractured through direct impaction of the calcaneus. For an accurate diagnosis, careful review of the x-rays is therefore necessary. On the ankle mortise view or Brodén view the dislocated lateral portion of the joint is visible abutting the fibula. On the lateral view there is a large overlap of the talus and calcaneus, which should be recognized.

This fracture pattern is unique among calcaneal fractures. Incision selection is important. A lateral extensile approach will make the procedure more difficult as the entire lateral portion of the calcaneus is intact. Viewing the articular surface as well as reduction of the posterior facet may prove exceedingly difficult if a lateral extensile approach is used.

Complications

Missed diagnosis

As these fracture patterns are atypical, occasionally they are unrecognized. This results in abutment of the laterally dislocated fragment against the distal end of the fibula and the talus. Patients will have no motion of the subtalar joint and will experience significant pain. The peroneal tendons will be chronically dislocated.

Chronic peroneal subluxation

The significance of the small osseous fracture off the posterior distal fibula may be unrecognized. It is important to understand that this is a bony avulsion of the superior peroneal retinaculum and must be treated to restore peroneal stability.

Posttraumatic arthritis

As in all calcaneal fractures, anatomical articular reconstruction is critical to decrease the risk of posttraumatic arthritis (**Fig 4.7-8**).

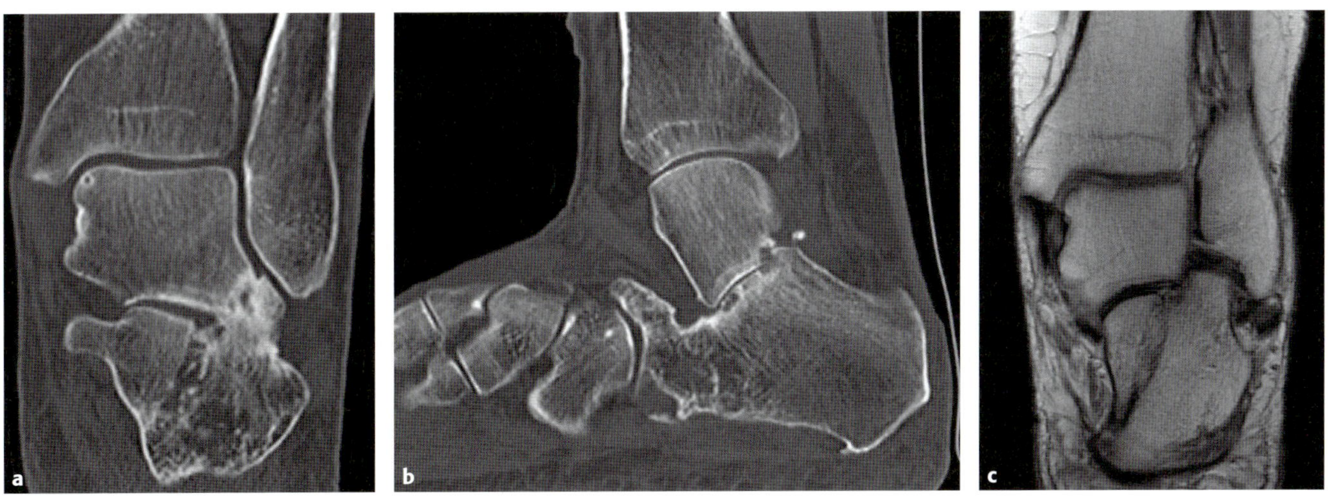

Fig 4.7-8a–c Example from a different case of an individual with late presentation after a missed fracture dislocation: axial and sagittal CT scans (**a–b**). Arthritis in the lateral portion of the calcaneus causes abutment to the talus and restricts motion. A magnetic resonance imaging of the same injury showing clear dislocation of the lateral calcaneus (**c**).

6 Alternative techniques

If the fracture is recognized early, a Schanz pin can be used to attempt percutaneous reduction. This must be done within 3 days. If reduction is achieved, percutaneous screws can be inserted.

In cases with delayed presentation, reduction of the dislocated segment can be a challenge. Calcaneal fibular abutment will alter hindfoot function and the peroneals will be chronically dislocated if the injury is not identified and treated. Osteotomy may be necessary in cases where the injury is missed, or early treatment is not performed. If the dislocated segment is a large portion of the articular surface, an intraarticular osteotomy and reconstruction are necessary. An osteotomy is performed including a medial shift of the displaced calcaneal body with stable fixation to the medial (sustentacular) fragment. A medial approach may be necessary to identify the original fracture line. The peroneal tendons are identified and freed of all adhesions. A Schanz screw or distractor may be necessary to assist in reduction, as soft-tissue contracture may be significant.

If the dislocated joint segment is small, it can be osteotomized and removed, provided that there is enough subtalar surface to provide joint stability.

With wide separation of the main fragments, a nonunion may develop if unrecognized. In these cases, the fibrous nonunion is resected and the former fracture debrided until good bleeding from the cancellous bone of the fragments is observed. Correction is carried out as described above.

If the dislocation is missed and the patient presents with long-standing deformity and arthritis, then arthrodesis, in addition to reconstruction, is necessary.

7 Postoperative management and rehabilitation

The patient is placed in a well-padded splint and the limb is elevated postoperatively. Sutures are removed at 2 weeks.

Functional exercises

The initiation of range-of-motion exercises is dependent on peroneal stability. Early exercises can be started if peroneal instability is not present at the time of surgical repair, which is rare. More commonly, peroneal instability exists at the time of surgical repair. Osseous repair of the posterior margin by minifragment plates or lag screws typically provides excellent stability, and range of motion is initiated at 2 weeks. If the peroneal retinaculum or peroneal tendons themselves are significantly injured and require repair, subtalar motion may need to be delayed until 4 weeks postoperatively.

Patients are followed up at 2 weeks for suture removal. X-rays are taken at 6 weeks and 9 weeks. Radiographic evidence of union is usually present by 9 weeks and weight bearing is advanced.

Implant removal

Implant removal is seldom necessary (**Fig 4.7-9** and **Fig 4.7-10**). Implants are removed only if symptomatic. Patients will experience irritation to the peroneal tendons if implants are bothersome.

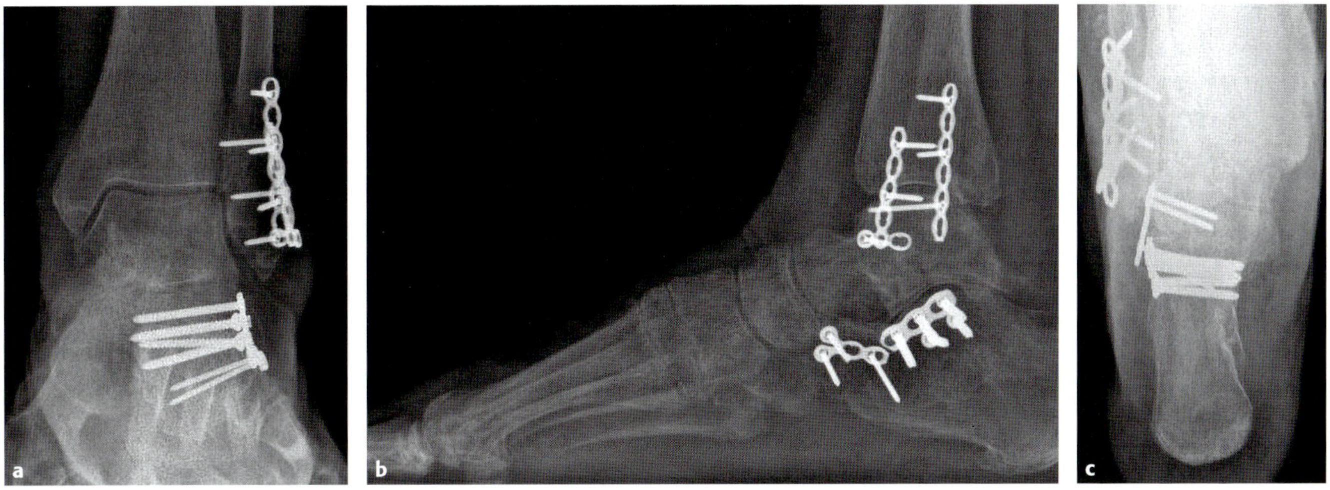

Fig 4.7-9a–c X-rays taken 1 year indicating a healed fracture with no arthritis and normal alignment.
a AP view.
b Lateral view.
c Axial view.

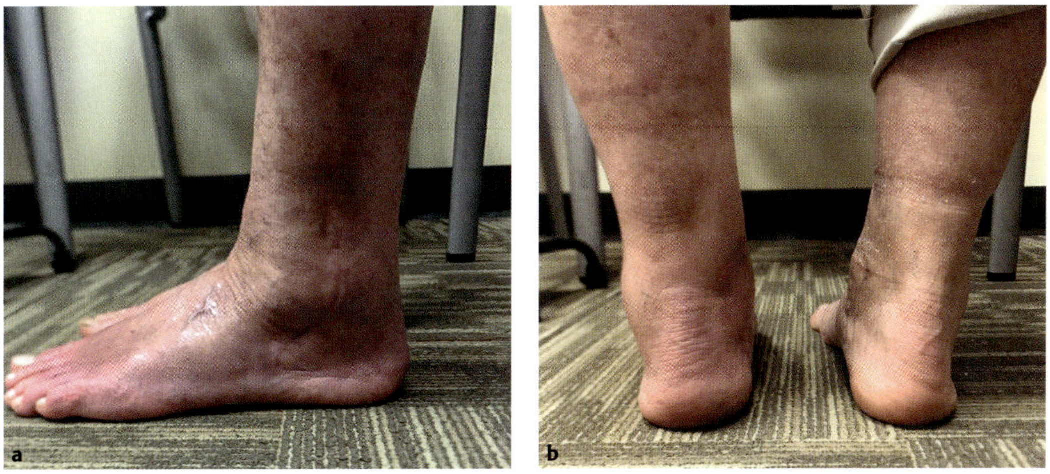

Fig 4.7-10a–b Clinical images taken 1 year postoperatively showing normal alignment with a healed incision from the dislocation approach.

8 Recommended reading

Biga N, Thomine JM. [Fracture-dislocation of the calcaneus. Apropos of 4 cases]. *Rev Chir Orthop Reparatrice Appar Mot.* 1977 Mar;63(2):191–202. French.
Merle d'Aubigné MR. Fracture isolée de la petite apophyse du calcanéum traitée par ostéosynthèse (Rapport de M. Wilmoth). *Mem Acad Chir Paris.* 1936;62:1155–1159. French.
Rammelt S, Zwipp H. Fractures of the calcaneus: current treatment strategies. *Acta Chir Orthop Traumatol Cech.* 2014;81(3):177–196.
Rammelt S, Grass R, Zwipp H. Joint-preserving osteotomy for malunited intra-articular calcaneal fractures. *J Orthop Trauma.* 2013 Oct;27(10):e234–238.
Rammelt S, Zwipp H. Corrective arthrodeses and osteotomies for post-traumatic hindfoot malalignment: indications, techniques, results. *Int Orthop.* 2013 Sep;37(9):1707–1717.
Zwipp H, Rammelt S, Barthel S. Calcaneal fractures: open reduction and internal fixation (ORIF). *Injury.* 2004 Sep;35 Suppl 2:Sb46–54.

5 Talus

Talus

5 Talar fractures and dislocations

Mandeep S Dhillon

1 Introduction

The talus derives its name from Greek 'Talos', which was an automaton created to protect Europe from invaders. Talos had one vein in his body running from neck to ankle; this vulnerability has been likened to the vulnerable blood supply of the talus.

The talus is unique as it is almost entirely covered by articular cartilage and has no muscular attachments. It participates in all movements of the ankle, midfoot, and hindfoot through its three important articulations: the talocrural (ankle) joint, the talonavicular joint, and the subtalar joint. Of these, the talocrural is the most mobile joint followed by the talonavicular joint; the subtalar joint has least mobility. Owing to these intricate articulations, it is easy to comprehend why injuries of the talus can have profound impact on biomechanics of the foot.

2 Anatomy and pathomechanics

The talus receives its blood supply from three important sources (**Fig 5-1** and **Fig 5-2**). The major blood supply of the talus is via the posterior tibial artery. The artery of the tarsal canal, a branch of the posterior tibial artery, supplies most of the talar body, whereas the deltoid branch of the posterior tibial artery supplies the medial portion of the talar body. Branches from the anterior tibial supply the talar head and neck. The perforating peroneal artery supplies the head and neck via the artery of the tarsal sinus. It is important to note that in talar fractures, the deltoid branch of the posterior tibial artery may be the only remaining source of blood supply; hence the surgeon should make every effort to preserve it.

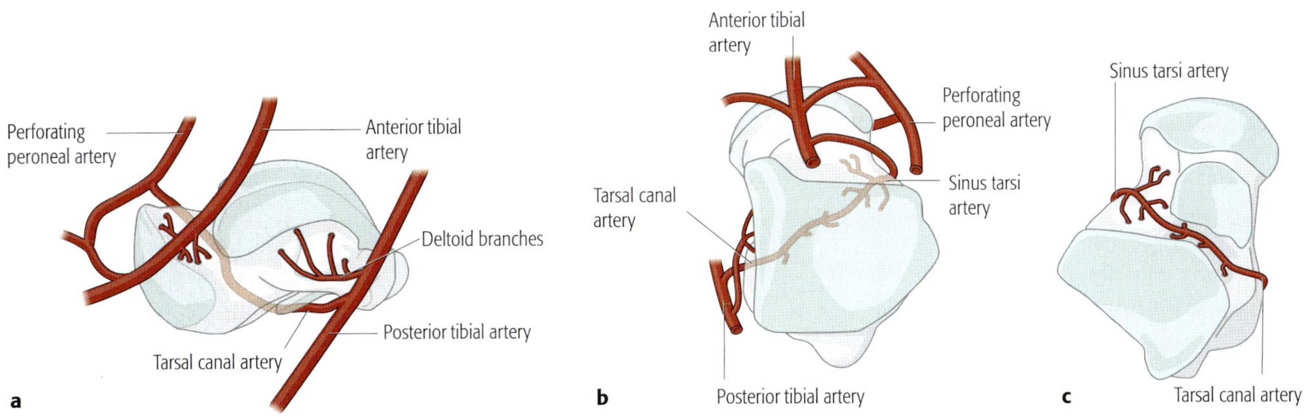

Fig 5-1a–c Blood supply of talus. Note the deltoid branches of the posterior tibial artery and the artery of the tarsal canal. A posteromedial approach to the body of the talus would destroy its blood supply. Therefore, if the body has to be exposed, one uses an osteotomy of the medial malleolus. (Image adapted from Patrick Cronier.)

The mechanism of injury for a talus neck fracture remains controversial. Forced dorsiflexion with inversion or eversion was thought to be the principal mechanism of injury that causes talus neck fractures. However, in 1977 cantilever bending of the talar neck, with the talus body wedged in between the plafond and calcaneus and an axial load applied from the plantar aspect resulted in talar neck fracture. By contrast talar body fractures are caused by axial loading, and invariably have varying degrees of comminution. Talar head fractures are rare and are caused by axial loading through the navicular. Fractures of the lateral process are thought to be produced by forced eversion and are often called "snowboarders injury". Fractures of the posterior process are produced by forced plantar flexion and, like lateral process fractures, are often associated with subtalar dislocations. Subtalar dislocations, on the other hand have different mechanisms of trauma; medial subtalar dislocations are caused by plantar flexion-inversion forces whereas lateral subtalar dislocations are caused by eversion forces. These forces could be aborted at any stage, with the end stage being pantalar/total talar dislocation or an extruded talus.

3 Fracture classification

Fractures of the talus can be classified anatomically as central and peripheral fractures. Central fractures include talar neck and body fractures. For the purpose of classification, fracture patterns anterior to the lateral process are classified as talar neck fractures whereas fracture patterns at or posterior to the lateral process are classified as talar body fractures. Peripheral fractures include fractures of the talar head, lateral and posterior process.

In the 2018 revised AO/OTA classification, fractures of the talus are denoted by "81". Fractures of the talus body are divided into three locations: body 81.1, neck 81.2, and head 81.3. Fractures of the lateral (81.1.A2) and posterior process (81.1.A3) are included as groups of talus body fractures. The body fractures could be simple avulsion fractures, partial articular fractures, or complex articular fractures. See the appendix for the AO/OTA classification of talus fracure.

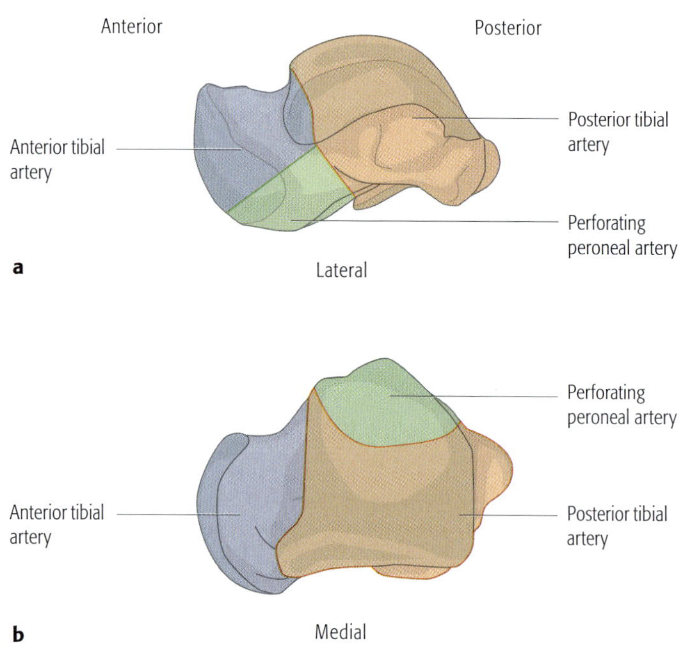

Fig 5-2a–b The deltoid branches are important to supply blood to the medial talar neck and talar body. Branches from the dorsalis pedis supply the talar head and most of the dorsal talar neck. The artery of the tarsal canal coming from branches off of the posterior tibial artery supply most of the talar body. The peroneal artery has the least contribution laterally.

Fractures of the talus neck have been classified by Hawkins into three types (**Fig 5-3**):

Type 1 Nondisplaced fracture of the talar neck.

Type 2 Fracture has displacement of the talar neck with or without subtalar dislocation.

Type 3 Fracture has a displaced talus neck fracture along with subtalar and tibiotalar dislocation.

Canale and Kelly described a type 4 variant, whereby there is subtalar, tibiotalar, and talonavicular (TN) dislocation in addition to the displaced talus neck fracture.

The Marti classification includes all peripheral and central talar fractures (**Fig 5-3**). There are four types:

Type 1 Perpipheral including talar process and head fractures

Type 2 Nondisplaced central (neck or body)

Type 3 Neck or body fracture with displacemnet at subtatar or ankle joint

Type 4 Neck or body fracture with displacement at subtatar and ankle joint, comminution of the taar body, and talonvicular joint displacement

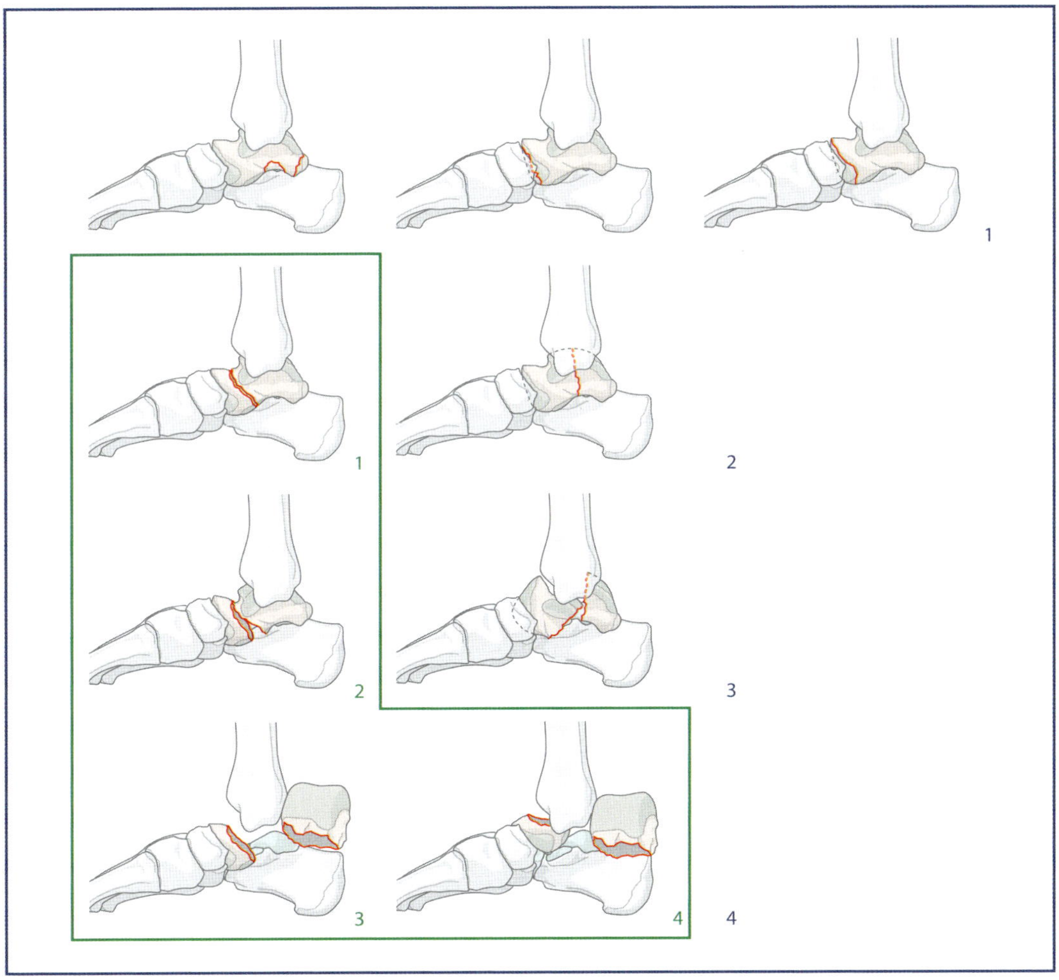

Marti classification (includes all peripheral and central talar fractures)

Hawkins classification (talar neck fractures only)

Fig 5-3 Marti and Harris classification of talar fractures. (Image adapted from Hans Zwipp and Stefan Rammelt.)

4 Subtalar dislocations

Talar dislocations may be subtalar, total talar, or peritalar. They may be open or closed injuries. Usually, a subtalar dislocation is defined as the simultaneous dislocation of the subtalar and TN joints although some injuries do not have TN dislocation. The ankle joint is not displaced. These injuries are often associated with peripheral talar fractures. Purely ligamentous dislocations have a better prognosis.

The dislocations may be medial or lateral, anterior or posterior, depending upon the direction the foot displaces in relation to the talus. If the deforming force continues the ankle joint also dislocates, leading to a total talar or peritalar dislocation. These dislocations may be closed or open and continuing force could even extrude the talus outside the skin (see chapter 5.9).

Medial dislocations result in a medially displaced heel, and an inverted and plantar flexed foot. The skin shows tenting over the prominent talar head and lateral malleolus, with associated swelling.

Lateral dislocations are often high-energy injuries and are frequently open injuries; these are less common (15–20% of cases) than medial subtalar dislocations, occur with an eversion force, and have a higher incidence of associated fractures.

The calcaneonavicular ligament is strong and does not easily rupture; the eversion force ruptures the weaker TN and talocalcaneal ligaments; the talus stays in place in the ankle, while calcaneus, navicular, and all distal foot bones move laterally and dorsally as a unit. Clinically, the heel is displaced laterally and the foot is everted and abducted. The talar head is prominent and palpable medially.

5 Preoperative assessment

Clinical assessment

Almost all talar fractures and dislocations are high-energy injuries. Soft-tissue injury may manifest as of swelling and ecchymosis. Medial subtalar dislocations present with an "acquired clubfoot" deformity, whereas lateral subtalar dislocation present with an "acquired flatfoot" deformity. Injuries of the lateral and posterior process can sometimes have minimal clinical findings and can be hard to detect, with associated delays in diagnosis.

Imaging

Standard projections of the ankle, including AP, lateral, and mortise views are necessary in all cases. The Canale and Kelly view (**Fig 5-4**) is useful for visualizing the talus neck. It is achieved by placing the foot plantigrade on the cassette, pronating the foot by 150° and cephalad angulation of the beam by 150° from the vertical.

A computed tomographic (CT) scan is invaluable for evaluating the fracture pattern and for detection of lateral and posterior process fractures, which can be difficult to detect on plain x-rays.

Magnetic resonance imaging is rarely, if ever, indicated in the acute injury.

6 Nonoperative treatment

Most displaced talaar fractures necessitate operative management and nonoperative treatment is rarely, if ever, indicated. Nondisplaced talus neck fractures (Hawkins type 1) can be managed nonoperatively; however, a CT scan is mandatory to prove that the fracture is indeed nondisplaced, and there is no associated comminution. Percutaneous fixation of such fractures has the advantage of allowing early range of motion without fear of displacement, and thereby less stiffness.

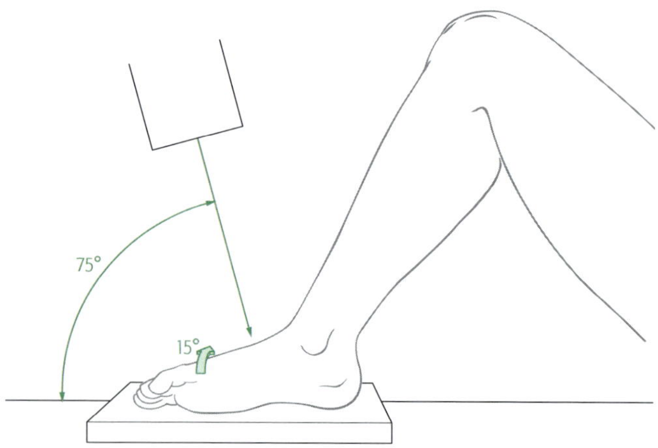

Fig 5-4 Canale and Kelly view.

7 Operative treatment

Patient positioning

The patients are usually positioned supine, with pillows under the ipsilateral buttock. Draping and positioning should take into account that most complex fractures need a dual approach. The foot is usually brought to the end of a radiolucent table, and the C-arm is positioned opposite to the surgeon for easy access. Tourniquet use is recommended.

Surgical approaches

Talar neck fractures are best addressed by dual surgical approaches. Use of two approaches has shown to improve the accuracy of reduction. The anteromedial and anterolateral approaches (**Fig 5-5**) are used to address the medial and lateral aspects of the talar neck, respectively. Utmost care should be taken to preserve the talar attachment of the deltoid ligament, as this may be the only remaining source of blood supply. Dissection dorsal to the talar neck should be avoided.

Talar body fractures are approached via osteotomy of the medial malleolus, which permits ready access to the talar dome (**Fig 5-6**).

The posteromedial aspect of the talar body can be approached via the posteromedial approach. In rare cases where the posterolateral part of the talar body needs to be approached, a posterolateral approach may be used or alternately, a fibular osteotomy may also be considered.

The lateral process of the talus can be approached via the direct lateral approach.

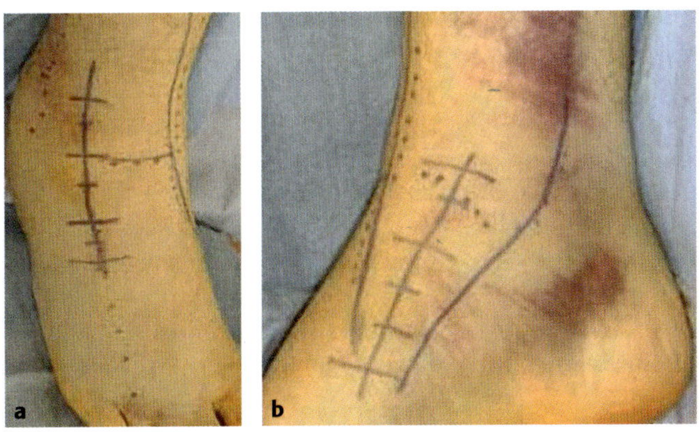

Fig 5-5a–b Surgical approaches.
a Anteromedial approach.
b Anterolateral approach.

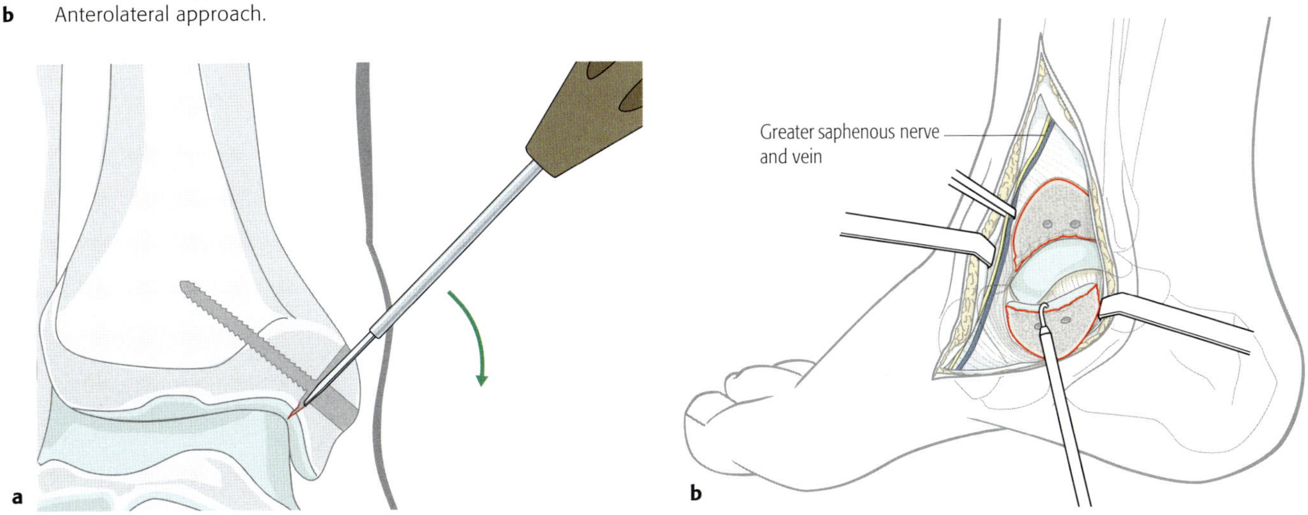

Fig 5-6a–b Malleolar osteotomy to improve exposure.
a Technique with predrilling of the screw holes.
b Retracted malleolus.

Considerations for surgery

Displaced talus neck fractures associated with dislocations need to be reduced on an emergent basis as this may worsen the soft-tissue insult and also compromise the precarious blood supply. Closed reduction can be attempted and need not be anatomical. In Hawkins 2 fractures of the neck, with no dislocation, surgical intervention can be delayed if the soft tissues are compromised. In some talar neck and body fractures, the talar body may have been extruded out of the ankle mortise posteromedially. This needs to be reduced imminently by closed or open means or skin necrosis will ensue, and chances of avascular necrosis (AVN) are multiplied. The key point to emphasize is that reduction is emergent, while definitive fixation can wait until all diagnostic modalities are in place and soft tissue swelling has subsided.

Once the decision has been made to operate, the surgeon should have a clear plan in mind, which should include the surgical approach to be used, reduction aids and the implants to be used. A femoral distractor with pins in the distal tibia and calcaneus can improve visualization of the talar body and also help in repositioning of the extruded talar body. K-wires placed as joysticks into the talar head can help in achieving reduction of the talar neck. Fixation is achieved by means of screws or plates. The medial side is usually comminuted; therefore a medial plate or fully threaded cancellous screw along with bone graft is necessary to prevent varus malreduction. The lateral side is usually non-comminuted and can be fixed by a compression screw. Headless screws can be used to fix smaller fragments and fractures of the lateral and posterior processes. The subtalar and talonavicular joint may need to be pinned with K wires to maintain reduction. In cases with severe comminution, an ankle spanning external fixator may be used to protect the fixation in the early phase.

Open fractures necessitate urgent wound debridement; however the principles of reduction and fixation remain the same. A joint spanning external fixator may be used if a soft tissue flap procedure is contemplated. Fractures with extrusion of the talar body and talar extrusions should be reduced as soon as possible. The management of talar extrusions remains controversial; however current literature favors primary replantation of the extruded talus.

8 Postoperative care

In general, early nonweight bearing and gentle range-of-motion exercises are started as soon as the incisions heal. A backslab, splint or cast may be used in the early phase to aid in soft tissue healing. Partial weight bearing in a removable CAM boot can be started around 4–6 weeks. Full weight bearing is delayed till union. In case of AVN, weight bearing should be delayed (**Fig 5-7**).

9 Complications and outcomes

Historically, talar fractures were reported to have poor outcomes. However, as our understanding of these complex fractures continues to evolve, the outcomes can be expected to improve. The common complications of talar fractures include avascular necrosis, arthrosis and malunion. Malunion is a disabling complication of talar neck fracture and is usually attributable to malreduction and shortening of the medial talar neck, resulting in varus deformity. Because of the unique anatomy of the talus, talar malunions almost uniformely will lead to direct or indirect joint incongruity. Avascular necrosis is the most dreaded complication of talar fractures, although its incidence seems to be reducing and the complications like collapse are becoming less common due to a better understanding. The Hawkins classification can be used to predict the incidence of avascular necrosis. If AVN develops, weight bearing should be delayed to prevent collapse of the talar dome. In many cases, the AVN is partial and involves the lateral part of dome as the intact deltoid artery supplies the medial aspect. However not all patients with AVN experience talar collaps with subsequent poor outcome. Arthrosis is a late complication of talar neck fractures and most commonly involves the subtalar joint.

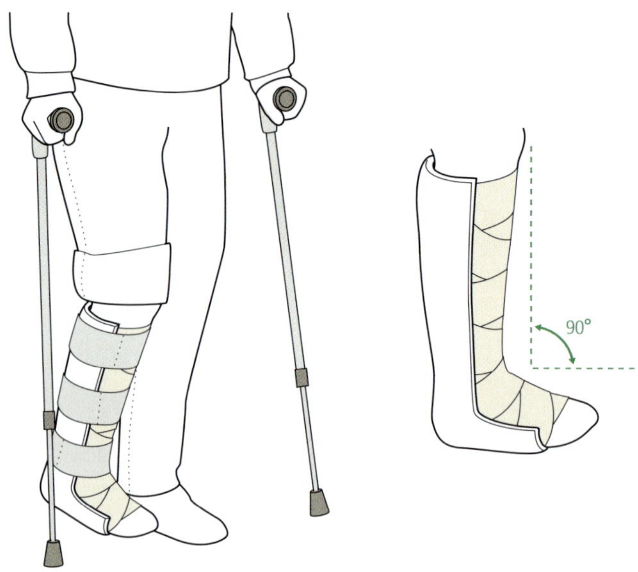

Fig 5-7 Postoperative rehabilitation. Nonweight-bearing crutch walking (**a**). The ankle should be maintained at 90° (**b**).

10 Recommended reading

Buza JA, 3rd, Leucht P. Fractures of the talus: Current concepts and new developments. *Foot Ankle Surg.* 2018 Aug;24(4):282–290.
Canale ST, Kelly FB Jr. Fractures of the neck of the talus. Long-term evaluation of seventy-one cases. *J Bone Joint Surg Am.* 1978 Mar;60(2):143–156.
Coltart WD. Aviator's astragalus. *J Bone Joint Surg Br.* 1952 Nov;34-b(4):545–566.
Gross CE, Haughom B, Chahal J, et al. Treatments for avascular necrosis of the talus: a systematic review. *Foot Ankle Spec.* 2014 Oct;7(5):387–397.
Cronier P, Talha A, Massin P. Central talar fractures—therapeutic considerations. *Injury.* 2004 Sep;35 Suppl 2:Sb10–22.
Hawkins LG. Fractures of the neck of the talus. *J Bone Joint Surg Am.* 1970 Jul;52(5):991–1002.
Jordan RK, Bafna KR, Liu J, et al. Complications of talar neck fractures by Hawkins Classification: a systematic review. *J Foot Ankle Surg.* 2017 Jul–Aug;56(4):817–821.
Penny JN, Davis LA. Fractures and fracture-dislocations of the neck of the talus. *J Trauma.* 1980 Dec;20(12):1029–1037.
Peterson L, Goldie IF, Irstam L. Fracture of the neck of the talus. A clinical study. *Acta Orthop Scand.* 1977;48(6):696–706.
Rammelt S, Zwipp H. Talar neck and body fractures. *Injury.* 2009 Feb;40(2):120–135.
Vallier HA, Nork SE, Benirschke SK, et al. Surgical treatment of talar body fractures. *J Bone Joint Surg Am.* 2003 Sep;85-a(9):1716–1724.
Vallier HA, Reichard SG, Boyd AJ, et al. A new look at the Hawkins classification for talar neck fractures: which features of injury and treatment are predictive of osteonecrosis? *J Bone Joint Surg Am.* 2014 Feb 5;96(3):192–197.

5.1 Osteochondral dome fracture

Omkar Baxi, Michael Yeranosian, Sheldon Lin

1 Case description

A 19-year-old man with no medical history injured his left ankle while playing basketball. He landed awkwardly on his forefoot and fell to the ground. He noted immediate pain and swelling of his ankle and was unable to bear weight.

On clinical examination, he experienced severe tenderness to palpation at the lateral malleolus and complained of a deep, dull ankle pain in the ankle while at rest. Abrasions were noted on the dorsal and lateral aspects of the ankle. The patient had intact distal vascular examination with strong dorsalis pedis and posterior tibial pulses. There were no neurological deficits.

X-rays obtained in the emergency department revealed a Weber B lateral malleolar fracture (AO/OTA 44B1, isolated transsyndesmotic fibular injury) and an ossific density on the lateral aspect of talus likely representing an osteochondral dome fracture (**Fig 5.1-1**). No talar subluxation or talar tilt was visualized.

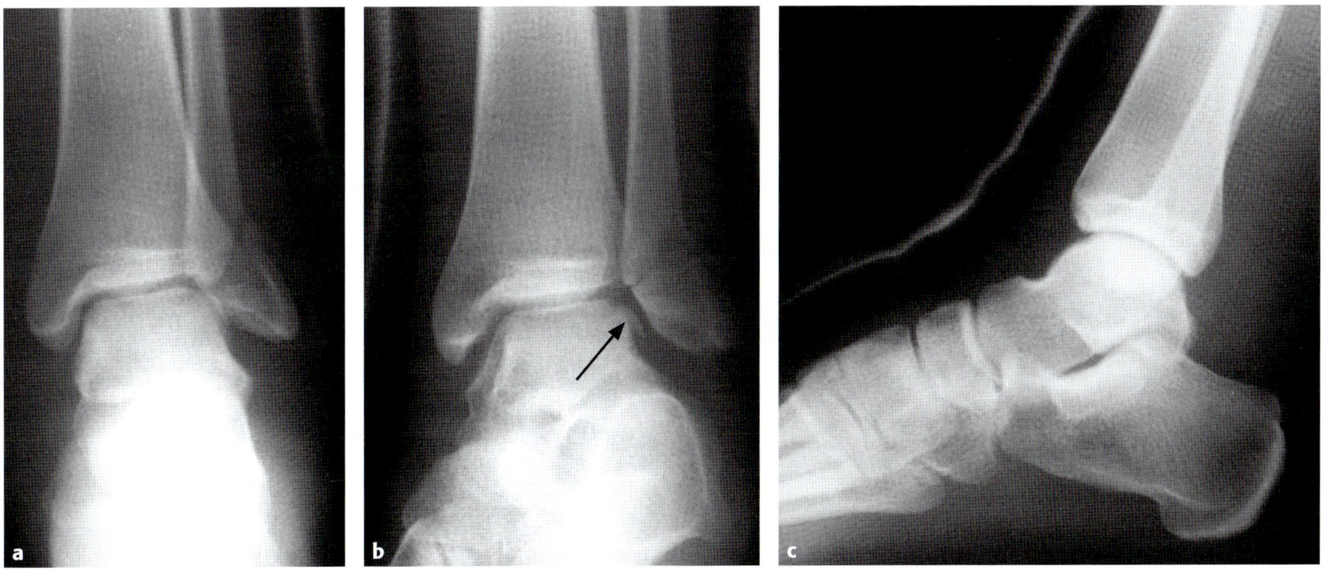

Fig 5.1-a–c X-rays of the left ankle revealing a Weber B lateral malleolar fracture. Careful assessment of the mortise view also reveals a small osteochondral fracture (arrow) of the lateral talar dome.

- **a** AP view.
- **b** Mortise view.
- **c** Lateral view.

The patient was placed into a short leg cast, and a post-cast computed tomographic (CT) scan (**Fig 5.1-2**) confirmed a fibular fracture and a small osteochondral fracture of the most lateral part of the talar dome.

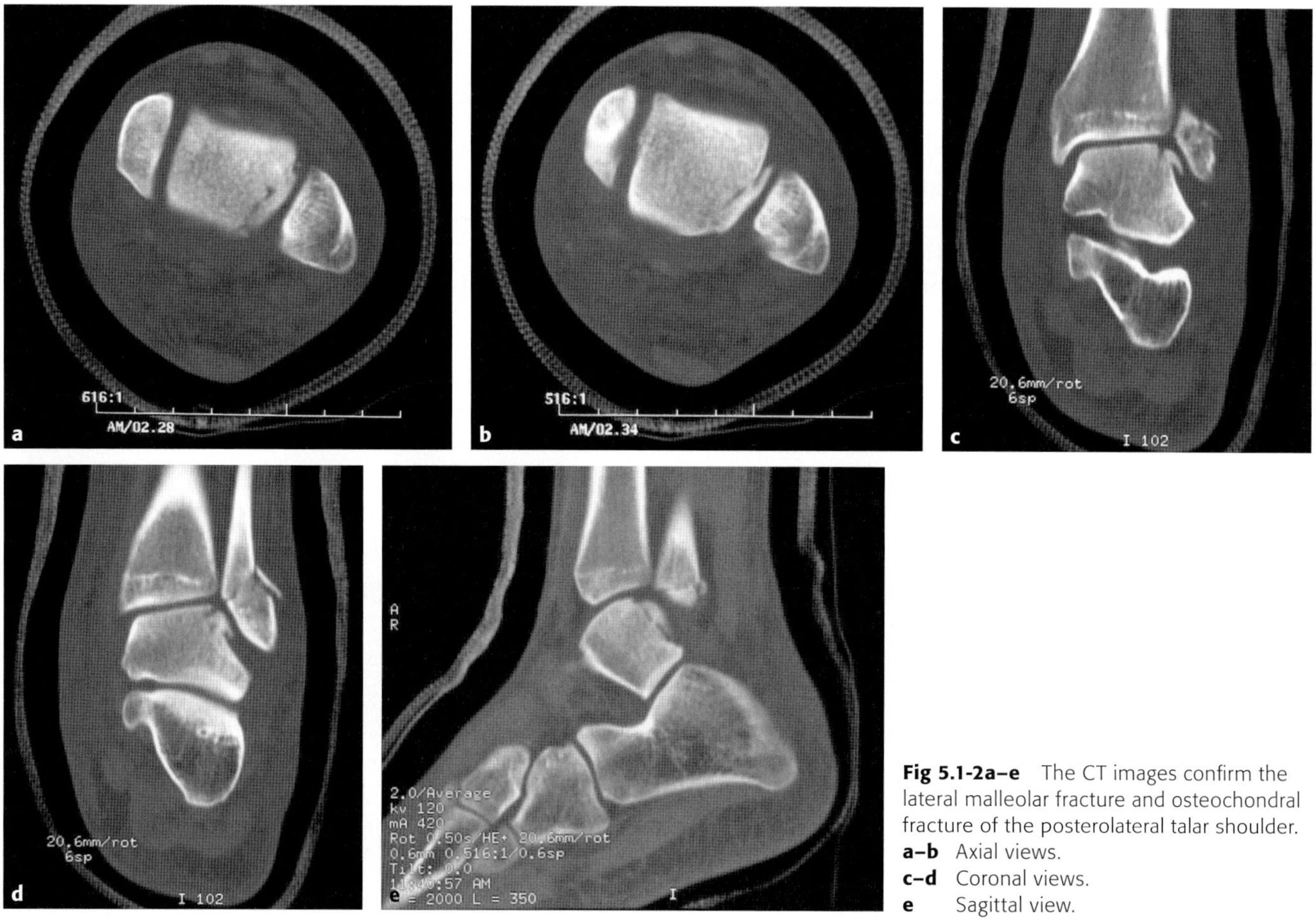

Fig 5.1-2a–e The CT images confirm the lateral malleolar fracture and osteochondral fracture of the posterolateral talar shoulder.
a–b Axial views.
c–d Coronal views.
e Sagittal view.

2 Preoperative planning

Indications for surgery

In the setting of an acute and radiographically evident talar osteochondral dome fracture, CT evaluation is necessary to evaluate the extent of the osseous component of the injury. Surgical treatment of osteochondral talar dome fractures is indicated if the fracture results in articular surface incongruity, or there is instability resulting in alteration of ankle alignment or if there are loose fragments.

Treatment options

Nonweight bearing and immobilization

If the talar osteochondral fragment is nondisplaced and stable, closed treatment is indicated. Nonweight bearing is often necessary. Range of motion (ROM) of the ankle is encouraged early to avoid stiffness.

Surgical excision of the fracture fragment

In the absence of enough bone necessary to allow for adequate fixation, the fragment should be excised to prevent it from acting as a loose joint body resulting in further articular injury. This may be done either by open or arthroscopic technique. In some cases, this will be a decision made intraoperatively based on operative findings.

Fracture fixation

If the osteochondral dome fracture fragment contains enough bone to obtain fixation and allow for bone-to-bone healing, acute fixation is advocated to maximize healing with articular (hyaline) cartilage and hopefully prevent or delay posttraumatic arthrosis. Various osteochondral fixation techniques have been described, though studies comparing long-term outcomes are lacking.

In this patient, the osteochondral dome fracture comprised the far lateral portion of the talar dome extending the entire anterior to posterior distance of the articular surface, thereby warranting reduction and fixation. Exposure of the lateral talar dome was to be accomplished by manipulation of the distal fibular fracture fragment. In the absence of a fibular fracture, a lateral malleolar osteotomy is typically performed. Fixation was planned with a bioabsorbable screw. Other options are also available: metal nonabsorbable screws should be used with caution as even with countersinking the screw, it may become prominent in the joint as the fragment settles; use of bioabsorbable pins is another fixation option.

3 Operating room setup

Patient positioning	• Supine on a radiolucent table with a bump under the ipsilateral hip to correct for the natural external rotation of the limb
Anesthesia options	• General or regional according to surgeon preference and the extent of injury. • Paralytic agents may be of benefit in cases where a distractor will be used, either as part of open or arthroscopic treatment.
C-arm location	• Positioned on the contralateral side of the table to be able to come into the field as needed. • The monitor of the C-arm should be positioned superiorly for ease of viewing by the primary surgeon.
Tourniquet	• May be used for improved visualization and reduction

For illustrations and overview of anesthetic considerations, see chapter 1.

Equipment

- Bone holding and bone reduction forceps
- Dental scaler
- K-wire set
- Bioabsorbable screws or pins
- Screws (headless screws or small diameter-headed screws amenable for countersinking)
- Ankle fracture fixation equipment per surgeon preference

4 Surgical procedure

The talar osteochondral fragment should be reduced and fixed under direct visualization. Approach selection must therefore consider the specific location of the osteochondral fracture on the talar dome. In the case of an isolated posterolateral talar injury, a lateral malleolar osteotomy is required to gain visualization of the lateral talar dome. For a concomitant fibular fracture, the lateral malleolar osteotomy principles can be applied through the fracture.

If the surgeon preference is using a tourniquet, the limb is exsanguinated and the tourniquet is inflated. A standard lateral approach to the fibula is planned with the incision shifted slightly anteriorly. The incision is carried out with care to avoid injuring the superficial peroneal nerve as it crosses the field. The nerve is generally located 5 cm proximal to the tip of the fibula but is variable and will occasionally cross the fibula quite low. For the remainder of the approach, the superficial peroneal nerve remains protected anterior to the dissection plane.

Dissection is then carried anteriorly to the level of the syndesmosis and the anterior inferior tibiofibular ligament is released to mobilize the distal fibula. Visualization of the lateral talar dome requires mobilization of the lateral malleolus, either through the fracture site or a planned osteotomy. If the fibula is intact, a transverse osteotomy is performed superior to the attachment of the syndesmotic ligaments (**Fig 5.1-3**). The osteotomy level must be proximal enough to allow for compression plating with enough distal fixation at the end of the procedure. For this patient with a fibular fracture, release of the anterior inferior tibiofibular ligament allowed adequate mobility of the distal fibula fracture and the fragment was rotated on its posterior soft-tissue hinge to allow visualization of the lateral talus.

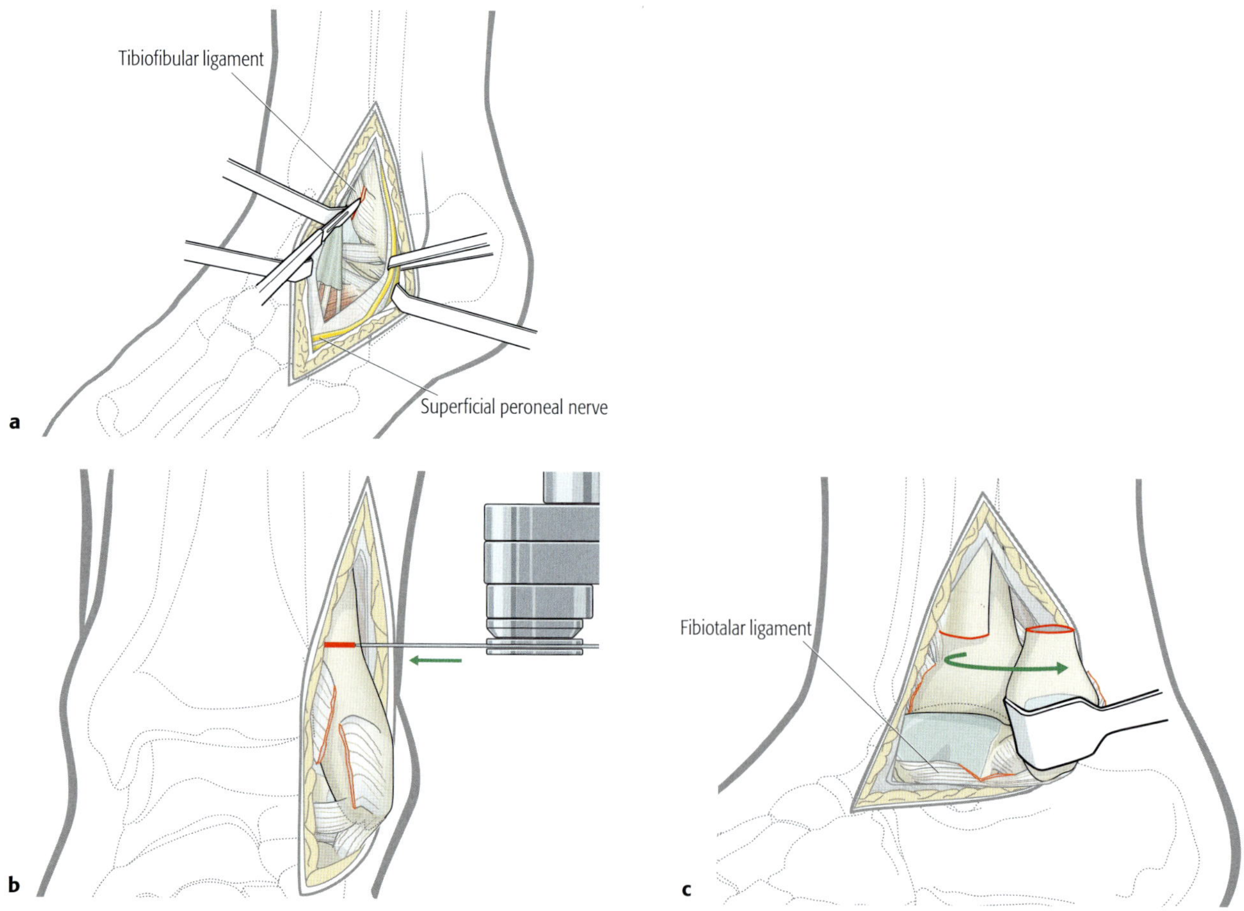

Fig 5.1-3a–c Visualization of the lateral talar dome.
a The anterior inferior tibiofibular ligament and the anterior talofibular ligament are sectioned with a cuff of tissue for future repair.
b–c If fracture is not present, a transverse osteotomy is performed (**b**), and the fibula is externally rotated to visualize the talus (**c**).

After the lateral aspect of the talus has been exposed, the osteochondral dome fracture can be directly addressed. Visualization can be improved by inverting the hindfoot and ankle. Additionally, a small distractor may be used to improve visualization.

If the fragment is large enough to accept screws, bioabsorbable screw fixation is used. The fragment can be directly manipulated and reduced with K-wire used as a joystick or with a dental instrument, and the reduction is held with a K-wire (**Fig 5.1-4**). Often, the variable which determines fixation stability is the amount of bone under the articular area of the fragment. If the fragment is too small to be held by bioabsorbable screws, a K-wire or bioabsorbable pin can be used for definitive fixation and left in place. Alternatively, the osteochondral fragment may be excised and cartilage restoration techniques, such as microfracture, osteochondral autograft transfer, or osteochondral allograft, may be used either on an acute or delayed basis. For this patient, the fragment was large enough to accept fixation. A small K-wire is inserted into the fragment and used as a joystick to reduce the fracture. Manual compression is held while two 2.7 mm biodegradable screws are inserted lateral to medial in the talar dome. Reduction is confirmed visually and with intraoperative C-arm views.

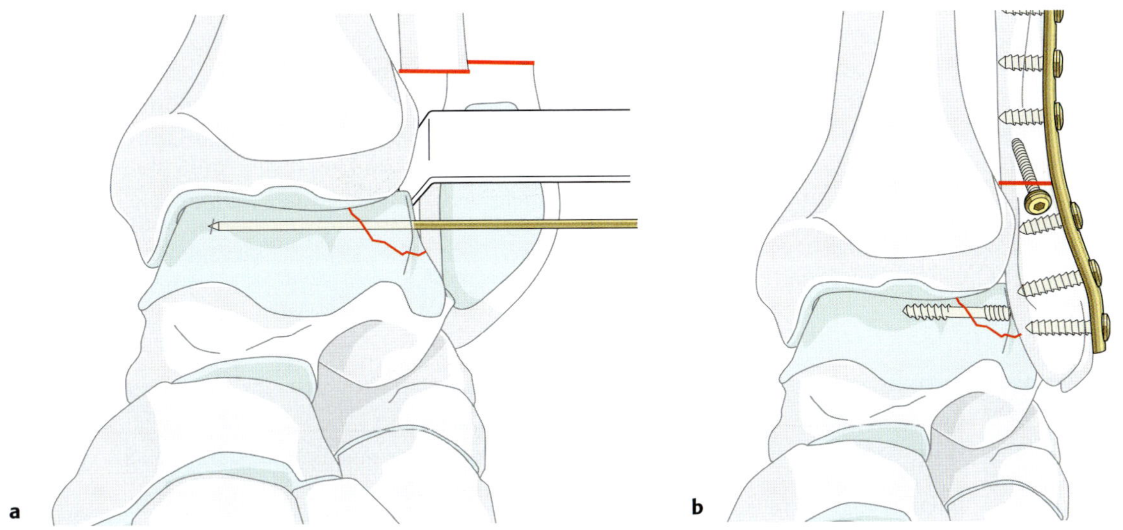

Fig 5.1-4a–b Talar osteochondral fracture fixation.

a Fibular osteotomy performed and retracted to visualize the fracture, which has been provisionally fixed with a K-wire.

b Definitive fixation of the osteochondral fracture performed with a headless compression screw and fibular osteotomy reconstructed with fibular plate fixation.

After talar fixation is completed, attention is turned back to the fibula. If an osteotomy was performed, compression plating with a one-third tubular or precontoured distal fibular plate is performed. For this patient with a fibular fracture, a precontoured distal fibular plate was chosen for fixation. Reduction of the fibula can be attempted with bone reduction forceps.

If the fibula cannot be adequately reduced, other reduction techniques may be necessary. A push screw technique may be necessary to restore length. Locking screws are placed unicortically through the plate in the distal fragment. An independent screw is then placed in bicortical fashion proximal to the plate. A lamina spreader is inserted between the screw and plate and opened, restoring length. After adequate reduction is obtained and confirmed with the C-arm, the proximal screws are inserted to complete fibular fixation (**Fig 5.1-5**). Alternatively, a small distractor may also be used to assist in gaining reduction. At this point, the previously sectioned anterior inferior tibiofibular ligament is identified and repaired with nonabsorbable suture. Stability of the syndesmosis is confirmed with external rotation stress testing and the hook test. If the ankle is unstable, transsyndesmotic screws should be inserted.

Medial talar osteochondral dome fractures

Medial talar osteochondral dome fractures are less common than lateral-sided injuries and often require medial malleolar osteotomy for adequate exposure. The osteotomy should be planned carefully, using a K-wire as a visual guide for the saw cut (**Fig 5.1-6**). The K-wire is inserted through the medial malleolus, penetrating the tibial plafond at the lateral margin of the talar fracture. A thin micro-sagittal saw or chisel is then used to osteotomize the medial malleolus to the level of the subchondral bone of the plafond. The osteotomy is completed with a thin, broad osteotome to avoid iatrogenic damage to the talus and minimize bone and cartilage loss from the kerf of the sawblade. The medial malleolus is then hinged on the deltoid ligament to expose the medial talar dome.

Reduction and fixation can then proceed using the same techniques described above. If a medial osteotomy is performed, make sure to include enough plafond to allow for good visualization. The osteotomy should enter the ankle joint along the plafond and not just include the medial malleolus, which might impair visualization of the osteochondral fracture.

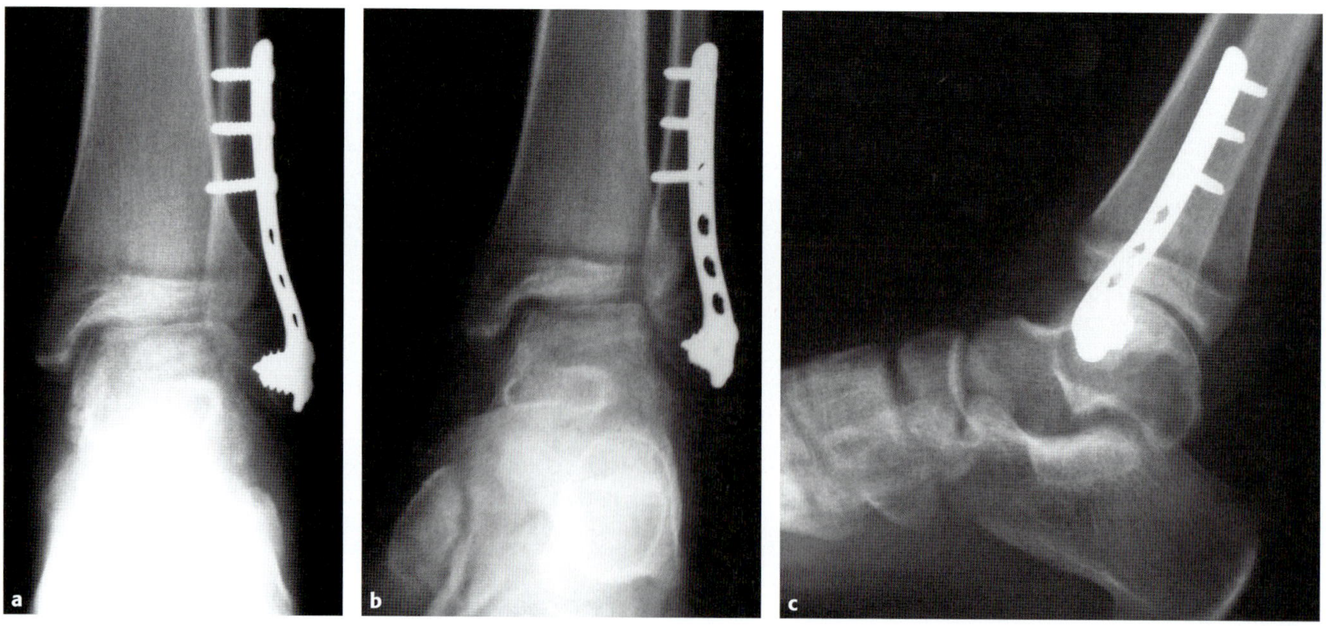

Fig 5.1-5a–c Postoperative x-rays demonstrate fixation of the lateral malleolar fracture with a locking plate after the talar osteochondral fragment has been fixed with radiolucent biodegradable headless screws.
a AP view.
b Mortise view.
c Lateral view.

5 Pitfalls and complications

Pitfalls

Missed diagnosis on initial presentation

A common pitfall in the treatment of osteochondral dome fractures is a missed diagnosis on initial presentation. The osseous piece of the fragment may be small and easily overlooked on the injury x-rays. A CT scan should be used in cases where plane x-rays are unclear or clinical suspicion for an osteochondral fracture remains high. Magnetic resonance imaging is useful to detect occult injuries but not as good as a CT scan in helping the surgeon see the injury in 3D.

Complications of the malleolar osteotomy

- In cases without an associated ankle fracture, malleolar osteotomies may be required for exposure. An incorrect osteotomy level will impede visualization of the talus. This can be avoided by inserting a K-wire under C-arm guidance to confirm the proper osteotomy trajectory.
- Improper fixation of the osteotomized malleolus may lead to nonunion and necessitate revision surgery.
- Finally, the osteotomy enters the ankle joint. Malreduction of the osteotomy or injury to the articular surface at the time of the osteotomy can lead to arthritis.

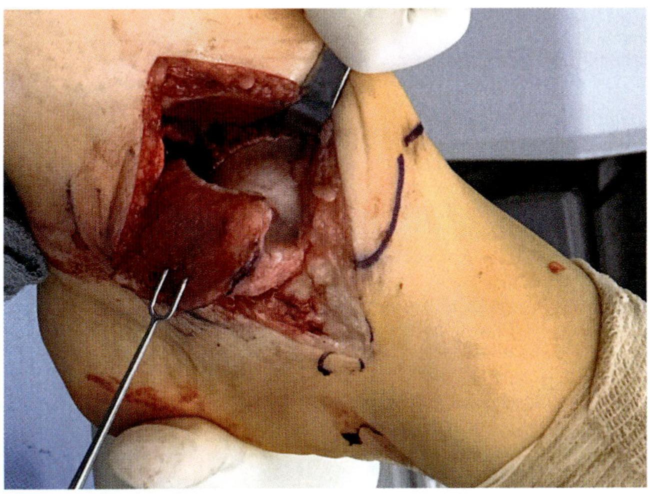

Fig 5.1-6 Example from a different case showing malleolar osteotomy performed to gain access to the medial talar dome. The malleolar piece is internally rotated to thoroughly evaluate the talar dome.

Loss of fixation of the osteochondral dome fragment

Loss of fixation of the osteochondral fragment may lead to a loose body within the tibiotalar joint and accelerate articular degeneration. Fixation should be confirmed intraoperatively. The technique of buried K-wires should be exercised with caution. If the osteochondral fragment resorbs, the buried K-wire will become prominent and can cause articular damage. If this technique is chosen, close follow-up is warranted to ensure the K-wire does not become prominent.

Complications

- Missed injury leading to loose body formation and accelerated articular degeneration
- Injury to the superficial peroneal nerve during the lateral exposure
- Articular damage to the talus with osteotomy creation
- Nonanatomical fixation of the medial or lateral malleolus following osteotomy
- Necrosis of the osteochondral fragment
- Secondary failure of fixation and loosening of the osteochondral fragment
- Articular injury from prominent hardware
- Posttraumatic ankle arthritis

6 Alternative techniques

Arthroscopic management of the osteochondral dome fracture is an alternative to open visualization with osteotomy techniques. Arthroscopic visualization is commonly used in cases without associated ankle fractures, but newer studies have also advocated arthroscopic-assisted open ankle fixation to assess the talar dome for osteochondral fractures that may have been missed on the x-rays. As these studies have not shown improved results over traditional techniques, it remains to be seen whether future studies establish a role for arthroscopy in ankle fracture management.

In cases of small osteochondral fragments not amenable to internal fixation, excision of the fragment may be the best alternative. After excision, cartilage restoration techniques frequently used in the knee may be used. Fibrocartilage production can be promoted with microfracture, antegrade drilling, or retrograde drilling of the lesion.

Larger osteochondral fracture fragments not amenable to fixation may leave a defect that may require osteochondral autograft or allograft transfer to promote healing via hyaline cartilage.

7 Postoperative management and rehabilitation

Most acute osteochondral fractures will be associated with ankle fractures and similar postoperative protocols will be used. Nonweight-bearing precautions for at least 6 weeks with progressive weight bearing thereafter are recommended. Since motion promotes cartilage healing, ROM exercises should be encouraged as early as possible, typically after the incision has healed at 2 weeks postoperatively. **Fig 5.1-7** shows the final follow-up x-rays of the patient with the medial osteochondral defect who underwent osteochondral autograft transfer.

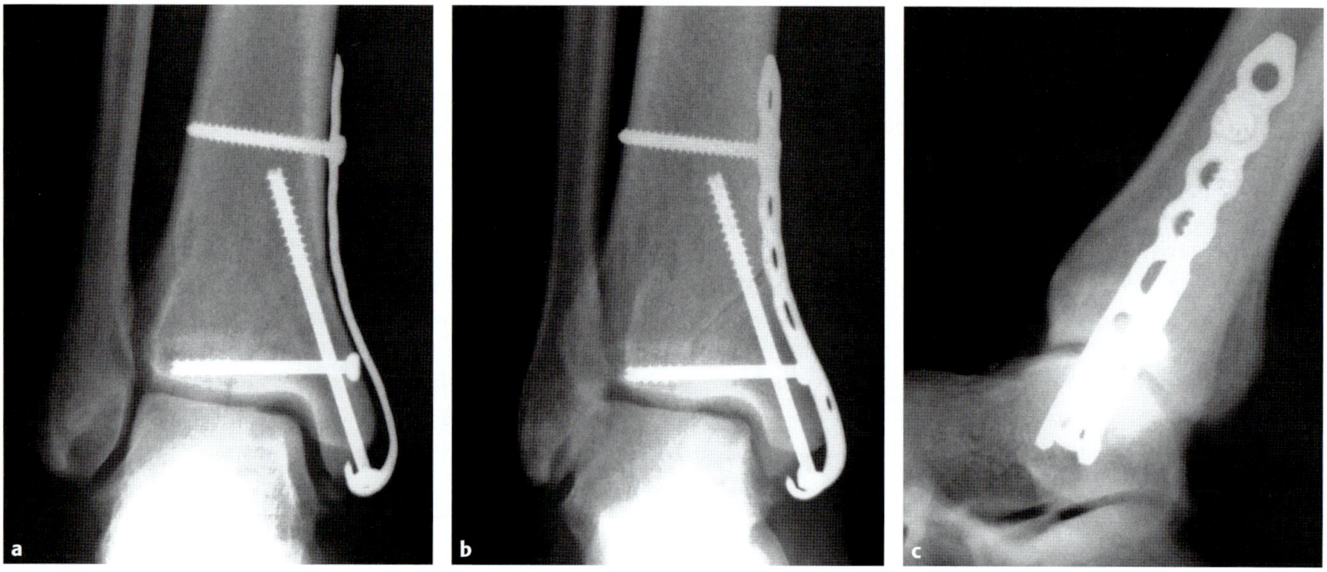

Fig 5.1-7a–c Example from a different case showing fixation of the medial malleolar osteotomy with a lag screw and a hook plate construct.
a AP view.
b Mortise view.
c Lateral view.

8 Recommended reading

Chan KB, Lui TH. Role of ankle arthroscopy in management of acute ankle fracture. *Arthroscopy.* 2016 Nov;32(11):2373–2380.
Choi WJ, Park KK, Kim BS, et al. Osteochondral lesion of the talus: is there a critical defect size for poor outcome? *Am J Sports Med.* 2009 Oct;37(10):1974–1980.
Dunlap BJ, Ferkel RD, Applegate GR. The "LIFT" lesion: lateral inverted osteochondral fracture of the talus. *Arthroscopy.* 2013 Nov;29(11):1826–1833.
Gonzalez TA, Macaulay AA, Ehrlichman LK, et al. Arthroscopically assisted versus standard open reduction and internal fixation techniques for the acute ankle fracture. *Foot Ankle Int.* 2016 May;37(5):554–562.
Hannon CP, Smyth NA, Murawski CD, et al. Osteochondral lesions of the talus: aspects of current management. *Bone Joint J.* 2014 Feb;96-b(2):164–171.
Leontaritis N, Hinojosa L, Panchbhavi VK. Arthroscopically detected intra-articular lesions associated with acute ankle fractures. *J Bone Joint Surg Am.* 2009 Feb;91(2):333–339.
Mitchell ME, Giza E, Sullivan MR. Cartilage transplantation techniques for talar cartilage lesions. *J Am Acad Orthop Surg.* 2009 Jul;17(7):407–414.
Nosewicz TL, Beerekamp MS, De Muinck Keizer RJ, et al. Prospective computed tomographic analysis of osteochondral lesions of the ankle joint associated with ankle fractures. *Foot Ankle Int.* 2016 Aug;37(8):829–834.
Pritsch M, Horoshovski H, Farine I. Arthroscopic treatment of osteochondral lesions of the talus. *J Bone Joint Surg Am.* 1986 Jul;68(6):862–865.
Regier M, Petersen JP, Hamurcu A, et al. High incidence of osteochondral lesions after open reduction and internal fixation of displaced ankle fractures: medium-term follow-up of 100 cases. *Injury.* 2016 Mar;47(3):757–761.
Salter RB, Simmonds DF, Malcolm BW, et al. The biological effect of continuous passive motion on the healing of full-thickness defects in articular cartilage. An experimental investigation in the rabbit. *J Bone Joint Surg Am.* 1980 Dec;62(8):1232–1251.
Takao M, Uchio Y, Naito K, et al. Diagnosis and treatment of combined intra-articular disorders in acute distal fibular fractures. *J Trauma.* 2004 Dec;57(6):1303–1307.
Vaghela KR, Clement H, Parker L. Syndesmosis preserving osteotomy of the fibula for access to the lateral talar dome. *Foot Ankle Surg.* 2016 Sep;22(3):210–213.

5.2 Lateral process fracture

Mandeep S Dhillon, Devendra K Chouhan

1 Case description

A 42-year-old man twisted his right ankle while participating in snow sports. Within an hour, he experienced pain and swelling in the ankle. He went to a nearby hospital where x-rays of the ankle showed a chip/avulsion fracture on the AP view. The lateral view did not show the fracture. The patient was diagnosed with a talar body fracture of the lateral process (AO/OTA 81.1.A2). A piece of bone was noted in the space between the fibula and the talus (**Fig 5.2-1**).

Due to the lack of facilities at the primary hospital, he was referred to a higher-level clinic for fracture management. A computed tomographic (CT) scan showed the fracture anatomy, ruling out any other associated injury. The coronal section showed the fracture of the lateral process of the talus with subtalar articular involvement (Funk type B1) and a small comminuted fragment in the subfibular space (**Fig 5.2-2**). The limb was splinted in a below-knee plaster slab and was elevated.

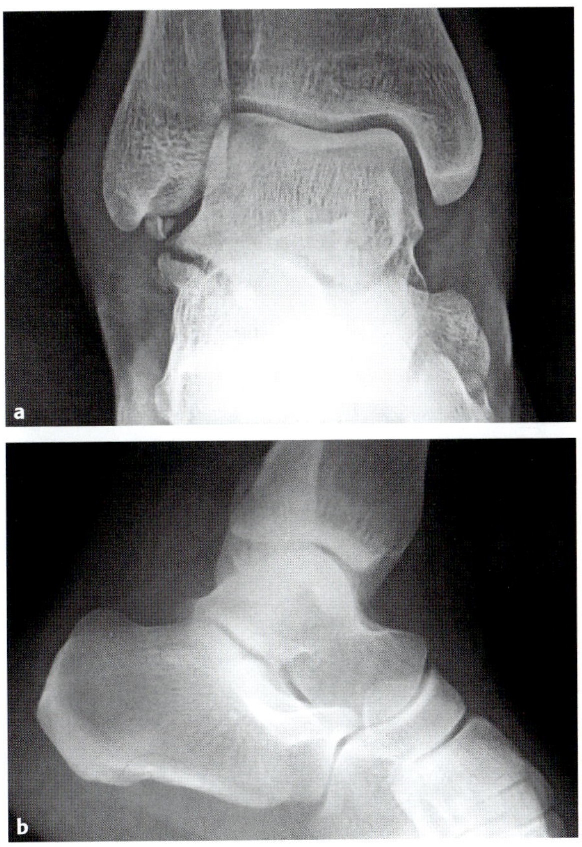

Fig 5.2-1a–b Injury x-rays.

a The AP view of ankle shows a fracture of the lateral process of the talus. Note the small piece in subfibular lateral gutter space.

b The lateral view of ankle can often be interpreted as normal.

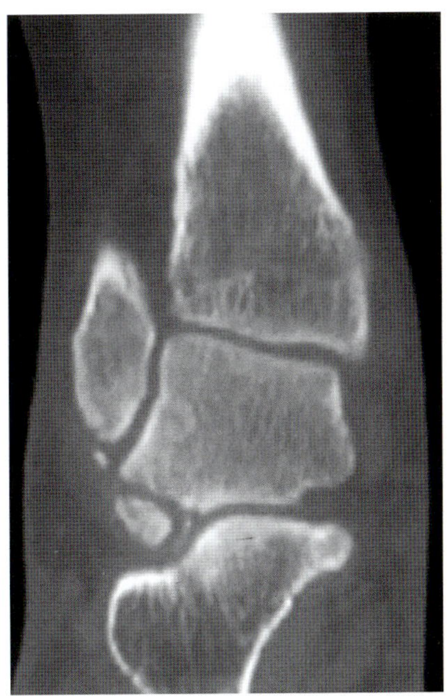

Fig 5.2-2 Coronal cut CT scan showing lateral process fracture.

2 Preoperative planning

Fracture classification

The AO/OTA classification code for this fracture is an avulsian fracture of the talar body (81.1.A2). However, the AO/OTA does not differentiate between different subtypes of fractures as described by Funk, where treatment may differ.

The Funk classification describes three types of fractures. Type A fractures do not involve articular surfaces. Type B1 or B2 are chip/avulsion or comminuted fractures involving only the subtalar joint. Type C1 or C2 fractures involve both subtalar and talofibular joints, with or without comminution.

Indications for surgery

The decision for open reduction and internal fixation (ORIF) was made due to the fragment size of > 1 cm, the significant displacement (> 2 mm), and involvement of the subtalar articular surface (> 10%) (Funk type B1).

Treatment options

The fracture is easily accessed using the sinus tarsi approach. Alternatively, an oblique lateral (Ollier) approach may be used. Displaced fractures of the lateral process should be treated operatively to reduce the likelihood of developing posttraumatic subtalar arthritis. Typically, large fragments (> 5 mm) are treated by open reduction and fixed with screws or a small plate. Comminuted injuries requiring fixation are generally treated with minifragment plating. Smaller fragments not amenable to internal fixation, loose pieces, and other debris in the lateral gutter should be removed. Data from biomechanical studies suggest that fragments up to 1 cm in length or 5 cm in size can be removed without risking ankle or subtalar instability. Therefore, if anatomical reduction cannot be achieved or fragmentation of the lateral process fragment occurs, the decision to excise the fragment rather than leaving an intraarticular step-off should be made generously.

Only incomplete fractures that are completely nondisplaced (on CT) should be treated nonoperatively.

3 Operating room setup

Patient positioning	• Supine on a radiolucent table, with a sand bag under the ipsilateral hip to tilt the patient 30–45° to the contralateral side. • The knee is bent and can be positioned with rolled towels or special supports (**Fig 5.2-3**)
Anesthesia options	• General or regional anesthesia
C-arm location	• The C-arm is positioned on the opposite side
Tourniquet	• Nonsterile tourniquet is applied in the thigh to achieve bloodless field at the time of reduction
Tips	• A headlight may be used to improve visualization

For illustrations and overview of anesthetic considerations, see chapter 1.

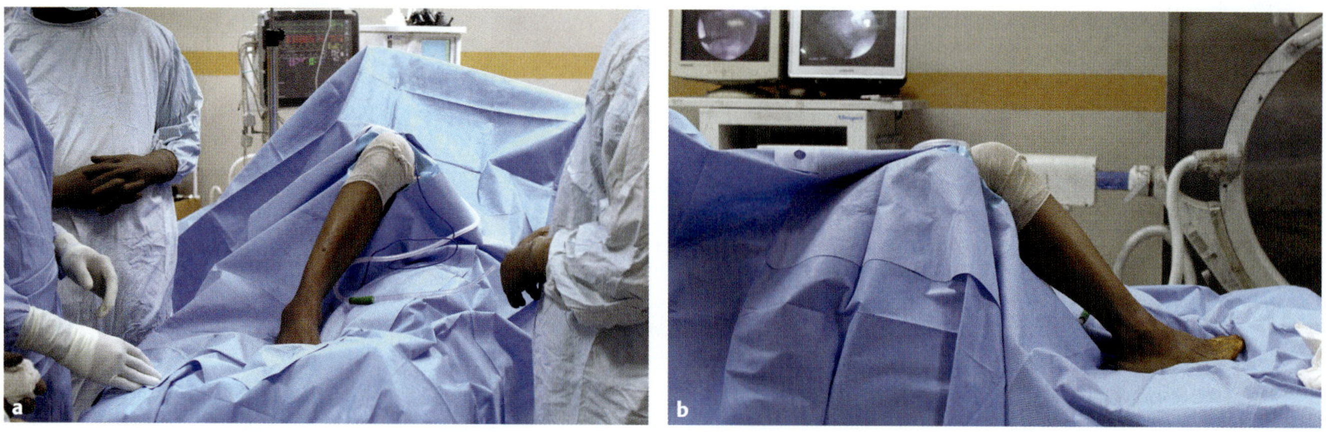

Fig 5.2-3a–b Patient positioning.
a Patient positioned supine and with a bump under the ipsilateral hip to internally rotate the limb by 30–45°.
b C-arm positioned on the opposite side of the operative table.

Equipment

- K-wire
- Headless or other screws as per surgeon preference
- Minifragment plates
- K-wires and drill bits
- Small distraction device to visualize the subtalar joint
- Reduction clamps for fracture reduction

4 Surgical procedure

For ORIF of the lateral process of the talus, a sinus tarsi approach is commonly used. Care should be taken to protect the anterior intermediate branch of the superficial peroneal nerve (**Fig 5.2-4**).

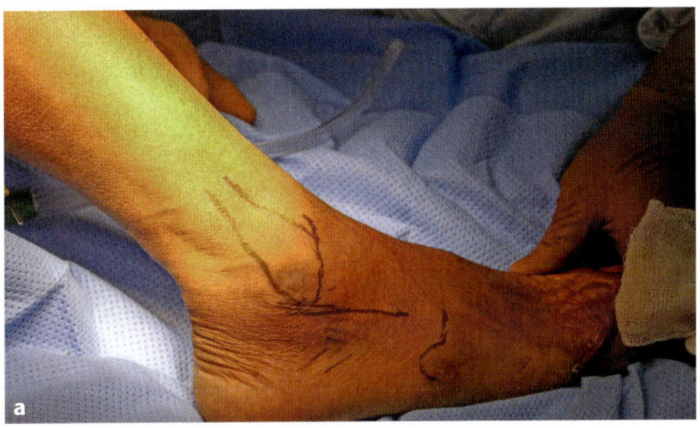

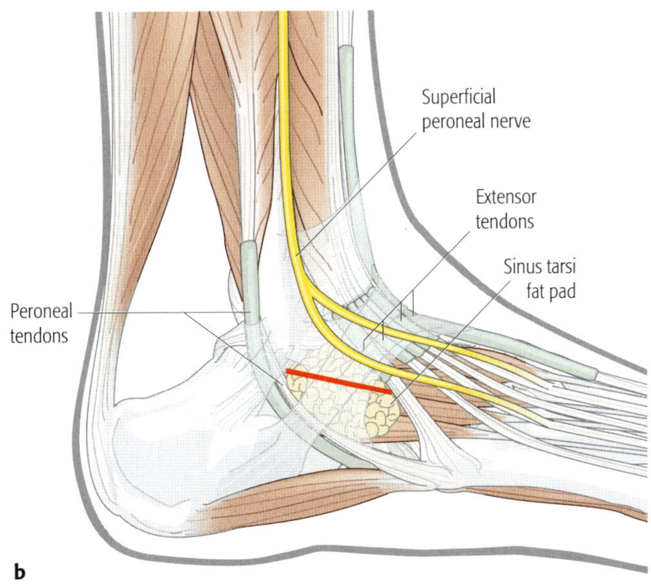

Fig 5.2-4a–b Skin marking. Note the superficial peroneal nerve is close to the anterior end of the incision.

The skin incision extends from the tip of the fibula, down toward the base of the fourth metatarsal, and is usually 3–4 cm long. The fat pad is incised, and extensor digitorum brevis muscle belly is elevated from the sinus tarsi to expose the subtalar joint. Subsequently release of the lateral talocalcaneal ligament exposes the fractured lateral process of talus. A foot retractor or additional K-wires used as joysticks, help in exposure. The anterior fibulotalar ligament can be elevated to improve the exposure (specifically in Funk type C fractures), after which the fragment is mobilized, and the joint debrided and cleared of fracture hematoma or fracture debris.

The lateral process fragment is reduced under direct visualization by using a K-wire as a joystick, and further stabilized by inserting a second K-wire which should be in the center of the fragment (**Fig 5.2-5**). The fragment size determines what size and type of screws, whether a headless or small fragment screw. If a headless screw is used, a second K-wire should be placed as the guide wire for this second screw. The appropriate drill bit is used over the centrally placed wire, and after depth measurement, the appropriate length screw is inserted. The second K-wire is left in place if there is doubt about rotational stability, or a second screw can be placed. If a screw is placed through the articular surface, the screw must be countersunk below the level of the joint surface.

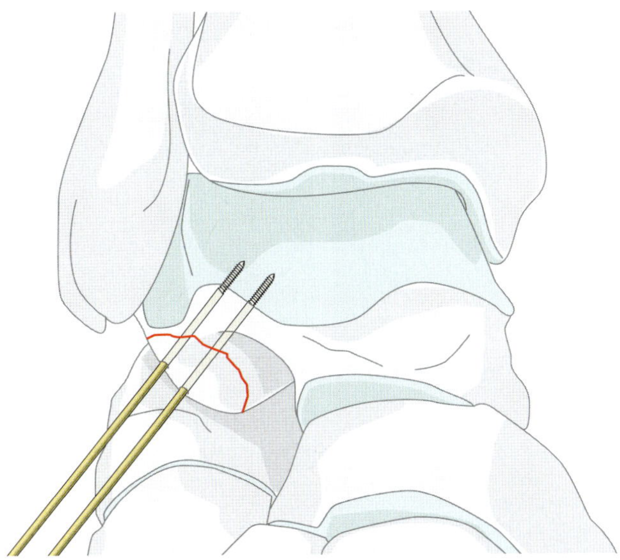

Fig 5.2-5 Fixation with K-wires before definitive screw fixation.

The accuracy of reduction is checked visually by distracting the subtalar joint, as well as with the C-arm using Brodén and reversed Brodén view. The sub-fibular piece of bone found in this case was under the middle bundle of the fibulotalar ligament and was removed.

For this patient, final stabilization of fragment was done with headless screws, and anatomical reduction reconfirmed visually and radiologically (**Fig 5.2-6**).

5 Pitfalls and complications

Pitfalls

- C-arm views are often difficult to obtain, and manual or instrumented distraction is the best way to inspect for the accuracy of the reduction. In cases of ankle joint involvement, release of the middle bundle of the talofibular ligament helps to improve exposure.
- Importantly, these fractures are often missed due to limited awareness of the injury and improper evaluation of available x-rays. A high index of suspicion must be maintained, and there should be a low threshold for ordering CT scans, especially after closed reduction of subtalar dislocations.
- Bony impingement may be seen, accompanied by pain, in neglected injuries.

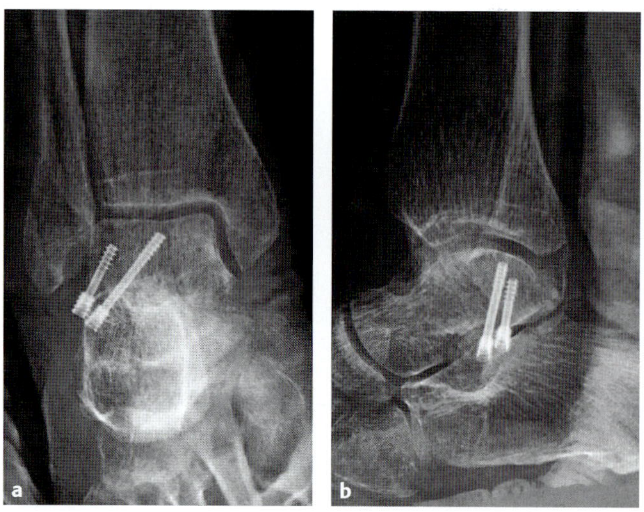

Fig 5.2-6a–b Fixation with two headless compression screws.
a AP view.
b Lateral view.

Complications

- Delayed or missed diagnosis
- Nonunion
- Delayed union
- Avascular necrosis
- Subtalar arthritis
- Stiffness

6 Alternative techniques

Fracture excision

Classifying the lateral process fracture is important, as it allows us to plan the surgical intervention. Funk type 1 fractures, which do not involve the subtalar or ankle joint can be excised, and the results are promising. Excision of fragments can also be done in the presence of significant comminution and in cases where the fracture is not reconstructable. As the lateral process forms a significant portion of the subtalar and ankle joints, even minor residual steps are poorly tolerated, and excision should be performed generously if perfect anatomical reduction cannot be achieved. For patients who present late, excision is the best option.

Arthroscopic-assisted fixation

Arthroscopic reduction and fixation of lateral process fractures has been advocated to minimize the surgical insult to talofibular and talocalcaneal ligaments. However, there is no evidence that use of the arthroscope alters healing time with return to full function nor does it decrease the complication rate.

Nonoperative treatment

Nonoperative treatment with cast immobilization and nonweight bearing is rarely indicated in lateral process fractures and is only indicated for fractures that are nondisplaced and incomplete on CT evaluation.

7 Postoperative management and rehabilitation

Postoperatively a below-knee splint or cast is applied for immobilization. Cooperative patients may be allowed early range-of-motion exercises outside the splint.

Subtalar joint stiffness is common after this injury and is less likely with early range of motion.

Patients are kept nonweight bearing but are made mobile with the aid of crutches. Brace or cast is removed at 6 weeks, and range of movement exercises are continued. X-rays in AP, lateral, and Brodén views of ankle are reviewed for confirmation of fracture healing. Gradually increasing weight bearing and strengthening exercises are now recommended (**Fig 5.2-7**).

Implant removal

This is not routinely done when headless screws are used, as they are difficult to remove and do not cause implant-related symptoms. Partially threaded screws are removed after fracture healing if they cause lateral impingement (but this should not happen if the proper countersink technique is used).

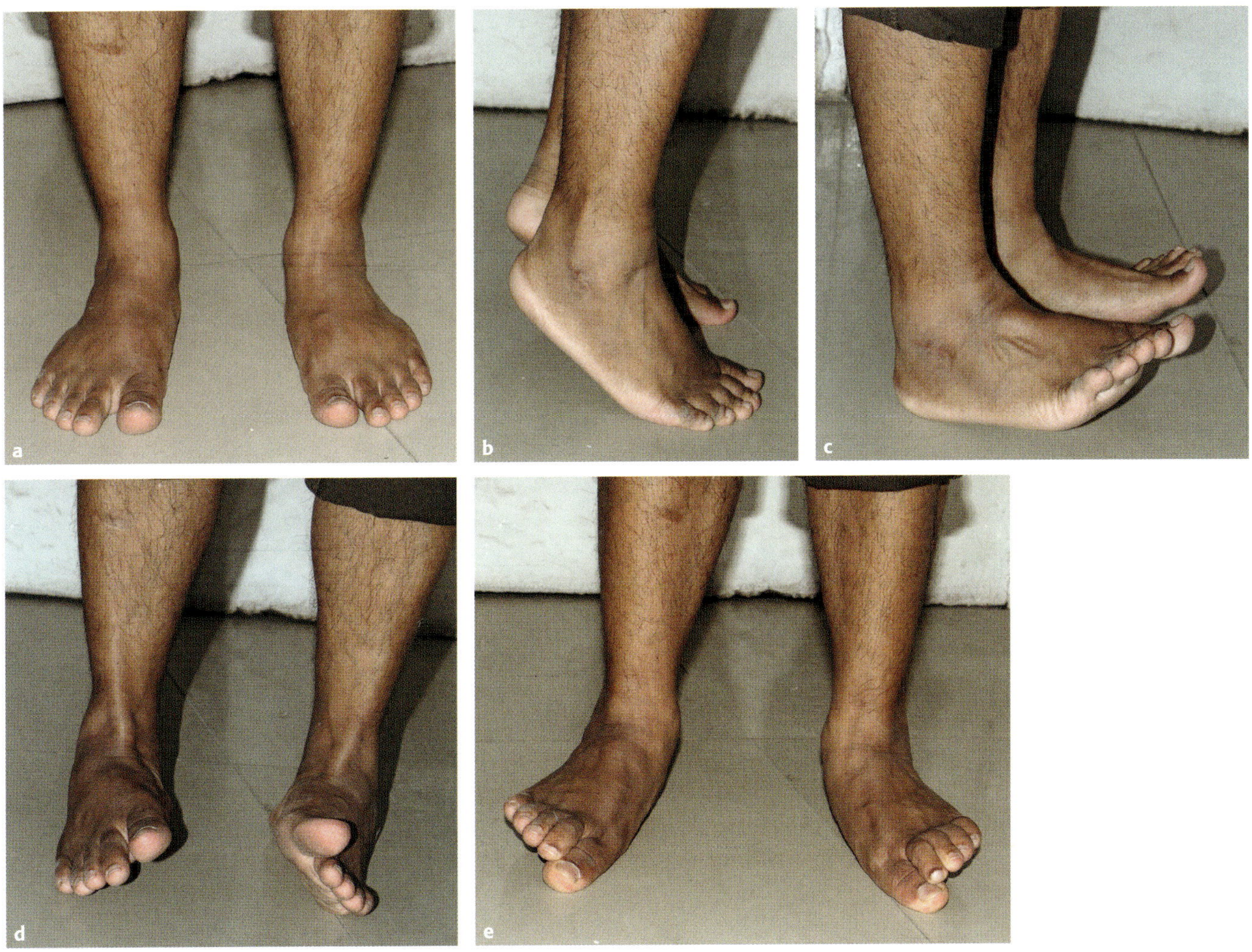

Fig 5.2-7a–e Foot function of the patient 16 weeks after surgery.
a Standing on both feet.
b Standing on toes.
c Standing on heel.
d Standing on lateral border.
e Standing on medial border.

8 Recommended reading

Funasaki H, Hayashi H, Sugiyama H, et al. Arthroscopic reduction and internal fixation for fracture of the lateral process of the talus. *Arthrosc Tech.* 2015 Feb;4(1):e81–86.

Funk JR, Srinivasan SC, Crandall JR. Snowboarder's talus fractures experimentally produced by eversion and dorsiflexion. *Am J Sports Med.* 2003 Nov–Dec;31(6):921–928.

Heckman JD, McLean MR. Fractures of the lateral process of the talus. *Clin Orthop Relat Res.* 1985 Oct(199):108–113.

Langer P, Nickisch F, Spenciner D, et al. In vitro evaluation of the effect lateral process talar excision on ankle and subtalar joint stability. *Foot Ankle Int.* 2007 Jan;28(1):78–83.

Perera A, Baker JF, Lui DF, et al. The management and outcome of lateral process fracture of the talus. *Foot Ankle Surg.* 2010 Mar;16(1):15–20.

Rammelt S, Bartonicek J, Park KH. Traumatic injury to the subtalar joint. *Foot Ankle Clin.* 2018 Sep;23(3):353–374.

Sands A, White C, Blankstein M, et al. Assessment of ankle and hindfoot stability and joint pressures using a human cadaveric model of a large lateral talar process excision: a biomechanical study. *Medicine (Baltimore).* 2015 Mar;94(11):e606.

Shank JR, Benirschke SK, Swords MP. Treatment of peripheral talus fractures. *Foot Ankle Clin.* 2017 Mar;22(1):181–192.

Tucker DJ, Feder JM, Boylan JP. Fractures of the lateral process of the talus: two case reports and a comprehensive literature review. *Foot Ankle Int.* 1998 Sep;19(9):641–646.

5.3 Posterior process fracture

John R Shank, Michael Swords

1 Case description

A 37-year-old woman sustained an injury to her left ankle after falling off a rock wall onto a beach. She presented with a chief complaint of ankle pain, swelling, and inability to ambulate.

On presentation, x-rays of the ankle revealed a fracture of the posterior medial body of the talus (**Fig 5.3-1**). A computed tomographic (CT) scan was performed, which confirmed a comminuted fracture of the posteromedial talar body with involvement of both the ankle and subtalar joints (**Fig 5.3-2**).

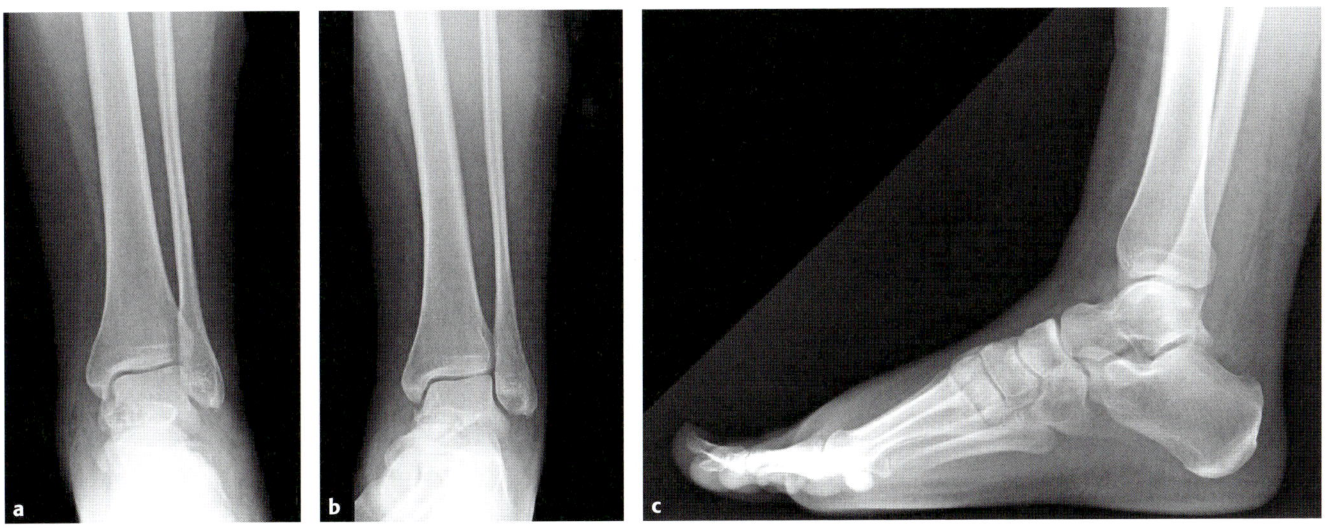

Fig 5.3-1a–c Postinjury x-rays of the ankle demonstrate a posteromedial fracture of the talar body. The fracture is noted on the AP image (**a**) and is difficult to visualize on the mortise (**b**) and partly seen on lateral (**c**) x-rays.

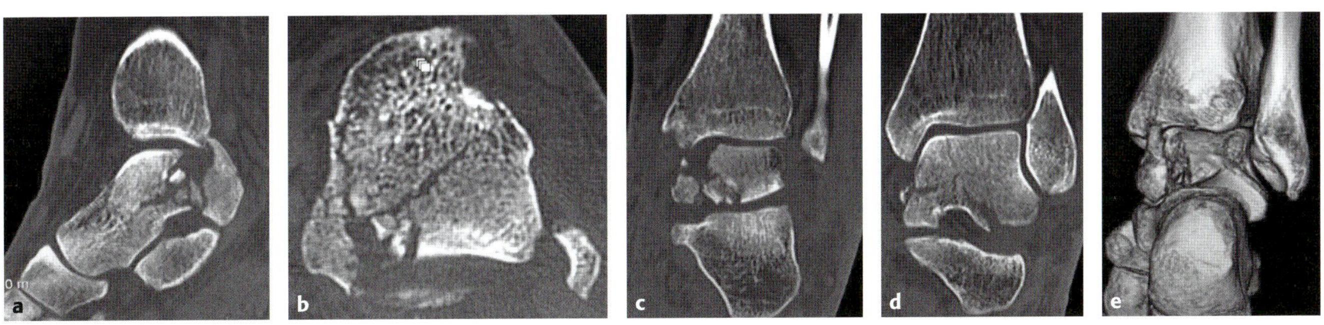

Fig 5.3-2a–e The CT images.
a–d The CT scan reveals a comminuted fracture of the posteromedial talar body involving both the ankle and subtalar joints.
e A 3D reconstruction view.

2 Preoperative planning

Indications for surgery

Surgical treatment of this injury is indicated based on the high incidence of nonunion, arthrosis, and avascular necrosis when these injuries are treated nonoperatively. The goal is to achieve anatomical reduction of the articular surface of the ankle and subtalar joints to minimize the risk of ankle arthrosis, subtalar arthrosis, and avascular necrosis (AVN).

Treatment options

The posteromedial talus is treated through a posteromedial approach with plate and screw fixation. Another treatment option is screw fixation for more simple fracture patterns. An external fixator placed medially can assist with visualization and reduction of these injuries. An appropriate preoperative plan should be made before proceeding with open reduction and internal fixation (**Fig 5.3-3**).

3 Operating room setup

Patient positioning	• Prone
Anesthesia options	• General anesthesia, often supplemented with a peripheral nerve block
C-arm location	• The C-arm is positioned on the ipsilateral side of the injury with the monitor placed near the head of the table.
Tourniquet	• Applied to the thigh, and all bony prominences are well padded
Tips	• A headlight may be used to improve visualization. • The C-arm often needs to be tilted toward the head of the patient to provide true AP and mortise views due to the bump under the operative leg when in the prone position.

For illustrations and overview of anesthetic considerations, see chapter 1.

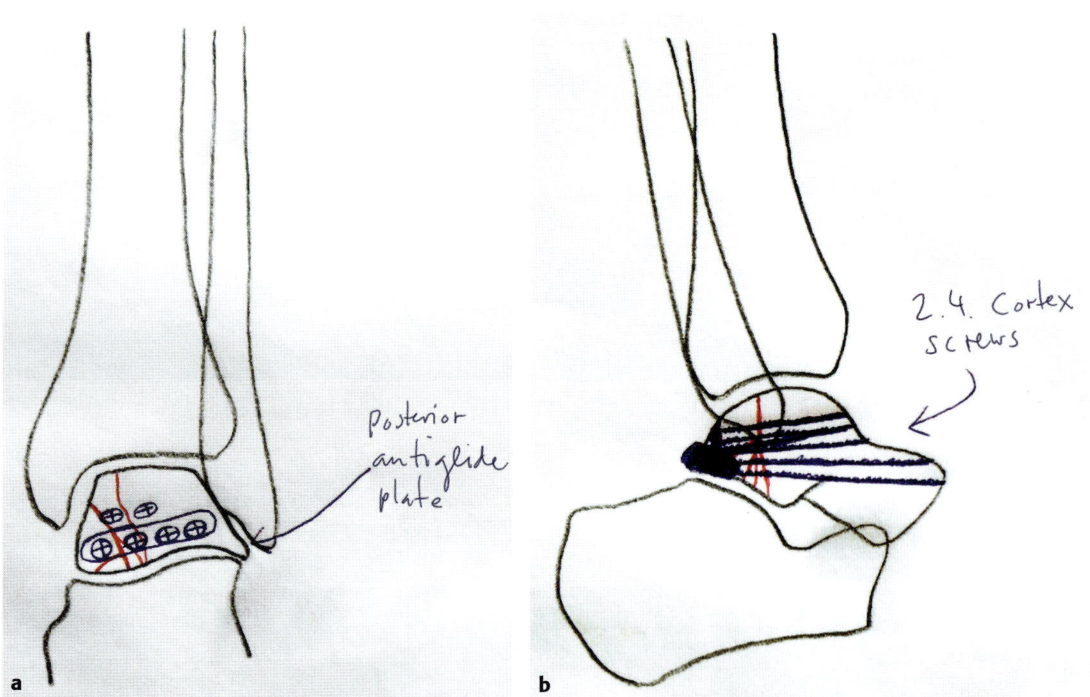

Fig 5.3-3a–b Preoperative plan.
a The posterior talar body is reduced temporarily with K-wires from posterior to anterior, reducing the articular surface of the ankle and subtalar joints. A small buttress plate is placed over the K-wires, which are exchanged for screws.
b The plate is contoured around the posteromedial talar body.

Equipment

- Headlamp for visualization
- Elevators and dental scalers
- External fixator or small distraction device
- K-wire set
- Modular implants with minifragment screws and small plates

The size of instruments and implants may vary according to the anatomy of the patient and to the unique anatomy of the fracture.

4 Surgical procedure

A posteromedial approach to the talus is used according to the preoperative plan. External fixation with distraction of the articular surface is performed to assist with visualization and reduction (**Fig 5.3-4**).

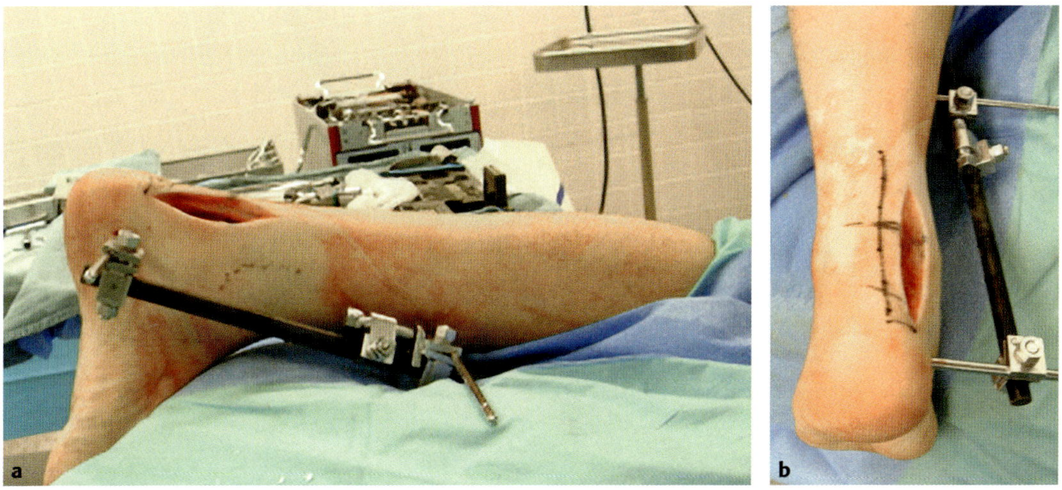

Fig 5.3-4a–b Medial external fixator placement allows for distraction and better visualization of the articular surfaces.

The incision for the posteromedial approach lies parallel to the medial aspect of the Achilles tendon with a gentle curve distally. Deep dissection is performed, after releasing the deep posterior compartment fascia between the Achilles tendon and the flexor hallucis longus (FHL) tendon (**Fig 5.3-5**). The neurovascular bundle is protected deep within the anterior flap, and often is not visible. The FHL retinaculum can be released for better exposure of the talar body. The posterior talar fracture is seen and cleared of hematoma. With maximum dorsiflexion of the ankle, the tibiotalar component of the fracture can be seen (**Fig 5.3-6**).

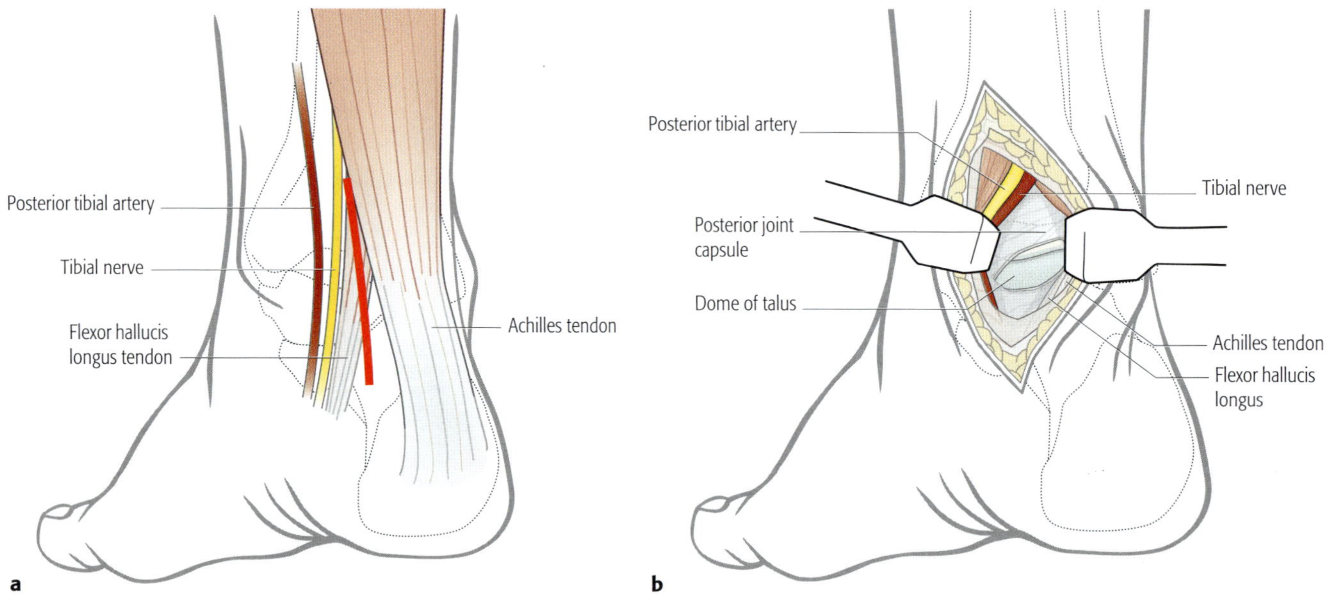

Fig 5.3-5a–b Posteromedial approach to the talar body.
a Landmarks for the skin incision.
b Intraoperative exposure of the posterior talar body and retraction of the FHL tendon.

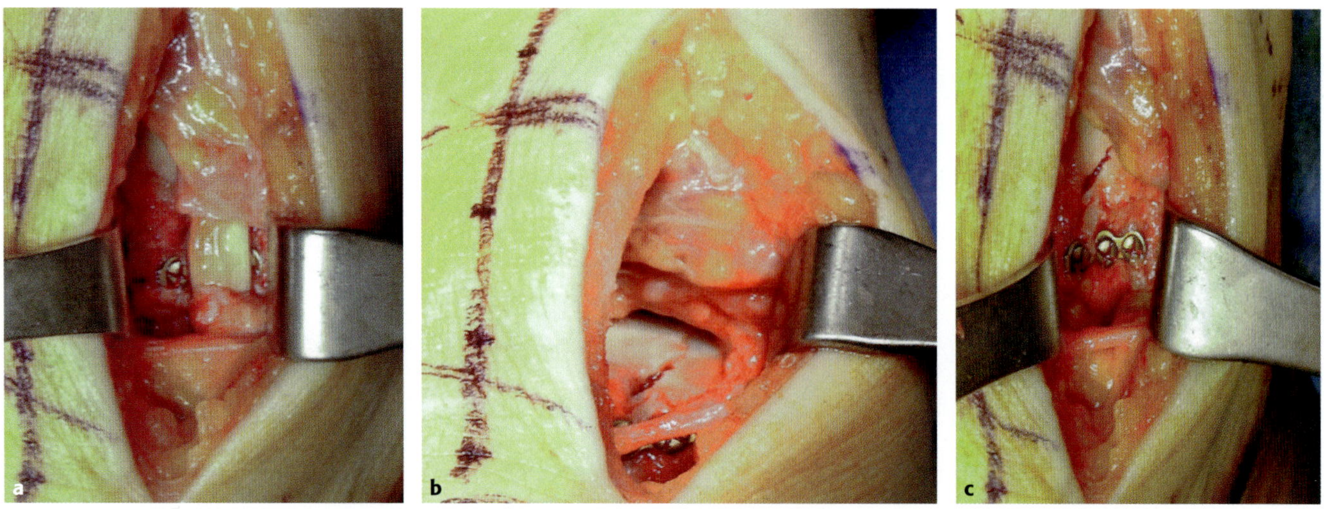

Fig 5.3-6a–c Posteromedial approach to the talar body.
a Exposure of the FHL.
b Retraction of the FHL to allow fracture visualization.
c Final fixation of the posteromedial talar body.

The intercalary fracture fragments are identified and assessed with a dental scaler. Comminuted injuries are evaluated for bone quality and cartilage viability. Reduction of major and minor fracture fragments is performed temporarily with K-wires (**Fig 5.3-7**). Bone grafting of large fracture defects can be performed; however, care must be taken to ensure that the

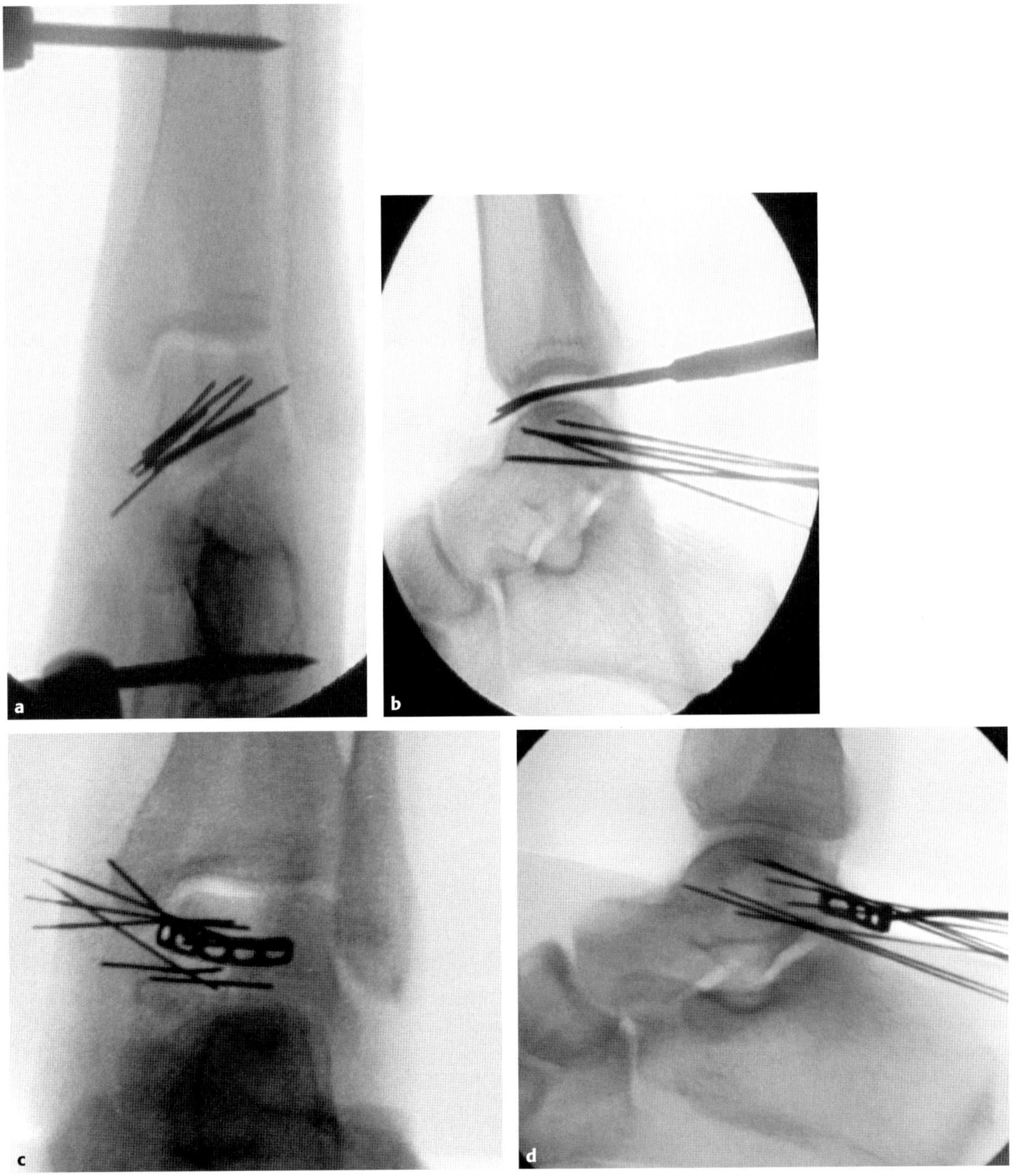

Fig 5.3-7a–d The external fixator is used for articular distraction, and articular reduction is performed with K-wires. The articular reduction of the ankle joint is assessed with an elevator or dental scaler. The plate is contoured around the posterior talar body and placed over and around the K-wires.

graft does not migrate into the joint surfaces or impinge within the ankle or subtalar joints. Definitive fixation can be achieved by sliding a contoured modular plate over the K-wires that are exchanged for screws (**Fig 5.3-8**). The FHL is carefully retracted for exposure and during placement of final fixation. K-wires can be cut and tamped flush with the posterior body of the talus. Anatomical reduction can be assessed under C-arm control and through assessment indirectly with a small (Freer) elevator palpation. The distractor assists in visualizing the joint surfaces. The C-arm is critical in assessing the quality of the subtalar reduction, as it is difficult to directly assess the reduction of the posterior facet.

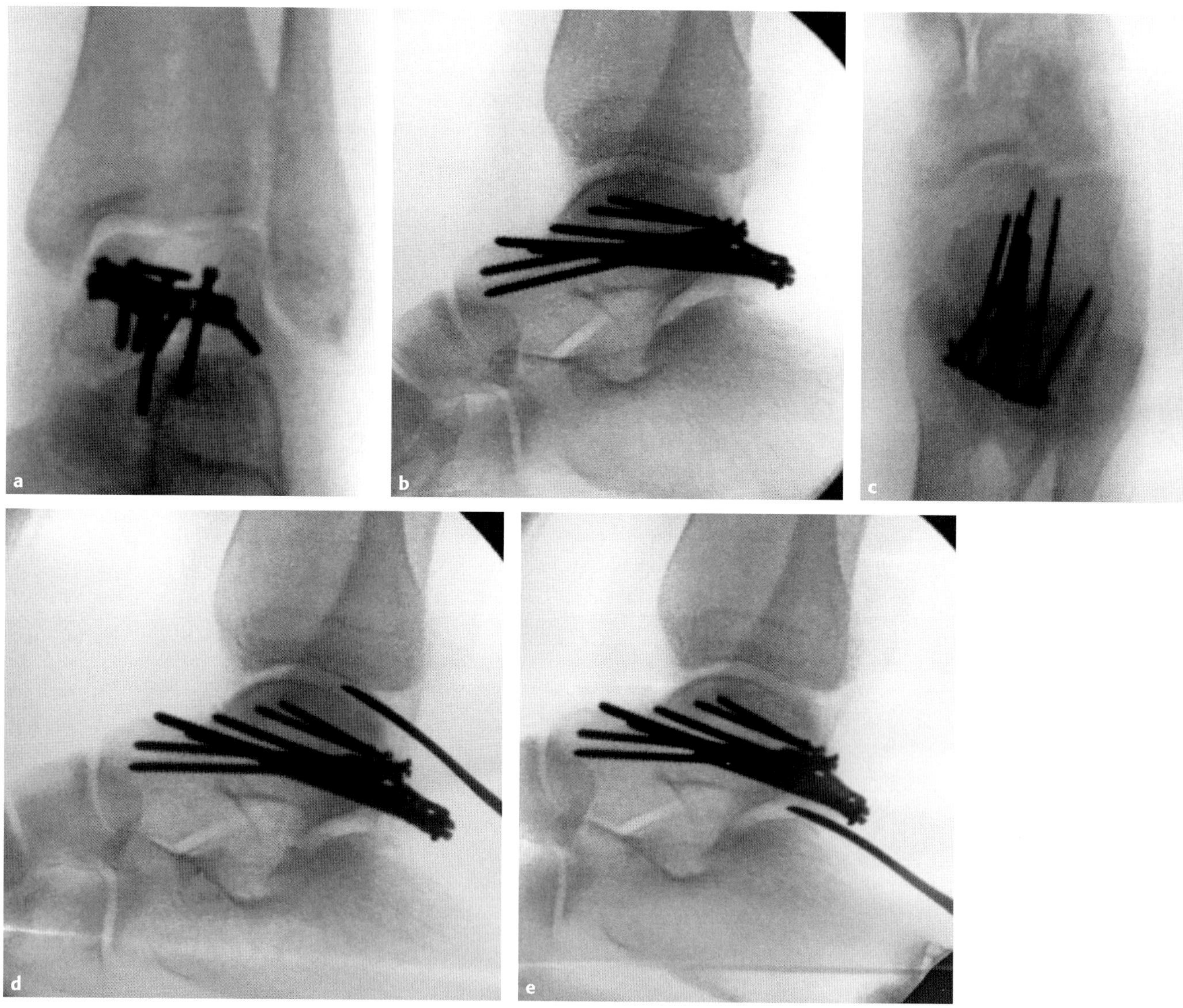

Fig 5.3-8a–e Intraoperative fixation.
a–c Intraoperative C-arm imaging demonstrating final hardware placement and assessment of the ankle and subtalar joints with a small (Freer) elevator.
d–e Articular reduction is assessed with a small (Freer) elevator to rule out articular step-off or displacement.

Care should be taken to ensure that implants are not impinging within the ankle or subtalar joints. The external fixator/distractor is removed at the end of the operative procedure. X-rays are performed at regular intervals postoperatively to assess healing (**Fig 5.3-9**).

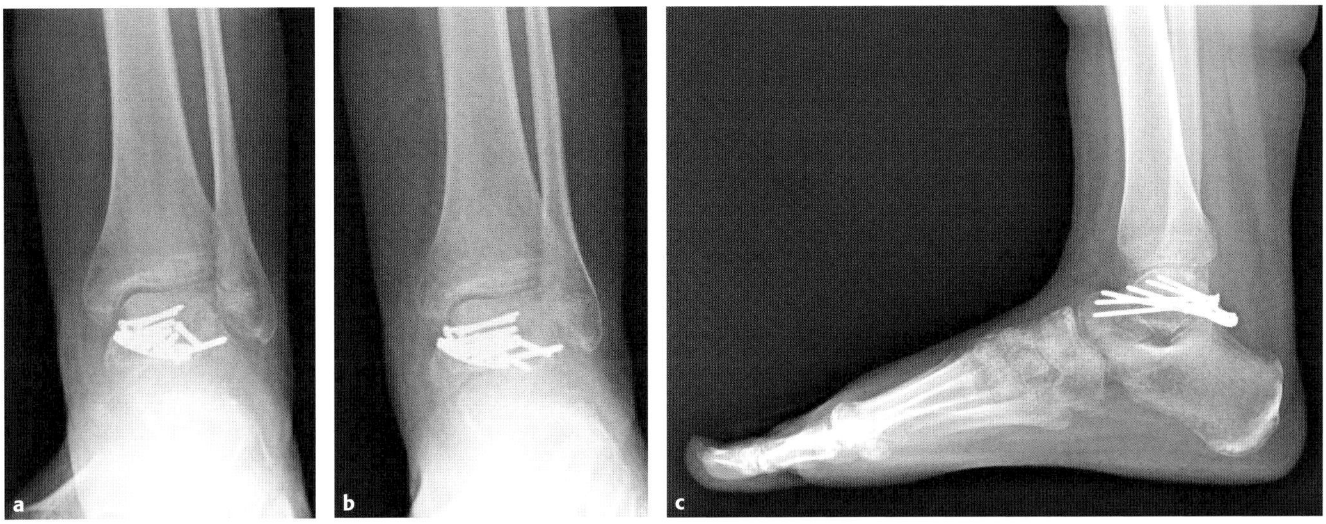

Fig 5.3-9a–c Postoperative AP and lateral images demonstrate anatomical reduction of the posteromedial talar body.

5 Pitfalls and complications

Pitfalls

Inadequate reduction and fixation of the posterior talus

The anterior approach to the posterior talus does not allow for adequate visualization of the fracture. Implants placed anterior to posterior do not provide adequate compression or buttress of the posterior talus and can result in malreduction and nonunion. Similarly, injuries treated nonoperatively have high rates of nonunion, a high potential for AVN and arthrosis (**Fig 5.3-10**).

Inadequate C-arm projections with the patient in a prone position

Fixation of the posterior talus with the patient in a prone position is less common than supine approaches to the talus. Care must be taken to achieve precise AP, mortise, and lateral images to achieve adequate reduction and to ensure implants are positioned appropriately. If the C-arm beam is not orthogonal to the patient's ankle, implants may be placed into the articular surface of the ankle or subtalar joints.

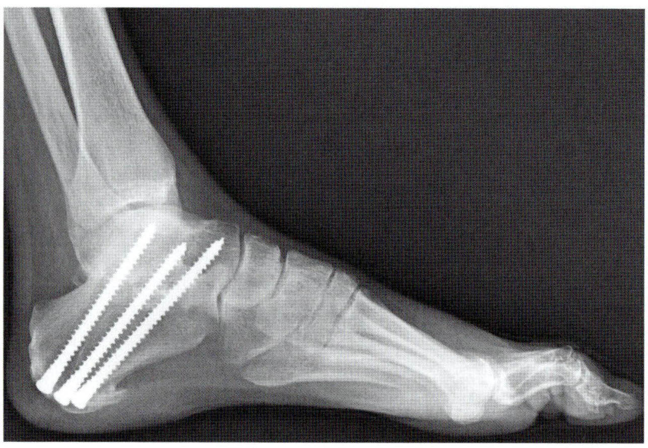

Fig 5.3-10 Example from a different case showing the lateral x-ray of a patient who underwent subtalar arthrodesis for posttraumatic subtalar arthrosis following nonoperative treatment of a posteromedial talar body fracture.

Irreducible intercalary fragments

Small intercalary fragments (ie, less than 5 mm in diameter) and fragments without adequate overlying cartilage should be removed rather than attempting fixation. These fragments do not contribute to joint congruity and may impede anatomical reduction or may displace into the joint as loose bodies.

Complications

- Injury to the posterior tibial neurovascular bundle
- Iatrogenic FHL injury
- Intraarticular placement of implants
- Loss of fixation
- Nonunion
- Malunion
- Avascular necrosis
- Posttraumatic arthritis
- Subtalar joint instability

6 Alternative techniques

Less comminuted injuries can be treated with 2.0 or 2.4 mm countersunk screws alone without plate fixation. An attempt to treat these injuries operatively should be performed. For irreparable fractures, failed fixation and nonunion, fragment excision can be performed.

7 Postoperative management and rehabilitation

Postoperatively, the ankle is immobilized in a 3-sided ("AO") splint with instructions to elevate the leg. Any applied suction drain is removed postoperative on day 1 or 2. Sutures are kept in place for 2–3 weeks and then removed.

Active and passive range-of-motion (ROM) exercise is initiated as soon as the incision is healed. Transition into a rigid boot or foot orthosis with the ankle held at 90° is performed at 2–3 weeks postoperatively. Nonweight bearing is recommended for 6–8 weeks postoperatively depending on fracture severity. Standard postoperative x-rays are obtained to ensure fracture union.

In cases of uncertainty in fracture healing, a postoperative CT scan can be performed. An active rehabilitation program is initiated at weight bearing to emphasize ROM, muscular balance, and gait training.

Implant removal

Removal of plates and screws for posterior process fractures is generally not necessary. If a patient experiences chronic posterior pain or impingement symptoms, implants can be typically removed at 1 year postoperatively using the same surgical approach.

8 Recommended reading

Giuffrida AY, Lin SS, Abidi N, et al. Pseudo os trigonum sign: missed posteromedial talar facet fracture. *Foot Ankle Int.* 2003 Aug;24(8):642–649.

Nyska M, Howard CB, Matan Y, et al. Fracture of the posterior body of the talus—the hidden fracture. *Arch Orthop Trauma Surg.* 1998;117(1–2):114–117.

Shank JR, Benirschke SK, Swords MP. Treatment of peripheral talus fractures. *Foot Ankle Clin.* 2017 Mar;22(1):181–192.

Swords M, Shank J, Benirschke S. Surgical treatment of posteromedial talus fractures: technique description and results of 10 cases. *Indian J Orthop.* 2018 May-Jun;52(3):269–275.

Thordarson DB. Talar body fractures. *Orthop Clin North Am.* 2001 Jan;32(1):65–77.

Young KW, Park YU, Kim JS, et al. Misdiagnosis of talar body or neck fractures as ankle sprains in low energy traumas. *Clin Orthop Surg.* 2016 Sep;8(3):303–309.

Zwipp H, Rammelt S. Secondary reconstruction for malunions and nonunions of the talar body. *Foot Ankle Clin.* 2016 Mar;21(1):95–109.

5.4 Displaced talar neck fracture (Hawkins 2)

Steven J Lawrence, Arun Aneja

1 Case description

A 48-year-old woman was involved in a motor vehicle accident in which her car was T-boned (a high-energy impact from side) by another car traveling approximately 65 km/h. She was transported by ambulance to the emergency department.

The medical history included poorly controlled type I diabetes, hypertension, and hypothyroidism.

The emergency department workup detected isolated orthopedic injuries, including an open left tibial plateau fracture and a closed left talar neck fracture with associated dislocation of the subtalar joint (AO/OTA 81.2B(b), Hawkins 2 fracture dislocation AO/OTA 81.2Bb) (**Fig 5.4-1**).

In the emergency department, a closed reduction of the talar injury was attempted with the patient sedated. A manipulation was performed with the knee flexed with axial traction on the calcaneus and plantarflexion of the ankle joint. However, the subtalar joint could not be successfully reduced (**Fig 5.4-2**).

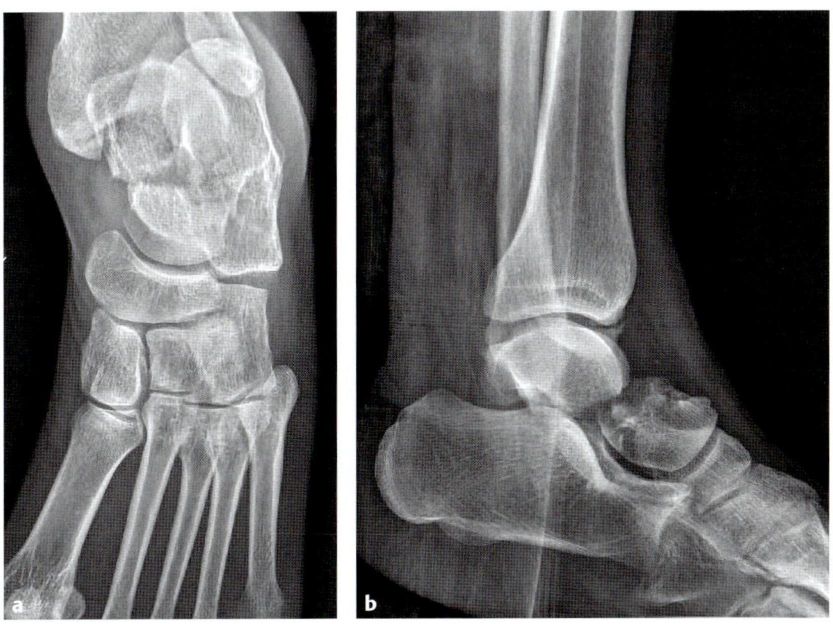

Fig 5.4-1a–b Preoperative x-rays.
- **a** AP x-ray of the foot showing shortening of the medial column of the talar neck fracture. Note varus alignment at the fracture site.
- **b** Lateral x-ray demonstrating displaced talar neck fracture with subtalar joint disruption.

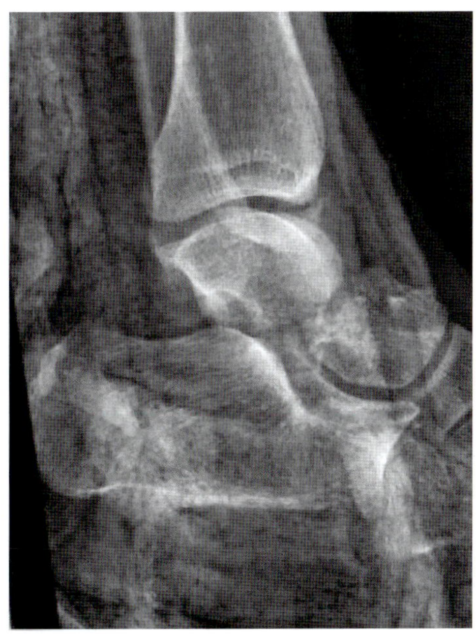

Fig 5.4-2 Lateral x-ray of foot demonstrating failed attempt of closed reduction.

Therefore, she was taken urgently to the operating room (OR) for closed reduction under general anesthesia, and splinting of her displaced talar fracture (**Fig 5.4-3**). The open tibial plateau fracture was irrigated and debrided, then open reduction and internal fixation (ORIF) was performed.

The definitive talar operative procedure was delayed for 9 days to permit hindfoot soft-tissue swelling to resolve and for medical optimization.

2 Preoperative planning

Indications for surgery

Displaced talar neck fracture dislocations require operative intervention. Initial management consists of a timely reduction, performed to restore bony, vascular, lymphatic, and soft-tissue continuity. A successful closed reduction of the fracture dislocation allows for delay in internal fixation. Should closed reduction fail, urgent ORIF is indicated. Long-term outcomes are dependent on initial injury, fracture displacement, and timely anatomical reduction.

Considerations for surgery

The anatomy of the talus is complex. Scrutiny of the injury x-rays and preoperative computed tomographic (CT) scans is essential to assess fracture displacement, comminution, and bone quality (**Fig 5.4-4**).

Concomitant fractures of the ankle or foot may also be present in these high-velocity injuries. The patient also presented with a medial malleolus fracture and a lateral process fracture.

Comminution is usually present on the dorsal and medial aspects of the talar neck. The fracture is addressed with dual incisions over the medial and anterolateral portions of the talus.

Extensive subcutaneous dissection as well as dissection over the dorsum of the talus should be avoided, as it may cause damage to any remaining blood supply.

With ORIF of a medial malleolus fracture, the malleolar fragment can be rotated downward hinging on the deltoid attachment (thus maintaining the blood supply to the distal medial malleolus); this allows better visualization of the medial talus. The medial malleolus can be fixed with two parallel 2.7 mm screws after ORIF of the talus.

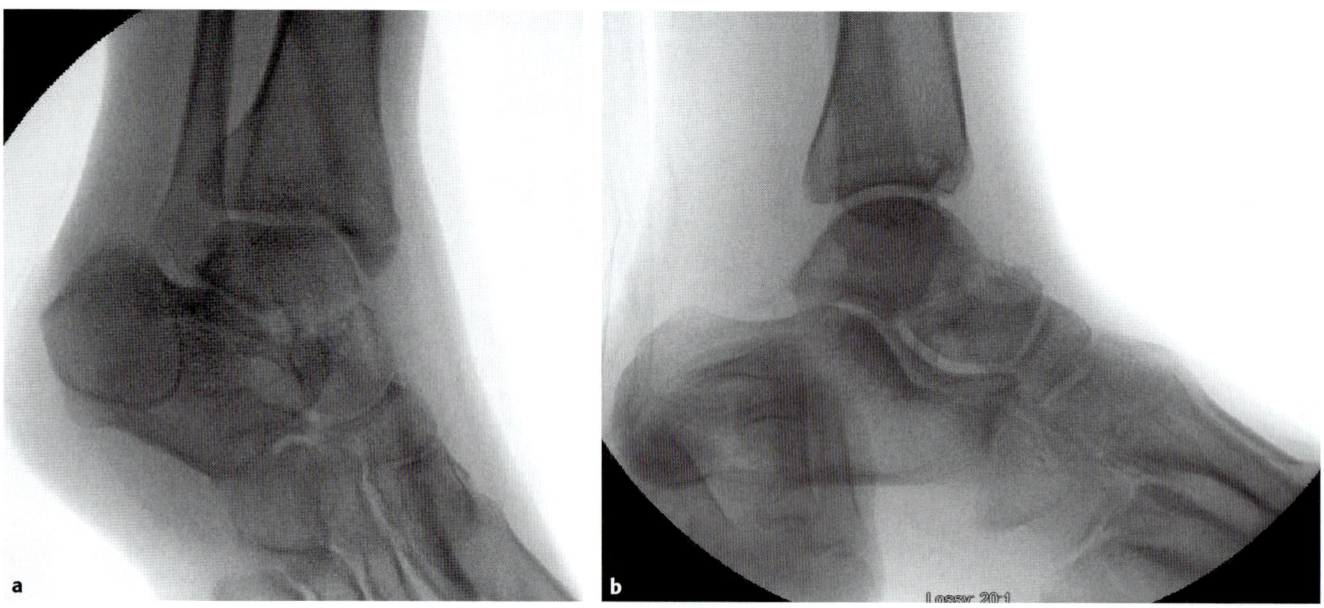

Fig 5.4-3a–b C-arm images after reduction.
a Canale view of successful closed reduction of Hawkins 2 fracture dislocation.
b Lateral foot x-ray revealing closed reduction of talar fracture dislocation.

3 Operating room setup

Patient positioning	• Supine with a bump under the ipsilateral buttock • Bony prominences are padded.
Anesthesia options	• General anesthesia with muscle paralysis is generally preferred when attempts at emergent reduction are performed. • Alternate forms of anesthesia can be undertaken based on medical comorbidities or surgeon preference. • This high-energy injury is commonly associated with polytrauma, and concomitant injuries may dictate patient intraoperative positioning.
C-arm location	• Positioned on the opposite side of the operative table.
Tourniquet	• A thigh tourniquet is recommended.
Tips	• The operative leg is placed on a foam wedge so lateral C-arm images can be performed without superimposition of the contralateral foot.

For illustrations and overview of anesthetic considerations, see chapter 1.

Equipment

- Smooth K-wires
- Minifragment plates 2.0 and 2.4
- 2.7–4.0 mm screws
- Juxtaarticular headed screws
- Oblique threaded K-wires or Steinmann pins to assist with reduction
- Reduction clamps
- Small distractor to facilitate visualization and removal of fragments from the subtalar joint

4 Surgical procedure

Treatment of talar fractures must be performed through a dual approach. Dual incisions provide medial and anterolateral windows to visualize the talar neck fracture. Many talar neck fractures have dorsomedial comminution, therefore, the best fracture reduction is usually obtained from the anterolateral window. However, utilization of both windows ensures optimal fracture alignment and avoids malrotation at the talar neck.

It is often helpful to have AP and lateral x-rays of the contralateral normal side in the OR as a reference for proper reduction.

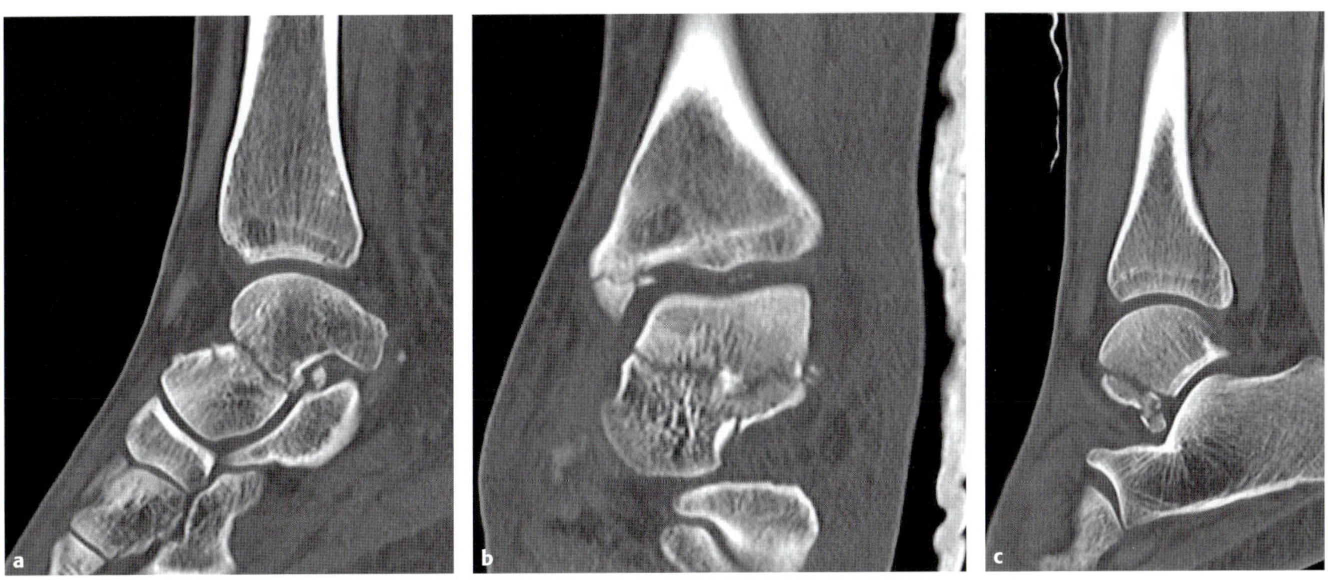

Fig 5.4-4a–c The CT scans.
a Sagittal cut indicating primary talar neck fracture. Some dorsal comminution is present.
b Coronal cut demonstrating the talar neck fracture as well as a minimally displaced medial malleolar fracture.
c Sagittal cut demonstrating the primary fracture line and a comminuted lateral process fracture.

Medial approach

The incision extends from the distal aspect of the medial malleolus to the navicular tuberosity (**Fig 5.4-5**). The interval is between posterior tibialis and anterior tibial tendon. Care should be taken to identify and retract the saphenous vein and the adjacent saphenous nerve. Without raising flaps, proceed with careful sharp dissection to the periosteum. Much of the dissection will have been done by the injury and resulting hematoma. The deltoid ligament must not be disrupted during fracture site exposure, as it is an important vascular source for the talar body and base of the talar neck.

Anterolateral approach

The skin incision is in line with the fourth metatarsal and extends proximally between the distal tibia and fibula to the inferior syndesmosis. Care should be taken to avoid the intermediate branches of the superficial peroneal nerve that may cross the field, as it will result in a painful bothersome neuroma. The extensor retinaculum is identified and incised and the anterior compartment tendons and neurovascular bundle are retracted medially. The extensor digitorum brevis (EDB) fascia is incised and the EDB muscle belly elevated and debris removed from the subtalar joint. This is facilitated by application of a small distractor from the tuber to the distal tibia. A small (Freer) elevator placed from anteromedial window can be used to identify the site of fracture at the anterolateral window. Care should be taken never to place the small (Freer) elevator or any distractor over the top of the talar neck, as it may damage the dorsal blood supply of the talus. Sharp knife dissection is used to expose the fracture site.

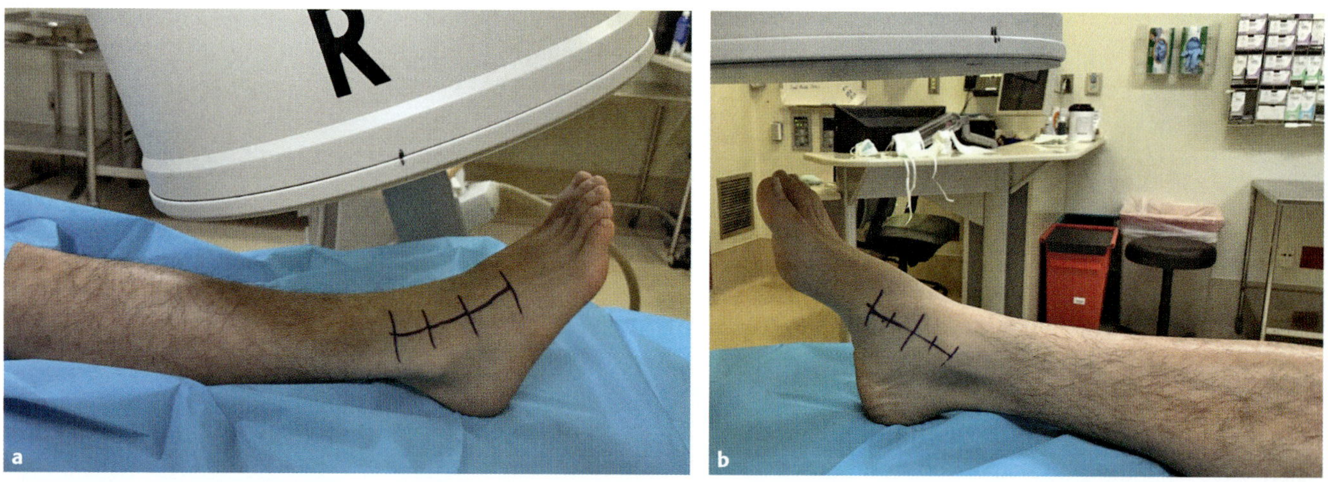

Fig 5.4-5a–b Intraoperative setup and position of portable C-arm imaging unit.
a The skin incision for the anterolateral incision.
b The skin incision for the medial incision.
(Photo courtesy of Ifeanyi Nzegwu, MD and Boshen Liu, MD.)

Provisional reduction

The fracture site is debrided and irrigated of hematoma and fibrous tissue, which may be impeding perfect reduction. Two windows are used to establish an adequate bilateral visualization of the fracture, which prevents malreduction in varus, valgus, and rotational planes (**Fig 5.4-6**). Provisional reduction is obtained with axial K-wires. The wires are cut short so that they do not block the definitive fixation (**Fig 5.4-7**).

A terminally threaded 2.0 mm K-wire placed in the proximal and/or distal segment can be used as a joystick to assist with reduction.

Anatomical reduction is usually obtained from the anterolateral window (but may vary based on the location of the comminution). Fracture compression can be accomplished by clamping the fracture fragments with a modified or small point-to point-reduction (Weber) clamps. Compressing across fracture comminution should be avoided, as this results in coronal plane malalignment.

The reduction is checked with the C-arm using the AP, lateral, and Canale views.

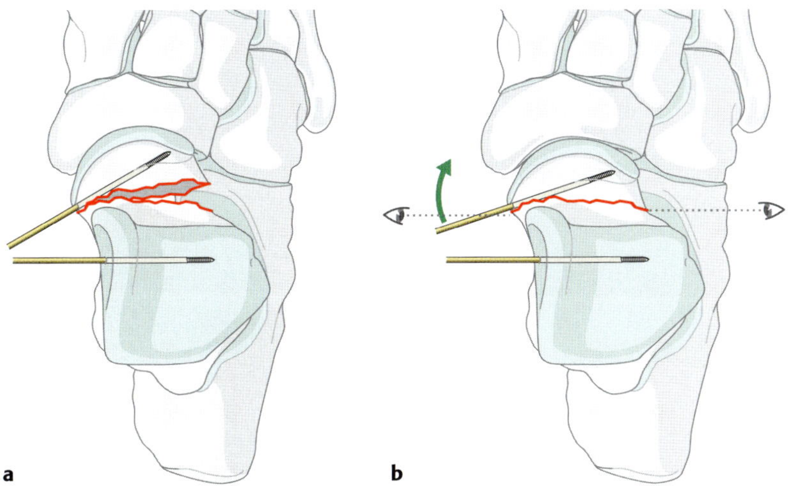

Fig 5.4-6a–b
a K-wires used as reduction tools for initial reduction of the fracture.
b The reduction should be confirmed visually from both sides.
(Images adapted from Stefan Rammelt, MD)

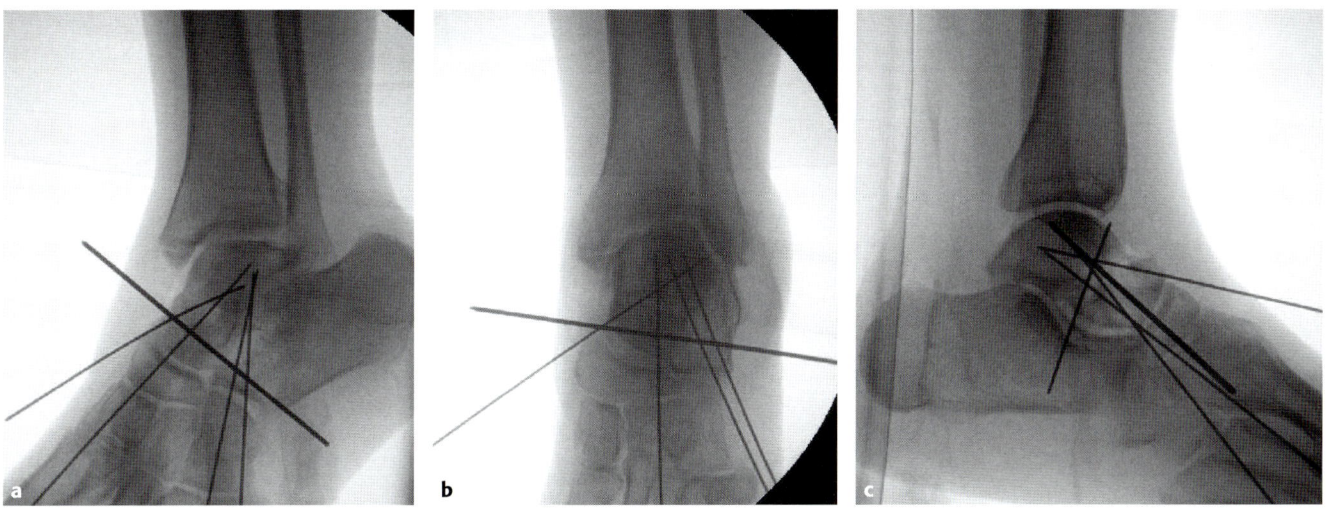

Fig 5.4-7a–c Intraoperative C-arm images.
a Canale view: provisional K-wire fixation of talar neck fracture and lateral process fracture. The transverse K-wire in talar neck is used as a joystick for fracture manipulation.
b AP view of hindfoot: provisional K-wire fixation of the talar neck fracture.
c Lateral view of hindfoot: provisional K-wire fixation of the talar neck fracture.

Definitive fixation and closure

After provisional fixation, the lateral column is stabilized first. The concomitant lateral process fracture is also addressed at this time (**Fig 5.4-8**).

Any small plate with small screws, whether mini or specific for the talus, can be used. A 4-hole T-plate with minifragment screws on the lateral aspect of the talus is often the best option. An appropriate contour to the lateral T-plate is created so that it is placed along the inferior aspect of lateral talus, just below the lateral process. Two proximal unicortical screws are placed while the two distal screws are bicortical. Screw penetration of the talonavicular joint should be avoided.

After stabilizing the lateral column of the talus, the forefoot can be abducted, which facilitates placement of screws from talar head in retrograde fashion while countersinking the screws (**Fig 5.4-9**). Countersunk or headless 2.4/2.7 mm screws can be used to function as struts. Alternatively, if there is significant dorsal medial comminution or bone loss, a 3-hole plate 2.0 can be strategically placed on the inferior medial aspect of the talar neck as so not to impinge against the medial malleolus. Care should be taken to not compress the medial screws as varus malreduction may occur. The medial screws must be placed below the equator of the talus as the deforming force is dorsiflexion. The screws are then better able to counter these forces which may also lead to malreduction.

The medial malleolar fracture is fixed with two compression screws (**Fig 5.4-10**).

After definitive fixation, scrutinize the final C-arm views to ensure anatomical reduction and ensure that the implants do not violate any adjacent joints. Final images should include AP foot, lateral foot, AP ankle, and Canale views. Failure to obtain all views may lead to unrecognized hardware penetration into the ankle joint.

The wound is then irrigated and closed in layers.

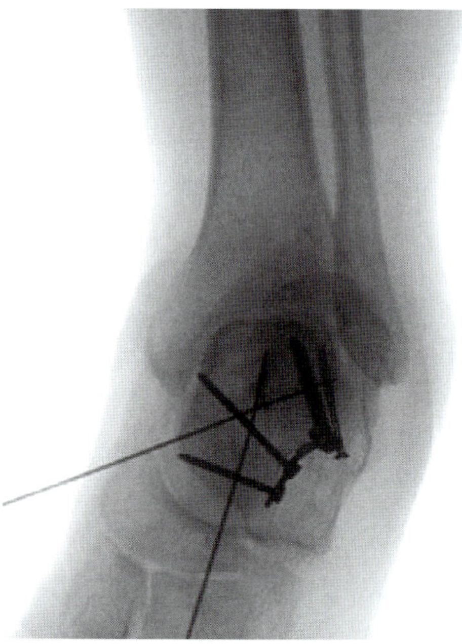

Fig 5.4-8 Intraoperative Canale view with fixation of the lateral talus with T-plate and screws and screw fixation of lateral process fracture.

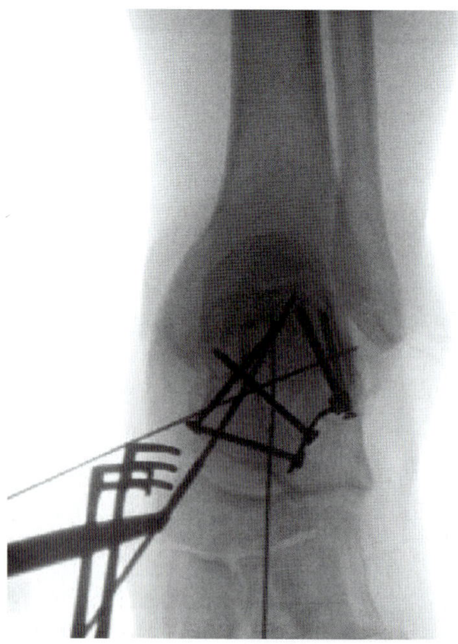

Fig 5.4-9 Intraoperative image of talus showing the placement of the medial column screws.

5 Pitfalls and complications

Pitfalls

Avascular necrosis

Avoid extensive subcutaneous dissection and dissection along the superior aspect of the talar neck and head as well as the deltoid ligament in order not to further violate blood supply to the talus.

Neuroma

Avoid the intermediate branches of the superficial peroneal nerve that may cross the field, as it may result in a painful neuroma.

Malunion

Where possible, be careful to place the medial screw below the equator to resist dorsiflexion forces. The medial screw should not be placed under compression in the presence of medial comminution to prevent varus malunion. In the case of comminution or bony defect, bone grafting is performed. An ORIF should be completed after which bone graft can be placed at the fracture site defects. Graft material is usually cancellous material, either autograft or allograft. If structural bone is used and inserted before ORIF is completed, it may "overstuff" the fracture resulting in deformity and malreduction of the subtalar joint.

Painful hardware

Implants are generally placed into the limited nonarticular portions off the talus—therefore, carefully check implant placement to avoid painful hardware impingement.

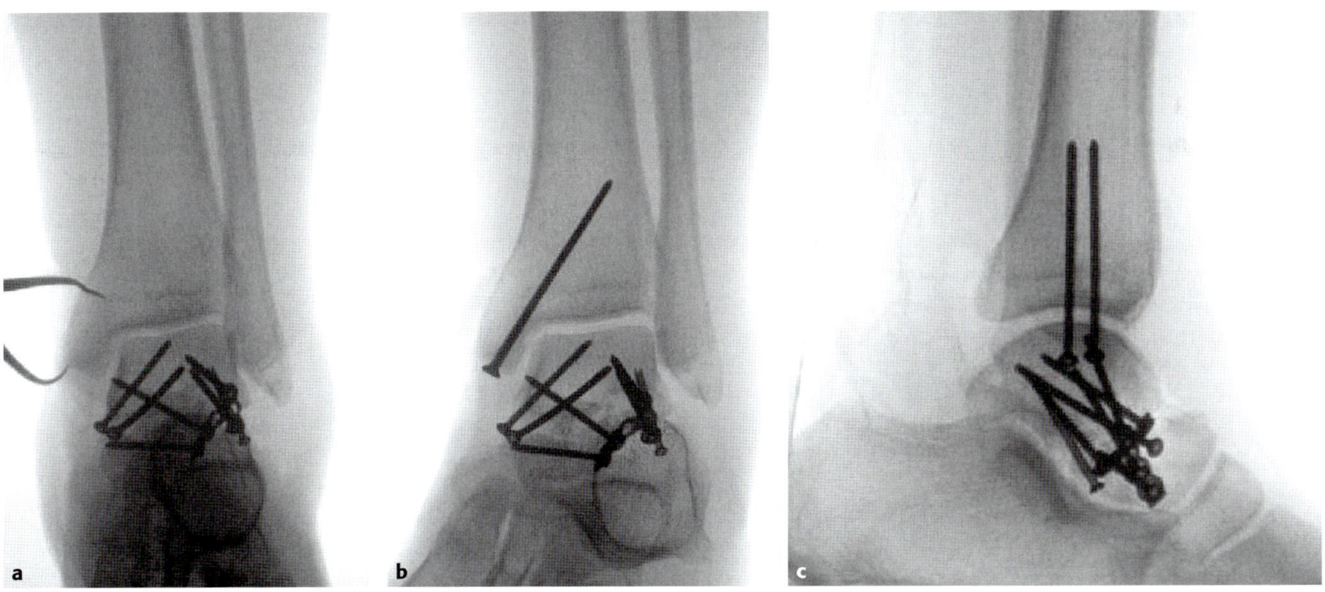

Fig 5.4-10a–c C-arm images showing reduction of the medial malleolus and the final construct.
a Mortise view of ankle: reduction of medial malleolar fracture.
b Mortise view of ankle: screw fixation of associated medial malleolar fracture and talar plate and screw fixation.
c Lateral view of ankle: fixation of talus and malleolar fractures.

Complications

- Avascular necrosis (AVN) is the most feared complication of talar fracture management. Prompt reduction and meticulous surgical dissection helps to minimize this devastating sequela.
- Wound breakdown with infection, as well as loss of fracture fixation may occur (**Fig 5.4-11**)
- Infection
- Malunion/nonunion—nonunion of this fracture dislocation is surprisingly rare, even in the presence of AVN. Malunion often leads to varus foot alignment and malfunction.
- Chondral injury—may occur in association with bony injury which will affect outcome (**Fig 5.4-12**)
- Posttraumatic arthritis

Long-term outcomes for this fracture subtype are reported to be excellent in only about 20% of cases. Arthrosis of adjacent joints occurs in approximately two-thirds of cases. The subtalar joint is the most common site of posttraumatic arthritis.

6 Alternative techniques

The medial column of the talus is short, therefore adequate plate fixation is difficult. Lateral column plating is commonly performed as two screws can be placed on either side of the fracture.

Screw fixation alone can be performed, if there is no comminution present and compression screw fixation does not result in shortening. Therefore in the presence of significant comminution, compression screws are best avoided, as iatrogenic shortening of the medial column of the talus may occur. Varus malunion will likely create a painful subtalar joint. Fully threaded screws can be used in this instance.

7 Postoperative management and rehabilitation

In the immediate postoperative period, the patient is immobilized in a splint or boot. Mild elevation of the hindfoot is recommended to augment lymphatic and venous outflow and to assist in wound healing. The hindfoot has a scant soft-tissue envelope with no muscle coverage. Excessive elevation may lead to compromise of circulation and necrosis.

Sutures are generally removed approximately 14 days postoperatively based on the soft-tissue healing. Serial x-rays are performed to monitor fracture healing and alignment. X-rays also may demonstrate a subchondral talar dome lucency (referred to as Hawkins sign) that indicates the presence of talar body perfusion (**Fig 5.4-13**). Hawkins sign is best appreciated at 6–8 weeks after injury and indicates intact vascularity resulting in resorption of subchondral bone. Increased bony density in the early phases or dome collapse subsequently indicates that AVN is present.

Once the soft-tissue envelope is healed and the fracture fixation remains secure, active and passive range of motion of the ankle, subtalar, and talonavicular joints are initiated.

X-rays taken 2 months after surgery demonstrate maintained fracture alignment, no hardware failure, and congruent joints without evidence of AVN (**Fig 5.4-14**).

Weight bearing is restricted until crossing trabeculae are visible on plain x-rays. If signs of radiographic healing are inconclusive, CT imaging can be useful.

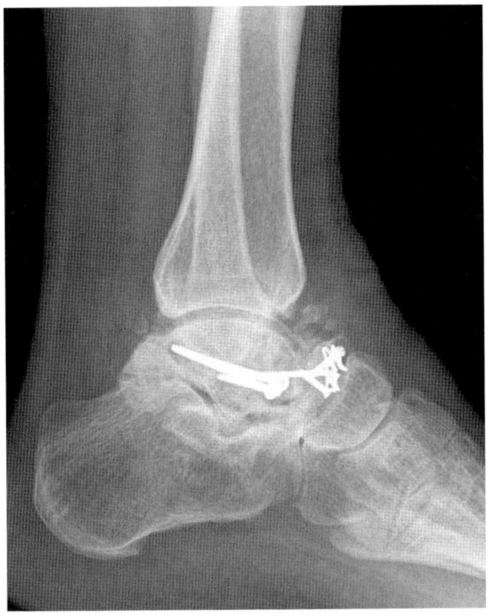

Fig 5.4-11 Example from a different case of a lateral x-ray view revealing hardware failure and loss of fixation after fixation of a talar neck fracture.

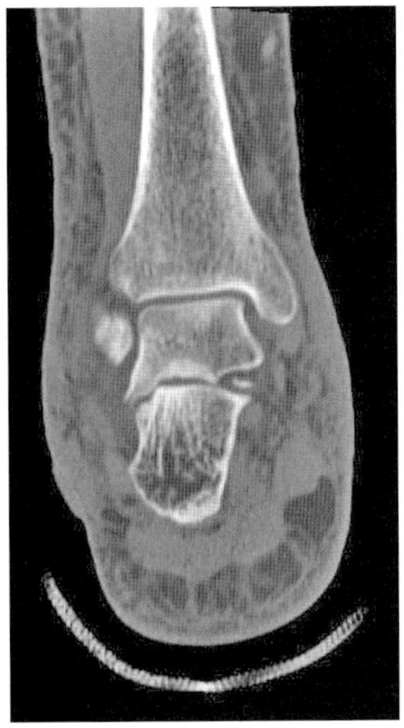

Fig 5.4-12 Example from a different case of a coronal CT cut showing a chondral injury to inferior articular surface of talar after closed reduction of a Hawkins 2 fracture dislocation.

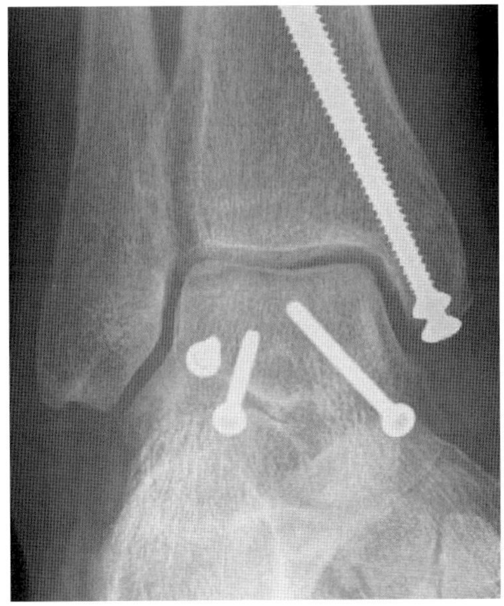

Fig 5.4-13 Mortise view of talus demonstrating subchondral lucency of talar dome (Hawkins sign). This bone resorption represents intact vascularity of the talar dome.
(Photograph courtesy of Justin Montgomery, MD Radiology Department, University of Kentucky, Lexington, KY, USA.)

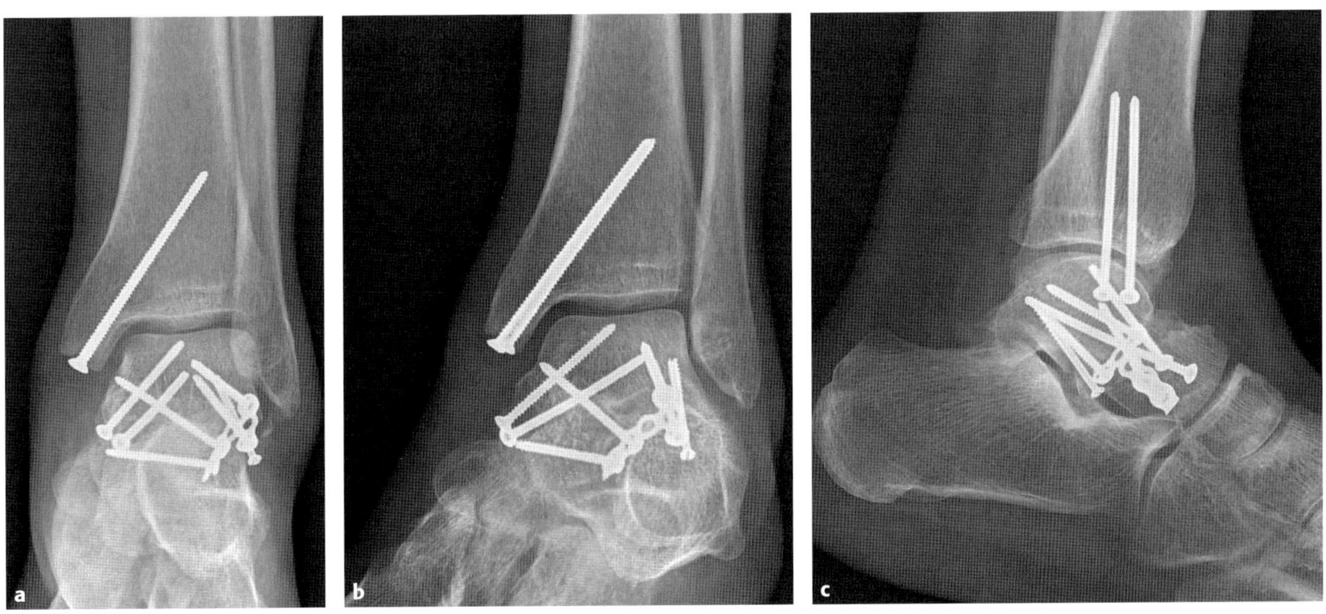

Fig 5.4-14a–c Postoperative x-rays.

a Mortise view: ankle and talar fixation. There is a minor gap in the lateral process after excision of a small fragment not amenable to fixation.
b Canale view of orthopedic construct.
c Lateral view of ankle: fracture fixation and associated orthopedic constructs.

8 Recommended reading

Bernirschke S, Kramer P. Talus fractures. *Tech Orthoped.* 2014; 29(1):13–19.

Charlson MD, Parks BG, Weber TG, et al. Comparison of plate and screw fixation and screw fixation alone in a comminuted talar neck fracture model. *Foot Ankle Int.* 2006 May;27(5):340–343.

Halvorson JJ, Winter SB, Teasdall RD, et al. Talar neck fractures: a systematic review of the literature. *J Foot Ankle Surg.* 2013 Jan–Feb;52(1):56–61.

Hawkins LG. Fractures of the neck of the talus. *J Bone Joint Surg Am.* 1970 Jul;52(5):991–1002.

Rammelt S, Winkler J, Zwipp H. Osteosynthese zentraler Talusfrakturen. *Oper Orthop Traumatol* 2013;25:525–541.

Vallier HA. Fractures of the talus: state of the art. *J Orthop Trauma.* 2015 Sep;29(9):385–392.

5.5 Displaced talar body fracture (Marti 3/4)

Michael Swords, Rajiv Shah, Sampat Dumbre Patil

1 Case description

A 24-year-old man was involved in a motor vehicle accident. He was transferred by ambulance to the emergency department with complaints of pain in the left foot and ankle. The patient had an obvious deformity to his foot and ankle. The injury was open on the lateral side of the forefoot without any neurovascular deficit. No associated injuries were noted.

X-rays of the foot and ankle in AP and lateral views showed a comminuted and displaced fracture of the talar body with dislocation of the subtalar and talonavicular (TN) joints. Additionally, fractures of the third, fourth, and fifth metatarsals (MTs) were noted (AO/OTA 8.1.1C3) (**Fig 5.5-1**).

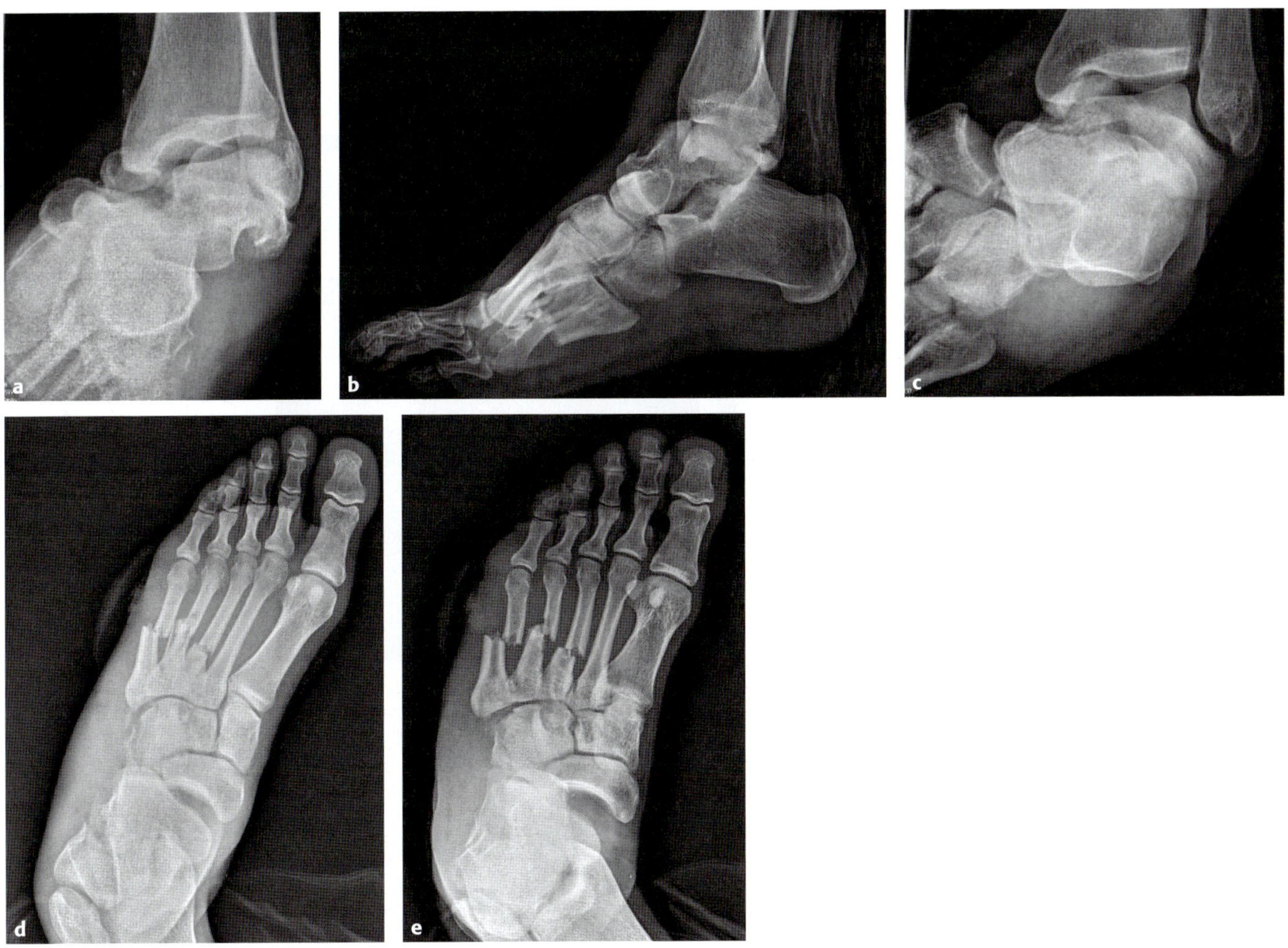

Fig 5.5-1a–e X-rays of the ankle and foot showing a comminuted displaced fracture of the body of the talus with dislocation of the subtalar and TN joint in AP (**a**), lateral (**b**), and mortise (**c**) images of the ankle; and of the foot in AP (**d**) and oblique (**e**) showing comminuted fracture of the talar body and fractures of the third to fifth MT shafts. There is also a cuboid fracture.

For this case, a computed tomographic (CT) scan was obtained (**Fig 5.5-2**). Surgery was undertaken emergently due to the dislocations and the open fracture of the fifth MT. The subtalar and TN dislocations were reduced with the patient under general anesthesia and an external fixator was applied. Irrigation, debridement, and plate fixation of the open fifth MT fracture was also performed (**Fig 5.5-3**).

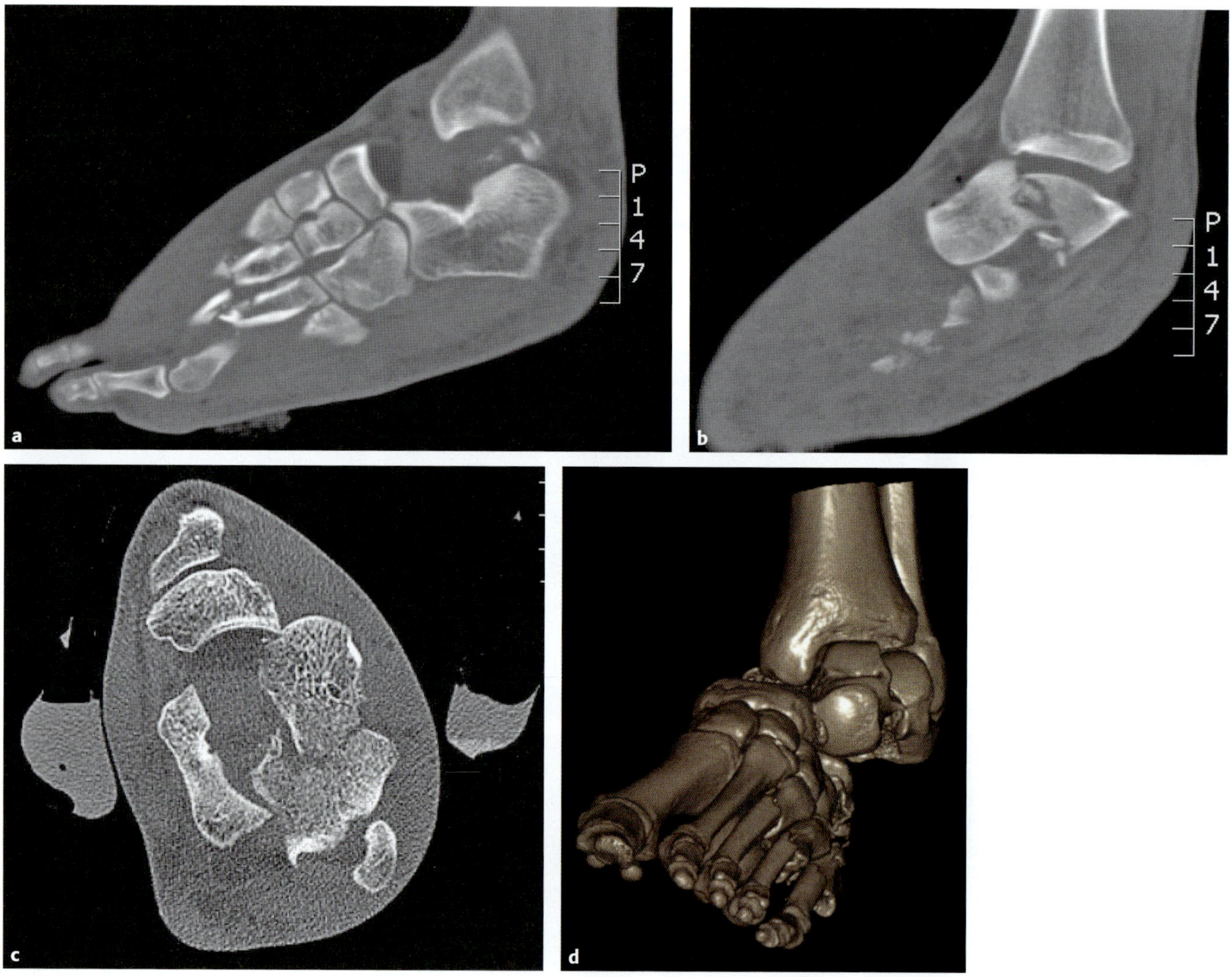

Fig 5.5-2a–d Injury CT scans showing the comminuted fracture of the talar body. The extent of injury is difficult to assess secondary to dislocation at the time of the CT.
a–b Sagittal views.
c Coronal view.
d 3D reconstruction.

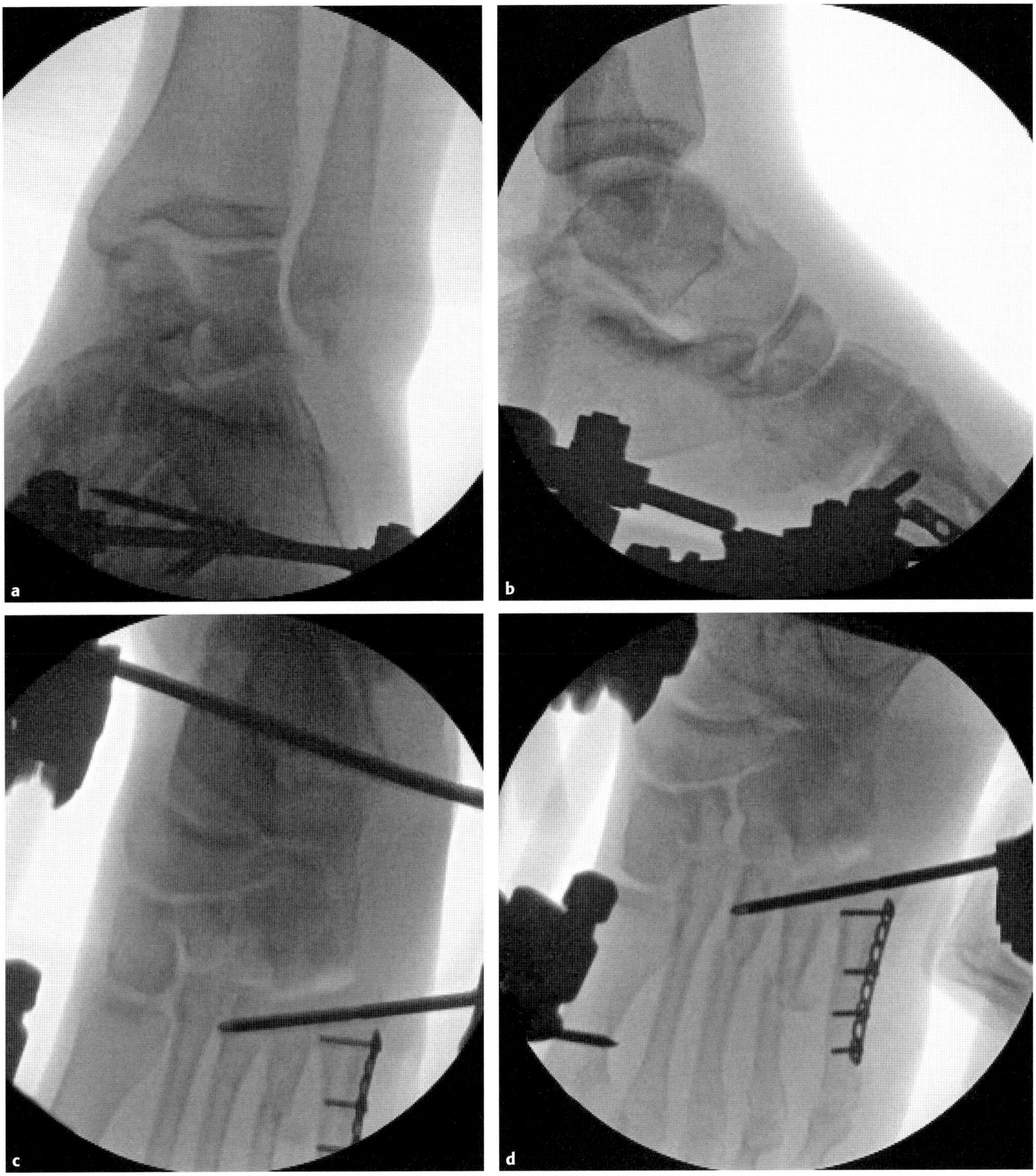

Fig 5.5-3a–d Intraoperative C-arm images demonstrating the reduction of the hindfoot. An external fixator has been placed to maintain general alignment of the ankle and subtalar joints. The external fixator is extended to the midfoot to maintain stability of the TN joint. The fifth MT has been plated.

a Mortise view.
b Lateral view.
c AP foot view.
d Oblique foot view.

2 Preoperative planning

Indications for surgery

A displaced and comminuted fracture of the talar body has to be managed surgically. If accurate repositioning of the fracture is not done, it leads to arthritis of the ankle and the subtalar joints. A comminuted talar body fracture treated without surgery will result in malalignment of the hindfoot, altering the position of the foot during stance and gait. Open reduction and internal fixation is necessary.

In cases with dislocation, prompt reduction is necessary.

Considerations for surgery

A CT scan after reduction is mandatory to understand the precise geometry of fracture fragments and their displacement (**Fig 5.5-4**).

Fracture fixation is achieved with screws and occasionally minifragment plates. All comminuted fragments require stabilization to restore joint congruity and stability.

The incisions required to approach fractures of the talar body are fracture specific. This fracture did not require an osteotomy as part of the approach. Occasionally a medial malleolar, or more uncommonly, a lateral malleolar osteotomy may be necessary. The surgical approaches required are dictated by the fracture pattern. This particular fracture pattern required three separate approaches to address the talar body fracture. Standard medial and lateral approaches are necessary to provide an accurate reduction of the talar body while the patient is supine. Later the patient will need to be placed prone to address the posterior comminution to the talar body. Care is taken to avoid placing hardware while the patient is supine, which may potentially block reduction of the posterior portion of the talus when the patient is in the prone position.

Surgery is performed after the swelling has resolved appropriately. Fixation of the talar body and posterior talus can be performed at one operative setting or alternatively, which may be performed in a staged manner.

For surgical fixation of multiple metatarsals see chapter 7.6.

3 Operating room setup

Patient positioning	• Supine on a radiolucent table with the operative limb elevated allowing full access to the hindfoot • Prone for reduction and fixation of the posterior portion of the talar body
Anesthesia options	• General, regional, or spinal
C-arm location	• From the contralateral side with the monitor placed towards the head of the table
Tourniquet	• Used at surgeon's discretion • Generally improves ability to visualize the fracture
Tips	• A headlight greatly improves the ability to see the fracture and assess the reduction.

For illustrations and overview of anesthetic considerations, see chapter 1.

For review of positioning for posterior talar fractures, see chapter 5.3.

Equipment

- K-wires (smooth and threaded)
- Steinmann pins
- Large external fixator set or small distractor set
- Screws as per surgeon preference
- Miniplates with 2.0 mm and 2.4 mm screws
- Reduction clamps
- Small fragment screws

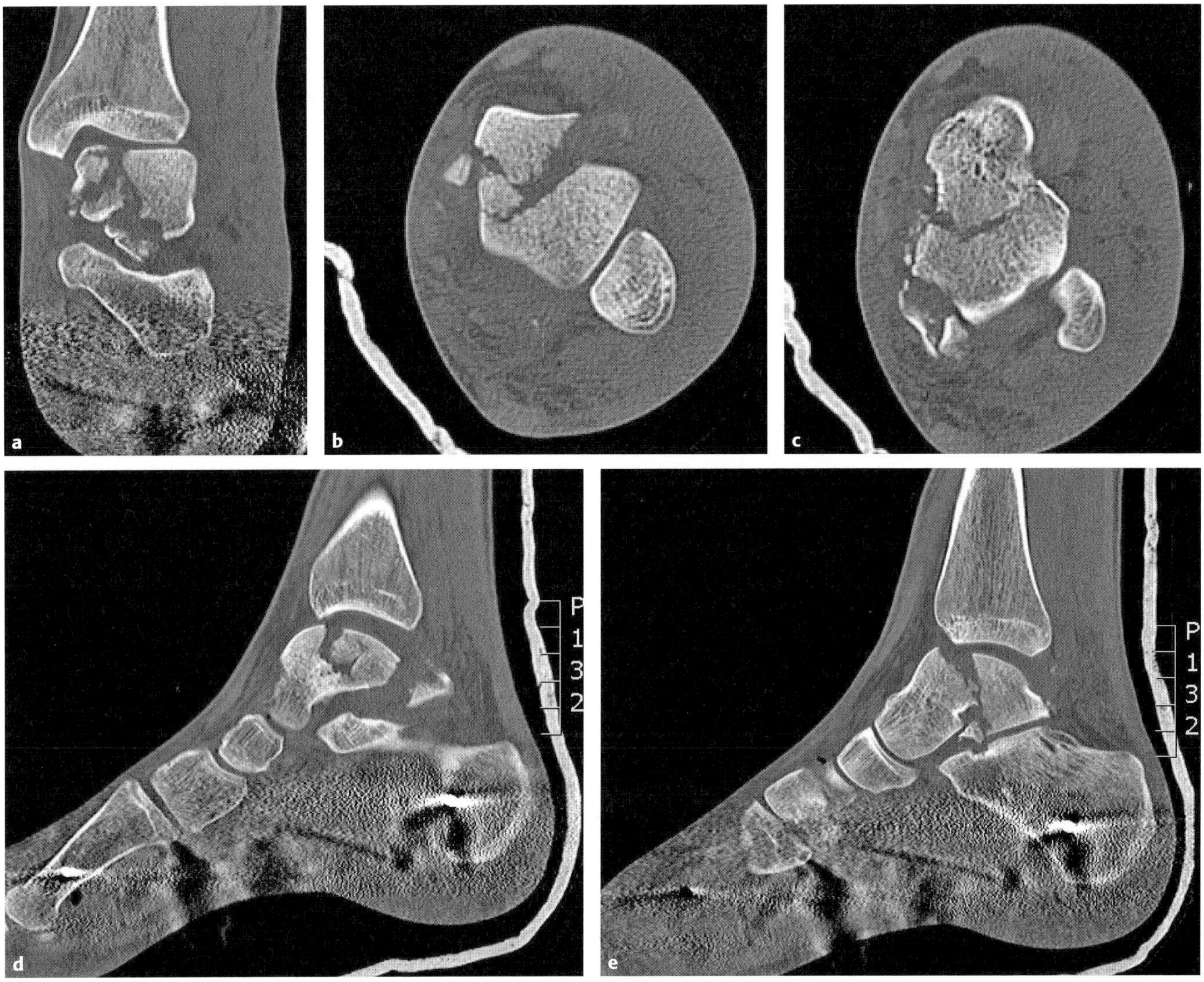

Fig 5.5-4a–e The CT scan after reduction and application of the external fixator provides more detail of the injury. The dominant fracture line is a sagittal split of the talar body. There is significant comminution present. The posterior portion of the talus is fractured and is comminuted (**c–d**).

a Coronal view.

b–c Axial view.

d–e Sagittal view.

4 Surgical procedure

Anatomical reduction of this fracture requires fixation to be performed in two stages. The first stage of the procedure will address the anterior portion of the talar body and will be done in the supine position. The second stage will address the posterior talar body and will require prone positioning. They may be performed sequentially as one surgical procedure or may be performed as two separate surgical procedures: Considerations for making this decision include overall patient health (can they tolerate prolonged surgery and prone positioning), soft-tissue swelling, and availability of surgical time to accommodate the longer surgery if both are performed at the same time.

The following approaches are used for each stage:

1. Medial and lateral approaches with the patient supine allow for reduction and fixation of the coronal split to the displaced body of the talus and address the central comminution.
2. Posteromedial approach with the patient prone allows for accurate reduction of the posterior portion of the displaced talar body fracture.

Medial approach

A medial approach is marked starting from the tip of the medial malleolus and extends distally in the interval between the anterior and posterior tibial tendons. The incision is deepened with care so as not to injure the greater saphenous vein and nerve, which are identified, isolated, and retracted out of the way. In most cases with associated dislocation no formal ankle arthrotomy is needed as the capsule tears during the trauma. Joint hematoma is evacuated allowing visualization of the fracture from the medial side.

In this case, as in most cases, a medial malleolar osteotomy was not necessary. If a medial malleolar osteotomy is necessary, the incision is extended 5 cm above the medial malleolus. The sheath of the tibialis posterior tendon is incised posteriorly and the posterior tibialis tendon is retracted with a small retractor. The malleolar osteotomy is marked with the electrocautery and its position is checked radiologically with the C-arm to make sure it is at the correct level for access to the talar fracture.

The screw paths that will be used later to repair the osteotomy should be predrilled to allow easy insertion of screws later and ensures anatomical reduction of the osteotomy.

Lateral approach

A lateral approach to the talus is performed. The incision extends from the tubercle of Chaput over the ankle and in line with the fourth MT. The superficial peroneal nerve may cross the proximal extent of the incision and must be protected. Dissection continues just lateral to the extensor tendons of the anterior ankle, which are retracted medially. Occasionally the extensor digitorum brevis may need to be elevated off the lateral aspect of the talus but is often detached with the trauma.

K-wires are introduced medially and laterally through the incisions (**Fig 5.5-5a**). The intercalary comminution is reduced while looking in the fracture plane from lateral, and the medial K-wires are advanced to hold these fragments in place. Care must be taken to not advance the K-wires out of the fragments and into the major coronal split because they will block the reduction. The medial and lateral portions of the displaced talar body fracture are reduced and held with a large articular reduction clamp. The fracture reduction is assessed using direct visualization and a small (Freer) elevator is used to confirm anatomical reduction. Once reduction is confirmed, the K-wires from medial and lateral are advanced across the major fracture line (**Fig 5.5-5b–f**). Screws are then placed from medial to lateral and lateral to medial for fixation (**Fig 5.5-5g–h**). All screws are countersunk below the articular surface. Additionally, care must be taken that the hardware does not project into the posterior portion of the body, which could block reduction of the posterior portion of the talus.

The K-wires and reduction clamp are then removed. The wound is closed in layers and a standard dressing is applied.

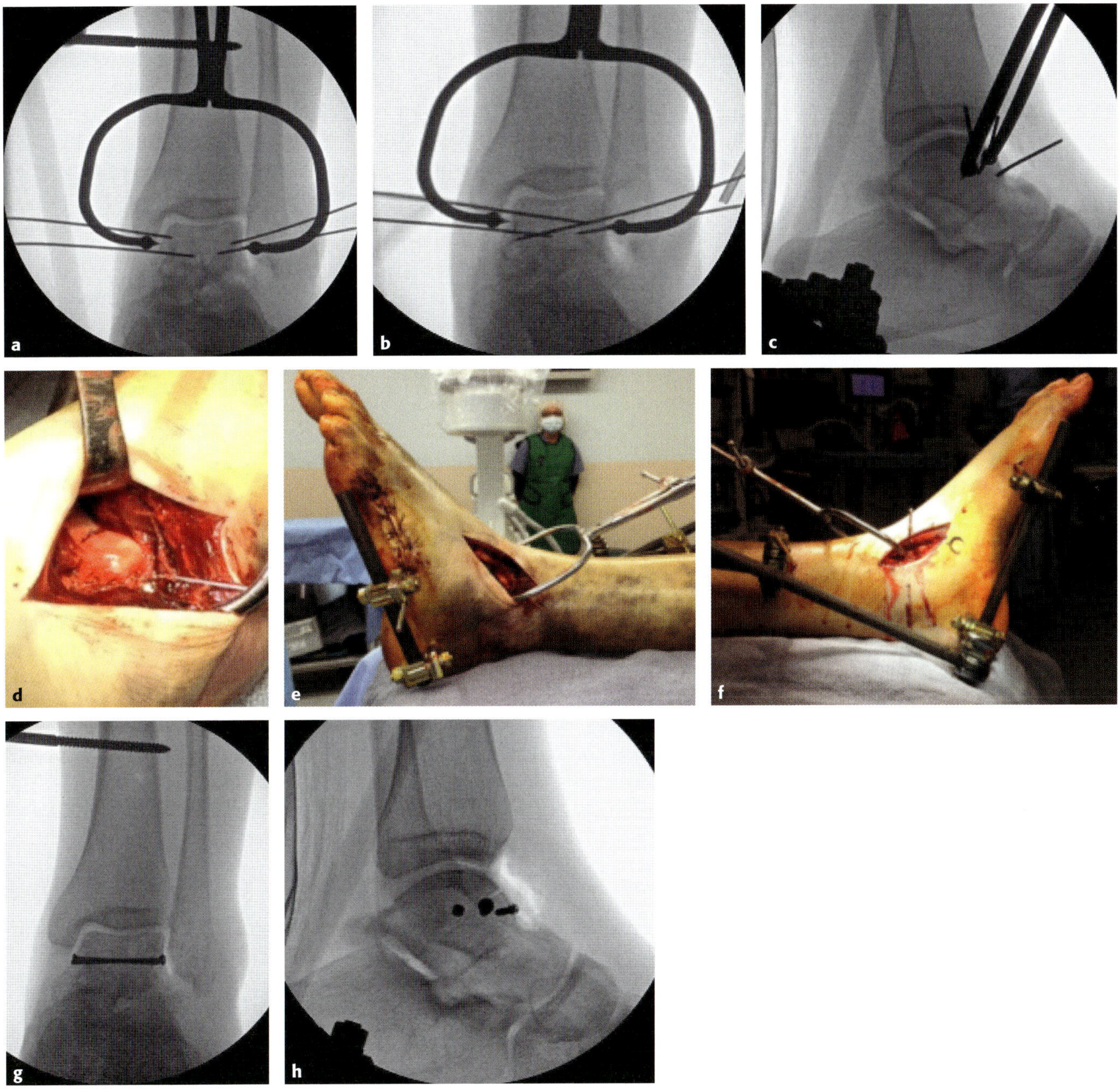

Fig 5.5-5a–h Fixation of the anterior portion of the body of the talus.

a–d The K-wires are inserted prior to reduction and advanced after reduction has been achieved. The fracture is held with a large point-to-point (periarticular) reduction clamp as seen on the C-arm mortise (**b**), lateral (**c**), and intraoperative (**d**) views.

e–f The provisional K-wires and reduction clamp as seen from the lateral and medial incisions.

g–h Mortise and lateral C-arm images show the screws placed for fixation of the talar body fracture.

Posteromedial approach

In this case, the posterior portion of the displaced talus body was addressed immediately following the above fixation. The patient was placed prone and a posteromedial approach to the ankle utilizing the interval between the Achilles and the flexor hallucis longus was used to approach the fracture. The posterior component of the fracture was reduced and stabilized with K-wires and subsequently plated with a minifragment plate 2.4 cut to appropriate length and 2.4 mm screws (**Fig 5.5-6**). See chapter 5.3 for details.

In this case, the portion of the external fixator spanning the ankle was removed after talar fixation was completed. The foot portion was maintained until the MT shaft and cuboid fractures were addressed which occurred roughly a week after the talar fixation.

The wounds are closed in layers and a well-padded splint is applied. The patient is instructed to elevate the limb postoperatively.

5 Pitfalls and complications

Pitfalls

Inadequate exposure

In order to reduce the fracture, it must be directly visualized. If this is not possible, a medial malleolar osteotomy may be necessary. The medial malleolar osteotomy must enter the joint at the top of the talus for adequate exposure. Correct angulation of the osteotomy is important for exposure, as well as avoiding damage to the distal tibial plafond. The medial malleolus should be predrilled for fixation prior to creating the osteotomy. If a medial malleolar fracture is present, then this may be used to allow visualization of the displaced talar body fracture.

Injury to associated structures

If a medial malleolar osteotomy is necessary, care must be taken not to injure the posterior tibialis tendon. A small (Hohmann) retractor is used to retract the tendon, and the tendon sheath must be repaired once the procedure is over.

Avascular necrosis

Unnecessary dissection and retraction causing injury to the remaining blood supply must be avoided. Excessive dissection should be avoided to prevent further damage to the remaining blood supply to the talus. All soft-tissue attachments should be maintained if possible.

If a medial malleolar osteotomy is performed, then aggressive retraction of the medial malleolar fragment must be avoided to prevent injury to vessels entering through the deep deltoid ligament. This may jeopardize the vascularity of the talar body and cause avascular necrosis.

Intraarticular hardware

Screws must be recessed below the articular cartilage to prevent injury to the articular cartilage with movement of the joint. Plates must be contoured and placed over the nonarticular surface so that they do not restrict range of motion (ROM) and cause further articular injury.

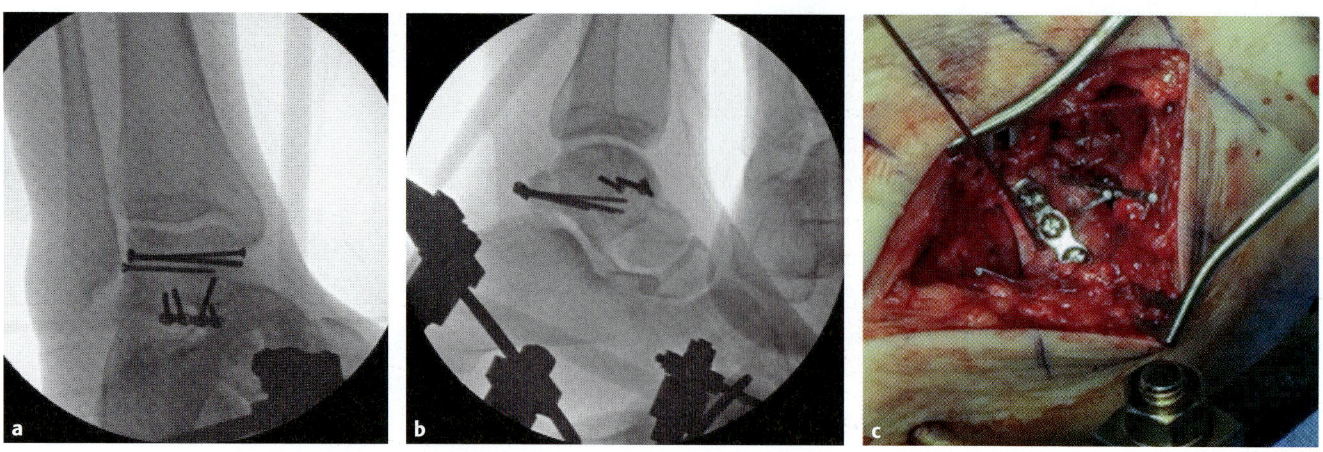

Fig 5.5-6a–c Fixation of the posterior portion of the body of the talus.
a–b Mortise and lateral C-arm images show the final fixation construct for the displaced body of the talus including fixation of the posterior talus.
c With the posteromedial surgical approach, the plate is placed on the small extraarticular portion of the posterior talus.

If significant comminution exists or bone loss is present, then the screws should be fully threaded and inserted as positional screws to avoid over compression resulting in altering the joint surfaces. This creates a malalignment between the talus and the corresponding articular surface.

Complications

- Malreduction
- Loss of reduction
- Posttraumatic arthritis of the ankle and/or subtalar joint
- Avascular necrosis of the talus
- Infection
- Stiffness
- Wound healing complications

6 Alternative techniques

For best outcomes comminuted talar body fractures require operative treatment with exact reduction. All other treatment techniques will lead to significant morbidity and should be avoided.

7 Postoperative management and rehabilitation

The patient remains in a splint for 2 weeks. Limb elevation and active toe movements are encouraged. At 2 weeks the splint is removed and the patient is placed in a removable fracture boot. If ankle and subtalar joint stability was present after surgical fixation, ROM exercises are initiated for the ankle and subtalar joints. If instability is present, ROM exercises are initiated at 6 weeks.

In this particular case a posterior plate was used to aid in fixation of the displaced talar body fracture. In this scenario it is important to engage in ROM exercises of the great toe beginning on postoperative day 1 to avoid the flexor hallucis longus tendon from scarring, resulting in poor ROM of the first metatarsophalangeal joint.

Weight bearing is started once fracture consolidation is noted on postoperative images, which usually takes 12 weeks. Posttraumatic stiffness of the ankle and particularly the subtalar joint are common after these injuries. The patient must actively engage in ROM exercises over time.

Final images of the patient at 3 years demonstrate anatomical alignment of the talus without evidence of posttraumatic arthritis (**Fig 5.5-7**), and fixation of the cuboid and MT injuries.

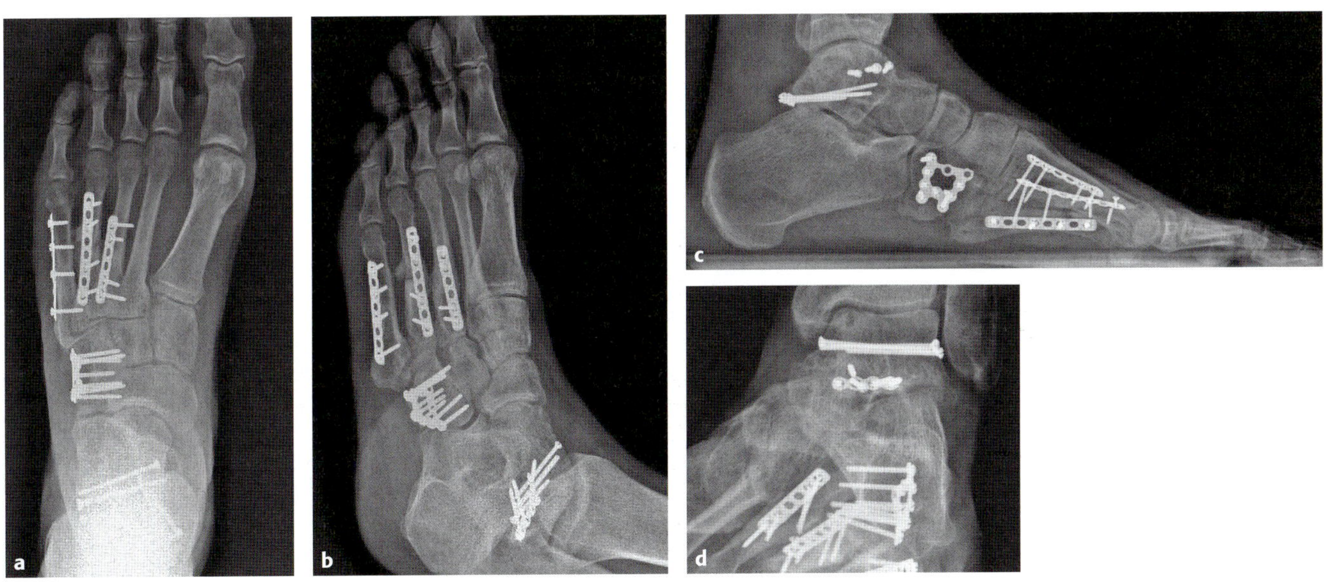

Fig 5.5-7a–d Final x-rays taken 3 years postoperatively showing the healed talar body. The cuboid and MT fractures have also healed in anatomical alignment.

- **a** AP view.
- **b** Oblique view.
- **c** Lateral view.
- **d** Mortise view.

8 Recommended reading

Ebraheim NA, Patil V, Owens C, et al. Clinical outcome of fractures of the talar body. *Int Orthop.* 2008 Dec;32(6):773–777.
Vallier HA. Fractures of the talus: state of the art. *J Orthop Trauma.* 2015 Sep;29(9):385–392.
Vallier HA, Nork SE, Benirschke SK, et al. Surgical treatment of talar body fractures. *J Bone Joint Surg Am.* 2004 Sep;86-A Suppl 1(Pt 2):180–192.

5.6 Talar neck fracture with dislocation of the body (Hawkins 3)

Keun-Bae Lee

1 Case description

A 43-year-old male pedestrian was hit by a car and sustained a closed fracture of his left talus and medial malleolus with posterior dislocation of the talar body.

X-rays of the ankle show a displaced vertical fracture of the talar neck with posterior dislocation of subtalar and tibiotalar joints (AO/OTA 81.2.C(b), Hawkins 3 AO/OTA 81.2.Cb) (**Fig 5.6-1**).

On day 2 after the injury, the foot had significant swelling and blisters (**Fig 5.6-2** and **Fig 5.6-3**).

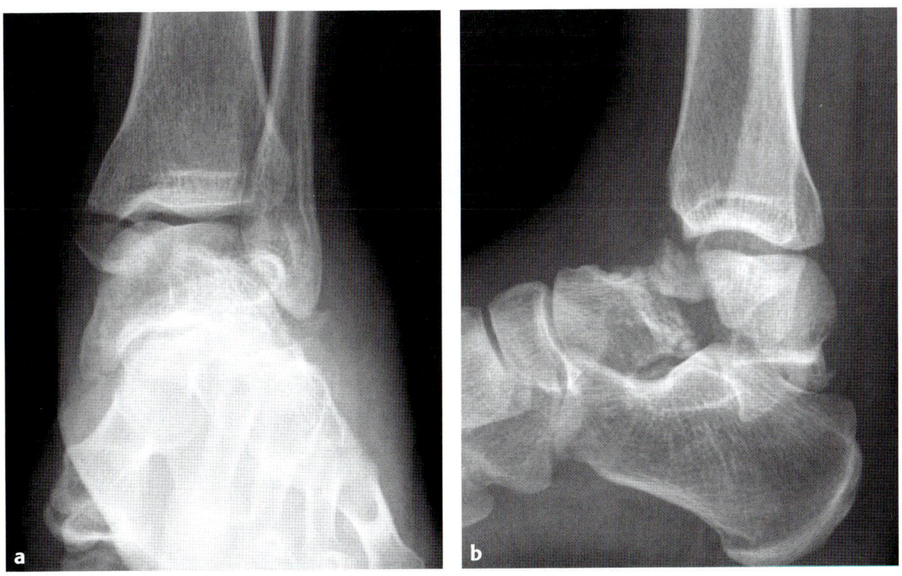

Fig 5.6-1a–b X-rays of a Hawkins 3 talar fracture dislocation; note the posteriorly displaced and rotated body of the talus, together with comminution of the neck and the medial malleolar fracture.
a AP view.
b Lateral view.

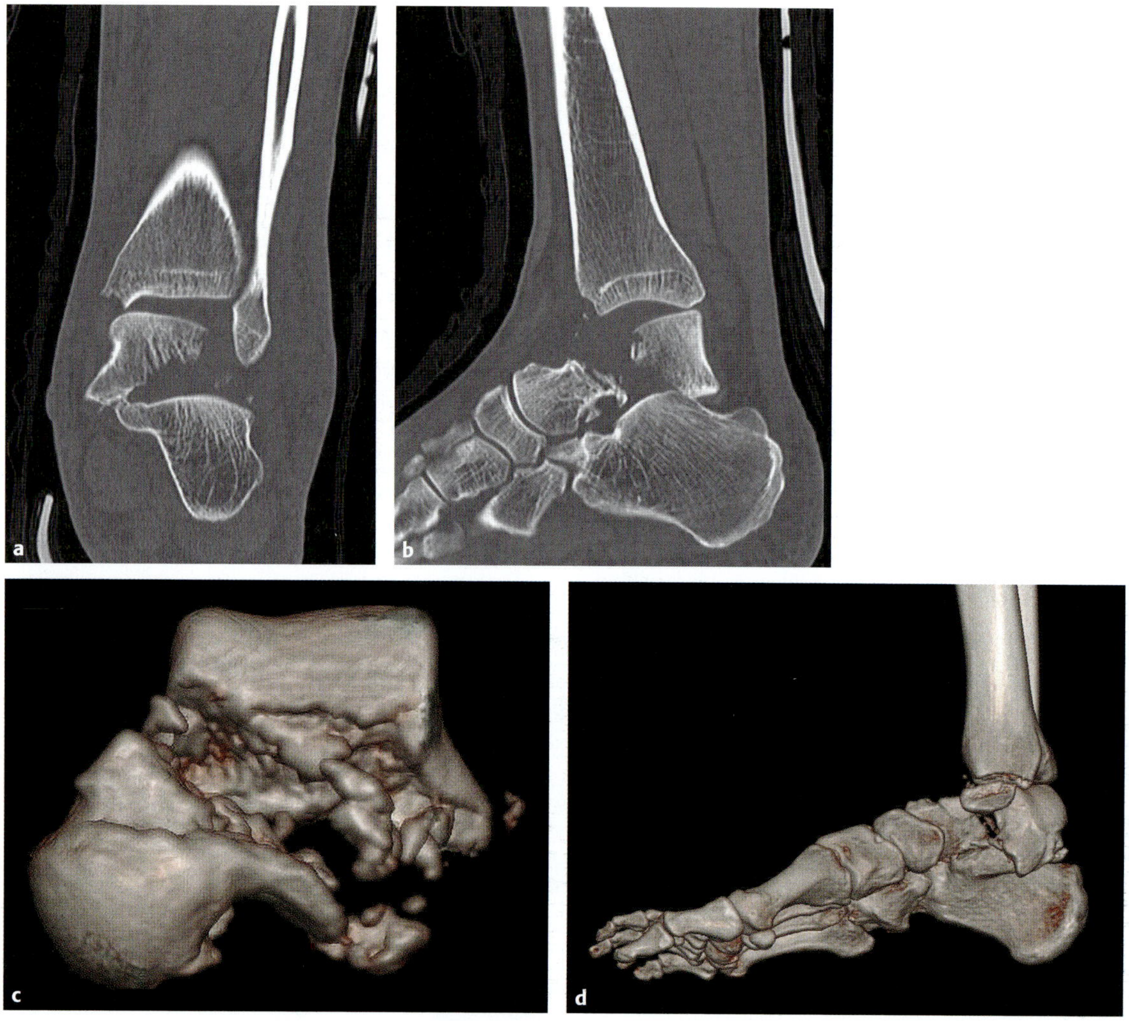

Fig 5.6-2a–d The computed tomographic images showing the comminuted talar neck fracture with posteromedial dislocation of the talar body.
a–b 2D reconstruction.
c–d 3D reconstruction.

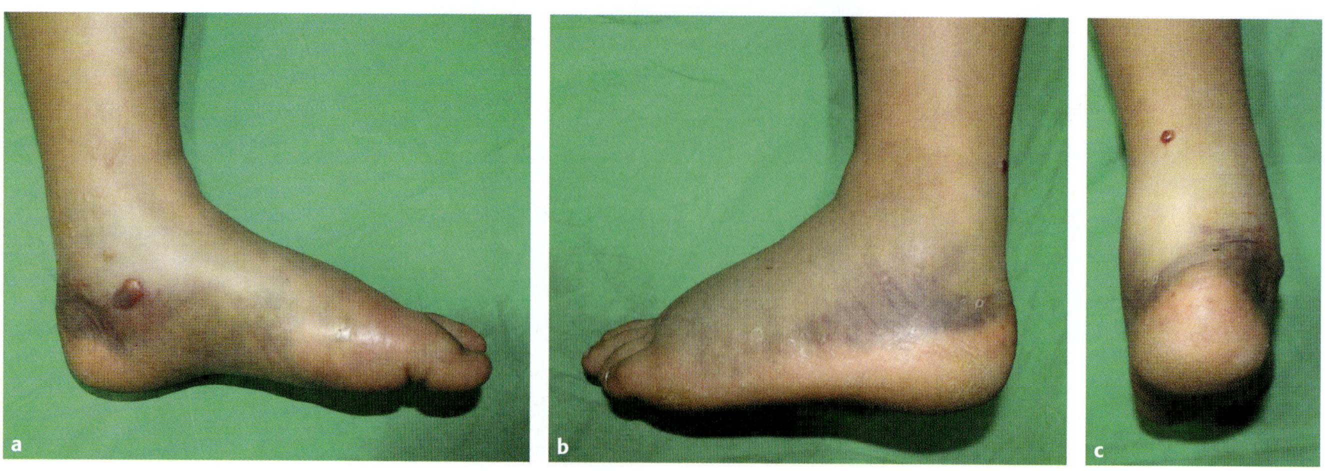

Fig 5.6-3a–c Deformity, swelling, and blisters on the left ankle.

2 Preoperative planning

Closed reduction should be attempted as soon as possible, under suitable anesthesia, to minimize soft-tissue and skin compromise, reduce the joints, and minimize further vascular insult to the talar body. This also aids in cartilage viability and reduces pain.

It was thought that the soft-tissue injury may alter the surgical approach and timing of surgical intervention. However, urgent open reduction and internal fixation (ORIF) should be performed, even in the presence of swelling, to achieve the anatomical reduction of the fracture dislocation if attempts at closed reduction fail. The goal of treatment is to relieve compression from the displaced body on the neurovascular bundle and skin medially and to minimize the occurrence of avascular necrosis (AVN).

3 Operating room setup

Patient positioning	• Supine on a radiolucent operating table extension with the foot brought to the end of the table
Anesthesia options	• General anesthesia is necessary as the reduction of the dislocation is difficult and requires muscle relaxation.
C-arm location	• Either the standard size or mini C-arm can be used. • The C-arm should be close to the foot of the table with the screen easily seen by the surgeon without having to turn around.
Tourniquet	• A well-padded tourniquet applied to the thigh (**Fig 5.6-4**)

For illustrations and overview of anesthetic considerations, see chapter 1.

Equipment

- K-wires
- Screws as per surgeon preference (3.5 mm cannulated screws, 4.0 mm cancellous screws can be used)
- Talus or minifragment plates as backup
- Point-to-point forceps
- Distractor
- C-arm and radiolucent table

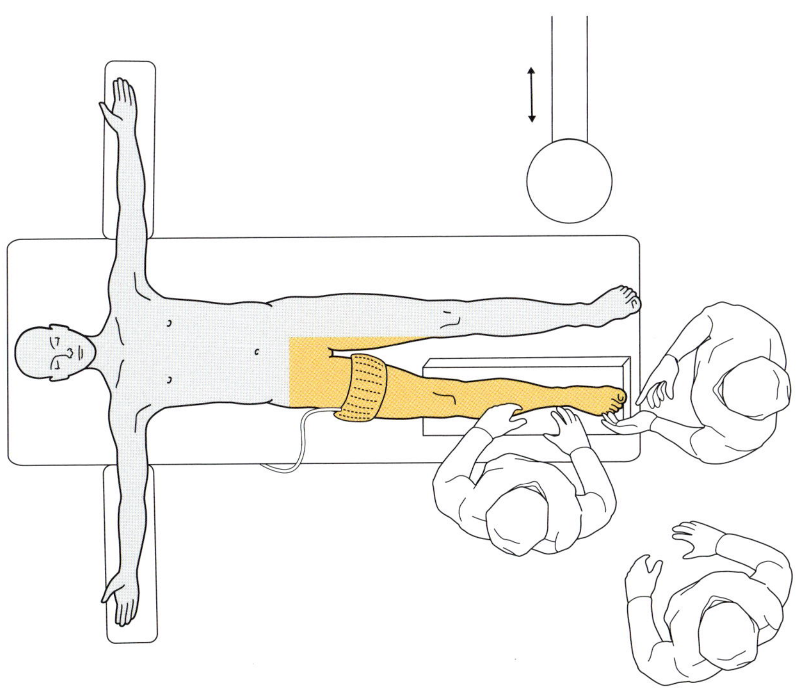

Fig 5.6-4 Patient in supine position, with thigh tourniquet in place. Note surgeon and C-arm positioning.

4 Surgical approach

A dual incision is essential for accurate reduction and stable fixation. The anteromedial incision runs from the medial malleolus proximally to the tuberosity of navicular distally. This is made directly over the talar neck and between the anterior and posterior tibial tendons. When fractures of the talar neck are associated with malleolar fractures, the placement of the medial incision facilitates reduction and fixation of the medial malleolar fragment and can help in better exposure of the body fragment after inferior retraction of the malleolus.

The medial malleolus and the medial talar body both receive their blood supply via the deltoid ligament. Therefore, care should be taken with a medial approach not to disturb this important blood supply. Once the skin and fascia are incised, the comminuted talar neck fracture and the posteromedially dislocated talar body with medial malleolar fracture, are visualized (**Fig 5.6-5**).

Reduction

The closed reduction maneuver is facilitated by longitudinal traction and reversal of the dislocation force (**Fig 5.6-6**). If successful, the talar body will reduce into the mortise. If this fails, open reduction is needed, that is facilitated by distraction aids. Care should be taken to preserve all soft-tissue attachments (blood supply) to the talar body, and all manipulations should be gentle (**Fig 5.6-6** and **Fig 5.6-7**). Occasionally, the medial tendons or neurovascular bundle may block reduction. The blocking structure will need to be carefully extricated before successful reduction.

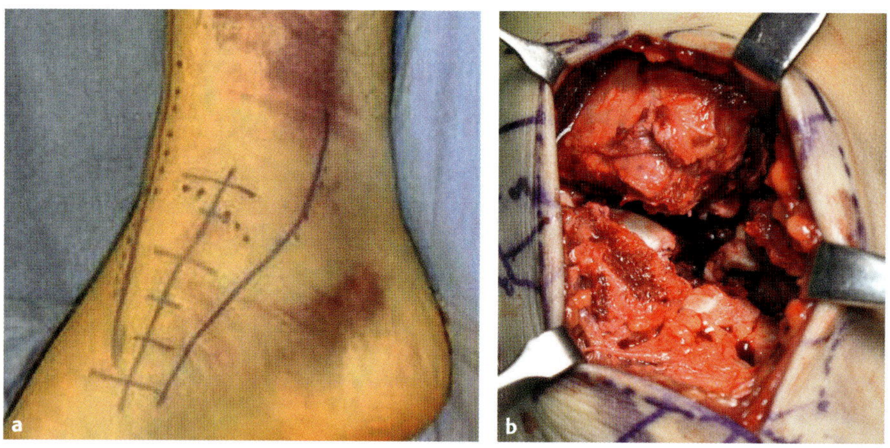

Fig 5.6-5a–b Placement of anteromedial incision (**a**). Direct exposure of the fractured neck (**b**) allowing the fracture to be well visualized.

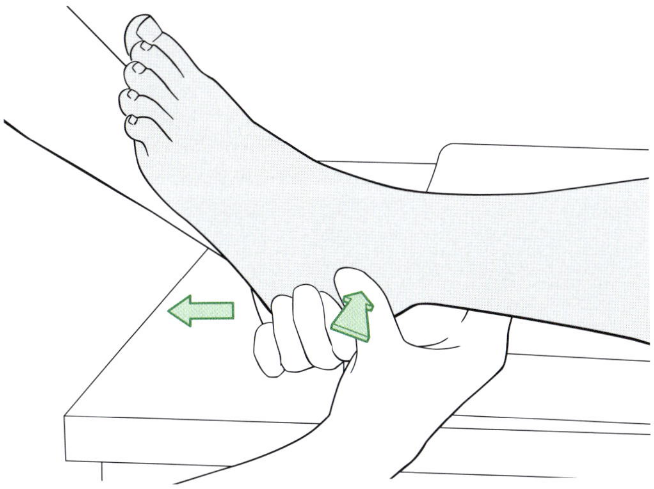

Fig 5.6-6 Method of closed reduction using manual traction and manipulation.

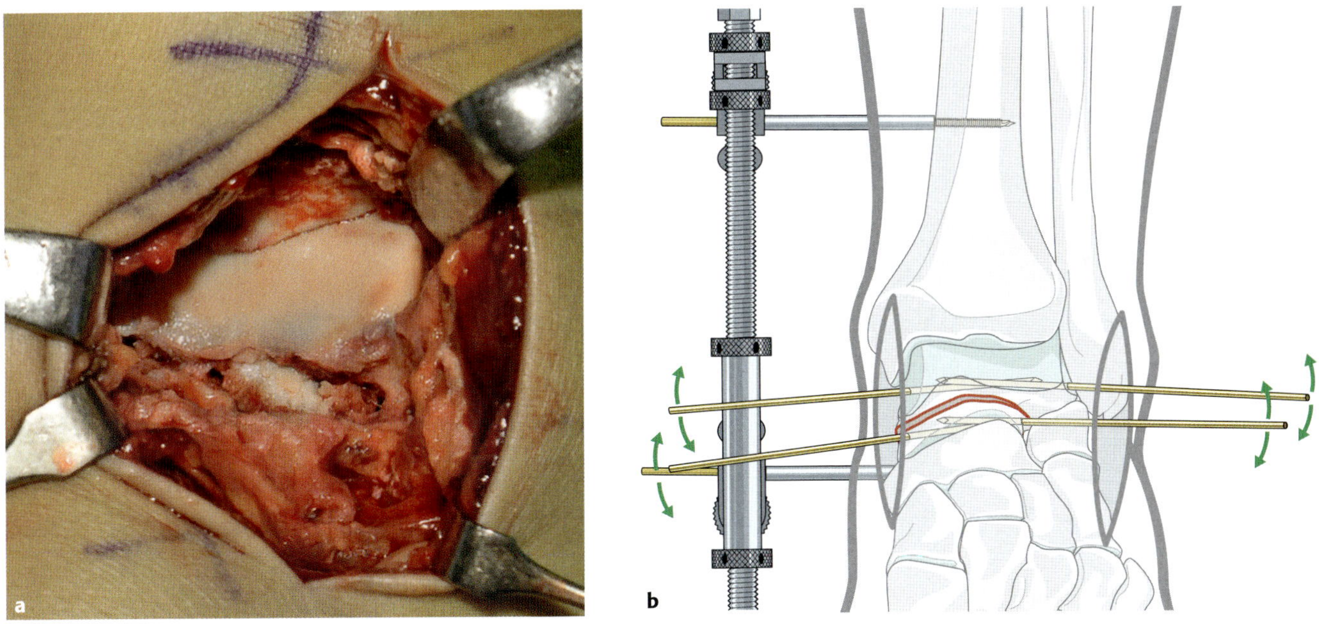

Fig 5.6-7a–b Additional anterolateral approach to expose the fracture (**a**). Reduction through combined approaches, using elevators, K-wires used as joysticks, and distractors (**b**).

Medial malleolar osteotomy

A medial malleolar osteotomy is performed by extending the anteromedial approach to provide access for the osteotomy. Remember that the deltoid ligament and the osteotomy fragment must be kept as one to preserve blood supply to the talar body. This patient had an associated medial malleolar fracture and did not require this technique as the fracture allowed easy access to the area of injury (**Fig 5.6-8**).

Internal fixation

X-rays of the normal side can be used as a template for ORIF of the injured talus, if necessary.

K-wire fixation after reduction is essential for preliminary fixation (**Fig 5.6-9a-b**). Provisional fixation with K-wires should be maintained until all screws are inserted to avoid loss of reduction. Stable fixation is then established with nonparallel screws. Since the lateral talar neck is not usually comminuted, screw fixation is first done in lag fashion on the lateral side. A comminuted medial talar neck can be stabilized by a 4.0 mm fully threaded cancellous screw, which is inserted in nonlag fashion. Screws should be placed plantar to the equator of the talus as the major deforming force is dorsiflexion. This placement helps to counter this force. As the medial screw is placed through the articular surface of the distal talus, it should be countersunk so as not to cause injury to the joint. A lag screw should be avoided on the medial side in the presence of comminution as it may lead to varus malunion; some cases may require bone grafting of superomedial defects which are seen after accurate reconstruction. The wounds are washed, and the medial malleolar osteotomy or fracture is stabilized using the appropriate method, which is usually two parallel screws (**Fig 5.6-10** and **Fig 5.6-11**).

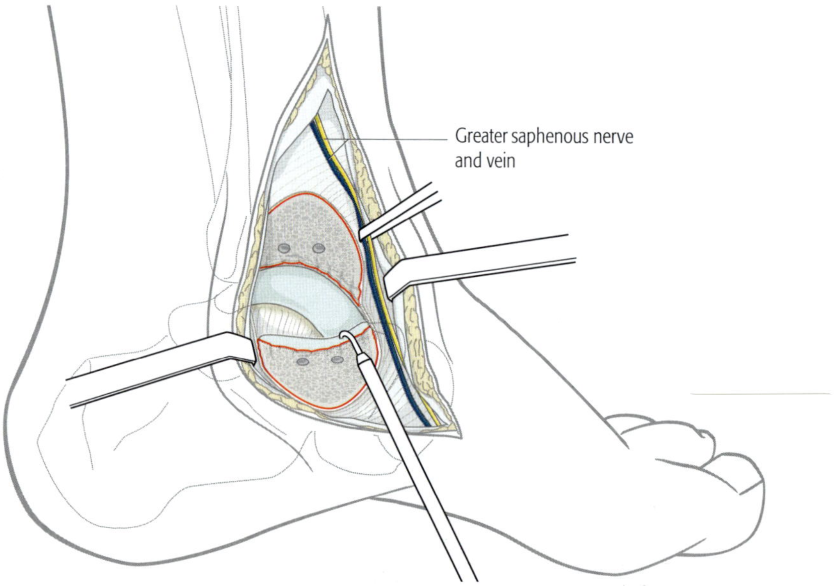

Fig 5.6-8 Exposure after retracted medial malleolar osteotomy.

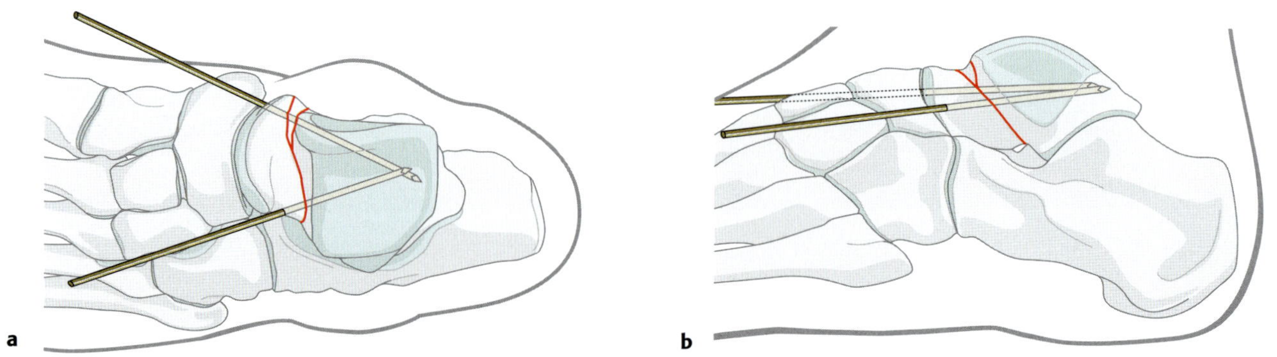

Fig 5.6-9a–b Preliminary K-wire fixation.

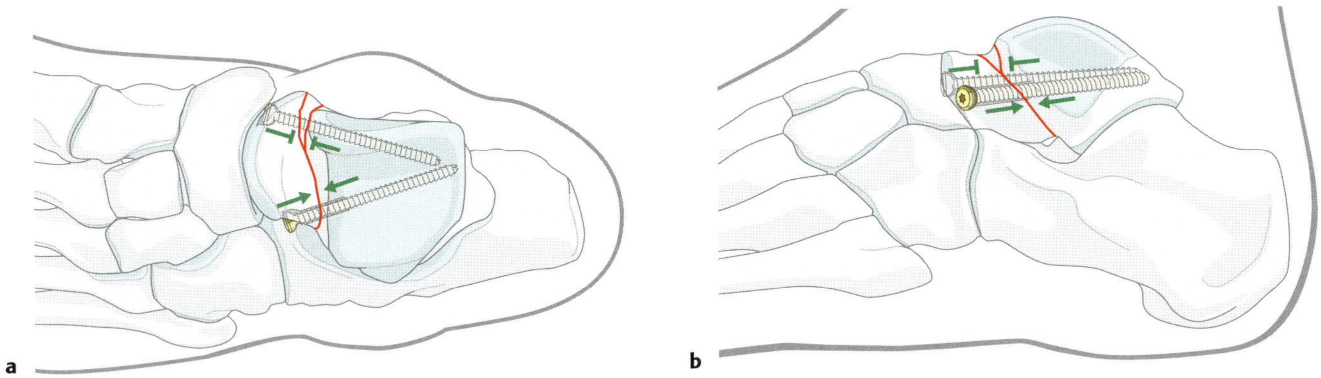

Fig 5.6-10a–b Cannulated screw fixation with the lag screw on the lateral side and the positional screw on the medial side.

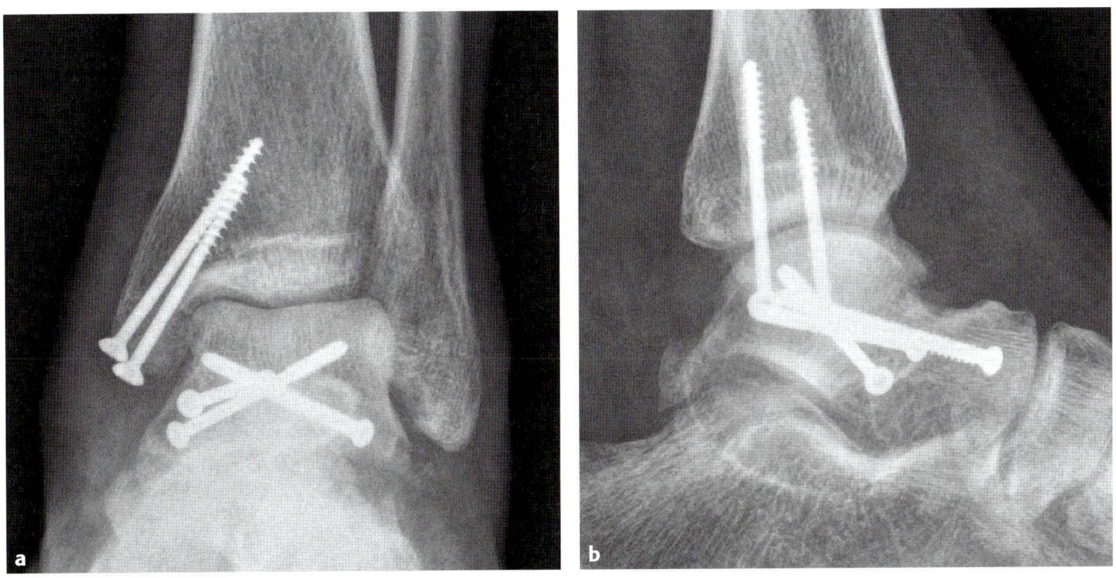

Fig 5.6-11a–b X-rays taken immediately postoperatively showing two 3.5 mm cannulated screws inserted on the medial side and one 4.0 mm cancellous screw on the lateral side. The accompanying medial malleolar fracture is fixed using partially threaded cannulated screws.

a AP view.

b Lateral view.

5 Pitfalls and complications

Pitfalls

- Failure to countersink screw heads may cause problems within the talonavicular joint.
- Failure to avoid the gutters may lead to the plates being placed into the ankle joint.

Complications

- Malreductions may lead to varus malalignment, a common problem with talar fractures.
- Talar neck fractures are at risk for development of AVN. The more displaced the fracture the greater the risk. Revascularization may take a long time and may ultimately be partial.

6 Alternative techniques

Minifragment plates may be used to augment fixation in more comminuted injuries. A combination of plates and screws can be used. As it is often difficult to place a screw through the distal lateral aspect of the talus, a lateral plate can be used.

In the case of a talar neck fracture, which laterally has a part of the talar body attached to the distal fragment, screws may be placed from the lateral extension of the talus into the talar body.

7 Postoperative management and rehabilitation

Aftercare

A splint or bivalved plaster cast is used with the ankle and foot in neutral position for early immobilization. When the patient is in bed, pillows should be used to keep the leg elevated to reduce swelling. Early range of motion (ROM) of the ankle and subtalar joint is advised (**Fig 5.6-12**).

Follow-up

The patient is evaluated by serial visits at postoperative weeks 2, 6, and 12. Sutures are generally removed at 2 weeks. Range-of-motion exercises for ankle and subtalar joints are important and should commence as soon as they are tolerated to restore a good ROM.

X-rays are taken at approximately 6 weeks to assess fracture union.

Patients with talar neck fractures should not begin weight bearing until union has occurred, which takes a minimum of 6 weeks. Because of the severity of these injuries and the poor vascularity of the talus, it is not unusual for weight bearing to be postponed until week 12. Weight bearing is initiated when fracture healing has occurred and progressed as tolerated. A computed tomographic scan is a good method to evaluate fracture union and joint congruity (**Fig 5.6-13**).

Follow-up for talar fractures should continue for a longer period (up to 1 year or more), as these fractures are at higher risk for arthritis as well as late complications related to AVN.

Follow-up at at 18 months postoperatively show good healing (**Fig 5.6-14** and **Fig 5.6-15**) and the function (ankle ROM and walking ability) at the 3-year follow-up was excellent (**Fig 5.6-16** and **Fig 5.6-17**).

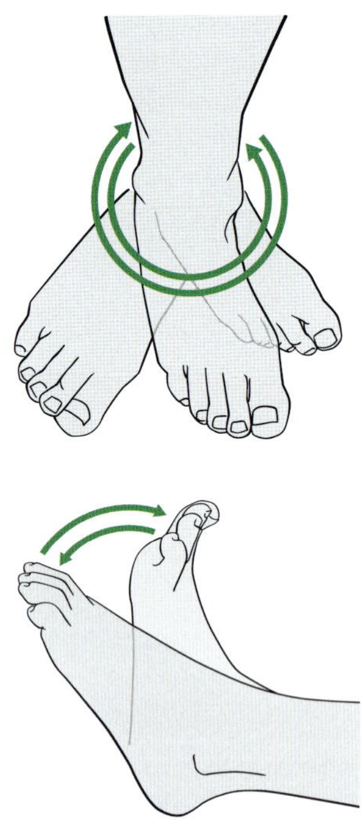

Fig 5.6-12 Subtalar and ankle joint ROM exercises.

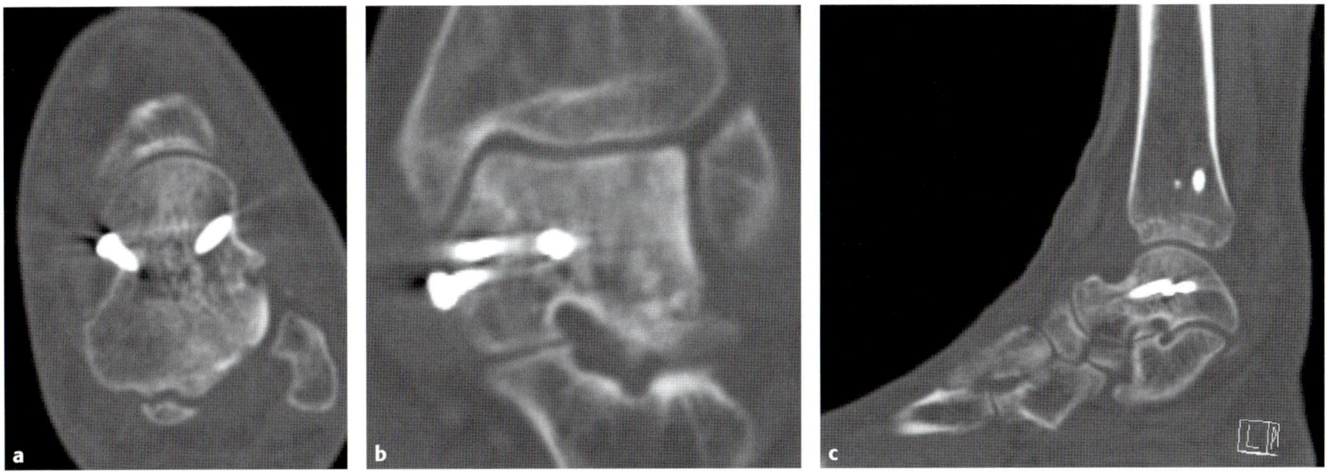

Fig 5.6-13a–c Follow-up computed tomographic scans taken 8 months postoperatively showing complete bony union with intact articular congruency.

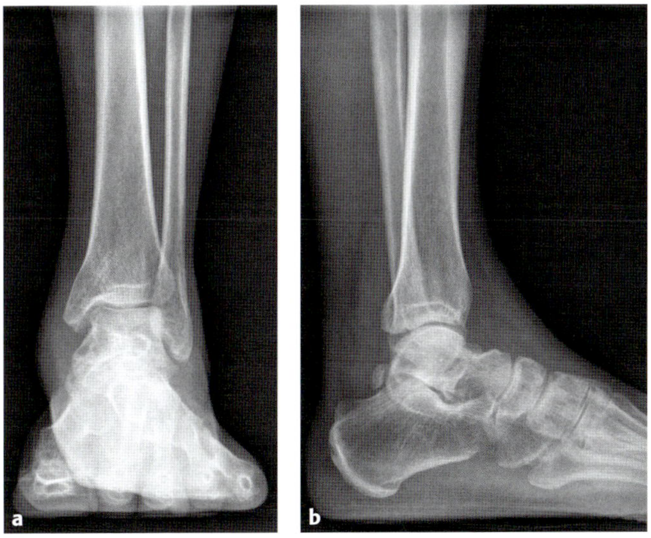

Fig 5.6-14a–b X-rays of the ankle at 18 months showing fracture healing and anatomical restoration of the joint congruency without AVN. The implants were removed 1 year postoperatively.

a AP view.

b Lateral view.

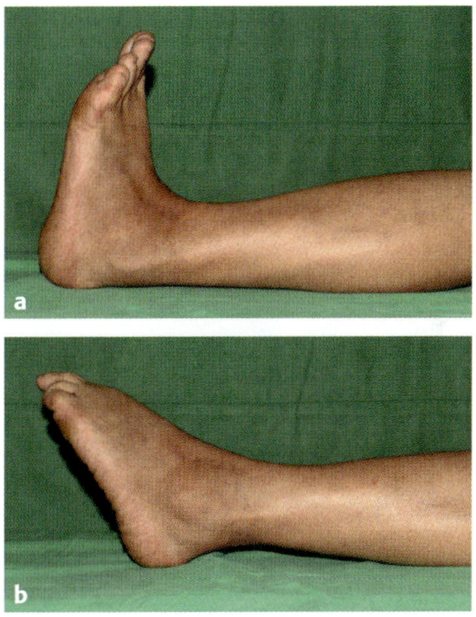

Fig 5.6-15a–b Views of the ankle 18 months postoperatively demonstrating well restored soft tissue with nearly full ROM.

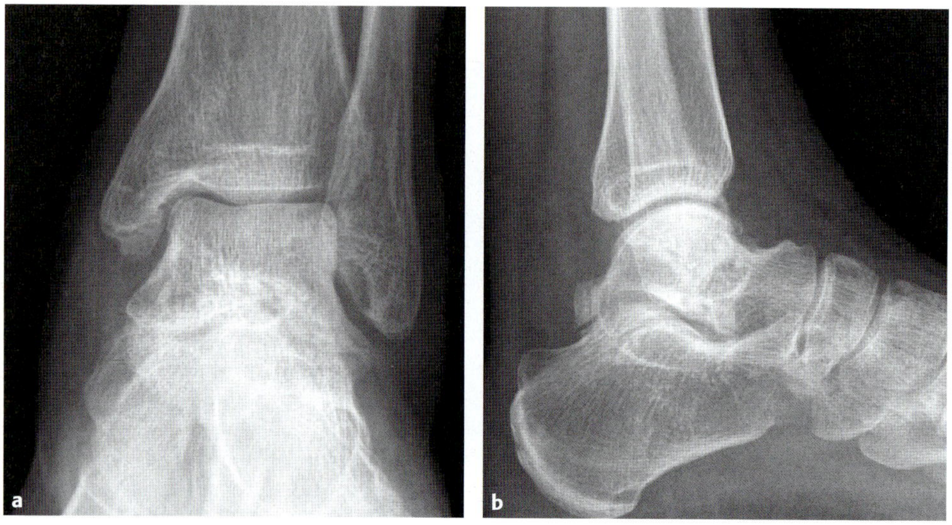

Fig 5.6-16a–b X-rays of the ankle showing anatomical restoration of the joint congruency after implant removal at the 3-year follow-up.
a AP view.
b Lateral view.

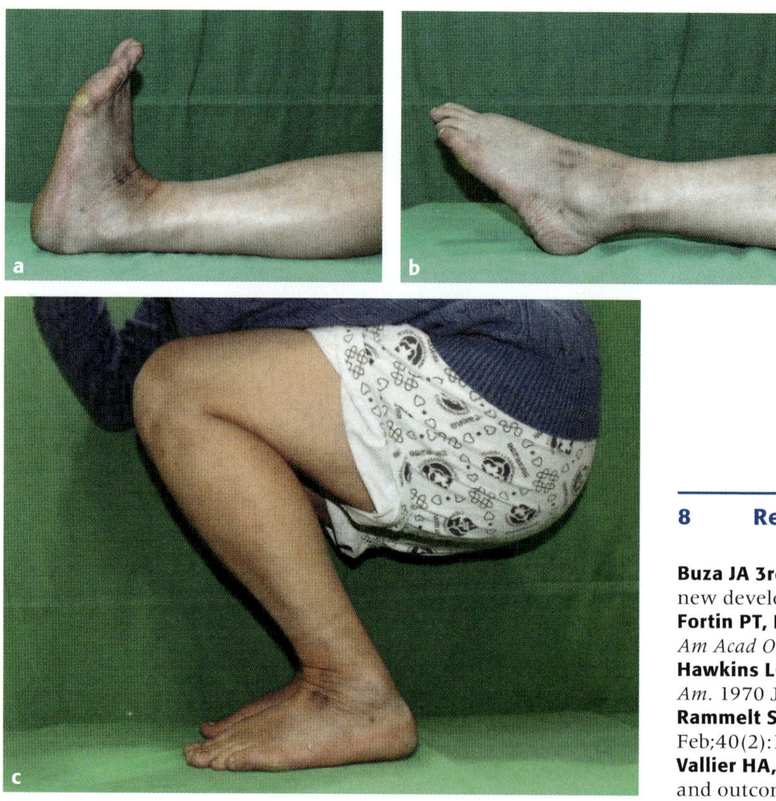

Fig 5.6-17a–c Views of the ankle at the 3-year follow-up demonstrating full ROM.

8 Recommended reading

Buza JA 3rd, Leucht P. Fractures of the talus: current concepts and new developments. *Foot Ankle Surg.* 2018 Aug;24(4):282–290.
Fortin PT, Balazsy JE. Talus fractures: evaluation and treatment. *J Am Acad Orthop Surg.* 2001 Mar–Apr;9(2):114–127.
Hawkins LG. Fractures of the neck of the talus. *J Bone Joint Surg Am.* 1970 Jul;52(5):991–1002.
Rammelt S, Zwipp H. Talar neck and body fractures. *Injury.* 2009 Feb;40(2):120–135.
Vallier HA, Nork SE, Barei DP, et al. Talar neck fractures: results and outcomes. *J Bone Joint Surg Am.* 2004 Aug;86(8):1616–1624.

5.7 Medial subtalar dislocation

Mandeep S Dhillon, Sharad Prabhakar

1 Case description

A 48-year-old man sustained an injury to his left foot in a road traffic accident while riding a motorcycle. Clinical examination showed the foot was deformed, with the forefoot inverted and plantar flexed, with swelling and bruising (**Fig 5.7-1**). X-rays revealed a medial subtalar dislocation with an intact ankle (**Fig 5.7-2**).

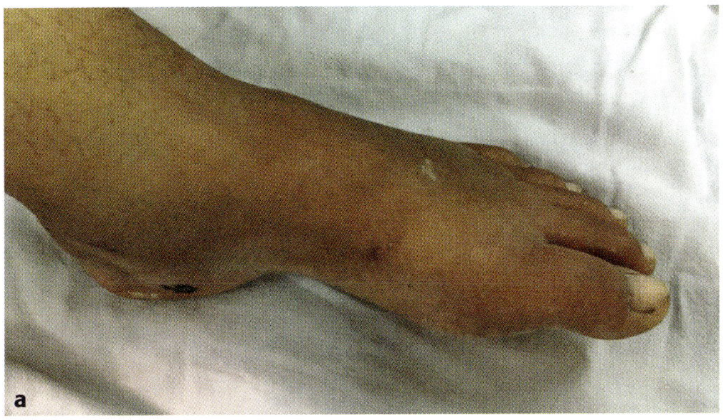

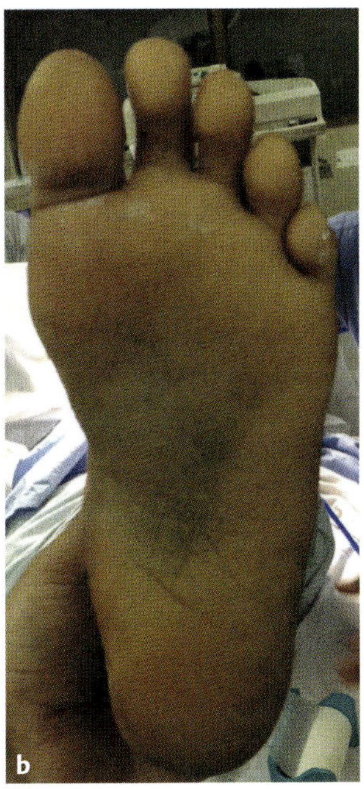

Fig 5.7-1a–b Injured foot revealing swelling, planter bruising with an inversion, and planter flexion deformity.

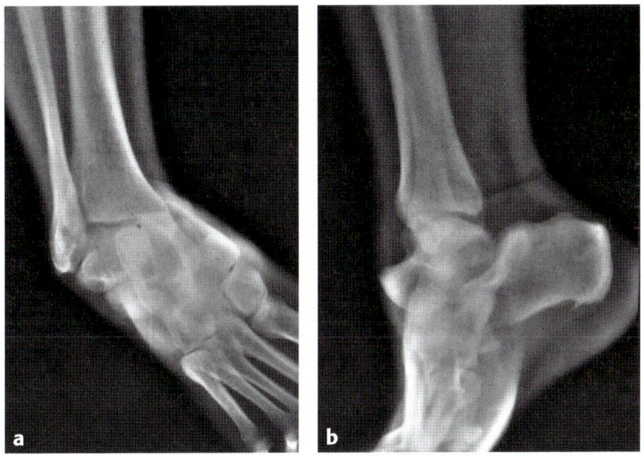

Fig 5.7-2a–b X-rays revealing a medial subtalar dislocation, with the ankle intact and the foot and heel inverted.

a AP view.

b Lateral view.

2 Preoperative planning

Surgical indications are rare, except for open dislocations or those that are irreducible by closed means.

Immediate reduction of subtalar dislocations in the emergency department with adequate sedation and muscular relaxation is required to minimize soft-tissue insult and neurovascular compromise.

Usually closed treatment of this injury is successful if reduction is done early and the appropriate steps are taken.

3 Operating room setup

Patient positioning	• Supine
Anesthesia options	• Reduction can be attempted with the patient under sedation if the dislocation is uncomplicated and recent, but provision for general anesthesia with maximum relaxation must be available.
C-arm location	• On the contralateral side of the injury with the screen of the C-arm positioned toward the head of the operative table to allow easy visualization by the surgeon
Tourniquet	• Not required
Tips	• Adequate relaxation is the key for ease of reduction

For illustrations and overview of anesthetic considerations, see chapter 1.

Equipment

No special equipment is needed as closed reduction succeeds in most cases. Closed reduction is often performed on the field by another athlete, or by emergency medical services upon their arrive.

4 Surgical approach

The knee is bent to 90° to minimize the pull of the gastrocnemius. Reduction for a medial dislocation follows the principle of traction in line of the deformity to disengage the talar head. The foot is then further plantar flexed and inverted, and distal traction is applied to unlock the talar head from the navicular. Direct pressure on the prominent talar head helps in reduction (**Fig 5.7-3**). The foot is subsequently dorsiflexed and everted with direct laterally directed pressure over the talar head. An audible click confirms reduction. Intraoperative C-arm evaluation helps ensure accuracy of reduction of the talar head.

For this patient, x-rays taken after closed reduction and below knee immobilization demonstrated anatomical reduction (**Fig 5.7-4**); indications for post reduction CT should be generous to exclude associated fractures of talar processes. Follow-up x-rays (**Fig 5.7-5**) at 1 year demonstrated normal subtalar joint with no evidence of arthritis. Excellent clinical outcome was demonstrated by no residual pain or limp and an unimpaired gait and good hindfoot motion (**Fig 5.7-6**).

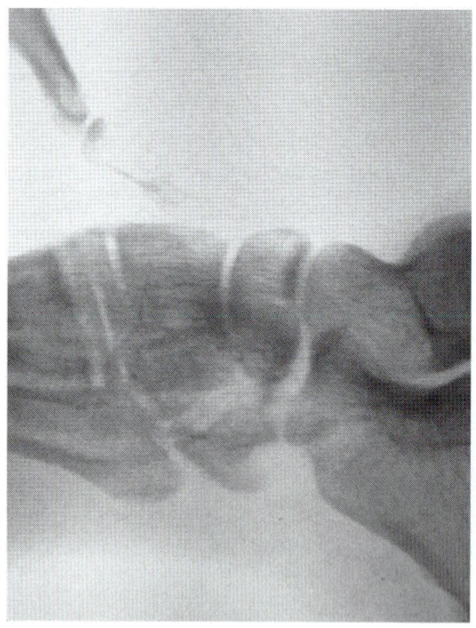

Fig 5.7-3 Intraoperative C-arm image showing pressure being applied to the talar head.

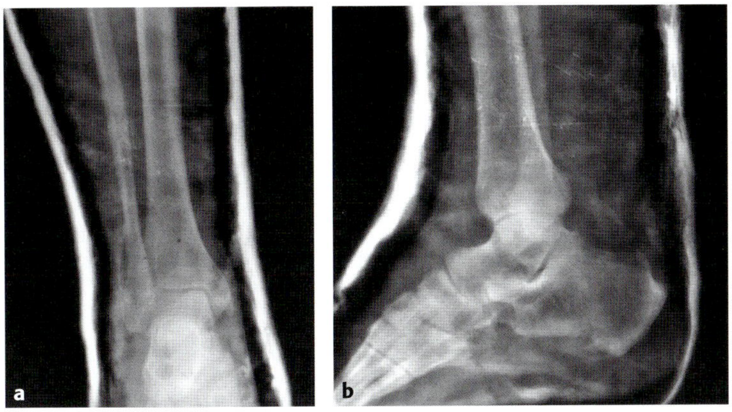

Fig 5.7-4a–b X-rays after closed reduction and application of a below-knee cast that was kept for 4 weeks.

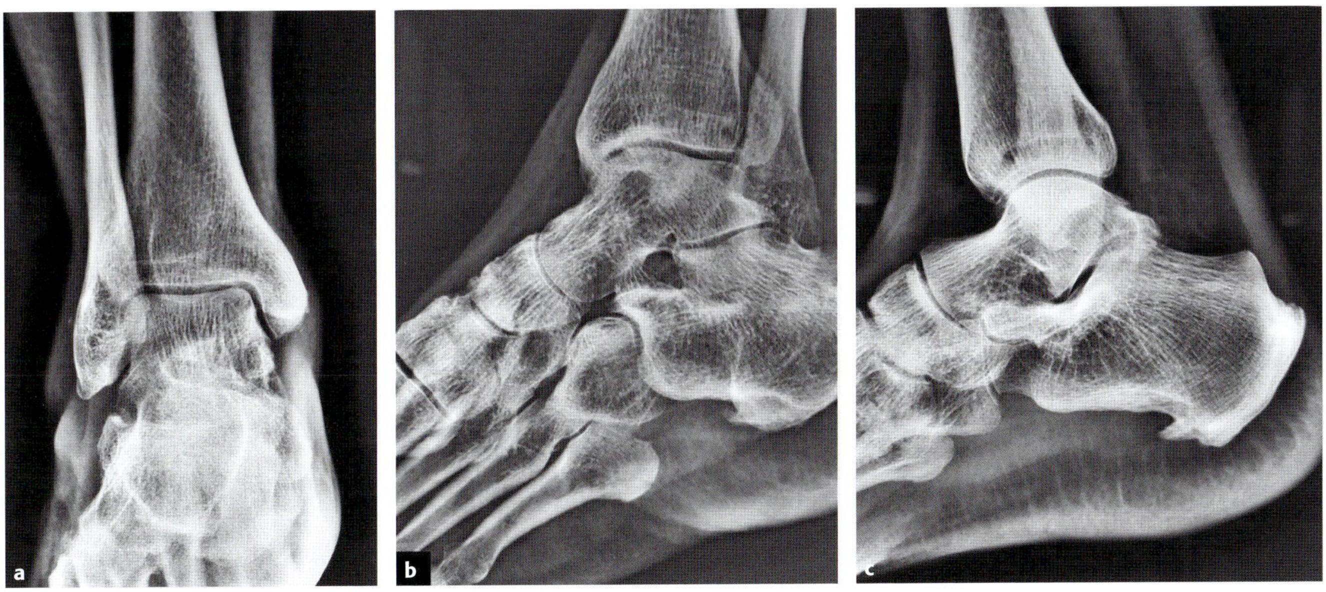

Fig 5.7-5a–c Follow-up x-rays at 1 year showing normal subtalar and talonavicular joints with no evidence of arthritis.

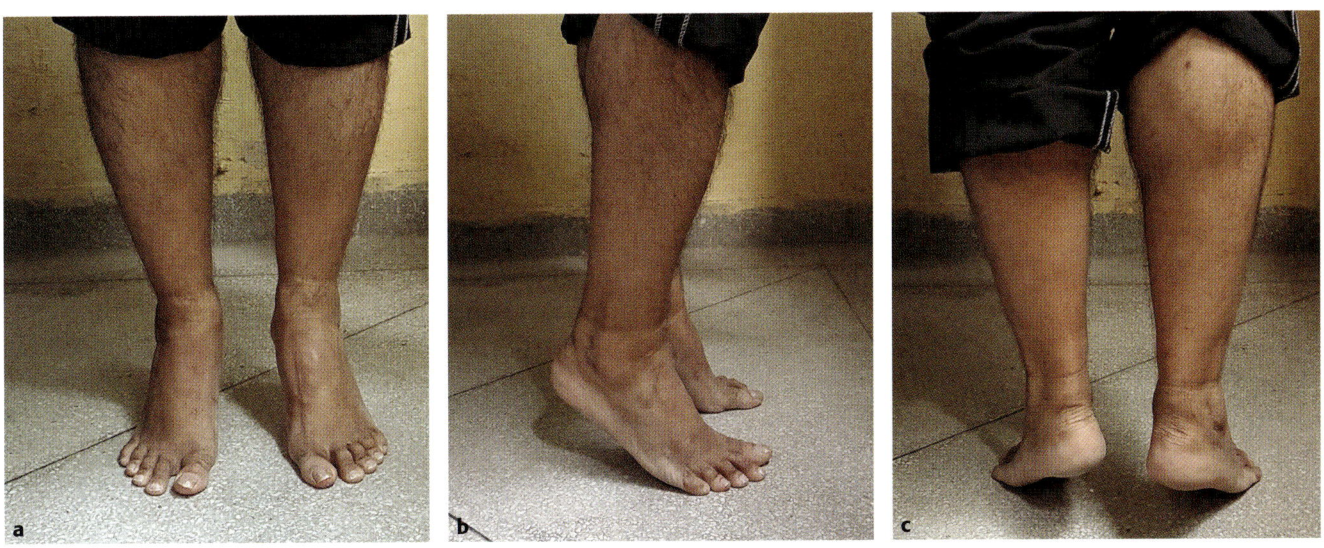

Fig 5.7-6a–c Excellent clinical outcome.

5 Pitfalls and complications

Pitfalls

- The talar head may be button-holed into the superior extensor retinaculum or the extensor digitorum brevis in up to 10% of these dislocations.
- Uncommonly, the talonavicular (TN) joint capsule, the deep posterior neurovascular bundle, or the peroneal tendons may interpose, preventing reduction and requiring open reduction via the anterolateral approach.
- Any associated fractures should be ruled out with a computed tomographic (CT) scan. However, the dislocation should be reduced as soon as possible, and the CT can be done after reduction to identify any peripheral fractures.

Complications

- Acute complications include skin necrosis, injuries to surrounding structures including the tibial nerve, posterior tibial vessels, periarticular fractures and tibialis posterior tendon rupture
- Infections, especially in open dislocations
- Avascular necrosis of the talar body
- Posttraumatic subtalar arthrosis with stiffness or degenerative joint disease or arthritis

6 Alternative treatment methods

If closed reduction is not possible, then open reduction is performed through an anterolateral approach, with manual reduction of the button holed talus head. If there is associated talar head fracture, then a dual approach (anteromedial plus anterolateral) may be needed for talar open reduction and internal fixation (**Fig 5.7-7**).

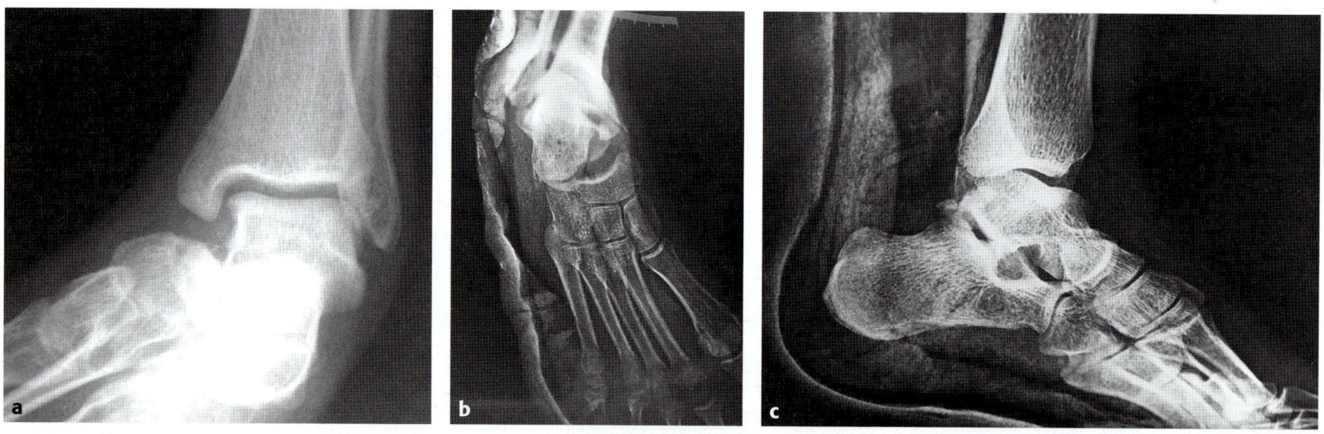

Fig 5.7-7a–q Example of a different case showing an alternative treatment using a dual approach.
a–c AP view of ankle, AP and lateral view of foot showing medial subtalar dislocation, unreduced by closed methods.

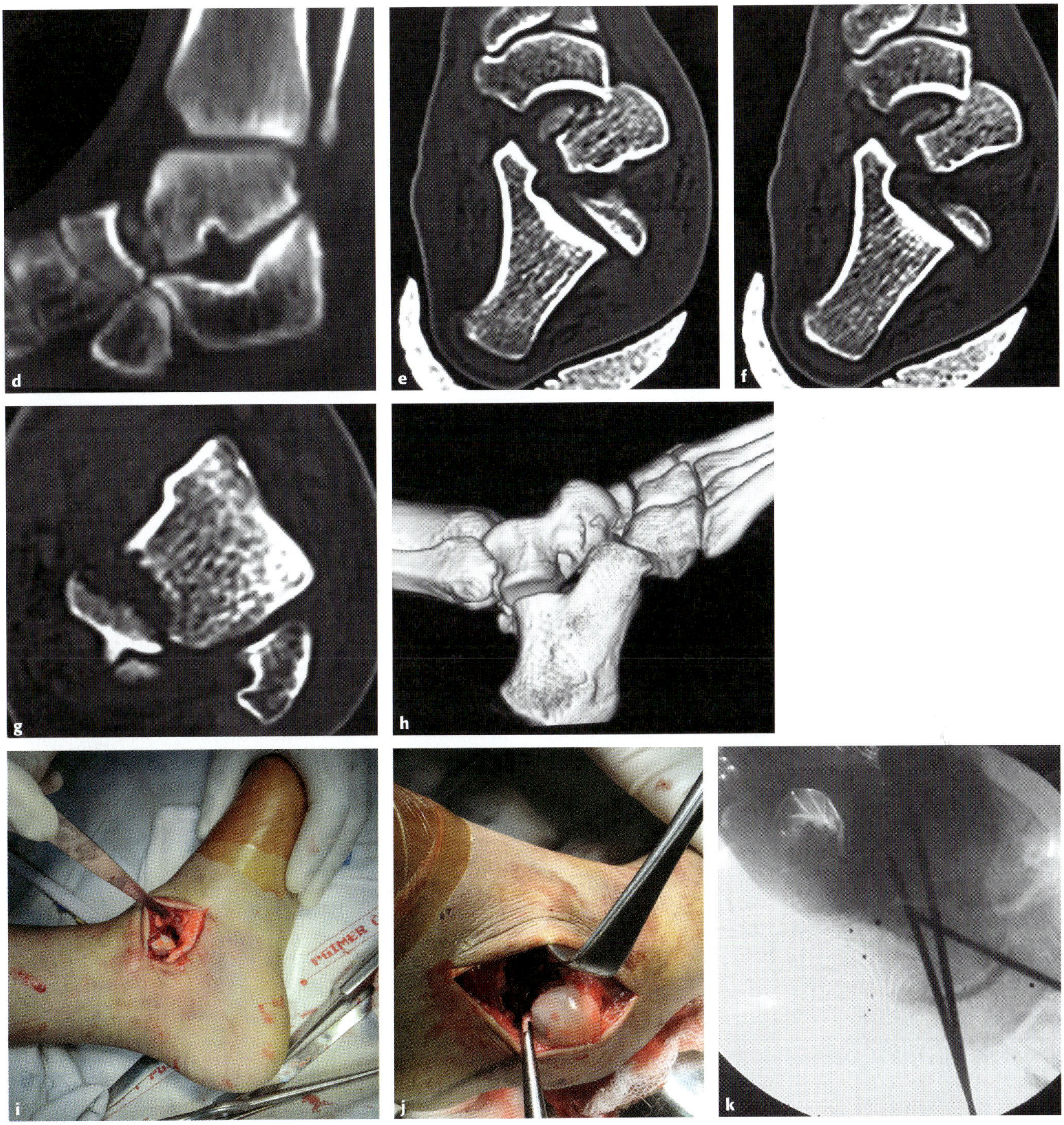

Fig 5.7-7a–q (cont) Example of a different case showing an alternative treatment using a dual approach.

- **d–g** A CT scan showing head of talus is missing from the TN joint. There is shearing/impaction fracture of the talar head which is laterally displaced. Notice the posterior process fracture.
- **h** A 3D CT reconstruction showing complete TN dislocation but partial subtalar subluxation. This was probably a Swivel dislocation.
- **i** Medial approach to the TN joint shows fractured talar head fragment with empty space at TN joint.
- **j** Lateral approach shows dislocated talar head fragment.
- **k** Intraoperative C-arm image shows good reduction and maintenance with K-wires.

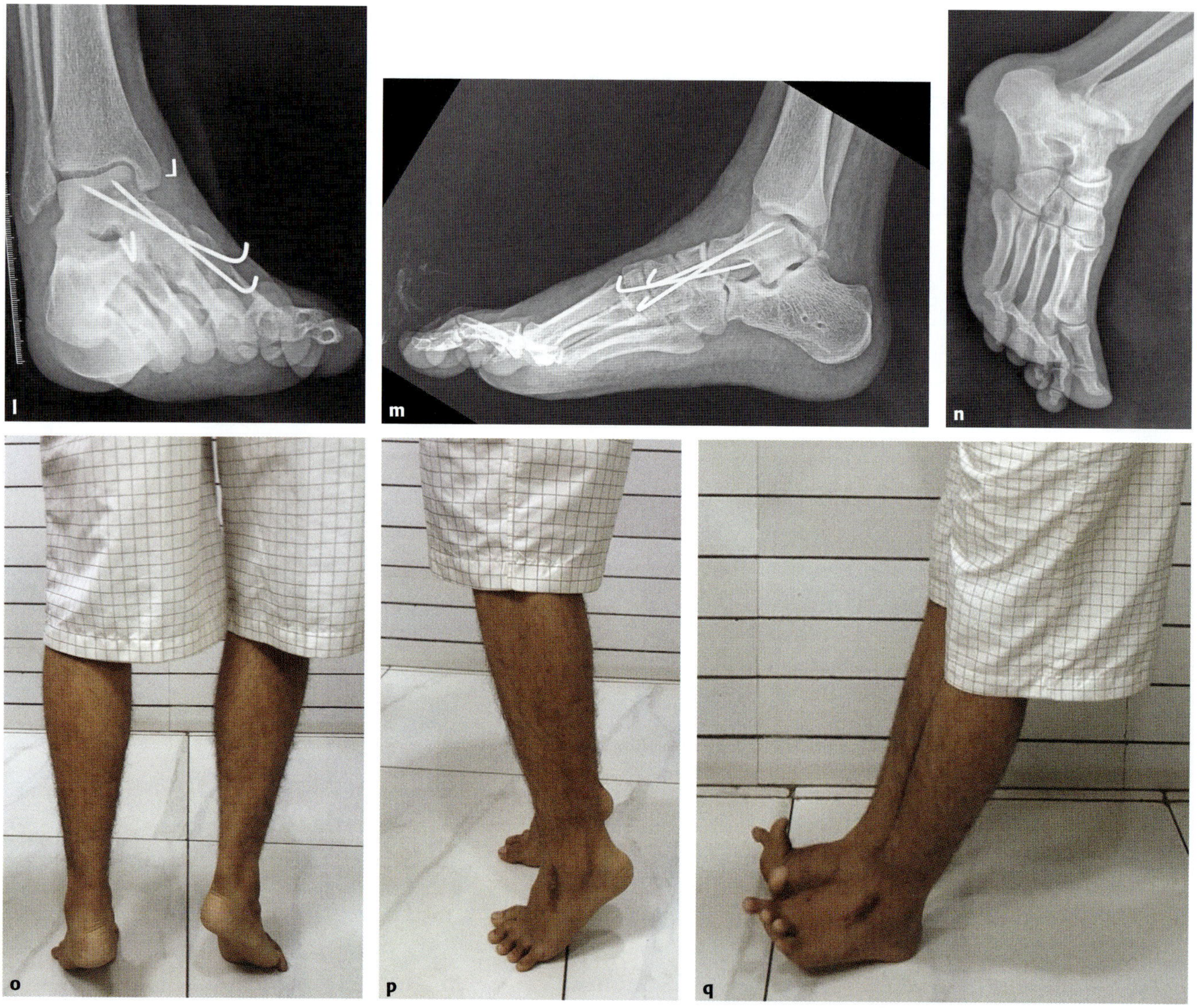

Fig 5.7-7a–q (cont) Example of a different case showing an alternative treatment using a dual approach.
l–m Postoperative AP and lateral x-rays of ankle and foot show good reduction and K-wire fixation.
n–q Follow-up at 1 year shows good outcome and function.

7 Postoperative management and rehabilitation

Nonweight-bearing immobilization is important with uncooperative patients. Emphasis should be on regaining early hindfoot motion to minimize hindfoot stiffness.

If K-wires have been used for stability, they are supplemented with external support and are removed by 3 weeks.

Graduated weight bearing is started in a protective brace.

8 Recommended reading

Datt N, Rao AS, Rao DV. Medial swivel dislocation of the talonavicular joint. *Indian J Orthop.* 2009 Jan;43(1):87–89.
Giannoulis D, Papadopoulos DV, Lykissas MG, et al. Subtalar dislocation without associated fractures: case report and review of literature. *World J Orthop.* 2015 Apr 18;6(3):374–379.
Goldner JL, Poletti SC, Gates HS 3rd, et al. Severe open subtalar dislocations. Long-term results. *J Bone Joint Surg Am.* 1995 Jul;77(7):1075–1079.
Rammelt S, Goronzy J. Subtalar dislocations. *Foot Ankle Clin.* 2015 Jun;20(2):253–264.

5.8 Lateral subtalar dislocation

Mandeep S Dhillon, Sharad Prabhakar

1 Case description

An 18-year-old woman presented after a road accident with a typical deformity of the foot. X-rays revealed a lateral subtalar dislocation, with complete dislocation of talonavicular (TN) joint and subluxation of the subtalar joint, with an intact ankle (**Fig 5.8-1**). A computed tomographic (CT) scan showed a dorsolaterally dislocated TN joint, and a subluxed subtalar joint (**Fig 5.8-2**).

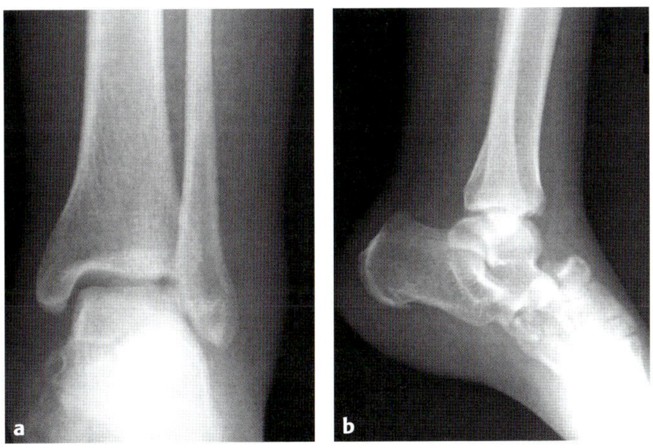

Fig 5.8-1a–b X-rays of the foot revealing dorsal dislocation of TN joint and subluxation of subtalar joint; AP view of the ankle reveals an intact ankle.
a AP view.
b Lateral view.

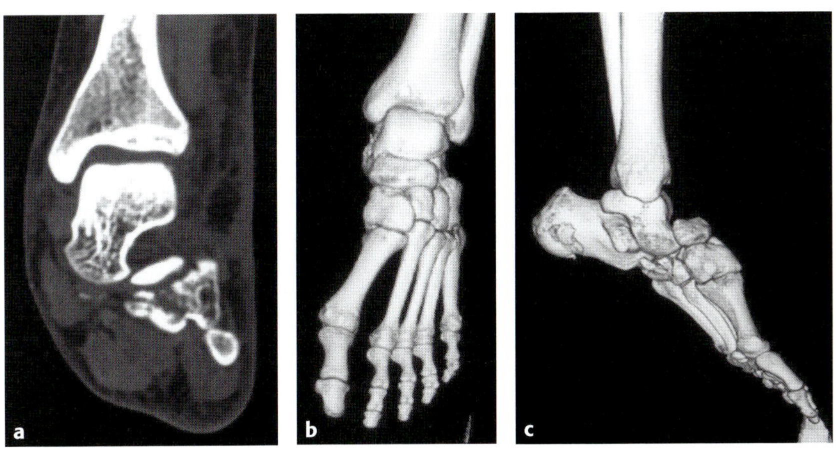

Fig 5.8-2a–c A CT scan with 3D reconstruction showing intact ankle joint but a dorsolaterally dislocated TN joint, and a subluxed subtalar joint.

2 Preoperative planning

Surgical indications are rare but are more common than in medial dislocations, as many lateral dislocations are open dislocations or are irreducible by closed means.

Most commonly, closed treatment of this injury is successful if reduction is done early and the appropriate reduction steps are taken. Pay close attention and understand the structures that can lead to irreducibility of the talar head.

Planning for failed reduction should include steps to immediately proceed with open reduction and internal fixation (ORIF). Open fractures need planning for external fixators if postoperative stability is in doubt.

3 Operating room setup

Patient positioning	• Supine
Anesthesia options	• Reduction can be attempted under sedation if the dislocation is uncomplicated and recent, but provisions for either regional or general anesthesia must be available.
C-arm location	• The C-arm is positioned on the contralateral side of the injury with the screen of position toward the head of the operative table to allow easy visualization by the surgeon.
Tourniquet	• Not required
Tips	• Adequate muscle relaxation is the key

For illustrations and overview of anesthetic considerations, see chapter 1.

Equipment

- No special equipment is needed if closed reduction is successful.
- For ORIF, standard equipment with K-wires and sometimes external fixation is all that is required.

4 Surgical procedure

For reducing lateral dislocations, the patient is placed supine, both the hip and knee are flexed to 90°; knee flexion relaxes the gastrocnemius. The foot is dorsiflexed and everted with distal traction, then reduction is completed with plantarflexion and inversion of the foot beneath the talus, while applying laterally directed pressure onto the talar head.

For this patient, subsequent intraoperative testing and evaluation with the C-arm showed some instability, and K-wires were percutaneously inserted across the reduced subtalar and TN joints (**Fig 5.8-3**), which were supplemented by an external fixator to increase stability of reduction.

Postoperative AP and lateral x-rays of the foot show well-reduced peritalar joints (**Fig 5.8-4**).

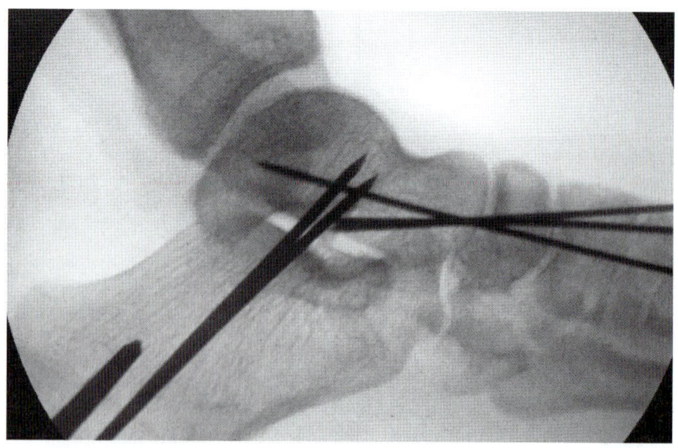

Fig 5.8-3 Intraoperative C-arm view displaying K-wires across the reduced subtalar and TN joints.

5 Pitfalls and complications

Pitfalls

Difficult reduction

In as many as 40% of cases, the tibialis posterior or the flexor digitorum longus tendon can displace around the head of the talus and prevent reduction. This may be associated with a rupture of the flexor retinaculum. An open approach over the prominent talar head may then be required to reduce the joint.

Associated fractures

After reduction CT scans can help to identify associated fractures, either of the talus head, lateral or posterior talar process and subtalar area; this identification at an early stage cannot be overemphasized, as missed injuries would lead to higher complication rates. Up to 60% of all subtalar dislocations, medial or lateral, have associated fractures. Lateral dislocations are not only uncommon but also require an abduction/dorsiflexion force, which could cause shearing off fractures of the talus head or nearby bones.

Complications

- Acute complications include skin necrosis, injuries to surrounding structures including the tibial nerve, posterior tibial vessels, periarticular fractures, and tibialis posterior tendon rupture
- The incidence of associated wounds is higher in lateral dislocations.
- Infections are a possibility in open dislocations
- Avascular necrosis of talar body
- Posttraumatic subtalar arthritis

6 Postoperative management and rehabilitation

- Nonweight-bearing immobilization is important in uncooperative patients. Emphasis should be focused on regaining early hindfoot motion to minimize stiffness.
- If K-wires have been used for stability, they are supplemented with external support and are removed by 3 weeks.
- Gradual weight bearing is started with a protective brace.

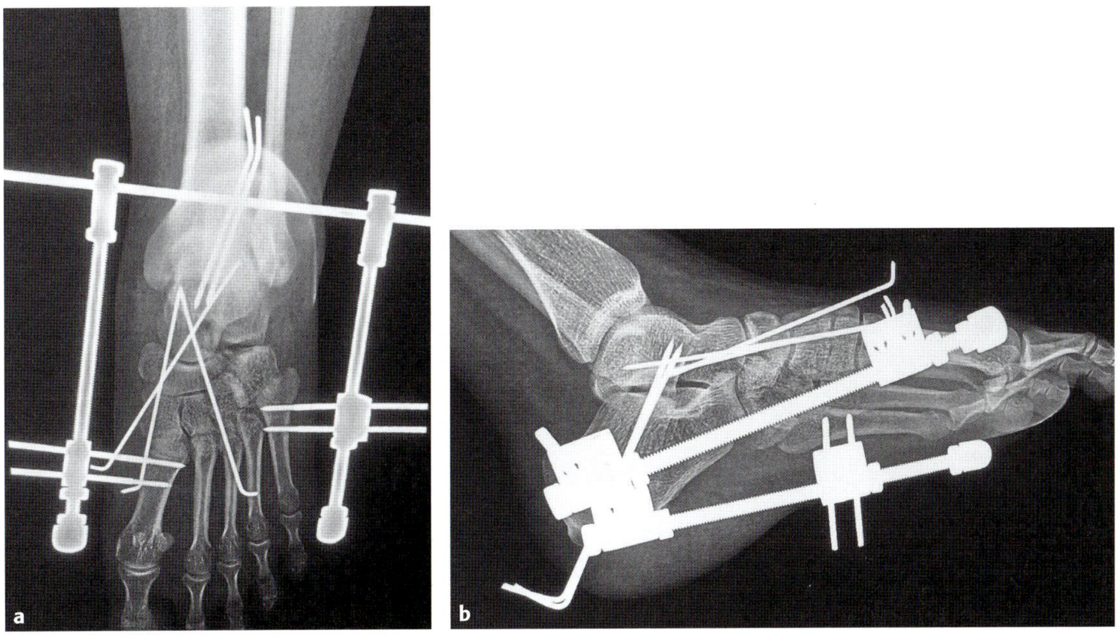

Fig 5.8-4a–b X-rays demonstrating well-reduced peritalar joints with no associated major fractures. An external fixator is used as a temporary stabilization device.

a AP view.

b Lateral view.

7 Recommended reading

Rammelt S, Goronzy J. Subtalar dislocations. *Foot Ankle Clin.* 2015 Jun;20(2):253–264.
Tucker DJ, Burian G, Boylan JP. Lateral subtalar dislocation: review of the literature and case presentation. *J Foot Ankle Surg.* 1998 May–Jun;37(3):239–247; discussion 262.
Veltman ES, Steller EJ, Wittich P, et al. Lateral subtalar dislocation: case report and review of the literature. *World J Orthop.* 2016 Sep 18;7(9):623–627.
Waldrop J, Ebraheim NA, Shapiro P, et al. Anatomical considerations of posterior tibialis tendon entrapment in irreducible lateral subtalar dislocation. *Foot Ankle.* 1992 Oct;13(8):458–461.

5.9 Extruded talus

Mandeep S Dhillon, Sampat Dumbre Patil, Siddhartha Sharma

1 Case description

A 34-year-old man was struck by a car. His right lower extremity was reportedly "run over". He presented to the emergency department 4 hours after the injury. Only his right lower extremity was injured.

The clinical examination revealed a laceration wound measuring approximately 10 x 6 cm, which extended from the distal anterior aspect of leg, across the front of ankle to the lateral aspect of the ankle. The talus was seen to be extruded from the wound as a glistening white structure.

The dorsalis pedis pulse was not palpable but the posterior tibial artery was normal to palpation. The foot was warm and well perfused.

On the AP and lateral ankle x-rays, the talus was seen to be dislocated from the ankle subtalar, and talonavicular (TN) joints—a luxatio talo totalis. A fracture of the posterior process of talus was also noted on lateral x-rays. A computed tomographic (CT) scan confirmed the diagnosis and did not reveal any additional fractures around the foot and ankle (**Fig 5.9-1**).

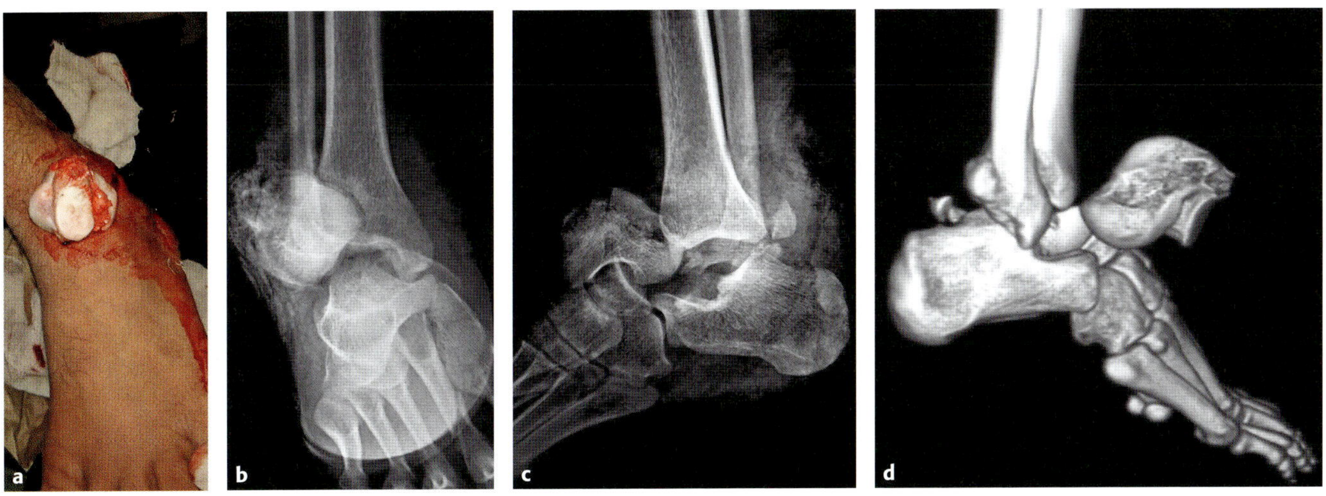

Fig 5.9-1a–d Preoperative images.
- **a** The extruded talus (glistening white structure) protruding from the lacerated wound over the anterior and aspect of ankle.
- **b–c** The AP and lateral x-rays of the ankle demonstrate lot of articulation of the talus from the talocrural, subtalar, and TN joint. The extruded talus lies anterolaterally and is rotated so that the head of talus faces the anterior surface of tibia. A fracture of the posterior process is seen on the lateral view.
- **d** The 3D CT confirms the diagnosis of talar extrusion. Fracture of the posterior process of talus can also be appreciated.

2 Preoperative planning

Indications for surgery

Talar extrusion through an open wound is an orthopedic emergency. The open nature of the injury necessitates urgent wound debridement.

Treatment options

The extruded talus should be serially washed and repositioned into the ankle, subtalar, and TN joints. Immediate talectomy with tibiocalcaneal arthrodesis is rarely indicated. Current literature seems to favor repositioning over excision, and calcaneotibial arthrodesis is hard to obtain with the complete talus missing. Repositioning has surprisingly low rates of infection and avascular necrosis (AVN) of talus, and often functional outcomes are satisfactory.

Adequate wound debridement is the key for preventing infection. The talus can usually be repositioned through the open wound after debridement. Smooth K-wires or pins, with or without ankle spanning external fixation, are needed to stabilize the reduced talocrural, TN and subtalar joints. Screws or K-wires are sometimes necessary to fix small osteochondral fragments of the extruded talus (**Fig 5.9-2**).

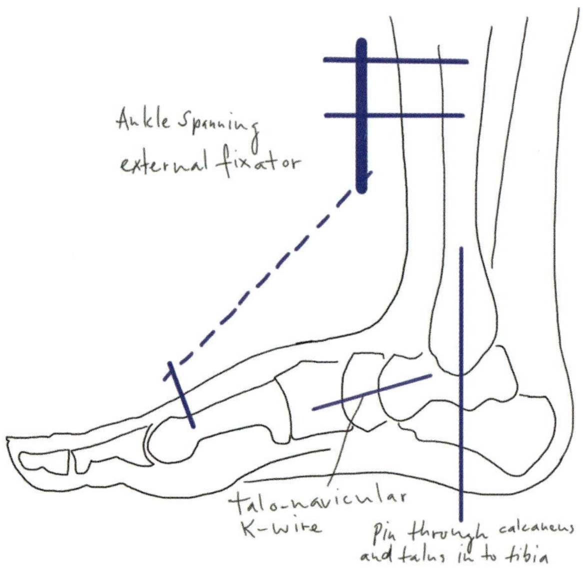

Fig 5.9-2 Preoperative plan.

In some cases, the extruded talus may be found at the scene of the injury. In such cases, if feasible, the talus should be washed with normal saline to remove dirt and grit, covered in wet saline gauges, placed in a sterile container, and transported in a cold box to the hospital. It should be placed on a cool bed but not immersed in an ice bath.

3 Operating room setup

Patient positioning	• Dictated by the location of the open wound. In most cases, the patient can be placed supine on a radiolucent table to permit unrestricted intraoperative C-arm imaging of the lower limb. • A sandbag can be placed under the ipsilateral buttock to aid in internal rotation, whenever access to the lateral aspect of ankle is required. • In case of a posterior wound, the lateral or prone positions may be preferred. When choosing the prone position, it is important to keep the abdomen free to avoid compression of the inferior vena cava. • Regardless of the position, all bony prominences should be well-padded.
Anesthesia options	• General or regional anesthesia; however, adequate muscle relaxation should be given to permit repositioning of the extruded talus. • Intravenous antibiotics are usually started as soon as the patient is admitted. • An additional single shot of cefuroxime is administered 30 minutes before surgery.
C-arm location	• The C-arm is brought in from the opposite side and the screen is placed at the head end. • A true lateral view of the ankle can be obtained by rotating the limb externally, placing the leg in a figure of four position, or by rotating the C-arm. • In the latter case, the injured limb should be elevated on a cushion or linen.
Tourniquet	• Applied but not necessarily inflated.
Tips	• The limb is draped keeping the knee free.

For illustrations and overview of anesthetic considerations, see chapter 1.

Equipment list

- K-wires, smooth and threaded
- Steinmann pins
- Large tubular external fixator
- 4.5 mm Schanz pins
- Tubular rods
- Universal clamps
- Tube-to-tube clamps
- Partially threaded cancellous screws
- Headless compression screws
- Large femoral distractor or small distractor

4 Surgical procedure

Wound debridement and lavage

The surgical procedure starts with thorough wound lavage and debridement. In most cases, the talus lies free, devoid of all soft-tissue attachments and can be removed from the wound and copiously irrigated with normal saline. Chlorhexidine (1% ChG solution) can be added to the irrigation solution. The washed talus can then be placed in a sterile container in saline solution containing 2 grams of vancomycin until it is repositioned (**Fig 5.9-3**).

It is important to check for any nondisplaced fractures of the extruded talus and to identify any missing osteochondral fragments or fragments of the medial, lateral or posterior process, which may be found within the bed of the wound. Nondisplaced fractures can be fixed in situ with screws. Osteochondral fragments and fractures of the talar processes can be fixed using screws or discarded if small and not amenable to fixation.

If the talus has any retained soft-tissue attachments, these must be carefully preserved as they may represent the only remaining blood supply to the talus.

The wound is meticulously debrided to remove all dead and devitalized tissues including the skin, fascia, soft tissues, and bone. It is thought that postoperative infection in repositioned talus stems from the unhealthy wound bed rather than the extruded talus; hence, it is imperative that the talus be repositioned only when the surgeon is satisfied that the wound bed is perfectly clean. If the talus was reduced/repositioned at the scene of the injury or immediately after, it can be redisplaced in the operating room for proper irrigation and debridement.

Intraoperative cultures may be obtained from deep tissues, although their role is unclear.

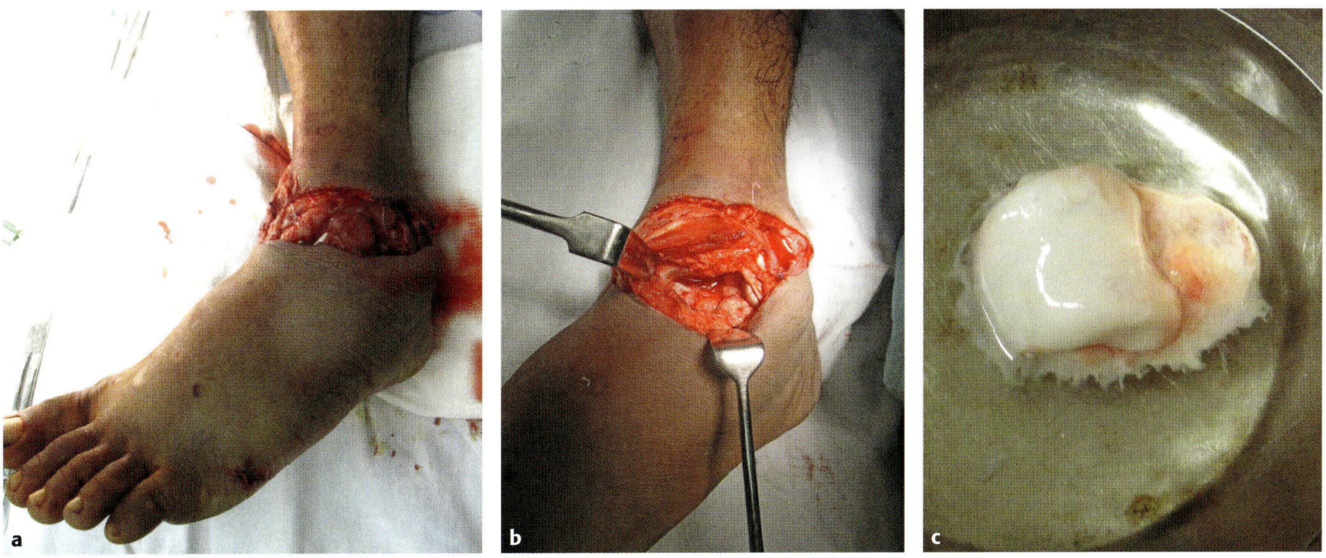

Fig 5.9-3a–c Wound debridement and lavage.
a The open wound on the ankle has been debrided.
b The talar bed is seen after retraction of the soft tissues.
c The extruded talus has been copiously lavaged and placed in antibiotic-saline solution as it awaits repositioning.

Talar repositioning

A distractor or an ankle spanning external fixator is used to open the vertical space between the ankle mortise and the calcaneus to facilitate repositioning of the talus (**Fig 5.9-4**). Traction on the first ray through the great toe distracts the navicular and permits the talar head to be reinserted. A K-wire placed into the dorsal surface of the talar neck can be used as a joystick to help reposition the talus. Once the talus is in position, reduction of the subtalar and talocrural joints is checked under C-arm imaging. If this is acceptable, a Steinmann pin is inserted from the plantar aspect of foot through the calcaneus across the body of talus and into the distal tibia. This stabilizes the talocrural and subtalar joints and can either be retained temporarily until an ankle spanning external fixator is applied or left in place for stability.

The TN joint reduction is checked next. Assessment of TN joint reduction on AP view may be difficult, as the medial border of navicular tuberosity protrudes medially and is not in line with the medial border of talar head. It is helpful to obtain x-rays of the contralateral, normal foot preoperatively to determine the relation of the navicular tuberosity to the medial border of talar head, to enable correct judgment of reduction on the AP view of the foot. Once reduction is confirmed on the AP and lateral C-arm views, one or two smooth K-wires are passed from the navicular to engage the talar head to stabilize the TN joint. It is of utmost importance that all three articulations of the talus are reduced anatomically.

Next an ankle spanning external fixator is applied. This is especially important if flap coverage is considered. A delta frame configuration, with two pins in the proximal tibial diaphysis and a Steinmann pin in the calcaneus can be used. Additionally, pins may be placed in the first and fifth metatarsals to hold the foot in a plantigrade position (**Fig 5.9-5**). The frame can be modified as per the wound and anticipated flap coverage, if necessary. The surgeon may choose to use pins, an external fixator, or the combination of both, as the situation demands.

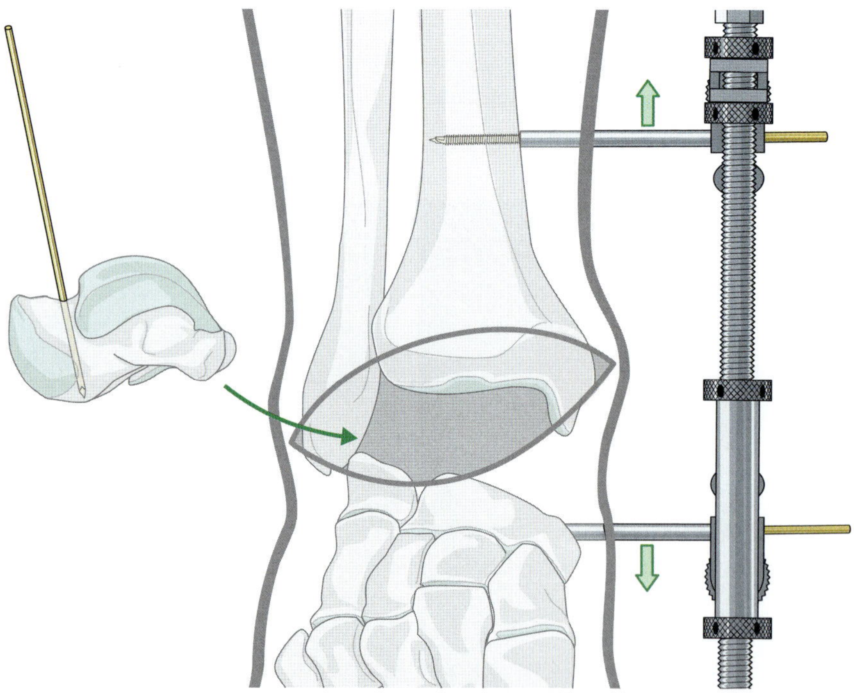

Fig 5.9-4 Use of a femoral distractor to aid in talar repositioning. A K-wire inserted in the talar neck can serve as a joystick to prevent slippage of talus and to manipulate the talus for repositioning.

Associated soft-tissue injuries

Attention is now turned to associated injuries of the foot and any tendon injuries. Wherever feasible, tendons must be primarily repaired using appropriate techniques. The wound is then assessed for closure. Closure is performed in layers and if possible, joint capsules of the talocrural and TN joints must be repaired. If possible, the extensor or the flexor retinaculum should also be repaired to prevent bowstringing of the tendons and adhesions. Subcutaneous closure is done ensuring that there is no undue tension on the skin margins. Skin is sutured by vertical tension relieving sutures (**Fig 5.9-6**).

If primary skin closure is not possible, primary or delayed flap coverage may be done, especially if the soft-tissue defect is significant.

Negative-pressure wound therapy may be used to aid in healing of the sutured wound or to achieve healing by secondary intention in cases where the soft-tissue cover is adequate, but the skin cannot be closed primarily.

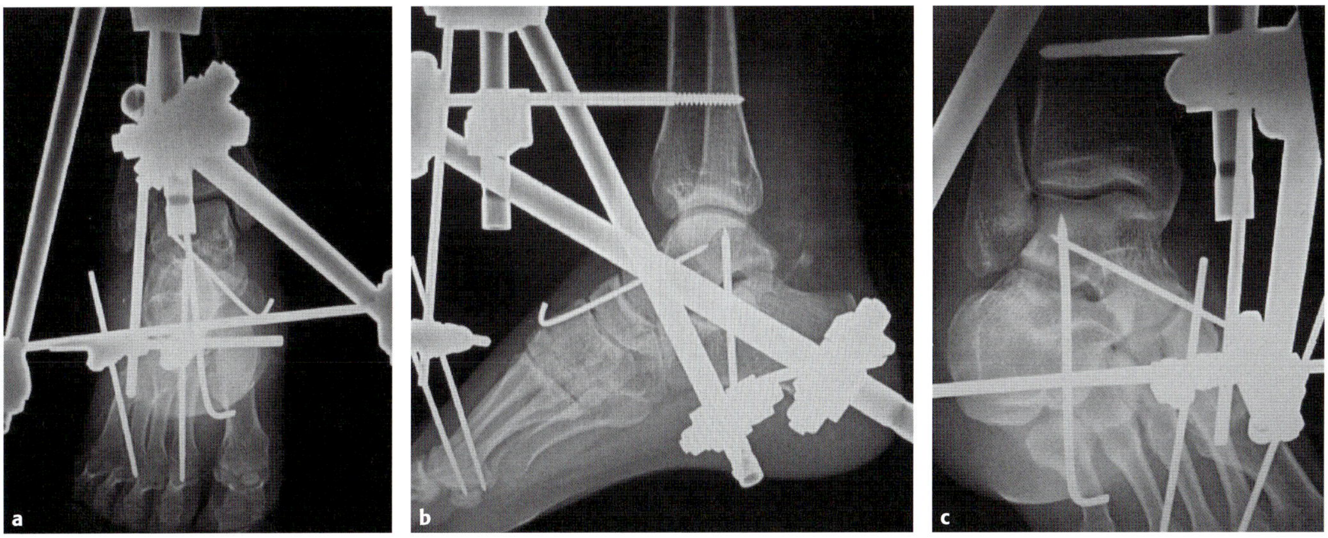

Fig 5.9-5a–c Postoperative x-rays showing concentric reduction of the repositioned talus.
a AP view.
b Lateral view.
c Mortise view.

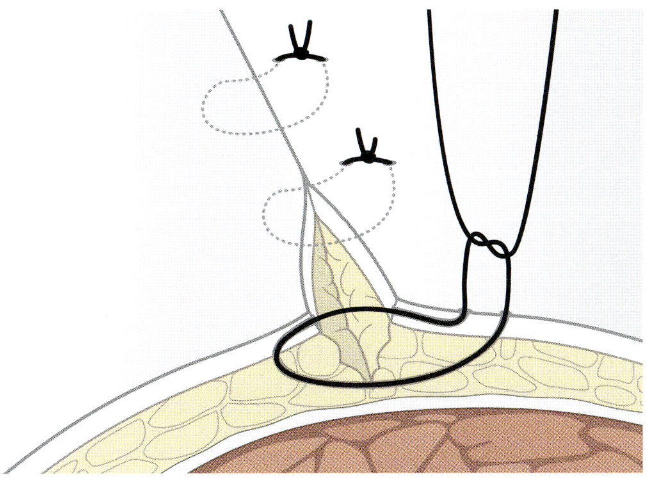

Fig 5.9-6 The modified Allgöwer suture.

5 Pitfalls and complications

Pitfalls

Inadequate visualization

Since the surgical approach is dictated by the open wound, the surgeon does not have a choice in the primary approach. The wound may need to be extended proximally or distally to permit adequate debridement as well as reduction of the extruded talus.

Difficulty in talus repositioning

It may be difficult to reposition the talus owing to proximal migration of the calcaneus. Therefore, axial traction through the calcaneus is necessary to open the space between the ankle mortise and calcaneus. In some cases, this can be simply achieved by manual traction with a Steinmann pin. However, repositioning is more easily performed if the surgeon uses a distractor, with pins inserted into the tibia and calcaneus. The pins in the tibia and calcaneus should be colinear so that distraction does not result in posterior or anterior angulation of the calcaneus. To facilitate reduction the talar head back into the navicular articular facet, manual traction through the first ray is helpful. A thorough search should be made for any osteochondral fragments within the bed of the wound before repositioning the talus, as these may obstruct reduction or result in nonconcentric reduction.

Nonconcentric reduction

Two-plane orthogonal x-rays of the ankle, subtalar and TN joints is required to ensure that these joints are concentrically reduced. It is especially important to have clear visualization of the subtalar joint in the Harris axial view or a Brodén view. The surgeon should determine before draping how this will be achieved and position the patient accordingly to avoid intraoperative problems.

Complications

Infection

Can be superficial or deep, early or late. Antibiotics alone can manage superficial infection whereas deep infection necessitates repeat wound debridement. Talectomy of the repositioned talus may be indicated if there is refractory osteomyelitis of the talus.

Avascular necrosis

Avascular necrosis of talus remains a major concern. However, not all cases with AVN fare poorly. A dead talus which does not fragment or collapse may be fully functional for ambulation. Remodeling of the talus can take up to 2 years after the injury.

Secondary arthritis

Arthrosis may develop at the ankle, the subtalar joints, or both. Avascular necrosis leading to collapse of the talar dome also results in ankle arthrosis. This is a late complication and will require arthrodesis (**Fig 5.9-7**). Fusion should be confined to the affected joint or joints.

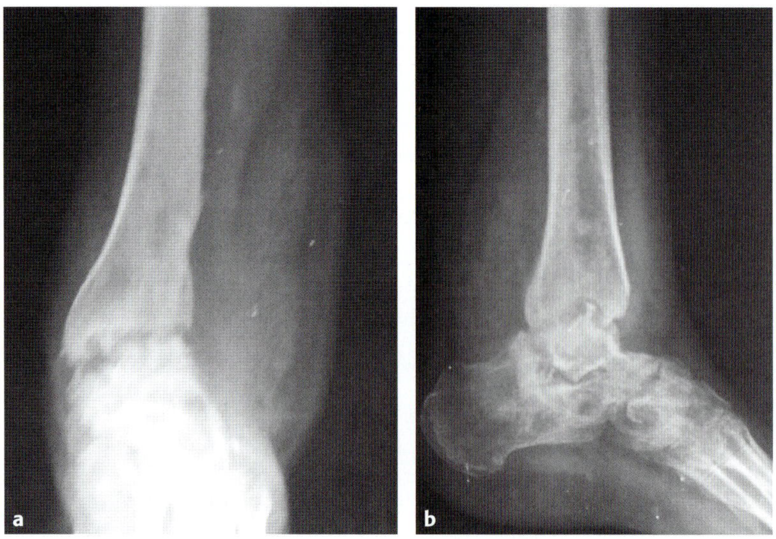

Fig 5.9-7a–b Example from a different case showing AVN with secondary osteoarthritis of the ankle and subtalar joints after talar reimplantation.
a AP x-ray.
b Lateral x-ray.

6 Alternative techniques

If the talus is lost at the scene of the injury or if there is gross contamination of the talus that is not amenable to lavage, tibiocalcaneal arthrodesis can be performed. The cartilage of the ankle mortise and the calcaneus are denuded of cartilage back to bleeding subchondral bone. The foot is placed in a plantigrade position with slight posterior translation and external rotation of the calcaneus. Compression arthrodesis can be achieved through many external fixation devices. Removal of the talus can result in up to 5 cm of shortening. Therefore, a fine-wire circular external fixator has the advantage of offering limb length equalization by lengthening through a proximal tibial corticotomy and transport (**Fig 5.9-8**).

Alternatively, a modified Blair fusion can be done with minimal loss in talar height. The anterior part of the distal tibia is slid down and fused to the calcaneus. Other secondary procedures include bulk allografting of corticocancellous bone blocks from the iliac crest. The talar head and thus the TN joint should be preserved whenever possible.

In cases that will be treated with arthrodesis secondary to loss of the talus, it is important to wait until the wound is deemed free of infection. An external fixator will maintain alignment until such time. This also allows the traumatic wound and injury-related swelling to recover.

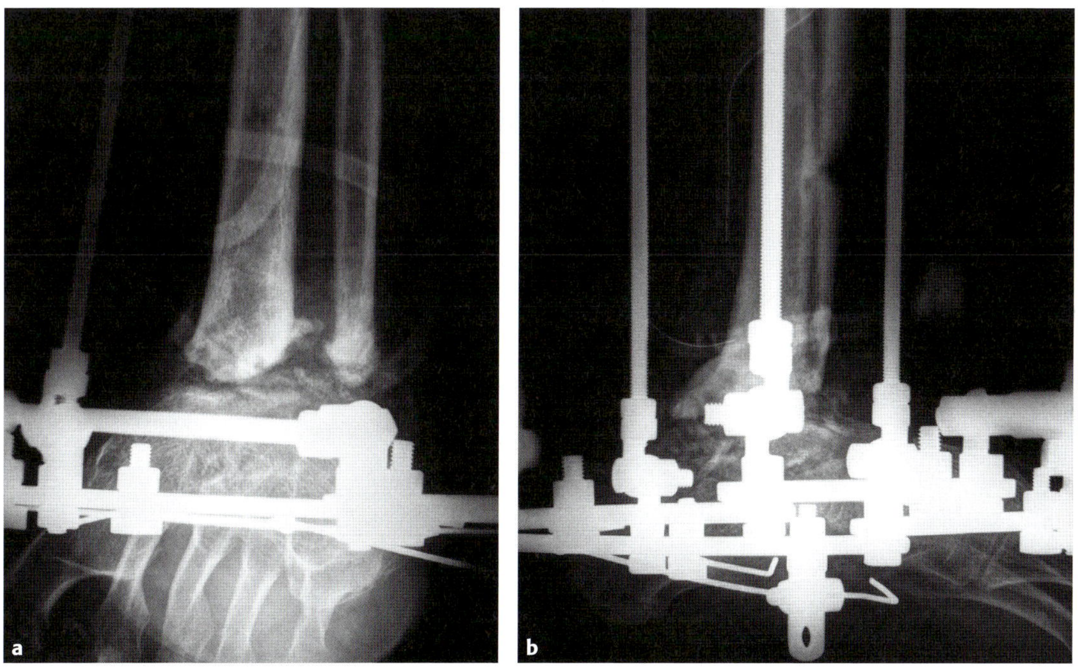

Fig 5.9-8a–b Example from a different case showing the technique for treatment of tibiocalcaneal arthrodesis using Ilizarov circular external fixator after extruded talus injury. Immediate postoperative AP (**a**) and lateral (**b**) x-rays.

7 Postoperative management and rehabilitation

Aftercare

The patient is observed closely for signs of infection. Serial blood counts and quantitative C-reactive protein measurements are done to rule out infection. Intravenous antibiotics can manage superficial infection; however, deep infection requires repeat surgical debridement and culture-specific antibiotics.

Functional exercises

There are no clear-cut guidelines on the rehabilitation of these patients. The external fixator and pins can be removed at approximately 6 weeks, once the skin and soft tissues have healed. The patient can then be placed in a below-knee cast or ankle foot orthosis to ensure plantigrade position of the foot. Range-of-motion exercises of the ankle can begin after 6–8 weeks. Full weight bearing is delayed for at least 3 months.

The patient should be counseled that this injury is severe and long-term stiffness of both the ankle and subtalar joint are to be expected. Risks of development of posttraumatic arthritis of the ankle and/or subtalar joint are exceedingly high (**Fig 5.9-9**).

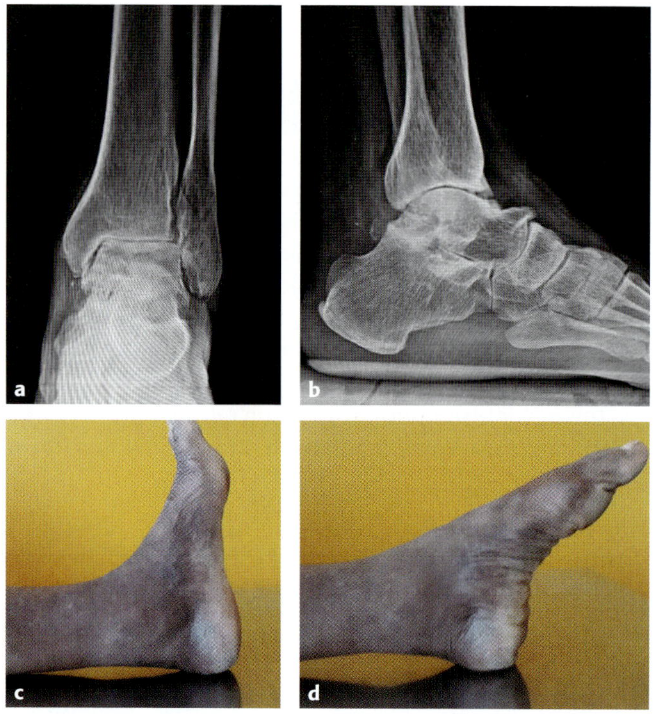

Figure 5.9-9a–d Example from a different case showing a 56-year-old man with a history of anterolateral extrusion of the talus. Follow-up images taken at 7 years demonstrate arthrosis of the ankle and subtalar joints.
a–b AP and lateral x-rays.
c–d The arthrosis notwithstanding, patient has good ROM at the ankle and is able to ambulate with minimal pain.

8 Recommended reading

Burston JL, Isenegger P, Zellweger R. Open total talus dislocation: clinical and functional outcomes: a case series. *J Trauma.* 2010 Jun;68(6):1453–1458.
Lee HS, Chung HW, Suh JS. Total talar extrusion without soft tissue attachments. *Clin Orthop Surg.* 2014 Jun;6(2):236–241.
Lee J, Hamilton G. Complete talar extrusion: a case report. *J Foot Ankle Surg.* 2009 May–Jun;48(3):372–375.
Smith CS, Nork SE, Sangeorzan BJ. The extruded talus: results of reimplantation. *J Bone Joint Surg Am.* 2006 Nov;88(11):2418–2424.
Vaienti L, Maggi F, Gazzola R, et al. Therapeutic management of complicated talar extrusion: literature review and case report. *J Orthop Traumatol.* 2011 Mar;12(1):61–64.
Weston JT, Liu X, Wandtke ME, et al. A systematic review of total dislocation of the talus. *Orthop Surg.* 2015 May;7(2):97–101.

6 Midfoot

Midfoot

6 Midfoot injuries

Andrew K Sands

1 Introduction

This section covers injuries of the Lisfranc and Chopart regions of the foot. The two regions are named after the surgeons who discovered and used these areas for rapid transfoot amputations. In an era before adequate anesthesia, surgeons who found a way to rapidly remove damaged areas of the foot often had their names associated with that surgical technique. The approach allowed a less painful resolution of the clinical problem.

2 Anatomy and pathomechanics

The two terms Lisfranc and Chopart in close association, since an injury to one may often extend into the other region. So practically, Lisfranc is the more distal of the two and involves the base of the metatarsals (MTs), the tarsometatarsal (TMT) joints, and the intertarsal (IT) joints involving the cuneiforms and cuboid. A Chopart injury would involve the midtarsal and IT joints from the cuneiforms through the navicular bone and cuboid, and into the distal part of the talus, which is often also called the coxa pedis. The talonavicular (TN) joint is responsible for much of the complex range of motion (ROM) of the foot and loss of normal TN motion results in loss of 90% or more of complex ROM of the hindfoot. Thus, the TN joint is often also known as the coxa pedis since foot and ankle surgeons think of it as the "hip" joint of the foot because of numerous functional and developmental analogies. Although the calcaneocuboid joint is less mobile than the TN joint, its motion is important for maintaining flexibility of the lateral column of the foot.

Biomechanically, the TN joint is extremely important for normal ROM and function. Loss of the TN joint also leads to loss of normal subtalar inversion and eversion, which leads to stressing of and future degeneration of the ankle joint. In contrast, the intratarsal or midtarsal joints as well as the first, second, and third TMT joints are not necessary for normal function and are labeled non-essential non-motion segment joints. An exception may be high-performance athletes where these joints exhibit some degree of vertical sliding (the normal plane of motion of these joints). But in non-athletes, these motion segments are not needed for normal function. Stiffness in this area without degenerative pain is not a deficit (**Fig 6-1**).

The TN joint is important in helping the foot to adapt to uneven surfaces, and to lock and unlock in the normal gait cycle. Loss of normal TN motion might also lead to a foot that is cavus or planus. While the most important part of the TN joint is motion, having a "shoe-able" foot is also important. Either extreme of foot deformity can lead to problems with wearing shoes.

On the other hand, in the case of the medial column (ie, first, second, and third TMT), the TMT and IT joints are flat joints with little anatomically necessary motion. They tend to slide without much rotation. If there is hypermobility in this area, such excessive motion leads to pathological deformity and tendon disruption, as seen in pes plano abductovalgus flatfoot deformity and hallux valgus. The fourth or fifth TMT joints are more mobile and move dorsal and plantar. This sliding motion is important in helping the foot to accommodate to uneven terrain. Arthritis of these joints is difficult to reconstruct. Fusion leads to abnormal stresses and is often difficult to obtain.

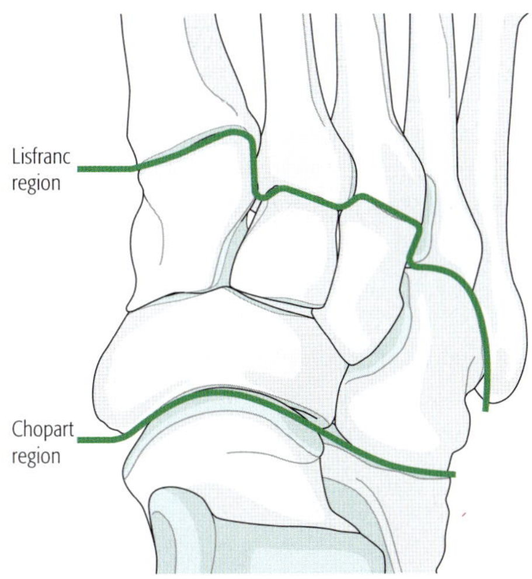

Fig 6-1 Lisfranc and Chopart regions of the foot.

These regions may be injured from axial loading and twisting of the foot:

- In low-energy sporting injuries, the injury may be subtle.
- In high-energy injuries, such as a pedestrian whose foot is run over or crushed, or a passenger injured by wheel well intrusion, the injury is more obvious.

3 Fracture classification

Classification of injuries in this area is difficult. Several systems have been proposed, however, as there are many joints and bones with resultant subluxations, dislocations, and fractures each in differing planes and directions; these classifications appear to be too complicated for practical use.

See appendix for details of AO/OTA fractures and dislocations of midfoot fractures.

4 Preoperative assessment

Clinical assessment

Clinical suspicion is important because patients with Lisfranc or Chopart injuries seen in the emergency department are often sent out with a diagnosis of a "sprained foot". This leads to missed injuries and misdiagnosis. Often patients with this injury have pain out of proportion to what should be expected. They describe the pain as being severe, often leading them to feel like "throwing up" or "passing out" (ie, visceral discomfort), and as much more severe than a regular sporting-type sprain. Often there will be a plantar medial ecchymosis on the foot.

Imaging

X-rays

The best and most cost-effective imaging is a three-view weight-bearing x-ray series. If the patient cannot bear any substantial weight, the injured foot should be placed on the flat plate to ascertain what the foot is doing in relation to the ground. Any weight bearing can allow for a displacement of the injury, which is the desired effect and a diagnostic tool which allows the surgeon to better appreciate any subtle injuries. Of course, more severe high-energy injuries may not be able to bear any weight.

Standard weight-bearing imaging of the foot includes:

- AP view: allows excellent view of the first TMT, medial column, and TN joint. The medial cuneiform and first TMT can be seen to be displaced if the injury has caused medial column disruption (**Fig 6-2a**).
- 30° and 45° oblique views: the base of the second MT can be seen to be displaced laterally from the intermediate cuneiform, and the third MT and fourth/fifth MTs can be seen to be displaced laterally from the lateral cuneiform and cuboid. Intertarsal and midtarsal injuries are also appreciated (**Fig 6-2b**).
- Lateral view: dorsal avulsions and dorsal displacement of the MT base on the cuneiforms can be appreciated on the lateral view (**Fig 6-2c**).

Beam angle for x-ray imaging

The x-ray head is tilted distally 20°, angled so that the beam is perpendicular to the dorsum of the foot. This allows for an ideal view of the TMT joints, with the foot in the simulated weight-bearing position. The TMT joints are not perpendicular to the sole of the foot, but rather to the dorsum of the foot. Oblique views (30° and 45°) are used to visualize the lateral TMT joints.

Computed tomographic (CT) scan

A CT scan can help define overlying double densities and 3D injuries, such as plantar bony avulsions that might not be apparent on plain films (**Fig 6-3**).

Magnetic resonance imaging (MRI)

An MRI is rarely if ever indicated in the acute injury. Some surgeons use MRI to document a tear in the medial cuneiform to medial base of second MT (Lisfranc) ligament, especially in pure ligamentous injuries (**Fig 6-4**).

Stress x-rays

Stress x-rays may be done in the emergency department or preoperatively in the operating room to confirm the instability pattern. However, these are painful and should be done under block if in the emergency department or after anesthesia has started if in the operating room (**Fig 6-5**).

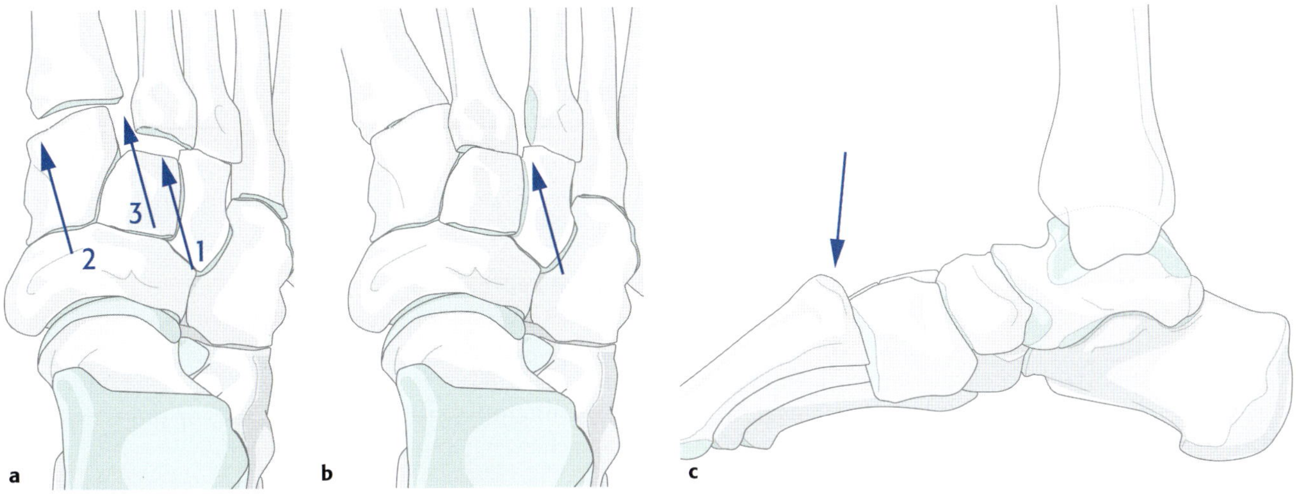

Fig 6-2a–c Common malalignments visible on x-rays (arrows indicate beam angles).
a AP view: lateral displacement of second MT on intermediate cuneiform (1); TMT disruption (2); gap between first and second MT (3).
b 30° oblique view: lateral displacement of third MT on lateral cuneiform.
c Lateral view: dorsal cortex of the MTs should be even with the dorsal cortex of the cuneiforms. Dorsal displacement of MT bases above the level of the cuneiforms is abnormal and an indication of a Lisfranc injury.

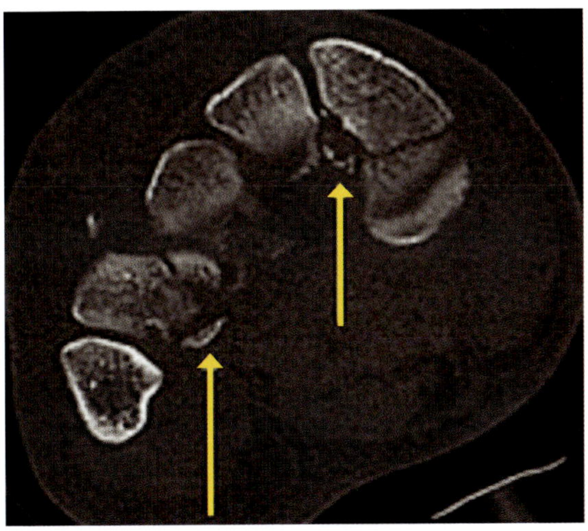

Fig 6-3 A CT scan is useful in identifying plantar comminution (arrows).

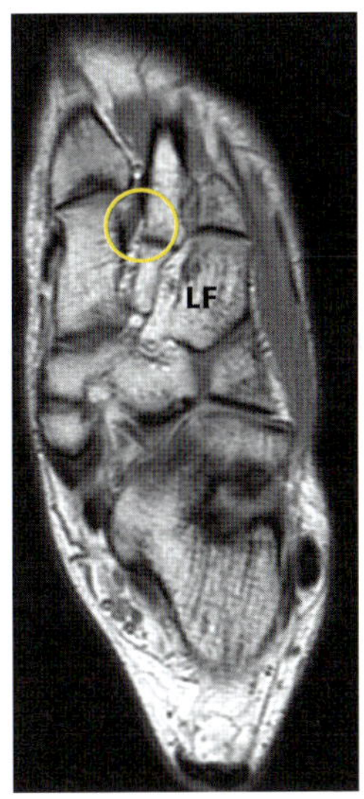

Fig 6-4 An MRI of the foot (coronal proton density) showing the Lisfranc ligament (LF) between the medial cuneiform and base of the second MT.

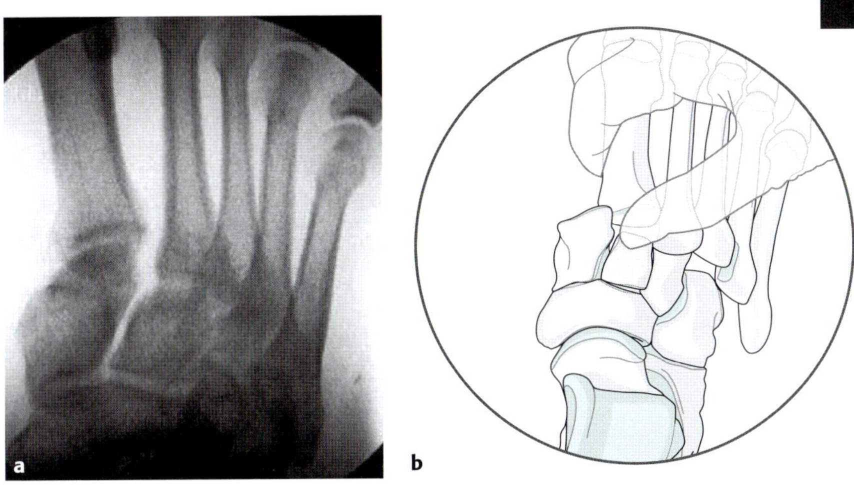

Fig 6-5a–b Stress x-rays are useful in identifying instability that may not be visible in static x-rays. Obtaining these can be painful for the patient, so these x-rays should be taken while the patient is under anesthesia, or if taken in the emergency department, an anesthetic block should be administered. X-ray protective gloves should be worn by the surgeon

5 Nonoperative treatment

It is possible to treat nondisplaced or minimally displaced TMT injuries by nonoperative means. There are times when surgery is not possible, such as in older, sicker patients, or patients who refuse surgery. In a severely injured patient, a midfoot injury may not be treated until the patient's more life-threatening injuries have been addressed. The foot injury is out of the acute phase and so might be considered to have been treated nonoperatively.

There is a variation where just the dorsal ligaments are injured but not the more structural plantar ligaments. While the pain is severe, there is little to no displacement of the anatomy. In these cases, nonoperative closed treatment can be performed. Cast or controlled-ankle-motion (CAM) boot treatment with strict nonweight bearing allows the tough midfoot ligaments to form scar tissue which is thick and strong enough to hold the adjacent bones in proper anatomical alignment. If they do so in the proper position, then there might be enough stability to prevent degenerative changes and subsequent deformity (in the form of a large dorsal bony prominence) or pain with walking. If the joints do not stabilize or in the case of a missed injury with early weight bearing or even minor displacement and instability, then any pain may lead to necessary reconstruction later. Fortunately, the later reconstruction fusion is performed with the same approach used for the acute injury. Unlike other foot injuries, later treatment might not cause increased loss of function.

6 Operative treatment

Patient positioning

For most cases supine with a bump under the ipsilateral buttock. Lateral positioning may be useful to access the anterior process of the calcaneus (see chapter 6.2). For more details, see chapter 1.

Surgical approaches

Typically, the double dorsal approach (dorsomedial and dorsolateral approaches) (**Fig 6-6**) and medial utility approach can be used (**Fig 6-7**). Higher-energy injuries might need compartment release (see chapter 6.8) or more extensile approaches.

Dorsomedial approach

The dorsomedial approach is over the first MT and first TMT. With foot compartment syndrome, it may be shifted over the second MT. The joint capsule is usually disrupted. The extensor hallucis longus and extensor hallucis brevis are retracted allowing access to the first TMT and the medial half of the second TMT as well as the IT joints. The proximal part of the incision may be extended allowing access to the dorsal navicular bone but care must be taken to avoid wide dissection, as the blood supply to the navicular comes from the dorsalis pedis artery.

Dorsolateral approach

The dorsolateral incision is roughly along the line of the fourth MT. The extensor digitorum communis muscle is retracted allowing access to the lateral part of the second TMT and the third TMT.

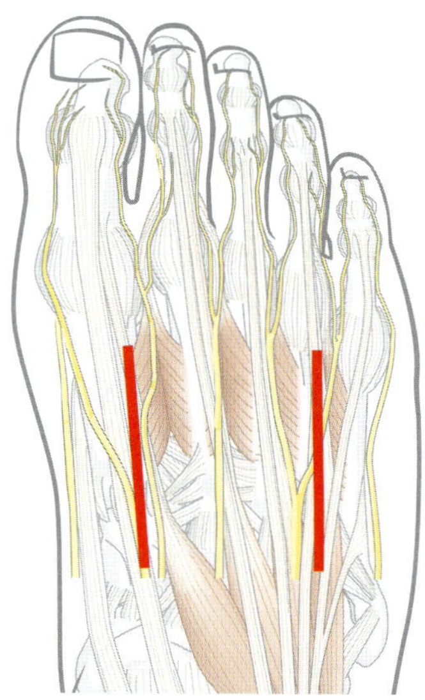

Fig 6-6 Dorsomedial and dorsolateral approaches.

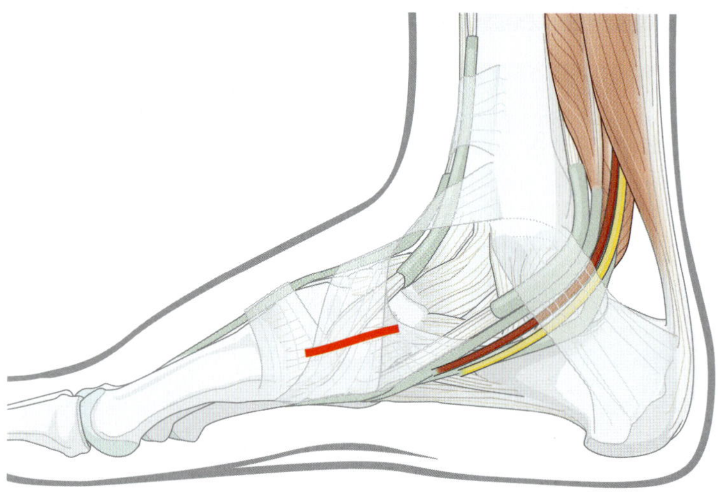

Fig 6-7 Medial utility approach.

Medial utility approach

The medial utility approach allows access to the medial aspect of the foot. It can be extended to allow access from the first MT shaft, across the TMT and IT joints, as well as the cuneiforms all the way across the TN to the distal talus. It can be used for placement of screws and plates if needed.

Lateral approach

The CC joint can be accessed via an oblique lateral approach above and parallel to the peroneal tendons.

Approach and reduction

Approach and reduction are performed by going back and forth between the two dorsal incisions without undermining the dorsal flap. This preserves the dorsalis pedis artery, on which the flap is based. The lateral base of the second TMT should be approached from the dorsolateral incision. If approached from the dorsomedial incision, there is the danger of damaging the blood supply of the dorsal flap.

In cases of a more proximal injury, the incisions may be extended. The medial utility incision is extended over the navicular prominence. The lateral axial hindfoot incision may be extended over the sinus tarsi roughly in line with the fourth MT. An oblique incision (Ollier incision) is preferred by some, but the axial incision allows extension proximally or distally for more soft-tissue relaxation or extended approach if a more extensive injury pattern is discovered intraoperatively.

Alternative approaches

Sometimes the injury pattern requires a single extensile dorsal approach to the foot. Care should be taken to avoid the dorsalis pedis artery which supplies the dorsal soft tissues as well as the bones. Percutaneous screws might be used in cases where incisions are not desired. However, a percutaneous approach does not mean that lack of anatomical reduction is acceptable.

Special considerations for surgery

The locking variable angle plating systems allow open reduction and internal fixation (ORIF) of the segments without using a dorsal approach. Long medial screws may be inserted from the medial incision across the TMT and IT joints stabilizing the medial (and intermediate) columns.

Often the nature of the injury is one which imparts a high amount of energy to the foot. This often results in displacement of these areas. In more severe injuries there may be a crush with comminution. Extensive dissection should be avoided. The reconstruction requires reestablishing the architecture of the foot. The medial and lateral columns must be realigned. The use of an external distractor and external frame can make this process less complicated. Then after several weeks, when the soft tissues have recovered, definitive ORIF can be performed. With severe comminution and/or instability, spanning plates are required, even across the TN joint. Spanning plates across the TN joint, which is an essential motion joint, should be removed as soon as the bones have healed enough to support the function of the foot. Plates or screws across the midtarsal IT joints and TMT joints can be left in place.

Finally, the fourth/fifth cuboid joint is a particularly difficult area to treat. These joints are needed for motion and enable the lateral foot to accommodate to uneven terrain. Rigid stabilization or later arthritis of these joints leads to problems. Therefore, fixation is often with a wire that is removed at 8 weeks. If a spanning plate is used to hold the lateral column out to length, then early removal once bony healing has occurred is desired. There have been no good options yet described for late postinjury arthritis of the fourth/fifth-cuboid joints.

Associated conditions

Patients with Lisfranc/midfoot injuries often have equinus contracture. It is unclear if this plays a role in the injury, but certainly it can compromise healing by exerting forces through the midfoot. Therefore, if equinus is present, a gastrocnemius or Achilles lengthening may be performed as an adjunct procedure at the time of surgery.

The contralateral side should be checked for gastrocnemius tightness via the Silfverskiöld test. If there is gastrocnemius tightness in the uninjured leg, then it is safe to assume it also exists in the injured leg. As such, a gastrocnemius release of some type should be performed as part of the acute operative treatment of Lisfranc, IT, and Chopart injuries. Equinus contracture/gastrocnemius contracture that goes unrecognized and untreated can lead to failure of operative care with early breakdown (**Fig 6-8**).

7 Postoperative care

In general, gentle early nonweight-bearing ROM is started as soon as the incisions heal. Weight bearing is delayed for 6 weeks and sometimes longer. Formal physiotherapy with a biomechanical ankle platform system (BAPS) board and ROM is delayed as well.

For the first 2 weeks, we recommend a 3-sided (AO) splint with fluffy padding. After that, once the wound has healed, a CAM boot provides protection while also allowing access to the foot for wound care and gentle ROM. If there is a question of patient reliability, then a cast can be used.

Spanning plates might be removed at 6 months. Formal physiotherapy with BAPS and gait training can allow the patient to return to normal activities of daily living and be fully functional. However, strenuous activities requiring the foot to accommodate to uneven ground might remain a challenge for many patients.

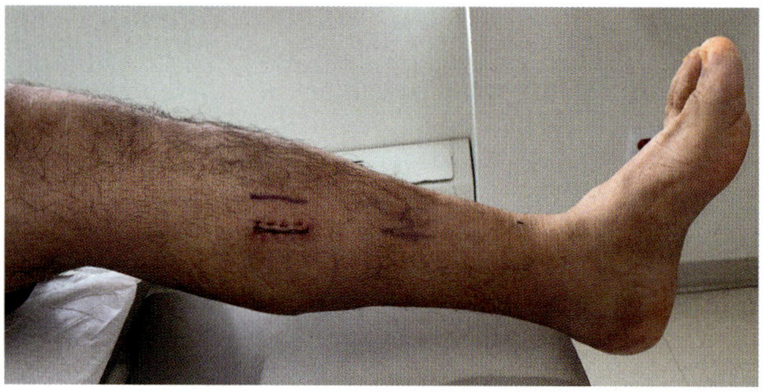

Fig 6-8 Gastrocnemius lengthening may be performed as an adjunct procedure to address equinus contracture/gastrocnemius contracture.

8 Complications and outcomes

Injuries treated nonoperatively may develop arthritis with deformity and pain, requiring reconstruction with osteotomy, realignment, and fusion.

If a careful approach is not made, there could be injuries to other structures on the dorsum of the foot including neurovascular structures. This will lead to of numbness or dysaesthesia in this area, which patients find extremely disturbing. If the dorsalis pedis is injured, then the dorsal flap between the two incisions can become compromised. Tendons may also be damaged leading to disability of the associated structures.

There is not much soft tissue on the dorsum of the foot, so any injury to the soft tissue must be allowed to recover before surgery is performed. If the soft tissue is lost, whether by the initial injury or through surgical misadventure, a free flap is often needed.

9 Recommended reading

Benirschke SK, Meinberg EG, Anderson SA, et al. Fractures and dislocations of the midfoot: Lisfranc and Chopart injuries. *Instr Course Lect.* 2013;62:79–91.

Chandran P, Puttaswamaiah R, Dhillon MS, et al. Management of complex open fracture injuries of the midfoot with external fixation. *J Foot Ankle Surg.* 2006 Sep–Oct;45(5):308–315.

Ellington JK, Bosse MJ, Castillo RC, et al. The mangled foot and ankle: results from a 2-year prospective study. *J Orthop Trauma.* 2013 Jan;27(1):43–48.

Kinner B, Tietz S, Muller F, et al. Outcome after complex trauma of the foot. *J Trauma.* 2011 Jan;70(1):159–168; discussion 168.

Kuo RS, Tejwani NC, Digiovanni CW, et al. Outcome after open reduction and internal fixation of Lisfranc joint injuries. *J Bone Joint Surg Am.* 2000 Nov;82(11):1609–1618.

Mulier T, Reynders P, Dereymaeker G, et al. Severe Lisfrancs injuries: primary arthrodesis or ORIF? *Foot Ankle Int.* 2002 Oct;23(10):902–905.

Rammelt S, Heineck J, Zwipp H. Metatarsal fractures. *Injury.* 2004 Sep;35 Suppl 2:Sb77–86.

Richter M, Thermann H, Huefner T, et al. Chopart joint fracture-dislocation: initial open reduction provides better outcome than closed reduction. *Foot Ankle Int.* 2004 May;25(5):340–348.

Rosenbaum AJ, DiPreta JA, Tartaglione J, et al. Acute Fractures of the Tarsal Navicular: A Critical Analysis Review. *JBJS Rev.* 2015 Mar 31;3(3).

Sands AK, Swords, MP. Open Reduction and Internal Fixation of Lisfranc/Tarsometatarsal Injuries. In: Pfeffer GB, Easley ME, Hinterman B, et al, eds. *Operative Techniques: Foot and Ankle Surgery.* Philadelphia: Elsevier; 2018:172–179.

Sharma S, Dhillon MS, Sharma G, et al. Nutcracker cuboid fractures are never isolated injuries. *J Foot Ankle Surg (Asia-Pacific).* 2014;1(1):9–11.

Thevendran G, Deol RS, Calder JD. Fifth metatarsal fractures in the athlete: evidence for management. *Foot Ankle Clin.* 2013 Jun;18(2):237–254.

van Dorp KB, de Vries MR, van der Elst M, et al. Chopart joint injury: a study of outcome and morbidity. *J Foot Ankle Surg.* 2010 Nov–Dec;49(6):541–545.

Welck MJ, Zinchenko R, Rudge B. Lisfranc injuries. *Injury.* 2015 Apr;46(4):536–541.

6.1 Talar head fracture

John R Shank

1 Case description

A 52-year-old man was involved in a motorcycle accident, at moderate speed, injuring his left foot. He presented to the emergency department with complaints of isolated ankle and midfoot pain. The clinical examination revealed swelling about the midfoot with tenderness isolated to the talonavicular joint. The ankle was neurovascularly intact. Diagnostic imaging, including x-rays and a computed tomographic (CT) scan, revealed an isolated, comminuted talar head fracture (**Fig 6.1-1**).

2 Preoperative planning

Indications for surgery

Surgical treatment of a talar head fracture is preferred because of the articular involvement of the fracture. There is an unacceptably high propensity for delayed union and arthrosis when these injuries are missed or treated nonoperatively. Overall foot function is dependent on appropriate alignment through the TN articulation making surgical treatment a requirement in virtually all fractures. Surgical fixation options are limited to small screws with implants coun-

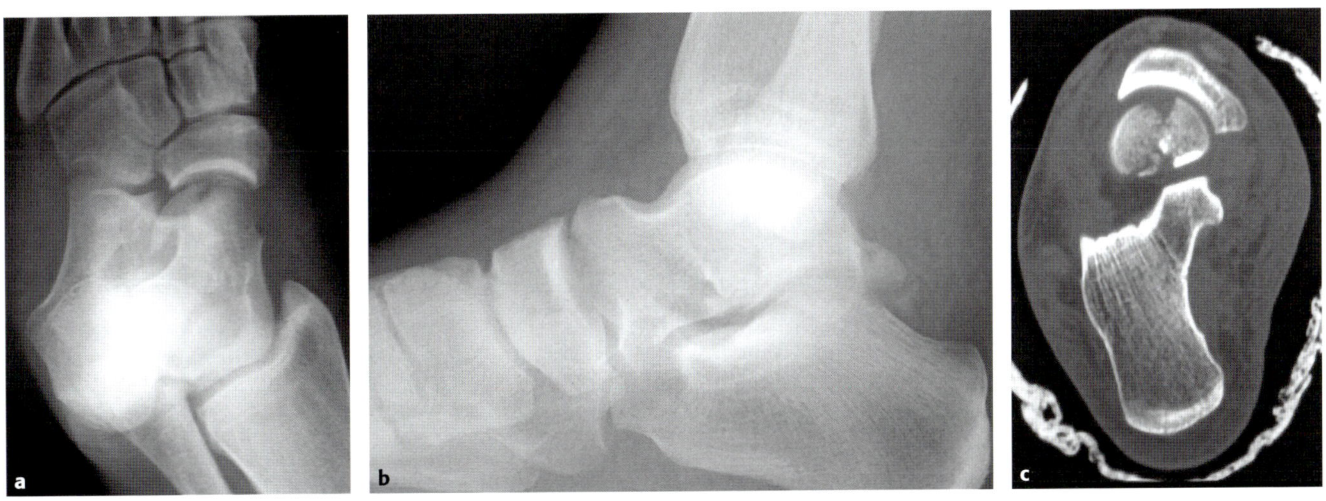

Fig 6.1-1a–c Comminuted talar head fracture with displacement of the TN joint.
a Oblique x-ray of hindfoot.
b Lateral x-ray of hindfoot.
c Computed tomographic image of the hindfoot.

tersunk beneath the articular surface. Schanz pins or distractors are commonly used for improved visualization of the talar head injury. An appropriate preoperative plan should be in place before proceeding with open reduction and internal fixation (**Fig 6.1-2**).

Nonoperative treatment is not recommended for talar head fractures.

3 Operating room setup

Patient positioning	• Supine
Anesthesia options	• General anesthesia, often supplemented with spinal or regional nerve block
C-arm location	• Same side as the injury allowing the surgeon a free view while performing reduction with the screen is positioned toward the foot of the operative table
Tourniquet	• Optional, applied to thigh
Tips	• Foot placed on a bump and slightly externally rotated, a position the limb assumes naturally on the operative table

For illustrations and overview of anesthetic considerations, see chapter 1.

Equipment

- Headlamp for visualization
- Elevators and dental scaler
- External fixator, femoral distractor or small distration device
- K-wire set
- Small and minifragment screws
- Plates
- Resorbable pins
- Any instruments needed to obtain autograft bone graft (surgeon choice)

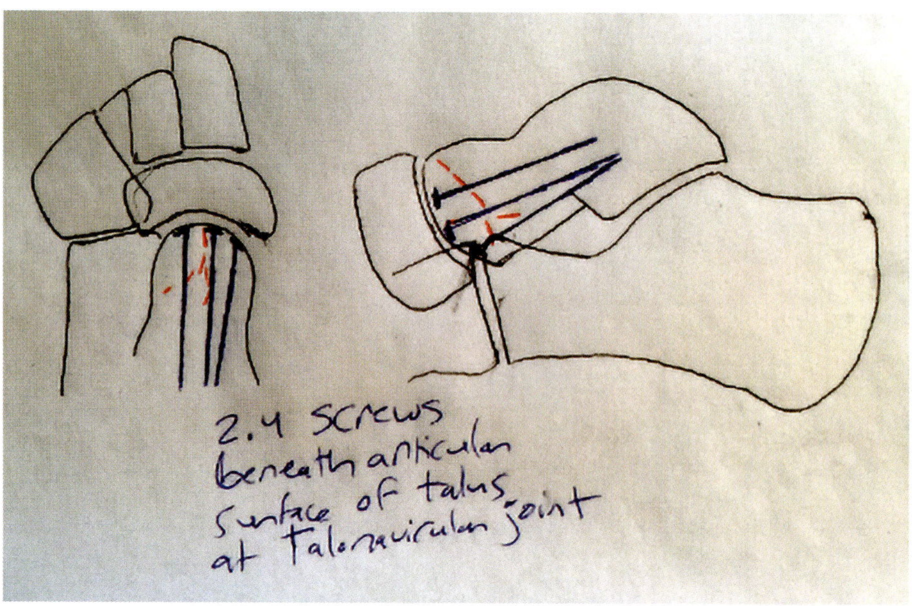

Fig 6.1-2 Preoperative plan.

4 Surgical procedure

For internal fixation, a medial utility incision can be used, located between the posterior tibial tendon and tibialis anterior tendon (**Fig 6.1-3**). The saphenous nerve and vessels should always be protected. An anterolateral approach, lateral to the neurovascular bundle and medial to the lateral branch of the superficial peroneal nerve can be performed as well, based upon the fracture anatomy.

A bone hook or Schanz pin can be used to displace the navicular away from the TN joint to visualize the talar head injury (**Fig 6.1-4**). Temporary K-wire reduction can be performed with bone grafting of any subchondral bony defects. Screw fixation with implants buried beneath the articular surface is favored (**Fig 6.1-5**). A spanning distractor is often helpful to distract the TN joint which improves intraarticular visualization.

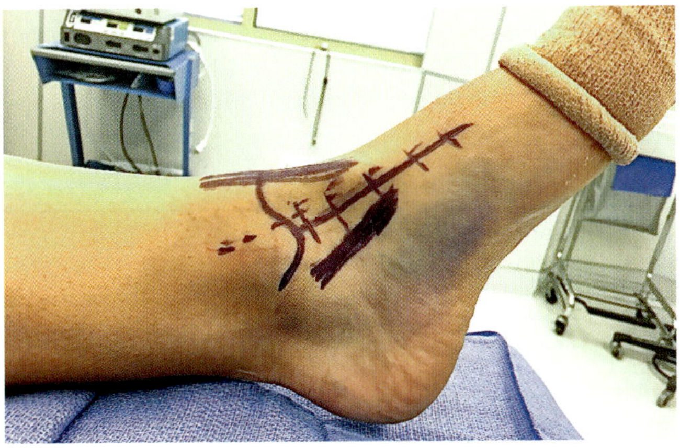

Fig 6.1-3 Medial approach to the midfoot, located between the anterior and posterior tibial tendons.

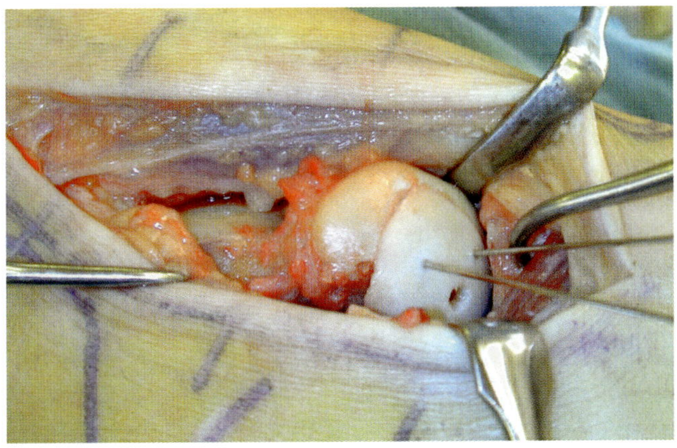

Fig 6.1-4 A bone hook is used to displace the navicular for visualization and fixation of the talar head injury.

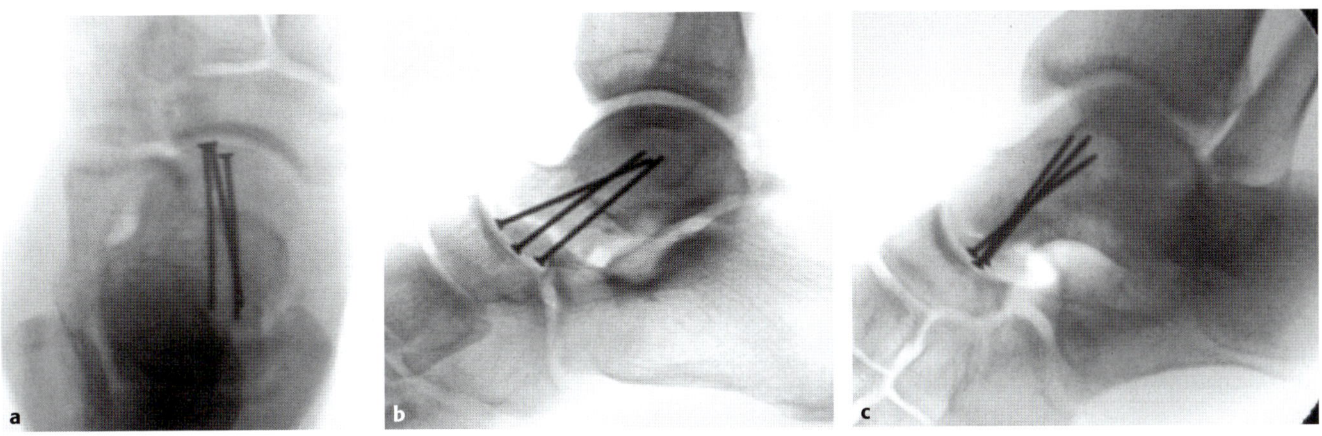

Fig 6.1-5a–c X-rays of the hindfoot showing the final fixation demonstrating anatomical reduction of the talar head. The screw heads are countersunk beneath the articular surface at the TN joint.
a AP view.
b Lateral view.
c Oblique view.

5 Pitfalls and complications

Pitfalls

Visualization of the talar head fracture

The challenge in open treatment of the talar head is adequate exposure at the TN joint. Either a bone hook or a Schanz pin is essential in providing visualization of the talar head injury. In cases with preexisting lateral peritalar subluxation (flatfoot), visualization of the talar head is improved. An anterolateral approach can be made for injuries with lateral talar head pathology. Use of a spanning distractor, as noted above, is often helpful.

Limited implant selection

The location of the injury limits implant selection and placement of screws countersunk beneath the articular surface. Implants placed through the cartilage surface can lead to more rapid arthrosis at the TN joint. Small plates for larger talar head fragments or resorbable pins for smaller osteochondral fragments can also be considered.

Complications

- Injury to the saphenous nerve (medial utility approach) and lateral branch of the superficial peroneal nerve (anterolateral approach)
- Injury to the dorsal neurovascular bundle through the anterolateral approach
- Wound complications from inadequate skin bridge between incisions
- Loss of fixation
- Malunion
- Nonunion
- Posttraumatic arthrosis

6 Alternative techniques

For severely comminuted injuries with shortening of the medial column, external fixation and/or bridge plating can be used to reduce the articular surface and to restore medial column length. Temporary K-wire fixation may be used as an alternative to screw fixation. Primary arthrodesis can be considered for severely comminuted injuries with major bone loss.

7 Postoperative management and rehabilitation

In suspected cases of delayed union, postoperative CT imaging can be performed for accurate fracture healing assessment.

An active rehabilitation program is initiated at weight bearing to emphasize range-of-motion, muscular balance, and gait training.

For further information about postoperative care see chapter 1.

Implant removal

Removal of implants from the talar head is generally not necessary. As implants are countersunk beneath the articular cartilage, removal can be difficult and can further injure the talar head cartilage.

8 Recommended reading

Early JS. Management of fractures of the talus: body and head regions. *Foot Ankle Clin.* 2004 Dec;9(4):709–722.
Early JS. Talus fracture management. *Foot Ankle Clin.* 2008 Dec;13(4):635–657.
Fortin PT, Balazsy JE. Talus fractures: evaluation and treatment. *J Am Acad Orthop Surg.* 2001 Mar–Apr;9(2):114–127.
Hood CR Jr, Miller JR, Hollinger JK. Defining talar head and neck pathology: the Malvern Classification System. *J Foot Ankle Surg.* 2018 Jan–Feb;57(1):131–139.
Ibrahim MS, Jordan R, Lotfi N, et al. Talar head fracture: a case report, systematic review and suggested algorithm of treatment. *Foot (Edinb).* 2015 Dec;25(4):258–264.
Kou JX, Fortin PT. Commonly missed peritalar injuries. *J Am Acad Orthop Surg.* 2009 Dec;17(12):775–786.
Lamothe JM, Buckley RE. Talus fractures: a current concept review of diagnoses, treatments, and outcomes. *Acta Chir Orthop Traumatol Cech.* 2012;79(2):97–106.
Rammelt S, Schepers T. Chopart injuries: when to fix and when to fuse? *Foot Ankle Clin.* 2017 Mar;22(1):163–180.
Shank JR, Benirschke SK, Swords MP. Treatment of peripheral talus fractures. *Foot Ankle Clin.* 2017 Mar;22(1):181–192.

6.2 Anterior calcaneal process fracture

John R Shank, Michael Swords

1 Case description

A 53-year-old man slid into second base during a softball game, forcefully twisting his right foot and ankle. He presented 3 days later with complaints of foot and ankle pain. He had multiple fracture blisters that were being treated with serial dressing changes. Clinically, the patient had swelling about the ankle and midfoot and was neurovascularly intact. X-rays of the right foot and ankle demonstrated no definitive fracture (**Fig 6.2-1**).

As the clinical examination was unclear as to the nature of the injury, a computed tomographic (CT) scan was obtained which demonstrated fractures through the anterior process of the calcaneus, posteromedial talar body, and medial aspect of the navicular (**Fig 6.2-2**). This chapter describes the anterior process calcaneal fracture, thus the other injuries will not be discussed.

This case emphasizes an injury to the calcaneus resulting from a laterally directed force at the midfoot, with corresponding medial column injuries.

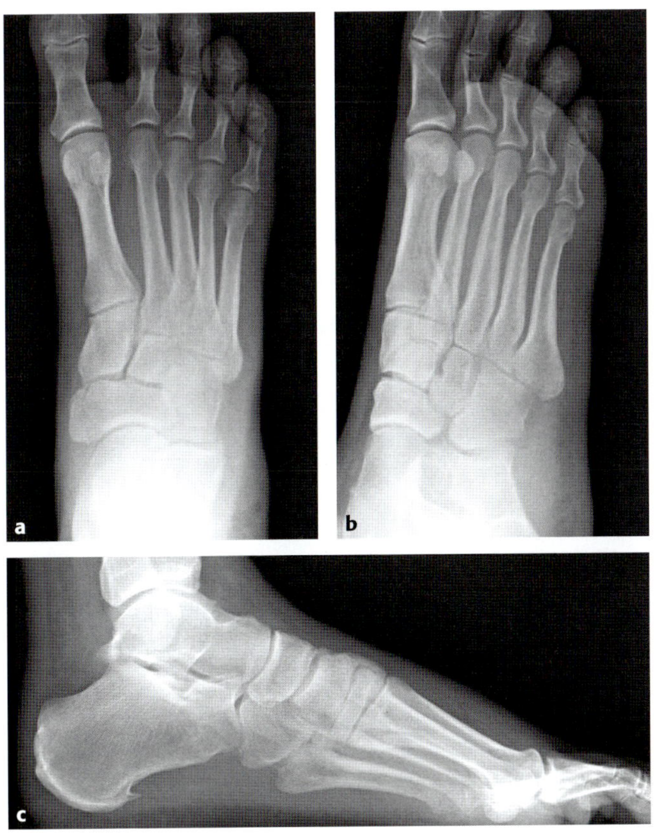

Fig 6.2-1a–c Postinjury x-rays.
a AP view.
b Oblique view.
c Lateral view.

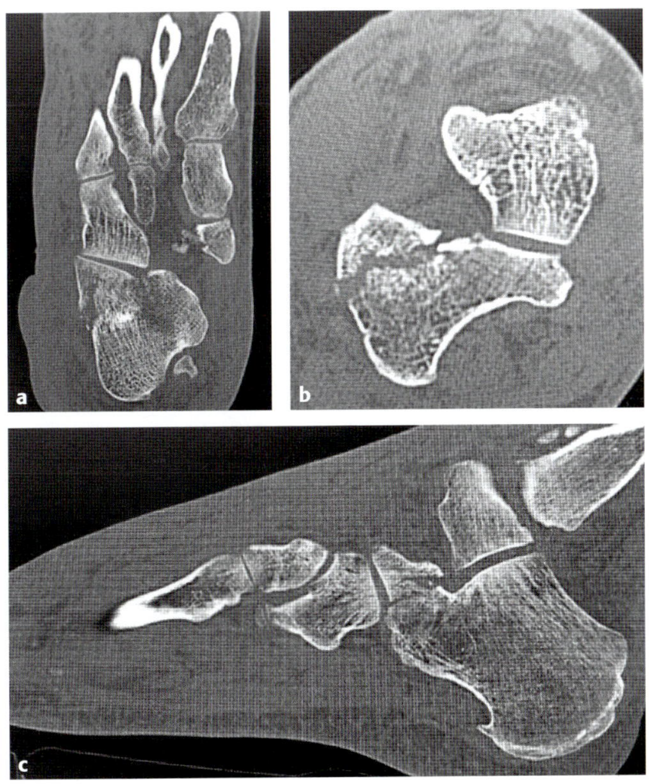

Fig 6.2-2a–c The CT scan demonstrating the anterior process calcaneal fracture and an incongruent calcaneocuboid joint.
a Axial view.
b Coronal view.
c Sagittal view.

2 Preoperative planning

Indications for surgery

Surgical indications include articular involvement and intraarticular incongruity of the calcaneocuboid (CC) joint in an otherwise healthy 53-year-old man, along with potential residual instability across the whole midfoot due to associated medial injuries. There is a high propensity for delayed union and posttraumatic CC arthrosis when these injuries are treated nonoperatively.

Treatment options

Nonoperative treatment is indicated in well-aligned injuries without joint incongruity or subluxation. Also, small extraarticular avulsion fractures can be treated nonoperatively.

Surgical fixation is indicated in cases with malalignment or joint subluxation, as in this case. Fixation options include small screw fixation or plate and screw fixation. For cases with significant anterior process involvement, concomitant cuboid fracture, or subluxation of the CC joint, an external fixator or bridge plating can be used to supplement fixation and to restore lateral column length. An appropriate preoperative plan should be made before proceeding with open reduction and internal fixation (**Fig 6.2-3**).

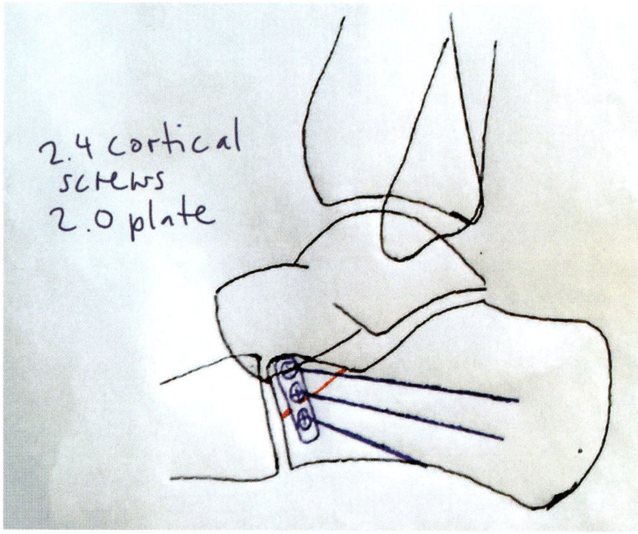

Fig 6.2-3 Preoperative plan.

3 Operating room setup

Patient positioning	• Lateral on a radiolucent table
Anesthesia options	• General anesthesia, often supplemented with spinal or regional nerve block
C-arm location	• Contralateral side of the injury with the screen positioned toward the foot of the operative table
Tourniquet	• Optional, applied to thigh
Tips	• Position may be supine when injury is part of more complex injury requiring access both medially and laterally. • The lateral position allows best visualization for the distal calcaneus or CC joint/lateral column (**Fig 6.2-4**).

For illustrations and overview of anesthetic considerations, see chapter 1.

Equipment

- Headlamp for visualization
- Elevators and dental scalers
- External fixator or distractor (small foot or femoral)
- K-wire set
- Modular implants with minifragment screws
- Bone graft instruments and equipment (surgeon choice)

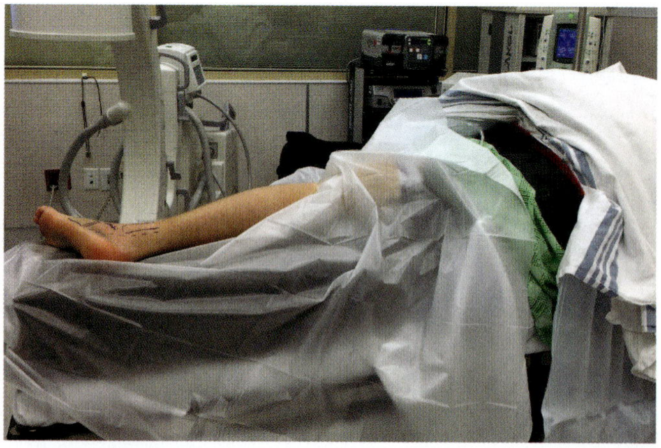

Fig 6.2-4 Lateral positioning allows for improved visualization of the anterior process of the calcaneus and CC joint.

4 Surgical procedure

For internal fixation, an anterolateral approach can be used directly over the region of the fracture site. The lateral branch of the superficial peroneal nerve should be protected in a dorsal flap and the peroneal tendons and sural nerve should be protected in a plantar flap. The extensor digitorum brevis is elevated subperiosteally and retracted superiorly, allowing visualization of the CC joint and associated fractures (**Fig 6.2-5**). An external fixator or small distraction device can be used in more complex injuries to distract the CC joint for articular visualization. Temporary K-wire fixation is then done, along with bone grafting of any subchondral bony defects. Screw fixation for simple fractures and plate and screw fixation for more complex injuries should be performed (**Fig 6.2-6**).

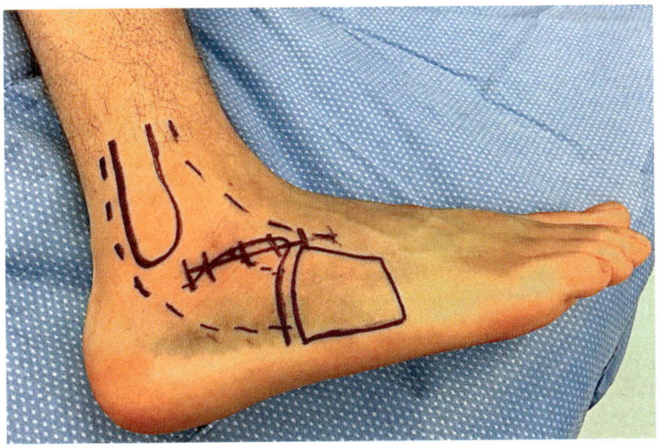

Fig 6.2-5 An anterolateral incision over the region of the fracture. The approach to the joint is dorsal to the peroneal tendons and sural nerve, and plantar to the lateral branch of the superficial peroneal nerve.

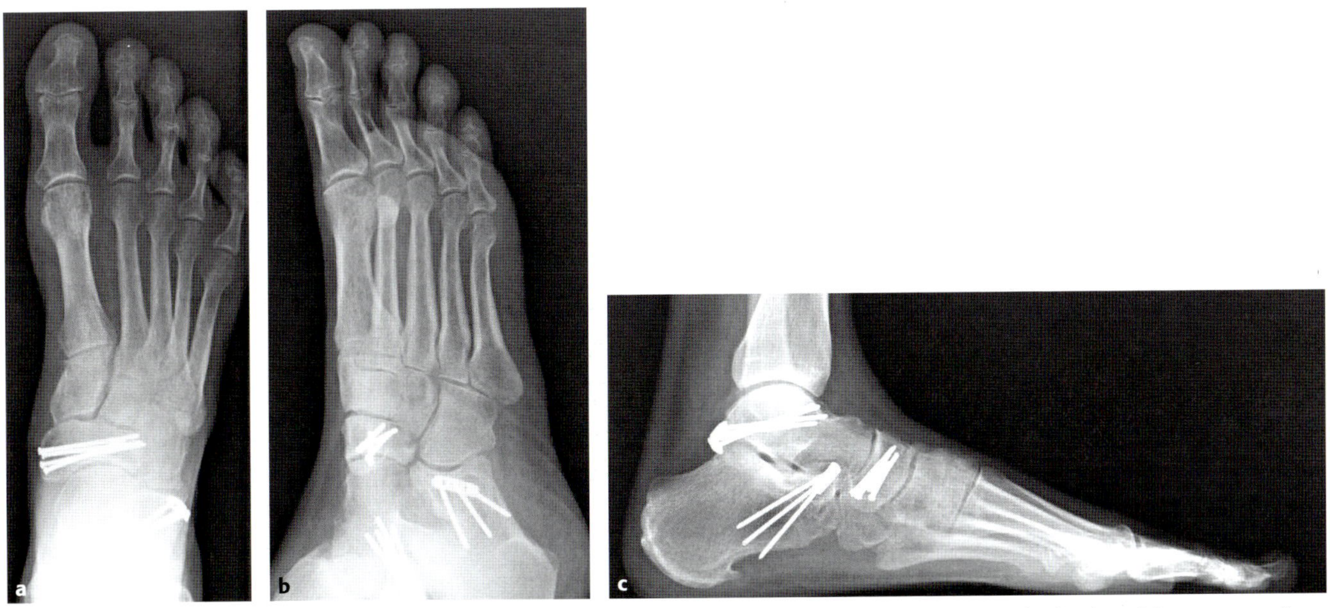

Fig 6.2-6a–c Final x-rays of the foot demonstrate reduction of the anterior process and the CC joint. Notice the fixation of the corresponding medial side injuries (see chapter 6.5).

a AP view.
b Oblique view.
c Lateral view.

5 Pitfalls and complications

Pitfalls

Inadequate reduction of calcaneocuboid joint

It can be difficult to reduce more comminuted injuries with standard plate and screw fixation. Often, an external fixator or bridge plating may be needed to adequately reduce the anterior process and CC joint. Articular incongruity or subluxation of the CC joint may lead to rapid arthrosis or malalignment and the need for arthrodesis.

Failure to recognize medial column injuries

Failure to recognize additional injuries in the Chopart joints, especially the medial column, leads to late deformity from inadequate treatment. Anterior process fractures should always raise the suspicion of a Chopart joint and medial column injury.

Complications

- Injury to the lateral branch of the superficial peroneal nerve or sural nerve
- Injury to the peroneal tendons
- Wound complications
- Loss of fixation
- Malunion
- Nonunion
- Posttraumatic arthrosis

6 Alternative techniques

For severely comminuted injuries, external fixation or locked bridge plating can be used to restore length and provide ligamentotaxis to the lateral column. Comminuted fractures may need to be distracted and bone grafted if screw fixation fails to maintain lateral column length. Excision can be considered for smaller fractures and for nonunions.

7 Postoperative management and rehabilitation

Postoperatively, sutures are kept in place for 2–3 weeks and then removed. If external fixation is used, removal should be planned at around 6 weeks postoperatively. Active and passive range-of-motion exercises are initiated as soon as the incision is healed. Transition into a rigid boot or foot orthosis with the ankle at 90° is performed at 2–3 weeks postoperatively or as soon as the external fixator device is removed. Nonweight bearing is recommended for a minimum of 6–8 weeks postoperatively, depending on injury severity and fracture type.

Standard postoperative x-rays are obtained to ensure fracture union. In cases of suspected delayed union or nonunion, postoperative CT imaging can be performed. An active rehabilitation program is initiated at weight bearing to emphasize range of motion, muscular balance, and gait training.

For more information about postoperative care, see chapter 1.

8 Recommended reading

Berkowitz MJ, Kim DH. Process and tubercle fractures of the hindfoot. *J Am Acad Orthop Surg.* 2005 Dec;13(8):492–502.

Degan TJ, Morrey BF, Braun DP. Surgical excision for anterior-process fractures of the calcaneus. *J Bone Joint Surg Am.* 1982 Apr;64(4):519–524.

Dhillon M, Khurana A, Prabhakar S, et al. Crush fractures of the anterior end of calcaneum. *Indian J Orthop.* 2018 MayJun;52(3):244–252.

Garvin EJ, Rominger CJ. Fractures of the anterior process of the calcaneus. *Am J Surg.* 1957 Sep;94(3):468–471.

Golder WA. Anterior process of the calcaneus: a clinical-radiological contribution to anatomical vocabulary. *Surg Radiol Anat.* 2004 Jun;26(3):163–166.

Halm JA, Schepers T. Resection of small avulsion fractures of the anterior process of the calcaneus for refractory complaints. *J Foot Ankle Surg.* 2017 Jan–Feb;56(1):135–141.

Jahss MH, Kay BS. An anatomic study of the anterior superior process of the os calcis and its clinical application. *Foot Ankle.* 1983 Mar–Apr;3(5):268–281.

Ouellette H, Salamipour H, Thomas BJ, et al. Incidence and MR imaging features of fractures of the anterior process of calcaneus in a consecutive patient population with ankle and foot symptoms. *Skeletal Radiol.* 2006 Nov;35(11):833–837.

Petrover D, Schweitzer ME, Laredo JD. Anterior process calcaneal fractures: a systematic evaluation of associated conditions. *Skeletal Radiol.* 2007 Jul;36(7):627–632.

Rammelt S, Schepers T. Chopart injuries: when to fix and when to fuse? *Foot Ankle Clin.* 2017 Mar;22(1):163–180.

Rammelt S, Zwipp H, Schneiders W, et al. Anatomic reconstruction of malunited Chopart joint injuries. *Eur J Trauma Emerg Surg.* 2010 Jun;36(3):196–205.

Renfrew DL, el-Khoury GY. Anterior process fractures of the calcaneus. *Skeletal Radiol.* 1985;14(2):121–125.

Roesen HM, Kanat IO. Anterior process fracture of the calcaneus. *J Foot Ankle Surg.* 1993 Jul-Aug;32(4):424–429.

Trnka HJ, Zettl R, Ritschl P. Fracture of the anterior superior process of the calcaneus: an often misdiagnosed fracture. *Arch Orthop Trauma Surg.* 1998;117(4–5):300–302.

Wang ZJ, Huang XL, Chu YC, et al. Applied anatomy of the calcaneocuboid articular surface for internal fixation of calcaneal fractures. *Injury.* 2013 Nov;44(11):1428–1430.

6.3 Navicular fracture

Juan Bernardo Gerstner Garces, Andrew K Sands

1 Case description

A 52-year-old man fell from his horse. He presented to the emergency department 24 hours after the injury. During the clinical examination he had increased pain and swelling of his right midfoot. His foot and leg were immobilized in a posterior splint, which relieved some of the pain. Comorbidities included hypertension controlled with medication.

There were dorsal, plantar, and medial midfoot ecchymoses (**Fig 6.3-1**). There was pain with movement of the Chopart and Lisfranc joints. There were no neurovascular deficits. The skin was intact with no open injuries, and there was no sign of compartment syndrome.

X-rays in weight-bearing (WB) AP, and lateral, as well as oblique views showed a comminuted navicular fracture and a Lisfranc medial column dislocation (**Fig 6.3-2**). Computed tomographic (CT) scans were ordered as part of the preoperative plan (**Fig 6.3-3**).

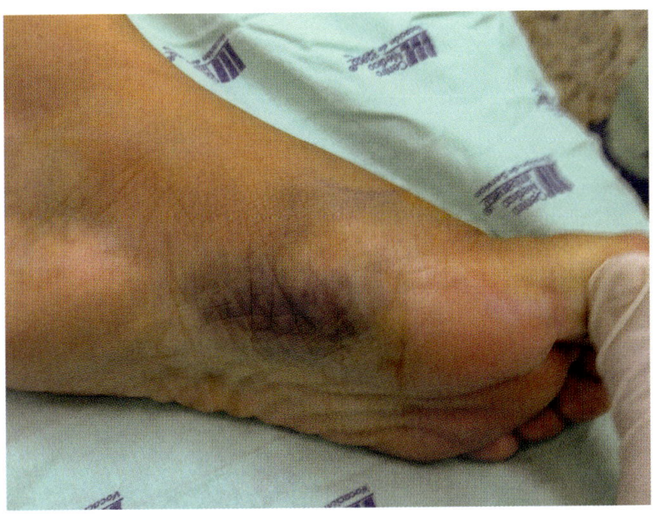

Fig 6.3-1 Plantar medial ecchymosis often is seen in these injuries.

2 Preoperative planning

Indications for surgery

This case shows a multifragmentary navicular fracture (AO/OTA 83C(b), Sangeorzan type I), and Lisfranc pure ligamentous medial and central column lesions in an otherwise healthy man. The injury was displaced and comminuted and there was a risk for nonunion or malunion. Therefore, surgery was indicated.

Treatment options

Closed treatment with immobilization and nonweight bearing

Closed treatment is chosen for individuals who are not candidates for surgical fixation because of excessive risk of complications. This includes patients who abuse tobacco, people with diabetes, or with peripheral vascular disease.

Open reduction and internal fixation (ORIF) may not be possible in patients with a complicated medical history with comorbidities. Stabilization of any subluxation or dislocation is essential even in high-risk individuals and may require percutaneous K-wire insertion for stability, after anatomical reduction has been performed.

Open reduction and internal fixation

The preferred treatment in patients with a navicular fracture with displacement or comminution is ORIF.

Because the injury in this case is displaced and comminuted, closed treatment with casting would lead to nonunion or malunion. This would result in an alteration of foot alignment. Therefore, the treatment chosen was ORIF.

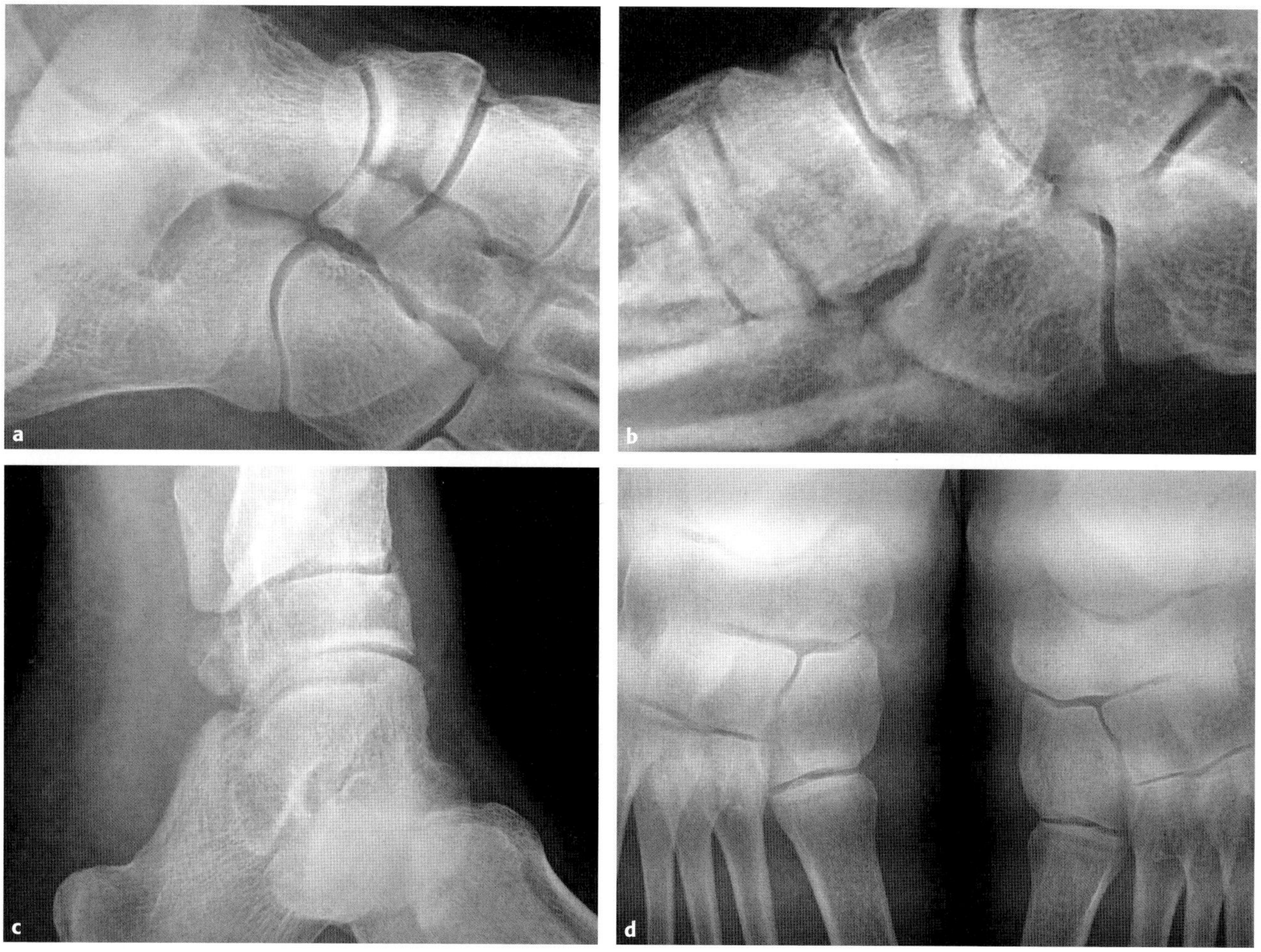

Fig 6.3-2a–d Multiple x-ray views of navicular fracture.

- **a** Internal oblique view.
- **b** External oblique view.
- **c** True lateral with WB.
- **d** True AP with WB

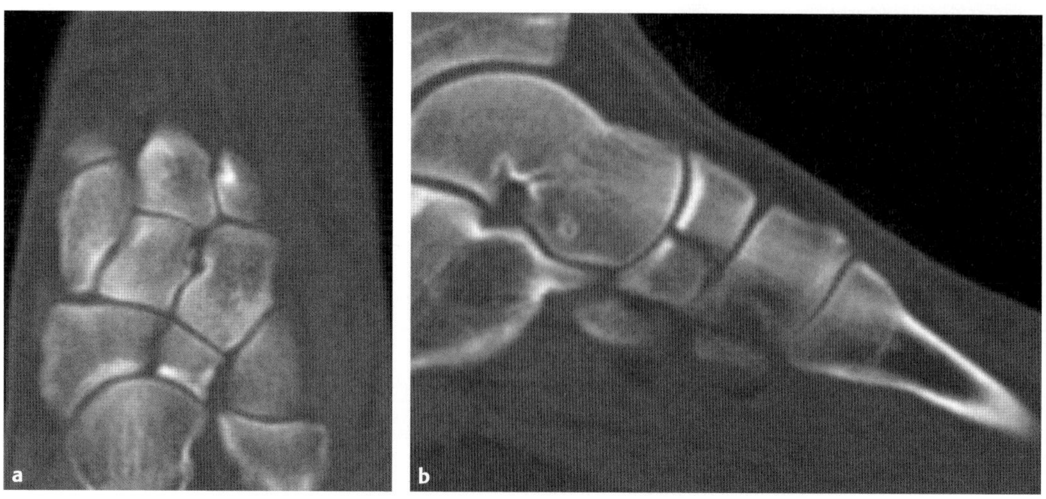

Fig 6.3-3a–b Computed tomographic images.

- **a** Axial view.
- **b** Sagittal view.

A preoperative plan is necessary (**Fig 6.3-4**). There should be a high degree of suspicion of lateral column fractures, such as cuboid fractures, fractures of the distal calcaneus, and Lisfranc fracture-dislocation. Isolated navicular fractures are rare. If dislocation occurs, peripheral talar fractures may also occur. A CT scan with 3D reconstruction (sagittal and coronal planes) is advisable to help evaluate for any additional injuries.

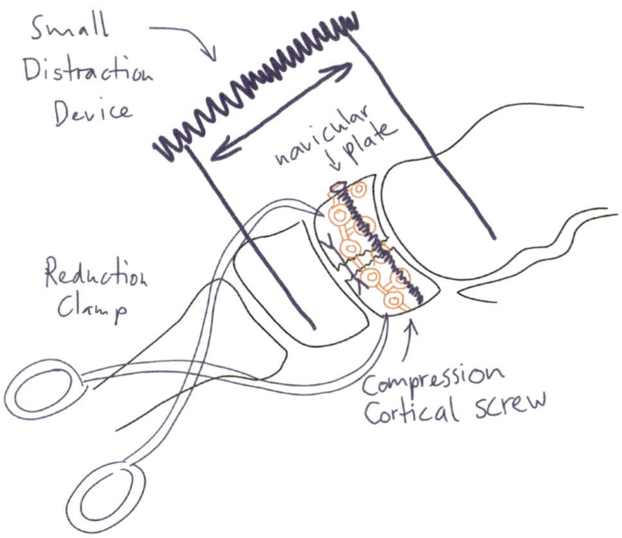

Fig 6.3-4 Preoperative plan.

3 Operating room setup

Patient positioning	• Supine
Anesthesia options	• General anesthesia, often supplemented with spinal or regional nerve block
C-arm location	• Placed on same side as the injury which allows the surgeon a free view while performing reduction. • The screen is positioned toward the foot of the operative table.
Tourniquet	• Optional, applied to thigh
Tips	• Foot is placed on a bump and slightly externally rotated, a position the limb assumes naturally on the operative table.

For illustrations and overview of anesthetic considerations, see chapter 1.

Equipment

- Smooth K-wires
- Small distraction device
- Point-to-point reduction (Weber) clamps
- Navicular locked compression plate (LCP) or variable angle locked compression plate (VA LCP) with 2.7 mm locking and cortex screws
- Bone harvesting set (including chisels, periosteal elevators, and bone trephines) or access to allograft or synthetic materials
- Retractors (Hohmann and self-retaining)
- Power equipment (corded or small battery)
- Minifragment locking and non-locking screws

4 Surgical procedures

The medial utility approach allows the surgeon to handle both navicular and Lisfranc pathologies with careful retraction of both the tibialis anterior and posterior tendons.

The incision for the anteromedial approach is made from the base of the first metatarsal (MT) to the neck of the talus (**Fig 6.3-5**). Careful dissection of the soft tissue is carried out, being cautious not to injure the branches of the medial dorsal cutaneous nerve. The tendons of the extensor hallucis longus and tibialis anterior are retracted dorsally and the tibialis posterior is retracted plantar. The talonavicular (TN) and navicular-medial cuneiform joint capsules are opened and distracted to allow careful inspection of both joint surfaces of the navicular, once the hematoma is cleared.

A small foot distraction device can be used to achieve proper length of the medial column and reduction of the fracture. It also helps to determine the exact reduction and can allow visualization of any screw penetration into any joints on either side of the navicular.

The foot distraction device is positioned so it does not interfere with the view of the reduction—it can be flipped to keep it out of the way as it works well in many different orientations. Once positioned, 3 mm pins from the distractor set are usually used. The proximal pin is placed into the neck of the talus just distal to the medial malleolus and must not enter the articular surface of the medial gutter of the ankle. The distal pin can be placed into the medial cuneiform or the medial base of the first MT.

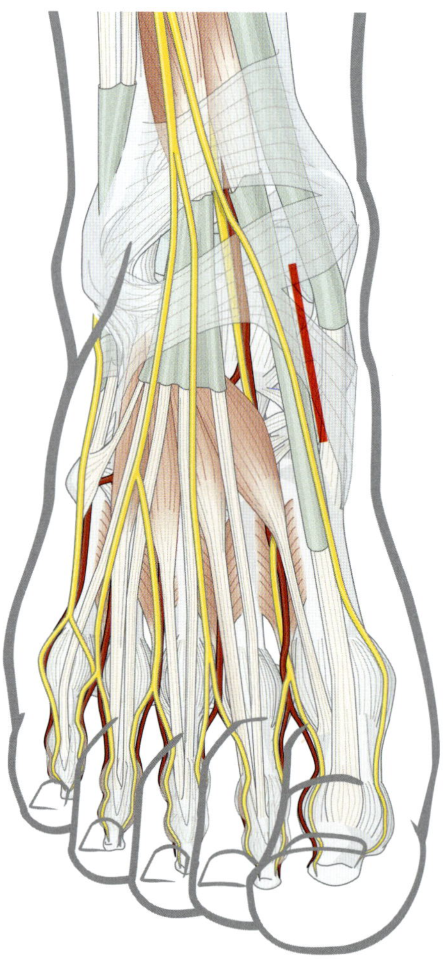

Fig 6.3-5 Dorsal approach.

Distraction is done smoothly and progressively allowing visualization of joint surfaces by ligamentotaxis. This permits improved visualization and a more accurate reduction (**Fig 6.3-6**).

Manipulation of the fragments can be performed with smooth K-wires used as joysticks. A point-to-point (Weber) reduction clamp can be used to reduce the space between fragments and assist in obtaining and maintaining reduction. Once final reduction is obtained, a curved reduction clamp is positioned and two smooth K-wires are directed across the fracture line providing temporary fixation. Multiple wires may be necessary in more comminuted injuries.

Comminution can now be evaluated and if defects are present, they may be filled with bone graft which can be obtained locally from the calcaneal tuber, or more remotely from the proximal tibia (which is draped into the surgical field). Allograft may also be used.

Dissection should be minimized to preserve as much of the blood supply to the navicular as possible. When possible, minimal approach with percutaneous screws should be used for ORIF. If a plate is needed, it can be positioned to assure the best place for restoration of anatomy (over the top and around the corners of the bone). The plate should be contoured to follow the shape of the bone, and then cut to the appropriate length. The first screw should compress the fracture line either through a hole in the plate or outside the plate. Care must be taken with lag fixation in comminuted injuries not to overcompress the navicular, which alters the spherical shape of the proximal navicular joint surface.

Once initial, gentle lag screw fixation is accomplished, the shape of the joint should be assessed to make sure it has not accidentally been squeezed out of the correct spherical shape.

Subsequent locking screws are then positioned to hold reduction and allow early mobilization. Additional skin incisions may be made to insert screws through the farthest holes of the plate.

Before removing the distraction device, careful inspection of both joints is made to ensure there is no intraarticular screw penetration of either joint (**Fig 6.3-7**). If any TN joint instability is noted after distraction is released, smooth K-wires can be placed across the joint for temporarily stabilization.

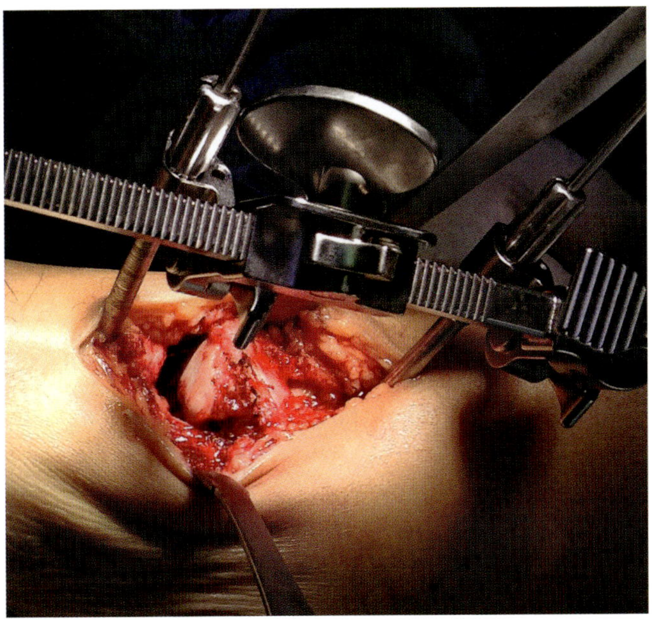

Fig 6.3-6 Distraction across the talonavicular joint allows excellent visualization of the injured area.

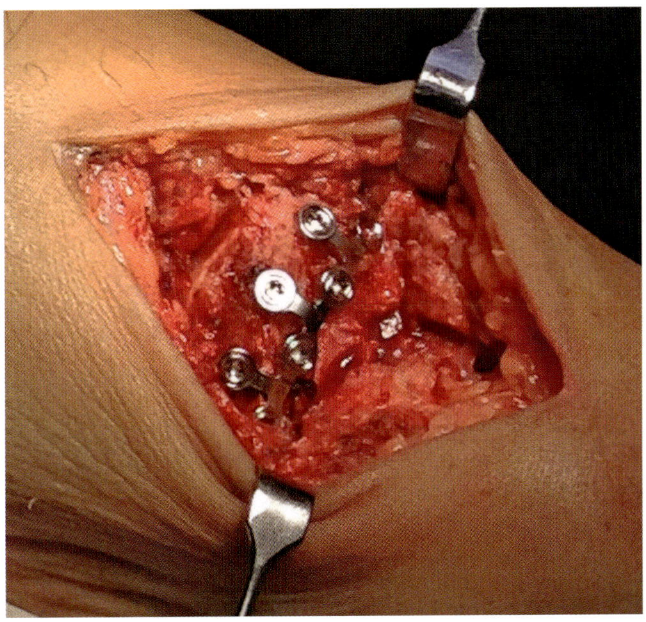

Fig 6.3-7 Surface inspection.

Final x-rays are obtained (**Fig 6.3-8**). After hemostasis is achieved, the wound is closed in layers with resorbable sutures. A splint is applied at the end of the procedure.

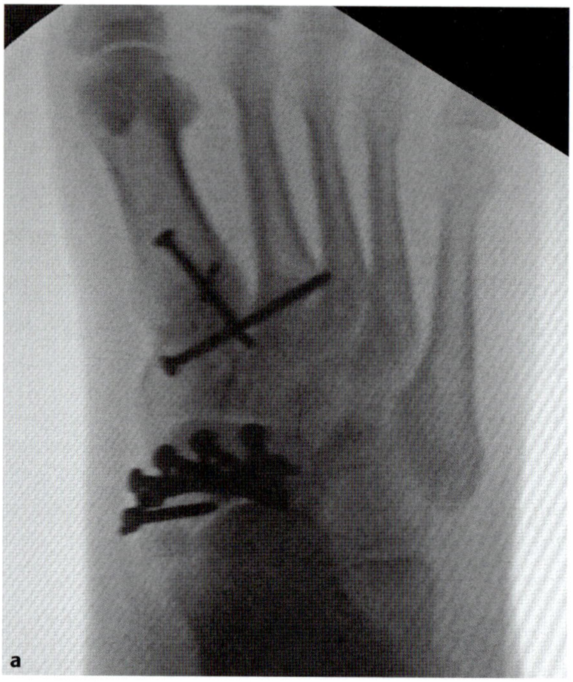

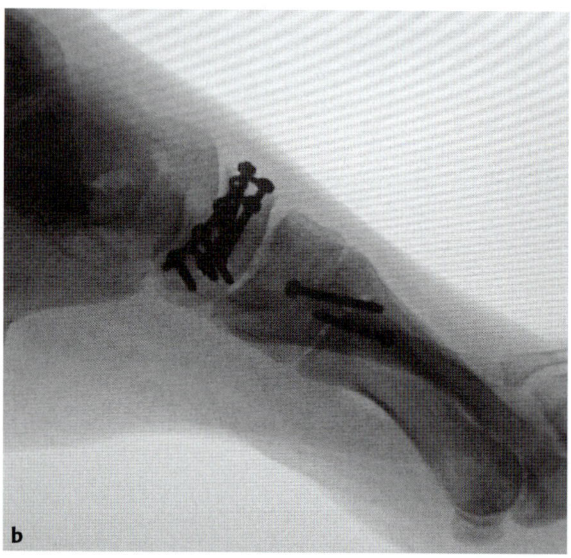

Figs 5.3-8a–b Intraoperative images.
a AP view.
b Lateral view.

5 Pitfalls and complications

Pitfalls

Intraarticular hardware

The foot distraction device can show both the navicular and talar joint surfaces within the TN joint. Proper intraoperative visualization of the joints avoids screw surface penetration into the joint.

Bone loss or bone defects

Navicular fractures are often high-energy injuries. Thus, bone loss or bone defects may be present. If not recognized and addressed, these may change the curvature of the articular surfaces, resulting in incongruity.

Overly compressed lag screws should be avoided in this fracture as overcompression leads to the change in the shape of the navicular side of the joint, from dome-shaped to peak-shaped.

Defects should be filled with bone graft, or composite material.

In cases of high-energy trauma and poor bone quality, comminution is expected. Locking plates should be available, as screws alone may not be able to maintain the shape and stability of the reduction. In cases of severe comminution or bone loss, an external fixator or bridge plate may be used to maintain length and stability during the healing period.

Joint subluxation

Navicular fractures may be associated with tarsal dislocations or subluxations. Careful assessment of joint congruity is necessary after surgical fixation of the navicular. If any subluxation or instability is present, temporary fixation of the joints with smooth K-wires should be performed to provide stability.

Extension of the fixation construct to the cuneiforms may be necessary and is often well tolerated, as the navicular-cuboid joints are not critical motion segments. Extension across the TN joint should be avoided where possible, as TN motion is vital for normal foot function.

Missed associated injuries

As navicular fractures rarely occur in isolation, careful review of x-rays and CT scans as well as a thorough physical examination of the foot should be performed to avoid missing associated injuries of the foot, as navicular fractures rarely occur in isolation.

Complications

- Posttraumatic arthritis
- Avascular necrosis and collapse of the navicular bone
- Malunion
- Nonunion
- Instability of the TN joint
- Injury to the saphenous nerve (anteromedial approach)
- Injury to the anterior tibial neurovascular bundle, if dissecting medially beyond the extensor digitorum longus tendon
- Irritation of the posterior tibial tendon with medial screw placement in the plate and the anterior tibial tendon running above the plate (**Fig 6.3-9**)
- Loss of fixation
- Screw penetration into the joint
- Missed associated injuries of the foot (**Fig 6.3-10**).

6 Alternative techniques

Single or double screw fixation can be used in simple fracture patterns (**Fig 6.3-11**). Comminuted fractures require locking plates and bridge plates as collapse is expected (**Fig 6.3-12**). In severe cases with comminution, external fixation can be left in place (along with internal fixation) for 6–8 weeks.

Percutaneous fixation can be used in nondisplaced or non-comminuted fractures. This has the advantage of not damaging the blood supply to the navicular, as the vessels enter the bone peripherally and could be injured in a severe injury or with extensive dissection.

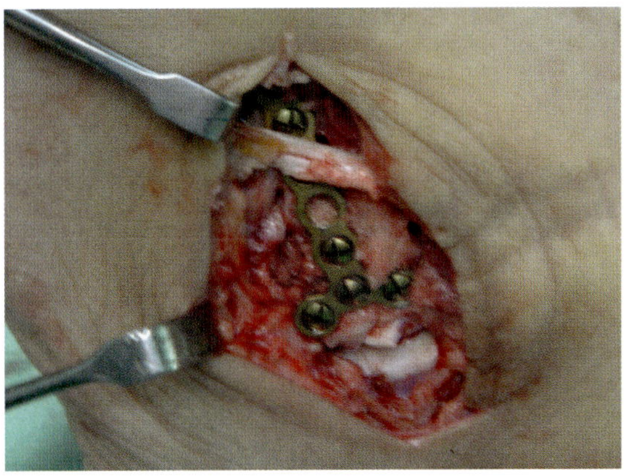

Fig 6.3-9 Anterior tibial tendon running above the plate.

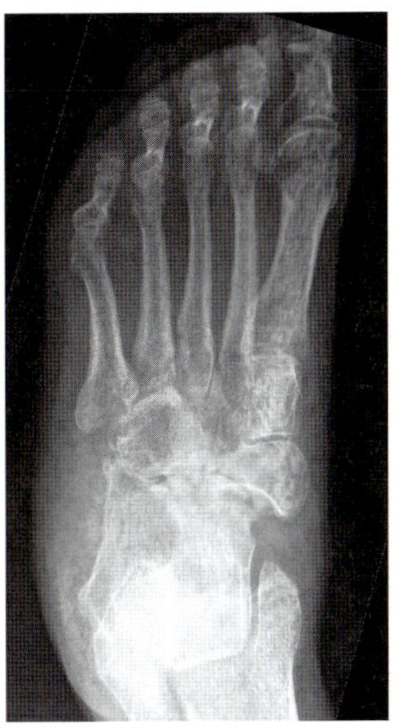

Fig 6.3-10 Example from a different case showing occult lesions associated with navicular fractures.

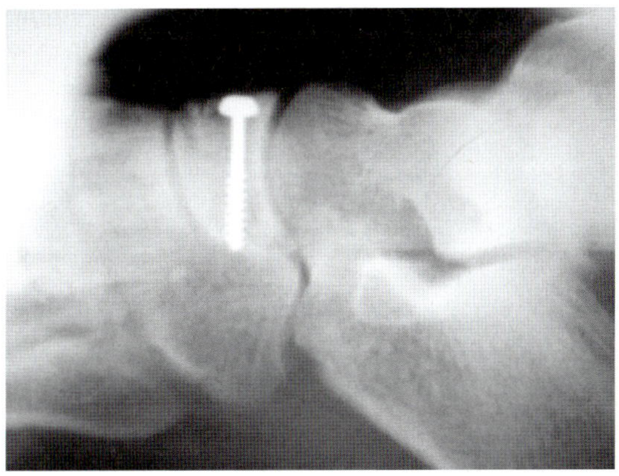

Fig 6.3-11 Example from a different case showing simple screw fixation.

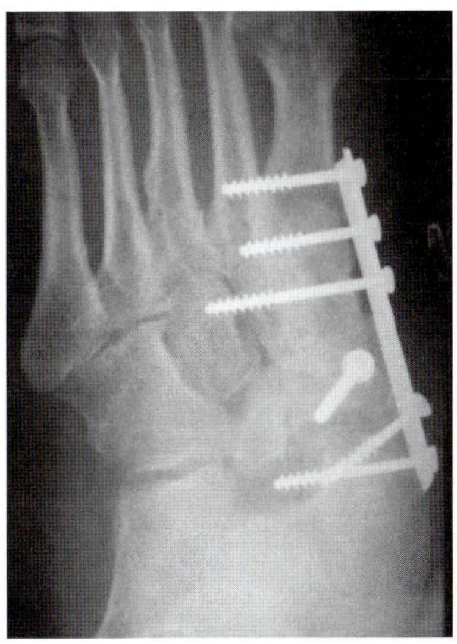

Fig 6.3-12 Example from a different case showing bridge plate.

Talonavicular fusion may be the best reconstruction option if comminuted compressed navicular fracture (with shortening) is not fixed acutely and a short medial column has resulted. The overall alignment of the foot must be restored. However, fusion of the TN joint leads to loss of motion at the TN joint (**Fig 6.3-13**) which results in significant loss of complex hindfoot and midfoot motion.

7 Postoperative management and rehabilitation

At the first postoperative visit (1–2 weeks) the splint is replaced with a nonweight-bearing Velcro boot until x-rays confirm fracture consolidation, which is usually seen at 6–8 weeks (**Fig 6.3-14**).

Physical therapy may begin in week 4 with gentle passive and active limited range of motion and pool exercises (assuming there are no K-wires left as stabilization hardware, in which case physical therapy should be delayed until the wires are removed).

Bridge plating and implant removal

If the need for added stability requires bridge plating of navicular fractures, early removal for rehabilitation and return of motion in the TN and adjacent joints for complex hindfoot motion is required.

Generally, bridge plates are removed 4–6 months postoperatively. In severely comminuted or unstable injury patterns requiring temporary external fixation, the external fixator is removed 6–8 weeks postoperatively.

With these injuries, there is a broad range of instability at the TN articulation. Despite a great deal of complexity of these injuries and a relatively high risk of complication, good outcomes are possible (**Fig 6.3-15**).

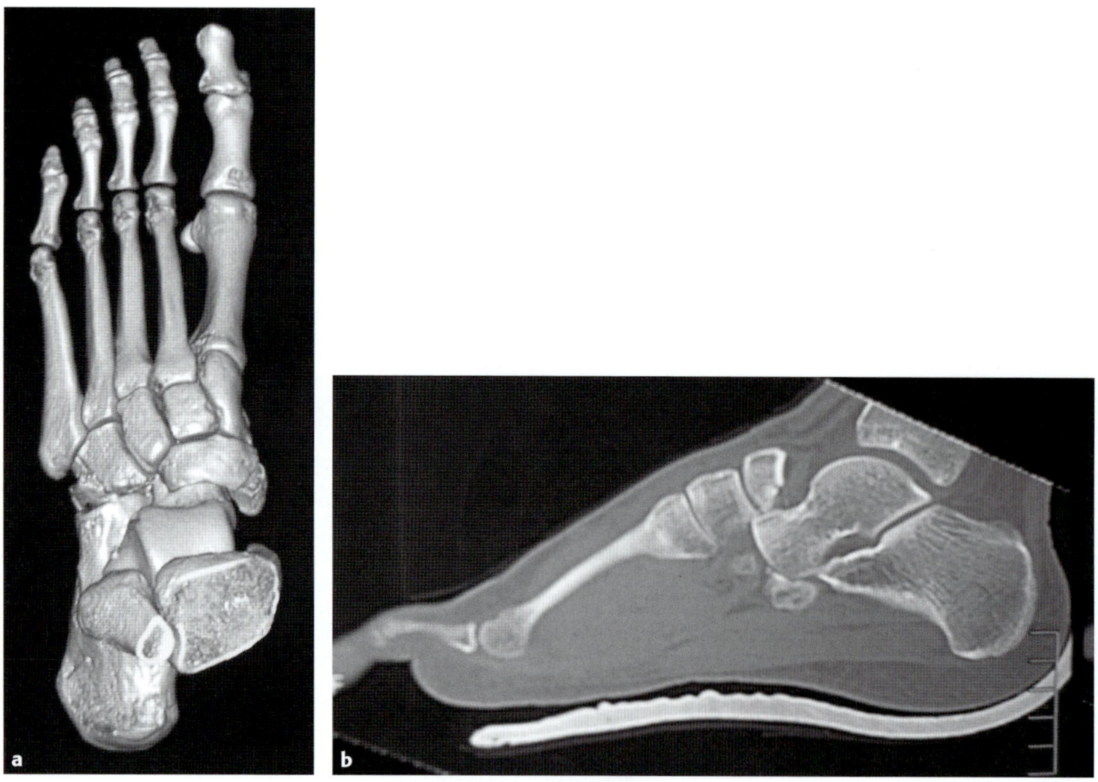

Fig 6.3-13a–b Example from a different case showing a neglected TN fracture dislocation and cuboid fracture at 6 weeks. Fusion was used to reconstruct the medial column and cuboid reconstruction.

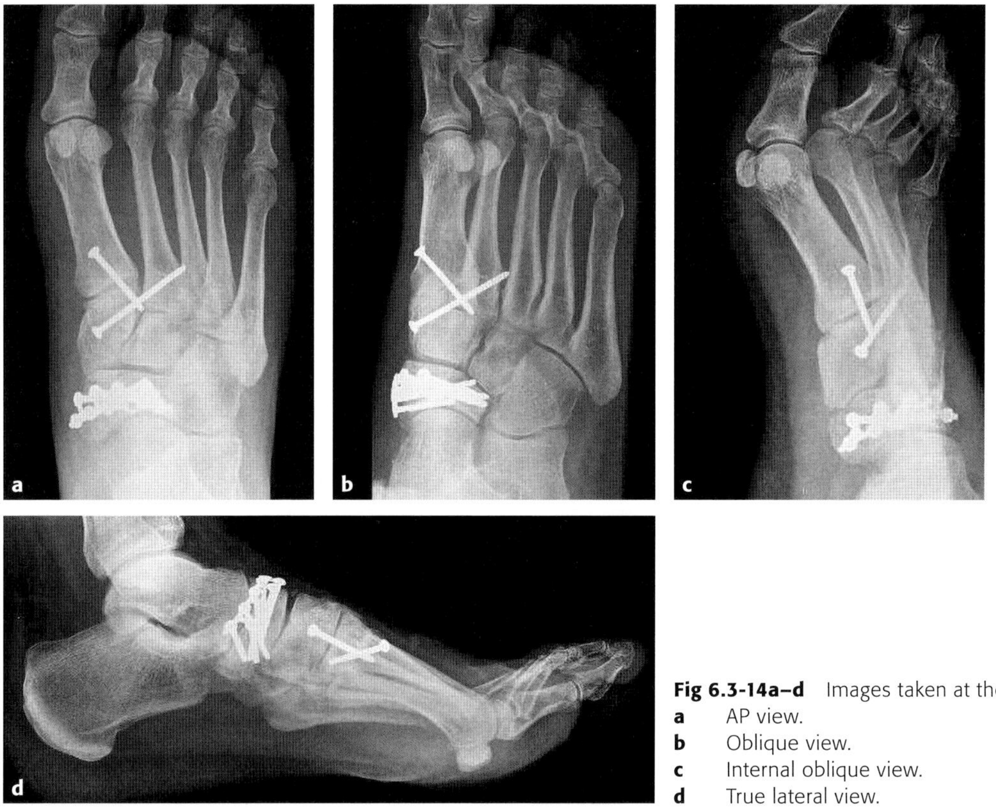

Fig 6.3-14a–d Images taken at the 6-week follow-up.
a AP view.
b Oblique view.
c Internal oblique view.
d True lateral view.

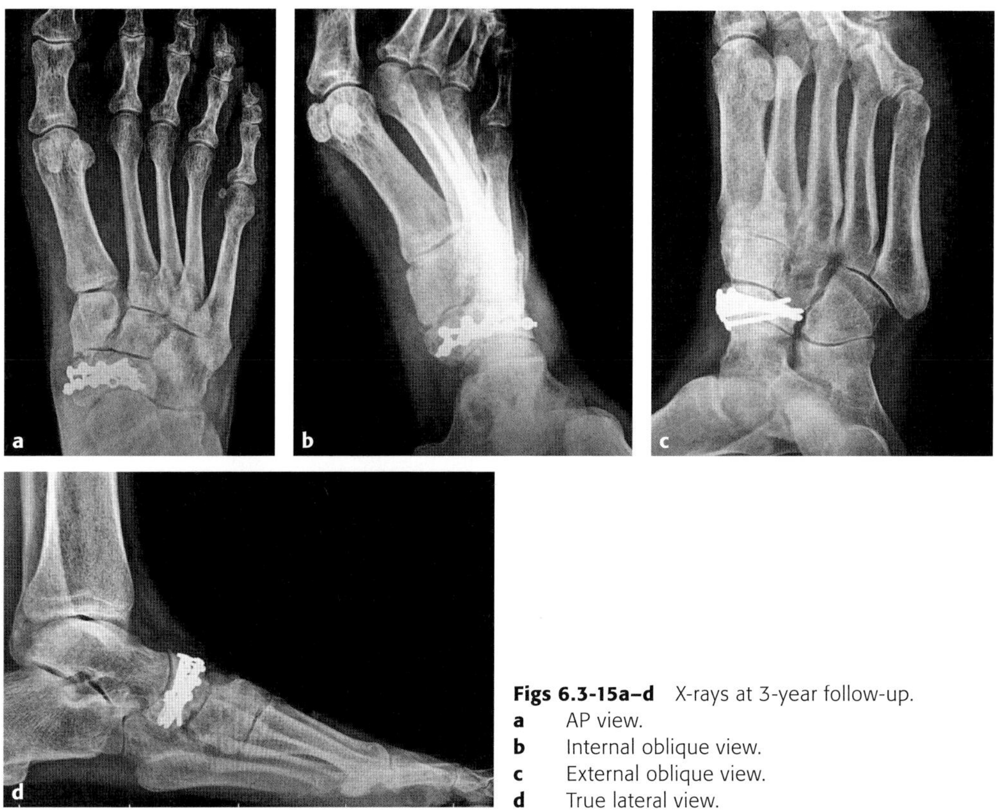

Figs 6.3-15a–d X-rays at 3-year follow-up.
a AP view.
b Internal oblique view.
c External oblique view.
d True lateral view.

8 Recommended reading

Penner MJ. Late reconstruction after navicular fracture. *Foot Ankle Clin.* 2006 Mar;11(1):105–119.

Pinney SJ, Sangeorzan BJ. Fractures of the tarsal bones. *Orthop Clin North Am.* 2001 Jan;32(1):21–33.

Rammelt S, Zwipp H. [Joint-preserving correction of Chopart joint malunions]. *Unfallchirurg.* 2014 Sep;117(9):785–790. German

Rammelt S, Schepers T. Chopart injuries: when to fix and when to fuse? *Foot Ankle Clin.* 2017 Mar;22(1):163–180.

Richter M, Thermann H, Huefner T, et al. Chopart joint fracture-dislocation: initial open reduction provides better outcome than closed reduction. *Foot Ankle Int.* 2004 May;25(5):340–348.

Sangeorzan BJ, Benirschke SK, Mosca V, et al. Displaced intra-articular fractures of the tarsal navicular. *J Bone Joint Surg Am.* 1989 Dec;71(10):1504–1510.

Schildhauer TA, Nork SE, Sangeorzan BJ. Temporary bridge plating of the medial column in severe midfoot injuries. *J Orthop Trauma.* 2003 Aug;17(7):513–520.

Simon JP, Van Delm I, Fabry G. Fracture dislocation of the tarsal navicular. *Acta Orthop Belg.* 1993;59(2):222–224.

Swords MP, Schramski M, Switzer K, et al. Chopart fractures and dislocations. *Foot Ankle Clin.* 2008 Dec;13(4):679–693.

6.4 Cuboid nutcracker fracture

Juan Bernardo Gerstner Garces, Andrew K Sands

1 Case description

A 51-year-old healthy man was involved in a motorcycle accident. He presented 3 days later to the clinic. Initial treatment was immobilization in a plaster splint and referral to a foot and ankle specialist. The physical examination revealed that he had a superficial wound over the distal part of the right posterior leg. The Achilles tendon was intact. There was edema about the foot, with plantar, medial and lateral ecchymosis at the midfoot, and excruciating pain with adduction/abduction movements (**Fig 6.4-1**). He also reported distal parasthesias along the cutaneous sensory zone of the superficial peroneal nerve.

X-rays showed a comminuted navicular fracture and a compression type cuboid fracture (nutcracker) (**Fig 6.4-2**). The injured leg was placed into a padded splint until the edema resolved. A computed tomographic (CT) scan was performed (**Fig 6.4-3**).

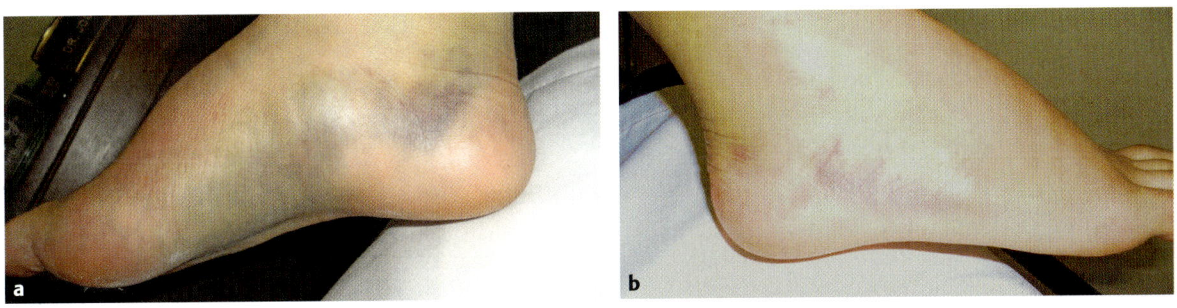

Fig 6.4-1a–b Ecchymosis indicative of a severe injury.
a Medial view.
b Lateral view.

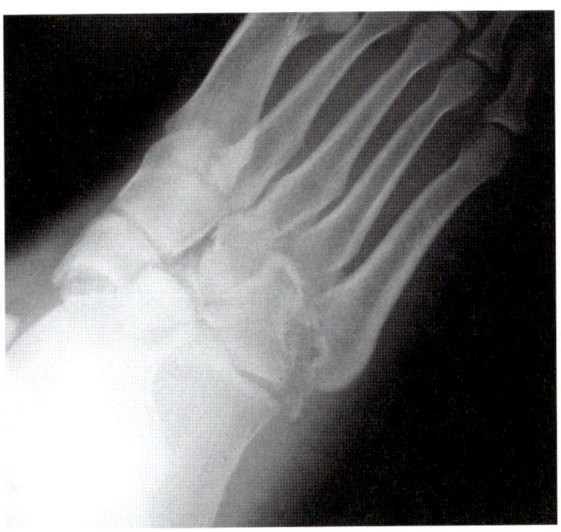

Fig 6.4-2 Preoperative AP x-ray of foot showing navicular and cuboid fractures.

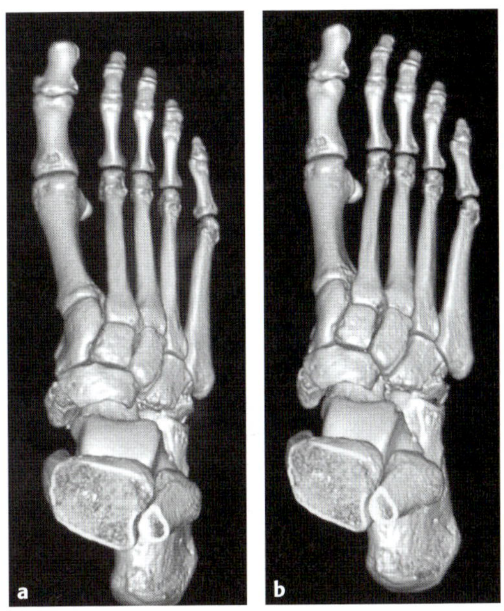

Fig 6.4-3a–b A 3D CT scans of the injuries. The navicular and cuboid fracture lines are clearly seen.

2 Preoperative planning

As cuboid fractures rarely occur in isolation, thorough examination of the whole midfoot is necessary. Most cuboid fractures are associated with medial column injuries.

Indications for surgery

Unstable injuries of both medial and lateral columns of the midfoot require surgery. Preoperative planning includes a sketch of the navicular (see chapter 6.3) and a sketch of the lateral column fracture (**Fig 6.4-4a**). The need for bone graft to fill any defect in the two bones can be estimated by evaluating the degree of compression or comminution (**Fig 6.4-4b–c**).

3 Operating room setup

Patient positioning	• Supine, with the operative leg elevated on a bump
Anesthesia options	• General anesthesia, often supplemented with spinal or regional nerve block
C-arm location	• Screen of the C-arm should be placed so the surgeon can monitor reduction from the medial and lateral side and obtain AP and lateral views
Tourniquet	• Optional, applied to thigh
Tips	• Foot is placed on a bump • A large bump should also be placed under the ipsilateral buttock which will internally rotate the foot, allowing easier access to the lateral column

For illustrations and overview of anesthetic considerations, see chapter 1.

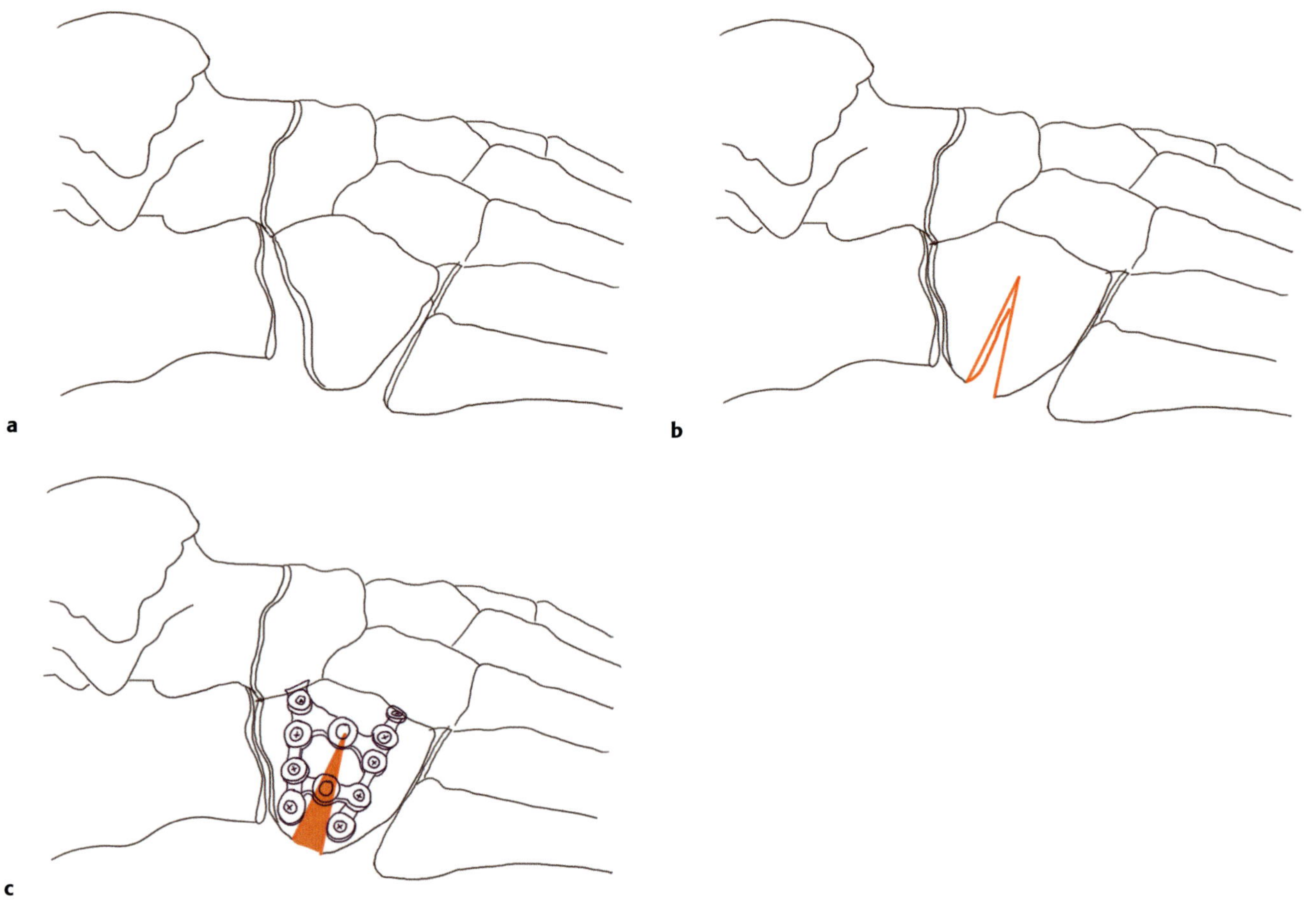

Fig 6.4-4a–c Preoperative plan.

Equipment

- Large curved clamp, useful to reduce the navicular fracture
- Smooth K-wires
- Foot distraction device (two devices if there are medial and lateral column injuries): to restore the exact length of each column and permit visualization of the articular surfaces to obtain an anatomical reduction
- Point-to-point reduction (Weber) clamps
- Lamina spreader
- Cuboid and navicular locking compression plates (LCP) or variable angle locking compression plate (VA LCP) with 2.7 VAL system and independent cortex screws
- Bone harvesting set (including chisels, periosteal elevators, and bone trephines)
- Power equipment (drill, wire driver, saw with smooth and thin sagittal blade)

4 Surgical procedure

Simultaneous approaches are made to the medial and lateral aspects of the foot:

- Direct lateral approach
- Dorsomedial approach

Fixation of the cuboid fracture

The cuboid injury is addressed using a direct lateral approach. Careful dissection of the subcutaneous tissue is made to avoid the sural and superficial peroneal nerves (**Fig 6.4-5**). The fascia over the extensor brevis muscle is released and the muscle belly is elevated. This allows access to the cuboid and the calcaneocuboid joint. In the case presented, dislocation of the calcaneocuboid joint can be seen (**Fig 6.4-6**).

The foot distraction device is placed with a pin in the distal area of the calcaneus and at the base of the fourth MT. Distraction is applied to restore the correct length of the lateral column. The articular surfaces are carefully reconstructed and held with a series of small K-wires. After the articular surfaces have been reconstructed the overall length of the cuboid is assessed.

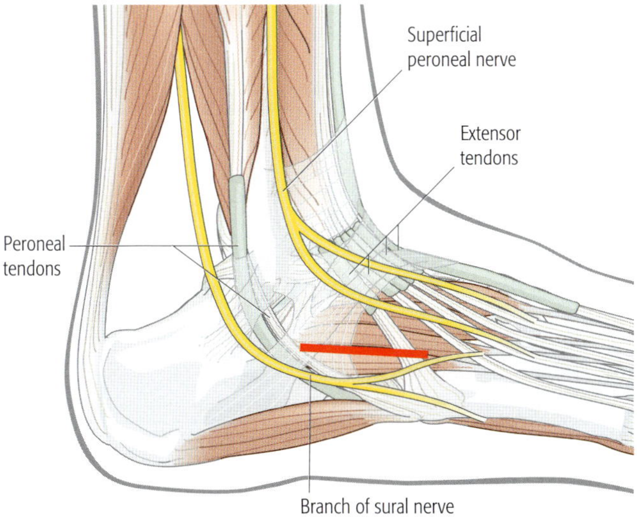

Fig 6.4-5 Anatomical outline of the lateral approach.

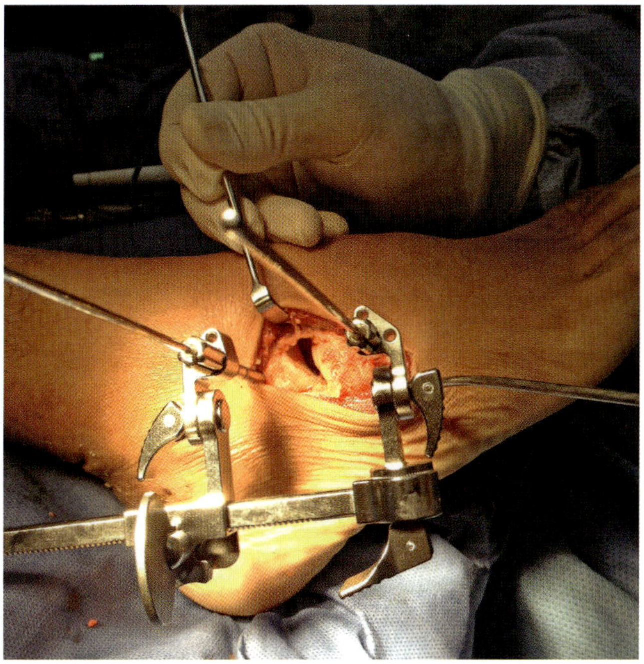

Fig 6.4-6 The cuboid fracture is visible through a lateral approach to the cuboid. A distractor is present providing improved visualization of the calcaneocuboid articulation and restores lateral column length.

As the cuboid fracture is a compression fracture, the bone is often impacted in the central body of the cuboid. If no fracture line is evident, an osteotome or sagittal saw cut can be used to divide the cuboid. A lamina spreader is placed into the created fissure and expanded gently. Care must be taken to avoid deforming the cuboid central region. This pushes the two articular portions of the bone outward to match the calcaneocuboid and metatarsal-cuboid articular surfaces (**Fig 6.4-7**). Two smooth K-wires can be inserted, and the spreader can be put through the middle part of the plate to hold the reduction while the cuboid locking plate is applied.

Often a large void is present in the body of the cuboid as a result of the injury compression forces. Once the plate is secured, the bone defect is filled with bone graft (**Fig 6.4-8**).

Any provisional external fixation is now removed. If the cuboid is highly comminuted, an external fixator may be left in place for 6 weeks postoperatively to maintain lateral column length during the early period of healing.

Intraoperative x-rays are obtained to ensure that reduction and hardware position are correct (**Fig 6.4-9**). The wound is closed in layers and a well-padded splint is applied.

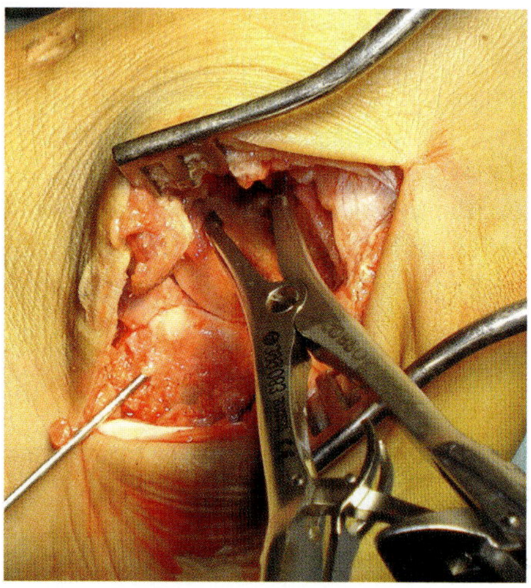

Fig 6.4-7 A lamina spreader is used as a reduction tool.

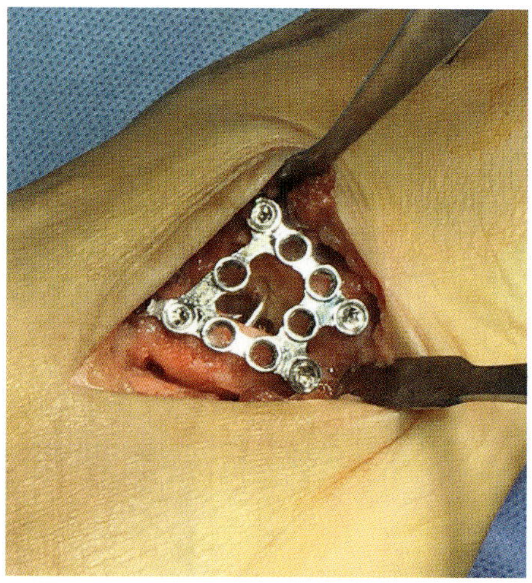

Fig 6.4-8 Plate in place on the cuboid.

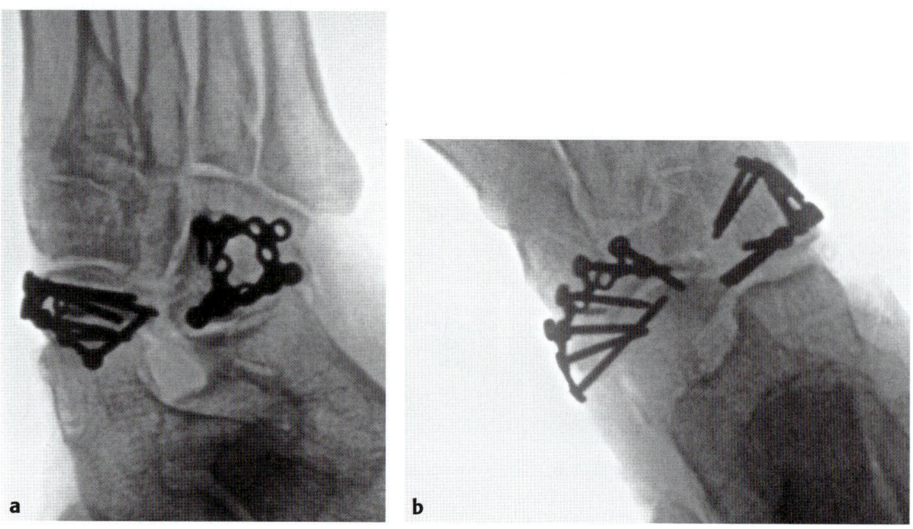

Fig 6.4-9a–b X-rays with plates in place.
a Oblique view.
b AP view.

Fixation of the navicular fracture

A dorsomedial approach from the base of the first metatarsal (MT) to the neck of the talus is used. Careful dissection of the nerves and vessels is carried out and retraction of the tendons of the extensor hallucis longus and brevis, tibialis anterior, and posterior are held by blunt (Hohmann) retractors. The talonavicular and navicular-medial cuneiform capsule is opened and retracted to carefully inspect the articular cartilage once the hematoma is cleared. Comminution is now evaluated and the need for bone graft (autograft from the calcaneal tuber or allograft) is added to the surgical plan.

The foot distraction device is placed so that it does not interfere with the view of the reduction. Distraction is done smoothly and progressively to ensure that ligamentotaxis occurs and perfect reduction of both joint surfaces is accomplished. Manipulation of the fragments can be done by using smooth K-wires as joysticks. Once final reduction is obtained, a curved reduction clamp is positioned and two smooth K-wires are directed to cross the fracture line as provisional fixation (**Fig 6.4-10**). Bone graft is added after final reduction and before the plate is placed, thus preventing the plate from impeding placement of the bone graft.

The navicular plate is cut to length, contoured, then positioned over the top and around the corners of the bone. The first screw may be through the plate or outside the plate and should be a compression screw. However, care must be taken to avoid overcompressing the lag screw. Excessive compression results in deformation of the spherical shape of the proximal navicular articular surface. After the first screw has been inserted, the remaining locking screws are positioned to hold reduction and allow early mobilization. Additional skin incisions can be made to insert screws through the farthest holes of the plate (**Fig 6.4-11**).

Before the distraction is released, careful inspection of all joints is made to ensure there has not been any screw penetration into the joint space. If any instability is noted after distraction is completed, a smooth K-wire is used as supplemental joint stabilization; or bridge plating may be used.

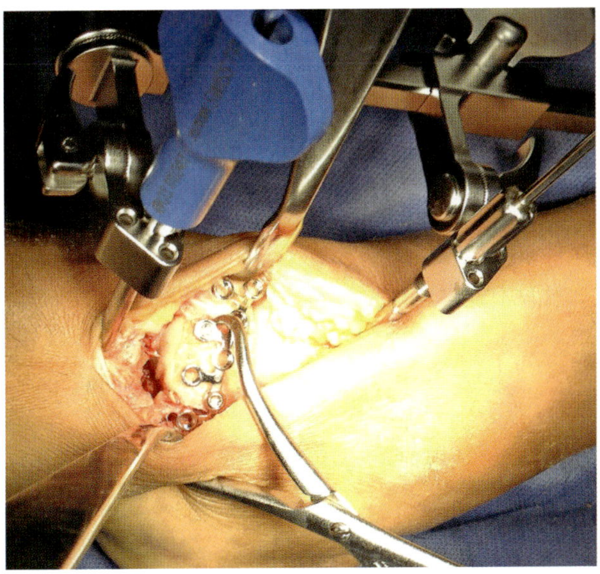

Fig 6.4-10 Dorsomedial approach with the foot distraction device in place.

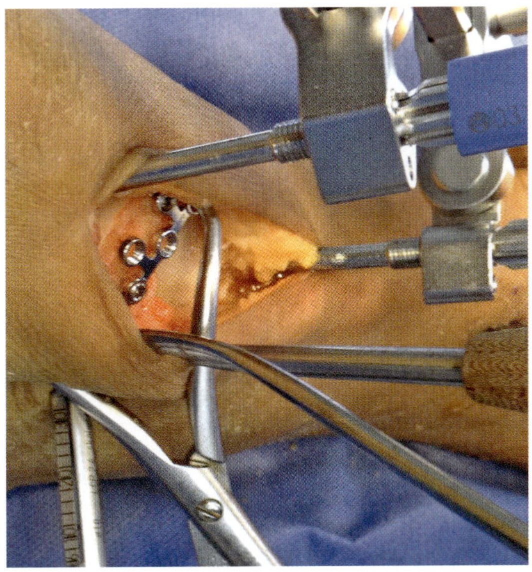

Fig 6.4-11 Dorsomedial approach with the plate in place.

5 Pitfalls and complications

Pitfalls

- Neglected cuboid fractures and medial column pathology leads to an abducted rigid foot, requiring medial and lateral column reconstruction (**Fig 6.4-12**).
- Malreduction of the articulation between the cuboid and the base of the fourth and fifth metatarsal. Anatomical reconstruction of this highly mobile joint is necessary, as no reliable salvage procedure for this complication exists.
- Lisfranc joint injury needs to be ruled out when treating cuboid fractures.
- Comminution is often seen but distraction and ligamentotaxis techniques usually stabilize small fragments that cannot be purchased by screws. If any instability is found after the distractor is released, K-wires through the joint are placed for temporary joint stabilization.
- Incorrect placement of incisions prevents proper access to both bones without damage to the intervening soft tissues (**Fig 6.4-13**).

Complications

- Injury to the sural and superficial peroneal nerve
- Damage to the extensor brevis muscle
- Irritation of the peroneal tendons
- Loss of fixation
- Malunion
- Nonunion
- Intraarticular hardware
- Posttraumatic calcaneocuboid joint arthritis
- Posttraumatic cuboid/MT joint arthritis
- Collapse of the cuboid
- Missed associated injuries of the foot

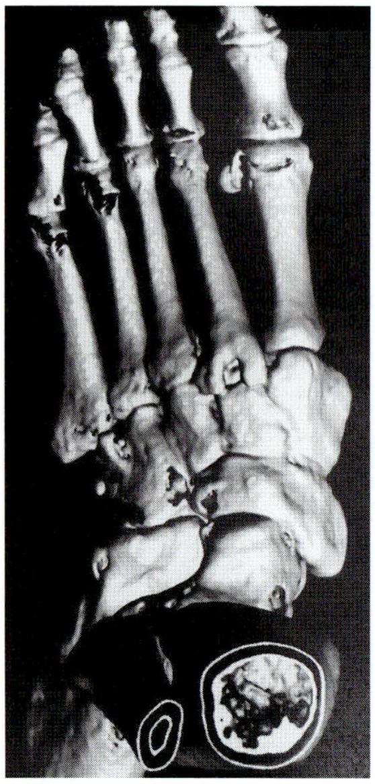

Fig 6.4-12 Example from a different case showing 3D image of a neglected hindfoot injury with displacement and abduction malalignment.

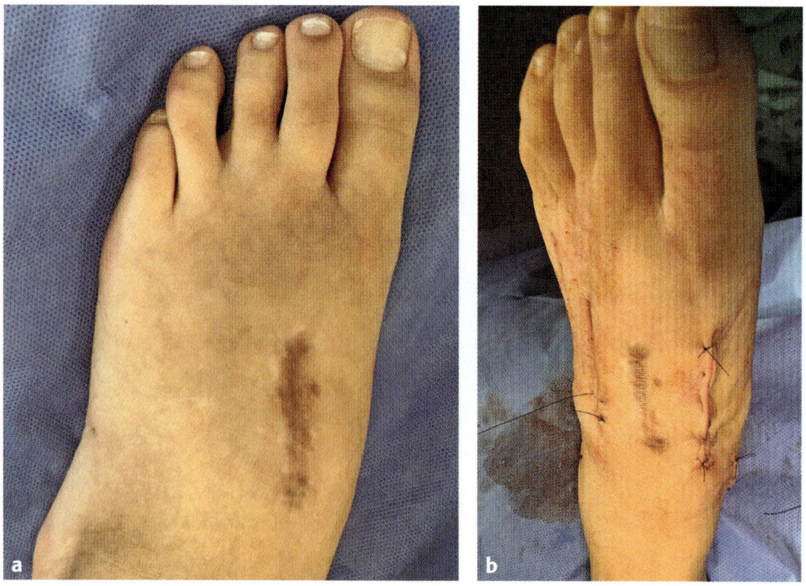

Fig 6.4-13a–b Example from a different case showing placement of incisions.

6 Alternative techniques

Bridge plates

When comminution is too severe to appropriately reconstruct, or bone quality is too poor to achieve appropriate fixation, bridge plates and supplementary K-wires should be used to maintain the length of the column (**Fig 6.4-14**).

External fixation

In the presence of severe soft-tissue injury including extensive fracture blisters or compartmental syndrome, medial and lateral external fixators can hold the length of the columns while the soft tissues recover. This may also be used as an alternative method to support the internal fixation and maintain the length until the fracture stabilizes.

7 Postoperative management and rehabilitation

If bridge plates are used, they are usually removed between 4 and 6 months after open reduction and internal fixation. If an external fixator is used to protect the reconstruction, it is usually removed 6–8 weeks postoperatively.

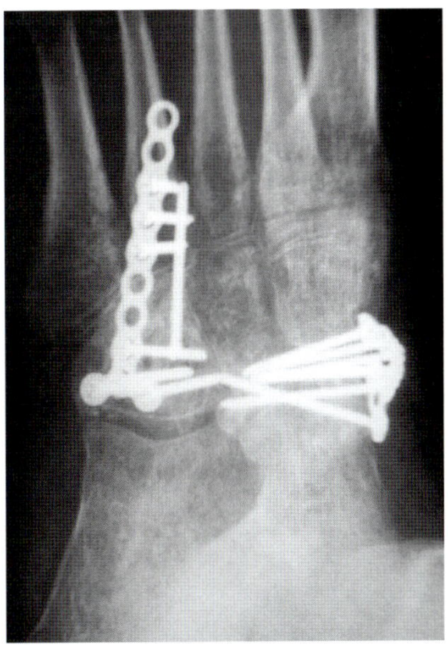

Fig 6.4-14 Example from a different case: X-ray showing alternative hardware arrangement with bridging plate in place across the cuboid/ MT joint.

8 Recommended reading

Benirschke SK, Meinberg E, Anderson SA, et al. Fractures and dislocations of the midfoot: Lisfranc and Chopart injuries. *J Bone Joint Surg Am.* 2012 Jul 18;94(14):1325–1337.

Fenton P, Al-Nammari S, Blundell C, et al. The patterns of injury and management of cuboid fractures: a retrospective case series. *Bone Joint J.* 2016 Jul;98-b(7):1003–1008.

Hermel MB, Gershon-Cohen J. The nutcracker fracture of the cuboid by indirect violence. *Radiology.* 1953 Jun;60(6):850–854.

Rammelt S, Schepers T. Chopart injuries: when to fix and when to fuse? *Foot Ankle Clin.* 2017 Mar;22(1):163–180.

Sangeorzan BJ, Swiontkowski MF. Displaced fractures of the cuboid. *J Bone Joint Surg Br.* 1990 May;72(3):376–378.

Swords MP, Schramski M, Switzer K, et al. Chopart fractures and dislocations. *Foot Ankle Clin.* 2008 Dec;13(4):679–693.

Weber M, Locher S. Reconstruction of the cuboid in compression fractures: short to midterm results in 12 patients. *Foot Ankle Int.* 2002 Nov;23(11):1008–1013.

6.5 Chopart dislocation with compromised soft tissue

John R Shank

1 Case description

A 42-year-old man attempted a 4.6 m jump on a motor-cross bike and landed forcefully on his left foot. He presented 5 days after the injury with complaints of left foot pain, deformity, and numbness. The clinical examination revealed a large fracture blister along the dorsum of his foot with fracture blisters and multiple abrasions noted medially (**Fig 6.5-1**). He had mild numbness along the superficial peroneal nerve (SPN) branches but was otherwise neurovascularly intact.

X-rays of the left foot showed a fracture dislocation of the talonavicular (TN) joint and a minimally displaced cuboid fracture (**Fig 6.5-2**). A computed tomographic (CT) scan was performed after initial external fixator placement for 3D assessment of the fractures of the Chopart joints (**Fig 6.5-3**).

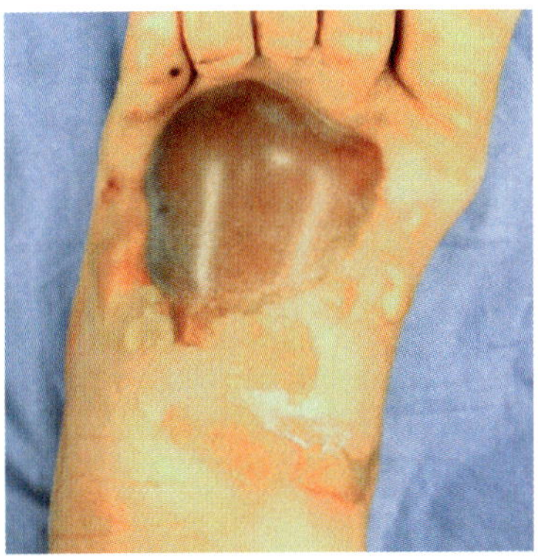

Fig 6.5-1 Clinical photograph obtained on initial presentation, 5 days following the injury, showing excessive swelling and fracture blisters.

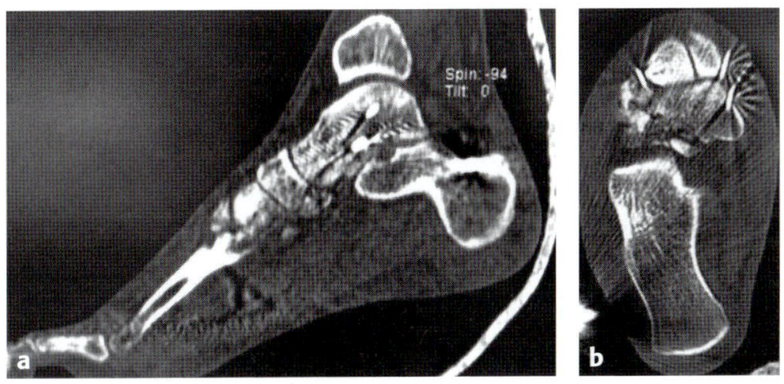

Fig 6.5-3a–b The CT images after external fixator placement.
a Sagittal view shows a congruent TN joint reduction with a displaced navicular body injury.
b Axial view shows lateral navicular comminution.

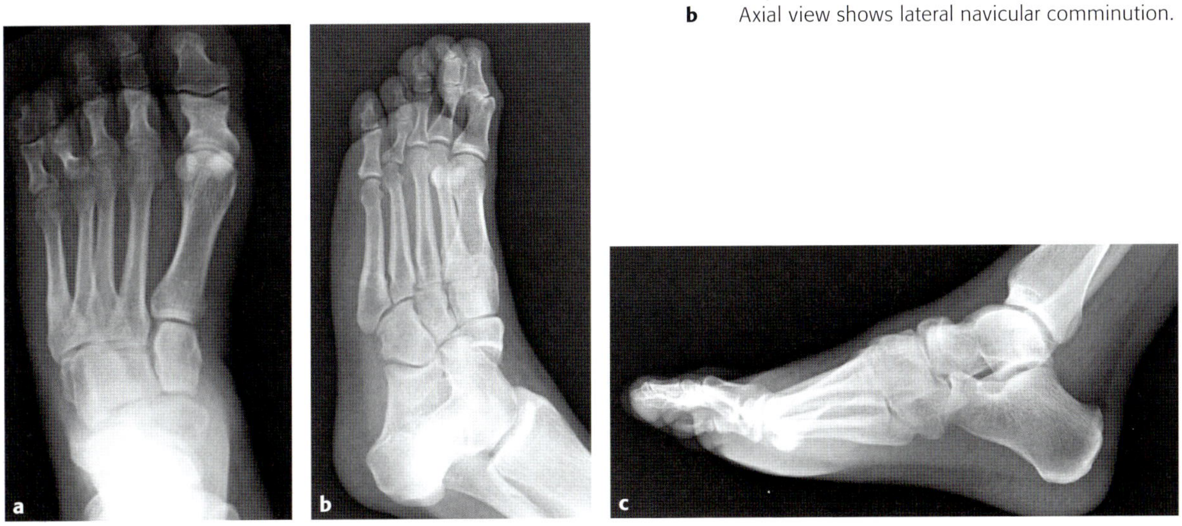

Fig 6.5-2a–c Postinjury images reveal a fracture dislocation of the TN joint and a minimally displaced cuboid fracture.
a AP view.
b Oblique view.
c Lateral view.

2 Preoperative planning

Indications for surgery

- Dislocation of the TN joint
- Multifragmentary fracture of the navicular
- Instability through Chopart joints
- Open injuries

Treatment options

Treatment options depend upon the severity of injury to the soft tissues and ability to maintain joint alignment.

External fixation

Based on the severity of the soft-tissue injury and the presence of fracture blisters, initial external fixation was favored for this injury. External fixation allows for restoration of column length and reduction of dislocations and provides stability while the soft tissues recover, allowing subsequent formal open surgical treatment. Generally, external fixation is used as part of a staged treatment plan.

Open reduction and internal fixation

Talonavicular joint alignment without subluxation and no soft-tissue damage allows for primary open reduction and internal fixation (ORIF) without the need for external fixation first. Typically, open reduction of the medial column injury precedes treatment of the lateral column injury. These surgeries are often performed in a staged fashion. An appropriate preoperative plan should be performed before proceeding with ORIF (**Fig 6.5-4**).

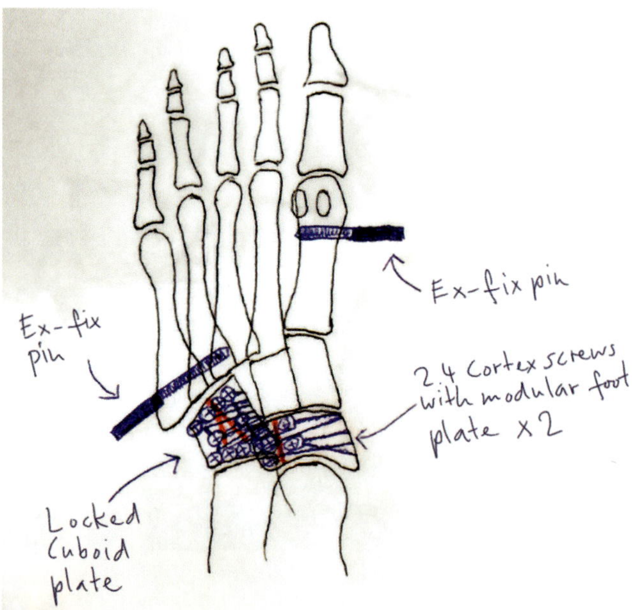

Fig 6.5-4 Preoperative plan.

In this case, there was excessive swelling and fracture blisters. Damage to the soft tissues required staged treatment. First, external fixation was placed and ORIF was delayed until the soft tissues had recovered.

3 Operating room setup

Patient positioning	• Supine with bump under the ipsilateral buttock
Anesthesia options	• General anesthesia, often supplemented with a peripheral nerve block
C-arm location	• Positioned toward the foot of the operative table to allow for easy visualization by the surgeon
Tourniquet	• Applied to the thigh
Tips	• Correction of the medial and lateral columns of the foot feature prominently in this fracture reconstruction

For illustrations and overview of anesthetic considerations, see chapter 1.

Equipment

- Headlamp for visualization
- Elevators and dental scalers
- External fixator or distractor
- K-wire set
- Modular implants with minifragment screws
- Locking plates and screws
- Allograft bone graft

Size of instruments and implants may vary according to the anatomy of the patient and the characteristics of the injury.

4 Surgical procedure

The patient is positioned toward the distal end of the OR table. An elevated foam ramp is placed under the leg. This allows access to both sides of the foot and improves the ability to obtain intraoperative x-rays.

The medial approach chosen is based on the fracture pattern and anatomy of the navicular. The approach to the medial column can be through a medial utility incision; through an anterolateral incision; or through dual approaches.

The medial utility incision is longitudinal and located between the posterior tibial and anterior tibial tendons (**Fig 6.5-5**). The saphenous nerve and vessels should be protected throughout this approach. Both the TN and naviculocuneiform joints can be visualized through this approach.

The anterolateral approach is longitudinal and located lateral to the dorsal neurovascular bundle and medial to the lateral branch of the SPN (**Fig 6.5-6**).

The lateral axial approach is used to expose the cuboid. It is longitudinal and located dorsal to the peroneal tendons and sural nerve with the extensor digitorum brevis elevated superiorly allowing visualization of the cuboid body (**Fig 6.5-7**). Both the calcaneocuboid and the articulations of the cuboid and the fourth and fifth metatarsal (MT) bases can be visualized through this approach.

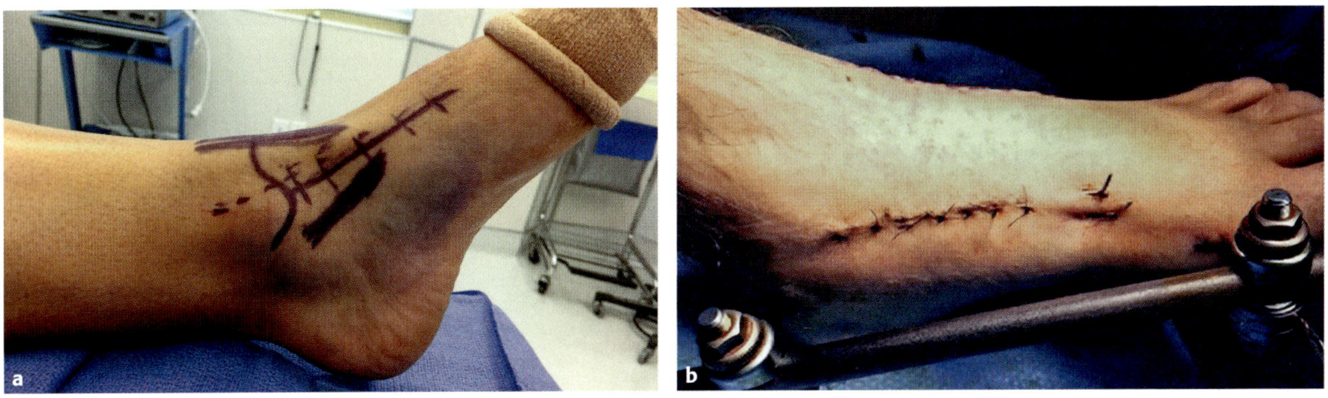

Fig 6.5-5a–b The medial side, approach to the medial column and navicular.
a The medial utility approach to the navicular located between the posterior tibial and anterior tibial tendons.
b If an external fixator or distractor is used, it is placed plantar to the incision, spanning from the calcaneus to the first MT.

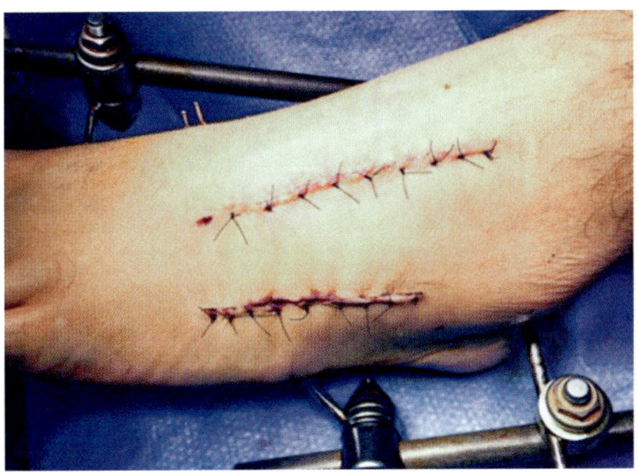

Fig 6.5-6 The anterolateral approach to the navicular located lateral to the dorsal neurovascular bundle and medial to the lateral branch of the SPN.

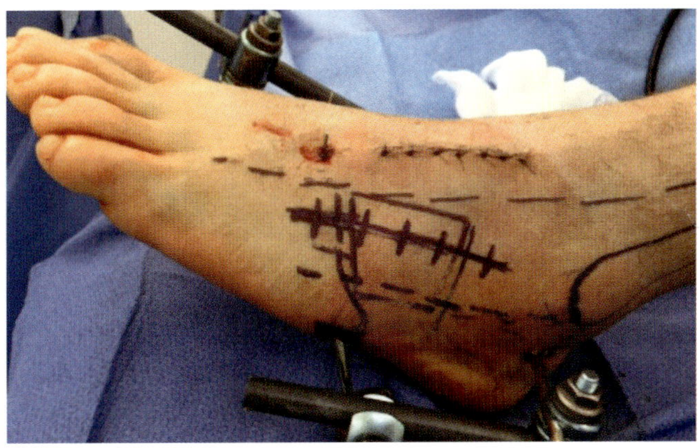

Fig 6.5-7 Approach to the cuboid, dorsal to the sural nerve and peroneal tendons and plantar to the lateral branch of the SPN.

For Chopart joint injuries with severe soft-tissue injury, a temporizing bicolumnar external fixator should be placed to allow for soft-tissue recovery before definitive ORIF (**Fig 6.5-8**). The fixator is a useful intraoperative tool to disimpact articular fragments, allowing for improved joint visualization and restoration of medial and lateral column length. An intraoperative distraction device can be applied at the time of definitive ORIF to assist in reduction. For this case, a bicolumnar external fixator was applied and the TN dislocation was temporarily reduced with K-wires (**Fig 6.5-9**). The soft tissues could then recover for several weeks.

Usually the medial column injury is addressed first. However, this patient had a significant soft-tissue injury medially which prompted treatment of the cuboid fracture first.

The lateral column and cuboid injury are approached through a longitudinal lateral incision over the cuboid body, dorsal to the peroneal tendons and sural nerve. The extensor digitorum brevis is subperiosteally elevated dorsally and protected with a blunt retractor. Following the preoperative plan, a lateral approach to the cuboid was performed with articular restoration of the joints between the cuboid and the fourth and fifth MTs (**Fig 6.5-10**). The external fixator is distracted and used for improved visualization of the lateral column. Next, the joints are reduced with K-wires under direct visualization. Care should be taken to restore the articular anatomy and length, rotation, and alignment of the lateral column. Bone grafting of the cuboid defect seen after distraction and reduction and is routinely performed before hardware is placed, as the hardware may block access to the defect. Finally, plate and screw fixation is performed and final reduction is confirmed under direct visualization and C-arm imaging. K-wires may be cut flush with the cortex and retained as needed to ensure articular reduction of smaller fragments (**Fig 6.5-11**).

In this patient, the navicular injury was treated 1 week after the lateral column injury due to the presence of a severe soft-tissue injury.

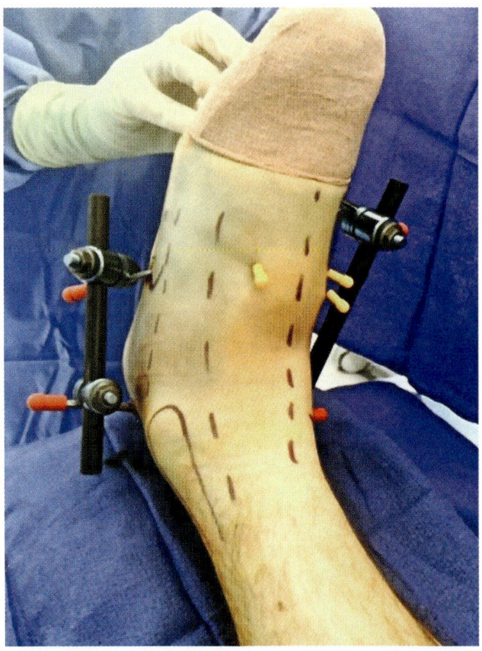

Fig 6.5-8 Bicolumnar external fixation allows for reduction of the medial and lateral column injury.

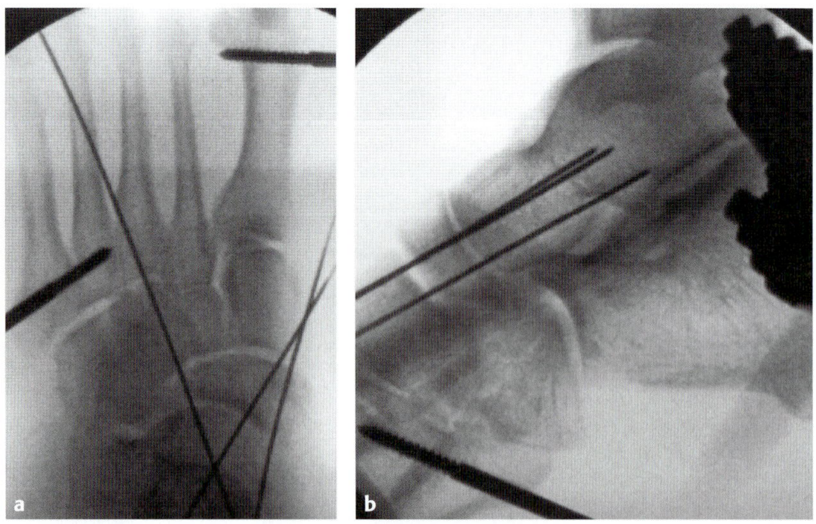

Fig 6.5-9a–b External fixator placement. External fixation and K-wires are used to reduce the TN fracture dislocation and to restore length and alignment of the medial and lateral columns.

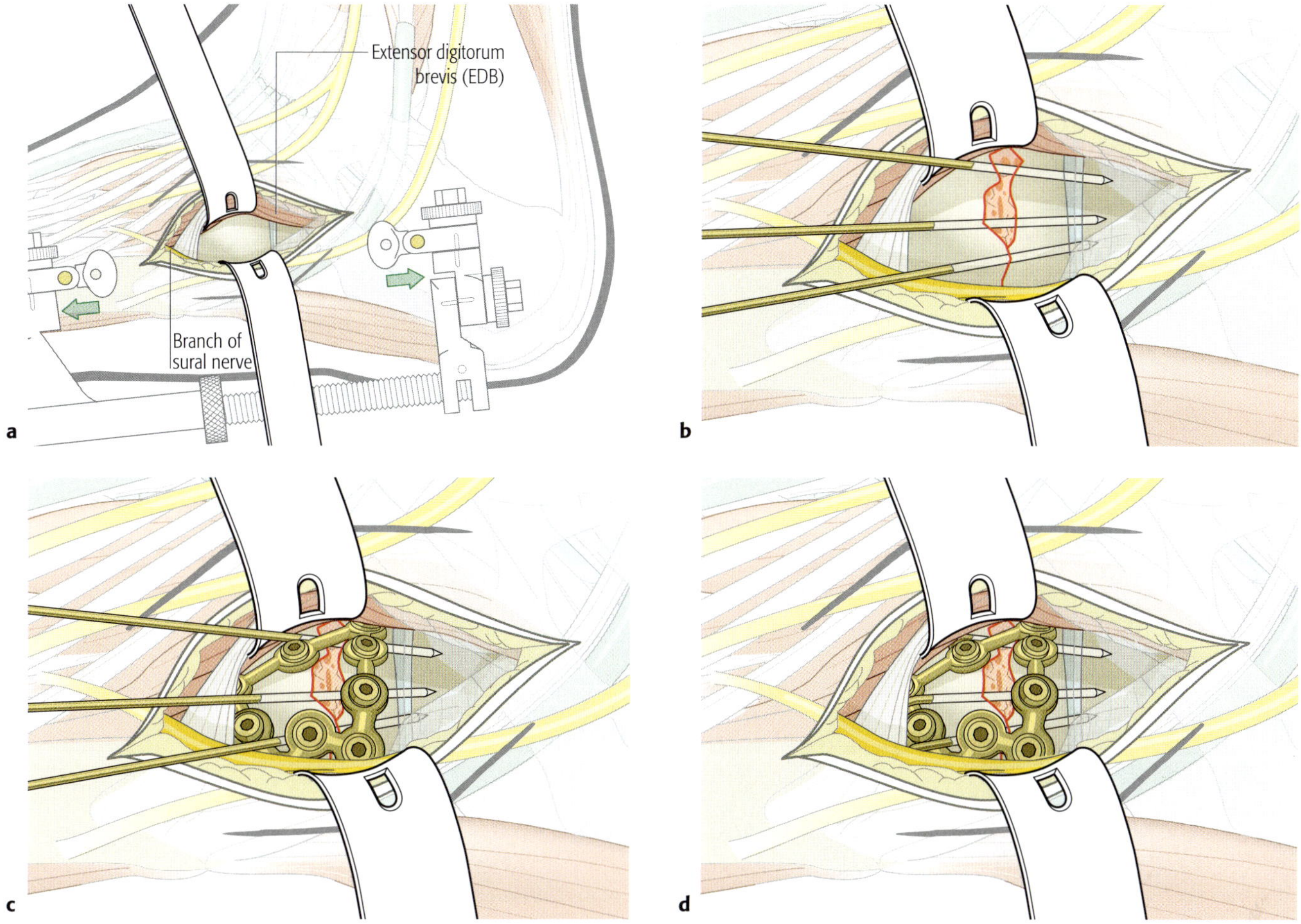

a b c d

Fig 6.5-10a–d Lateral approach to the cuboid.

a The incision is located dorsal to the peroneal tendons and sural nerve and plantar to the lateral branch of the SPN.

b The articular surface of the cuboid. The fourth and fifth MT joints are reduced with K-wires and defects are bone grafted.

c A cuboid plate is placed proximal to or over the K-wires.

d The K-wires are cut and contoured around the plate.

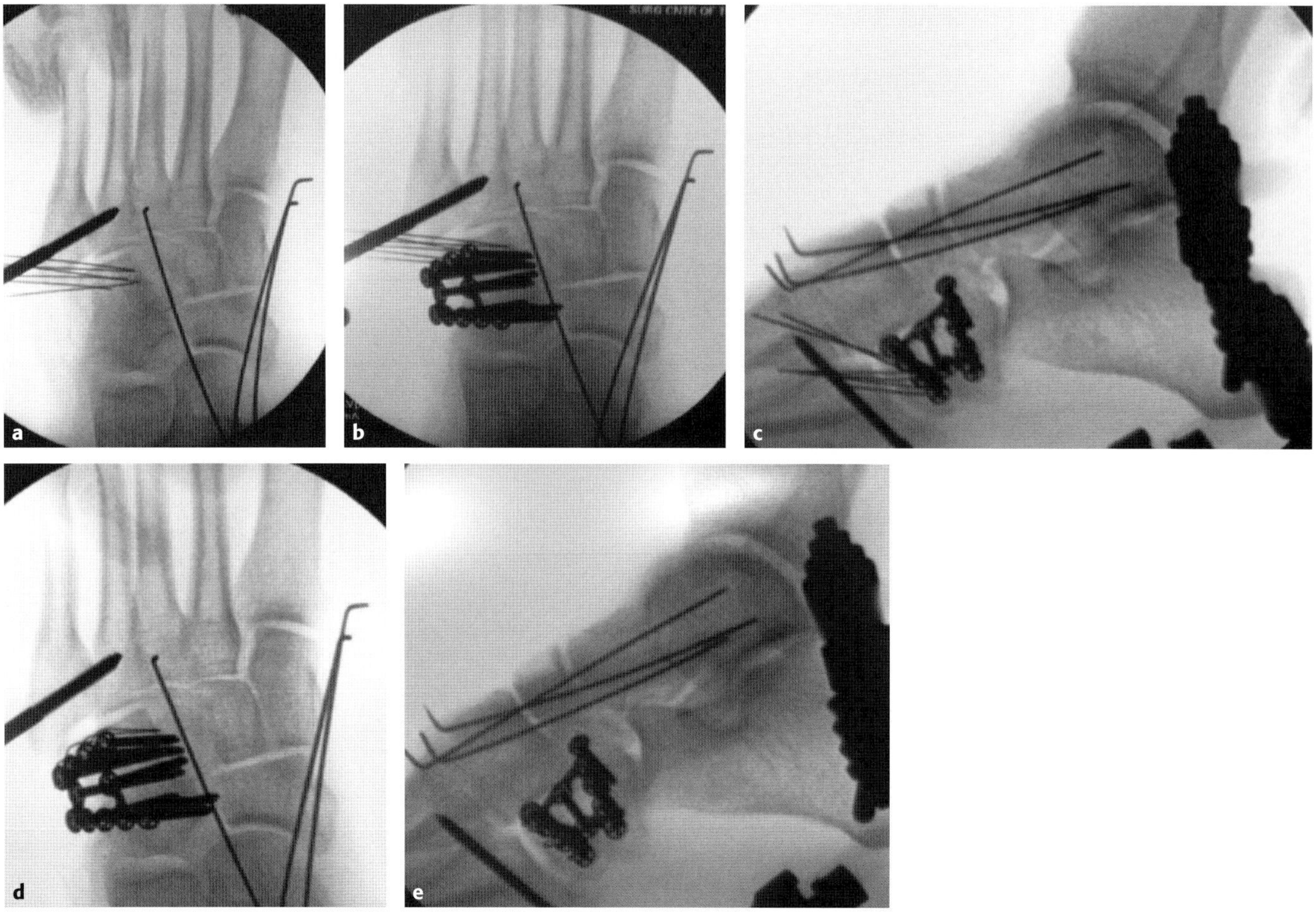

Fig 6.5-11a–e Intraoperative C-arm images demonstrating reduction sequence of the lateral column.

- **a** The external fixator is used to restore lateral column length and the articular surface is reduced with K-wires.
- **b–c** A VAL cuboid plate 2.7 is used for fracture fixation.
- **d–e** The K-wires are bent and cut to maintain the articular reduction.

An anterolateral approach to the navicular was performed with articular restoration of both the TN and naviculcuneiform joints (**Fig 6.5-12**). The major lateral fragment was reduced to the medial fragment with a reduction clamp and stabilized with K-wires. Both the TN and naviculocuneiform joints were reduced under direct visualization and secured with multiple K-wires. Finally, plate and screw fixation was performed from dorsolateral to plantarmedial with reduction of the navicular confirmed under direct visualization and C-arm imaging (**Fig 6.5-13**). K-wires can be retained, as needed, to ensure articular reduction of smaller fragments.

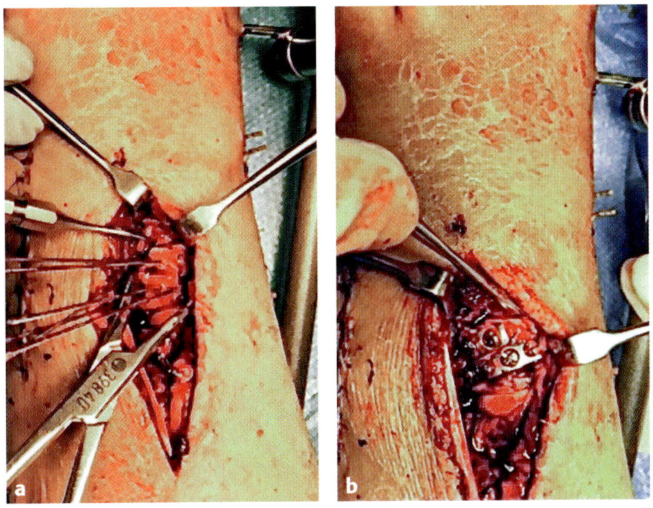

Fig 6.5-12a–b Reduction of the navicular through an anterolateral approach.
a Articular reduction of the TN and naviculcuneiform joints with K-wires.
b Plate fixation of the navicular fracture.

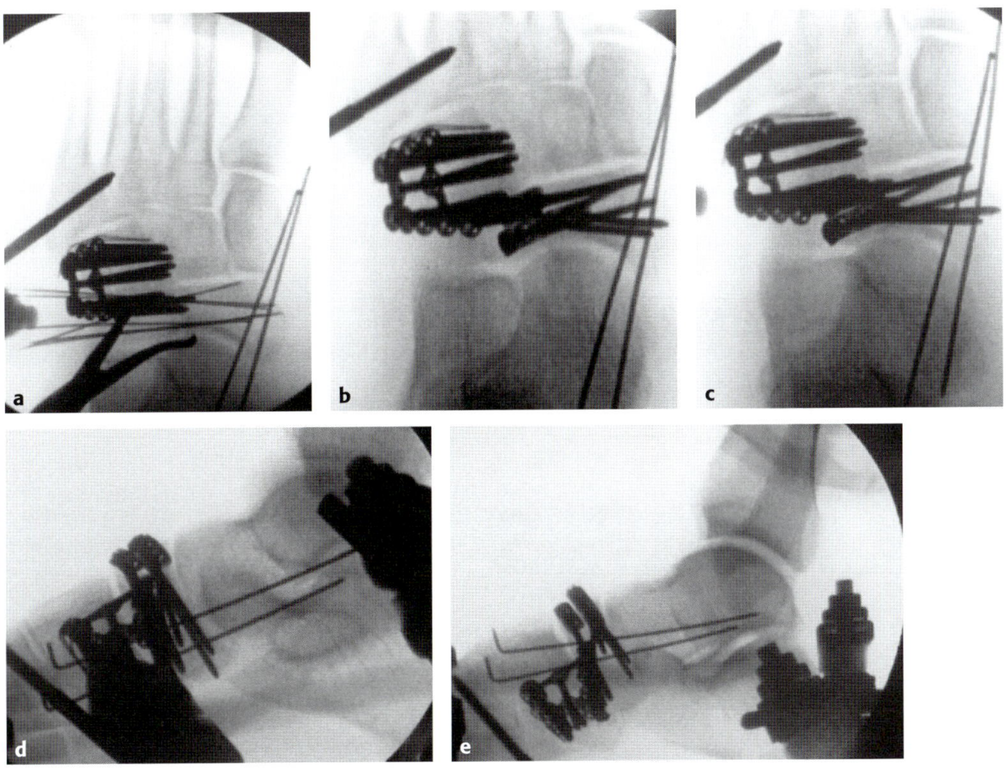

Fig 6.5-13a–e Intraoperative C-arm images demonstrating the reduction sequence of the medial column. The K-wires and external fixator were kept in place for 6 weeks to maintain reduction.
a The external fixator is used to restore medial column length and the articular surface is reduced with K-wires.
b–e Two modular buttress plates are used for fracture fixation.

The external fixator should be kept on for 6 weeks postoperatively in cases of severe Chopart injuries. This helps to protect the medial and lateral column reductions. It is removed at 6–8 weeks, when soft tissue and bony healing has occurred (**Fig 6.5-14**).

5 Pitfalls and complications

Pitfalls

Inadequate reduction of the medial and lateral columns

Severe injuries treated without initial external fixation are often malreduced with a shortened medial and/or lateral column. Initial distraction is important in disimpacting articular fragments and restoring length and alignment of the medial and lateral columns. Step-off and inadequate restoration of the talar-first MT axis (Meary) line can lead to rapid arthrosis and a poor outcome. The importance of the external fixator and a staged approach to these injuries cannot be over emphasized.

Complications

- Posttraumatic arthrosis
- Nonunion
- Malunion
- Loss of fixation
- Wound complications from inadequate skin bridge between incisions
- Injury to the dorsal neurovascular bundle through the anterolateral approach
- Injury to the SPN (anterolateral approach), and the sural nerve (lateral approach)
- Injury to the saphenous nerve (medial utility approach)

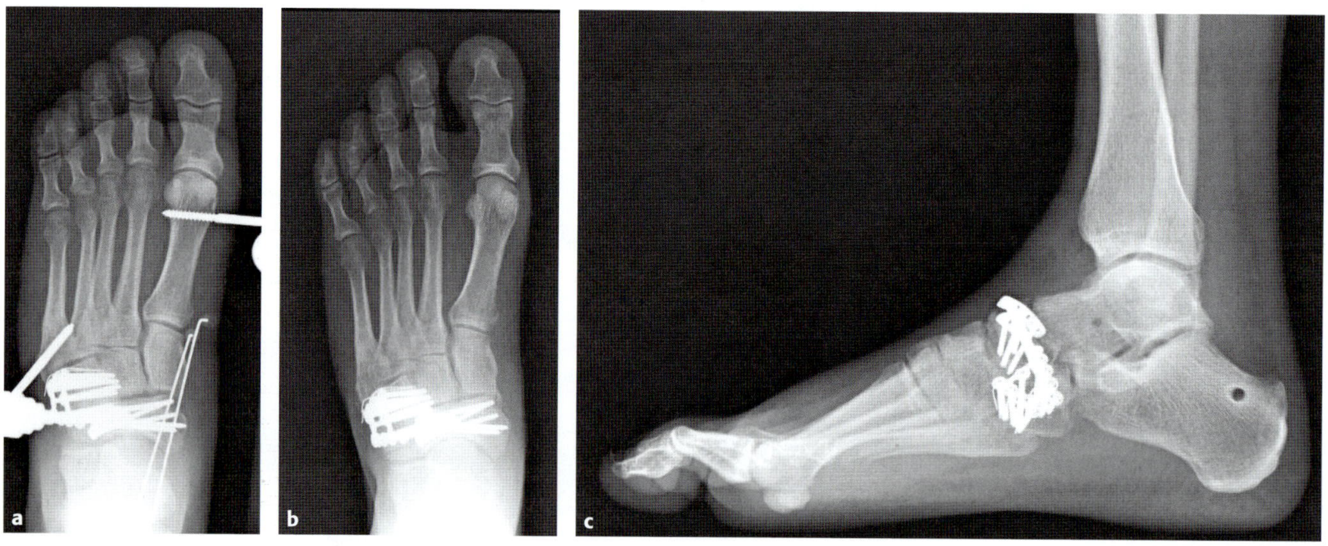

Fig 6.5-14a–c Final postoperative images demonstrating maintenance of reduction.
a The external fixator was kept in place for 6 weeks postoperatively.
b–c Final AP and lateral x-rays demonstrate anatomical reduction of the medial and lateral columns.

6 Alternative techniques

Severe midfoot fracture dislocations with extensive comminution or bone loss can be treated with bridge-plating techniques with locked bridge plating, particularly in osteoporotic bone. Primary arthrodesis should be reserved for severe injuries. If primary arthrodesis is performed, reestablishing appropriate column length is critical to a successful outcome.

7 Postoperative management and rehabilitation

If external fixation is left in place postoperatively, removal should be planned at around 6 weeks after surgery. Active and passive range-of-motion exercises are initiated as soon as the incisions are healed.

Implant removal

Removal of plates and screws from the midfoot may be required to minimize pain and prominence. If a patient experiences chronic pain or prominence, implants can typically be removed at 1 year using the same approaches. Implant removal is accompanied by arthrolysis in case of fibrous adhesions and restricted range of motion at the midtarsal joints. In the case of posttraumtic arthritis, fusion with column realignment may be needed.

Bridge plates, if used, are generally removed after bony healing is confirmed on standing x-rays. This is usually performed around 12 weeks postoperatively. Motion exercises are then performed.

8 Recommended reading

Bayley E, Duncan N, Taylor A. The use of locking plates in complex midfoot fractures. *Ann R Coll Surg Engl.* 2012 Nov;94(8):593–596.

Benirschke SK, Meinberg E, Anderson SA, et al. Fractures and dislocations of the midfoot: Lisfranc and Chopart injuries. *J Bone Joint Surg Am.* 2012 Jul 18;94(14):1325–1337.

Chandran P, Puttaswamaiah R, Dhillon MS, et al. Management of complex open fracture injuries of the midfoot with external fixation. *J Foot Ankle Surg.* 2006 Sep–Oct;45(5):308–315.

Kadow TR, Siska PA, Evans AR, et al. Staged treatment of high energy midfoot fracture dislocations. *Foot Ankle Int.* 2014 Dec;35(12):1287–1291.

Klaue K. Treatment of Chopart fracture-dislocations. *Eur J Trauma Emerg Surg.* 2010 Jun;36(3):191–195.

Rammelt S, Schepers T. Chopart injuries: when to fix and when to fuse? *Foot Ankle Clin.* 2017 Mar;22(1):163–180.

Richter M, Thermann H, Huefner T, et al. Chopart joint fracture-dislocation: initial open reduction provides better outcome than closed reduction. *Foot Ankle Int.* 2004 May;25(5):340–348.

Richter M, Wippermann B, Krettek C, et al. Fractures and fracture dislocations of the midfoot: occurrence, causes and long-term results. *Foot Ankle Int.* 2001 May;22(5):392–398.

Swords MP, Schramski M, Switzer K, et al. Chopart fractures and dislocations. *Foot Ankle Clin.* 2008 Dec;13(4):679–693.

van Dorp KB, de Vries MR, van der Elst M, et al. Chopart joint injury: a study of outcome and morbidity. *J Foot Ankle Surg.* 2010 Nov–Dec;49(6):541–545.

6.6 Tarsometatarsal injury—percutaneous reduction and fixation

Matthew Tomlinson

1 Case description

A 20-year-old woman twisted her foot when she missed a step. Clinical findings included difficulty with weight bearing, swelling of the midfoot, and a plantar ecchymosis. X-rays showed incongruency of the tarsometatarsal (TMT) joints with lateral subluxation of the base of the second metatarsal (MT) on the AP view. Subluxation was further demonstrated on the oblique view. No significant subluxation was seen on the lateral view.

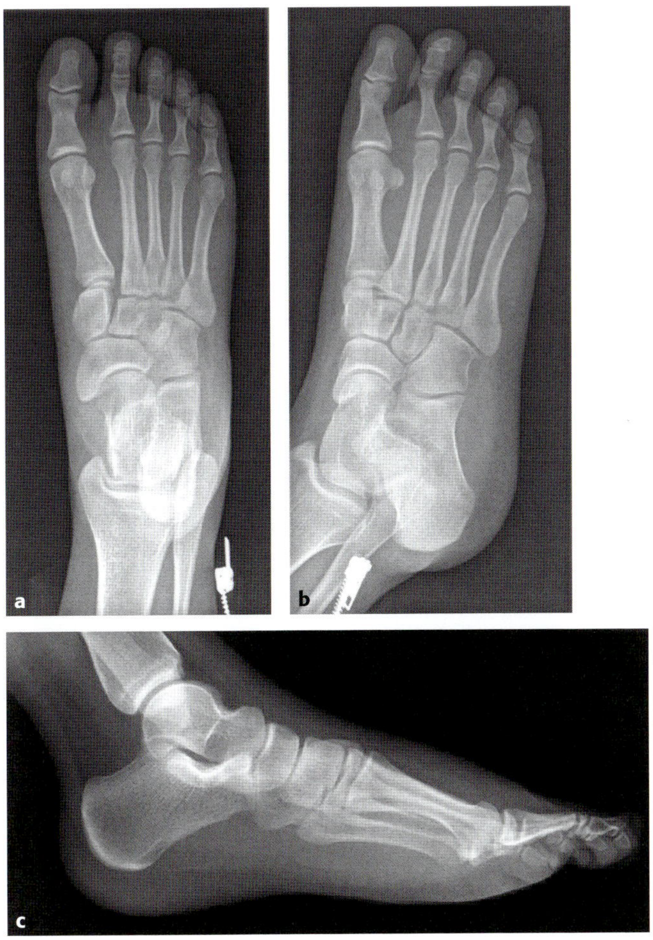

Fig 6.6-1a–c Preoperative x-rays.
a AP view (WB).
b Oblique view (WB).
c Lateral view (NWB).

2 Preoperative planning

Indications for surgery

Weight-bearing (WB) AP and oblique, and nonweight-bearing (NWB) lateral x-rays (**Fig 6.6-1**) confirm a subtle Lisfranc injury with subluxation. Further confirmation of the deformity is seen on computed tomographic (CT) scanning (**Fig 6.6-2**). Surgical stabilization is indicated.

General considerations for surgery

Untreated Lisfranc injuries can be associated with a poor outcome because of progressive deformity and secondary osteoarthritis of the midfoot joints. Surgical treatment in anatomical reduction and internal fixation has been associated with superior outcomes compared with nonoperative treatment. In subtle Lisfranc injuries this can be accomplished using a percutaneous technique, provided that anatomical reduction can be achieved.

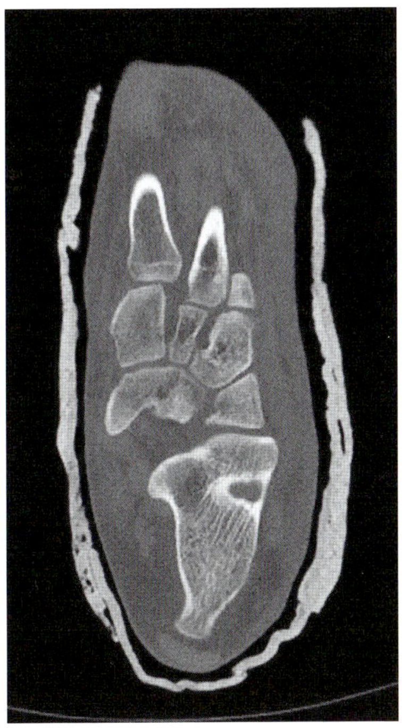

Fig 6.6-2 A CT scan showing subluxation of the first and second TMT joints.

When to use percutaneous reduction and fixation

Preoperative planning involves an assessment of the instability pattern and determination of the ideal construct to achieve stable internal fixation. The surgeon must decide whether the percutaneous method is safe to use. This is done through analysis of x-rays and CT scans. The most suitable cases are usually the homolateral type where there is only minor subluxation of the TMT joints. In cases with more severe displacement and gross instability, formal open reduction and internal fixation (ORIF) should be used. In this case it was decided that a percutaneous technique can be used (**Fig 6.6-3**).

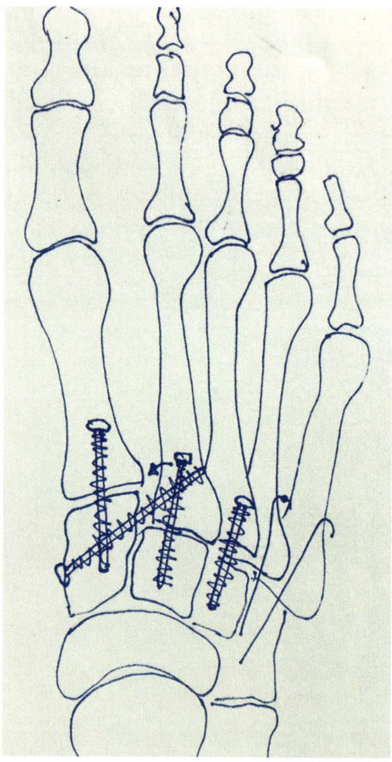

Fig 6.6-3 Preoperative plan. The direction of reduction of the second TMT joint and screw and wire placement. Wires are only necessary if the fourth and fifth TMT joints are unstable.

When planning the procedure, the surgeon should ensure that the patient can be positioned on a radiolucent table and that a high-quality C-arm is available for imaging each step of the reduction and fixation. A thorough knowledge of the normal radiographic anatomy of the Lisfranc complex is mandatory.

The percutaneous technique requires the use of reduction clamps, K-wires, and screws. It is preferable to use 4 mm solid fully threaded cortex screws for all the joints whenever possible, but certainly for the first TMT joint fixation and the Lisfranc screw (from medial cuneiform to base of second MT). If the anatomy is too tight for 4.0 mm screws, then 3.5 mm solid cortex screws can be used for the smaller joints. K-wires are used for the fourth and fifth TMT joints. In children and adolescents the K-wires are used in combination with screws. Some surgeons may prefer to use cannulated screws for fixation although these may not be as strong as solid screws, potentially leading to early fixation failure and hardware breakage.

3 Operating room setup

Patient positioning	• Supine • It is desirable to keep the foot positioned vertically. An ipsilateral buttock bump can be used to internally rotate the affected limb (**Fig 6.6-4**).
Anesthesia options	• General, with regional supplementation
C-arm location	• The C-arm should be placed on the same side as the injury. • The screen should be placed so the surgeon can easily view the images. Usually this is near the patient's head.
Tourniquet	• Applied to the proximal thigh but not inflated unless needed. • If the surgery is converted to standard open technique and there is bleeding which obscures the surgeon's view, then the tourniquet is inflated.
Tips	• The limb is draped free to allow mobility at the hip and knee necessary for simulated weight-bearing views.

For illustrations and overview of anesthetic considerations, see chapter 1.

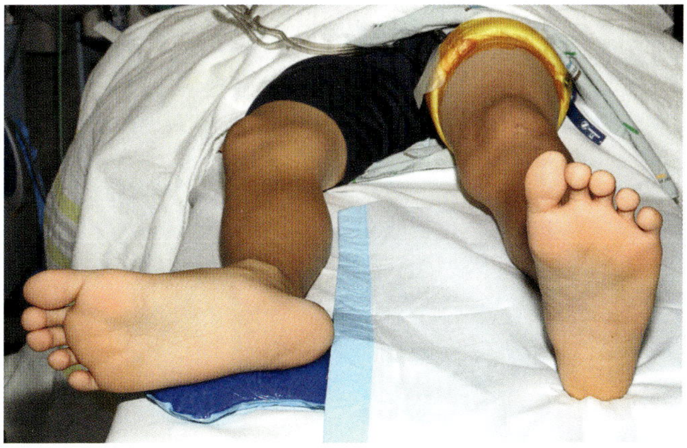

Fig 6.6-4 Typical intraoperative setup for percutaneous Lisfranc fixation, in this case for a left foot injury. A bump has been placed under the ipsilateral hip to position the foot appropriately.

Equipment

- Scalpel (#15 blade)
- Small, medium, and large point-to-point reduction (Weber) clamps
- Wire driver
- K-wires (assorted sizes)
- Drill with drill bits (2.5 mm, 2.9 mm, and 4.0 mm)
- Long drill bits are better as they allow the bits to lay flatter and the drill chuck to be more distal and to not grind on the toes.
- A longer bit screwdriver allows insertion of the screws without the handle hitting the top of the foot.

4 Surgical procedure

Under C-arm control and using palpable surface anatomy, the shape of the TMT joints is marked out with a sterile marking pen.

There are several reduction and fixation techniques. For this patient, reduction started with the first TMT joint. By applying manual force while abducting the first MT, lateral subluxation of the first TMT joint can be reduced and if necessary, any dorsal or plantar subluxation reduced as well. Reduction is aided by placing a thumb or finger over the medial cuneiform medially and applying gentle pressure. A small incision is made 2–3 cm distal to the first TMT on the dorsal surface. A K-wire is driven across the joint to stabilize it temporarily. Reduction is confirmed on simulated WB views using the C-arm. It is essential to obtain anatomical reduction of the first ray. This first step serves as the guide to allow subsequent reduction of the other MTs.

In most injuries, the second MT is subluxated laterally. The base of the second MT must be reduced to sit into the corner against the lateral base of the first MT and the lateral facet of the medial cuneiform. The reduction is achieved by placing a medium reduction clamp percutaneously from the medial cortex of the medial cuneiform and the lateral base of the second MT (**Fig 6.6-5**). This reduces the torn Lisfranc ligament or the small avulsion fragment attached to the Lisfranc ligament, if present. If reduction of the second MT cannot be achieved and it is suspected that fragments of bone or soft tissue are interposed, the percutaneous technique is stopped and an open reduction is necessary. In most cases, however, anatomical reduction can be achieved.

Once the second MT is reduced and reduction is confirmed radiographically on both AP and 30° oblique views, a small incision is made 2–3 cm distal to the second TMT joint dorsally and a K-wire driven across the joint (**Fig 6.6-6**).

The third TMT joint is reduced with manual manipulation and a point-to-point reduction (Weber) clamp. A K-wire is placed across the third TMT joint once it is reduced. The reduction can be checked using a 45° oblique view with the C-arm. In many cases the third TMT joint sits anatomically after reduction of the first and second TMT joints and a separate screw is not always necessary.

After the first, second, and third TMT joints are anatomically reduced and provisional fixation has been achieved with K-wires, a "Lisfranc" screw can be placed from the medial cuneiform to the base of the second MT. This screw is placed through a small axial incision over the medial cuneiform while the reduction clamp is still in place between the medial cuneiform and the lateral base of the second MT. Under C-arm guidance, the drill is aimed toward the second MT base distal to the second TMT joint and crossing the facet between the medial cuneiform and the medial base of the second MT (**Fig 6.6-7**). The screw extends from the medial aspect of the medial cuneiform to the lateral cortex of the proximal second MT, thus locking the second MT into its anatomic position.

The next step is definitive fixation to the first, second, and, if necessary, the third TMT joints (**Fig 6.6-8**). The 4 mm cortex screws are used rather than 3.5 mm screws or cannulated screws because they are stronger and less likely to break. However, 3.5 mm screws or cannulated screws may be adequate in lighter patients. If cannulated screws are

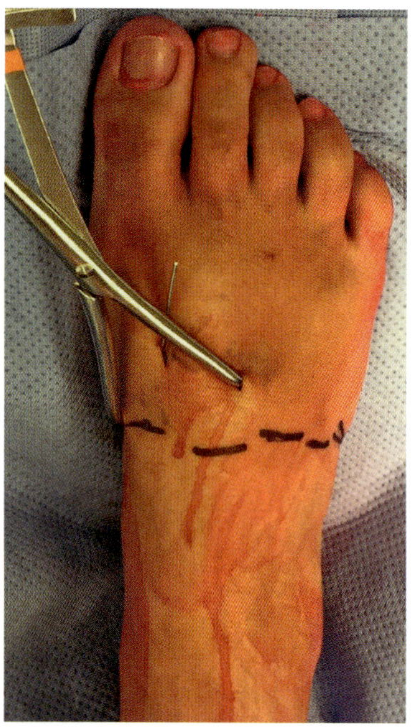

Fig 6.6-5 K-wire stabilization of the first TMT joint and reduction of the second TMT joint using a clamp between the base of the second metatarsal and the medial cuneiform.

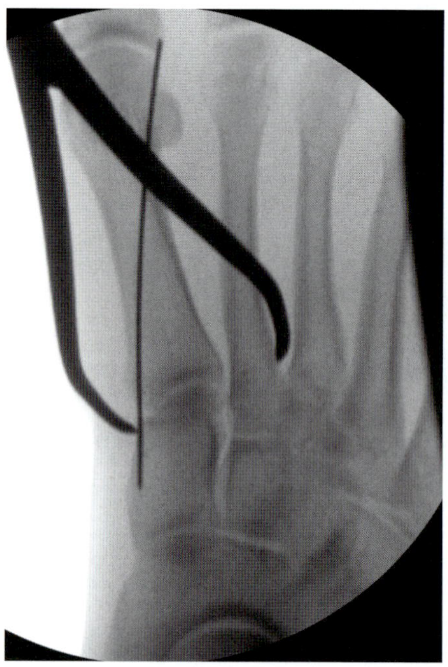

Fig 6.6-6 Confirmation of anatomical reduction using the C-arm.

used, they can be placed over the K-wires; but if solid screws are used, they must be placed beside the K-wires already in situ. Once the screws are placed across the TMT joints and proper placement is confirmed with the C-arm, the K-wires can be removed (**Fig 6.6-9** and **6.6-10**).

If there is persistent instability of the fourth and fifth TMT joints, they should be reduce and stabilized using K-wires rather than screws. As the lateral column is supposed to be mobile, the K-wires are removed at 6 weeks to maintain maximum motion through the lateral column.

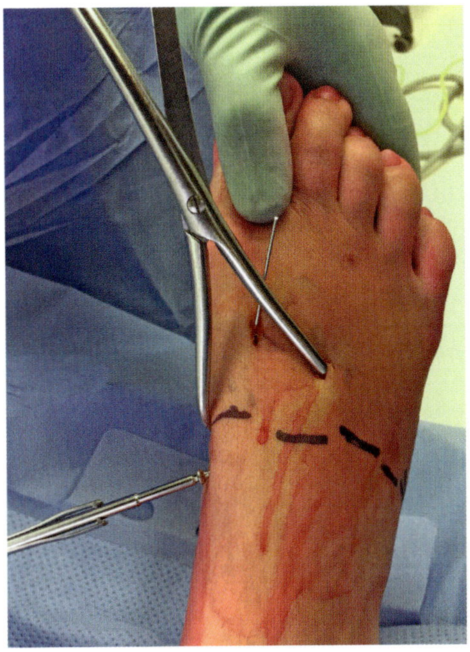

Fig 6.6-7 Placement of the Lisfranc screw between the medial cuneiform and second TMT joint.

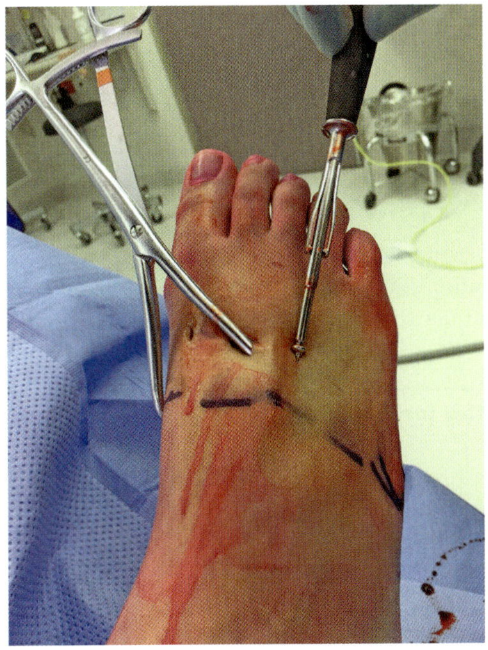

Fig 6.6-8 Percutaneous placement of the third TMT screw.

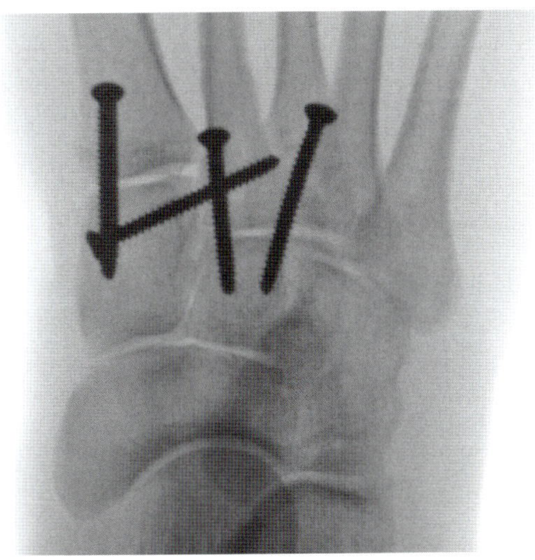

Fig 6.6-9 The final construct.

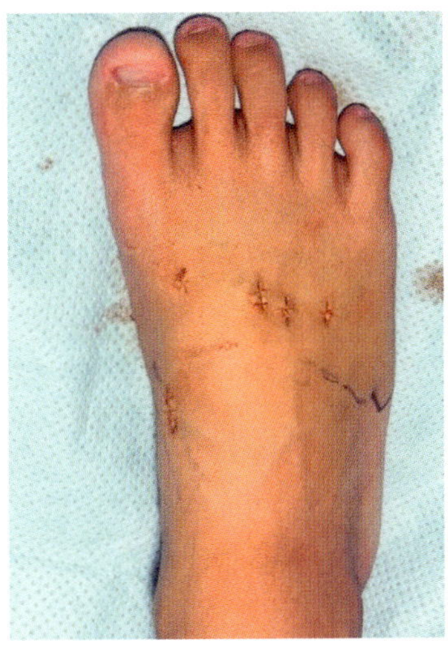

Fig 6.6-10 Postoperative appearance showing the final placement of the small incisions.

5 Pitfalls and complications

Pitfalls

- The percutaneous technique may not be able to achieve an anatomical reduction of the Lisfranc injury. In this situation ORIF is a better option.
- Accurate interpretation of the C-arm views obtained during the procedure, so a thorough knowledge of the normal anatomy of the Lisfranc complex is essential.
- Understanding and interpreting the oblique views will aid with proper placement of the wires and screws, otherwise misplacement of the implants may occur.

Complications

- Malreduction
- Superficial peroneal or deep peroneal nerve injury
- Extensor tendon injury
- Late onset osteoarthritis

6 Alternative techniques

Closed treatment in a cast or boot, ORIF, and primary arthrodesis are alternative techniques that may be used for treatment of TMT injuries.

The use of lag screw technique by drilling a 4.0 pocket (starting) hole, helps with reduction of the joints. Standard screw technique may sometimes cause diastasis across the area to be fixed.

7 Postoperative management and rehabilitation

Postoperative elevation is used to reduce swelling and aid in wound healing. Weight bearing is not permitted for 6 weeks and a cast or boot is used to immobilize the foot and ankle. If x-rays at 6 weeks show satisfactory position of hardware and anatomy, then gradual progressive return to WB by 12 weeks is allowed.

Implant removal

Screws may be removed as per surgeon preference and local custom. For this patient, screws were removed after 6 months.

If wires are used in the fourth and fifth MTs, they are removed after 6 weeks. Following removal of the screws, unrestricted activity is allowed.

8 Recommended reading

Myerson MS, Fisher RT, Burgess AR, et al. Fracture dislocations of the tarsometatarsal joints: end results correlated with pathology and treatment. *Foot Ankle.* 1986 Apr;6(5):225–242.
Perugia D, Basile A, Battaglia A, et al. Fracture dislocations of Lisfranc's joint treated with closed reduction and percutaneous fixation. *Int Orthop.* 2003;27(1):30–35.
Puna RA, Tomlinson MP. The role of percutaneous reduction and fixation of Lisfranc injuries. *Foot Ankle Clin.* 2017 Mar;22(1):15–34.

6.7 Tarsometatarsal injury—open reduction and internal fixation

Andrew K Sands, Michael Swords

1 Case description

A 24-year-old recreational sportsman injured his left foot when it was planted into the turf toes down. Another player fell onto his heel, driving the foot into the ground and causing immediate severe pain. There was a noticable deformity at the midfoot.

He was transported by ambulance to the emergency department where x-rays were taken, which demonstrated a displaced Lisfranc injury (**Fig 6.7-1** and **Fig 6.7-2**).

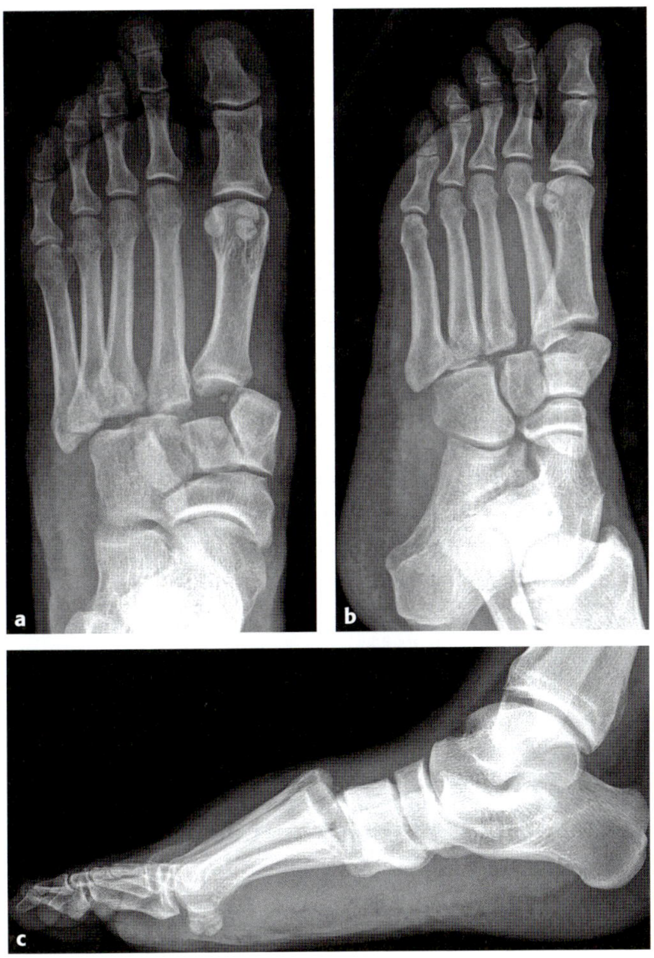

Fig 6.7-1a–c The x-rays show a homolateral and dorsally displaced Lisfranc injury pattern. All five MT bases are displaced.

- **a** AP view.
- **b** Oblique view.
- **c** Lateral view.

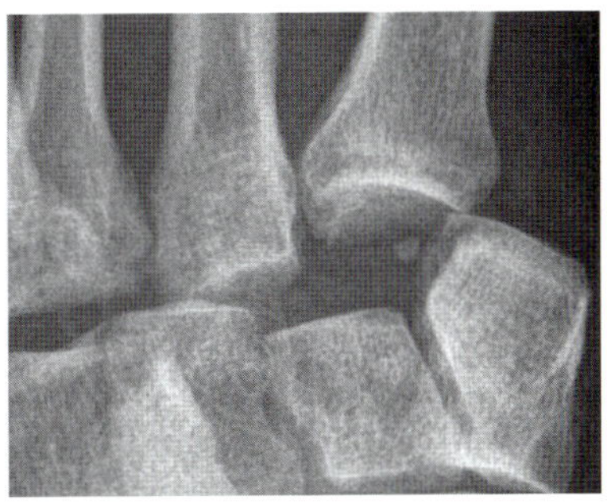

Fig 6.7-2 Magnified view of the Lisfranc region showing multiple small avulsion fractures.

2 Preoperative planning

Indications for surgery

While some minimally displaced Lisfranc injuries may be treated nonoperatively, injuries with displacement of more than 2 mm are treated surgically due to a high risk of disability and/or late instability leading to deformity. This injury has significant displacement and gross malalignment of the midfoot requiring surgical fixation. There is no acceptable nonoperative treatment for the injury in this case.

Planning of approaches

These injuries are frequently associated with significant soft-tissue swelling. Most injuries, including this case, are treated with dual incisions on the dorsum of the foot (**Fig 6.7-3**). In severe cases, temporizing external fixation may be necessary to maintain alignment prior to definitive treatment. Surgical management should be delayed until soft-tissue swelling has resolved.

In most cases, surgical management is performed using the dorsomedial approach and dorsolateral approach.

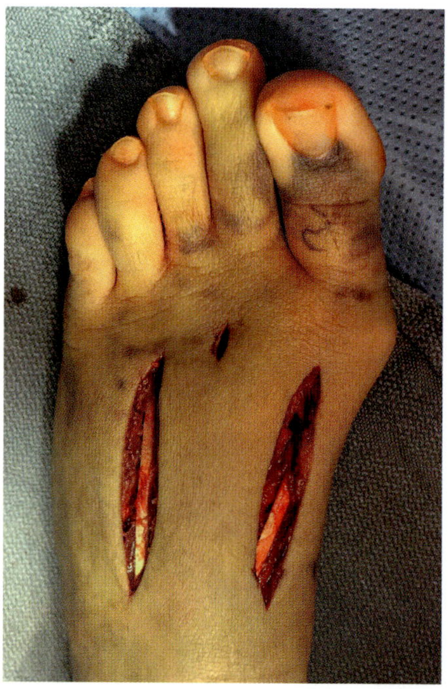

Fig 6.7-3 Dorsomedial and dorsolateral incisions are shown. Appropriate spacing of the two incisions is necessary to maintain a viable skin bridge and avoid complications. A small medial incision can be used to assisit in reduction and insertion of hardware. Surgery should be delayed until the swelling has resolved.

The dorsomedial incision is centered over the tarsometatarsal (TMT) area, between the extensor hallucis longus (EHL) tendon and extensor hallucis brevis (EHB). The dorsolateral incision is centered over the TMT area, roughly in line with the fourth metatarsal (MT).

The skin bridge between the two incisions should be kept as wide as possible. The medial incision can be placed more medial and the lateral incision can be shifted more lateral as needed. The skin bridge between the two incisions must be respected and excessive retraction, undermining, or dissection should be avoided.

A small medial incision in the line of the medial utility incision can be used to allow placement of reduction clamps and insertion of screws.

Considerations for surgery

Injuries in this region are varied in presentation and may be homolateral or divergent. They may be pure ligamentous injuries with disruption of the joints. There may be small plantar avulsions at the MT base or more extensive MT fractures. A thorough evaluation of the injury is required as the type of injury dictates the technique employed. Injury patterns associated with MT comminution are treated with bridge plating.

Primary arthrodesis may be considered for treatment of injuries with significant intraarticular injury, for elderly patients, and for purely ligamentous injury. In this case while small fractures are present, there is no significant comminution allowing for rigid fixation with large diameter screws inserted in a lag screw fashion.

Fixation implant choices

Fixation may be done with a variety of implants.

K-wires

K-wires are useful in holding temporary reduction of injuries. Where possible they should be replaced with screws during the procedure. Rarely, K-wires may be left in place as definitive fixation and even cross to the next joint for added stability. While K-wires are inexpensive, they do not provide sufficient stability for definitive fixation in most cases around the midfoot area.

Screws

The midfoot screw is recommended for any fixation across the TMT area. This is a solid 4.0 mm screw with a larger core and is more resistant to bending, torque, and failure. These screws are fully threaded and can be used statically or in a lag screw fashion. If 4.0 mm screws are not available, then 3.5 mm screws can be used. However, there is an increased risk of breaking. Smaller diameter solid screws can be used for intertarsal area instability as they are usually placed transversely.

Plates

Small, low profile plates (standard or locking) can be used instead of or in conjunction with screws. If plates are used, the surgeon must keep in mind that, to avoid screw head interference, the screws must be placed outside the plane where the plate is placed. Plates can be used to span comminuted areas or as secondary stabilization implants over the top of screw fixation.

In the case presented, screw fixation using 4.0 mm midfoot screws was ideal due to the lack of comminution.

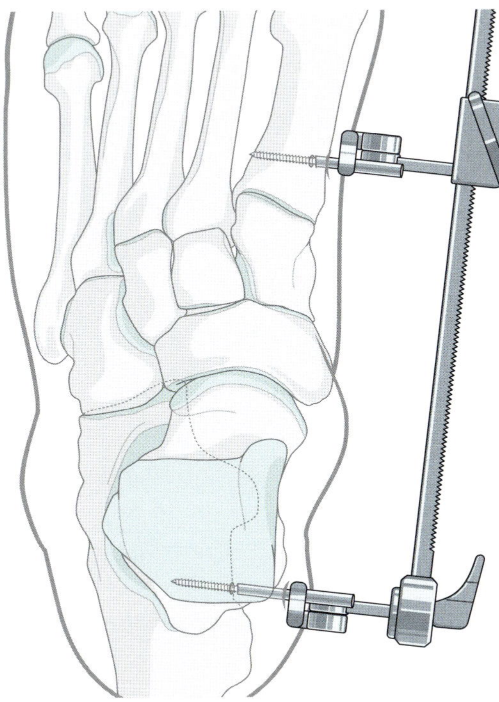

Fig 6.7-4 A small distraction device can be useful to restore length and maintain column length during reconstruction of the midfoot.

3 Operating room setup

Patient positioning	• Supine with large ipsilateral bump under the buttock
Anesthesia options	• General, spinal, or regional
C-arm location	• The C-arm is positioned so that the screen is easily visible to the surgeon. • If the mini-C-arm is used, it is helpful to move the patient all the way down to the end of the operative table. This allows for easy rotation of the C-arm from lateral foot to AP foot, without having to adjust the foot position. Simulated dorsiflexion can be accomplished by gently pushing up on the forefoot with a large mallet with the C-arm in the lateral position. Use of the mini-C-arm allows less radiation exposure to the operating room team and obviates the need for larger lead barriers.
Tourniquet	• Used at the surgeon's discretion • Generally improves ability to visualize the reduction
Tips	• A foam ramp placed under the affected leg lifts the leg and operative area above the unaffected leg allowing easier cross table imaging. • Surgical stools allow the operative team to reposition around the operative table with ease to address various injuries to the foot.

For illustrations and overview of anesthetic considerations, see chapter 1.

Equipment

- 4.0 mm cortex screws (3.5 mm if unavailable)
- K-wires
- Point-to-point reduction (Weber) clamps
- Small distraction device (to restore column length if needed **[Fig 6.7-4]**)
- Midfoot plates 2.0, 2.4, 2.7 (locking and nonlocking)
- Dental scaler
- Elevators

Implant size may vary based on the individual anatomy.

4 Surgical procedure

Surgery is performed after appropriate preoperative evaluation and resolution of soft-tissue swelling. A dorsomedial incision is made and dissection is carried down in the interval between the EHL and EHB. A second incision is made on the dorsolateral foot in line with the fourth MT. Care is taken to identify and protect the terminal branches of the superficial peroneal nerve in the proximal extent of the incision.

The intertarsal area is inspected to ensure there is no associated injury. If an intertarsal injury is present, it must be reduced and stabilized prior to TMT reduction and fixation. The joint disruptions present at the first and second TMT joints are identified. The disrupted joints are cleaned of hematoma and small bony debris, allowing visualization of the articular surfaces and accurate reduction. If necessary, the first TMT joint is reduced and held provisionally with K-wires to restore the medial column.

Lisfranc reconstruction begins at the medial base of the second MT. The second MT is reduced against the lateral base of the first MT and lateral edge of the medial cuneiform. Care must be taken to clean out the corner of any debris and soft tissue. Reduction is then performed with a point-to-point reduction (Weber) clamp with one tip placed in the medial cuneiform through a small medial incision, while the other tine of the reduction clamp is placed through the lateral incision along the lateral base of the second MT (**Fig 6.7-5**). If the lateral tine of the point-to-point reduction (Weber) clamp is placed on the lateral base of the second MT through the medial incision instead of through the lateral incision, it results in excessive dissection across the neurovascular bundle of the dorsal foot flap and may compromise the soft tissue of the dorsum of the foot. The base of the second MT is reduced and held with K-wires, and then screwed into place with a lag screw from the medial cuneiform into the base of the second MT. The first TMT is then reduced and secured with K-wires. A lag screw is placed from a pocket hole on the dorsal base of the first MT into the medial cuneiform, aimed at and possibly exiting, the plantar medial corner of the cuneiform (**Fig 6.7-6**). A screw, if needed, can then be placed from the second MT base to the middle cuneiform (**Fig 6.7-7**). The third TMT is reduced by placing the point-to-point reduction (Weber) clamp from the medial cuneiform to the lateral base of the third MT. The reduction is secured with a K-wire then a lag screw placed into the lateral cuneiform. The fourth and fifth MT bases usually move medial with the reduction and fixation of the other TMT joints. Smooth K-wires can be used to secure the base of the fourth and fifth MT to the cuboid if instability or displacement is still present after fixation of the first, second,

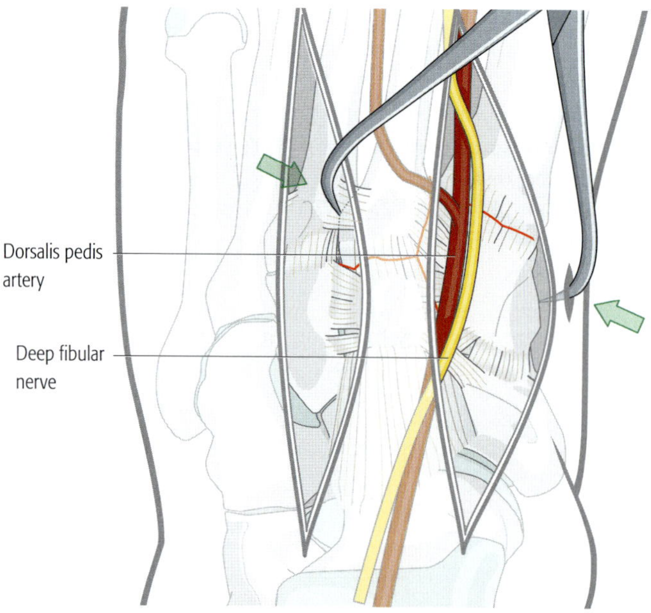

Fig 6.7-5 Reduction is performed with a point-to-point reduction (Weber) clamp.

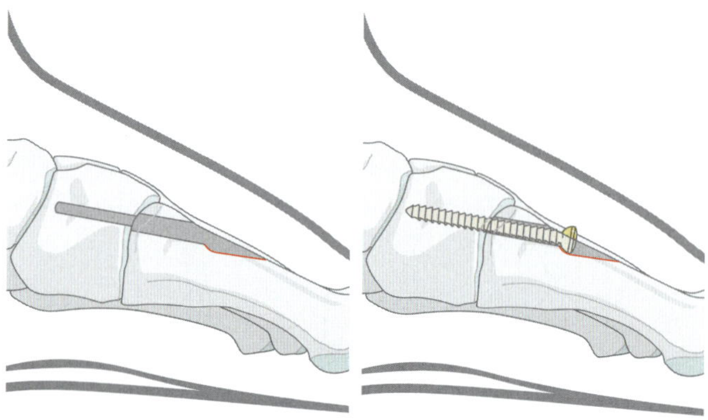

Fig 6.7-6 Longitudinal screws should be inserted after a pocket hole is created in the dorsal cortex. If the screw is inserted without a pocket hole the plantar portion of the screw head will abut the dorsal cortex and create a fracture from the drill hole extending to the articular surface at the base of the first MT.

and third TMT joints. The lateral border of the foot is mobile since the fourth-fifth cuboid joints are mobile joints (**Fig 6.7-8**). At the conclusion of the procedure, final C-arm images are taken in AP, lateral, and oblique views to confirm anatomical reconstruction.

Wounds are closed in a normal fashion with absorbable sutures for deep closure followed by superficial closure. Nonadherent dressings are applied to the incisions. The patient is placed in a well-padded short leg splint.

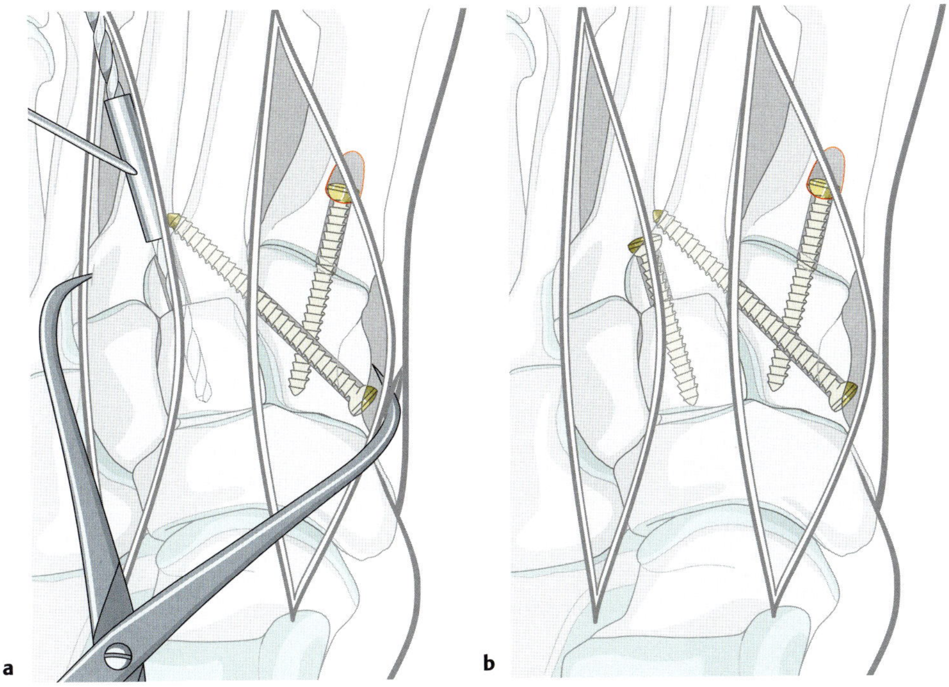

Fig 6.7-7a–b After the first TMT joint and second MT base have been secured with screw fixation. If needed, a third screw is placed longitudinally running from the second MT base to the middle cuneiform.

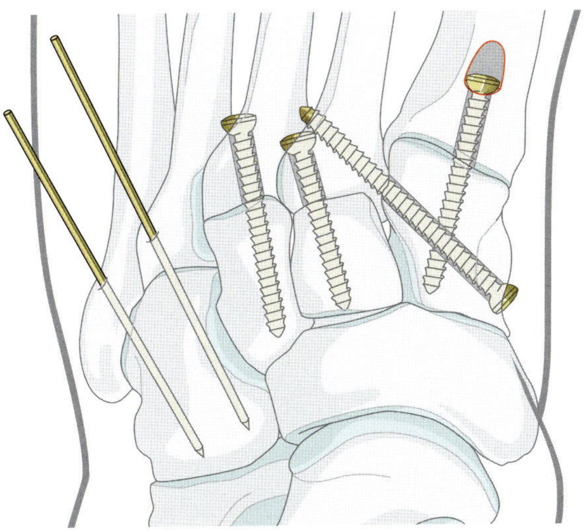

Fig 6.7-8 Final construct demonstrating anatomical reduction and rigid screw fixation of the first to third TMTs and K-wire fixation of the more mobile lateral TMT joints. K-wire fixation is typically removed at 6–8 weeks postoperatively prior to initiation of weight bearing.

5 Alternative techniques

Nonoperative treatment

Nonoperative treatment may be appropriate in injuries that are purely ligamentous without displacement. Repeated evaluation is necessary to ensure stability is maintained over time and no late displacement occurs. Nonweight bearing is advised for 6 weeks and return to sport is allowed at around 6 months.

Plate fixation

Bridge plating can be performed using dorsal spanning plates to secure articular alignment without violating the cartilage (**Fig 6.7-9**). Plates are also indicated when there is associated comminution or MT fractures present, compromising the stability of screw fixation.

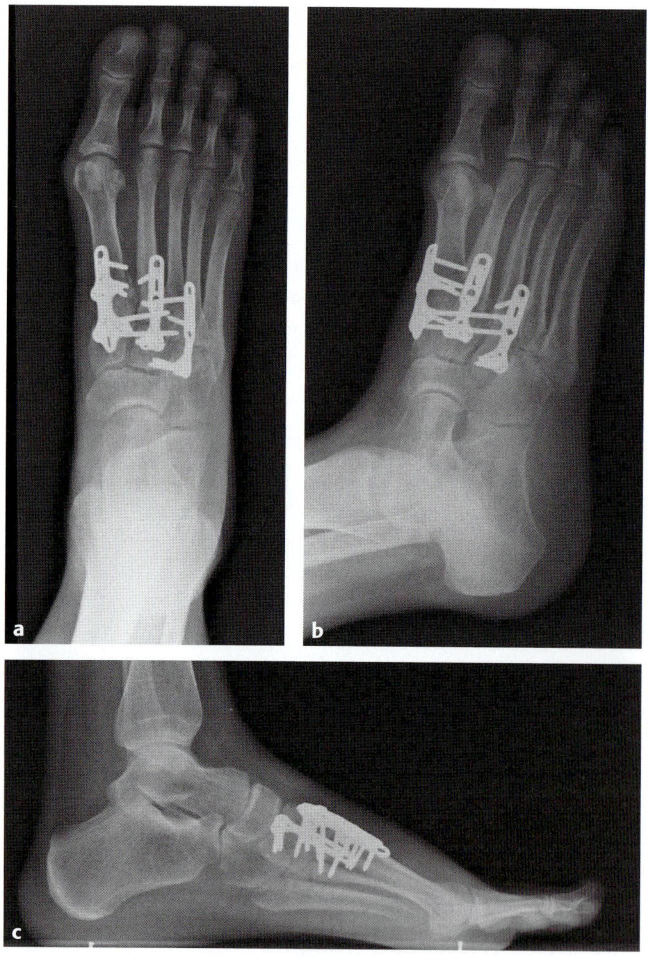

Fig 6.7-9a–c Example from a different case of bridge plate fixation. This is an alternative fixation strategy that does not require intraarticular hardware. Plating is also indicated in injuries with associated comminution.

Primary arthrodesis

Primary arthrodesis is becoming a more acceptable way of treating these injuries. Elderly patients, purely ligamentous injuries, and those with extensive articular injury are good candidates for primary arthrodesis. Exact reduction is necessary for arthrodesis to have the best results.

6 Postoperative management and rehabilitation

The patient is placed in a splint postoperatively. Activity is limited to prevent swelling. The patient is seen roughly 2 weeks postoperatively for suture removal (**Fig 6.7-10**). After suture removal the patient is typically placed in a fracture boot. Range-of-motion exercises for the metatarsophalangeal joint, subtalar joint, and ankle are encouraged as soon as the injury allows. Nonweight bearing is typically necessary for 6–8 weeks but may be longer based on other concomitant injuries to the foot. X-rays are taken at 6–8 weeks (**Fig 6.7-11**). If K-wires were used to stabilize the fourth-fifth cuboid-MT articulations, they are removed at around 6–8 weeks. K-wires across the fourth and fifth TMT joints should be removed prior to initiation of weight bearing. If the pins are left out of the skin, they may be removed in the outpatient setting. Pins that are buried will often require removal as a separate surgical procedure. Weight bearing is progressed once healing has occurred.

Nicotine cessation is critical to avoid problems with incisional or osseus healing. Stiffness of the metatarsophalangeal joints is not unusual after this injury, particularly in plantarflexion.

Implant removal

Hardware removal is controversial. Some surgeons advocate removal at around 4–6 months, while others only remove the hardware if it becomes symptomatic (**Fig 6.7-12**).

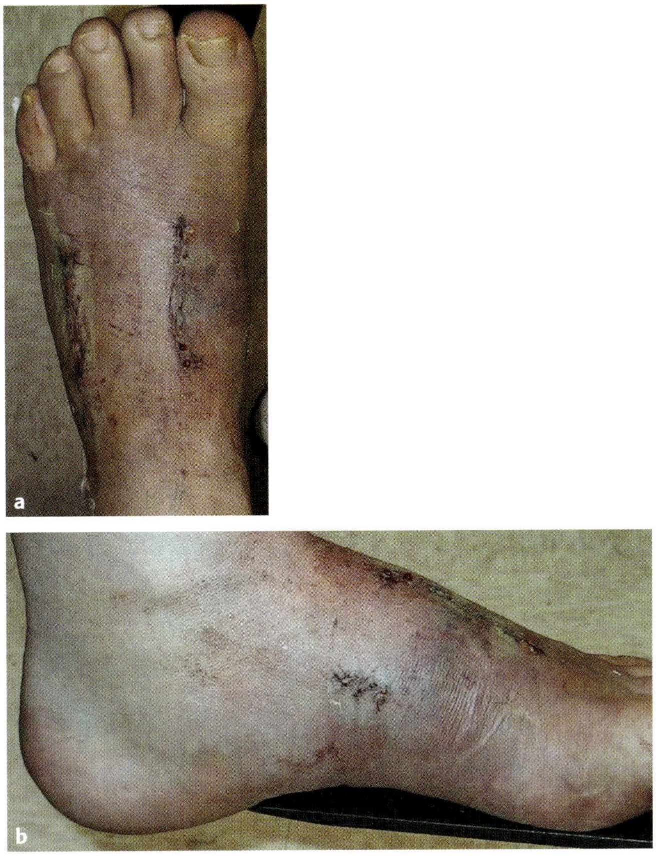

Fig 6.7-10a–b The patient is seen 2 weeks after surgery. All incisions are healed and the sutures have been removed from the two dorsal incisions (**a**) and the small medial incision (**b**).

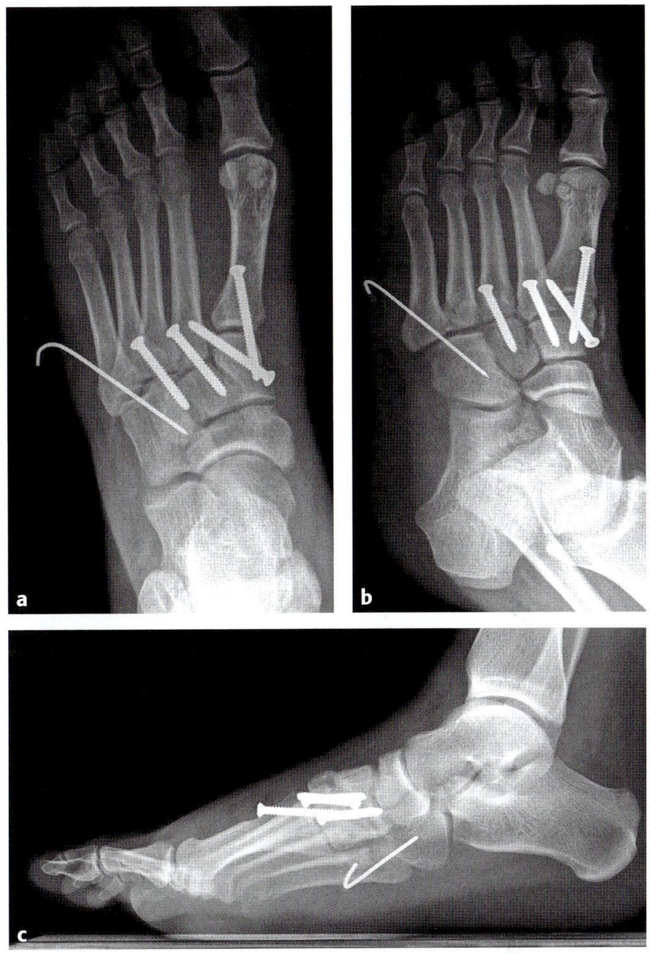

Fig 6.7-11a–c Postoperative x-ray at 6 weeks showing anatomical reduction and appropriate position of all implants. The K-wires are removed prior to the initiation of weight bearing.

- **a** AP view.
- **b** Oblique view.
- **c** Lateral view.

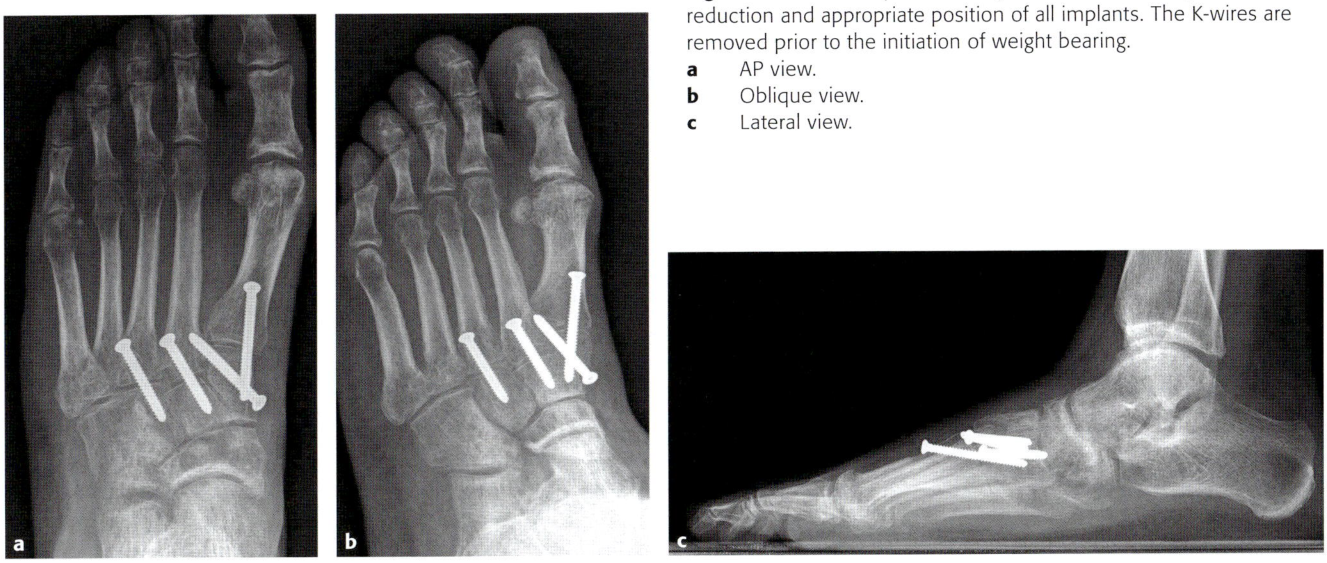

Fig 6.7-12a–c X-rays show anatomical reconstruction of the midfoot at 1-year postinjury. The K-wires were removed from the lateral joints prior to initiation of weight bearing. The screws were asymptomatic so they were not removed.

- **a** AP view.
- **b** Oblique view.
- **c** Lateral view.

7 Pitfalls and complications

Pitfalls

Poor visualization

The incisions are made axially in line with the foot. This gives the surgeon the opportunity to extend the incisions more proximal or distal for increased visualization of the area to be addressed. Transverse incisions do not allow for increased visualization. Additionally, these injuries are often part of a multiply injured foot, which require the ability to extend the incisions.

Making the incisions too close together

Try to space the incisions out as much as possible to prevent damage to the dorsal soft tissue of the foot and the central flap, which contains the dorsalis pedis artery. Avoid overly vigorous dissection, as it can damage the artery and possibly compromise the flap. Additional incisions on the dorsum of the foot will likely result in wound complications.

Unrecognized fractures or instability

It is possible that a fracture or instability is missed and then unexpectedly found intraoperatively. Stress evaluation for stability should be performed at the beginning of the procedure and repeated prior to closure. The surgeon should have plates available at the time of surgery. The plates may be necessary for spanning the fracture or instability. If screws are used and the dorsal cortex fails when the screw head engages the dorsal cortex, then plates must be available for spanning the dorsal cortex breakout area to salvage the now broken area.

Complications

- Wound complications
- Failure of hardware
- Nonunion
- Arthritis
- Infection
- Stiffness
- Instability

8 Recommended reading

Benirschke SK, Meinberg E, Anderson SA, et al. Fractures and dislocations of the midfoot: Lisfranc and Chopart injuries. *J Bone Joint Surg Am.* 2012 Jul 18;94(14):1325–133.

Ly TV, Coetzee JC. Treatment of primarily ligamentous Lisfranc joint injuries: primary arthrodesis compared with open reduction and internal fixation. A prospective, randomized study. *J Bone Joint Surg Am.* 2006 Mar;88(3):514–520.

Myerson MS, Fisher RT, Burgess AR, et al. Fracture dislocations of the tarsometatarsal joints: end results correlated with pathology and treatment. *Foot Ankle.* 1986 Apr;6(5):225–242.

Main BJ, Jowett RL. Injuries of the midtarsal joint. *J Bone Joint Surg Br.* 1975 Feb;57(1):89–97.

Welck MJ, Zinchenko R, Rudge B. Lisfranc injuries. *Injury.* 2015 Apr;46(4):536–541.

6.8 Tarsometatarsal injury with compartment syndrome

Stefan Rammelt, Arthur Manoli II, Andrew K Sands

1 Case description

A 30-year old construction worker's left foot was run over by a cart. Despite having worn protective shoes, he immediately had severe pain in the midfoot. His foot was immobilized in a temporary splint at the site and he was brought to the emergency department by emergency services. The splint was removed to allow for an adequate physical examination then a soft splint was placed which did not compress the foot.

On admission to the hospital there was moderate swelling of the left midfoot and forefoot, presumably from an expanding internal hematoma (**Fig 6.8-1**). The patient was unable to bear weight on the injured foot.

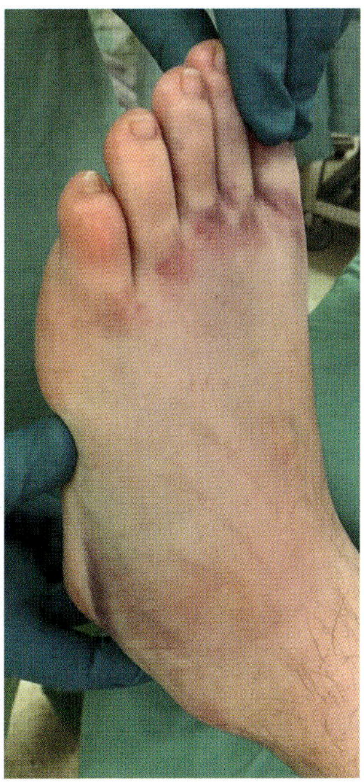

Fig 6.8-1 Dorsal aspect of the injured left foot with moderate swelling at the midfoot and subcutaneous hematoma at the forefoot.

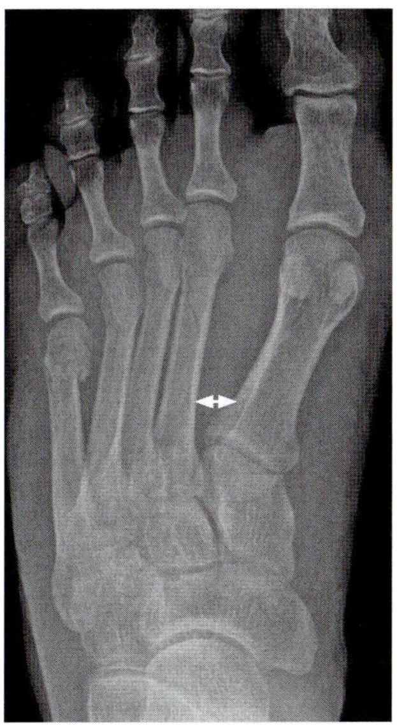

Fig 6.8-2 The AP (dorsoplantar) x-ray of the injured left foot reveals an enlarged distance between the first and second MT bases (double arrow). The contour of the second and third MT bases appears blurred; thus suspicious of a basal fracture. This image is highly suspicious of a TMT (Lisfranc) joint injury warranting further investigation.

Examination of the left foot revealed that sensory and motor functions were intact and normal. It was a closed injury. There were no clinical signs which might indicate presence of a compartment syndrome (CS), such as massive swelling, loss of skin wrinkling, and pain on passive stretch of toes.

As this is a clinically obvious midfoot injury, standard AP (dorsoplantar), oblique, and lateral x-rays of the whole foot were obtained revealing a disruption of the medial tarsometatarsal (TMT; Lisfranc) joint with increased distance between the first and second metatarsal (MT) bases and suspected fractures of the second and third MT bases (**Fig 6.8-2**).

As an injury to the TMT joint was suspected, a computed tomographic (CT) scan was performed (**Fig 6.8-3a**). Axial CT imaging revealed a fleck sign (bony avulsion between the first and second MT bases). This is highly indicative of an injury to the Lisfranc ligament, running from the medial cuneiform to the second MT base. Interestingly, there was no lateral shift of the second MT base which commonly occurs when the Lisfranc ligament is disrupted. There was also a fracture of the third MT base. Sagittal CT reconstruction revealed an additional bony avulsion of the second MT base dorsal to the first TMT joint (**Fig 6.8-3b**). No bony injuries to the fourth and fifth TMT joints were seen.

As there was bony injury with minimal displacement, no emergent surgery was warranted. The patient was admitted to the hospital for soft-tissue monitoring. A splint was carefully applied taking care to not cause any compression of the soft tissues of the foot, and the left leg was placed on pillows. Cold therapy was applied to the foot, and the soft-tissue pressures were monitored hourly by clinical examination.

At 05:00 the following morning the patient reported increasing pain of the left foot despite rest, elevation, pain medication, and the cooling pack. Repeat clinical examination revealed massive swelling of the whole foot with loss of skin wrinkling and the formation of blisters along both the dorsal and plantar areas (**Fig 6.8-4**). Without further diagnostic tests, the patient was taken to the operating room (OR).

When the presence of CS is highly suspected, waiting to find and use the electronic measuring device is unnecessary. Manual examination, such as pain with passive stretch of the toes and increased tissue tightness, should be the surgeon's main guide to the need for urgent surgery. Prolonged delay can lead to extensive soft-tissue damage and loss of function.

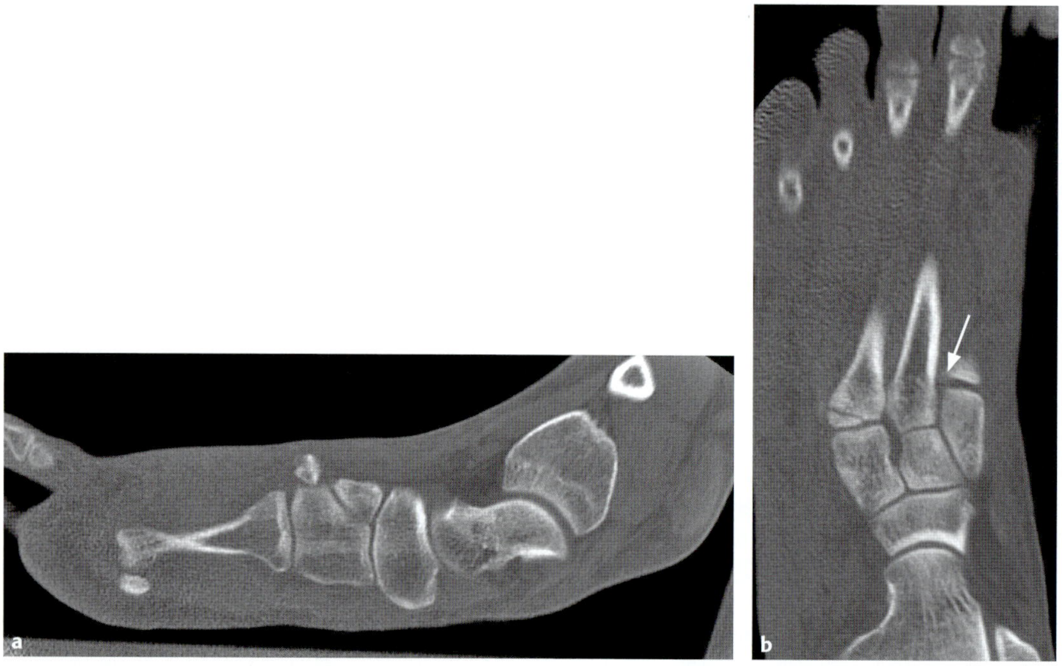

Fig 6.8-3a–b Computed tomographic scans.
a Axial view revealed a fleck sign between the first and second MT base (arrow) and a wide joint space at the first TMT joint. In addition, a fracture was seen at the third MT base confirming a relevant injury to the TMT joint.
b Sagittal view showed a dorsally displaced avulsion fragment from the second MT base at the first TMT joint.

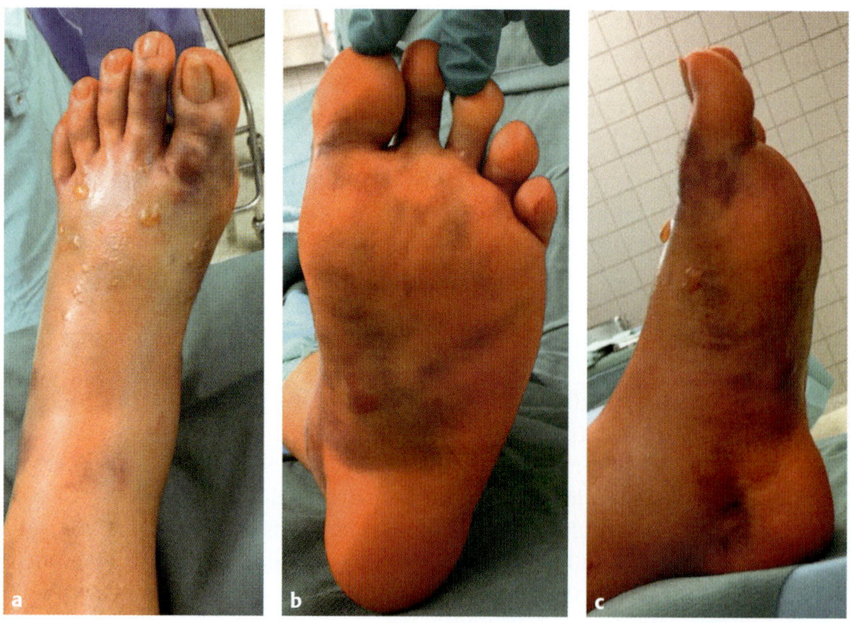

Fig 6.8-4a–c Soft-tissue status approximately 10 hours after admission. Notice the severe swelling of the whole foot, complete loss of skin wrinkling, and the formation of blisters at the dorsal and plantar aspect which are typical signs of an acute foot compartment syndrome. In the presence of these clinical symptoms, no further diagnostic tests are needed. Also note the plantar ecchymosis (**b**) as a pathognomonic sign of a severe disruption of the strong plantar ligaments at the midfoot indicating a relevant injury to the Chopart and/or Lisfranc joint.

2 Preoperative planning

Compartment release

Compartment syndrome is caused by increasing pressure within one or more of the muscular compartments, secondary to hemorrhage or edema, resulting in impaired venous outflow. Local tissue pressures exceed capillary perfusion pressure, resulting in ischemia and subsequent necrosis followed by fibrosis and contracture of the compartment's contents. After 4–6 hours of ischemia, muscles and peripheral nerves undergo irreversible damage. Early compartment release prevents long term damage to these structures.

Therefore, for this case, after the clinical diagnosis of a foot compartment syndrome (FCS) was made, emergent surgical decompression (compartment release) was performed. Also, as the calcaneal compartment of the foot communicates with the deep posterior compartment of the leg, there is a possibility of a FCS extending into the leg, with resulting severe higher injuries.

There are nine foot compartments (**Fig 6.8-5**):

1 The medial compartment contains the abductor hallucis and flexor hallucis brevis muscles.
2 The superficial plantar compartment contains the flexor digitorum longus and brevis muscles.
3 The lateral compartment contains the abductor digiti minimi and flexor digiti minimi brevis.
4 The adductor compartment contains the oblique head of the adductor hallucis muscle.
5–8 The four interossei compartments are dorsally located between each of the MTs, and each includes dorsal and plantar interosseus muscles. Due to the small size of its muscles, both the adductor and interossei compartment exist in the forefoot only.
9 The calcaneal (deep central) compartment contains the quadratus plantae muscle. It exists only in the hindfoot but has a communication with the deep posterior compartment of the lower leg. Therefore, a CS involving the deep posterior compartment may lead to a FCS of the calcaneal compartment.

The dorsal compartment is confined by the dorsal skin and fascia. It contains the short extensor muscles which are sometimes considered as a tenth compartment.

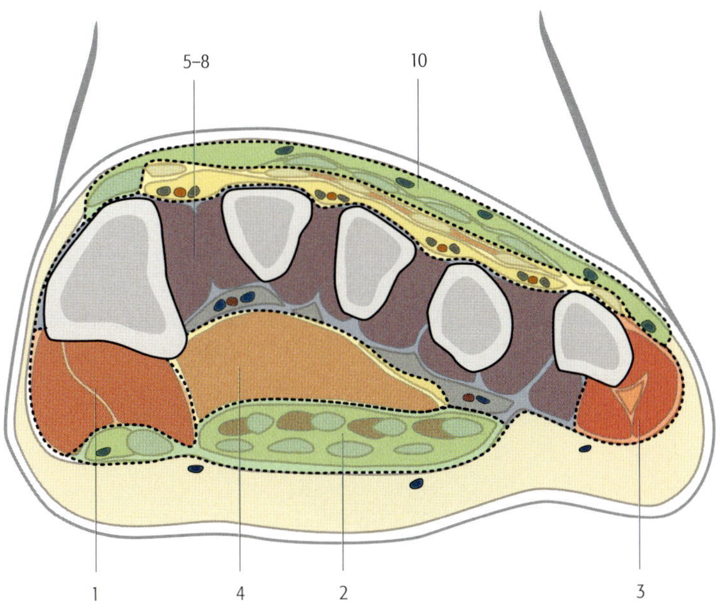

Fig 6.8-5 The foot compartments at the level of the TMT joint.
1 Medial
2 Superficial (central)
3 Lateral
4 Adductor (forefoot only)
5–8 Four interossei (forefoot only)
10 The dorsal aspect of the foot is sometimes considered a tenth compartment.

The approaches for compartment decompression generally include two dorsal incisions (**Fig 6.8-6a**) for access to forefoot or interossei compartments, and one medial incision for decompression of the calcaneal, medial, lateral and superficial compartments (**Fig 6.8-6b–c**). Alternatively, a single long central dorsal incision (Hannover incision) can be used. In the presence of a Lisfranc injury, the same incision is used for reduction and fixation of the TMT fractures and dislocations.

The deep posterior (calcaneal) compartment can be released via a medial incision. The number and location of incisions needed must be tailored to the individual pattern of injury and amount of soft-tissue damage.

Open reduction and internal fixation of the Lisfranc injury

For this active and healthy 30-year-old patient, stabilization of the Lisfranc joint was indicated for TMT instability secondary to injury of the Lisfranc ligament between the first cuneiform and the second MT base.

Nonoperative treatment of unstable Lisfranc injuries can lead to chronic instability with progressive arthritis and an acquired pes-plano-abducto valgus (flatfoot) deformity (posttraumatic flatfoot).

With only minimal displacement of the first TMT joint and instability of second and third TMT joints and fracture of the third MT base, open reduction and internal fixation can be performed via the approaches provided by the compartment release. The approaches may be extended for better surgical exposure. Any intertarsal instability is addressed first. Then the first to third TMT joints can be stabilized temporarily with K-wires. A "Lisfranc screw" can be placed between the medial cuneiform and second MT base along the course of the ruptured Lisfranc ligament.

Usually, the fourth and fifth MT bases will realign to the corresponding cuneiforms after reduction of the first to third MT bases. The surgeon should be prepared to stabilize the fourth and fifth TMT joints with K-wires if these remain displaced after fixation of the first to third TMT joint.

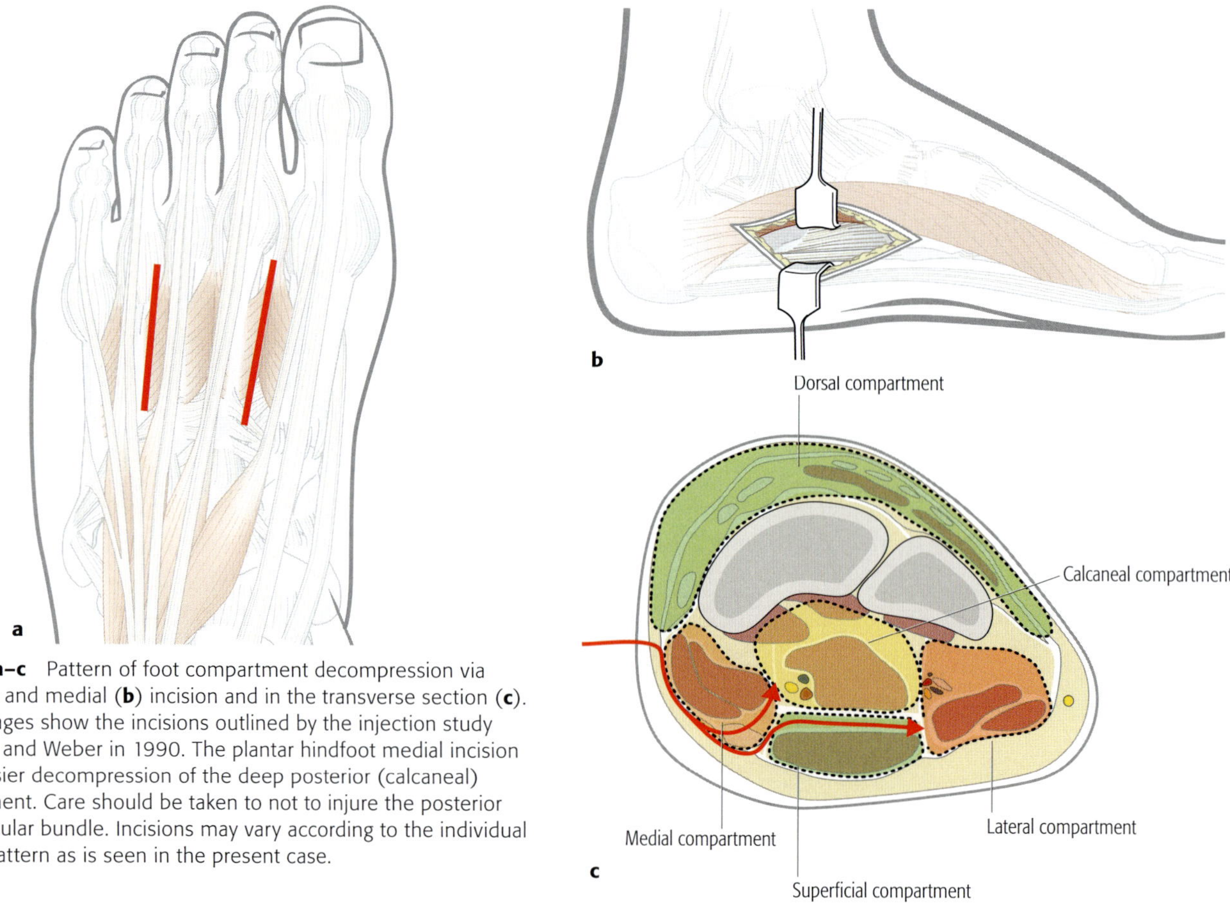

Fig 6.8-6a–c Pattern of foot compartment decompression via dorsal (**a**) and medial (**b**) incision and in the transverse section (**c**). These images show the incisions outlined by the injection study by Manoli and Weber in 1990. The plantar hindfoot medial incision allows easier decompression of the deep posterior (calcaneal) compartment. Care should be taken to not to injure the posterior neurovascular bundle. Incisions may vary according to the individual fracture pattern as is seen in the present case.

3 Operating room setup

Patient positioning	• Supine on a radiolucent table with the foot draped free and mobile to allow easy C-arm imaging. • The leg should be placed on a foam ramp or a full-length bump made out of extra sheets folded lengthwise to raise the affected foot above the contralateral foot. This allows easier cross table imaging.
Anesthesia options	• General and/or regional anesthesia
C-arm location	• The C-arm and screen are placed to allow the surgeon an unobstructed view in all positions • The C-arm should be easily rotated for AP, oblique, and lateral imaging
Tourniquet	• Optional. Applied to the proximal thigh. If good blood pressure control is possible by anesthesia, then the cuff need not be inflated.
Tips	• When using a large C-arm, the foot is placed flat on the operative table for simulated weight bearing (WB). An assistant holds the knee bent at 90–100°. The leg can then be rotated internally to obtain a 45° oblique view, or externally to obtain a lateral view of the foot. • If a mini-C-arm is used, the flat imaging side of the unit can be placed against the sole of the foot for simulated WB views.

For illustrations and overview of anesthetic considerations, see chapter 1.

Equipment

- Point-to-point reduction (Weber) clamp
- 3.5–4.0 mm cortex screws and drill bits
- K-wires

Size of system, instruments, and implants may vary according to anatomy.

4 Surgical procedure

Forefoot compartment decompression is carried out via two dorsal incisions for access to the forefoot and interossei compartments (**Fig 6.8-7a**). The dorsomedial incision is placed over the second MT shaft and the dorsolateral incision is placed over the fourth MT shaft or web space. The first and second web spaces are accessed from the medial incision and the third and fourth web spaces from the lateral incision.

The fasciae of the interosseous muscles are released through the dorsal incisions. The adductor compartment is opened deep within the first interspace. The interosseus muscles should be stripped off the second MT shaft, then the adductor fascia is found deep to the interosseus muscles and opened bluntly in the direction of the muscle fibers. A blunt clamp is spread to release the hematoma. Care should be taken not to injure the perforating branch of the dorsalis pedis artery to the plantar arch that crosses between the bases of the first and second MT.

For this patient swelling and palpable tension were still present after dorsal decompression, so an additional medial incision was made to decompress the calcaneal, medial, superficial and lateral compartments at the midfoot and hindfoot (arrow in **Fig 6.8-7b**).

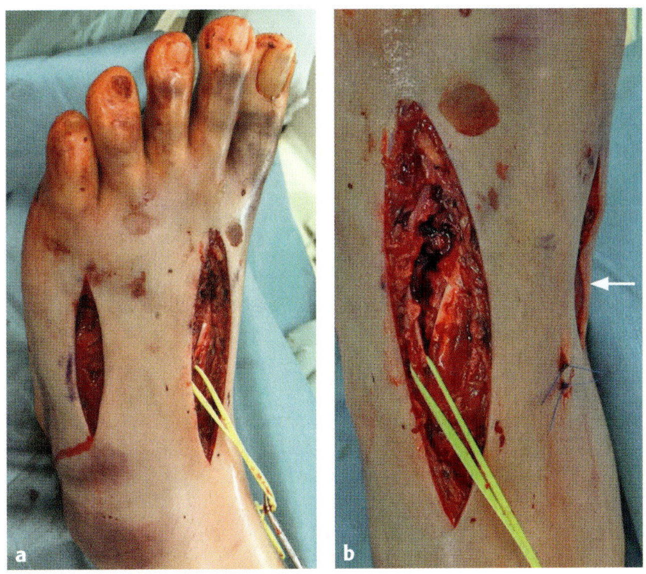

Fig 6.8-7a–b Forefoot compartment decompression was carried out via two parallel dorsal incisions (**a**). An additional medial incision was performed for hindfoot decompression (arrow **b**). The dorsomedial incision was extended proximally for the exposure of the TMT joints.

The Lisfanc joints are cleared of intervening bone or soft tissues. In this case, the unstable first and second TMT joints were approached through the dorsomedial incision. The TMT joints are reduced and fixed with K-wires. A stab incision is made over the medial aspect of the medial cuneiform. Reduction of the second MT to first cuneiform is then achieved with a point-to-point reduction (Weber) clamp (**Fig 6.8-8a**).

Anatomical reduction of the first and second TMT joint is confirmed with the standard AP, oblique, and lateral C-arm projections.

Next, the third TMT joint is fixed with a K-wire. For this patient the small, nondisplaced fracture at the third MT base was not fixed separately, as it did not displace with TMT transfixation.

After anatomical reduction has been confirmed, a drill bit is introduced into the small incision at the medial cuneiform and aimed toward the second MT base. The drill bit is directed distally and slightly upward. Fixation along the course of the avulsed Lisfranc ligament is achieved with a 4.0 mm cortex screw ("Lisfranc screw"). Correct screw and K-wire position and length are checked again with the three standard C-arm projections (**Fig 6.8-8**). It is sometimes possible to place this same screw across to the third MT as well. Care must be taken to not cause any further gapping if this technique is chosen.

For this patient, the fourth and fifth TMT joints were aligned anatomically after fixation of the first to third TMT joints; thus no need for separate reduction and fixation was seen.

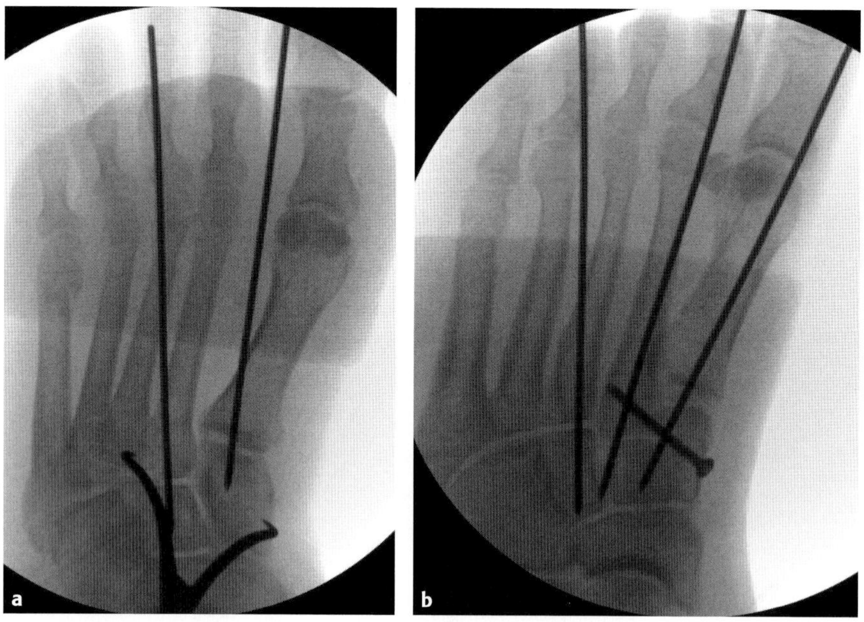

Fig 6.8-8a–b

a Reduction of the Lisfranc injury started with reduction of the unstable first and second TMT joints and K-wire transfixation. The first and second ray are reduced with a point-to-point reduction (Weber) clamp.

b Next, the third TMT joint was fixed with a K-wire and the correct position of the third to fifth TMT joints was verified with a 45° oblique C-arm view of the midfoot. A screw ("Lisfranc screw") from the medial cuneiform to the second metatarsal base was introduced via a medial stab incision.

The K-wires used for fixation of the first to third TMT joints are then bent and cut within the subcutaneous tissue to facilitate later removal (**Fig 6.8-9**). Alternatively, the K-wires can be replaced by screws for definitive internal fixation.

Anatomical reduction is mandatory, as even minor malalignment at the TMT joint can result in painful arthritic deformities. Correct screw position and length is checked again at the end of surgery with the standard AP, oblique, and lateral C-arm projections.

After internal fixation the fasciotomy wounds can be covered temporarily with a collagen membrane as artificial skin cover, if primary closure is not possible. Vacuum-assisted closure may be used to assist in wound closure (**Fig 6.8-10**).

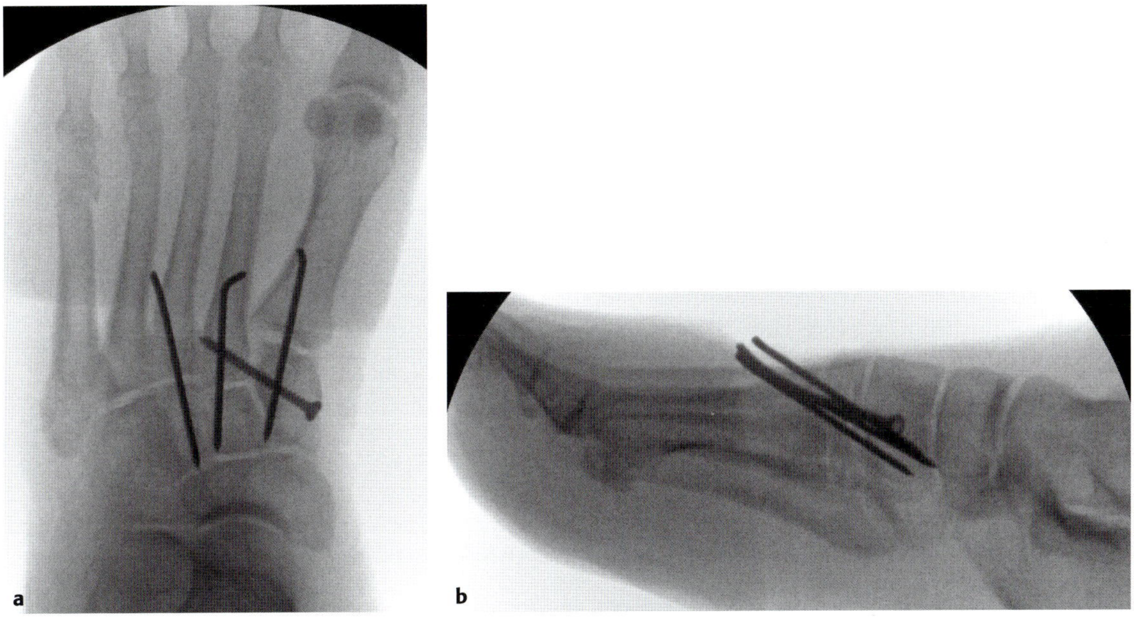

Fig 6.8-9a–b The K-wires introduced into the first through third tarsometatarsal joints were bent and cut under the skin the subcutaneous tissue to facilitate later removal.

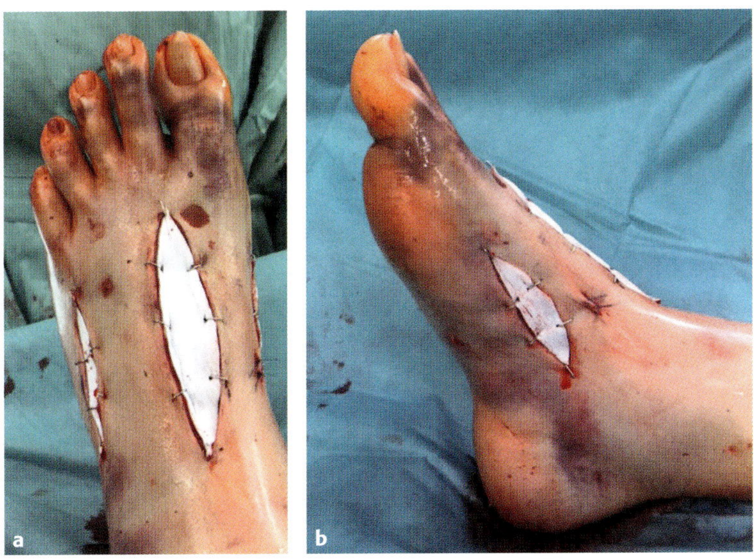

Fig 6.8-10a–b Temporary wound closure without applying any tension was achieved with a collagen-based artificial skin substitute.

5 Pitfalls and complications

Pitfalls

Overlooked FCS

Lisfranc fracture-dislocations are among the most frequent causes of FCS. Delayed fasciotomy or untreated FCS regularly leads to stiffness, chronic disability, deformity, and pain. The intrinsic foot muscles appear to be more susceptible to elevated pressure than the larger muscles of the thigh or leg. Necrosis of the intrinsics can lead to ischemic contractures which result in lesser toe deformities and pes cavus deformity. Neurovascular compromise due to elevated compartment pressures can also cause chronic pain and an insensate foot with secondary neuropathic pathology (eg, chronic ulceration or joint destruction).

For this patient, a direct trauma with a relatively subtle injury to the TMT joint was accompanied by CS which developed within 10 hours. A high level of suspicion is required not to miss the window of opportunity in which the compartment release can still performed to prevent later contracture.

The existence of an FCS and the severity of its sequelae are still debated. However, direct pressure measurements have revealed high compartmental pressures of the foot of up to 90 mm Hg. Aside from painful, slowly developing hammer toes, contracture of the intrinsic foot muscles can lead to a painful deformed foot. As discussed previously, a CS of the deep compartment of the leg can be accompanied by a FCS due to the connection between the two compartments.

Inadequate treatment

Nonoperative treatment of unstable Lisfranc injuries regularly leads to chronic instability with progressive arthritis and deformity. Subtle Lisfranc injuries—such as in the present case—with minimal displacement or isolated diastasis between the first cuneiform and second MT base are frequently overlooked with deleterious consequences for the patient.

Inadequate reduction

Anatomical reduction is the single most important prognostic factor in the treatment of Lisfranc injuries. Even minor incongruities may lead to painful midfoot deformities and secondary forefoot and hindfoot malpositioning. Adequate exposure of the TMT joints, particularly the first and second, is helpful in avoiding intervening ligament or bony debris, gross instability, or further fragmentation of a fractured MT base.

Great care should be taken to obtain the three standard C-arm projections intraoperatively to reliably control reduction and screw position.

Complications

- Injury to the dorsalis pedis artery and deep peroneal nerve
- Injury to the anterior tibial tendon
- Injury to the medial plantar nerve and vessels (with medial compartment release)
- Loss of reduction or fixation
- Malunion
- Nonunion
- Chronic instability after implant removal
- Posttraumatic arthritis

6 Alternative techniques

Instead of K-wires, screws can be used for TMT joint transfixation.

For highly unstable injuries with comminution of the MT base (most likely the second), small dorsal bridging plates can be used for stabilization.

Some surgeons prefer primary fusion of purely ligamentous Lisfranc injuries, as they have a greater risk of developing posttraumatic arthritis necessitating secondary fusion.

7 Postoperative management and rehabilitation

Postoperatively, the leg is immobilized in a splint and elevated to a level position. Cold therapy can be applied to the foot. The compartment status is monitored at least twice daily.

For this patient, the swelling of the foot and pain had subsided by postoperative day 6. He was returned to the OR where the wounds were primarily closed without tension on the skin (**Fig 6.8-11**). After complete wound closure, active and passive range-of-motion exercises of the ankle, subtalar, and midtarsal (Chopart) joints and the toes were initiated on postoperative day 1. A rigid-soled shoe (or removable fracture boot) was applied and he was restricted to partial WB (up to 20 kg, ie, foot flat in a compliant patient) on the injured leg for 6 weeks. Standard postoperative x-rays 1 week after mobilization of the patient revealed anatomical reduction.

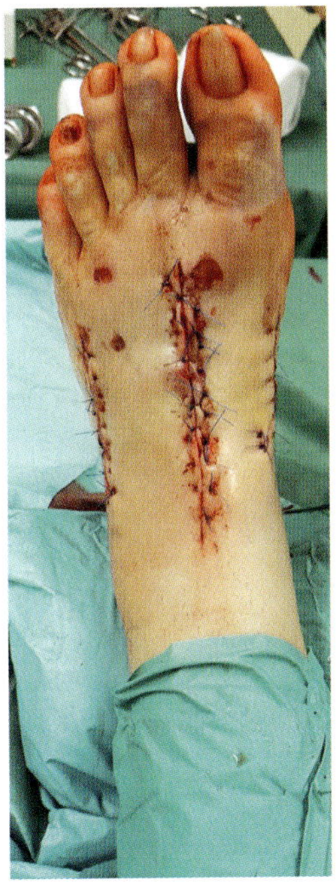

Fig 6.8-11 Delayed primary closure of wounds.

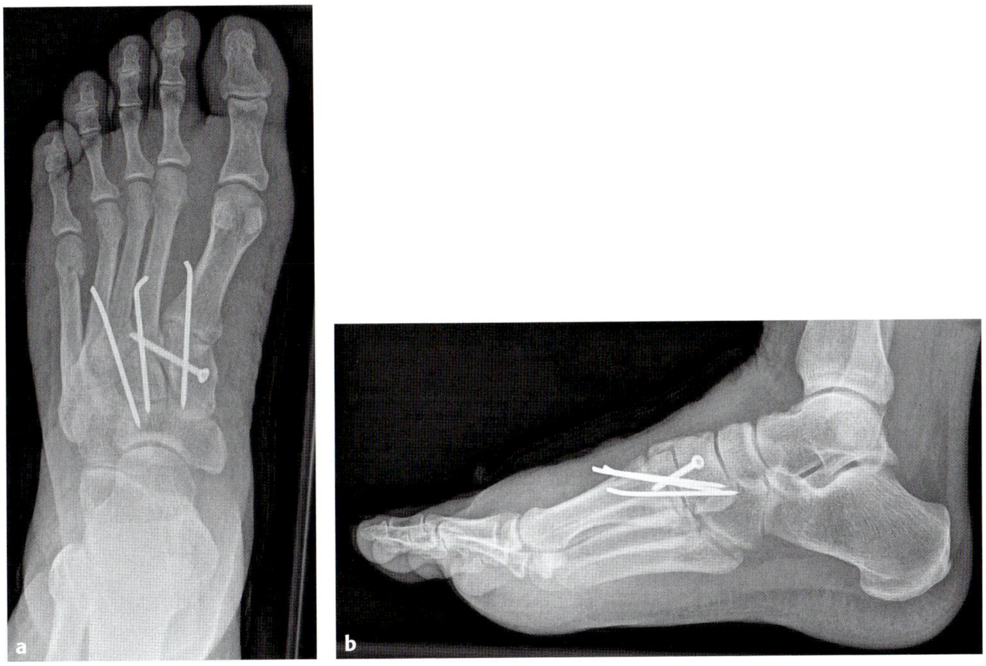

Fig 6.8-12a–b Lateral and AP views showing postoperative reduction of the Lisfranc joints.

Implant removal

For this patient K-wires and screw were removed via small incisions 8 weeks postoperatively.

Alternatively, screws in the first to third TMT joints can be left in place. If one elects to remove the screws after 4–6 months, the TMT joints are checked for stability with forced abduction and adduction of the forefoot, after screw removal (**Fig 6.8-12** and **Fig 6.8-13**). After stability is confirmed, WB is increased gradually after implant removal. A more active rehabilitation protocol is then initiated including muscular balancing and gait training.

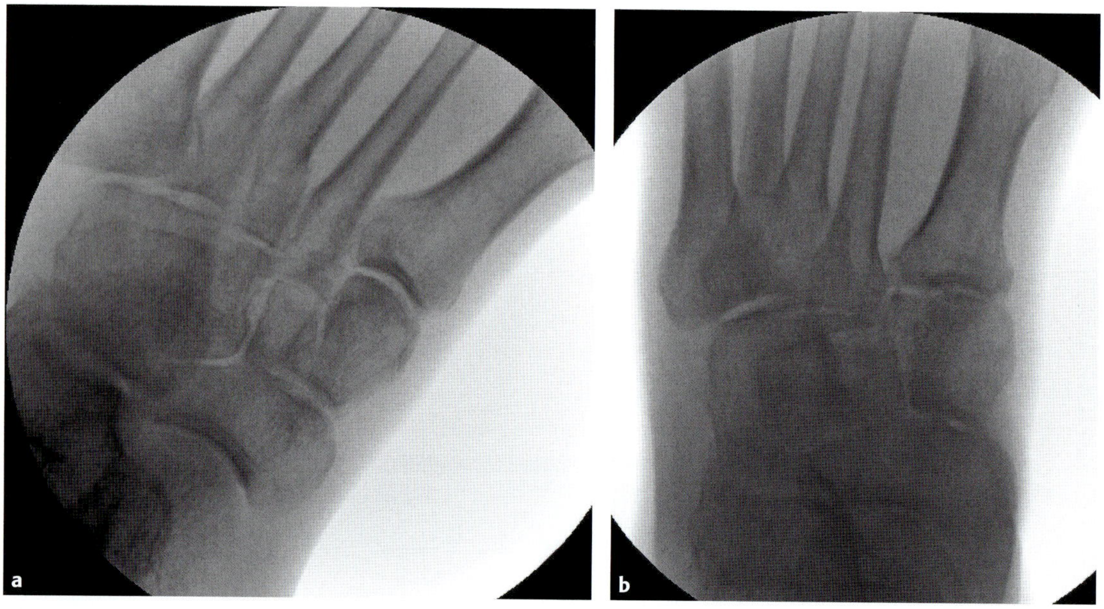

Fig 6.8-13a–b Stress views with forefoot adduction/abduction after implant removal showing no instability.

8 Recommended reading

Castro M, Melao L, Canella C, et al. Lisfranc joint ligamentous complex: MRI with anatomic correlation in cadavers. *AJR Am J Roentgenol.* 2010 Dec;195(6):W447–455.

Faciszewski T, Burks RT, Manaster BJ. Subtle injuries of the Lisfranc joint. *J Bone Joint Surg Am.* 1990 Dec;72(10):1519–1522.

Kuo RS, Tejwani NC, Digiovanni CW, et al. Outcome after open reduction and internal fixation of Lisfranc joint injuries. *J Bone Joint Surg Am.* 2000 Nov;82-a(11):1609–1618.

Ly TV, Coetzee JC. Treatment of primarily ligamentous Lisfranc joint injuries: primary arthrodesis compared with open reduction and internal fixation. A prospective, randomized study. *J Bone Joint Surg Am.* 2006 Mar;88(3):514–520.

Manoli A 2nd. Compartment syndromes of the foot: current concepts. *Foot Ankle.* 1990 Jun;10(6):340–344.

Manoli A 2nd, Weber TG. Fasciotomy of the foot: an anatomical study with special reference to release of the calcaneal compartment. *Foot Ankle.* 1990 Apr;10(5):267–275.

Myerson MS. The diagnosis and treatment of injury to the tarsometatarsal joint complex. *J Bone Joint Surg Br.* 1999 Sep;81(5):756–763.

Nunley JA, Vertullo CJ. Classification, investigation, and management of midfoot sprains: Lisfranc injuries in the athlete. *Am J Sports Med.* 2002 Nov–Dec;30(6):871–878.

Rammelt S. Chopart and Lisfranc joint injuries. In: Bentley G, ed. *European Surgical Orthopaedics and Traumatology. The EFORT Textbook.* Berlin Heidelberg New York: Springer; 2014:3835–3857.

Rammelt S, Schneiders W, Schikore H, et al. Primary open reduction and fixation compared with delayed corrective arthrodesis in the treatment of tarsometatarsal (Lisfranc) fracture dislocation. *J Bone Joint Surg Br.* 2008 Nov;90(11):1499–1506.

Ross G, Cronin R, Hauzenblas J, et al. Plantar ecchymosis sign: a clinical aid to diagnosis of occult Lisfranc tarsometatarsal injuries. *J Orthop Trauma.* 1996;10(2):119–122.

Sands AK, Grose A. Lisfranc injuries. *Injury.* 2004 Sep;35 Suppl 2:Sb71–76.

Sands AK, Rammelt S, Manoli A 2nd. Foot compartment syndrome—a clinical review. *Fuß Sprunggelenk.* 2015 March;13(1):11–21.

6.9 Tarsometatarsal/intertarsal complex midfoot injury

Andrew K Sands

1 Case description

A 62-year-old man was standing in the street when his foot was run over by a truck. He was brought to the emergency department by ambulance where a full evaluation was performed. He had no associated skeletal or internal injuries, or any associated medical comorbidities. There was no head injury or loss of consciousness. The injury was closed with no loss of skin. His foot was swollen but there was no evidence of leg or foot compartment syndrome. There was valgus deformity. Capillary refill was intact. Sensory examination showed minimal decrease to light touch related to the injury.

X-rays revealed complex injuries including the metatarsals(MTs), the cuneiforms, and tarsal bones with intertarsal (IT) joint injuries (**Fig 6.9-1a–c**).

A computed tomographic (CT) scan with reconstructions was obtained demonstrating the 3D nature of the injury and revealing secondary injuries hidden by double density overlaps within the image (**Fig 6.9-1d–e**).

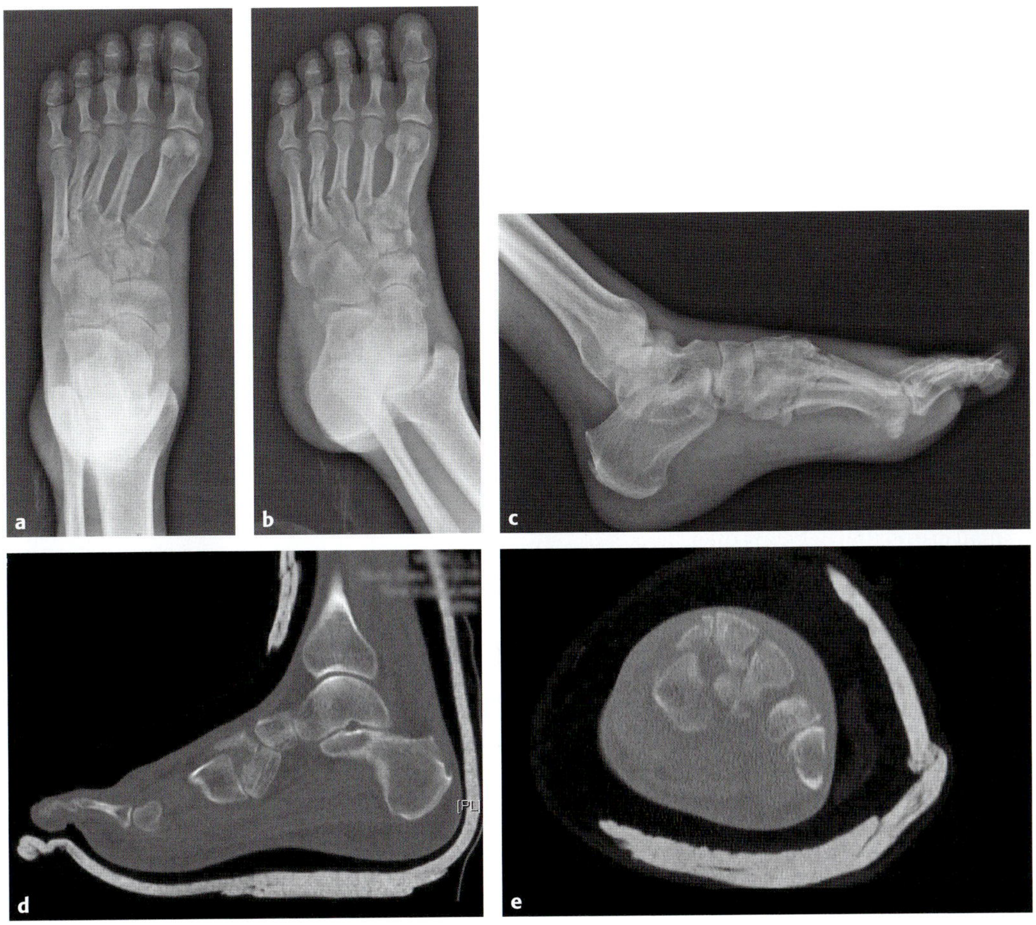

Fig 6.9-1a–e Emergency department injury x-rays (**a–c**), and CT images (**d–e**) showing the splinted foot.

- **a** AP view.
- **b** 30° oblique view.
- **c** Lateral view.
- **d** Sagittal reconstruction.
- **e** Coronal reconstruction.

2 Preoperative planning

Indications for surgery

In the case of a complex midfoot injury, the foot may be injured from the bases of the MTs, through Lisfranc joints and IT area, and include the Chopart joint area. These injuries can be difficult to treat as they are unstable and may include a soft-tissue injury as well. In these cases, immediate open reduction and internal fixation (ORIF) will lead to soft-tissue compromise and breakdown. Staged treatment is therefore required.

Considerations for surgery

As with any midfoot injury, attention to form and biomechanics of the foot is paramount. The medial and lateral columns must be realigned allowing the soft tissue to relax.

Avoid incisions or many percutaneous wires along the dorsum of the foot.

Imaging

Emergency department x-rays often are not clear due to double density overlap hiding the complex injuries (**Fig 6.9-1a–c**). Often, external fixation is placed in the operating room which achieves general but not final reduction. Then a CT scan for 3D representation of the injury is performed (**Fig 6.9-1d–e**).

Stage 1: Realignment of the columns of the foot

This involves placement of external fixation along the mid-medial and mid-lateral axes of the foot. Distraction with a small distraction device on each side allows for proper realignment of the columns. Often, any dorsal displacement corrects sufficiently to avoid undue pressure on the soft tissues.

Depending on the injury and amount of spanning needed, two pins can be placed; one in the middle of the first MT and the other in the medial talar neck, just anterior to the medial malleolus. The medial small distraction device is then assembled.

The lateral pins can be placed in the distal calcaneus and the fourth or fifth MT midshafts. The lateral small distraction device is then assembled.

The small distraction devices are then adjusted under C-arm guidance to achieve reduction and alignment of the columns. Occasionally, percutaneous wires are needed for reduction assistance.

Once the alignment has been achieved, the small distraction devices should be replaced by carbon fiber rods. Semicircular cross-rods between the small distraction devices can also be used for further stability.

Stage 2: Definitive reduction and fixation

After the soft tissue has recovered from the initial injury (usually 2–3 weeks), definitive ORIF can be performed. The external fixation device can be used as an intraoperative reduction tool. The small distraction device can be reapplied to the pins and over-distraction performed. This allows for better visualization into the fractures.

After ORIF, the external fixation device is usually removed. However, in the case of a potentially unreliable patient or in osteoporotic bones, the external fixation can be left in place as supplementary fixation for as long as the surgeon deems necessary (usually 6–8 weeks).

3 Operating room setup

Patient positioning	• Supine, moved down to the end of the operative table with an ipsilateral bump under the buttock. • The leg is placed on a foam ramp and the heel is placed on a towel bump as needed for imaging.
Anesthesia options	• General anesthesia, often supplemented with a peripheral nerve block
C-arm location	• Placed on the ipsilateral side of the injury with the C-arm screen positioned towards the foot
Tourniquet	• Placed on the upper thigh and inflated at the surgeon's discretion. • Generally improves fracture visualization
Tips	• A foam ramp under the affected leg lifts the leg and operative area above the unaffected leg allowing easier cross table imaging. • A towel bump under the heel lifts the foot off the ramp a bit more which allows easier positioning of the mini-C-arm around the end of the table.

The same OR setup can be used for both surgical stages.

For illustrations and overview of anesthetic considerations, see chapter 1.

Equipment

Stage 1: Realignment of the columns of the foot

- Mini/small external fixator system
- Small distraction devices (two; one for medial column, one for lateral column)

Stage 2: Definitive reduction and fixation

- Reduction tools, such as dental tools
- Elevators
- Two small distraction devices (one for medial column, one for lateral column)
- Plates, preferably mesh plate (for wide area coverage, customization, variable angle locking [VAL] screw aiming)
- Screws of appropriate size
- Olive wires
- K-wires for temporary fixation

4 Surgical procedure

Stage 1: Realignment of the columns of the foot

These cases are not usually considered emergencies and usually do not have to be taken to the OR immediately. The case can be delayed until the more experienced day crew is available.

As soon as possible the patient is taken to the OR where, under general anesthesia with adequate muscle relaxation, the medial and lateral distraction devices are placed under C-arm guidance.

Once the pins are in place medially and laterally, and the small distraction devices are assembled and in place, the columns of the foot are brought out to length and realigned using the two distraction devices (**Fig 6.9-2a–b**).

When the foot is properly aligned, the distraction devices are swapped for external fixation bars and locked in place (**Fig 6.9-2c**). It should be noted that the distraction devices are instruments and should not remain on the foot during the hospital stay or when the patient returns home between stage 1 and stage 2 of the procedure. The patient should be educated on how to properly care for the pins and the skin on the dorsum of the foot. The patient is advised to keep the foot elevated to horizontal at all times. The patient returns to the clinic after 1–2 weeks so that the soft tissues can be evaluated. Based on the clinical findings, surgery for definitive reduction and fixation is then planned.

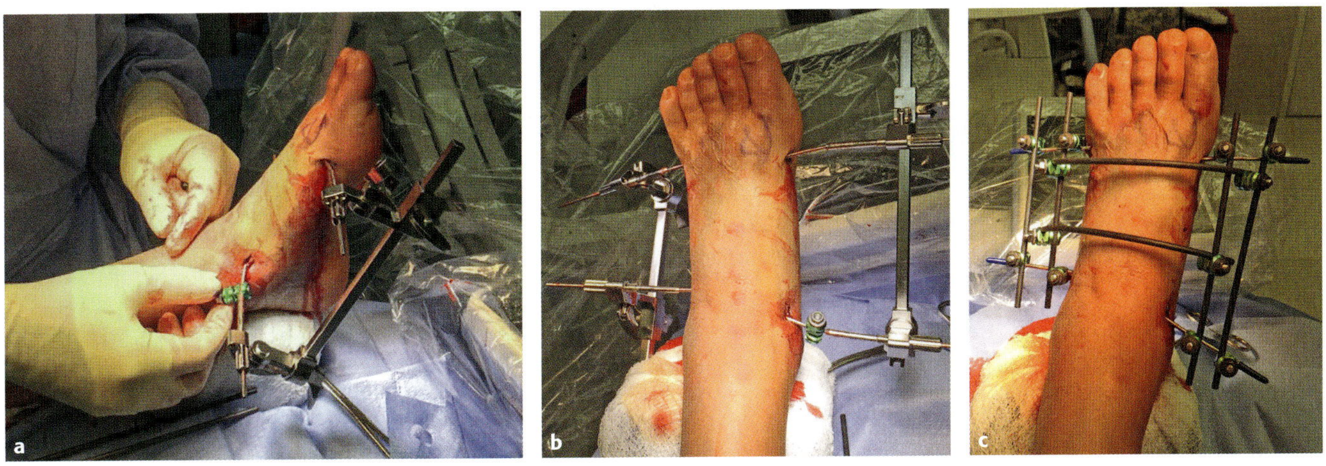

Fig 6.9-2a–c Placement of external fixator with reduction using a small distraction device.
a Placement of the medial small distraction device under mini-C-arm guidance.
b Medial and lateral small distraction devices in place. Length and reduction are adjusted under mini-C-arm guidance.
c Carbon fiber rods are placed so that the small distraction device can be removed.

Stage 2: Definitive reduction and fixation

The medial and lateral external fixators from stage 1, when overall foot realignment was done under anesthesia (**Fig 6.9-3**), can be removed for patient preparation and for the incisions.

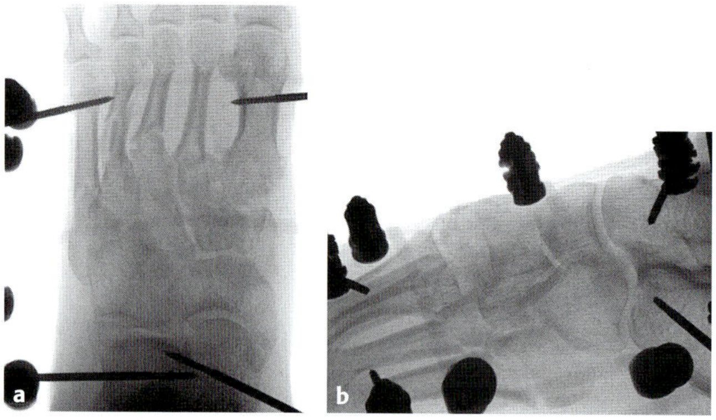

Fig 6.9-3a–b Intraoperative images showing preliminary reduction with the external fixator in place after the stage 1: realignment of the columns of the foot.

- **a** AP view.
- **b** Lateral view.

Medial approach

A medial utility incision is made 1 cm below the tip of the medial malleolus extending over the medial navicular prominence, out toward the medial eminence of the first MT head, roughly along the glabrous line. Usually the incision is extended to include the base of the first MT to the medial talar neck, but incision length depends on the extent of the injury (**Fig 6.9-4a–b**).

Lateral approach

An axial incision is made over the superior part of the distal calcaneus, extending distally over the cuboid and along the fourth ray toward the fourth toe (**Fig 6.9-4c–d**).

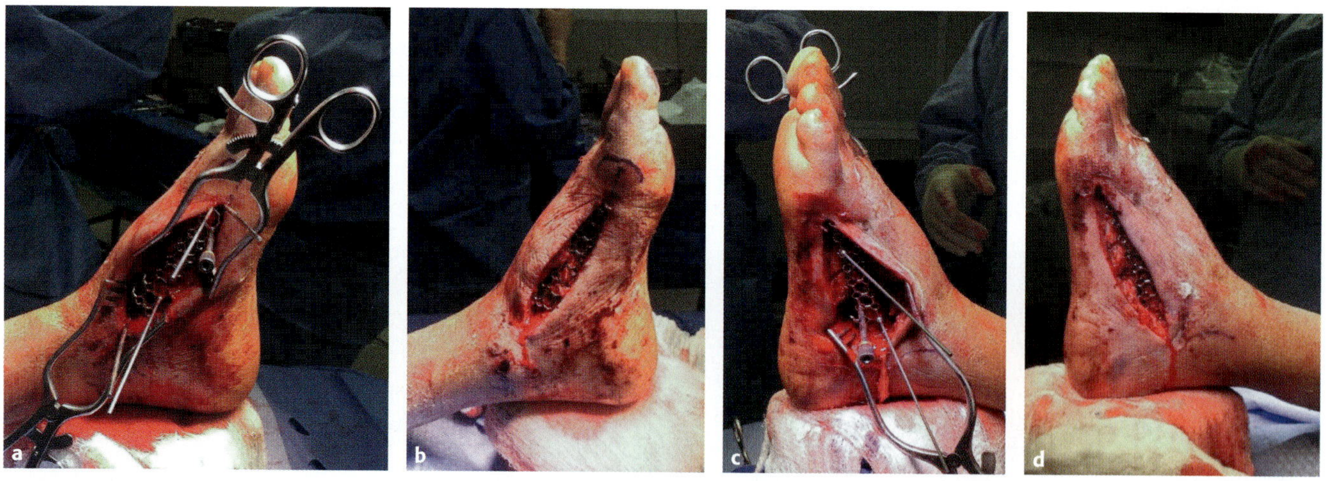

Fig 6.9-4a–d Intraoperative images showing definitive ORIF with plates: medial and lateral reduction, plate adaption, placement of VAL screws, and final construct.

- **a** Medial axial incision. The plate has been snipped into shape, contoured and secured temporarily with an olive wire.
- **b** Medial plate in place and secured with screws.
- **c** Lateral axial incision. The plate has been cut to shape, contoured, and temporarily secured with an olive wire.
- **d** Lateral axial incision with plate in place and screws placed.

Any dorsal approach over the foot should be avoided as the soft tissue and blood supply have been injured (**Fig 6.9-5**). The newer VAL plates with longer screws allow for indirect reduction with the distraction devices and ORIF through the medial and lateral incisions.

Fixation

The mesh plate is cut to shape. Usually, one plate is enough for both medial and lateral columns. The general shape is cut with the gross cutters. The cut arms are smoothed using the hole cutter (**Fig 6.9-6**). The sections of plate can then be contoured. The concave nature of the plate usually fits perfectly along the medial column without much bending needed. The lateral plate needs to be manually twisted so that the it sits flat on the midfoot. Any contouring must be done with the proper 2.7 plate hole benders. If these are not used, then the VAL nature of the holes is ruined.

The two plates are then placed along the incisions and provisionally secured with small olive wires. Position is checked on AP, 30° oblique, and lateral C-arm views. If the middle MTs or cuneiforms are displaced dorsally, a small incision may be needed to push them into place. A K-wire can then be used to secure them until screws are placed.

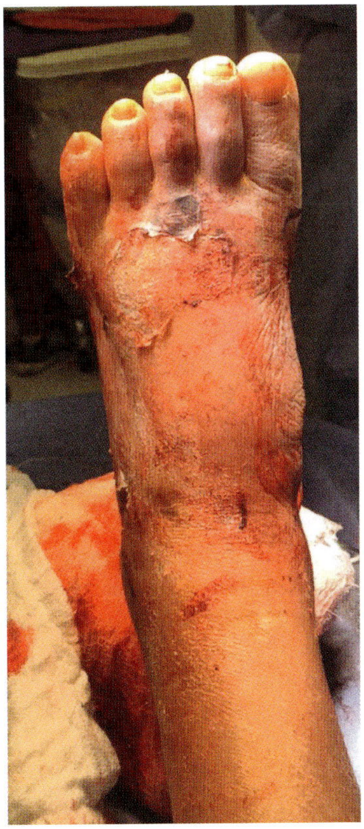

Fig 6.9-5 No incisions are needed along the dorsum of the foot as the plates are placed medially and laterally. The central region is reduced and secured indirectly. The skin on the dorsum of the foot has been traumatized with visible healing fracture blisters.

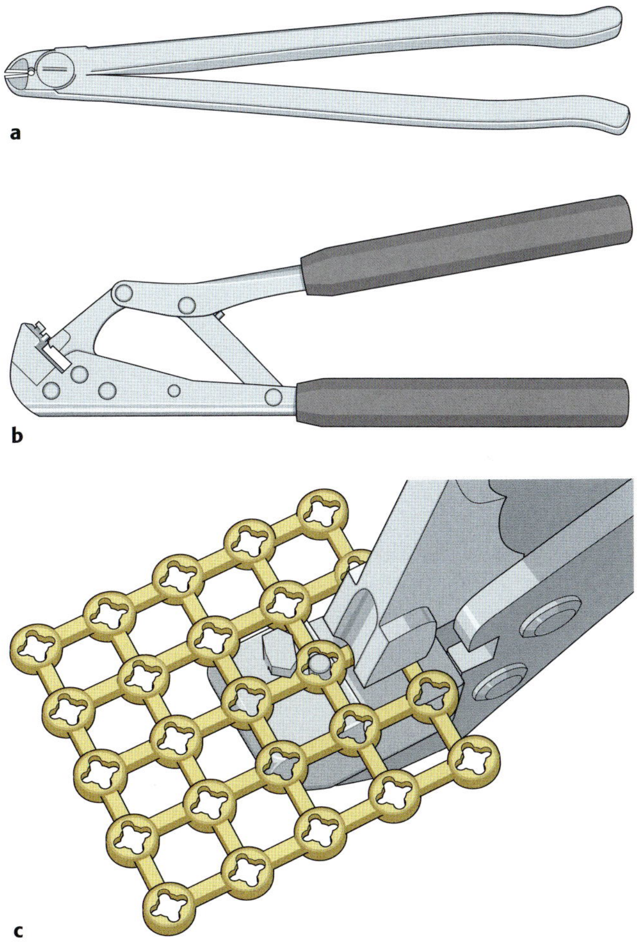

Fig 6.9-6a–c Mesh plate cutters.

a The wire cutter can be used to cut the general shape of the plate through the small connector arms. This, however, leaves small metal burrs on the holes.

b–c The cutting pliers are placed into the hole and the descending cutter is placed so that it removes the metal burr but does not cut into the VAL hole.

Once the columns, TMT, and IT joints are reduced and the plates are in the correct position, the 2.7 mm VAL screws are placed. The nature of the VAL screws (15° off axis in each plane) allows for aiming of the screws across many segments, which allows for stable locking of these segments, both medially and laterally (**Fig 6.9-7**).

Care must be taken to aim the screws dorsally when screws are placed across segments as the area under the second and third TMTs are where the neurovascular structures traverse the foot toward the toes.

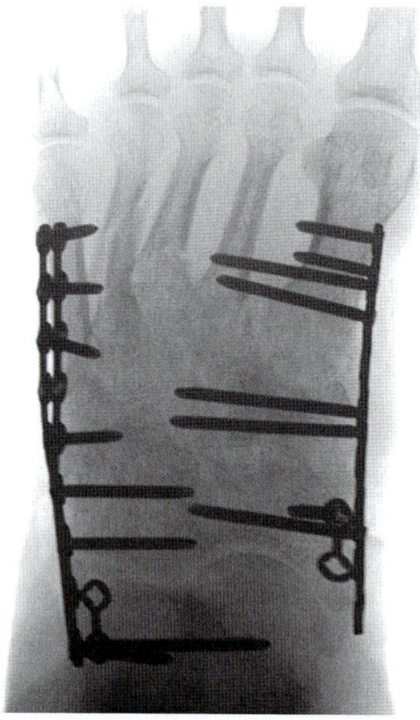

Fig 6.9-7 Postoperative AP x-ray showing ORIF with mesh VAL plate 2.7.

5 Pitfalls and complications

Pitfalls

Failure of anatomical reduction

If the TMT and IT joints remain displaced, then a small dorsal incision can be made as long as care is taken to protect the dorsalis pedis artery. Percutaneous wires can also be used to manipulate and fix displaced bones. However, since the five midfoot bones move as a block, they tolerate small malreductions. Provided that the talonavicular (TN) joint and Lisfranc joints are reduced, the other articulations are secondary in importance.

Overcompression of the navicular facet facing the distal talus

For the navicular and the TN joint, particular care must be taken to avoid over compression of the navicular facet facing the distal talus. This facet is normally spherical. If medial to lateral screws are over tightened, this may lead the spherical shape changing to one that is more acutely peaked. Joint mechanics and range of motion would then be adversely affected.

Complications

- Over-vigorous dissection of the soft tissue can lead to a breakdown of the dorsal flap and wound complications.
- Failure of reduction leading to deformity, arthritis, loss of function, and possible difficulty wearing shoes.
- Incorrect placement of incisions leading to inability to obtain reduction and placement of hardware.
- Timing of surgery: If the soft tissue has been damaged, then surgery must be delayed until the soft tissue recovers. Surgery performed too soon after injury leads to wound complications, such as breakdown.
- Failure to recognize an associated compartment syndrome. See chapter 6.8 for more details.

6 Alternative techniques

If external fixation is used to allow the soft tissues to recover after injury, then it can be used as the definitive treatment without ORIF, assuming anatomical alignment is achieved. It is left in place for 8 weeks until the midfoot bones are stable. In cases with severe soft-tissue injury, initial treatment with an external fixator followed by delayed arthrodesis is necessary.

Percutaneous K-wires can be used if closed manipulation is able to obtain reduction. This technique can also be used if the dorsal foot soft tissues have been compromised.

7 Postoperative management and rehabilitation

If the external fixator has been left in place, it can be removed after 6–8 weeks. Be sure to have the correct tools or wrenches ready in the clinic or as an outpatient surgical procedure.

Gentle ankle and first metatarsophalangeal motion can be started immediately while weight bearing is delayed.

If spanning plates are needed to stabilize the TN or calcaneocuboid joint, these should be removed once the fractures have healed (typically 3–6 months) so that range-of-motion exercises can be started. Talonavicular stiffness causes 90% loss of complex hindfoot motion, which is important to maintain (**Fig 6.9-8**).

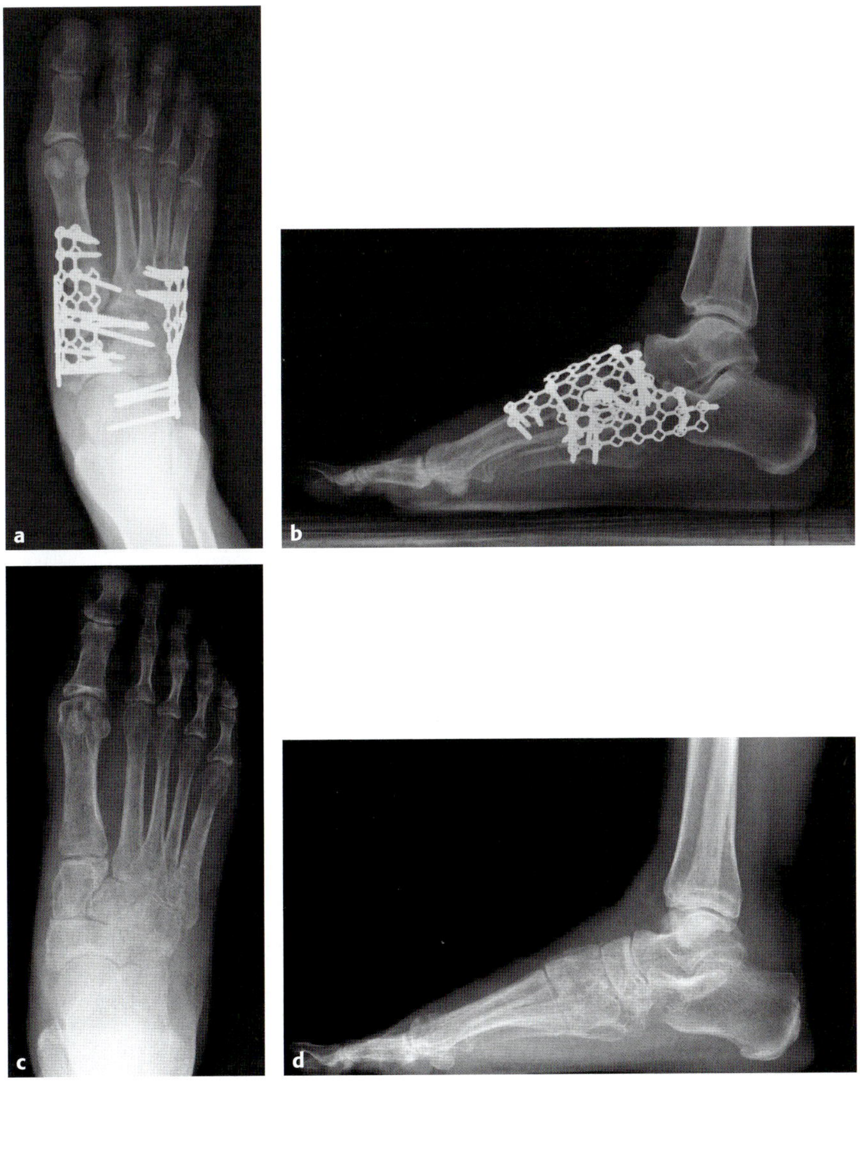

Fig 6.9-8a–d Example from a different case showing the same principle of medial and lateral plating with long crossing screws and indirect reduction and stabilization of the IT areas. The spanning plates were removed 6 months after injury, which facilitated restoration of complex hindfoot motion.
a–b AP and lateral views of the mesh plates in place.
c–d AP and lateral views after mesh plates were removed.

8 Recommended reading

Benirschke SK, Meinberg EG, Anderson SA, et al. Fractures and dislocations of the midfoot: Lisfranc and Chopart injuries. *Instr Course Lect.* 2013;62:79–91.

Chandran P, Puttaswamaiah R, Dhillon MS, et al. Management of complex open fracture injuries of the midfoot with external fixation. *J Foot Ankle Surg.* 2006 Sep-Oct;45(5):308–315.

Dhillon MS, Nagi ON. Total dislocations of the navicular: are they ever isolated injuries? *J Bone Joint Surg Br.* 1999 Sep;81(5):881–885.

Kadow TR, Siska PA, Evans AR, et al. Staged treatment of high energy midfoot fracture dislocations. *Foot Ankle Int.* 2014 Dec;35(12):1287–1291.

Richter M, Thermann H, Huefner T, et al. Chopart joint fracture-dislocation: initial open reduction provides better outcome than closed reduction. *Foot Ankle Int.* 2004 May;25(5):340–348.

Richter M, Wippermann B, Krettek C, et al. Fractures and fracture dislocations of the midfoot: occurrence, causes and long-term results. *Foot Ankle Int.* 2001 May;22(5):392–398.

Swords MP, Schramski M, Switzer K, et al. Chopart fractures and dislocations. *Foot Ankle Clin.* 2008 Dec;13(4):679–693.

7 Metatarsals

Metatarsals

7 Metatarsal fractures

Mandeep S Dhillon, Siddhartha Sharma

1 Introduction

This section discusses injuries of the five metatarsals (MTs). Lisfranc injuries and phalangeal injuries are discussed in chapter 6 and chapter 8.

2 Anatomy and pathomechanics

The first MT is shorter and wider compared with the other four MTs. It receives two important insertions; the tibialis anterior tendon inserts on the plantar medial surface of its base that elevates and dorsiflexes the bone, and the peroneus longus inserts on the plantar lateral surface of the base and produces plantarflexion. However, the first MT has no ligamentous connections with the second MT and is therefore relatively mobile.

On the plantar aspect of the first MT head are the two sesamoids, both of which take part in weight bearing (WB). The heads of the other four (lesser) MTs each provide a WB point. Therefore, it is easy to understand that the first MT, having two of the six total contact points, bears 50–65% of the total body weight.

The central three MTs have no extrinsic muscle attachments, however, they provide attachment to the plantar and dorsal interosseous and lumbrical muscles. The thick transverse tarsal ligament connects the plantar plates of the metatarsophalangeal (MTP) joints of the lateral four MTs. This results in an increasing cascade of motion in the sagittal plane, which increases as one moves from the second to the fifth MTP joint. This also explains why stress fractures are more common in the second and third MTs, as these bones are relatively long and less mobile.

The fifth MT has important structures attached to it. The plantar surface of the tubercle of the fifth MT provides attachment for the lateral band of the plantar fascia. The dorsolateral surface of this tubercle provides attachment for the peroneus brevis, whereas the peroneus tertius tendon attaches on the dorsal aspect of the proximal metaphyseal-diaphyseal junction.

The MT shafts are mainly supplied by a single nutrient artery that enters from the medial aspect, at the junction of the proximal and middle thirds. Secondary epiphyseal and metaphyseal arteries supply the MT bases.

The normal alignment of the MT heads is referred to as the "MT cascade" (or "Maestro curve"). This alignment is important for normal foot biomechanics. In the AP view of the foot, the MT heads are arranged in a curve, also known as the Lélièvre's parabola. However, sagittal alignment of the MT heads is of utmost importance. In the axial or tread view, all MTs lie in a straight line (**Fig 7-1**). When determining this relationship on x-rays, it is important to remember that for the first MT it is the sesamoids rather than the MT head that bear weight.

Mechanisms of injury

Metatarsal fractures may be caused by direct or indirect mechanisms. Direct injury, such as a heavy object falling onto the foot or direct impact on the foot, results in a comminuted fracture pattern. Twisting injuries result in spiral fracture patterns.

Fractures of the fifth MT can be produced by various mechanisms. Fractures involving the base (zone 1) are usually the result of an inversion mechanism, wherein the lateral band of the plantar fascia may cause avulsion of the tuberosity (**Fig 7-2**). Zone 2 fractures are produced by an adduction force, which leads to a bending moment at the metaphyseodiaphyseal junction. This fracture line starts laterally and propagates medially towards the intertarsal joint. Zone 3 injuries at the proximal metaphysis are essentially stress fractures, which are the result of repetitive loading. The patient may have had pain for several weeks before the fracture line is noted on x-rays. Zone 2 and zone 3 fractures are prone to delayed union and nonunion.

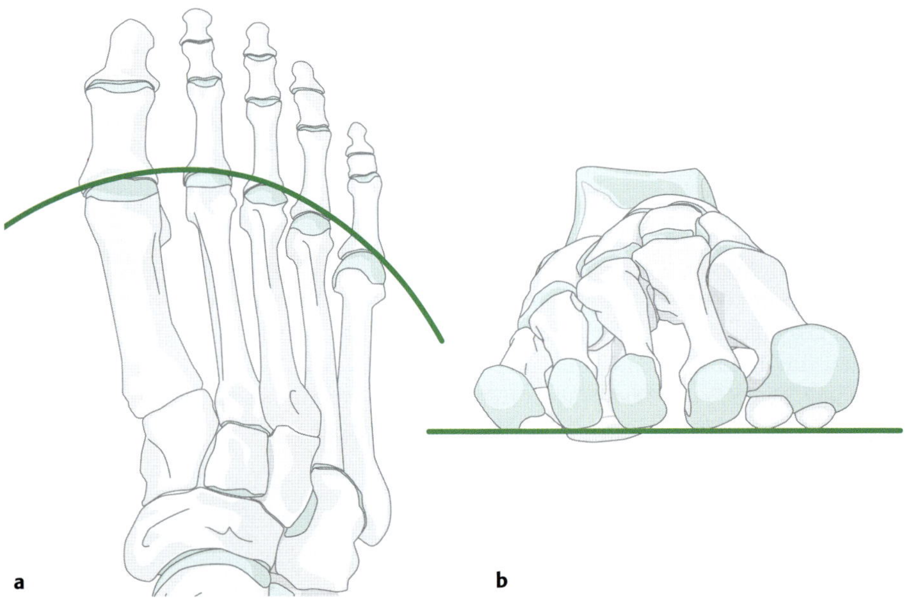

Fig 7-1a–b Normal MT cascade (ie, Maestro curve, Lelièvre parabola).
a On AP view, the MT heads are arranged in a parabola.
b Looking at the foot from front (tread view), the MT heads lie in a straight line.

3 Fracture classification

Metatarsal fractures can be divided into base, shaft, and head fractures. In case of an MT base fracture, instability at the tarsometatarsal (TMT, also called Lisfranc) joint has to be ruled out.

See the appendix for information on the AO/OTA Classification of MT fractures.

Lawrence and Botte`s fracture classification of the proximal fifth MT can be described occurring in one of three zone (**Fig 7-2**):

- Zone 1 injuries involve the base and may or may not involve the TMT articulation.
- Zone 2 injuries (Jones fractures) involve the proximal metaphyseodiaphyseal junction and the fracture line exits into the fourth to fifth intermetatarsal joints.
- Zone 3 injuries involve the proximal 1.5 cm of the MT shaft.

4 Preoperative assessment

Clinical assessment

Patients with MT factures present after direct blows or impact, or when they are involved in major accidents when these fractures are associated with other injuries. There is pain and swelling, but in cases with isolated fractures patients can often walk on the foot. Clinical evaluation reveals tenderness on palpation and irregularity or break in continuity of the bone; there is significant swelling and in cases of multiple fractures care must be taken to look for compartment syndrome.

Imaging

The diagnosis of MT shaft fractures can be readily established on plain x-rays. A standard trauma series of the foot should include AP, lateral, and 45° angle oblique views of the foot, in order to visualize all MTs and their articulations. In case of isolated fractures, WB or stress x-rays are sometimes necessary to rule out instability and help define the extent of shortening or displacement. A computed tomographic scan may be indicated when the fracture involves the TMT joint, or if there is a suspicion of associated injury to the Lisfranc or Chopart articulations. Magnetic resonance imaging or a 3-phase bone scan may be indicated if there is a suspicion of stress fracture.

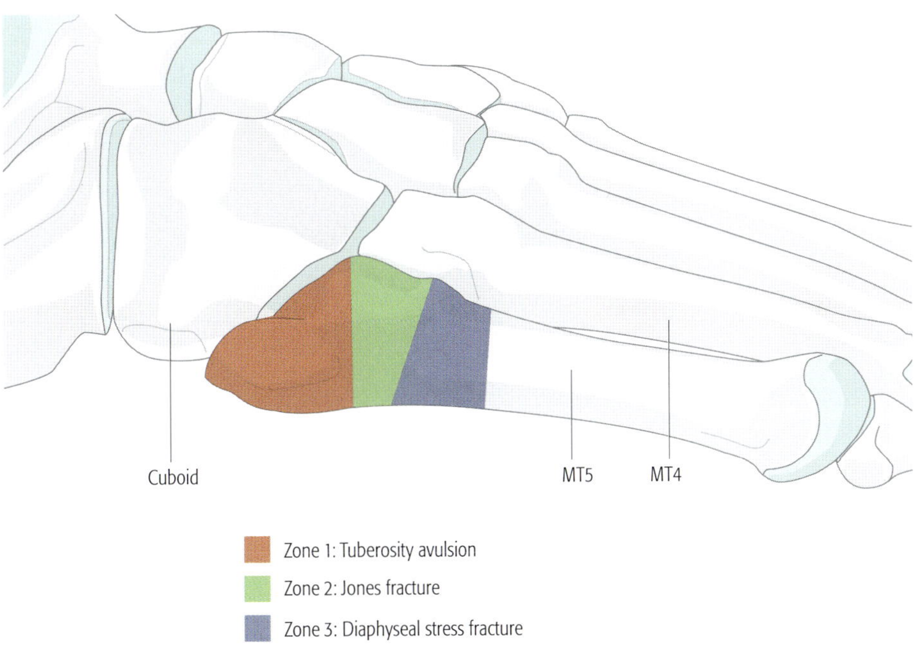

Fig 7-2 Classification of the proximal fifth MT according to Lawrence and Botte.

5 Nonoperative treatment

The key to management of MT fractures is to maintain the normal cascade of the MT heads in order to preserve the biomechanics of the foot.

Any shortening of the first ray is poorly tolerated as it bears about 50% of the total body weight. It is thus imperative to rule out instability or shortening if nonoperative treatment is planned. Weight-bearing views and stress x-rays should be done to rule out TMT instability. Stable fractures with no shortening can be managed in a well-padded below-knee cast, with the foot in a plantigrade position for 4–6 weeks.

Significant shortening of the central (second to fourth) MTs can also alter the normal WB pattern of the foot and result in transfer metatarsalgia. In case of isolated fractures of the central MTs, it is imperative to rule out instability of the TMT joint, especially if the fracture line is near the base. If there is any doubt, stress or WB x-rays must be obtained. Isolated fractures with no TMT joint instability and with less than 10° of angulation in the sagittal plane and less than 4 mm of shortening can be managed nonoperatively in a cast or hard-soled shoe. Isolated fractures with more than 10° of sagittal angulation and more than 4 mm of shortening can be considered for closed reduction and casting.

Metatarsal head and neck fractures tend to displace in the dorsal or plantar direction and are amenable to closed reduction by traction on the affected digit and manipulation. The reduction can be held in a well-molded cast shoe.

Fractures with significant shortening, sagittal angulation, multiple fractures, and those involving the TMT joints require operative intervention.

Fracture management of the fifth MT base depends on their anatomical location. Zone 1 injuries can be managed nonoperatively in a hard-soled shoe, with WB as tolerated by the patient. With displacement of more than 3 mm and/or joint incongruity to the cuboid, open reduction and internal fixation is preferred. Zone 2 injuries can be managed in a WB device such as a cast or fracture boot for 8–10 weeks. Zone 3 injuries should be managed on the lines of stress fractures and a full workup is indicated to rule out any underlying metabolic or endocrinological abnormalities that may have predisposed to the injury. Nonoperative treatment in a nonweight-bearing device such as a cast or fracture boot may be needed for up to 3 months. Screw fixation of zone 2 and zone 3 injuries in professional dancers and athletes results in faster return to sports.

6 Operative treatment

Patient positioning

Generally supine with a bump under the ipsilateral buttock. For more details, see chapter 1.

Surgical approaches

Fractures of the first MT shaft can be approached via a medial or dorsal approach (**Fig 7-3**). For fractures involving the base or head of the MT, or those associated with extensor tendon injury, TMT or MTP dislocation, the dorsal approach may be preferable.

Medial approach

A straight incision is made over the medial aspect of the first MT, from medial cuneiform to the first MTP joint. The abductor hallucis muscle is reflected in a plantar direction. If exposure of the first TMT joint is needed, the distal part of the tibialis anterior tendon can be elevated.

For the dorsal approach, a straight incision is made medial to the extensor hallucis longus tendon. The tendon is retracted laterally to expose the shaft. The incision can be extended proximally or distally to expose the first TMT or the first MTP joint. Visualization of the MT head can be improved by plantarflexion of the great toe.

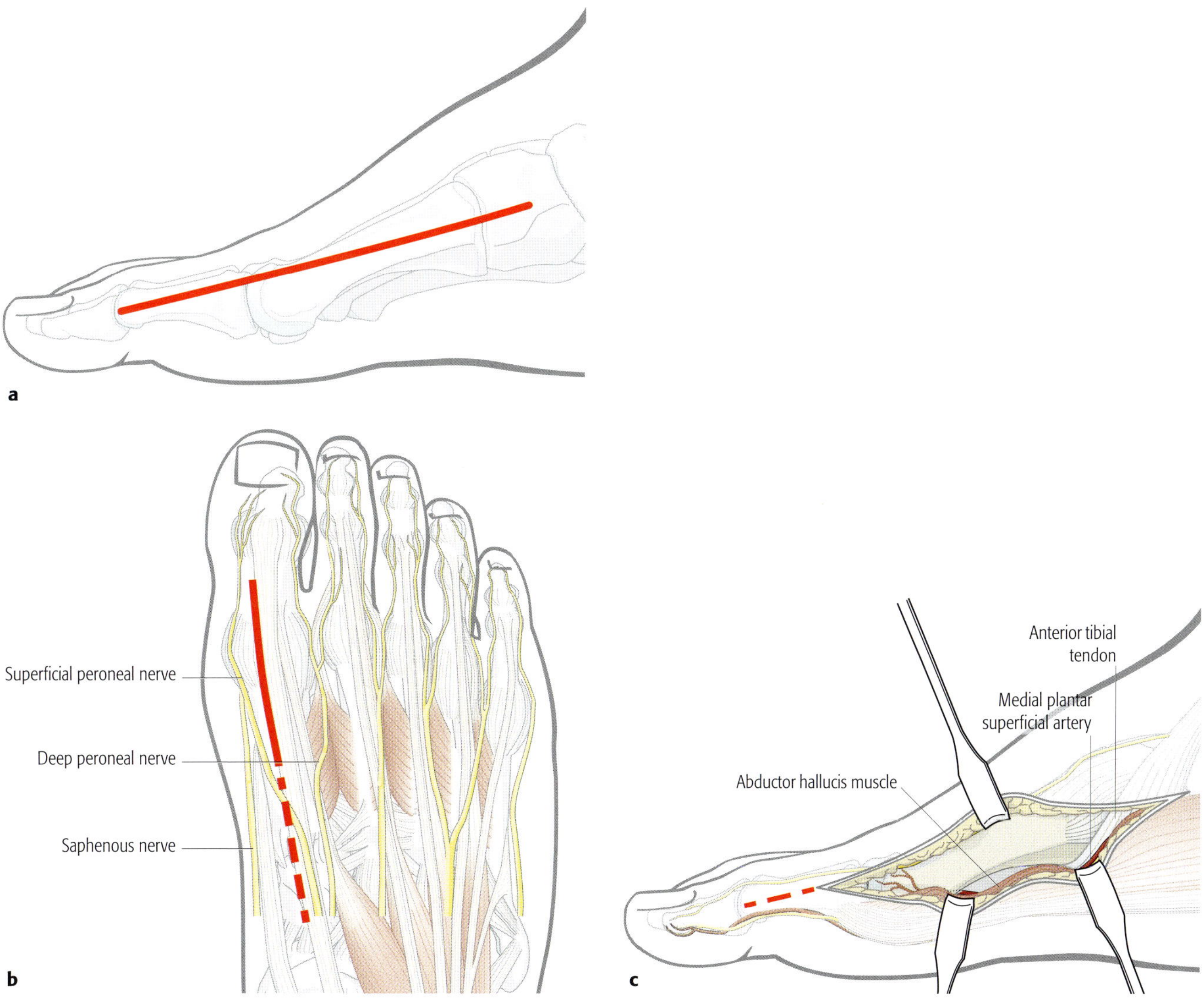

Fig 7-3a–c Medial (**a–b**) and dorsal (**c**) approach to the first MT.

The central MTs can be exposed via the dorsal intermetatarsal approaches (**Fig 7-4**). When considering these approaches, a few key points must be remembered. First, it is important to preserve the superficial veins of the foot, especially those that run along the long axis of the MT. Second, intermetatarsal branches of the deep peroneal nerve that supply the dorsum of the toes should be carefully preserved. Third, the plane of dissection should be between the long and short extensor tendons, staying lateral to the extensor digitorum longus tendon. Finally, the surgical dissection should be extensile enough to permit fracture reduction and fixation; extensive dissection should be avoided. The interosseus muscle may need to be detached to provide exposure, but this should be kept to a minimum. The second and third MTs can be exposed by an incision placed between these two; a skin incision lateral to it can expose the fourth MT. If all central MTs must be exposed, three incisions can be used: the first incision is between the second and third MTs, the second incision between the third and fourth MTs, and the third incision between the fourth and fifth MTs. Extreme care must be taken not to forcefully retract the soft tissues.

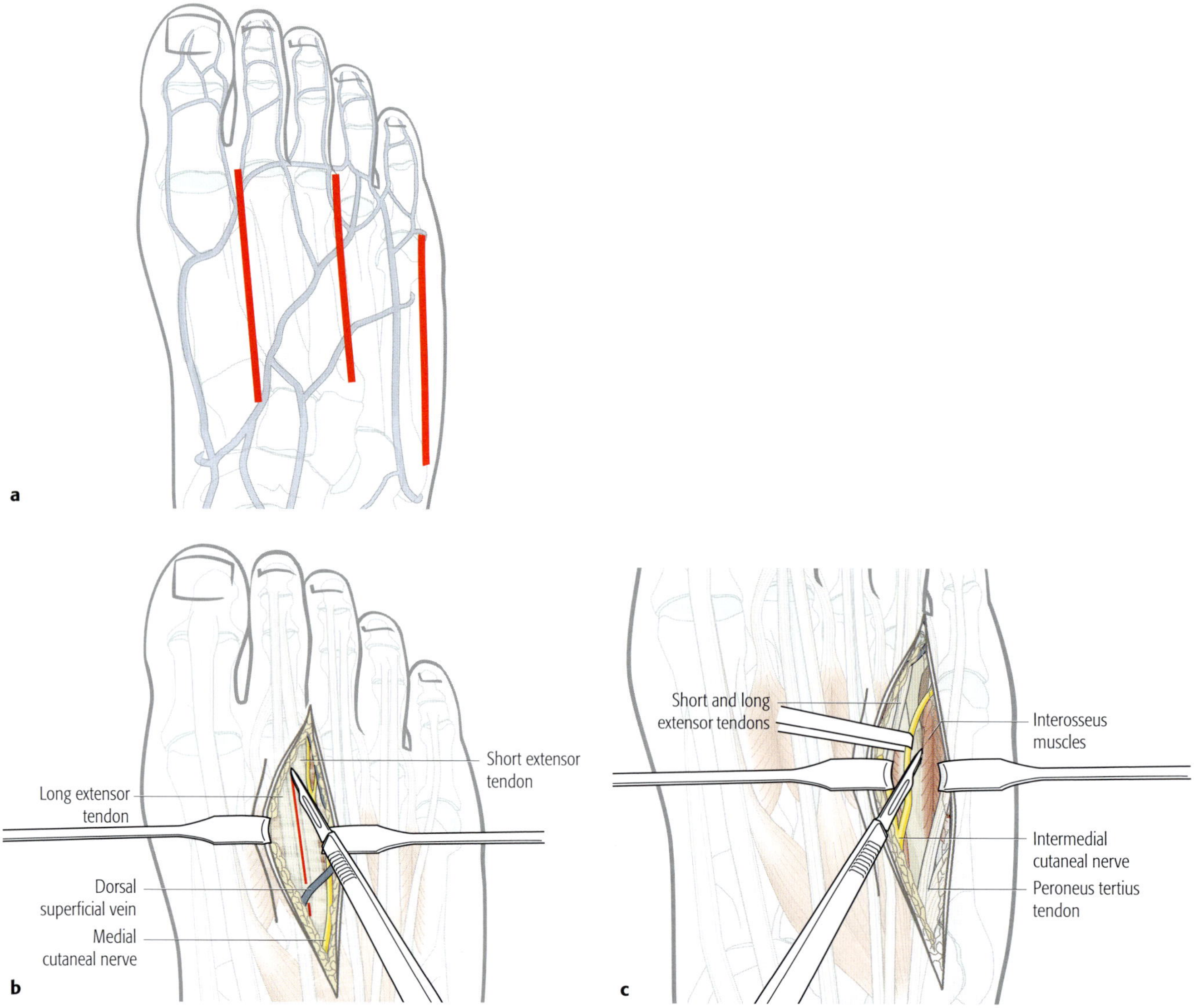

Fig 7-4a–c Dorsal intermetatarsal approach to the central MTs.
a Skin incisions for multiple central MT fractures.
b Access to the second and third MTs.
c Access to the fourth MT.

Lateral approach

The fifth MT can be approached through a lateral approach (**Fig 7-5**). The skin incision lies at the junction of the dorsal and plantar skin, starts proximal to the tuberosity of the fifth tuberosity, runs along the lateral aspect of the shaft of the MT, and may be extended distally as needed. The short saphenous vein is identified and preserved. Cutaneous branches of the sural nerve must also be protected. Next, the fascia over the abductor digiti quinti is incised and the muscle retracted in a plantar direction. The dorsal skin along with the soft tissues is retracted dorsally to expose the MT. As with all other approaches, careful dissection and avoidance of undue retraction is essential.

Surgical techniques

Once the decision has been made to manage the fracture operatively, the choice of fixation modality is dictated by the fracture pattern. It is important to assess the status of soft tissues before planning surgery. Sometimes it may be necessary to wait several days for the soft tissues to recover.

The first MT is broad, and fractures in this location are best managed with plates. Diaphyseal fractures should be fixed under compression (**Fig 7-6**). Lag screws may be used in case of spiral or oblique fracture patterns. For diaphyseal fractures of other MTs, either plates or K-wires may be used. If open reduction is planned, a K-wire can be introduced into the distal fragment, drilled out through the MT head after dorsiflexion of the toe, and then driven back into the proximal fragment after reducing the fracture (**Fig 7-7**).

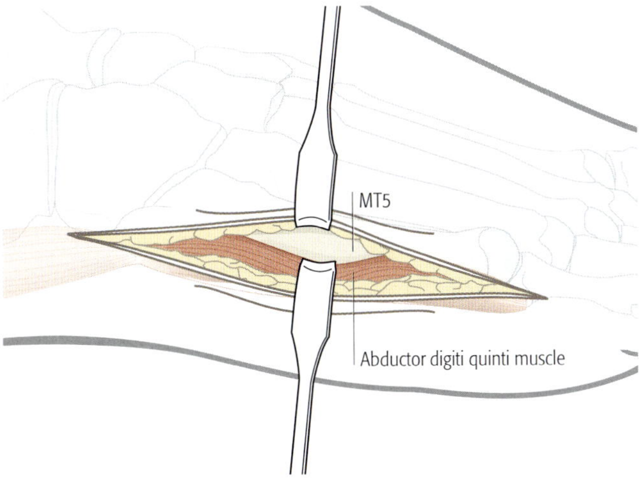

Fig 7-5 Lateral approach to the fifth MT.

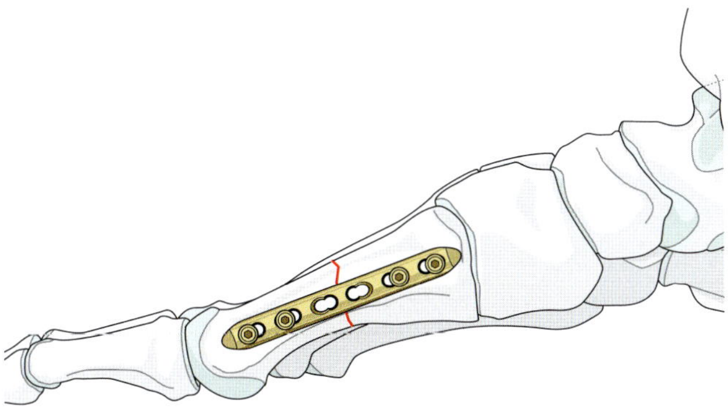

Fig 7-6 Compression plating of a first MT diaphyseal fracture.

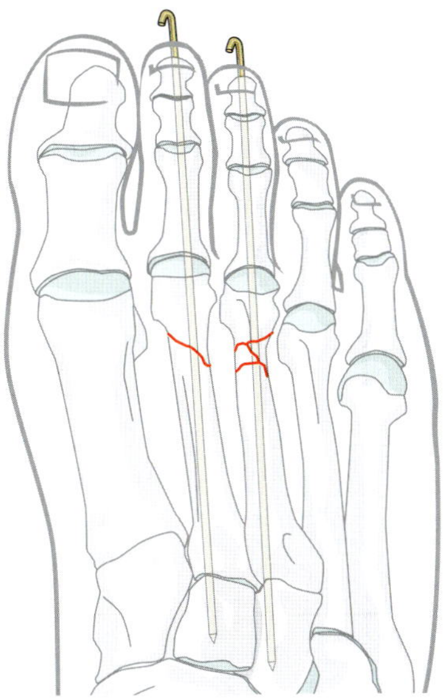

Fig 7-7 K-wire fixation of second and third MTs.

For fractures near the base special plate designs that permit insertion of variable angle locking screws can be used (**Fig 7-8**).

Fracture of the MT neck can be reduced by closed or open means and stabilized with K-wires or plates. Specially designed T-plates or L-plates can be used for subcapital fracture patterns, especially if it is necessary to bridge comminuted fractures (**Fig 7-9**).

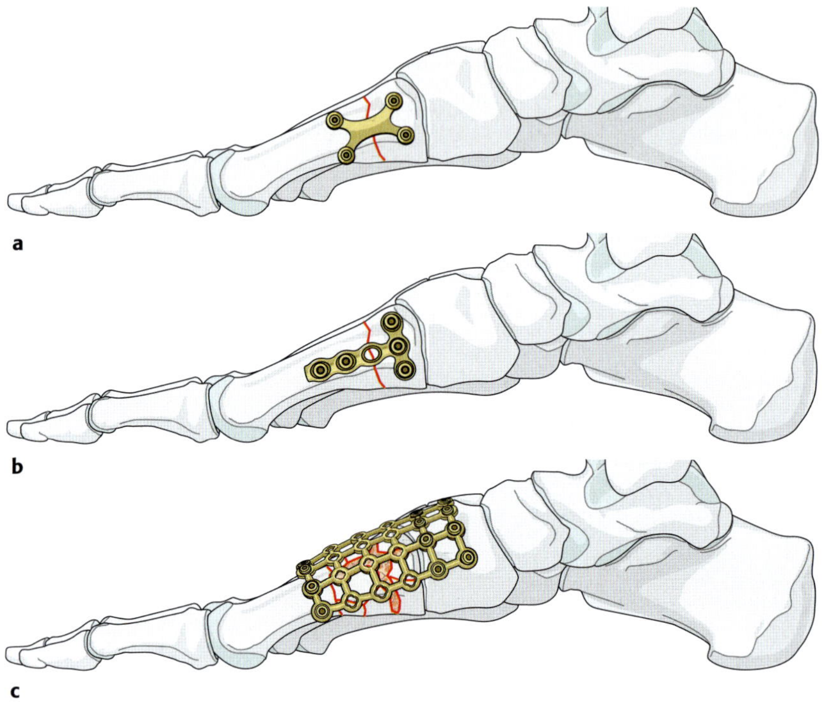

Fig 7-8a–c Specially designed, variable angle locking plates can be used to stabilize fractures near the MT base.

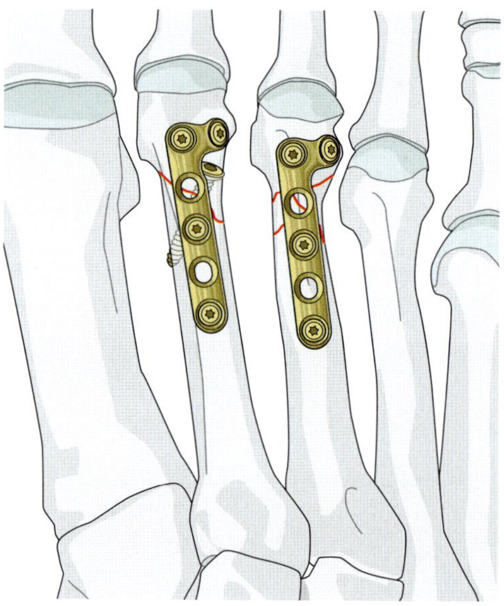

Fig 7-9 L-plates can be used to stabilize comminuted subcapital fractures.

Intraarticular fractures of the MT head can be fixed using 2.0 mm or 2.4 mm lag screws (**Fig 7-10**). At times, the avulsed plantar plate may be interposed, which prevents reduction. This needs to be sought out and cleared in order to obtain reduction.

For fractures of the fifth MT base and proximal metaphysis, a lag screw technique is used. Depending on the size of the bone, a 3.5 mm or 4.0 mm screw is inserted. A reduction clamp is used to reduce the fracture. The proximal cortex is overdrilled and the screw inserted perpendicular to the fracture line; the screw usually engages the strong medial cortex of the distal fragment in this position (**Fig 7-11**). Alternatively, displaced tuberosity avulsion fractures can be fixed with tension band wiring. Fifth MT shaft fractures are fixed with K-wires or with plates if multifragmentary.

Associated issues

Multiple MT fractures are the result of high-energy mechanisms. It is imperative to rule out and address instability of the Lisfranc and midfoot joints, as discussed earlier. With multiple fractures, there is generally a lower threshold for surgical management as the normal MT cascade is usually disrupted. Great care must be taken when planning surgical incisions to minimize soft-tissue trauma.

Open MT fractures can be devastating, especially when they involve crushing and soft-tissue loss. Prompt administration of antibiotics and wound lavage, early surgical debridement, and stabilization followed by appropriate wound coverage are the cornerstones of management. Since soft-tissue reconstructive options around the foot are limited, such cases are best managed in conjunction with the plastic surgery team. The patient must be counseled about the possible long-term consequences.

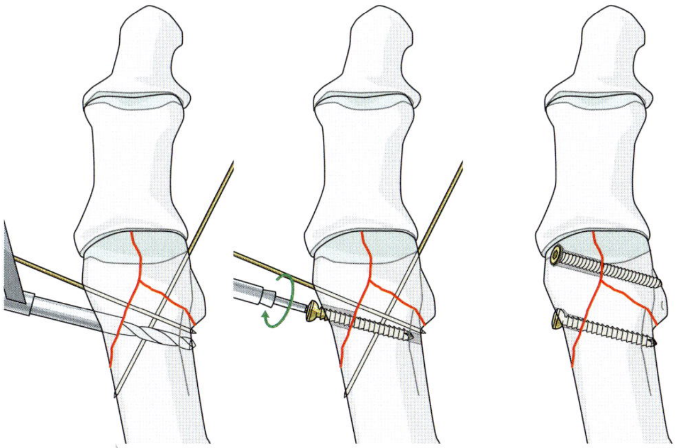

Fig 7-10 Lag screw fixation of juxtaarticular fractures of the MT head.

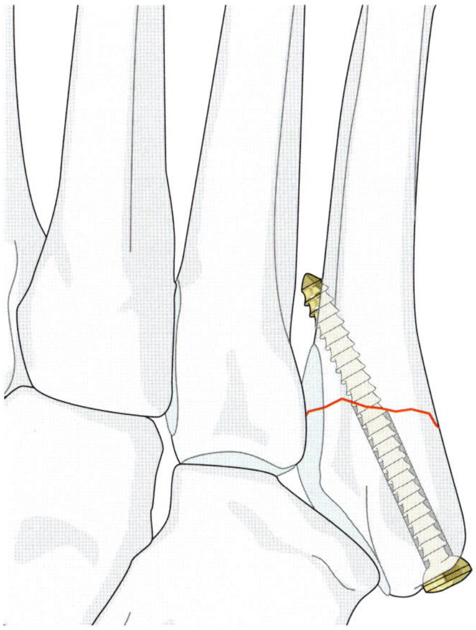

Fig 7-11 Lag screw fixation of the proximal fifth MT fracture (zone 2).

7 Postoperative care

Postoperative care depends on the fracture pattern and the type of fixation chosen and needs to be individualized. If the soft tissues are precarious, the limb must be elevated to the level of the heart and active movements of the toes encouraged. Immobilization can be achieved with a well-padded cast or a removable boot that permits easy wound inspection.

Partial or heel WB can be started if the surgeon deems that the fixation is stable. Sutures are generally removed at 2 weeks. Radiographic examination is done on a 4–6 weekly basis. Full WB is permitted once the fracture has healed completely.

8 Complications and outcomes

Foot compartment syndrome (FCS) is perhaps the most devastating complication of any foot injury. The diagnosis of FCS is primarily clinical, although measurement of compartment pressures can be used. Treatment of FCS is discussed in chapter 6 and chapter 6.8.

Most isolated MT fractures can be expected to have excellent outcomes if the MT cascade is maintained well by operative or nonoperative means. Loss of the normal cascade can significantly alter the biomechanics of the foot and lead to significant functional impairment.

Recommended reading

Cheung CN, Lui TH. Proximal Fifth Metatarsal Fractures: Anatomy, Classification, Treatment and Complications. *Arch Trauma Res.* 2016 Dec;5(4):e33298.
Lawrence SJ, Botte MJ. Jones' fractures and related fractures of the proximal fifth metatarsal. *Foot Ankle.* 1993 Jul–Aug;14(6):358–365.
Le M, Anderson R. Zone II and III fifth metatarsal fractures in athletes. *Curr Rev Musculoskelet Med.* 2017 Mar;10(1):86–93.
Meinberg EG, Agel J, Roberts CS, et al. Fracture and Dislocation Classification Compendium-2018. *J Orthop Trauma.* 2018 Jan;32 Suppl 1:S1–s170.
Rammelt S, Heineck J, Zwipp H. Metatarsal fractures. *Injury.* 2004 Sep;35 Suppl 2:Sb77–86.
Reid JJ, Early JS. Fractures and dislocations of the midfoot and forefoot. In: Bucholz RW, Heckman JD, Court-Brown CM, et al, eds. *Rockwood and Green's Fractures in Adults.* 7th ed. Philadelphia: Lippincott Williams and Wilkins; 2010:2111–2172.

7.1 Metatarsal head fracture

Michael Swords, Mandeep S Dhillon, Stefan Rammelt

1 Case description

A 23-year-old man was injured when he fell from a tree. The patient experienced severe pain and inability to bear weight. He was transferred to the emergency department by ambulance. His only injuries were to the right foot. The injury was closed with associated severe swelling. He had altered sensation to the dorsum of his foot. The entire forefoot was deformed.

X-rays were obtained which showed comminuted and displaced fractures of the second, third, and fourth metatarsal (MT) heads. The patient also had a dislocation of the fifth MT cuboid joint and a beak-type calcaneal fracture (**Fig 7.1-1**).

He was treated initially with surgical fixation of the calcaneal fracture to prevent skin breakdown of the posterior soft tissues. His foot was then placed in a splint to allow swelling to resolve prior to surgical fixation of the MT head fractures.

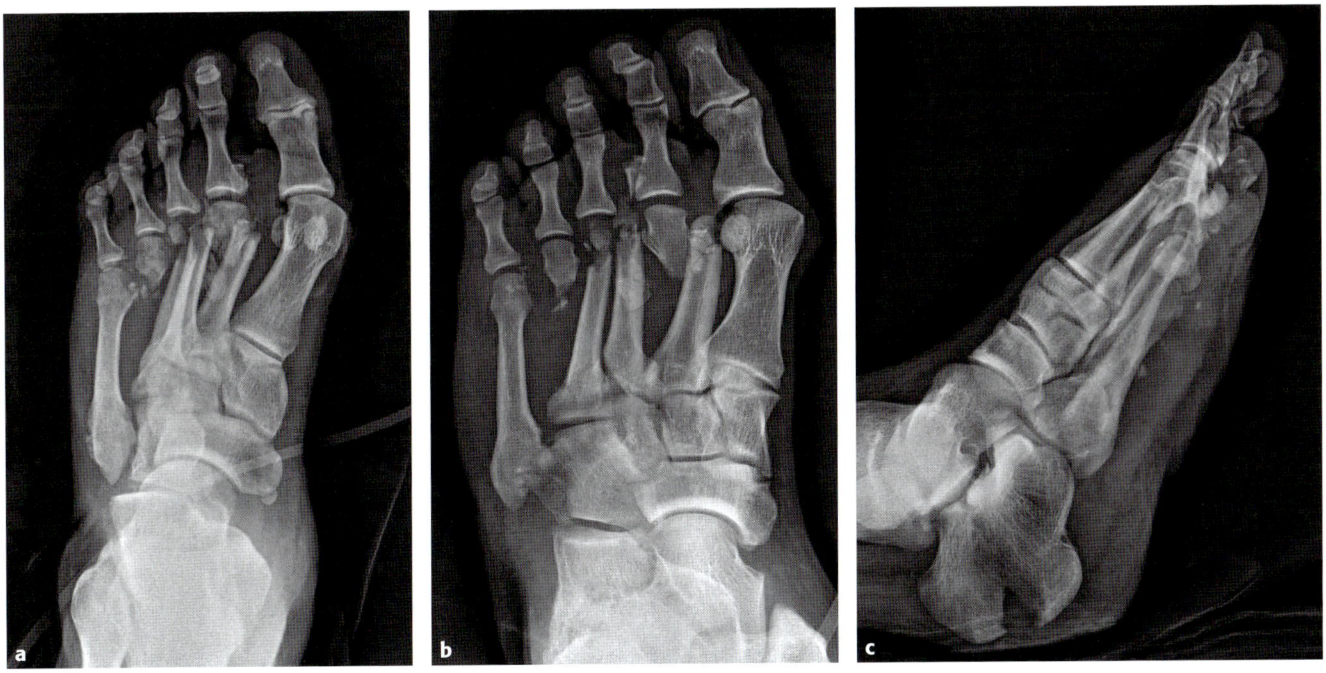

Fig 7.1-1a–c Injury x-rays showing comminuted MT head fractures of the second, third, and fourth MTs. The patient also has an avulsed calcaneal fracture and dislocation of the fourth and fifth MT bases at the cuboid.

a AP view.
b Oblique view.
c Lateral view.

2 Preoperative planning

Considerations for surgery

Isolated MT head fractures are not commonly seen. Distal MT fractures usually involve multiple bones and are often associated with more proximal injuries in the same foot.

Accurate reduction of any sagittal displacement is essential to maintain painless weight bearing (WB). Other indices such as WB parabola and ray length are of lesser concern, but still require consideration.

Minimally displaced fractures of the MT heads with the hallux in acceptable alignment are usually treated nonoperatively. However, displaced fractures may be associated with first metatarsophalangeal (MTP) joint dislocation or shortening of an individual ray, making reduction of the articular surface and alignment important.

Tip: Look for damage to the plantar plate and flexor complex by assessing sesamoid position on an AP x-ray. If there is proximal migration of the sesamoids, then injury to the plantar plate or flexor complex should be evaluated.

Indications for surgery

Surgery was indicated because of the marked malalignment of the MTs and the gross instability of the first MTP joint. Additionally, the base of the fifth MT was dislocated from the cuboid and required reduction and fixation. Surgery was delayed to allow for appropriate resolution of the soft-tissue swelling.

A computed tomographic (CT) scan should be performed when the injury is more severe or comminuted as is often the case in high-energy injuries. The CT also allows for evaluation of other injuries to the foot which may not be recognized on an x-ray. A CT was performed in this case due to comminution and to evaluate the rest of the foot (**Fig 7.1-2**).

Treatment options

Management options depend on the degree of displacement and the amount of comminution present.

Percutaneous fixation is an option in displaced fractures that can be reduced by closed manipulation. However, closed manipulation and reduction may not result in acceptable reduction and stabilization.

Open reduction and internal fixation is required when acceptable reduction and stabilization cannot be achieved by closed means.

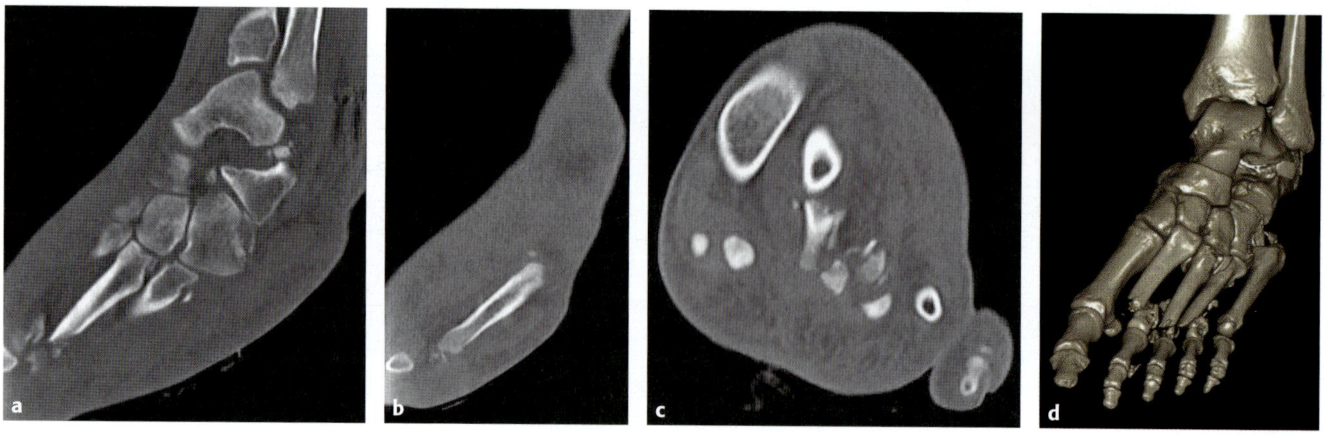

Fig 7.1-2a–d Computed tomographic scan revealing a severe injury to the MT heads.
a Sagittal view: comminution of the third MT head.
b Sagittal view: comminution of the fourth MT head.
c Coronal view: severe comminution of the third MT head.
d Three-dimensional reconstruction showing the severity of the MT head fractures and the injury at the cuboid fourth and fifth MT articulation.

3 Operating room setup

Patient positioning	• Supine, at the foot end of the operative table • A bump can be placed under the distal tibia to allow for clearance of the foot from the operating table and for foot manipulation.
Anesthesia options	• General anesthesia, regional spinal anesthesia, or a combination, as per surgeon preference
C-arm location	• When the mini-C-arm is used, it is positioned on the same side as the injury. • When a full-sized C-arm is used, it can be positioned to come across the table from the other side.
Tourniquet	• A thigh tourniquet can be placed and inflated if bleeding obscures visualization.
Tips	• Placing two small folded towels under the forefoot allows easier insertion of longitudinal K-wires into the toes without interference from the operative table.

For illustrations and overview of anesthetic considerations, see chapter 1.

Equipment

- Point-to-point reduction (Weber) clamp
- Two T-handle chucks to insert and manipulate the wires
- K-wires of various diameters as per surgeon preference (single-ended or double-ended sharp tips according to the technique chosen)
- Pliers and wire cutter
- Small-fragment screw set
- Plates, as required
- Dental scaler

4 Surgical procedure

Open reduction and retrograde K-wire fixation

The patient is placed supine on a radiolucent table and positioned with the feet at the end of the bed. An attempt at reduction is performed by closed means. If this is successful, the fractures can be pinned by introducing intramedullary K-wires from the plantar base of the proximal phalanx of the adjacent toe and across the MTP joint into the fractured head segment and then into the MT shaft. Generally, the fracture that appears easiest to reduce is attempted first and then the reduction progresses to the more comminuted fractures.

In this case, closed reduction was not possible, so open reduction and retrograde K-wire fixation was performed. A small incision was made medially along the extensor tendon exposing the second MTP joint and the distal portion of the MT. Using a dental scaler, the MT head is reduced at the MTP joint. A K-wire is driven from the tip of the toe longitudinally out through the base of the phalanx. The wire is then advanced into the MT head. Finally, the MT head is reduced to the shaft of the MT and the wire is advanced down the MT shaft (**Fig 7.1-3**).

In cases of multiple fractured MT heads more than one incision may be needed. Generally, careful incision placement between the second and third MTs will allow fixation of both MT heads. An incision can be placed between the fourth and fifth MT heads to allow fixation of the two lateral MT heads. Alternatively, a small incision can be made lateral to each individual MT head allowing for appropriate management.

To address the lateral column injury, a longitudinal incision is made to reduce dislocation at the cuboid, fourth, and fifth MT articulation. Due to gross instability, this is treated with reduction and plate fixation.

The surgical wounds are closed at the end of the procedure in a normal fashion. The pins are cut and bent.

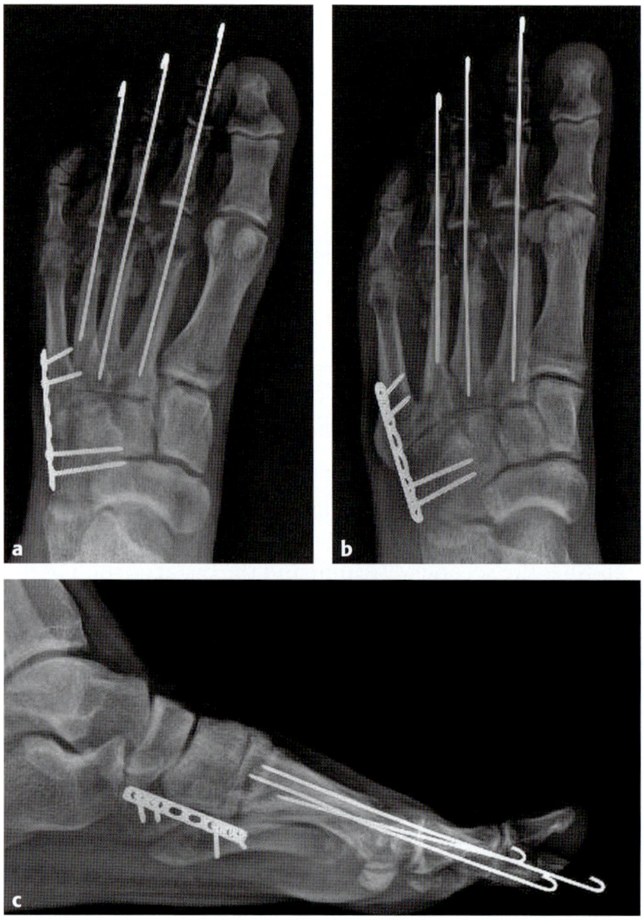

Fig 7.1-3a–c Postoperative images showing K-wire fixation of the MT heads. The dislocation of the fourth and fifth MT bases at the cuboid has been reduced and stabilized with a plate due to gross malalignment and instability.

- **a** AP view.
- **b** Oblique view.
- **c** Lateral view.

Fixation of a large articular fragment with resorbable pins

A dislocated or displaced large osteochondral articular fragment may not be large enough for screw fixation and not amenable to K-wire transfixation because of its size, shape, and location.

Case example: **Fig 7.1-4a–c** shows an isolated fracture of the fifth MT head in a 29-year-old male patient after a stubbing injury. The whole articular surface is displaced plantarly and rotated leaving the fifth MTP joint completely dysfunctional (**Fig 7.1-4d**).

In such a case, the fifth MTP joint is accessed via a small lateral approach. The capsule is opened from lateral. The joint and the displaced fragment are cleared from hematoma. The large osteochondral fragment is then reduced onto the remaining MT head. It is held temporarily with a small (1.4 mm) K-wire. The shell-like fragment containing the whole articular surface of the fifth MT head could not be fixed with screws or a small plate. Therefore, a second K-wire is used as a drill at an oblique angle to the first one and a 1.3 mm resorbable pin (polydioxanone) is introduced into the drill hole and cut flush to the joint surface. The first K-wire is then exchanged with a second resorbable pin (**Fig 7.1-4e**). Correct alignment of the metatarsal head is confirmed with intraoperative C-arm imaging (**Fig 7.1-4f–g**).

Aftertreatment consists of restricted WB (sole contact) in a hard-soled cast shoe for 6 weeks. After radiographic confirmation of solid bone healing, WB is gradually increased.

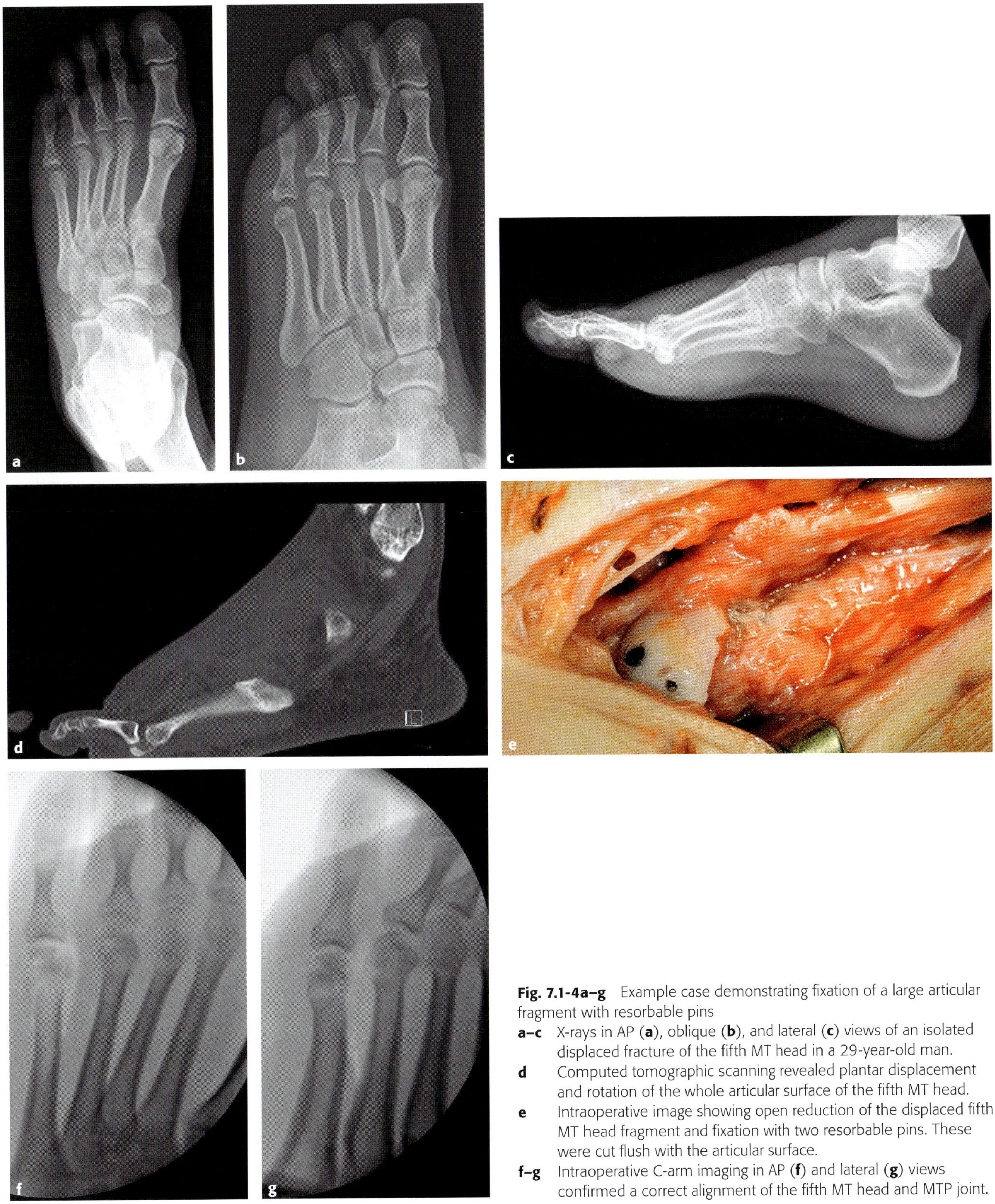

Fig. 7.1-4a–g Example case demonstrating fixation of a large articular fragment with resorbable pins

- **a–c** X-rays in AP (**a**), oblique (**b**), and lateral (**c**) views of an isolated displaced fracture of the fifth MT head in a 29-year-old man.
- **d** Computed tomographic scanning revealed plantar displacement and rotation of the whole articular surface of the fifth MT head.
- **e** Intraoperative image showing open reduction of the displaced fifth MT head fragment and fixation with two resorbable pins. These were cut flush with the articular surface.
- **f–g** Intraoperative C-arm imaging in AP (**f**) and lateral (**g**) views confirmed a correct alignment of the fifth MT head and MTP joint.

Treatment of first metatarsal head fractures

The skin is incised over the medial aspect of the MT shaft, in line with medial cuneiform to the first MTP joint; any part of this medial utility incision can be used, depending on the area to be fixed.

The dorsal margin of the abductor hallucis muscle is retracted plantar. The fracture is disimpacted and reduced with an elevator and the fracture reduction performed with point-to-point reduction forceps.

Fixation is performed by placing a small screw across the fracture.

The approach to the lateral first MT head through the first web space is often difficult. For fractures on the lateral aspect of the head, the screws can be placed from the medial incision or percutaneously from the lateral side. A second screw can be placed for long oblique fractures (**Fig 7.1-5**).

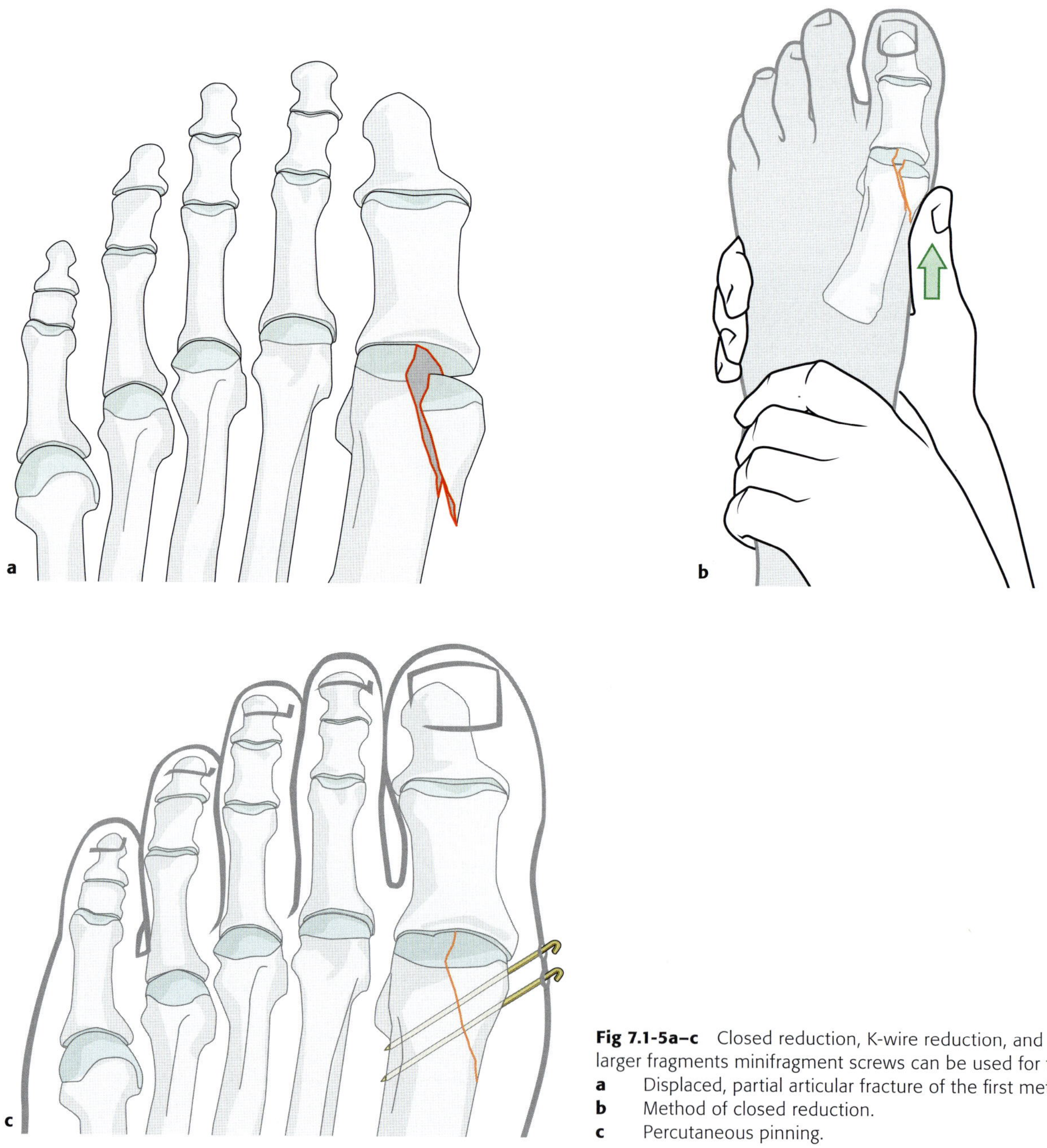

Fig 7.1-5a–c Closed reduction, K-wire reduction, and fixation. In larger fragments minifragment screws can be used for fixation.
a Displaced, partial articular fracture of the first metatarsal head.
b Method of closed reduction.
c Percutaneous pinning.

5 Alternative techniques

Closed reduction and pinning

Closed reduction and percutaneous pinning is recommended when the fracture is reducible by closed means, without compromising anatomical reduction of the MT head (**Fig 7.1-6**).

After appropriate alignment of the fragment is achieved by closed reduction, a K-wire can be placed percutaneously, perpendicular to the fracture plane, and a second parallel wire is placed to prevent rotation of the small fragment. Reduction is confirmed with intraoperative imaging.

Tips and tricks

Double-tipped K-wires may be used. The wire is inserted through the fracture site and drilled out distally. The driver is then moved to the exposed end of the wire which has exited the skin distally at the end of the toe. The fracture is reduced and the K-wire is drilled back across the fractured MT head and retrograde into the MT shaft.

Care should be taken when using K-wires to protect the tips so that no member of the operative team is injured by exposed sharp tips. A tip guard should always be used even if the tip is only temporarily exposed. Risk of injury increases when a double-tipped wire is used.

Nonoperative treatment

Minimally displaced fractures with the hallux and toes in good alignment are treated nonoperatively. Adjacent toes can be used for alignment and stabilization using tape or Velcro strapping (**Fig 7.1-7**). Footwear modification using a rigid-soled shoe is also helpful. In more severe injuries, a controlled-ankle-motion walking boot or nonweight-bearing (NWB) can be used.

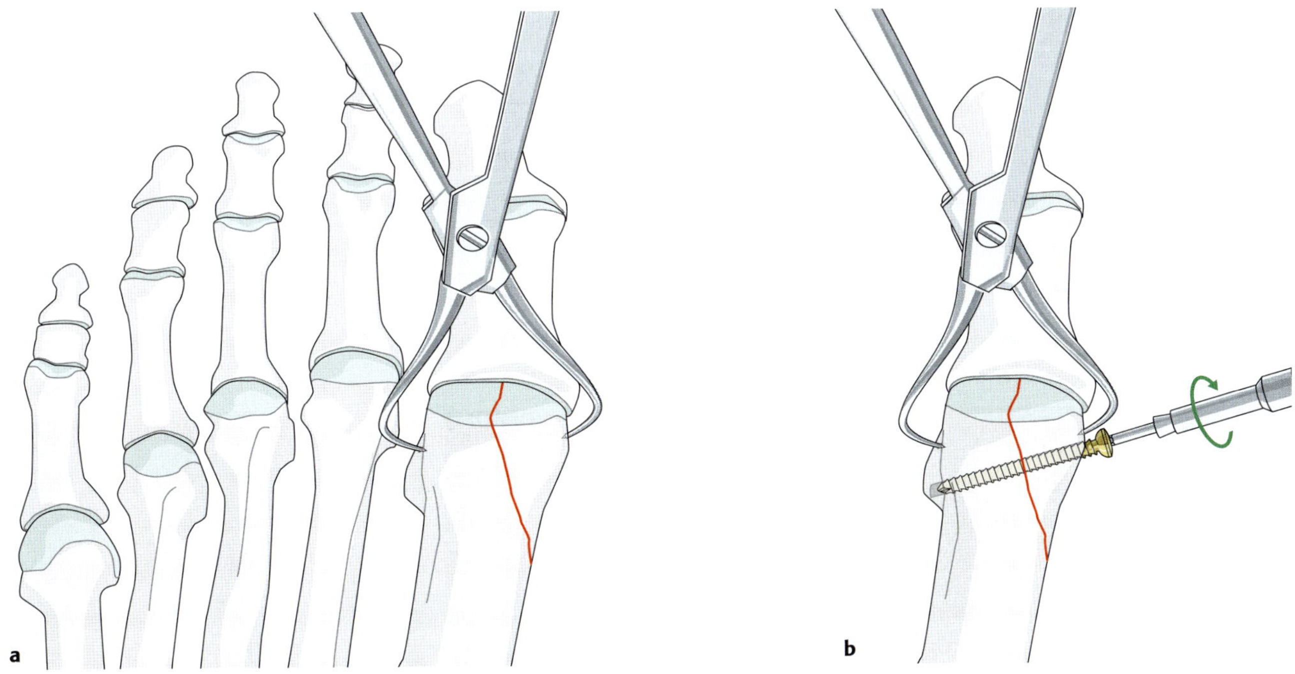

Fig 7.1-6a–b Open reduction and internal fixation.
a Reduction with clamp, either percutaneously or by a minimally invasive approach allowing visualization of the articular reduction and insertion of the fixation.
b Screw insertion.

6 Pitfalls and complications

- Inadequate reduction and maintenance of MT length
- Intraarticular screw penetration
- Persistent metatarsalgia
- Toe stiffness
- Arthritis
- Chronic instability of the MTP joints

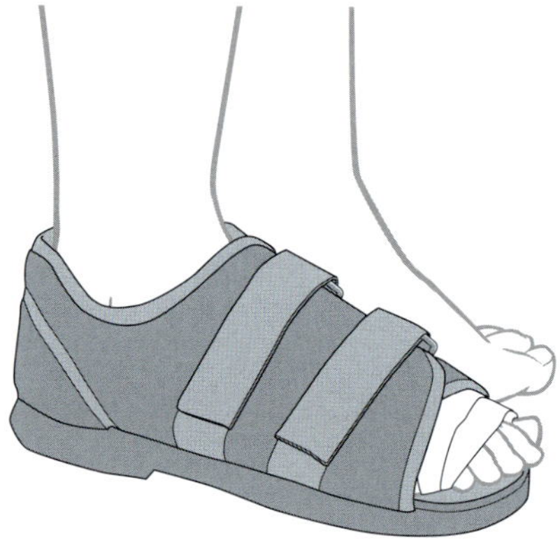

Fig 7.1-7 Buddy taping and a rigid-soled shoe. This treatment is generally indicated for nondisplaced or incomplete fractures. The patient is allowed full range of motion of the hindfoot and heel WB while the fracture is healing.

7 Postoperative management and rehabilitation

Elevation is important to prevent swelling. If no other injuries are present in the foot the patient may be heel WB in a flat rigid-soled shoe or hard cast until the K-wires are removed at 6 weeks. For this patient, the plate across the cuboid fifth MT articulation was removed at the same time. The ankle and subtalar joints are exercised to maintain motion. Aggressive range-of-motion exercises and stretching of the toes are initiated as soon as the K-wires are removed to optimize long-term function (**Fig 7.1-8**).

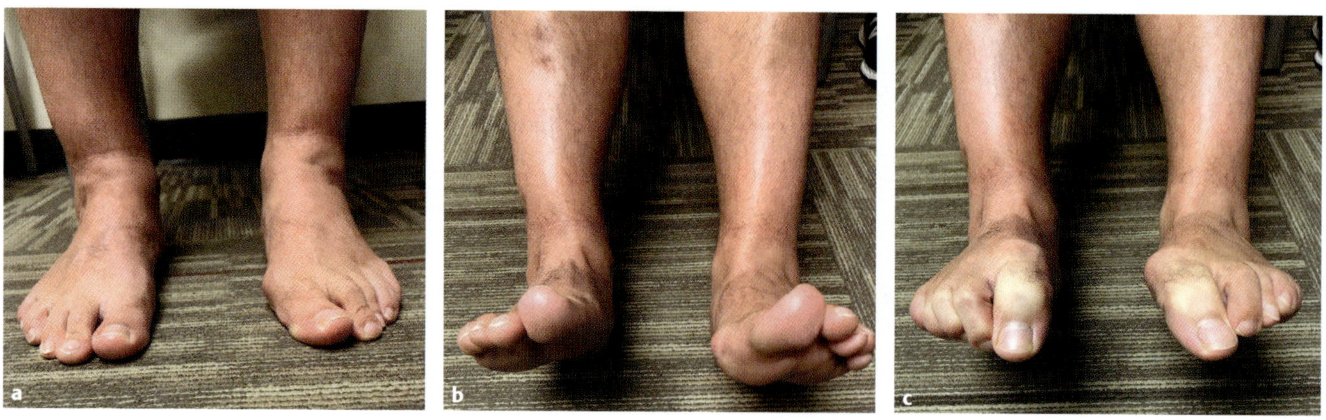

Fig 7.1-8a–c Final clinical images demonstrating acceptable clinical alignment of the forefoot. There is slightly decreased MTP flexion on the left (injured) foot when compared to the right (uninjured) foot (patient from **Fig 7.1-1–Fig 7.1-3**).
a Standing.
b Toe extension.
c Toe flexion.

Other injuries in the foot may alter the postoperative care. In this case, the patient was NWB with the ankle immobilized for 8 weeks due to the calcaneal injury. For isolated MT head fractures the patient is advanced to full WB as tolerated and transitions into normal footwear as able once the K-wires have been removed (**Fig 7.1-9**).

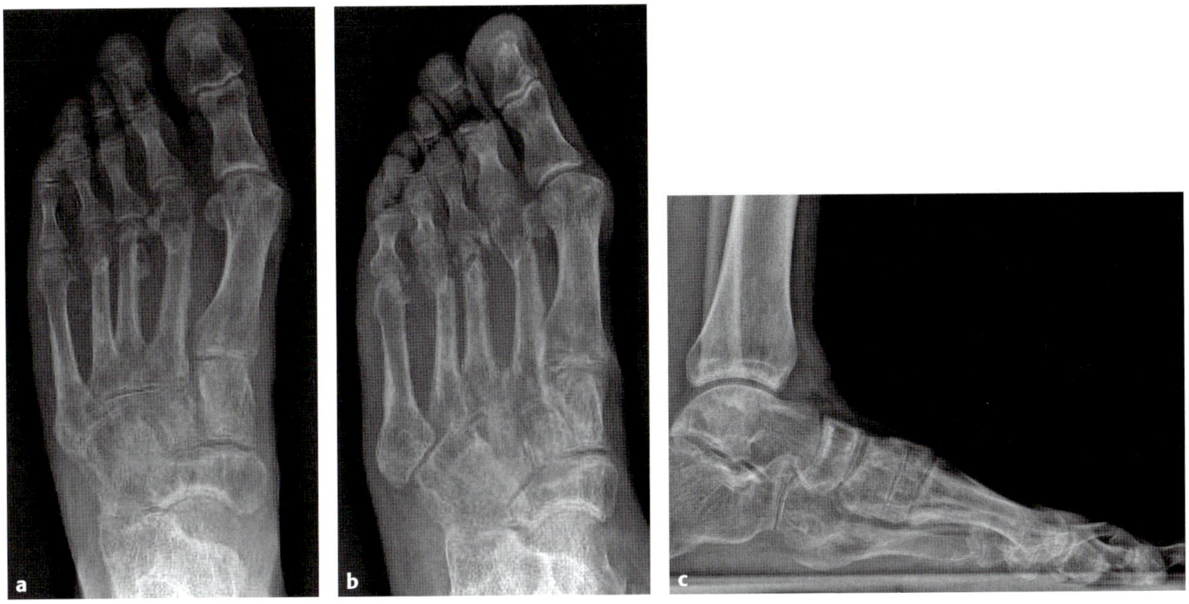

Fig 7.1-9a–c X-rays at 1 year demonstrate acceptable alignment of the forefoot with all K-wires removed. The plate has been removed from the lateral column.

a AP view.
b Oblique view.
c Lateral view.

8 Recommended reading

Lui TH. Isolated osteochondral fracture of the metatarsal head of lesser toes. *Foot Ankle Surg.* 2015 Jun;21(2):e40–44.

Mereddy PK, Molloy A, Hennessy MS. Osteochondral fracture of the fourth metatarsal head treated by open reduction and internal fixation. *J Foot Ankle Surg.* 2007 Jul–Aug;46(4):320–322.

Silver SA, Mizel MS. Open reduction and internal fixation of a simultaneous lesser metatarsal fracture and MPJ dislocation. *Foot Ankle Int.* 2000 Jun;21(6):520–521.

7.2 Simple first metatarsal diaphyseal fracture

Richard E Buckley, Jitendra Mangwani

1 Case description

A 35-year-old man fell down some stairs while walking barefoot. X-rays showed a distal diaphyseal fracture of the first metatarsal (MT) with some shortening of the first ray (**Fig 7.2-1**).

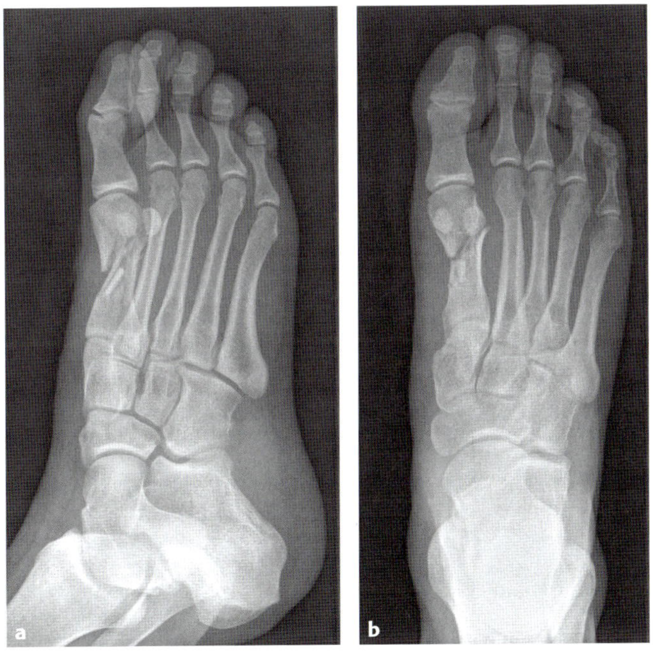

Fig 7.2-1a–b Preoperative x-rays showing a significantly displaced first MT fracture.
a AP view.
b Oblique view.

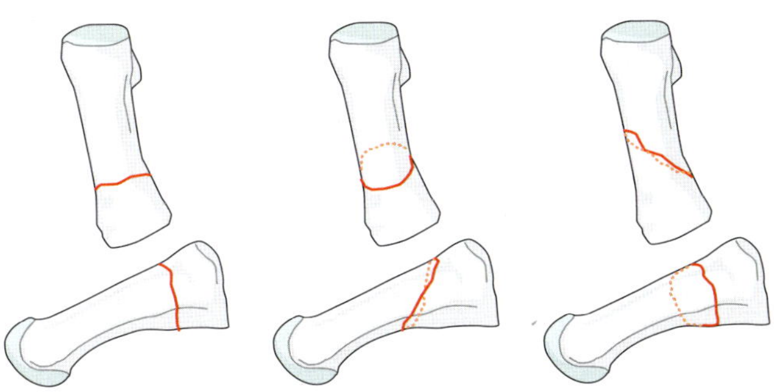

Fig 7.2-2 Minimally displaced fractures that can be treated nonoperatively.

2 Preoperative planning

Indications for surgery

A significantly displaced transverse diaphyseal fracture with comminution and shortening is an indication for surgery. Medial column alignment and weight bearing (WB) properties are affected, requiring an open reduction and internal fixation (ORIF) for reconstruction. If this fracture is accompanied by dislocations of the lesser metatarsophalangeal (MTP) joints, the fracture should be treated with ORIF to maintain reductions of the joints and to reconstruct the medial column of the foot. Other indications include: open fractures, multiple intraarticular fractures, and a combination of Lisfranc and MT displaced fractures.

Treatment options

Minimally displaced nonarticular fractures may be treated nonoperatively (**Fig 7.2-2**). If the fracture is unstable and significantly displaced, then rigid internal fixation is required. (**Fig 7.2-3**).

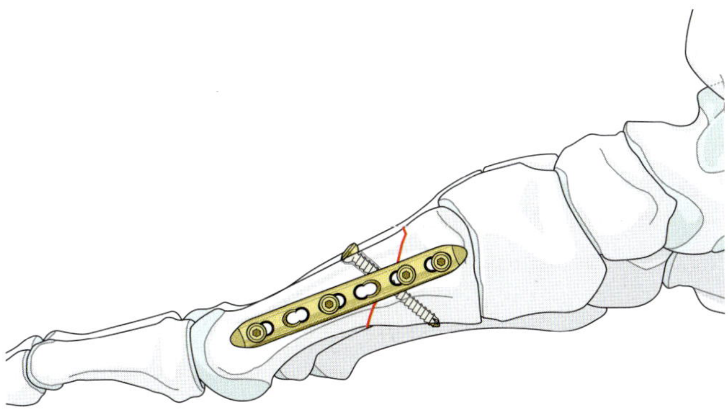

Fig 7.2-3 Example of fixation with a lag screw and neutralization plate for a metadiaphyseal fracture of the first MT.

3 Operating room setup

Patient positioning	• Supine with a sterile toe glove to cover the toes
Anesthesia options	• General anesthesia
C-arm location	• Positioned on the opposite side of the operative room table
Tourniquet	• Not needed
Tips	• A well-padded foam ramp or bolster placed under the affected side brings the foot and ankle above the other foot for improved access for visualization.

For illustrations and overview of anesthetic considerations, see chapter 1.

Equipment

- K-wires (1.2, 1.6, and 2.0 mm)
- Modular foot plates 2.4 and 2.7
- Small fragment set
- Point-to-point reduction (Weber) clamps

4 Surgical procedure

The medial approach to the first MT is used for fixation of most fractures of the first MT (**Fig 7-3a–b**). A dorsal approach may be useful for ORIF of distal fractures of the first MT and first MTP dislocations that are irreducible (**Fig 7-3c**). Dorsal placement of a plate or joint reduction is often possible through a medial utility incision.

Reduction

Reduction is performed using longitudinal traction to reduce any MTP dislocations and pressure over the MT shaft. If it is reduced in an open fashion, point-to-point reduction (Weber) clamps are useful followed by provisional fixation with K-wiring (**Fig 7.2-4**). Stripping of the periosteum should be avoided.

Fixation

Proper alignment of the MT heads is a critical goal in restoring the pathomechanics of the forefoot. The normal length of the MT must be restored as MTs always shorten when they are fractured (or if they are accompanied by lesser MTP dislocations) (**Fig 7-1**). If closed reduction is chosen, then length, rotation, and alignment must be anatomically restored before it is pinned with K-wires. This is difficult to do but mandatory to establish normal foot biomechanics.

If anatomical reduction is not possible in a closed fashion, ORIF with small plates should be performed (**Fig 7.2-5**). When a plate is used, fixation is adequate with two screws (3.5 mm) or three screws (2.7 mm or 2.4 mm) through the plate on either side of the fracture (depending upon the size of the fractured bone segment).

Compression should be applied if it is a simple transverse fracture.

5 Pitfalls and complications

The most common pitfalls involve obtaining and maintaining accurate anatomical reduction. This occurs because of malreduction in length, rotation, or angulation. X-rays of the contralateral foot may serve as a template. Malreductions may result in metatarsalgia at the level of the first or second MT head (**Fig 7.2-6**).

Complications include symptomatic malunion, which may require an osteotomy to correct the plantarflexed, shortened or malangulated MT.

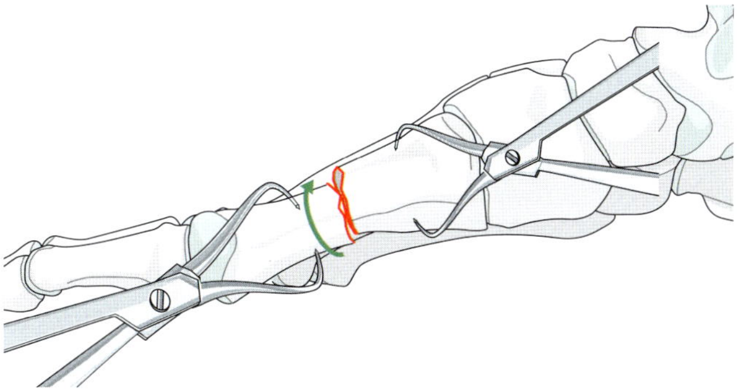

Fig 7.2-4 Reduction is obtained by manipulating the fracture fragments with point-to-point reduction (Weber) clamps, paying careful attention to the rotation of the distal fragment.

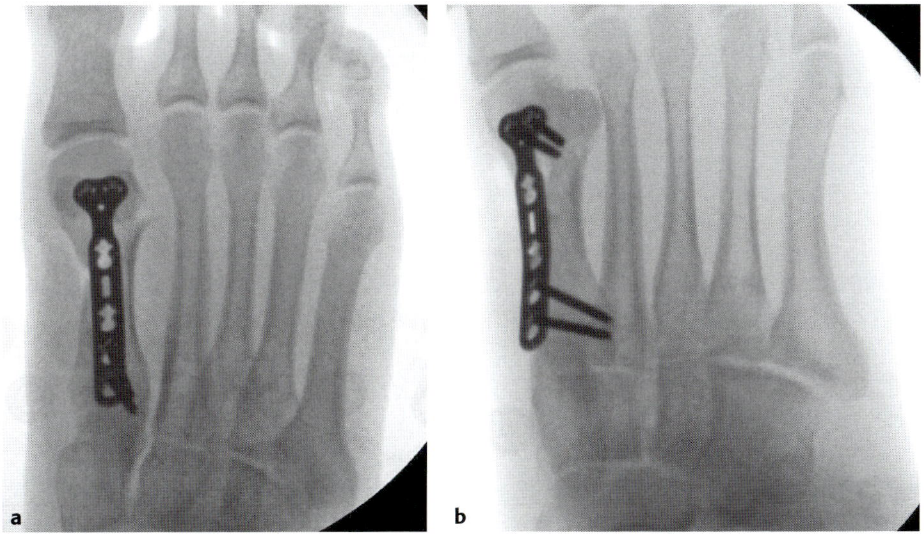

Fig 7.2-5a–b Intraoperative x-rays showing a bridging plate for the comminuted fracture of the first MT.

a AP view.
b Oblique view.

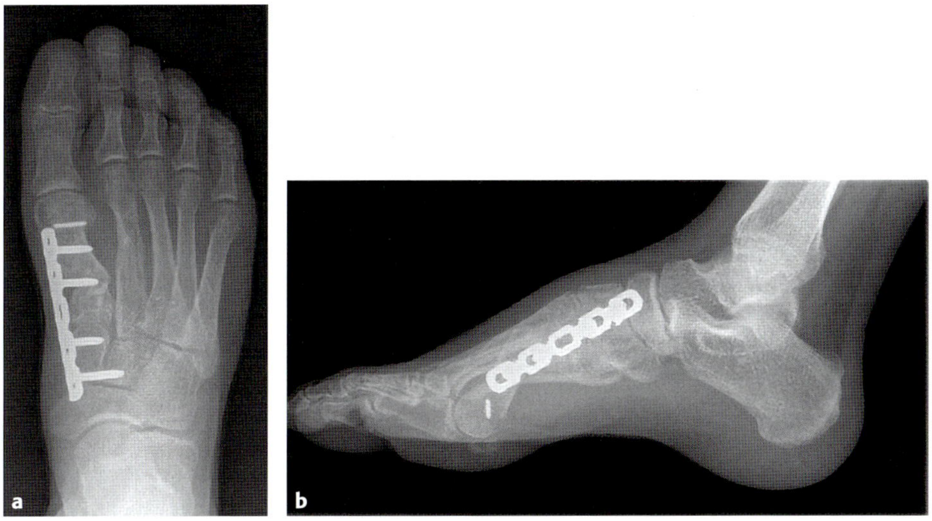

Fig 7.2-6a–b Example from a different case showing x-rays of a plantar flexed, shortened, distal first MT head. Open reduction and internal fixation has resulted in a malreduced, shortened, plantar flexed, first MT with severe first plantar metatarsalgia.

a AP view.
b Lateral view.

6 Alternative techniques

Nonoperative treatment may be used for minimally displaced fractures. If the fracture is displaced, then closed reduction with multiple K-wire fixation or minimally invasive surgery is an option.

7 Postoperative management and rehabilitation

Depending on the patient's body habitus and reliability, nonweight bearing is maintained for 6 weeks. Before discontinuation of nonweight bearing, there must be evidence of fracture union (**Fig 7.2-7**). If stable reduction has been achieved with ORIF, then partial WB may be possible with a flat, rigid-soled shoe after 3 weeks until evidence of bony union is present.

Full return to work was achieved by this patient using a rigid, soled high-top work boot at 3 months.

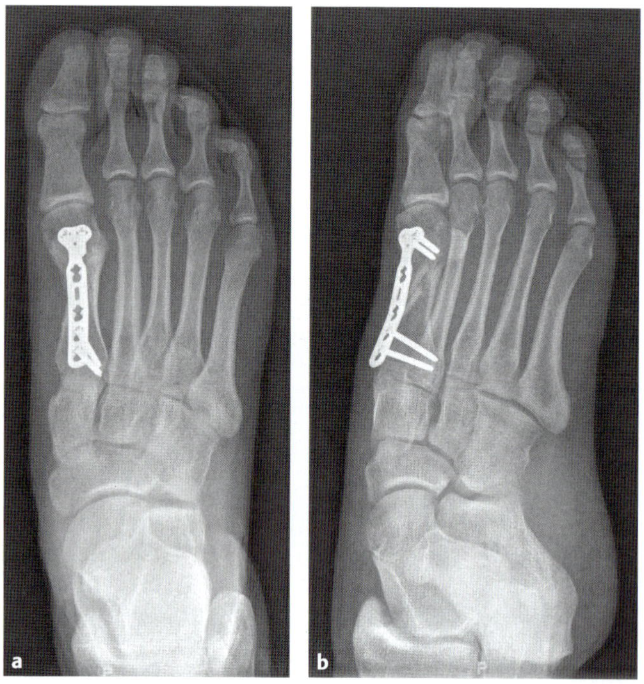

Fig 7.2-7a–b X-rays showing fracture union.
a AP view.
b Oblique view.

Implant removal

Implant removal is not recommended unless the implant causes significant pain with activity or is infected. Removal should not be performed before 9–15 months.

8 Recommended reading

Buckley RE, Moran CG, Apivatthakakul T. *AO Principles of Fracture Management.* 3rd ed. Stuttgart: Thieme; 2017.
De Boer P, Buckley R, Hoppenfeld S. *Surgical Approaches in Foot and Ankle Surgery: the anatomic approach.* Baltimore: Lippincott; 2012.

7.3 Comminuted first metatarsal diaphyseal fracture

Kartik Hariharan, Richard E Buckley, Kar Hao Teoh

1 Case description

A 25-year-old man jumped from a bridge overpass and fell 10 m. He sustained a complex, closed, comminuted first metatarsal (MT) fracture with an associated fracture dislocation of the base of the first MT and additional fractures of the second and third MTs (**Fig 7.3-1** and **Fig 7.3-2**).

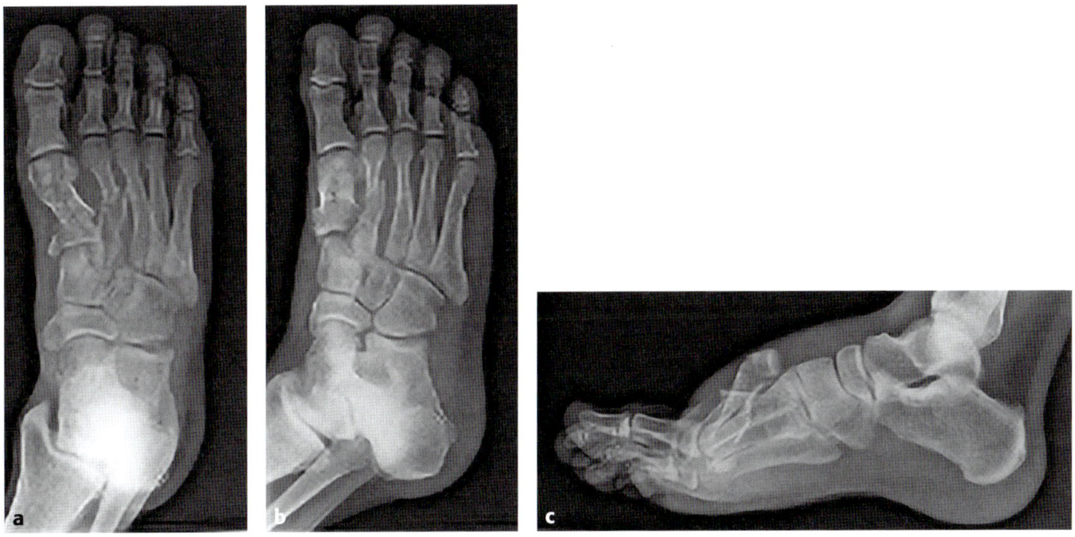

Fig 7.3-1a–c Preoperative x-rays revealing a complex closed, comminuted first MT fracture (and fracture dislocation into the base of the first MT) with additional second and third MT fractures.
a AP view.
b Oblique view.
c Lateral view.

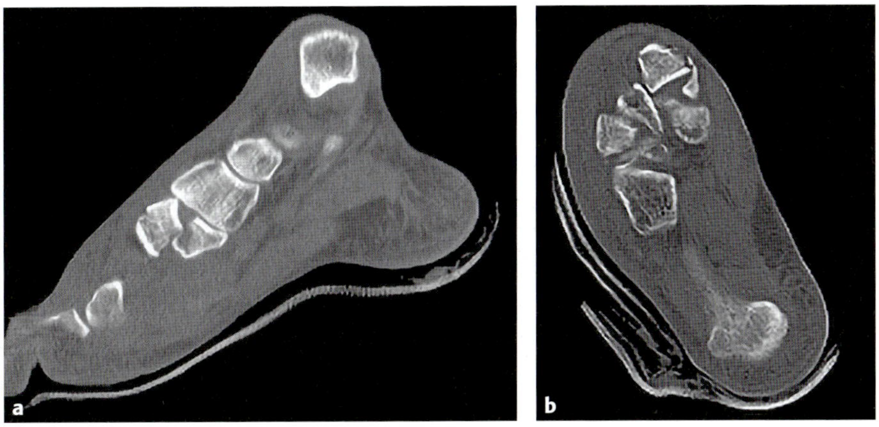

Fig 7.3-2a–b Preoperative computed tomographic scans confirming the comminution into the first MT joint.
a Sagittal view.
b Coronal view.

2 Preoperative planning

Indications for surgery

Open reduction and internal fixation (ORIF) is indicated for diaphyseal fractures with displacement more than 2 mm, distal or proximal joint involvement, comminuted fractures, and in crush injuries (with or without additional MT fractures).

A comminuted fracture with displacement more than 2 mm requires ORIF to reconstruct the anatomy of the foot. If this fracture is accompanied by fractures of other MT shafts, or dislocations of the lesser metatarsophalangeal (MTP) joints, then the first MT fracture should be fixed in order to maintain reductions of the joints and to reconstruct the medial column of the foot.

Other indications include open fractures, multiple intraarticular fractures, and a combination of Lisfranc (tarsometatarsal [TMT]) injury and displaced MT fractures.

Considerations for surgery

The original length of the first ray must be achieved to recreate the forefoot parabola's ("Lélièvre parabola" or "Maestro curve") normal MT head weight-bearing (WB) pattern (**Fig 7-1**). In a crush injury of the first MT, apart from restoring the length and alignment of the first MT, it is also important to reduce the subluxed or dislocated first TMT joint and reconstruct or fuse the articular surface of the first TMT joint.

Primary fusion might be indicated for multifragmentary fractures (ie, more than three pieces) where the articular surface is not reconstructible.

Nonoperative treatment may be indicated for low-demand patients where the fracture is in reasonable alignment.

3 Operating room setup

Patient positioning	• Supine on a radiolucent table • A well-padded bump is placed under the affected side for improved access and visualization. • A sandbag or blanket roll is placed beneath the buttock of the affected side to counteract the natural external rotation of the leg and bring the foot into a neutral position.
Anesthesia options	• General, regional, or spinal
C-arm location	• Placed on the opposite side of the operative table
Tourniquet	• Can be used to improve visualization during articular reconstruction

For illustrations and overview of anesthetic considerations, see chapter 1.

Equipment

- 1.2, 1.6, and 2.0 mm K-wires
- Modular foot plates 2.4 and 2.7
- Point-to-point reduction (Weber) clamps
- Small distractors to visualize first TMT joint in crush injuries

4 Surgical procedure

The medial approach (**Fig 7-3a-b**) is used for the fixation of certain fractures of the first MT. The dorsal approach is useful for ORIF of distal fractures of the first MT and first MTP dislocations that are irreducible. It may be easier to apply a plate dorsally over the first MT, as the tibialis anterior tendon inserts on the medial surface of the medial cuneiform and adjoining part of base of the first MT of the foot.

There is no internervous plane available for use in the medial approach. The dissection is directly down to the bones, which are located in the subcutaneous region where there is little or no subcutaneous tissue or fat. After the skin incision, dissection is continued down directly to the periosteum without elevating flaps, taking care to avoid, any cutaneous nerves that can be identified. The tendons of the extensor hallucis longus (EHL) are identified. It is possible to work between the window of the EHL and tibialis anterior tendon. The neurovascular bundle lies laterally. The approach is deepened in the line of the skin incision to expose the joint between the first MT and the medial cuneiform. The incision can be extended distally to access the rest of the MT and proximally to access the first TMT joint. Structures at risk are the EHL and the dorsomedial cutaneous nerve of the superficial peroneal nerve.

If a dorsal approach is used, the dissection is between the EHL and extensor hallucis brevis (**Fig 7-3c**). The dorsalis pedis neurovascular bundle lies just lateral to the approach and care must be taken to avoid injury during this approach.

Comminuted fractures are often open injuries, some of which have bone loss that requires restoration of length and bone grafting.

Reduction

Reduction is performed through a combination of manual longitudinal traction to reduce any MTP dislocations and pressure over the MT shaft. If open reduction is performed, point-to-point reduction (Weber) clamps are useful, followed by provisional fixation with K-wires placed transversely to more stable, intact adjacent MTs. Stripping the periosteum should be avoided. In the rare case of complete traumatic stripping, dead bone pieces should be removed and the space can be filled with bone graft if the fracture is closed, or an antibiotic spacer for subsequent bone grafting if the fracture is open.

It is critical to restore the MTs in their axial or horizontal plane, so that in the axial or tread view all the MT heads are on the same level. If the correct height of the first MT head in the WB surface is not recreated, weight will be transferred to the second MT head causing pain.

Fixation

Proper alignment of the MT heads is a critical goal in restoring the pathomechanics of the forefoot. The normal length of the MT must be restored as MTs always shorten when they are fractured or if they are accompanied by lesser MTP dislocations. Fixation with two screws (3.5 mm) or three screws (2.7 or 2.4 mm) on either side of the fracture is adequate when a plate is used (depending upon the size of the bone). The bridging technique should be used if there is comminution or bone loss at the MT base (**Fig 7.3-3** and **Fig 7.3-4**). Postoperative images in AP, lateral, and oblique projections are obtained to verify anatomical reconstruction of the forefoot geometry and implant placement.

In more severe injuries the use of 90°-90° plating may be considered. A plate is placed dorsally under the EHL along the dorsal aspect of the first MT. A second plate is placed medially via the medial utility incision, further maintaining alignment and resisting EHL dorsiflexion forces and increasing strength of the fixation construct. Subcapital fractures of the lesser MTs may be subjected to closed reduction and antegrade or retrograde percutaneous pinning (**Fig 7.3-5**).

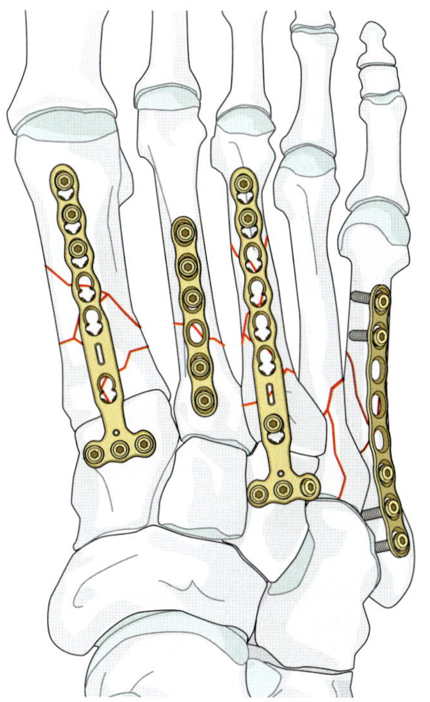

Fig 7.3-3 Areas and arrangement of plate placement.

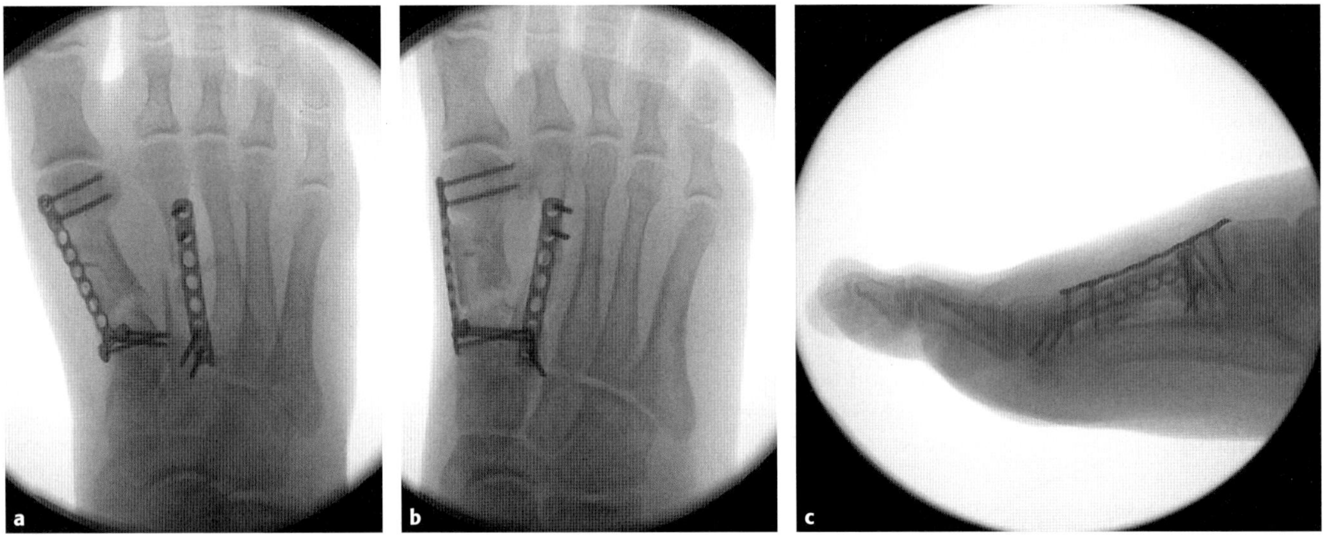

Fig 7.3-4a–c Postoperative images of the injury with the plated first MT and second MT.
a AP view.
b Oblique view.
c Lateral view.

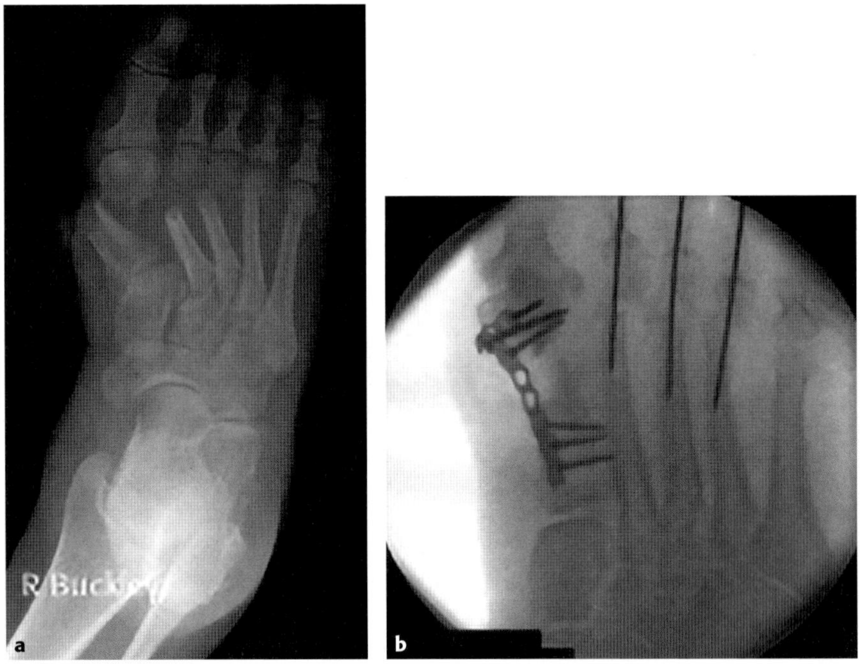

Fig 7.3-5a–b Example from a different case of a crushed foot. X-rays taken before (**a**) and after (**b**) K-wire fixation (with plate fixation of the first MT).

5 Pitfalls and complications

Pitfalls

- Not obtaining an accurate reduction is a common problem which can occur because of malreduction in length, rotation, or angulation. Careful reductions and x-rays of the other unaffected foot showing the physiological forefoot variants like index plus/index minus may enhance the surgeon's ability to obtain an excellent surgical result.
- Inadequate visualization of the articular surface in crush injuries involving the first TMT joint can lead to inadequate reduction. The use of a small distractor can be helpful to visualize the joint.
- Inadequate strength of fixation may cause late displacement of the fracture. Using plates that are too weak can lead to plate deformation and dorsiflexion at the fracture.

Complications

Malreduction

Malreductions may manifest as delayed metatarsalgia at the level of the first or secondary MT heads. A "dorsal bunion" is seen at the apex of the deformity. This results in a malreduced, shortened, and plantarflexed first MT with overload of the first MT head and subsequent severe first plantar metatarsalgia.

If a patient manifests a malreduction, then an osteotomy may need to be performed to create a more anatomical situation by correcting the plantarflexed, shortened, or malangulated MT.

6 Alternative techniques

This fracture is not amenable to closed treatment. For comminuted fractures where there is good bone at either end of the diaphysis, plating is the best technique. For crush injuries with intraarticular involvement, joint-spanning plating can be considered.

Joint-spanning plating

Example case: A 47-year-old woman sustained a hyperplantarflexion injury to her left foot when she tripped over a cable and a heavy object fell onto her foot. On presentation, she had an obvious dorsal prominence over the base of her first MT with a swollen midfoot (**Fig 7.3-6a**). X-rays showed an impacted crushed base of first MT fracture with dorsal subluxation of the first TMT joint (**Fig 7.3-6b–c**). This was reduced in the emergency department and her foot was placed into a splint. Computed tomographic (CT) scanning was performed to evaluate reconstruction options of the articular surface (**Fig 7.3-6d–e**).

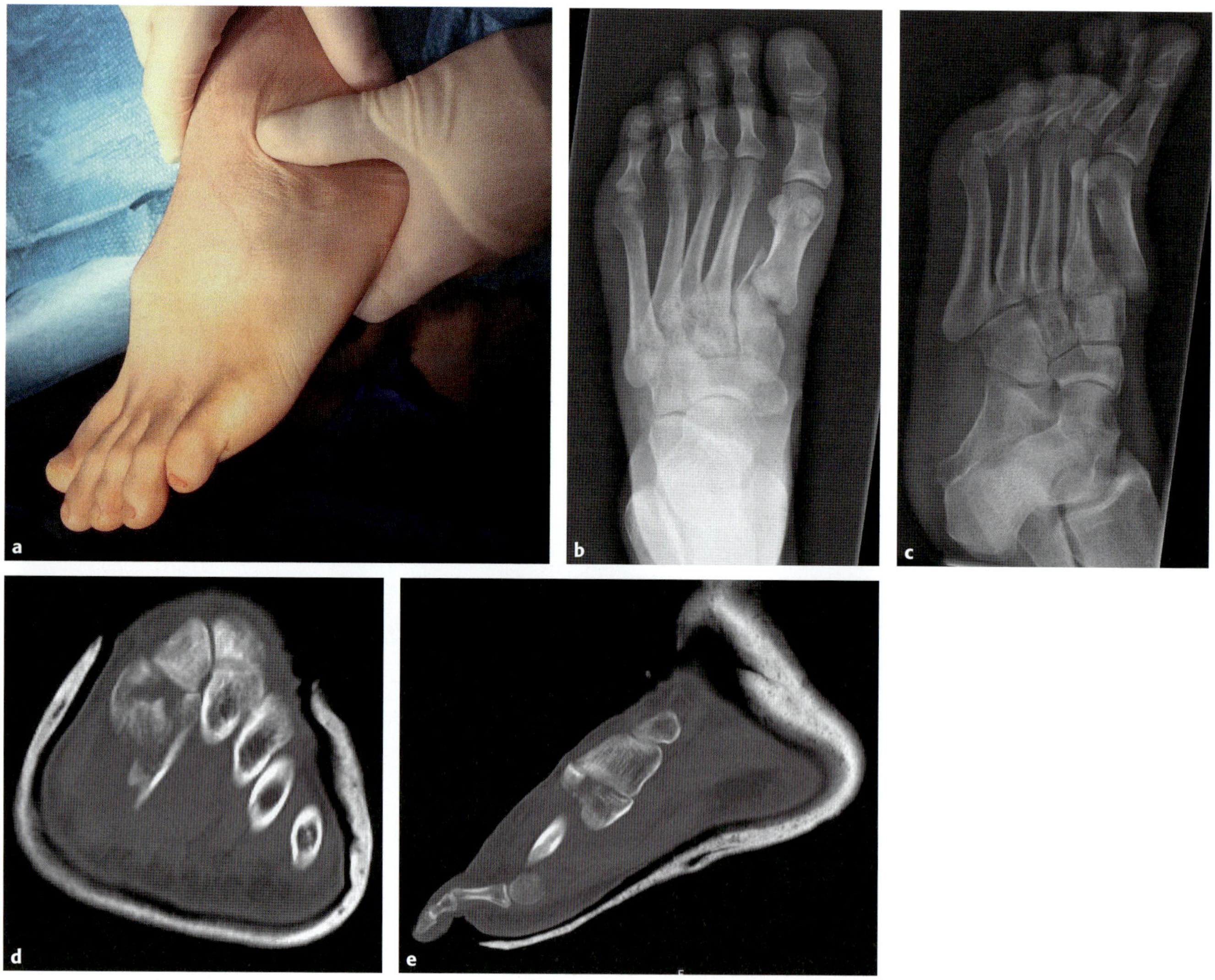

Fig 7.3-6a–i Example case showing the alternative technique using joint-spanning plating.

a The dorsal prominence from a subluxed first TMT joint.

b–c AP (**b**) and oblique (**c**) x-rays showing an impacted and crushed base of the first MT fracture, with dorsal subluxation of the first TMT joint.

d–e Axial and sagittal CT slices show a multifragmentary crush injury of the base of first MT with intraarticular extension. A central fragment of approximately 6 mm is depressed by 10 mm. The medial and middle cuneiform, the Lisfranc joint, and the remaining MT are intact.

A dorsal approach was used (**Fig 7.3-6f**). The first TMT joint was exposed, and the articular surface was inspected using a small distractor (**Fig 7.3-6g**). The die-punch fragment was rotated to the correct position, elevated, reduced, and held with a K-wire; subsequently the dorsal subluxation and plantar spike were reduced. A dorsal plate spanning the joint was applied (**Fig 7.3-6h–i**). A lag screw was placed through the plate to secure the plantar fragment.

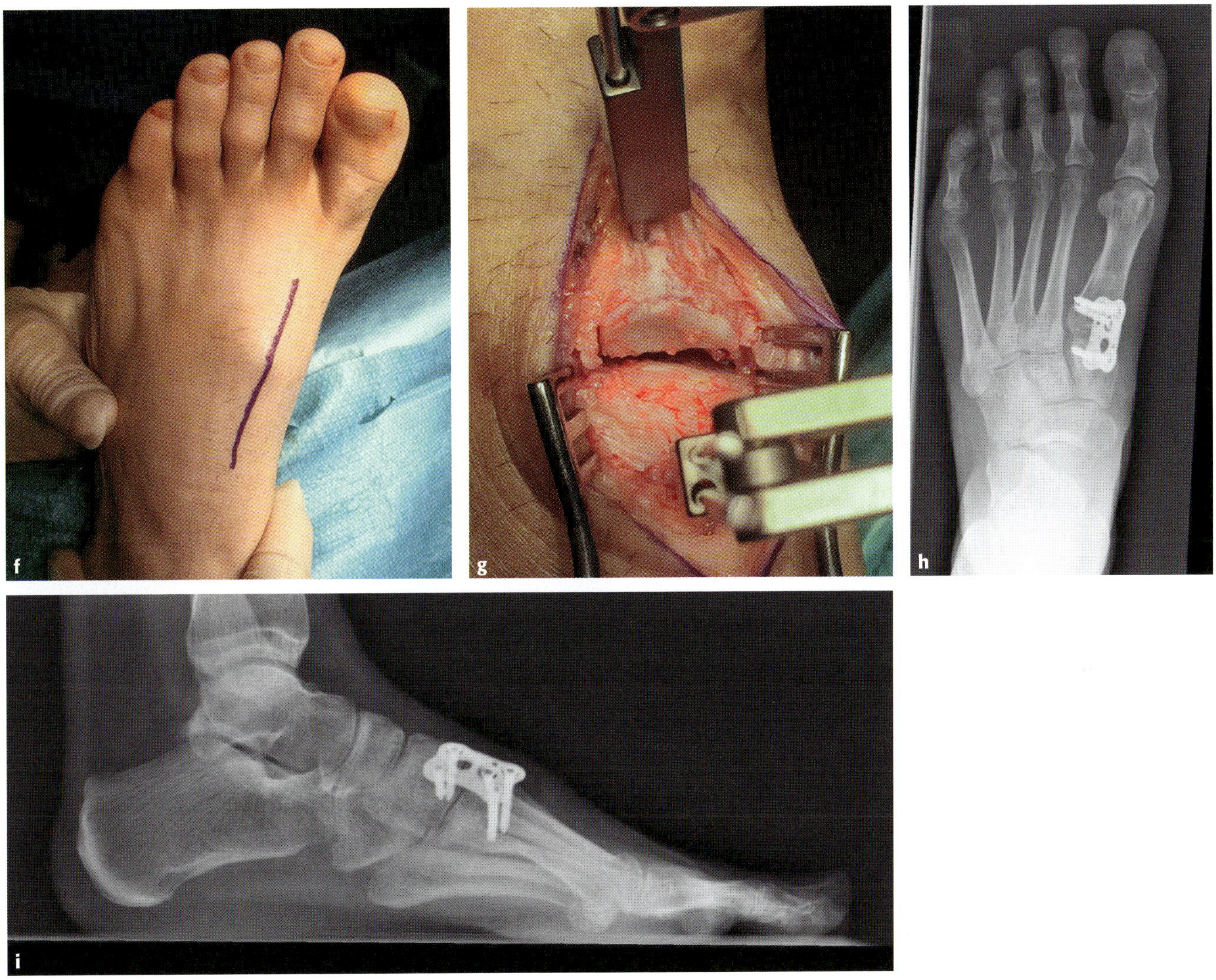

Fig 7.3-6a–i (cont) Example case showing the alternative technique using joint-spanning plating.
f The incision for the dorsal approach.
g The impacted articular surface of the first TMT joint with a K-wire distractor.
h–i Postoperative x-rays in AP (**h**) and lateral (**i**) showing the joint-spanning fixation following reduction of the die-punch fragment and plantar fragment held with a lag screw.

Open reduction and internal fixation with lag screws

Example case: A 50-year-old man dropped a roof truss onto his left foot sustaining extensive comminution of the first MT with intraarticular extension (**Fig 7.3-7a–c**). A CT scan revealed two main fracture lines (**Fig 7.3-7d–e**). Open reduction and internal fixation (ORIF) was performed with two lag screws (**Fig 7.3-7f–h**).

External fixation

Occasionally, these complex comminuted fractures are open and include bone loss. In these instances, a temporary external fixator can be used. The Masquelet technique is also useful when there is diaphyseal bone loss. With very severe open fractures, an external fixator is sometimes necessary until definitive healing occurs.

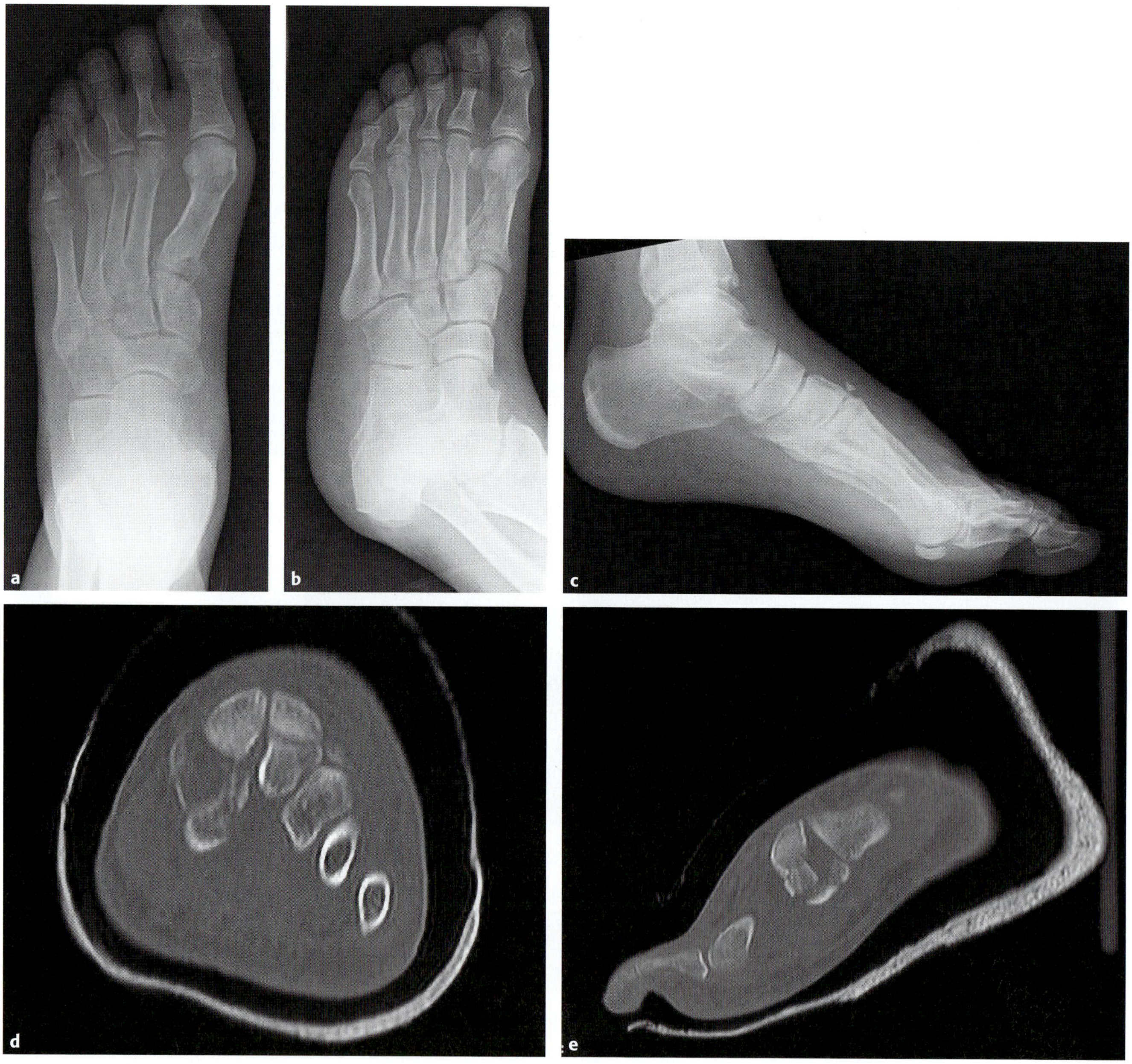

Fig 7.3-7a–h Example case showing the alternative technique of ORIF with lag screws.
a–c X-rays in AP (**a**), oblique (**b**), and lateral (**c**) views showing extensive comminution of the first MT with intraarticular extension.
d–e A CT scan confirms the finding but reveals two main fracture lines.

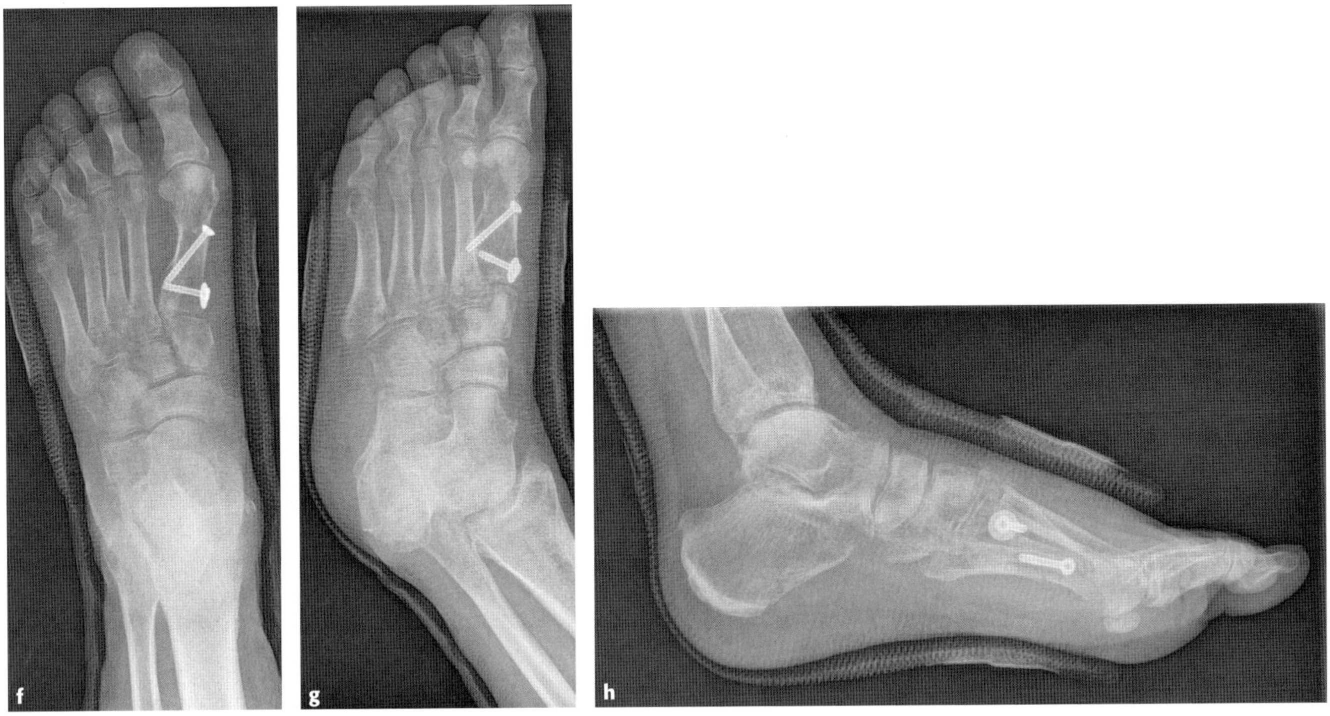

Fig 7.3-7a–h (cont) Example case showing the alternative technique of ORIF with lag screws.
f–h A medial approach was used in this case. The two main fracture lines were reduced with the aid of a point-to-point reduction (Weber) clamp and held with K-wires. Open reduction and internal fixation was performed with two lag screws.

7 Postoperative management and rehabilitation

Aftercare

The patient should be seen at 2 weeks to inspect the wound and remove sutures. X-rays should be taken to confirm that no secondary displacement has occurred.

The patient is seen at 6 weeks for further x-rays. Mobilization starts in a fracture boot once x-rays show adequate bone healing. Occasionally, delayed healing occurs, and in such cases, WB is delayed. Some cases may also require delayed bone grafting (**Fig 7.3-8** and **Fig 7.3-9**).

Functional exercises

For compliant patients in a fracture boot, early ankle range-of-motion (ROM) exercises should be started 2 weeks after surgery to prevent stiffness. However, patients should not bear weight until 6 weeks postoperatively.

For patients in a below-knee cast for 6 weeks, physiotherapy should start once the cast is removed. They can then gradually mobilize in a fracture boot. Use of a below-knee cast may result in stiffness in all joints of the foot and ankle. If ORIF is done with appropriately strong hardware, early nonweight-bearing ROM exercises should be started as soon as the wound is healed and certainly after the first postoperative follow-up appointment.

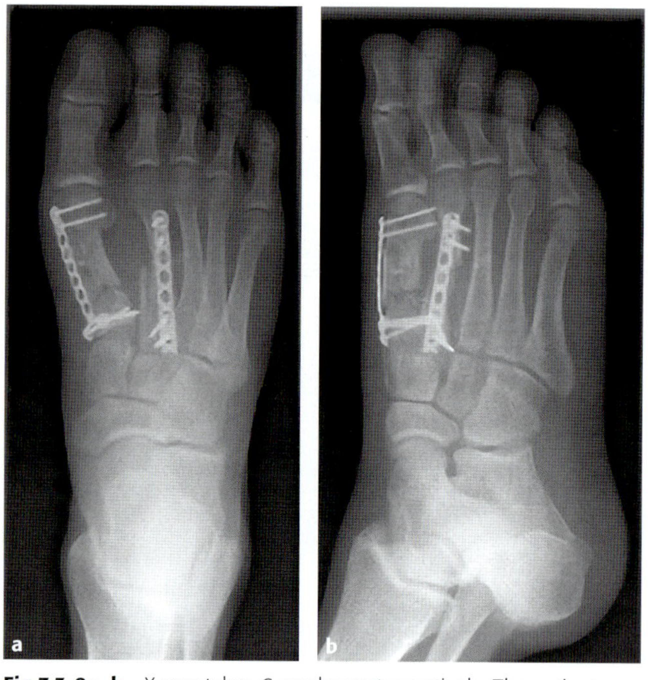

Fig 7.3-8a–b X-rays taken 6 weeks postoperatively. The patient still experienced tenderness over the fracture site and required bone grafting. The first MT is also a few millimeters short.
a AP view.
b Oblique view.

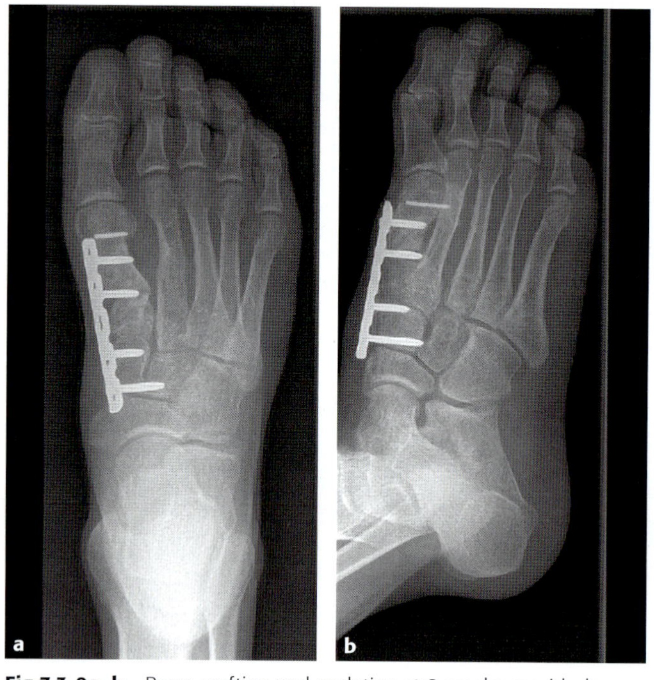

Fig 7.3-9a–b Bone grafting and replating at 8 weeks provided healing by 16 weeks. The second MT plate was removed as it was prominent under the skin. The first MT is still a few millimeters short.

Implant removal

Implant removal is recommended at 3–6 months if the implant is bridging a joint (**Fig 7.3-10**). Hardware removal is otherwise performed only if bothersome or when tendon irritation occurs. Plates spanning the first TMT do not need to be removed if arthrodesis of the joint was performed and the hardware is asymptomatic.

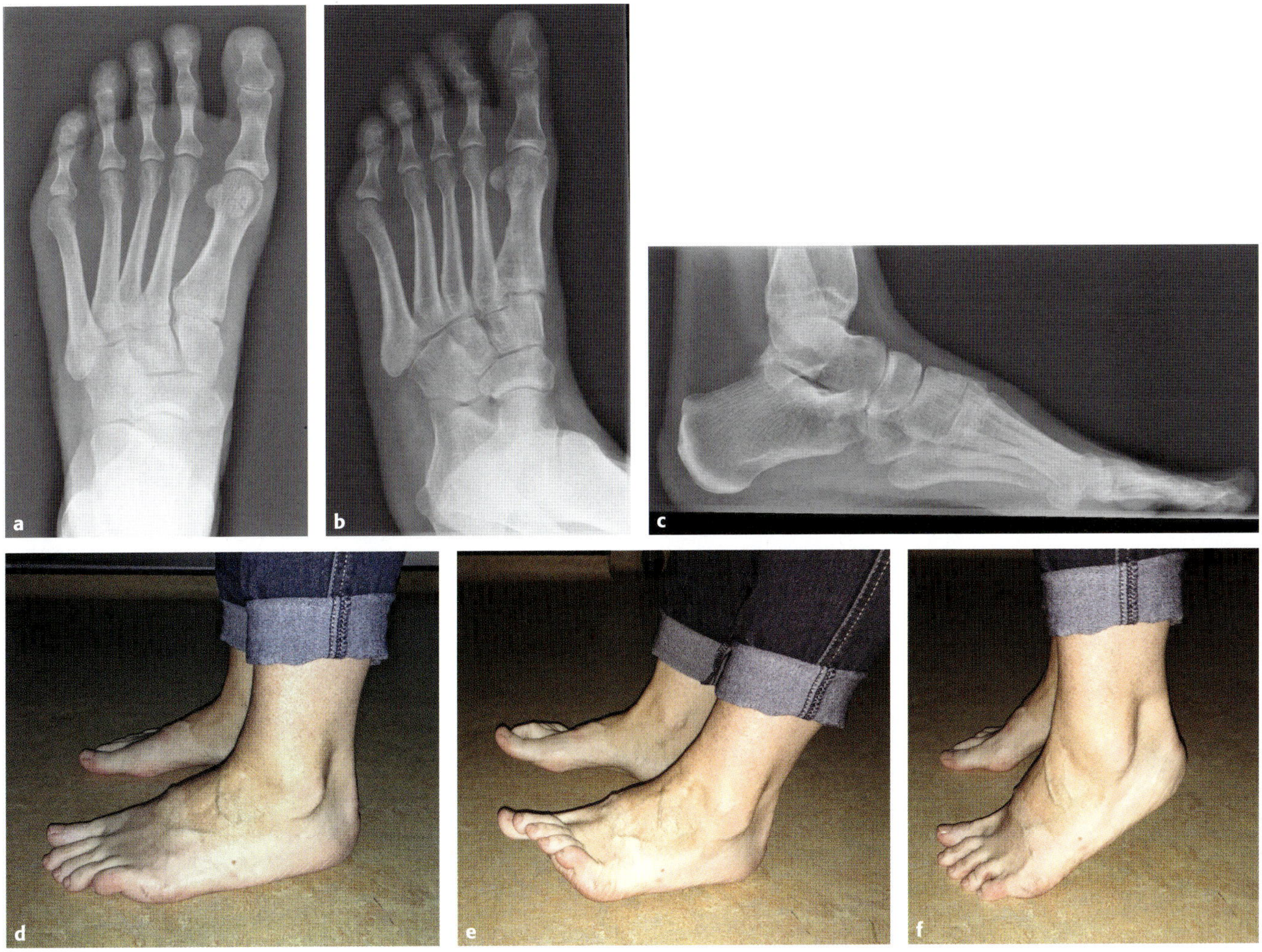

Fig 7.3-10a–f Patient from case example of joint-spanning plating (**Fig 7.3-6**).
a–c Removal of joint-spanning plate was performed at 5 months.
d–f Follow-up at 2.5 years shows well-preserved ROM. The patient experienced occasional swelling after long walks but otherwise had no functional problems.

8 Recommended reading

Buckley RE, Moran CG, Apivatthakakul T. *Principles of Fracture Management.3rd ed.* Stuttgart: Thieme; 2017.
De Boer P, Buckley R, Hoppenfeld S. *Surgical Exposures in Foot and Ankle Surgery—the Anatomic Approach.* Baltimore: Lippincott Williams & Wilkins; 2012.

7.4 Proximal first metatarsal fracture with joint involvement

Khairul Faizi Mohammad

1 Case description

A 28-year-old man sustained a direct blow to the left foot resulting in a twisting injury during a motorcycle rally. He experienced a sharp pain to the foot and was unable to bear weight. After postinjury x-rays were taken (**Fig 7.4-1**), K-wires were inserted and the patient returned home with the foot immobilized in a vacuum splint. Afterwards, x-rays revealed a malreduced, unstable, intraarticular fracture subluxation of the proximal first metatarsal (MT) and fracture of the base of the fifth MT (**Fig 7.4-2**).

Initial treatment involved elevation, a modified Jones bandage for swelling control, and observation for compartment syndrome (**Fig 7.4-3**).

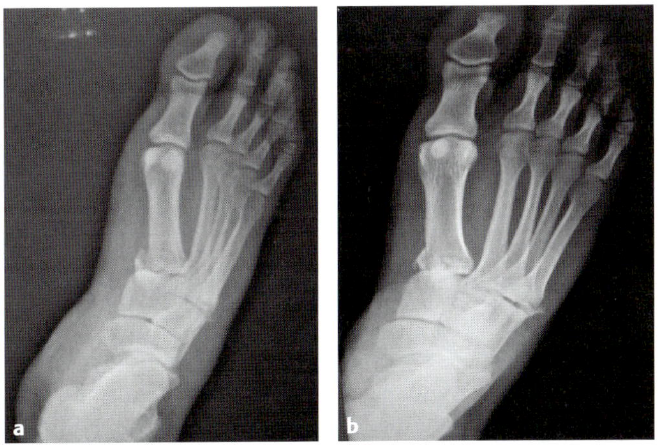

Fig 7.4-1a–b Postinjury x-rays.
a Intraarticular fracture subluxation of the first MT with an intraarticular fracture of the base of the fifth MT.
b Note the instability of the first TMT joint.
(Images courtesy of Amir Adham Ahmad, MD.)

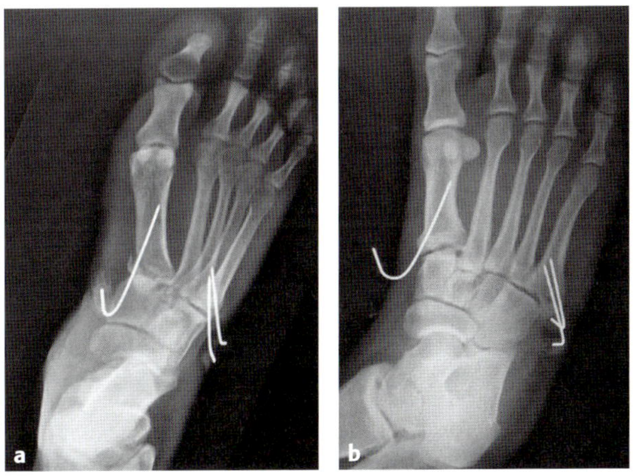

Fig 7.4-2a–b X-rays taken after stabilization with K-wires, showing a malreduced and unstable first TMT joint.
(Images courtesy of Amir Adham Ahmad, MD.)

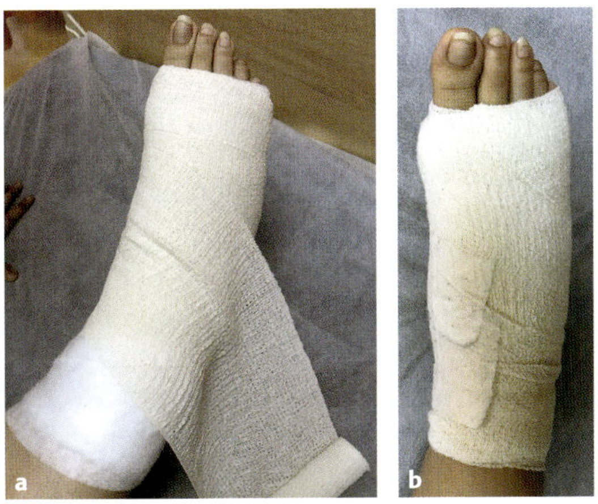

Fig 7.4-3a–b Application of a modified Jones bandaging to the foot. This involves using alternating layers of cotton and crepe bandage in a cross-layering method.

2 Preoperative planning

Indications for surgery

A displaced intraarticular fracture of the proximal first MT needs accurate reduction and rigid fixation to achieve a stable and congruent first tarsometatarsal (TMT) joint (AO/OTA 87.1.1). Treatment for the base of the fifth MT is discussed in chapter 7.9.

Treatment options

Tarsometatarsal joint stabilization can be achieved with a plate spanning the joint from the medial cuneiform to the shaft of the first MT. The articular fragment is typically reduced and maintained with interfragmentary screws (if fragment size allows). Other options include external fixation along the medial column and intraarticular reconstruction with interfragmentary screws.

A medial utility approach to the medial column allows adequate exposure of the medial column and appropriate placement of the plate with adequate soft-tissue coverage (**Fig 7.4-4**).

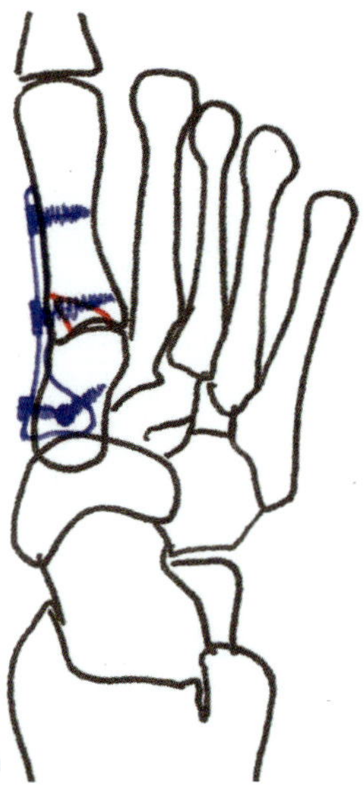

a

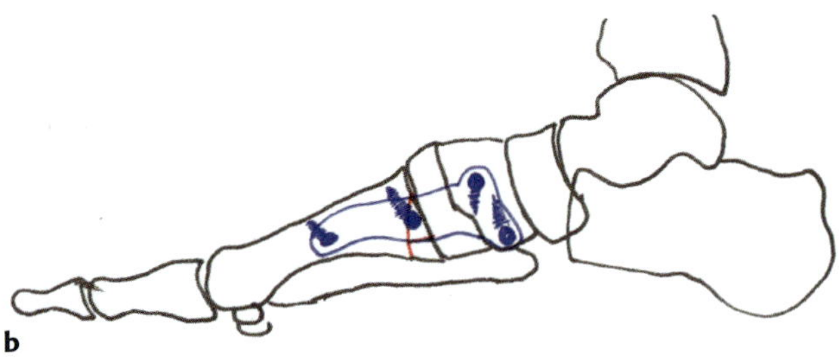

b

Fig 7.4-4a–b Preoperative plan.
a AP view. The intraarticular fragment will be held with an interfragmentary screw either independent of the plate or from within the plate. This will depend on the bone stock after removing the K-wires.
b Lateral view. A 3.5 mm plate will be used to span the first TMT joint to regain length and alignment. Placement will be on the inferomedial aspect of the medial arch, spanning from the first MT to the medial cuneiform.

3 Operating room setup

Patient positioning	• Supine on a radiolucent table • The foot is draped free to the level of the knee to allow rotation internally and externally (**Fig 7.4-5**).
Anesthesia options	• General anesthesia, regional spinal anesthesia, or a combination as per surgeon preference
C-arm location	• The C-arm is placed at the foot of the operative room table with the screen placed opposite the surgeon for clear viewing.
Tourniquet	• Thigh tourniquet can be placed and inflated if bleeding obscures visualization.

For illustrations and overview of anesthetic considerations, see chapter 1.

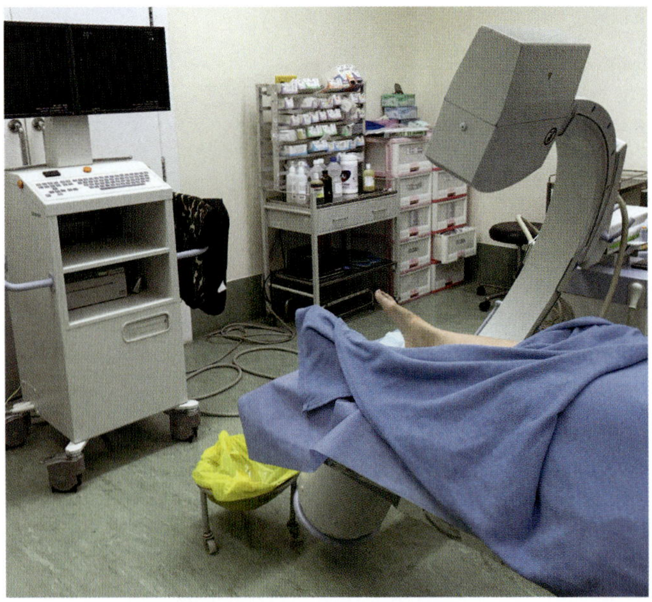

Fig 7.4-5 The C-arm is located on the ipsilateral side of the affected foot with the screen placed at the foot of the patient.

Equipment

- Buttress locking compression plate 2.4–3.5
- 2.4–3.5 mm cortex screws
- 2.4–3.5 mm locking head screws
- Small external fixator set with 3.5 or 4.0 mm Schanz pins
- Reduction clamps
- Small distractor

The equipment used will vary in accordance with varying anatomy of the fracture configurations. A combination of the equipment can also be used.

4 Surgical procedure

The incision is centered on the first TMT joint, parallel to the inferior border of the medial column (**Fig 7.4-6a**). The surgical plane between the abductor hallucis muscle and the inferior border of the first MT is developed proximally and distally. At this point, the fracture and TMT ligaments can be assessed (**Fig 7.4-6b**). The first TMT joint is reduced and secured with temporary transfixion K-wires.

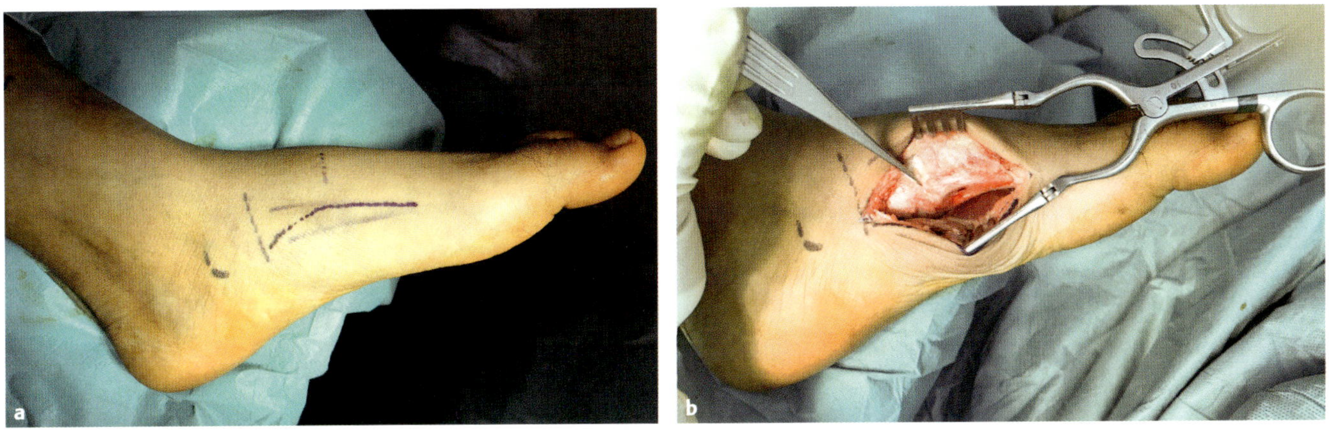

Fig 7.4-6a–b Surgical approach.
a Landmarks for the skin incision showing a variation of the medial utility approach along the inferior border of the medial bony arch and centered on the first TMT joint.
b Intraoperative exposure of the first TMT joint. Note the thicker soft-tissue coverage on the medial plantar side.

Tarsometarsal stabilization is achieved by applying a contoured buttress locking compression plate 3.5 on the medial plantar aspect of the joint to achieve adequate soft tissue cover (**Fig 7.4-7a**). Alignment of the first MT and the stability of the first TMT joint can then be reassessed under C-arm guidance (**Fig 7.4-7b**). Definitive fixation of the articular fracture is achieved with interfragmentary screws through the plate (**Fig 7.4-7c–d**).

The tourniquet is released. Hemostasis is secured and closure is performed in layers. A well-padded modified Jones bandage is applied.

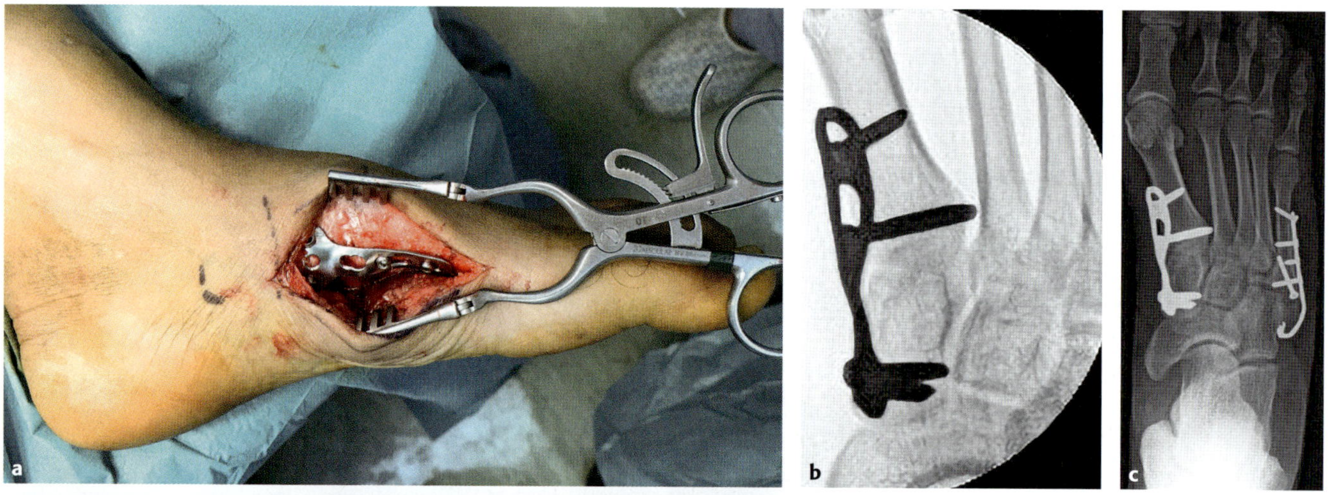

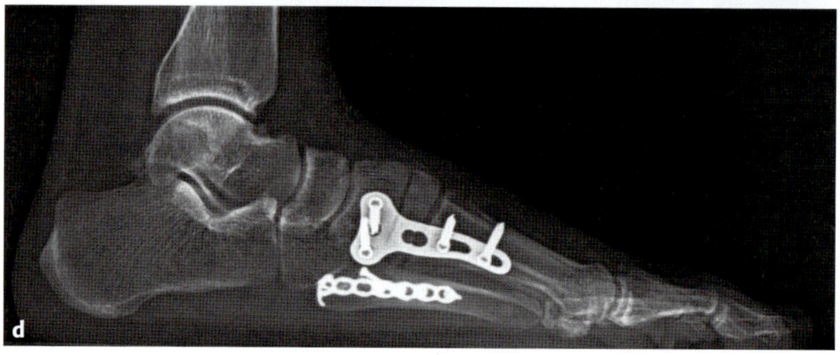

Fig 7.4-7a–d Plate application.
a–b The plate has been contoured and applied to the plantar medial aspect of the medial arch.
c Postoperative AP x-ray.
d Postoperative lateral x-ray.

5 Pitfalls and complications

Pitfalls

Irreducible intraarticular fragments

Very small intraarticular fragments (< 5 mm) devoid of articular cartilage and not attached to soft tissue should be removed rather than attempting fixation (**Fig 7.4-8**).

Unstable and shortened medial column

An unstable and shortened medial column can occur if adequate stability and length is not achieved between the MT and medial cuneiform. In addition to application of a T-plate, which increases the fixation to the medial cuneiform, a small fragment external fixator could be applied from the distal end of the MT to the calcaneus. This will achieve alignment of the medial column and distraction to length (**Fig 7.4-9**).

Complications

- Compartment syndrome is a surgical emergency. A single, extended medial utility incision allows decompression of the all compartments including the calcaneal compartment near the knot of Henry malunion.
- Nonunion
- Malunion
- Posttraumatic arthritis
- First TMT instability
- Wound dehiscence

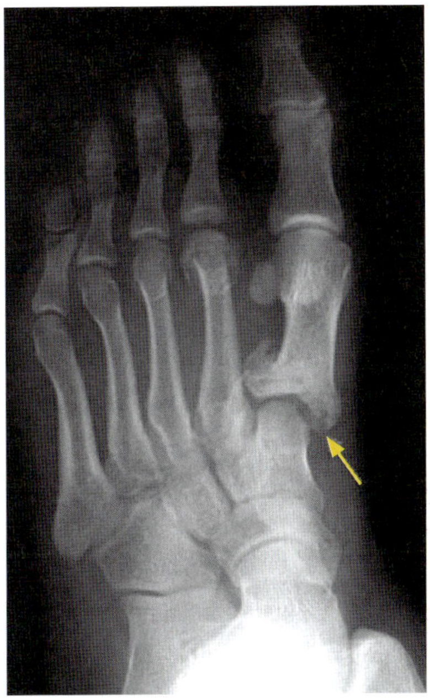

Fig 7.4-8 Example from a different case showing irreducible intraarticular fragments (yellow arrow). Small intraarticular fragments can be difficult to reduce and fix. Stability of the joint may be compromised after removal. Additional stabilization is therefore required.
(Image courtesy of Sean E Nork, MD.)

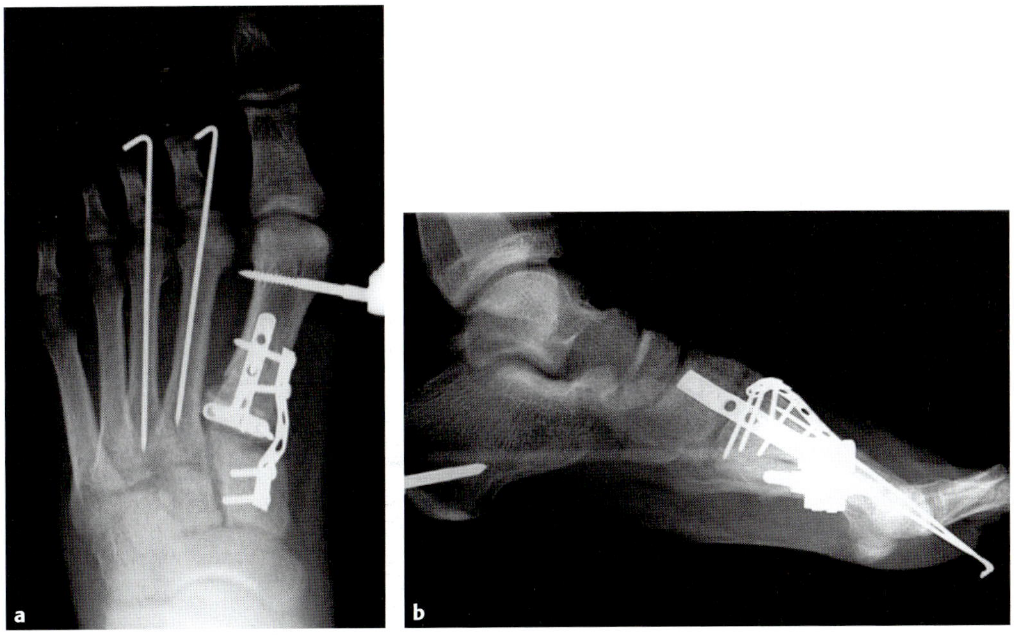

Fig 7.4-9a–b Example from a different case of an unstable and shortened medial column after reduction and spanning fixation.
a X-ray AP view.
b X-ray lateral view.
(Images courtesy of Sean E Nork, MD.)

6 Alternative techniques

Intraarticular interfragmentary fixation can be performed with 2.4–3.5 mm screws. Plates may be used to buttress the articular fragments provided the first TMT joint is stable and accurately reduced.

If the first TMT joint is unstable, it should be spanned in addition to achieving articular congruency. Spanning can be achieved with a bridge plate or with a small external fixator (**Fig 7.4-10**).

Cross-joint fixation with screws or K-wires can also be done to stabilize the first MT after joint articular reconstruction.

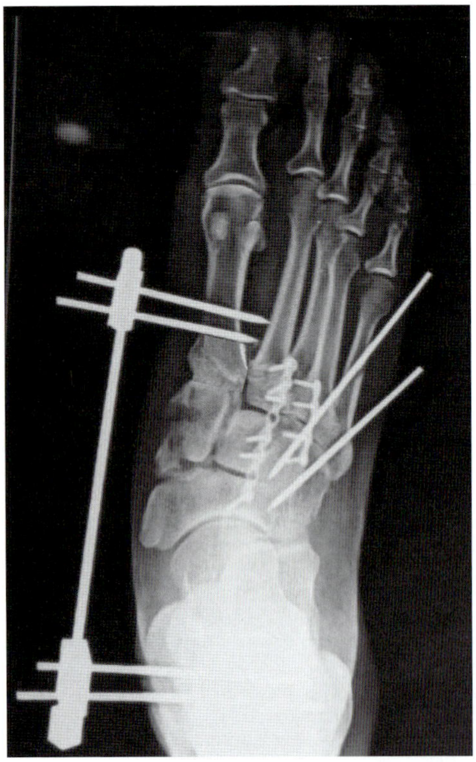

Fig 7.4-10 Example case showing the alternative technique for spanning the first TMT joint with a small external fixator.
(Image courtesy of Ravinder Sidhu, MD.)

Open reduction and internal fixation without joint bridging

In first MT base fractures without comminution or gross instability, fracture fixation need not be supplemented by a plate bridging the joint (**Fig 7.4-11a–c**). Depending on the size and number of fragments, fixation can be achieved with screws, K-wires, or a small plate.

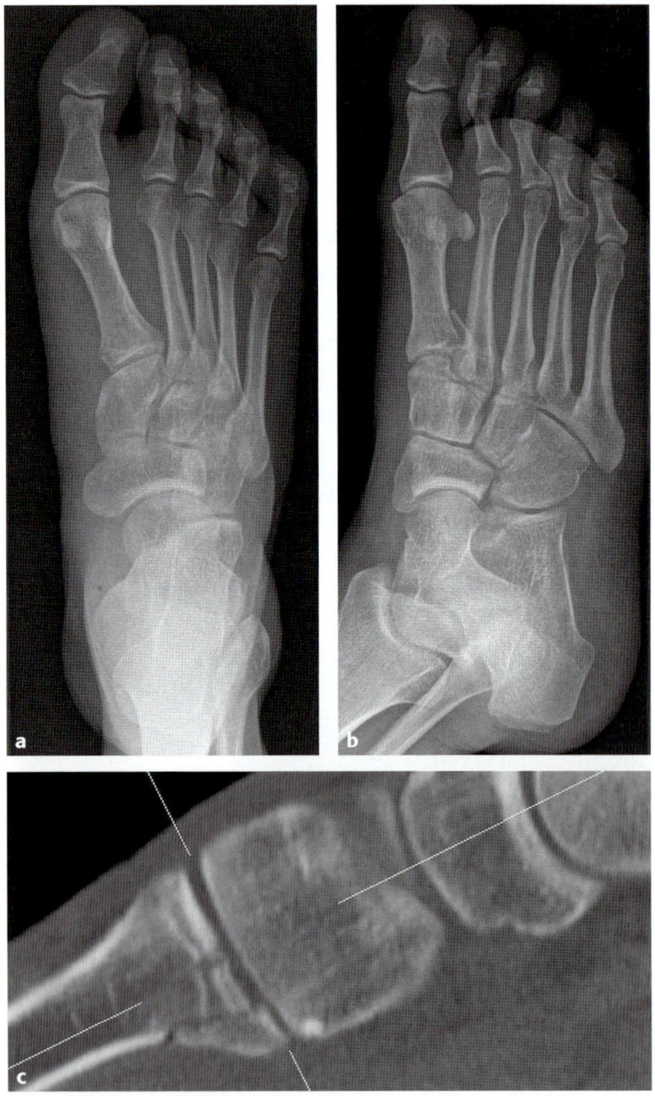

Fig. 7.4-11a–f Example from a different case showing open reduction and internal fixation without joint bridging.
a–c Lateral (**a**) and oblique (**b**) x-rays of a 31-year-old male patient show an intraarticular first MT base fracture without signs of a dislocation at the TMT (Lisfranc) joints. The computed tomographic scan reveals a multifragmentary fracture of the joint facet to the medial cuneiform (**c**).
(Case courtesy of Stefan Rammelt, MD.)

Open reduction is achieved via a small medial approach over the first TMT joint. The articular fragments are reduced to each other and the proximal first metatarsal shaft using the joint surface of the medial cuneiform as a template. Fragments are temporarily fixed with K-wires. Definite fixation is achieved with screws (**Fig. 7.4-11d–f**). If the first TMT joint is stable after fixation of the first MT base fracture, transfixation, or bridging of the first TMT joint is not necessary.

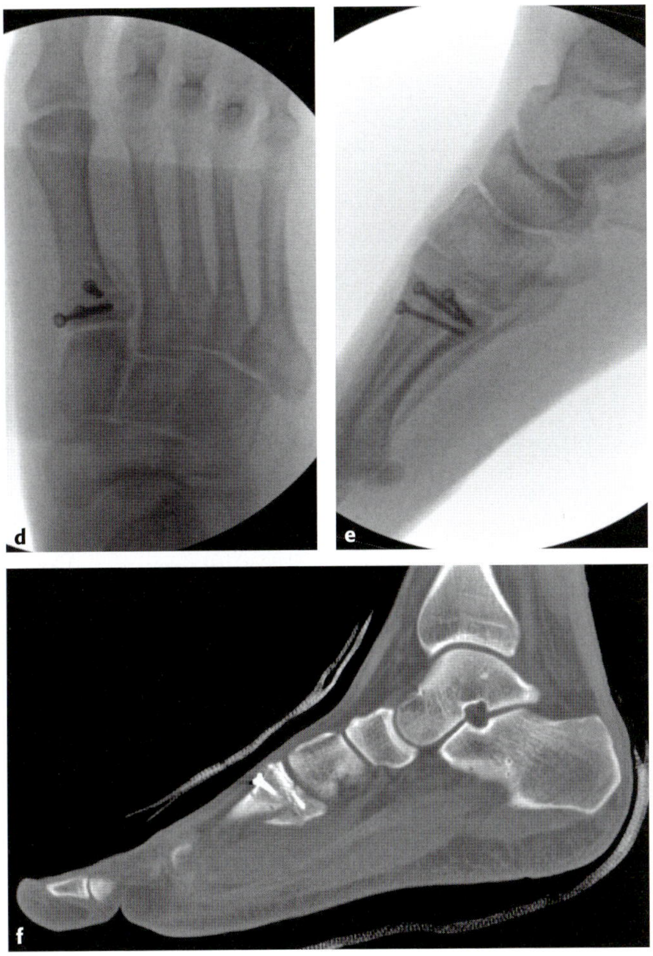

Fig. 7.4-11a–f (cont) Example from a different case showing open reduction and internal fixation without joint bridging.

d–e Open reduction and screw fixation is achieved via a small medial approach. The first TMT joint is stable after fracture fixation, thus obviating the need for joint transfixation or bridging.

f Postoperative CT scanning demonstrates anatomical reduction of the articular surface and a stable, congruent first TMT joint.

(Case courtesy of Stefan Rammelt, MD.)

7 Postoperative management and rehabilitation

A well-padded 3-sided plaster splint wrapped in elastic bandages is applied at the conclusion of surgery. Nonabsorbable sutures are removed once the wound has healed. The 3-sided plaster splint is then exchanged with a postoperative surgical boot. Early range-of-motion exercises of the ankle and toes are started as tolerated. The patient is allowed full weight bearing after 6 weeks (**Fig 7.4-12**). If an external fixator was applied, full weight bearing can be started after it is removed.

Active rehabilitation regime is then initiated including functional exercises (gait training to running), balancing, and proprioception.

Implant removal

Spanning external fixators are removed between 6 weeks to 3 months and spanning internal plates at 6 months.

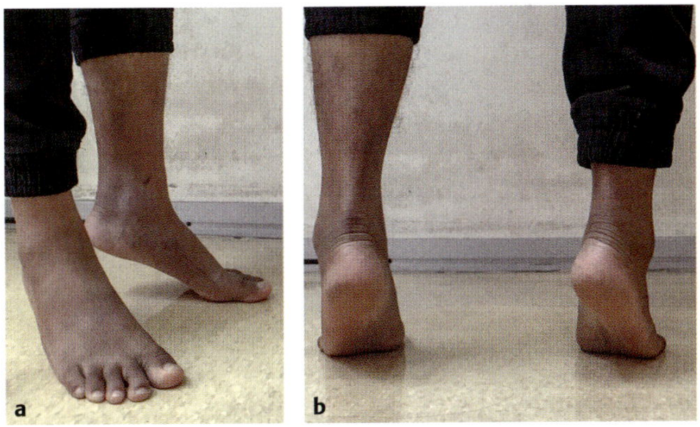

Fig 7.4-12a–b Clinical condition at 1 year postoperatively.

a Stability of the first TMT joint seen in a patient performing painless double leg heel rise (right foot).

b Range of motion of the foot and the ability to stress the TMT joint (right foot).

8 Recommended reading

Ballmer FT, Hertel R, Ballmer PM, et al. Other applications of the small AO external fixator to the lower limb. *Injury.* 1994;25 Suppl 4:S-d69–76.
Boutefnouchet T, Budair B, Backshayesh P, et al. Metatarsal fractures: A review and current concepts. *Trauma.* 2014;16(3):147–163.
Frink M, Hildebrand F, Krettek C, et al. Compartment syndrome of the lower leg and foot. *Clin Orthop Relat Res.* 2010 Apr;468(4):940–950.
Rammelt S, Heineck J, Zwipp H. Metatarsal fractures. *Injury.* 2004 Sep;35 Suppl 2:Sb77–86.

7.5 Multiple metatarsal neck fractures—K-wire fixation

Rajiv Shah, Mandeep S Dhillon, Shivam Shah

1 Case description

A 41-year-old man was involved in a road traffic accident and sustained an injury to his right foot. He was admitted to the emergency department within 3 hours of the injury with pain and swelling of the foot. His foot was immobilized in a below-knee plaster slab, elevated, and appropriate analgesics were given.

X-rays of his foot in AP, oblique, and lateral view showed displaced and comminuted fractures of all four lesser metatarsals (MTs), involving the distal shafts of second and third MTs, the neck of the fourth MT, and head of the fifth MT (**Fig 7.5-1**).

2 Preoperative planning

Multiple fractures involving the MT head, neck, and shaft, with displacement and shortening are indications for surgical intervention. If accurate length, rotation, and sagittal alignment of the MTs are not restored, the consequence is the loss of the parabolic arch of the foot, leading to painful plantar corns and callosities with direct or transfer metatarsalgia.

The surgical options are either open reduction and internal fixation, or closed manipulative reduction and minimally invasive stabilization. The patient had significant soft-tissue swelling; so the need arose to preserve biology, and a minimally invasive procedure using closed manipulative reduction followed by intramedullary K-wire fixation was selected.

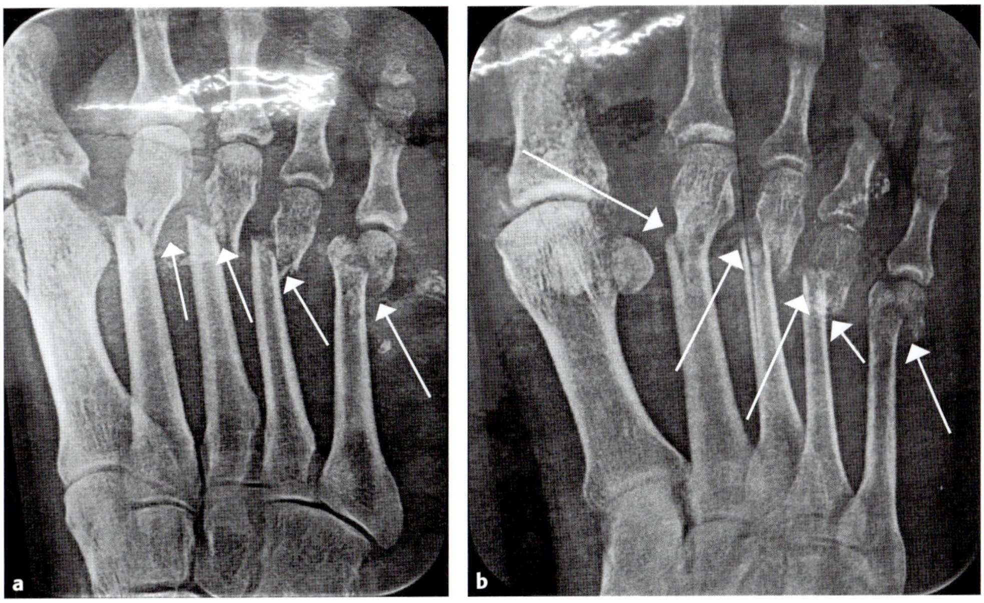

Fig 7.5-1a–b Injury x-rays showing multiple displaced neck shaft fractures (arrows) of all four lesser MTs.
a AP view.
b Oblique view.

3 Operating room setup

Patient positioning	• Supine • The foot can be brought to the edge of the operative table, with the knee flexed and kept over support used for tibial interlocking nailing, and can then be rested over the flat camera side of the reversed image intensifier, which is positioned from the opposite side (**Fig 7.5-2a**).
Anesthesia options	• Regional or spinal anesthesia is preferred.
C-arm location	• Screen of C-arm is positioned at the foot end of the operative table for easy image visualization.
Tourniquet	• Thigh tourniquet is applied and inflated.
Tips	• After appropriate cleaning and draping, a rolled towel is placed under the foot providing a better position for manipulation and wire insertion (**Fig 7.5-2b**).

For illustrations and overview of anesthetic considerations, see chapter 1.

Equipment

- T-handle with chuck
- 1.0–2.5 mm K-wires
- K-wire bender

4 Surgical procedure

With a 2.5 mm K-wire mounted on a T-handle, an oblique pilot hole is made starting 5 mm distal to the articular surface of the metatarsal base to be operated. This entry avoids the ligaments of tarsometatarsal joints (**Fig 7.5-3a**). A pilot hole is made either over the medial or over the lateral surface of MT base, avoiding injury to the extensor tendons (**Fig 7.5-3b**). For a medially displaced distal fragment, the pilot hole is made on the medial surface and vice versa.

A 1.5 mm K-wire is bent at the tip and in the middle to create a curve, and the sharp tip of bent K-wire is cut to make it blunt. Use of blunt-tipped K-wire avoids cortical penetration while driving it inside the medullary canal (**Fig 7.5-4**). The wire thickness varies from 1.0 to 1.8 mm according to medullary canal size.

The wire is mounted on a T-handle and is advanced under C-arm guidance with gentle rotatory movements up to the fracture site (**Fig 7.5-5**).

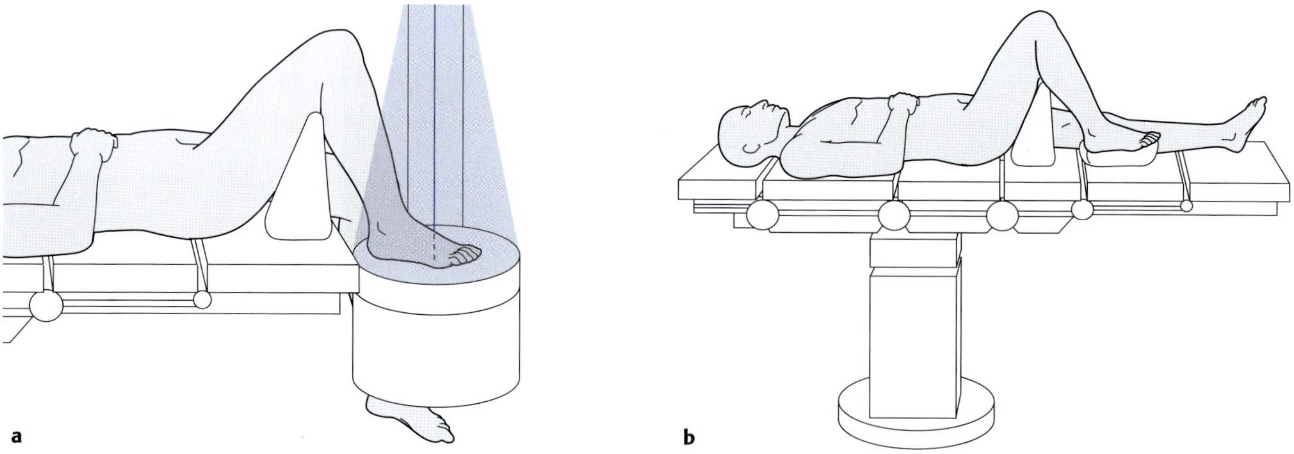

Fig 7.5-2a–b Foot positioning.
a Position of foot over reversed image intensifier.
b Positioning of a towel bump under the foot to be operated.

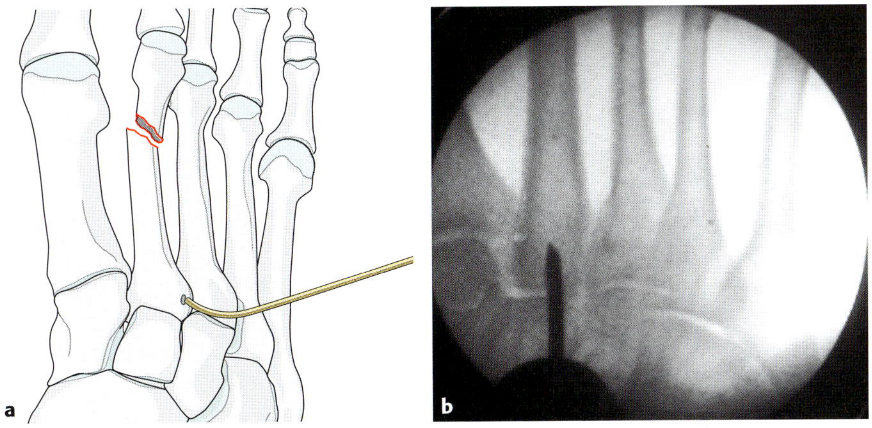

Fig 7.5-3a–b
a The pilot hole for K-wire entry.
b Intraoperative image of pilot hole entry at the base of MT.

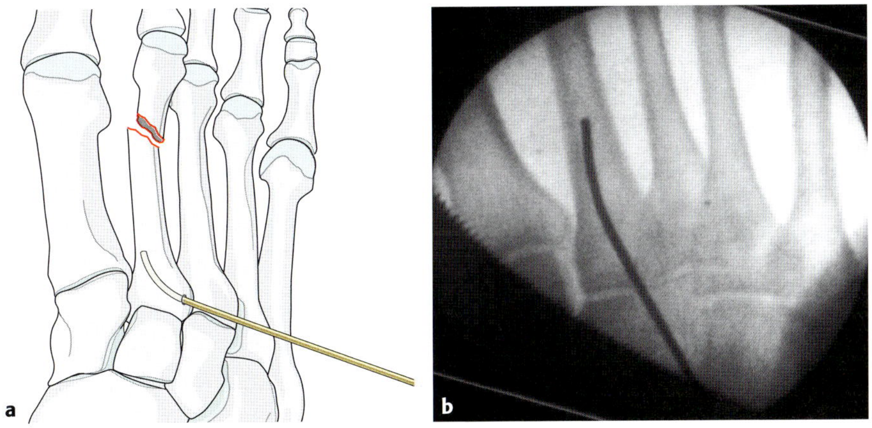

Fig 7.5-4a–b The passage of K-wires.
a Passage of bent K-wire in a medullary cavity of MT with flattened tip.
b Passage of K-wire with rotatory movements along the MT shaft.

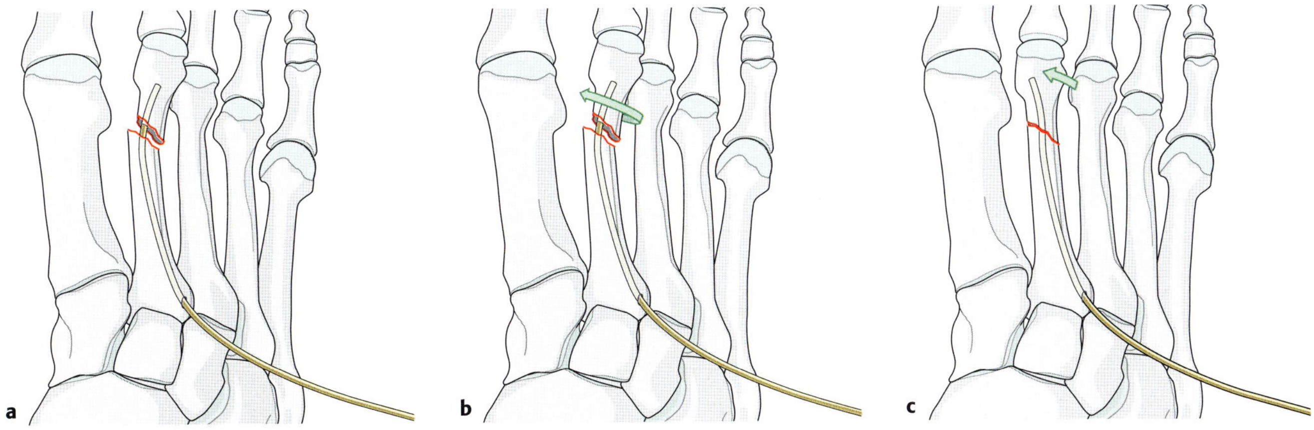

Fig 7.5-5a–c The rotation of bent K-wire aids in achieving the reduction.

Fracture reduction is achieved by an assistant applying traction over the toe. Once reduction is achieved, the wire is advanced through the fracture site into the distal fragment (**Fig 7.5-6**). If a satisfactory reduction is not achieved, the wire is pushed further into the distal fragment and rotated; the rotatory movement of the bent K-wire in the cancellous bone of distal fragment helps to reduce the fracture (**Fig 7.5-7**). This blunt K-wire is now advanced up to subchondral bone. This maneuver maintains the length of metatarsal, thereby restoring the parabolic transverse arch of the foot.

In some fractures, traction alone is insufficient to reduce the fracture. In such cases a 2.0 or 2.5 mm K-wire placed percutaneously can be used as a joystick to manipulate the metatarsal shaft (**Fig 7.5-8**).

In case of wide fragment separation and/or soft-tissue interposition, open reduction via a small direct incision over the fracture may be needed. For an MT with wide medullary cavity, a second wire should also be passed in similar fashion from opposite side of the MT base; this gives a 3-point fixation and rotational stability to the fixation The proximal ends of K-wires are bent and kept outside the skin for subsequent removal (**Fig 7.5-9**).

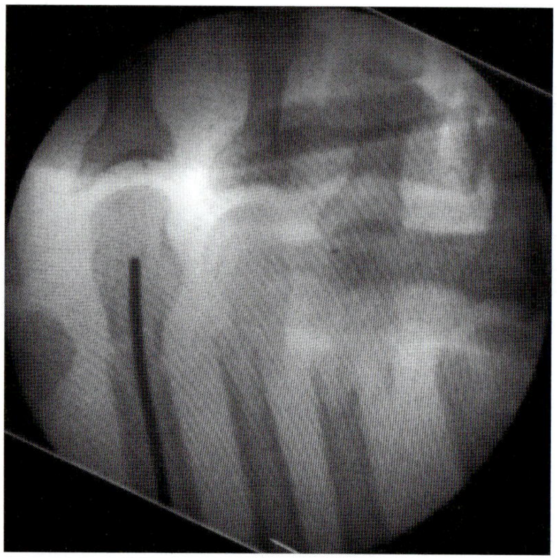

Fig 7.5-6 Intraoperative image showing the reduced fracture.

5 Pitfalls and complications

Pitfalls

Incorrect entry point

- Incorrect entry for K-wire causes irritation of extensor tendon and joint invasion, leading to stiffness. Repeated checking for the correct entry with C-arm helps prevent this.
- Entry too distal may not provide the proper trajectory making manipulation difficult and may not provide good fixation. Introducing the curved or bent K-wire from the side of displacement of the distal fragment helps the K-wire conform to the shape of the medullary canal, and the curve allows easier passage into the displaced distal fragment.

Cortex perforation

- The wire may breach or pierce the opposite cortex earlier than desired, creating a wrong tract. This can be avoided by cutting the sharp tip of the wire to make it blunt; introducing the wire with rotatory movements only. Frequent imaging also helps.
- Distal articular perforation can occur by excessive hammering of the wire up to the subchondral bone. If this happens, the wire is removed, and a new wire is reintroduced.

Complications

- Loss of reduction
- Distal migration of wires
- Wire backout
- Infection at pin-tract site
- Nonunion

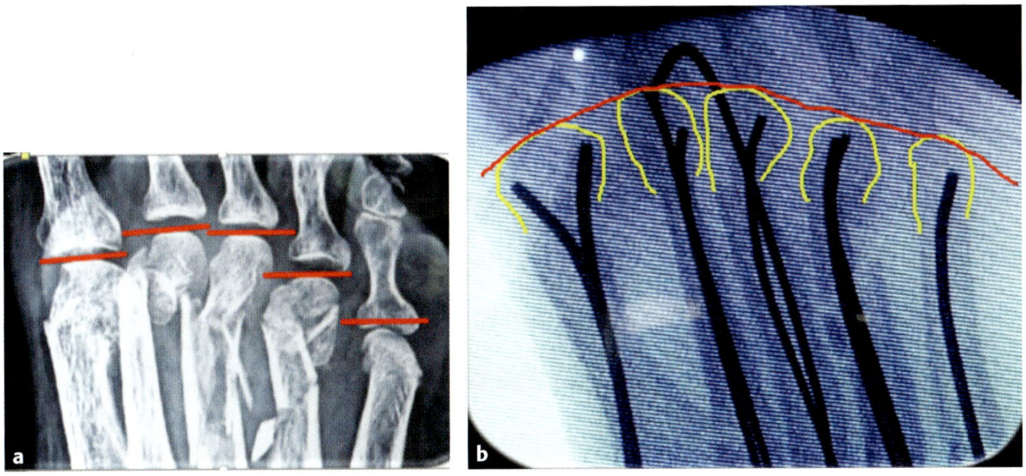

Fig 7.5-7a–b AP X-rays showing multiple MT fractures and restoration of parabolic arch following percutaneously placed K-wires, which aided reduction.

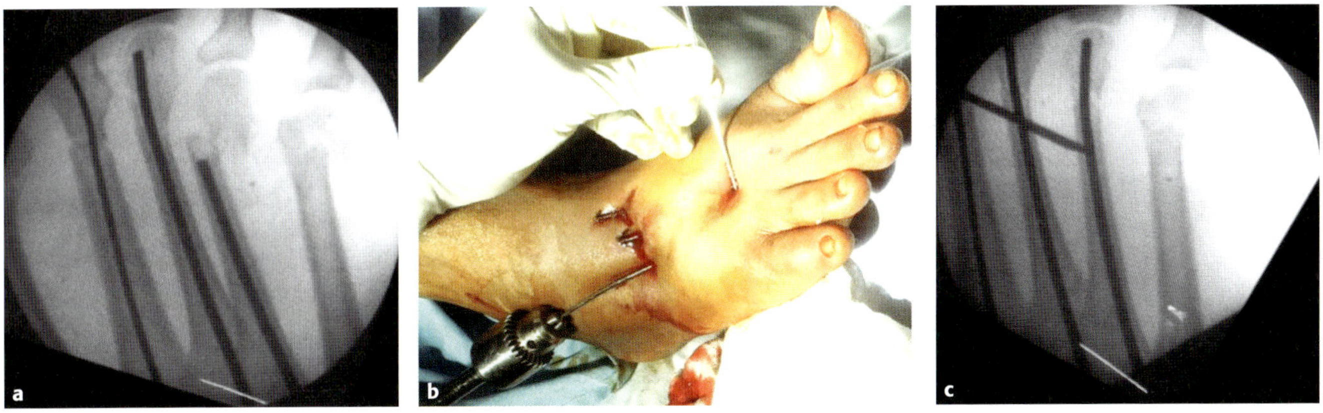

Fig 7.5-8a–c Intraoperative image showing shortened and displaced metatarsal neck fracture, which is difficult to reduce (**a**). The second K-wire inserted percutaneously is being used as a reduction tool (**b**) to achieve final reduction (**c**).

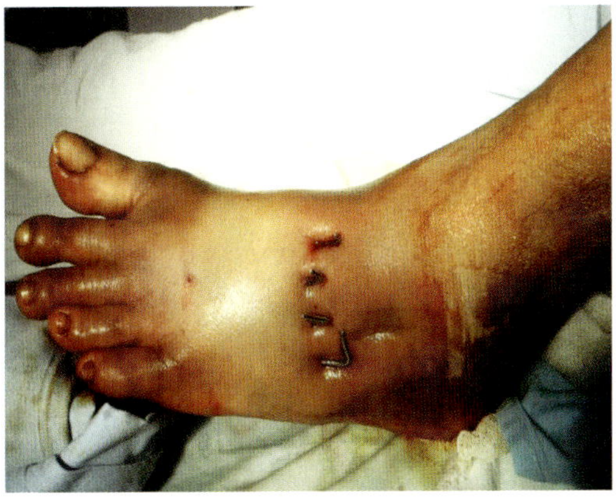

Fig 7.5-9 At the end of the surgery, the bent proximal ends of K-wires are kept outside the skin to ease later removal.

6 Alternative techniques

Open reduction and retrograde wiring

This technique, although easier to use has some disadvantages: complications related to opening the fracture site surgery and violation of MT joints leading to joint stiffness may be significant.

Plate fixation

Multiple MT fractures can also be treated with plate fixation. The incisions are generally spaced between two fractured MTs allowing fixation of both from one incision. In cases when plate fixation is the preferred treatment and all MTs are fractured, incisions can be placed between the first and second MT and the third and fourth MTs. If the fifth MT requires plate fixation, the incision can be placed along its lateral aspect.

Fractures that can benefit from plate fixation are those with unstable patterns, especially long oblique and comminuted fractures or those with significant displacement. Surgery should be done after soft-tissue swelling has been reduced. Care should be taken to avoid excessive soft-tissue undermining to prevent wound complications, see chapter 7.6.

7 Postoperative management and rehabilitation

K-wire entry sites are covered with sterile dressings and a compression bandage is applied. Postoperative imaging is done (**Fig 7.5-10**). The limb is elevated over two pillows and active toe and foot movements are encouraged. The patient is discharged after 48 hours with advice of nonweight-bearing ambulation with a pair of crutches.

X-rays are taken at the end of 6 weeks and K-wires are removed. Weight bearing is started from this point onward and is progressively increased as tolerated. Final images are obtained at the end of 8 weeks and the patient can perform all activities by this time (**Fig 7.5-11**).

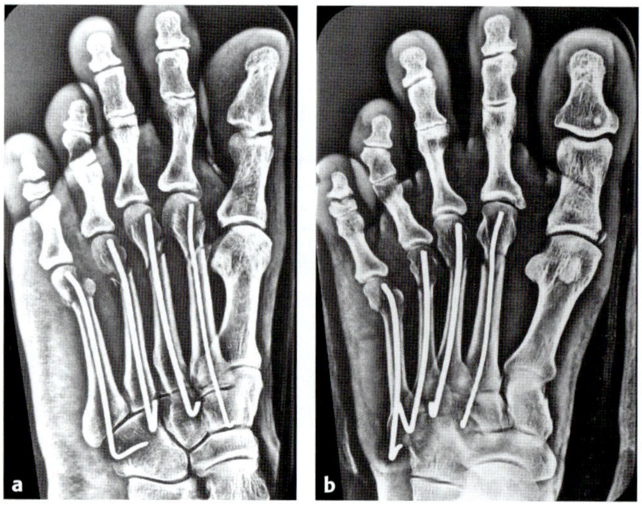

Fig 7.5-10a–b Immediate postoperative x-rays.
a AP view.
b Oblique view.

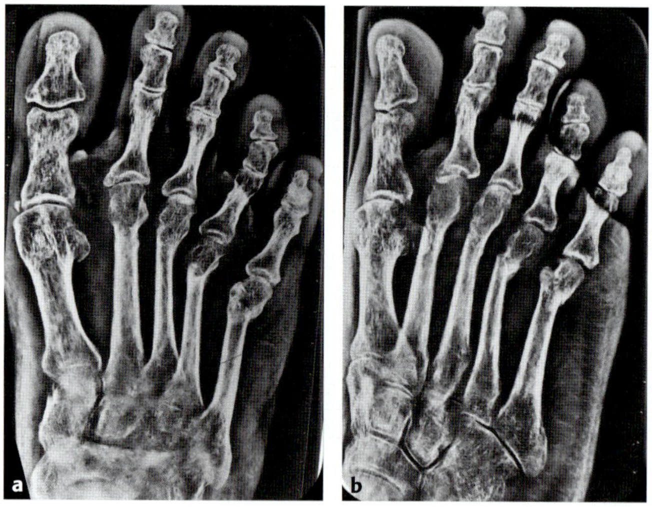

Fig 7.5-11a–b Final x-rays at the end of 10 weeks after K-wire removal.
a AP view.
b Oblique view.

8 Recommended reading

Bryant T, Beck DM, Daniel JN, et al. Union rate and rate of hardware removal following plate fixation of metatarsal shaft and neck fractures. *Foot Ankle Int.* 2018 Mar;39(3):326–331.
Kim HN, Park YJ, Kim GL, et al. Closed antegrade intramedullary pinning for reduction and fixation of metatarsal fractures. *J Foot Ankle Surg.* 2012 Jul-Aug;51(4):445–449.
Lee SK, Kim KJ, Choy WS. Modified retrograde percutaneous intramedullary multiple Kirschner wire fixation for treatment of unstable displaced metacarpal neck and shaft fractures. *Eur J Orthop Surg Traumatol.* 2013 Jul;23(5):535–543.
Rammelt S, Heineck J, Zwipp H. Metatarsal fractures. *Injury.* 2004 Sep;35 Suppl 2:Sb77–86.

7.6 Multiple metatarsal neck fractures—plate fixation

Jitendra Mangwani, Georgios Datsis, Georgina Wright, Michael Swords

1 Case description

A 42-year-old man was injured at work in an automobile factory when a large piece of industrial steel weighing approximately 450 kg fell onto his right foot. He was wearing protective steel toe work boots. He experienced severe pain and was transferred to the emergency department by ambulance. The only injuries were on the right foot. It was a closed injury associated with severe swelling, with altered sensation to the dorsum of his foot. The medial forefoot area was deformed.

X-rays showed a dislocation of the first metatarsophalangeal (MTP) joint as well as multiple metatarsal (MT) fractures. He was treated initially by closed reduction of the dislocation to the first MTP joint. Surgery was delayed to allow appropriate resolution of the soft-tissue swelling (**Fig 7.6-1**).

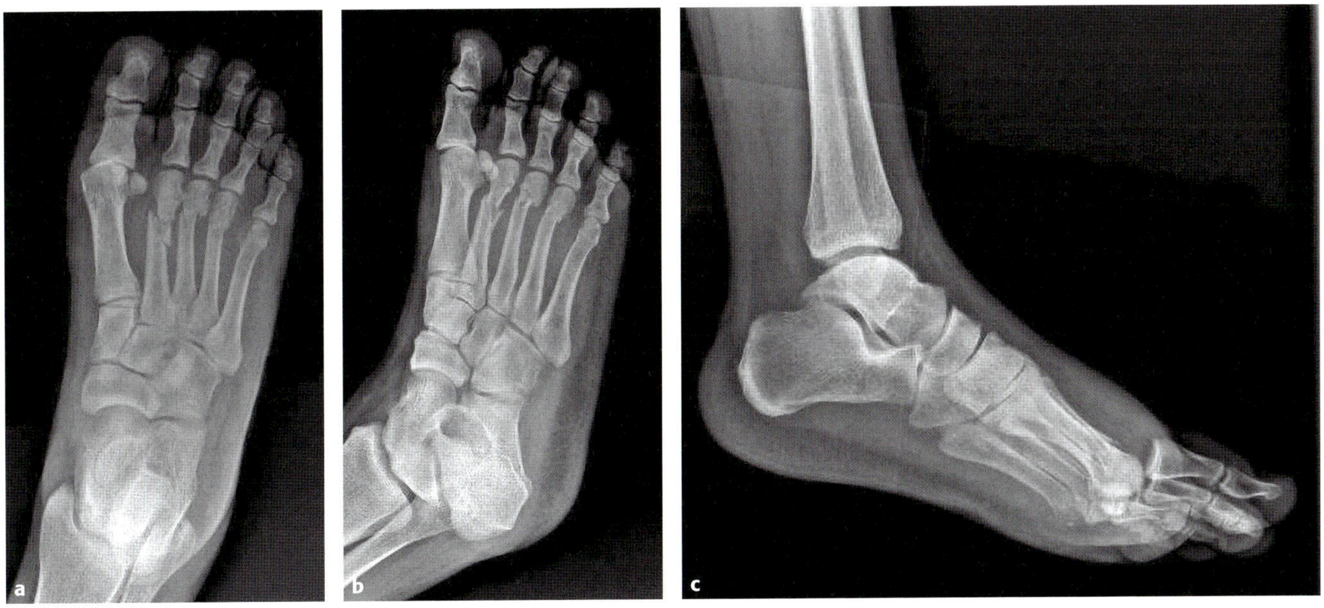

Fig 7.6-1a–c Injury x-rays demonstrating a dislocation of the first MTP joint and MT neck fractures of the second, third, and fourth MTs. Notice the extensive swelling seen on the lateral view over the dorsum of the foot.

a AP view.
b Oblique view.
c Lateral view.

2 Preoperative planning

Indications for surgery

Surgery was indicated due to marked malalignment of the MTs as well as gross instability of the first MTP joint and comminution of the second MT.

Indications include:

- Deformity in sagittal plane of more than 10°
- > 4 mm translation
- Multiple unstable MT neck fractures

Considerations for surgery

The second to fifth MTs bear approximately 40% of the body weight when walking. Restoration of their alignment in the sagittal plane is therefore an important consideration in preventing transfer metatarsalgia because of malunion.

In the absence of sagittal displacement, these fractures can be managed nonoperatively with immobilization in cast. Surgery should be timed to allow soft-tissue swelling to settle to avoid wound-healing problems.

Consideration must be given to stability, comminution, and the number of fractures of the MT neck before deciding which implant to use. For plating, preoperative planning should consider the number of screws that the size of the distal fragment would allow, and implants should be ordered appropriately (**Fig 7.6-2**).

Simple MT neck fractures can be alternatively treated with antegrade or retrograde K-wire fixation.

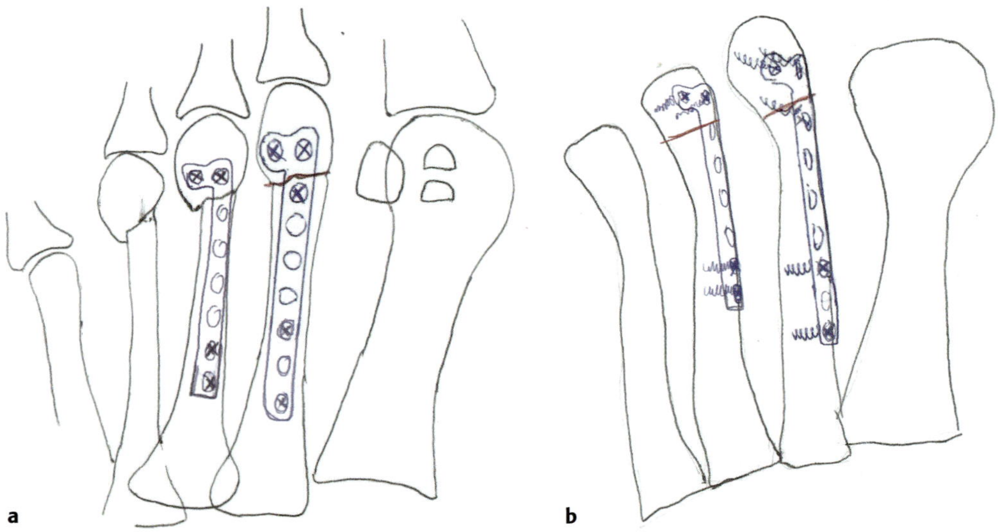

Fig 7.6-2a–b Preoperative plan for fixation.

3 Operating room setup

Patient positioning	• Supine
Anesthesia options	• General anesthetic is suggested for ease of patient positioning and comfort and can be supplemented by spinal or regional techniques. • The use of local blocks should be avoided due to the risk of compartment syndrome, as occurs in many trauma situations.
C-arm location	• Mini-C-arm: at the foot of the table, so that it can easily be moved alongside the patient for both AP and lateral views obtained intraoperatively. • Standard C-arm: on the contralateral side of the patient with the screen visible at the foot end of the operative table.
Tourniquet	• Used to improve fracture visualization

For illustrations and overview of anesthetic considerations, see chapter 1.

Equipment

- Small fragment set
- Small point-to-point reduction (Weber) clamps
- K-wires (1.1 or 1.4 mm)
- Standard and variable angle locking compression plates
- 2.4 and 2.7 mm screws (as per surgeon preference)
- 2.4 and 2.7 mm locking cortex screws (should be available if bone quality is poor)
- Finger trap device for toe traction

4 Surgical procedure

Approach

Care must be taken to avoid injury to the extensor tendons, sensory nerves, and dorsalis pedis artery on the dorsum of the foot (**Fig 7.6-3**). Appropriately placed dorsal incisions can be used, either directly over the MT for a single fracture or between the two MTs to allow access to adjacent MTs (**Fig 7-3a–b**). The length of the incision should be adequate to allow access and to prevent unnecessary stretching of the soft tissues.

Superficial veins should be identified and preserved if possible. Where it is not possible to preserve these veins, it is important to ensure that adequate hemostasis is achieved to prevent postoperative hematoma formation.

Branches of the deep and superficial peroneal nerve supplying the toes are also present in the area and must be preserved during dissection.

The extensor digitorum brevis and extensor digitorum longus tendons run longitudinally and can be retracted medially or laterally as appropriate to allow access to the MT below them.

The MT neck is exposed by locally detaching the interossei muscles sufficiently to allow adequate visualization and reduction of the fracture as well as placement of the plate; the intermetatarsal ligament should be preserved.

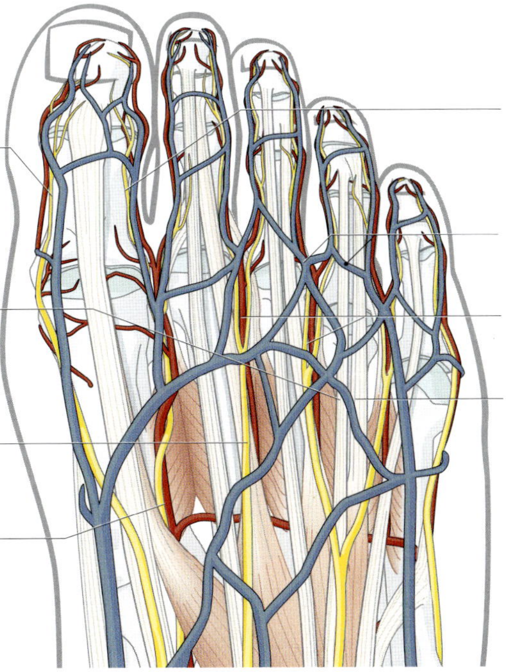

Fig 7.6-3 Pertinent anatomy and surgical approaches. The dorsal anatomy of the foot is complex and veins, nerves, and tendons have to be identified and protected.

Reduction and temporary fixation

Manual traction of the toe is often sufficient to allow reduction of the fracture fragments (**Fig 7.6-4a**). Finger traps may be used to apply axial traction on each ray.

In simple fracture patterns, reduction with small point-to-point reduction (Weber) clamps can be achieved (**Fig 7.6-4b**). If the fracture is comminuted, then temporary fixation with K-wires may be necessary. The K-wire can be driven into the intramedullary shaft of the MT or, in cases of severe comminution, the MT head can be pinned to the neighboring MT head until the plates have been provisionally placed. The articular cartilage of the MT head should be protected.

Reduction position should be confirmed on both AP, oblique, and lateral x-rays.

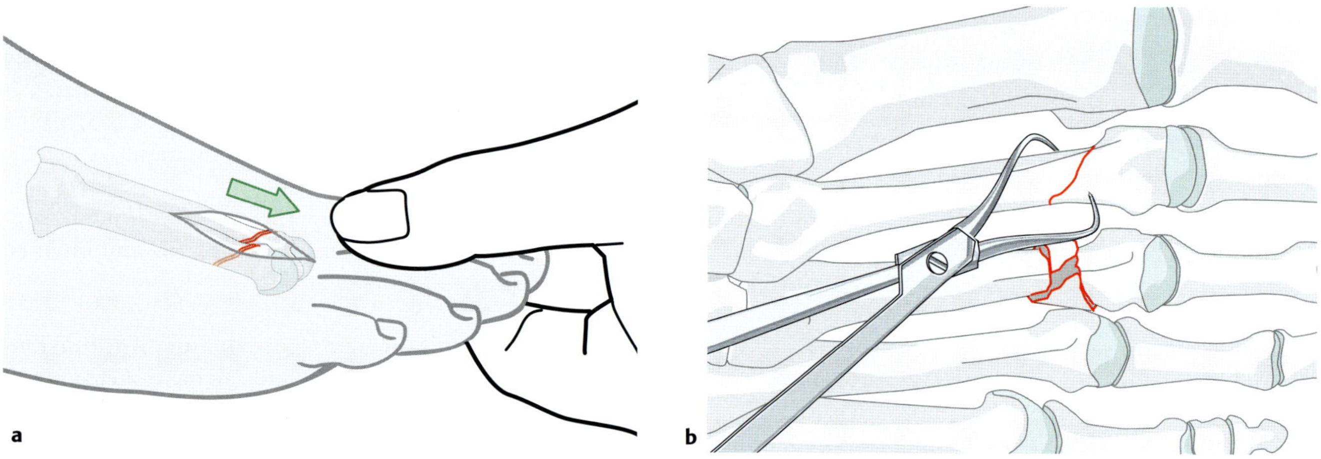

a b

Fig 7.6-4a–b Reduction maneuvers.
a Manual traction through the toe is generally enough to correct length and rotational alignment of the distal segment.
b Reduction can be held with point-to-point reduction (Weber) clamps or with K-wires and checked for accuracy with the C-arm in two planes.

Fixation

An L-plate or T-plate (**Fig 7.6-5**) of appropriate size is chosen to maintain the reduction. Distal fixation is improved with the addition of more screws. Locked screws also aid stability. With a simple fracture pattern, the plate can be used in compression with the addition of a lag screw. If the fracture is comminuted, then the plate can be used as a bridging device to restore the length and alignment. Care should be taken to ensure the screws are of the correct length to gain adequate fixation without breaching the articular surface of the MT head (**Fig 7.6-6**).

When multiple fractures are fixed, they are held in position with K-wires while each is fixed with the plate (**Fig 7.6-7a**). If comminution is present, definitive plate fixation should be in bridging mode, thus ensuring accurate length and rotation of fragments (**Fig 7.6-7b**).

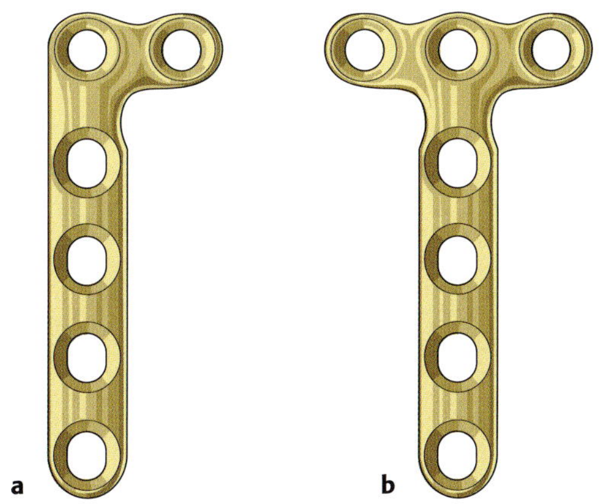

Fig 7.6-5a–b Screw purchase in the MT head is difficult and the L-plate or T-plate is typically used for improved fixation. Locking screws and/or plates provide angular stability.

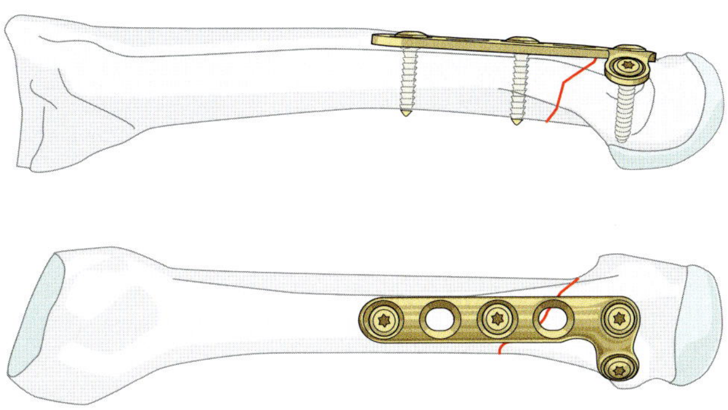

Fig 7.6-6 Screw length must be carefully measured to avoid plantar protrusion.

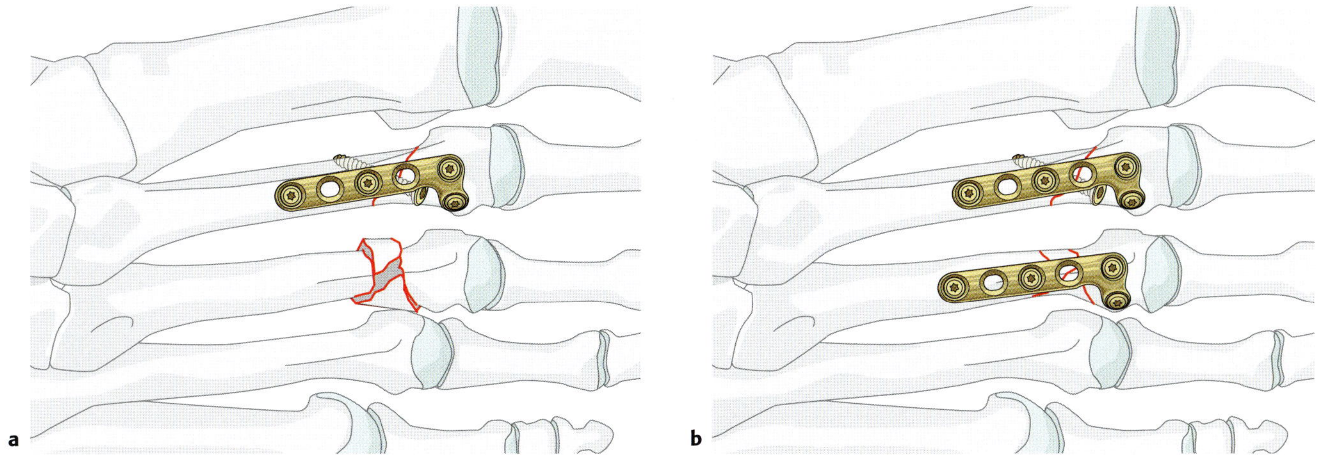

Fig 7.6-7a–b Fixation methods.

a Multifragmentary fractures may be too small to be maintained with temporary K-wire fixation.

b Definitive fixation is done with the L-plate or T-plate, used in a bridging mode, to maintain length and rotation.

For this patient, the first MTP joint was reduced and pinned. For the second and third MTs, a standard T-plate 2.0 was cut to form an L-plate and placed on the second and third MTs. The plate was first secured to the distal fragments, allowing the plate to be used as a reduction aid. The position of the plates and overall reduction were aligned and then screws were inserted proximally, bridging the comminuted area. The fourth MT alignment improved when the third MT was plated, as a result of indirect reduction. The intact intermetatarsal ligament allowed the fourth MT to be treated in a closed manner (**Fig 7.6-8** and **Fig 7.6-9**).

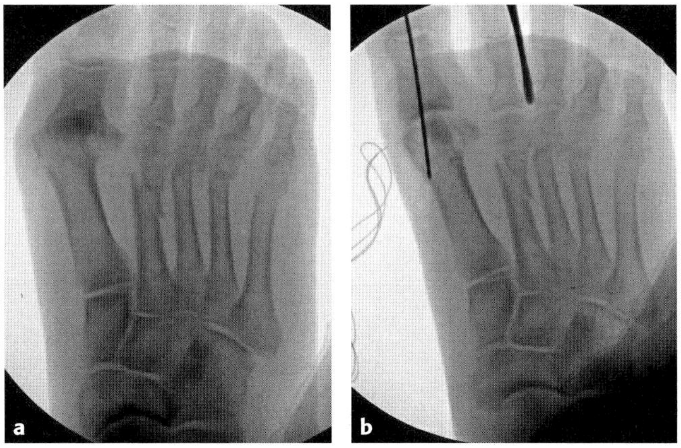

Fig 7.6-8a–b Intraoperative C-arm images.
a AP view demonstrating the dislocated first MTP joint as well as fractures of the second, third, and fourth MT necks. The second has extensive comminution.
b AP view showing the first MTP joint has been reduced and stabilized with a K-wire. A small (Freer) elevator is used in percutaneous fashion to aid in reduction of the second MT head.

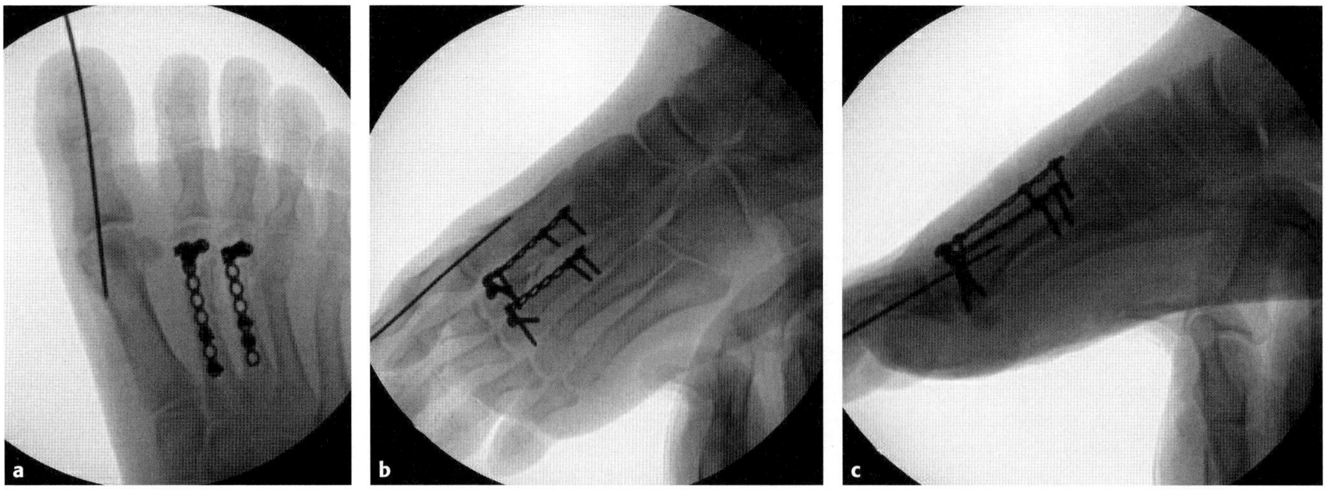

Fig 7.6-9a–c Final intraoperative C-arm images demonstrating anatomical alignment with plate fixation of the second and third MTs. The fourth MT was in acceptable alignment so no fixation was necessary.
a AP view.
b Oblique view.
c Lateral view.

5 Pitfalls and complications

Pitfalls

Inadequate reduction or malunion

It is important to restore the alignment of the foot and the relation of the MTs to one another. Ensuring the correct sagittal alignment prevents transverse metatarsalgia of the adjacent areas. While length is important, it is most important to correct the sagittal position.

Inadequate distal fixation

Fixation in the MT head can be difficult to obtain due to its small size and poor bone quality. Using a plate with two (locking) screws inserted into the head can improve fixation. It is important to ensure that the position of the screw is correct at the first attempt to prevent drilling multiple holes.

Complications

- Wound healing complications, such as delayed healing or contraction of the scar
- Stiffness of MTP joints
- Chronic regional pain syndrome
- Injury to the branches of the deep or superficial peroneal nerve
- Malunion
- Nonunion
- Transfer metatarsalgia
- Irritation from metalwork

6 Alternative techniques

Simple MT neck fractures may alternatively be treated with antegrade or retrograde K-wire fixation. If the fracture is too comminuted or too distal, or the condition of the soft tissues does not allow open reduction and fixation, K-wires can be used as definitive fixation restoring the alignment of the MTP joint (**Fig 7.6-10**). This technique is not reliable in maintaining the MT length and has the possible disadvantage of wires crossing joints resulting in stiffness.

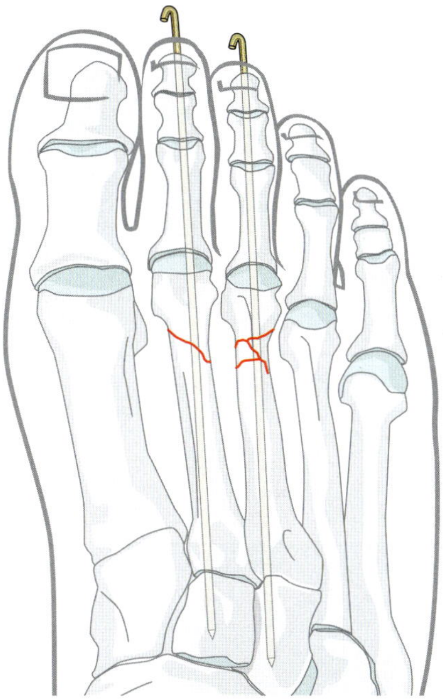

Fig 7.6-10 An alternative method using K-wire fixation. The K-wires can be inserted percutaneously. Proximally they could enter the cuneiforms or exit metatarsal shafts for better stability.

Ideally, K-wire fixation should be performed percutaneously. With the antegrade technique, the K-wire is introduced from the MT base and the tip bent to increase stability (see chapter 7.5). With the retrograde technique, the K-wire is introduced from plantar through the head of the MT (rarely through the base of the corresponding toe and MTP joint to avoid dorsal angulation of the MT and clawing of the toe) (**Fig 7.6-11a–b**). Small incisions can be made to assist with reduction. The wires are removed when union is achieved, typically at 6 weeks postoperatively (**Fig 7.6-11c–e**).

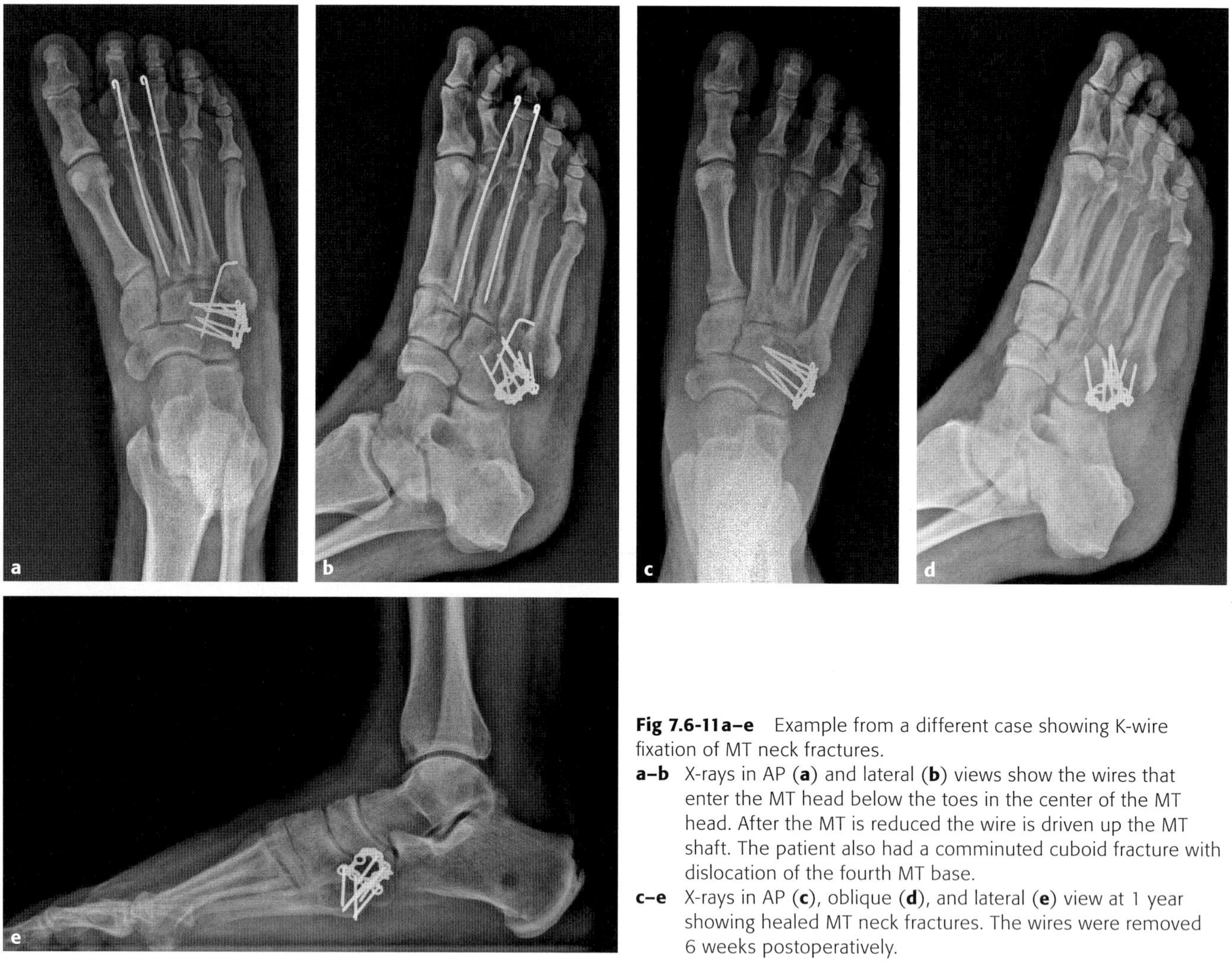

Fig 7.6-11a–e Example from a different case showing K-wire fixation of MT neck fractures.

a–b X-rays in AP (**a**) and lateral (**b**) views show the wires that enter the MT head below the toes in the center of the MT head. After the MT is reduced the wire is driven up the MT shaft. The patient also had a comminuted cuboid fracture with dislocation of the fourth MT base.

c–e X-rays in AP (**c**), oblique (**d**), and lateral (**e**) view at 1 year showing healed MT neck fractures. The wires were removed 6 weeks postoperatively.

7 Postoperative management and rehabilitation

The foot is dressed in bulky bandages and a heel weight-bearing shoe or controlled-ankle-motion boot, which is worn for 6 weeks. If the surgeon believes that the fixation and bone quality allow it, the patient can walk, heel weight-bearing, as comfort allows. Elevation of the foot is recommended for the first 2 weeks; subsequent elevations is as per surgeon preference to allow soft-tissue swelling to abate.

Range-of-motion exercises for the lesser MTP joints can start once wound healing is satisfactory, usually around 2 weeks postoperatively, unless there are K-wires crossing the MTP joints that are removed from the dislocated MTP joint at 6 weeks.

X-rays are taken at 6 weeks and the patient can weight-bear at this stage if union is satisfactory.

Implant removal

Plates can be left in situ unless any specific local irritation occurs. K-wires are usually removed at 6 weeks (**Fig 7.6-12**).

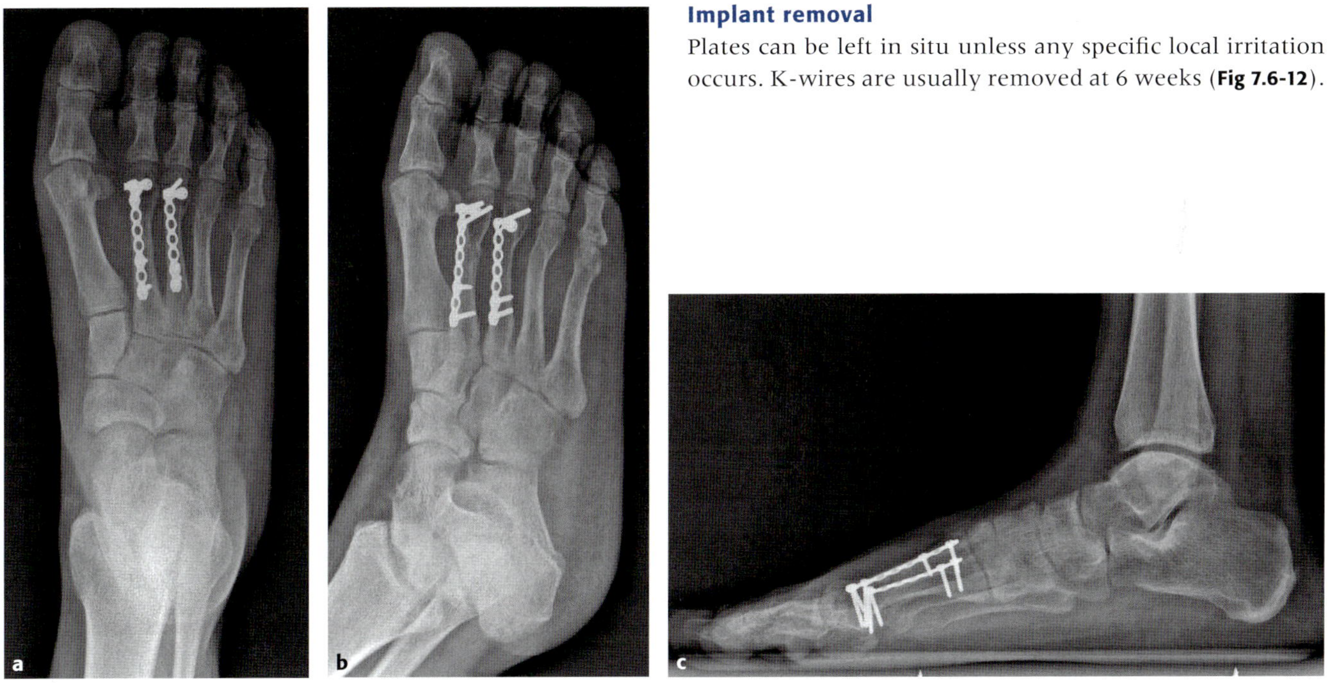

Fig 7.6-12a–c Follow-up x-rays at 1 year showing healed fractures of the MT necks in acceptable alignment. The K-wire was removed from the first MTP joint 6 weeks after surgery. The first MTP joint is reduced and congruent.

a AP view.
b Oblique view.
c Lateral view.

8 Recommended reading

Clements JR, Schopf R. Advances in forefoot trauma. *Clin Podiatr Med Surg.* 2013 Jul;30(3):435–444.

Kim HN, Park YJ, Kim GL, et al. Closed antegrade intramedullary pinning for reduction and fixation of metatarsal fractures. *J Foot Ankle Surg.* 2012 Jul–Aug;51(4):445–449.

Petrisor BA, Ekrol I, Court-Brown C. The epidemiology of metatarsal fractures. *Foot Ankle Int.* 2006 Mar;27(3):172–174.

Rammelt S, Heineck J, Zwipp H. Metatarsal fractures. *Injury.* 2004 Sep;35 Suppl 2:Sb77-86.

Sánchez Alepuz E, Vicent Carsi V, Alcantara P, et al. Fractures of the central metatarsal. *Foot Ankle Int.* 1996 Apr;17(4):200–203.

Shereff MJ. Fractures of the forefoot. *Instr Course Lect.* 1990;39:133–140.

7.7 Multiple metatarsal shaft fractures

Sampat Dumbre Patil, Mandeep S Dhillon, Michael Swords

1 Case description

A 24-year-old man fell from a motorcycle and sustained an injury of his right foot. The injury was closed with intact soft tissues, with no associated injuries. He was taken to a local hospital where x-rays were taken and a well-padded below-knee splint was placed. The patient was subsequently referred to the hospital for further management.

The injury was reevaluated clinically and radiologically on day 2 after injury; there was significant soft-tissue swelling in the foot. X-rays of the right foot in AP, oblique, and lateral views showed fractures of the second and third metatarsal (MT) shafts and the fourth MT neck (**Fig 7.7-1**).

The below-knee splint was left in place for 3 more days, with the leg elevated to heart level, and the patient was prepared for subsequent surgery to be performed as an outpatient. Surgery (open reduction and internal fixation) was performed 5 days after the injury.

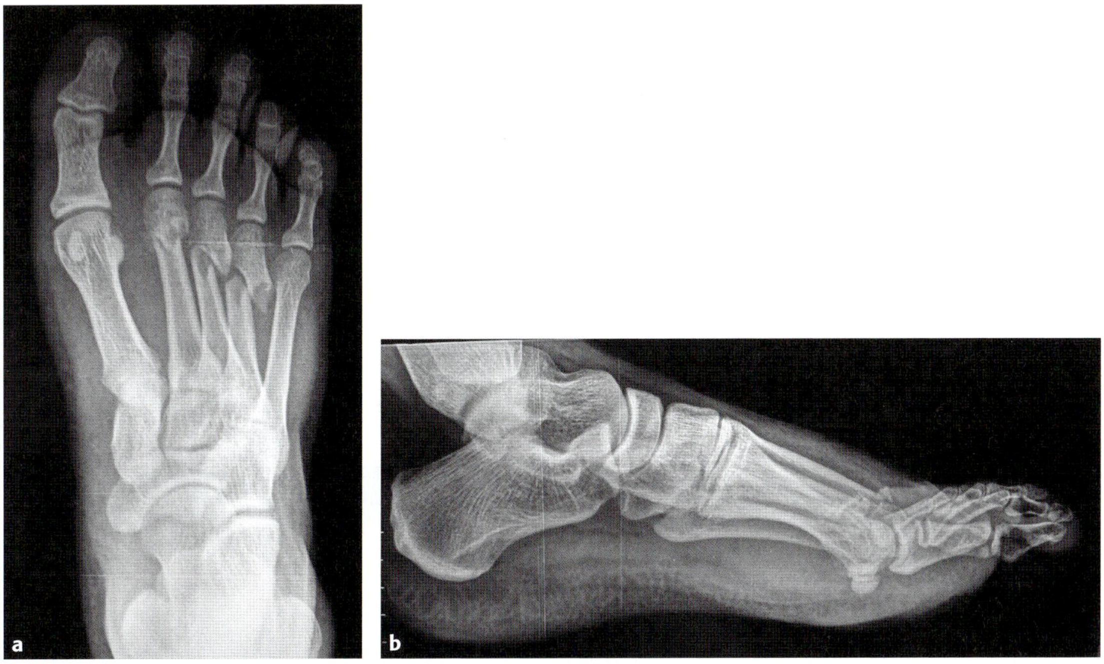

Fig 7.7-1a–b X-rays of the right foot showing fractures of the third and fourth MT shaft and of the second MT neck.
a AP view.
b Lateral view.

2 Preoperative planning

Indications for surgery

Surgical stabilization was indicated due to the presence of multiple, significantly displaced MT fractures. For fractures of the distal shaft and MT neck, closed reduction and intramedullary wire fixation of the MTs was planned.

Treatment options

X-ray assessment of the medullary canal of all MTs was done and it was deemed satisfactory for intramedullary fixation with 1.8 mm or 2 mm wires. For this patient, the fourth MT was reduced and fixed first, as it was thought that the reduction of the fourth MT shaft would achieve appropriate length, which in turn would assist the reduction of the shaft of the third and the neck of the second MTs (**Fig 7.7-2**). A single dorsal approach for the third and fourth MTs was planned with a separate one for the second MT.

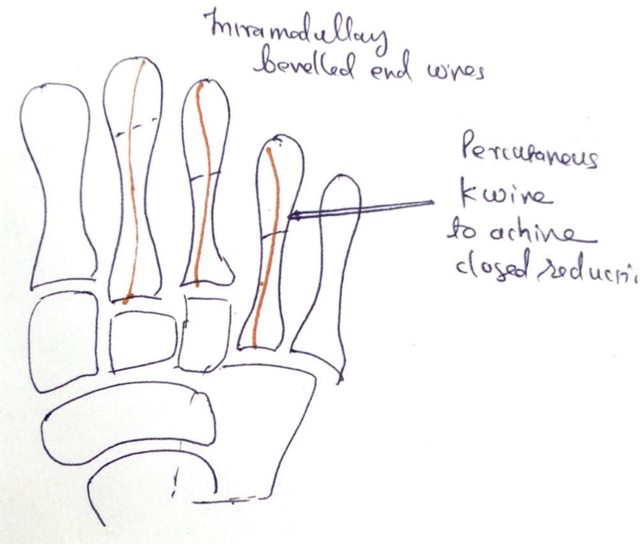

Fig 7.7-2 Preoperative plan.

3 Operating room setup

Patient positioning	• Supine with a sand bag under the right buttock (injured side) to keep the lower limb slightly internally rotated.
Anesthesia options	• Spinal (general, peripheral nerve block)
C-arm location	• Positioned on patient's contralateral side while the surgeon operates from the affected side.
Tourniquet	• Applied to the mid-thigh • Inflate if needed

For illustrations and overview of anesthetic considerations, see chapter 1.

Equipment

- Two T-handles to mount the wires
- 1.8 mm K-wires
- Plier and wire cutter

4 Surgical procedure

Two dorsal incisions are planned: the first for the entry point of the third and fourth MTs, and the second as entry point for the second MT (**Fig 7.7-3**). The first entry point is identified using the C-arm, with the 1.8 mm K-wire having sharp, pointed ends mounted on a T-handle used to mark this entry point (**Fig 7.7-4a**). The beveled, blunt-ended 1.8 mm K-wire is mounted on a T-handle and bent at two places, which will aid subsequent fracture manipulation and reduction (**Fig 7.7-4b**).

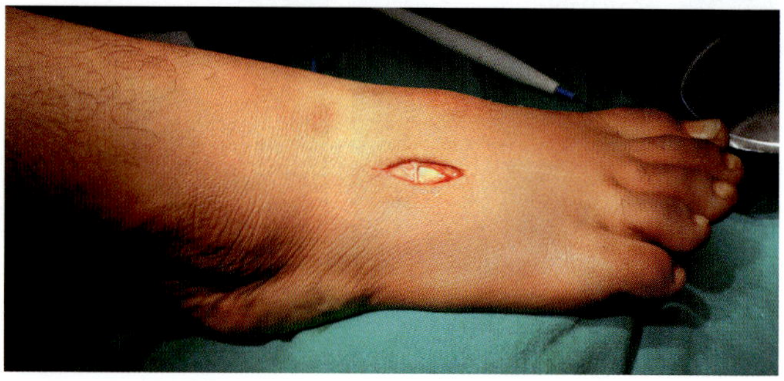

Fig 7.7-3 Dorsal incision for the entry point of the fourth and third MT fractures.

This bent wire is then passed antegrade into the medullary canal through the entry point previously created at the base of the fourth MT. Closed reduction is performed with longitudinal traction to the toes, while percutaneously manipulating the shaft with a separate K-wire mounted on another T-handle. Under C-arm guidance the bent and beveled 1.8 mm wire is now passed into the distal fragment, and the bent tip rotated to improve the reduction (**Fig 7.7-4b–e**).

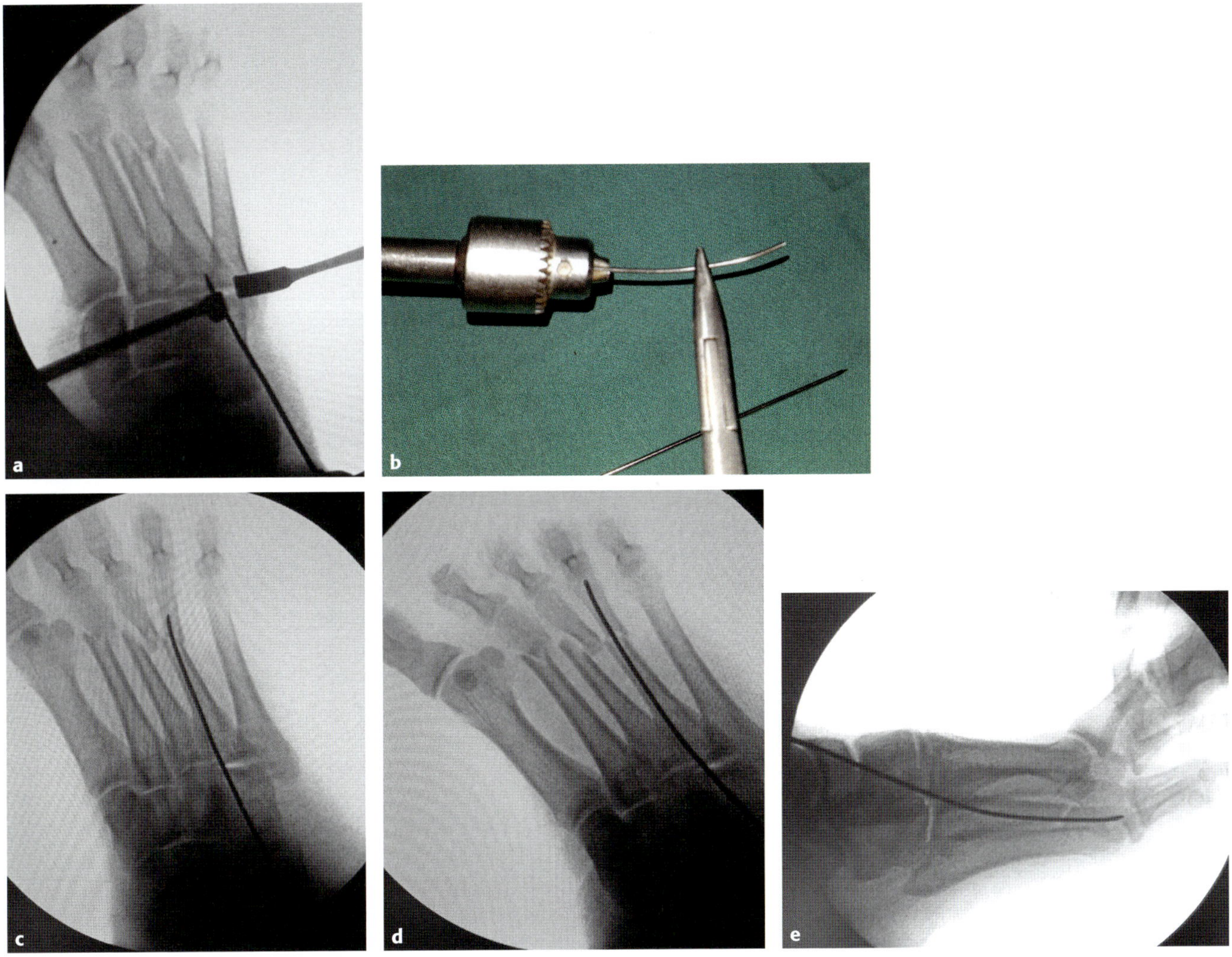

Fig 7.7-4a–c Steps in fixation of the fourth MT fracture.
a The entry point is identified.
b Bending the wire prior to insertion.
c K-wire in the proximal fragment.
d–e K-wire in the distal fragment after the reduction.

It is better to fix the least comminuted MT first, as this helps to restore length (of the fourth MT in this case), and helps indirectly to bring the other MTs out to length.

The same procedure is repeated on the third MT, using the same incision.

The second MT is approached through a separate incision at the base of the second MT, and the same procedure of intramedullary fixation is repeated (**Fig 7.7-5**).

All reductions are checked in AP, oblique, and lateral C-arm views (**Fig 7.7-6**).

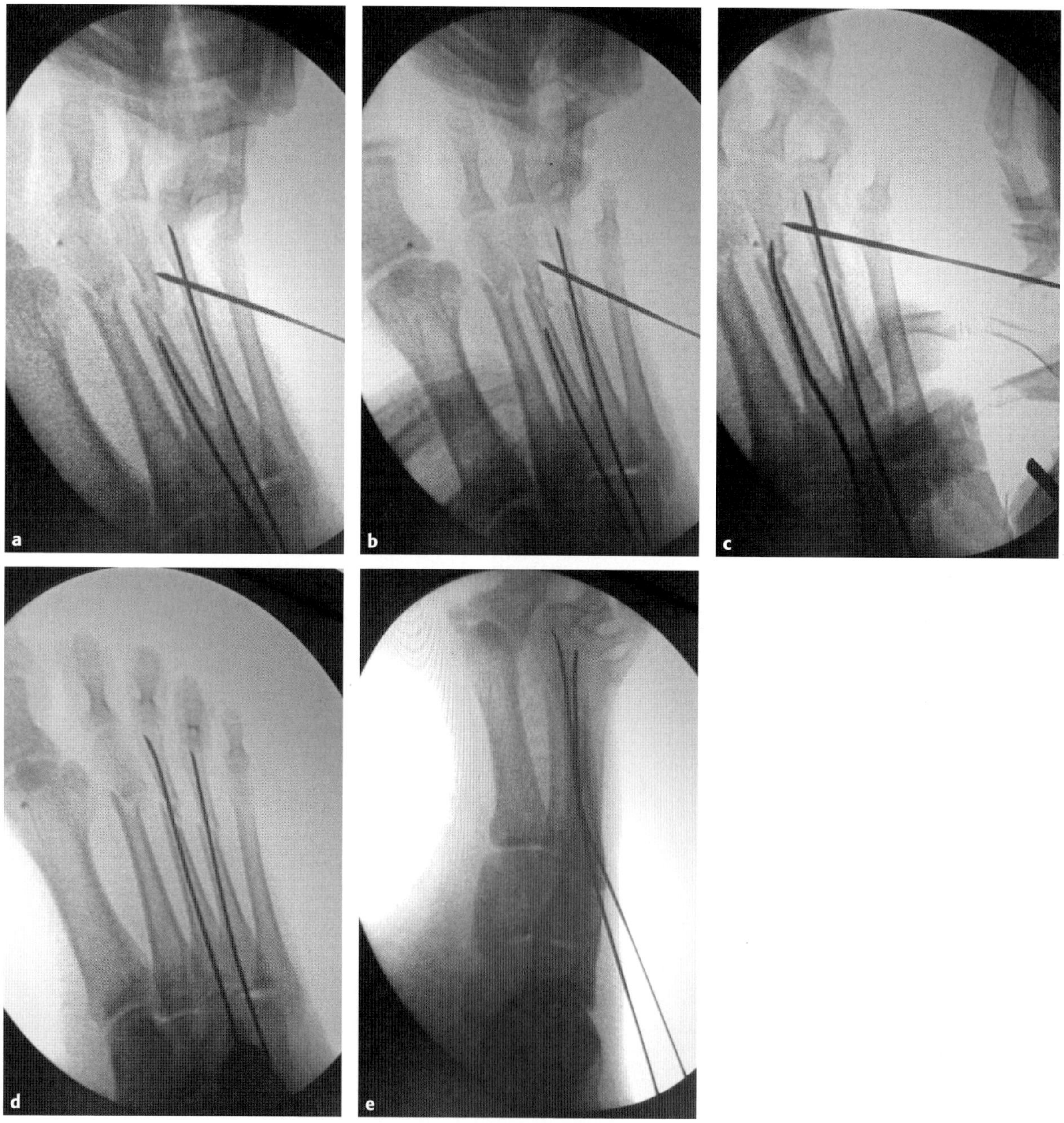

Fig 7.7-5a–e Steps in fixation of the third MT fracture. Note manipulation of the distal fragment with a separate percutaneous K-wire mounted on a T-handle (**a–b**).

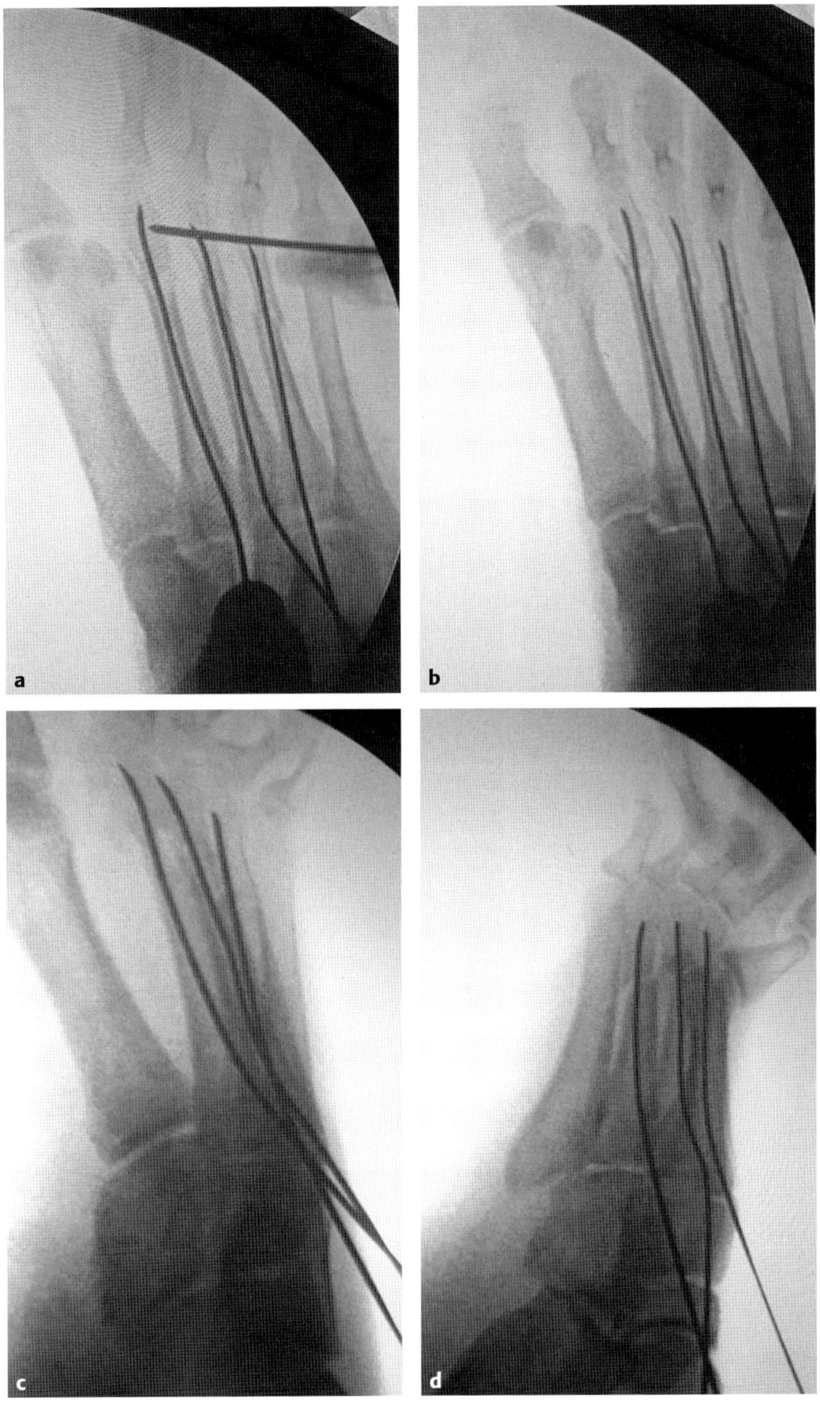

Fig 7.7-6a–d Steps in the fixation of the second MT fracture. The reduced fractures are shown with K-wires in place. The long ends are then cut off and bent over to avoid extensor tendon irritation.

The distal bent tips of the wires are rotated in such a manner that they help to obtain the closed reduction and fine tune if inadequate. The proximal ends of the wires are bent and cut flush to the bone (**Fig 7.7-7**). Care should be taken to avoid irritating extensor tendons with the wires.

Hemostasis is confirmed, and the wound is closed. A below-knee splint is applied, or a controlled-ankle-motion walking boot can be applied.

Postoperative x-rays should reconfirm a satisfactory reduction and alignment. The normal cascade of the length of MTs from first to fifth was restored (**Fig 7.7-8**).

5 Pitfalls and complications

Pitfalls

Small medullary canals of the MTs may not allow intramedullary wire insertion. Hence the medullary canal should be assessed preoperatively, and alternative method of fixation should be readily available.

Complications

- Extensor tendon irritation due to the cut proximal ends of the wires or if plates are used
- Loss of length of the MT in the presence of comminution
- Injury to cutaneous nerves at the entry point incisions

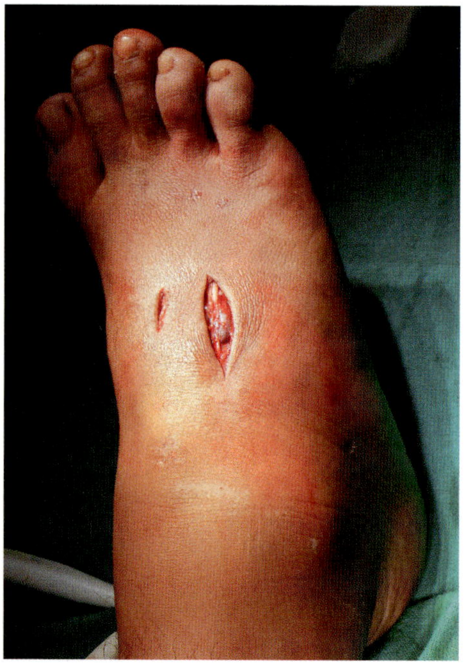

Fig 7.7-7 Dorsal incisions after cutting the wires flush.

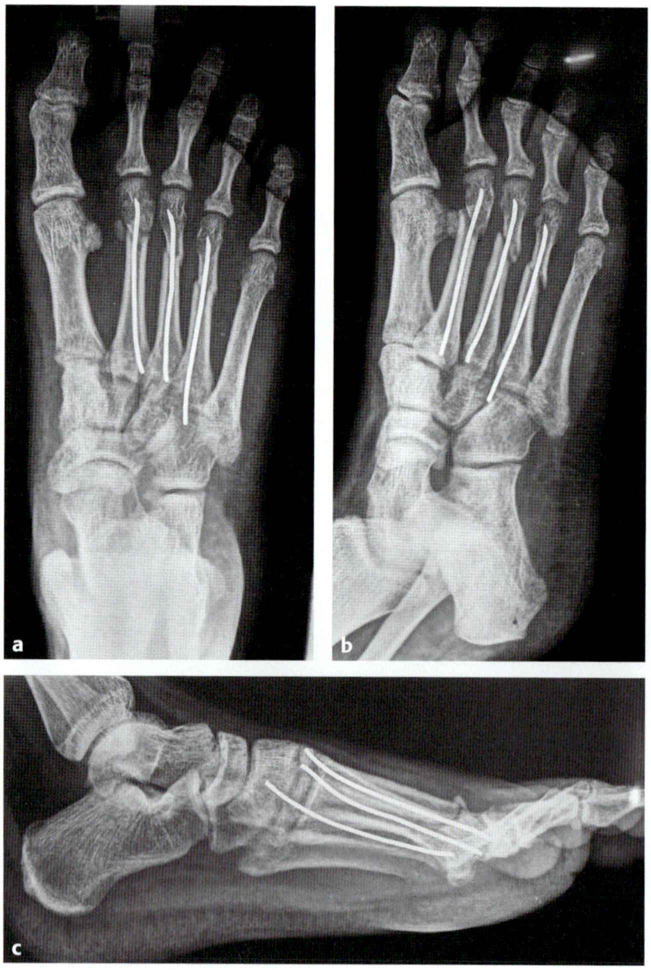

Fig 7.7-8a–c Postoperative x-rays of the right foot showing the fixation.
a AP view.
b Oblique view.
c Lateral view.

6 Alternative techniques

Most isolated MT fractures can be treated without surgery. Surgery is indicated in cases with more than 10° of angulation or 3 mm of displacement in the sagittal plane. Nonoperative treatment in these cases may result in metatarsalgia from uneven heights of the MT heads.

For the patient in this case, the wires were inserted intramedullary in an antegrade fashion, from the base to the head of the MT.

The intramedullary K-wire fixation can also be done through a retrograde approach. The wire is introduced from the plantar aspect of the head of the MT by extending the metatarsophalangeal (MTP) joint. The K-wire is passed across the fracture site towards the base, and the reduction needs to be checked with the C-arm.

Plate fixation

Metatarsal shaft fractures can also be managed surgically by open reduction and internal fixation with plates. Fractures of the second to fourth MT shafts (**Fig 7.7-9a–c**) can be exposed through a dorsal incision, or multiple incisions, depending on fracture geometry. Fractures are reduced and plated using minifragment plates and screws (low profile) to avoid extensor tendon irritation (**Fig 7.7-9d–f**). Follow-up x-rays show excellent healing and a normal foot (**Fig 7.7-9g–i**).

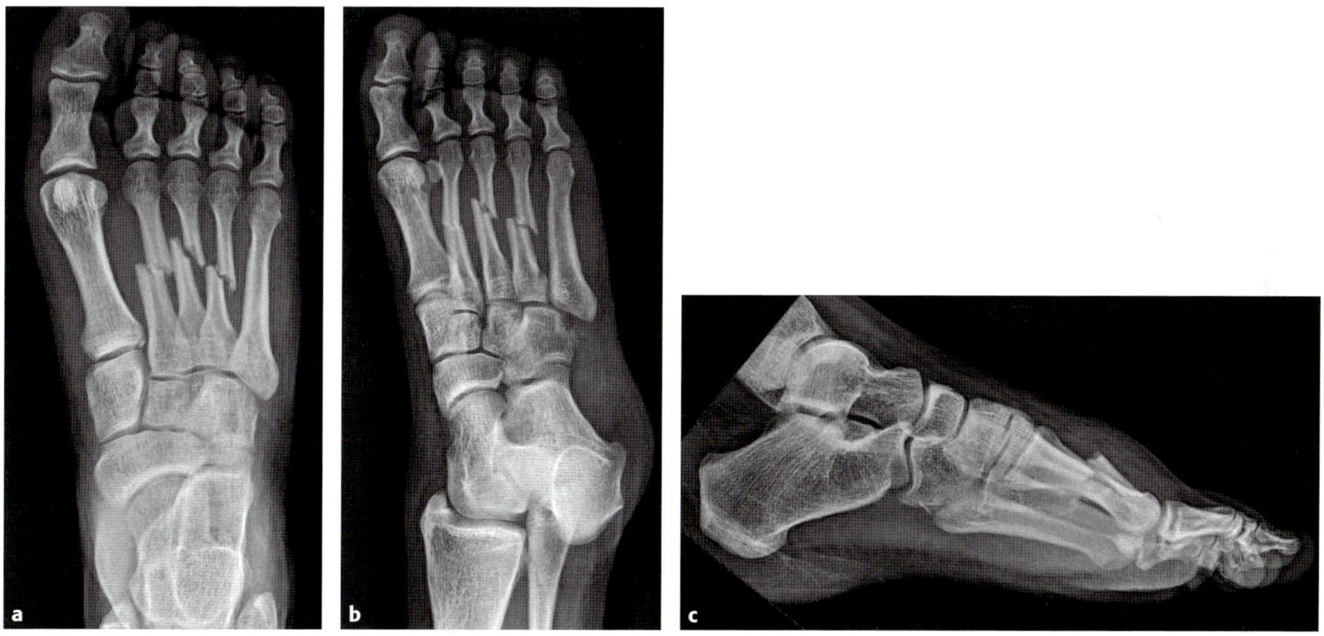

Fig 7.7-9a–i Example from a different case demonstrating plate fixation.
a–c X-rays in AP (**a**), oblique (**b**), and lateral (**c**) views showing fractures of the second to fourth MT shafts.

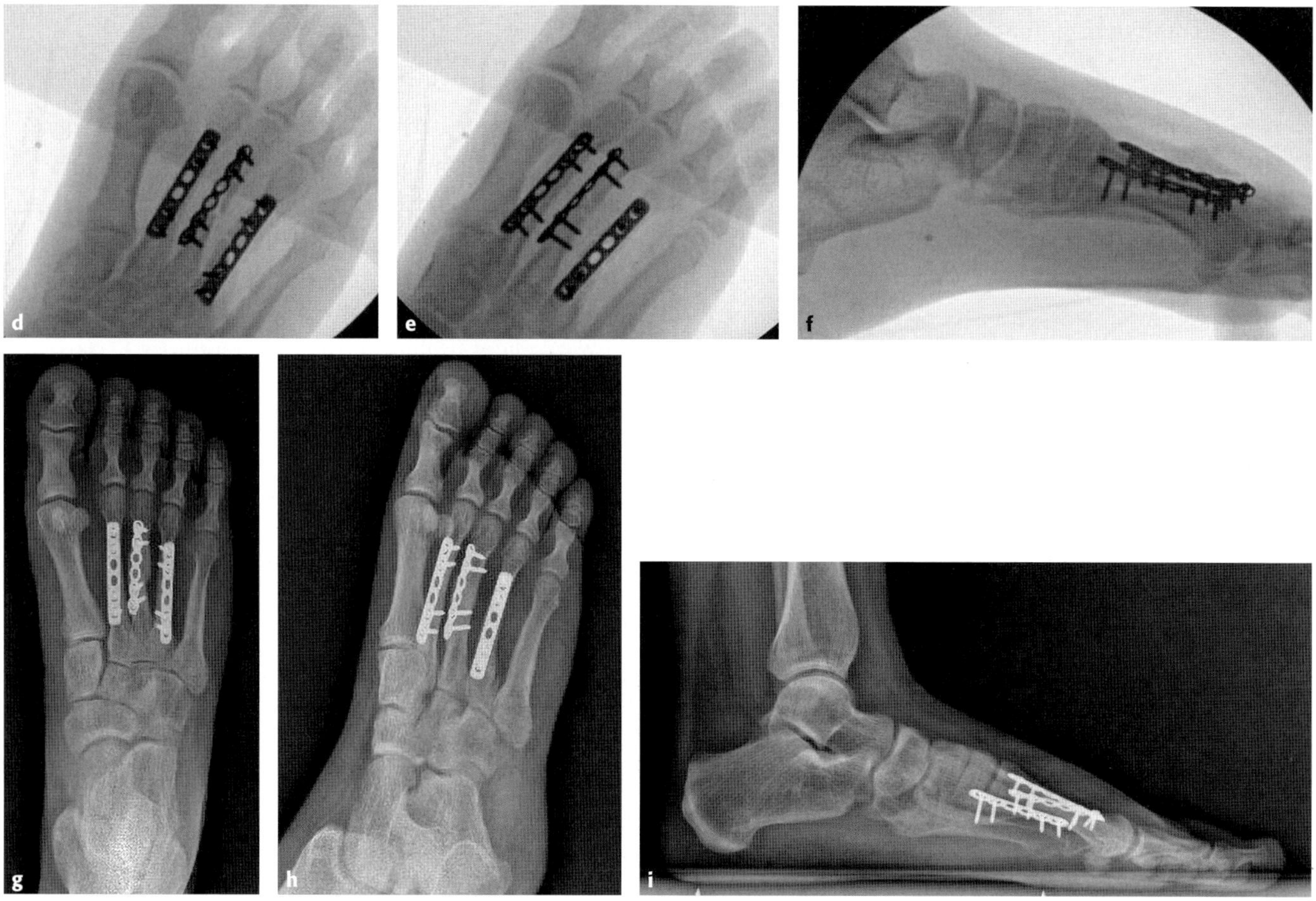

Fig 7.7-9a–i (cont) Example from a different case demonstrating plate fixation.
d–f Fractures are reduced and plated using small fragment plates and screws
g–i Follow-up x-rays show excellent healing and a normal foot.

7 Postoperative management and rehabilitation

Short-leg splint of any kind (3-sided ["AO"] splint, plaster-of-Paris) is used for 4 weeks postoperatively; the sutures are removed after 3 weeks. Partial weight bearing can be started after 6 weeks with a controlled-ankle-motion boot. Bone healing is checked every month with x-rays. In this case bony union was achieved in 3.5 months (**Fig 7.7-10**) and the patient was able to return to his duties and sporting activities.

Implant removal

Implant removal is not routinely recommended. If the proximal end of the wire backs out and causes irritation to the skin or the extensor tendon, then wire removal should be done. Plates should be removed if they irritate the extensor tendons.

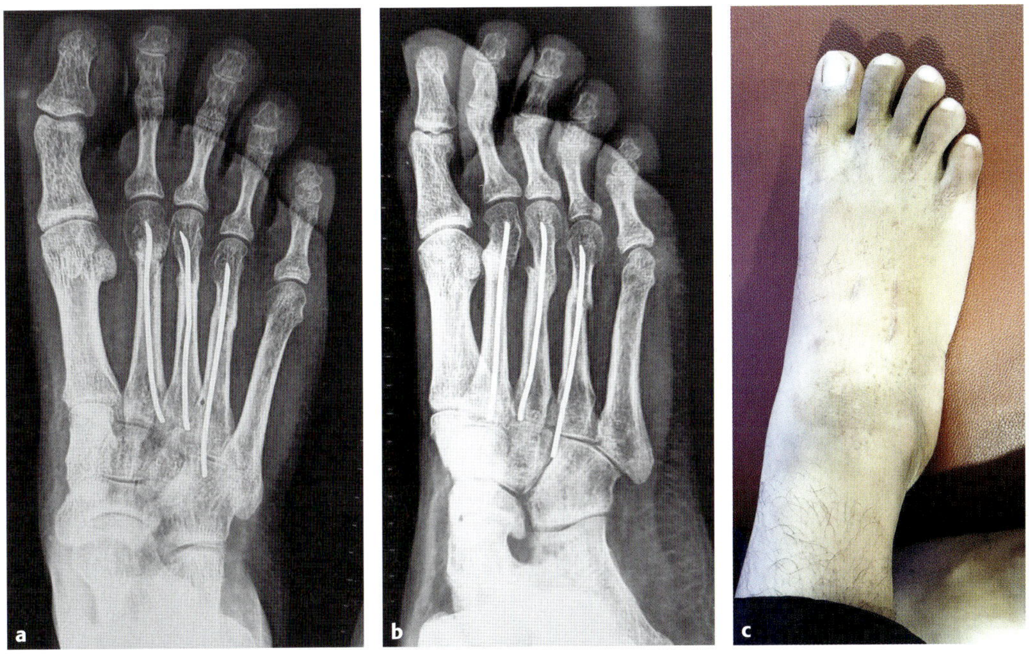

Fig 7.7-10a–c Follow-up x-rays showing bony union at 3.5 months.

8 Recommended reading

Baumfeld D, Macedo BD, Nery C, et al. Anterograde percutaneous treatment of lesser metatarsal fractures: technical description and clinical results. *Rev Bras Orthop.* 2012;47(6):760–764.

Court-Brown CM, Caesar B. Epidemiology of adult fractures: a review. *Injury.* 2006 Aug;37(8):691–697.

Petrisor BA, Ekrol I, Court-Brown C. The epidemiology of metatarsal fractures. *Foot Ankle Int.* 2006 Mar;27(3):172–174.

Rammelt S, Heineck J, Zwipp H. Metatarsal fractures. *Injury.* 2004 Sep;35 Suppl 2:Sb77–86.

Sánchez Alepuz E, Vicent Carsi V, Alcántara P, et al. Fractures of the central metatarsal. *Foot Ankle Int.* 1996 Apr;17(4):200–203.

7.8 Proximal central metatarsal base fracture with joint involvement

Arun Aneja, Steven J Lawrence

1 Case description

A 17-year-old woman was involved in a high-energy motor vehicle collision as a restrained passenger. The vehicle struck a telephone pole. She was transported to the trauma center. She sustained multiple orthopedic injuries, including: multiple foot fractures, ipsilateral forearm, tibial, and ankle fractures, and a contralateral femoral fracture. All injuries were closed. Urgent stabilization of her long-bone injuries was performed.

Her left foot injury, which included comminuted fractures of the first to third metatarsal (MT) bases (**Fig 7.8-1**), was initially reduced and splinted. Due to swelling of the soft tissues, definitive fixation was delayed.

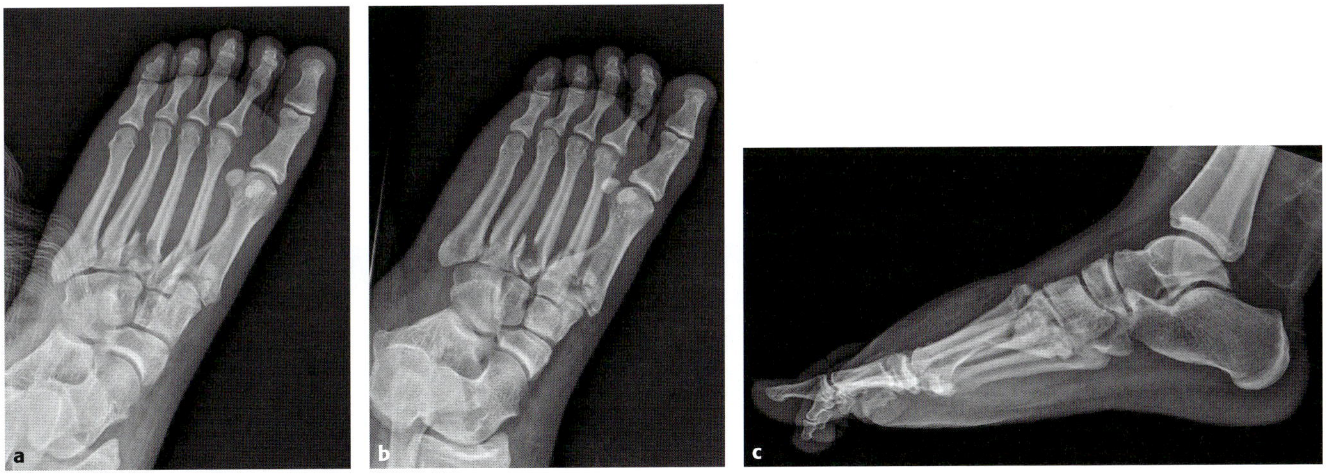

Fig 7.8-1a–c Preoperative x-rays of the foot.
a Fractures of the first to third MT bases (AP view).
b Intraarticular involvement of the third MT (oblique view).
c Dorsal step-off of the Lisfranc joint complex (lateral view).

2 Preoperative planning

The anatomy of the midfoot is complex. Isolated traumatic injury to the central MT bases is uncommon and occurs with direct dorsal crush injuries. Multiple MT base fractures usually occur following indirect trauma. Intraarticular MT base fractures are commonly associated with concomitant injuries to chondral and ligamentous elements resulting in a complex Lisfranc fracture-dislocation. Management of the triad of injury (ligamentous, chondral, and osseous) is a challenging task.

Indications for surgery

- Open fractures
- Intraarticular MT base fractures with significant displacement
- Fractures which result in instability of the midfoot.

Considerations for surgery

Advanced imaging (eg, computed tomographic [CT] scan or magnetic resonance imaging [MRI]) can be useful to determine specific injury characteristics. Computed tomography demonstrates fracture displacement, comminution, and subtle joint incongruity, as well as subtle avulsion fractures of the plantar cuneiforms (**Fig 7.8-2**). Lisfranc ligament integrity and chondral impaction injury can be best captured by MRI. Stress radiographic studies under the C-arm or weight-bearing x-rays are useful to determine if ligamentous disruption is present.

A preoperative plan must be formulated to manage the fractures and joint injuries (**Fig 7.8-3**). With extensive fracture comminution and adjacent joint instability, spanning the injury with dorsal bridge plating of the fracture and joint is a viable treatment option. Furthermore, this technique limits soft-tissue dissection to preserve vascularity of the fracture fragments with use of a single implant. If no Lisfranc injury is present, start with the first MT base fracture and proceed laterally. For simple fractures, consider anatomical reduction with primary bone healing. For comminuted fractures, consider relative stability with bridge plating.

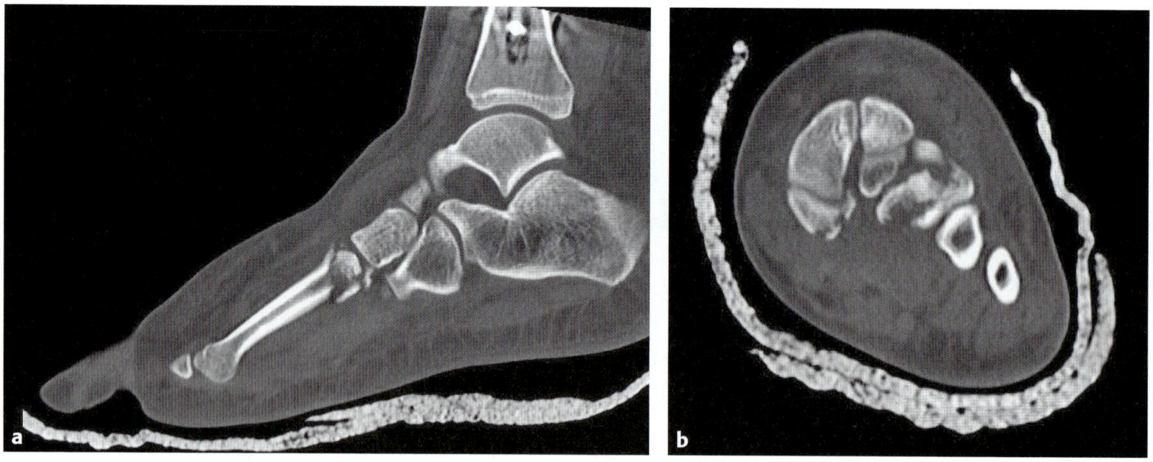

Fig 7.8-2a–b Preoperative CT scan.
a Sagittal cut of the third MT showing comminution and articular disruption of the base.
b Coronal cut of the comminuted third MT base fracture.

3 Operating room setup

Patient positioning	• Supine with a bump under the ipsilateral buttock so that the patella points straight upward
Anesthesia options	• General anesthesia is generally preferred. • Other forms of anesthesia may be dictated by associated injuries or medical comorbidities.
C-arm location	• The C-arm is positioned at the side of the operative table opposite to the involved extremity.
Tourniquet	• A thigh tourniquet is applied.
Tips	• Place the ipsilateral knee in flexion over a tibial triangle or foam wedge to facilitate lateral C-arm imaging of the foot. This also assists in positioning the foot for dorsal plantar views.

For illustrations and overview of anesthetic considerations, see chapter 1.

Equipment

- K-wires
- Minifragment screws, low profile small fragment plates and screws
- Dental scaler
- Point-to-point reduction (Weber) clamps
- Small distraction device—may be necessary for restoration of length

4 Surgical procedure

The patient had injuries of the first to third MTs. Emphasis will be on the process of the third MT injury stabilization.

Approach

The surgical incision is centered over the first and second tarsometatarsal (TMT) joint. This can be confirmed under the C-arm to mark the site of incision (**Fig 7.8-4**). The involved leg is elevated, exsanguinated, and the tourniquet is inflated.

After skin incision, careful dissection is undertaken to the level of extensor hallucis longus (EHL) tendon with full-thickness soft-tissue flaps. The EHL tendon sheath is incised dorsally and retracted medially. The neurovascular bundle is identified and protected throughout the procedure. The neurovascular bundle is mobilized and can be retracted medially or laterally based on the MT joint addressed. The floor of the tendon sheath is then incised and subperiosteal dissection is undertaken medially to the medial margin of the first TMT joint, and laterally to the lateral aspect of the third TMT joint, while protecting and mobilizing the neurovascular bundle as needed.

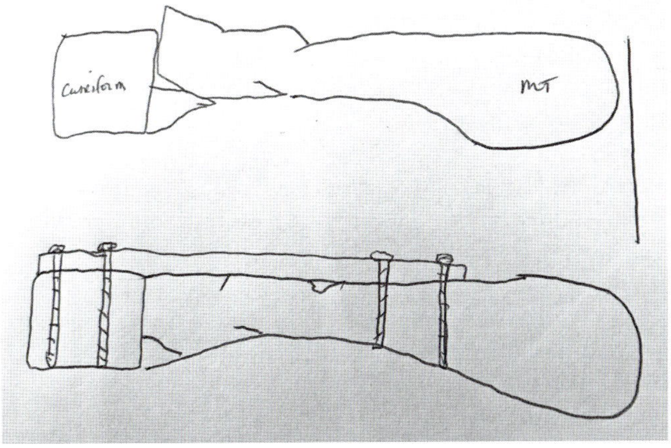

Fig 7.8-3 Preoperative plan showing the bridge plating technique for second and third MT fractures. The plating bridges the fracture and the tarsometatarsal joints.

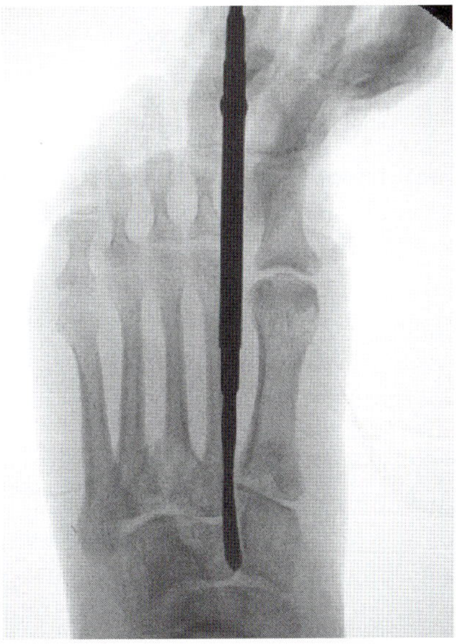

Fig 7.8-4 Intraoperative planning of surgical incision with the C-arm.

Fixation of first metatarsal fracture-dislocation

After exposure, provisional reduction of the first MT base fracture-dislocation is performed. The first MT shaft is typically externally rotated relative to the medial cuneiform. Pulling to restore length and internal rotation of the MT shaft reduces the fracture dislocation. A point-to-point reduction (Weber) clamp and provisional K-wires are placed outside the path for dorsal plating. A minifragment plate 2.7 is used as a bridge plate to span the fracture and the first TMT joint (**Fig 7.8-5a**). The plate is appropriately contoured to prevent plantar gapping of the fracture. Screws of appropriate size are applied proximally and distally to create a friction interface between the plate and the bone. Once the first TMT joint is reduced, reduction of the remaining midfoot joints becomes easier.

Fixation of the second metatarsal

Next, the extraarticular second MT base fracture is addressed. In the case presented, it consisted of a short metaphyseal segment and a simple transverse fracture line, so anatomical reduction with absolute stability under direct fracture visualization was chosen.

The fracture is reduced and provisionally stabilized with K-wires outside the path of definitive plate placement. Next, a minifragment plate 2.4 is contoured and applied in compression mode to achieve primary bone healing of this simple fracture pattern (**Fig 7.8-5b**). Intraoperative imaging is performed with a C-arm to ensure that the medial border of the middle cuneiform is aligned with the medial aspect of the second MT.

Fixation of the third metatarsal

Finally, the third TMT and the third MT base fractures are exposed. For this patient, given the extensive comminution with intraarticular involvement, relative fracture stability was achieved with a dorsal bridge plating technique. While reducing the first and second TMT joints and MT bases, the intermetatarsal ligaments provide indirect reduction, if the fourth and fifth TMT joints are not violated. The third TMT joint is reduced and provisionally stabilized with K-wires that are strategically placed away from the planned location of the dorsal plate. An appropriately sized minifragment plate is applied dorsally in bridging fashion (**Fig 7.8-3** and **Figs 7.8-5c–d**). At least two bicortical screws are required to be placed proximal and distal to the zone of comminution. C-arm oblique imaging of the foot should show that the medial aspect of the fourth MT is aligned with the medial aspect of the cuboid.

Final intraoperative C-arm imaging including AP, lateral, and oblique views are scrutinized to assure correct fracture reduction, joint alignment, and hardware position (**Figs 7.8-5c–e**).

Intraoperative stress testing of the midfoot under direct visualization and stress views is recommended after fixation to rule out occult intracuneiform or fourth or fifth TMT instability. The final surgical construct is demonstrated in **Fig 7.8-6**.

5 Pitfalls and complications

Pitfalls

Most MT base fractures, have good healing potential and nonunions are uncommon. However, intraarticular MT base fractures have, by definition, have an associated chondral injury. Posttraumatic TMT arthrosis is not uncommon. Fortunately, the second and third TMT joints have limited sagittal motion compared to the adjacent motion of the first, fourth, and fifth TMT joints. Therefore, joint stability, bone length, alignment, and rotation are essential for normal midfoot function. Lisfranc fracture-dislocation must be ruled out in the presence of multiple MT base fractures.

Severe fracture comminution with bone loss may require bone grafting to prevent a nonunion. With severe comminution, a bridge plating technique can be performed. Indirect reduction minimizes periosteal stripping and restores length, alignment, and rotation. Soft-tissue injury may occur with midfoot surgical repair, especially the dorsalis pedis and the adjacent deep peroneal nerve. They are found just dorsal to the lateral aspect of the second MT base and must be carefully protected. Furthermore, the superficial peroneal nerve is also prone to iatrogenic injury with fixation of the central MT bases.

Persistent pain following initial open reduction and internal fixation due to joint arthrosis or persistent joint instability may be salvaged with a TMT fusion.

Complications

- Malunion or nonunion
- Posttraumatic TMT arthrosis
- Neurovascular injury
- Metatarsophalangeal joint stiffness
- Wound healing delay
- Wound infection

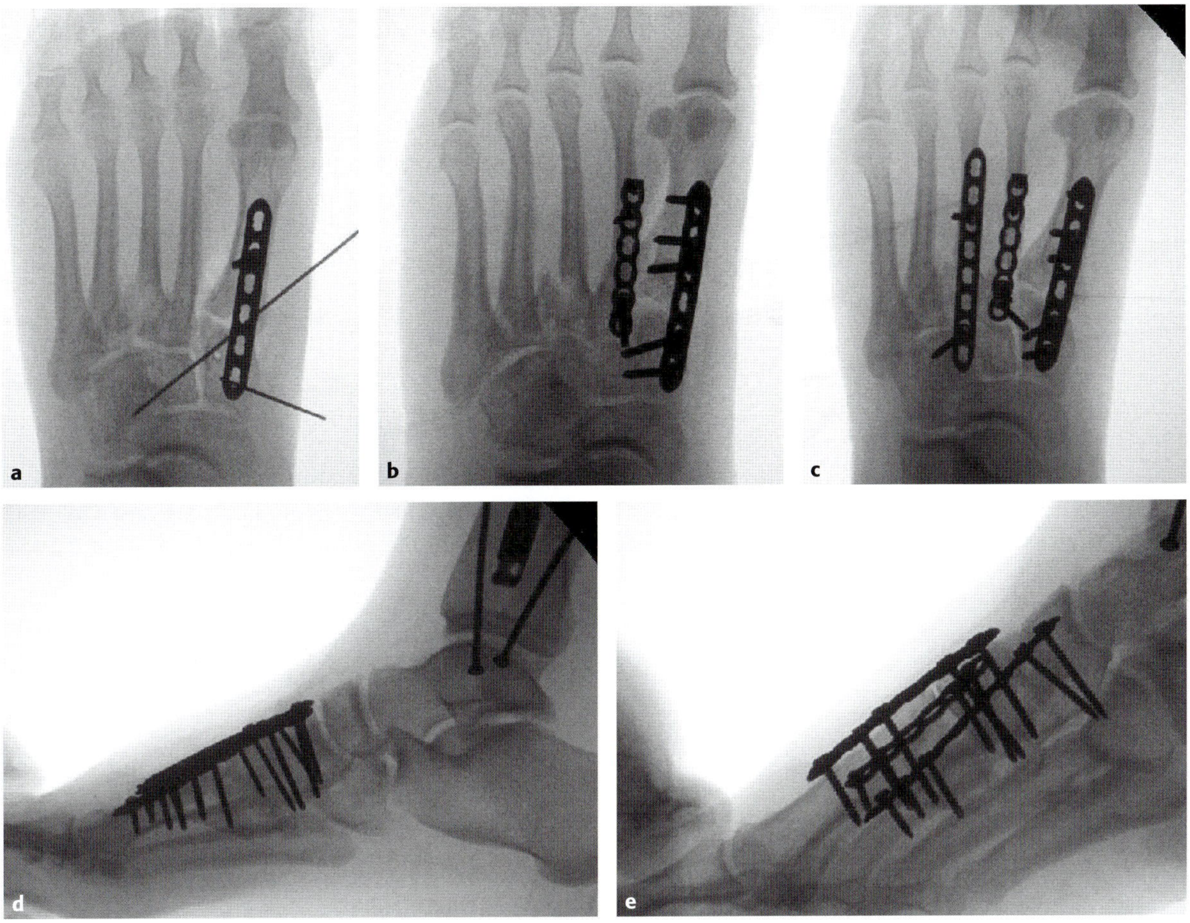

Fig 7.8-5a–e Intraoperative C-arm images of the foot.

a Provisional K-wire fixation of the first MT fracture and subsequent bridge plate fixation of the first MT and first joint (AP view).
b Sequential bridge plate fixation of the second MT (AP view).
c Bridge plate fixation of the third MT and third TMT joint (AP view).
d Final bridge plate construct of the first to third MT bases (lateral view).
e Screw and plate construct outlining the MT bases, and dorsal plate and screw fixation (oblique view).

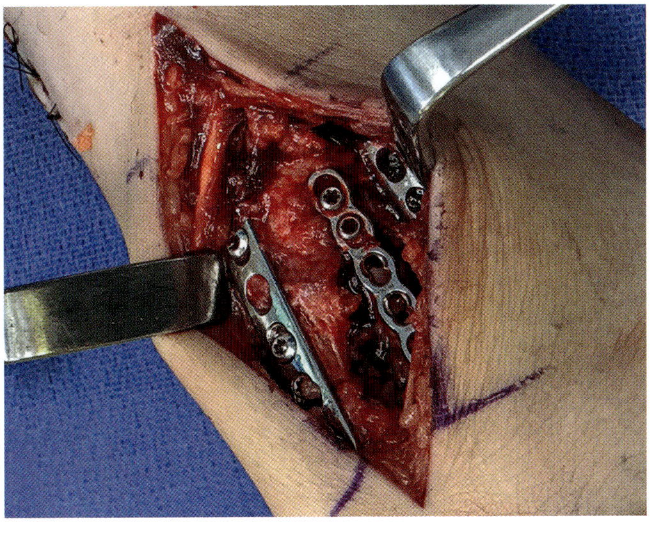

Fig 7.8-6 Intraoperative photograph of surgical exposure and dorsal implants.

6 Alternative techniques

Single, dual, or triple strictly parallel dorsal midfoot incisions can be used based on the number of MTs involved. An appropriate skin bridge is necessary to prevent skin necrosis.

Fracture and joint fixation with K-wires as permanent fixation is discouraged since adequate stability is rarely achieved. The use of mini-external fixation devices may be helpful in provisional fixation in select instances, especially with severe, open injuries with significant bone loss and/or infection.

When severe osteoporosis is present, locking plates can be used. Special dorsal Lisfranc joint plates that span two or three joints may be used in select instances.

Suture buttons have been used to stabilize midfoot ligamentous disruption; however, in the presence of high-energy comminuted fractures, they have limited indications.

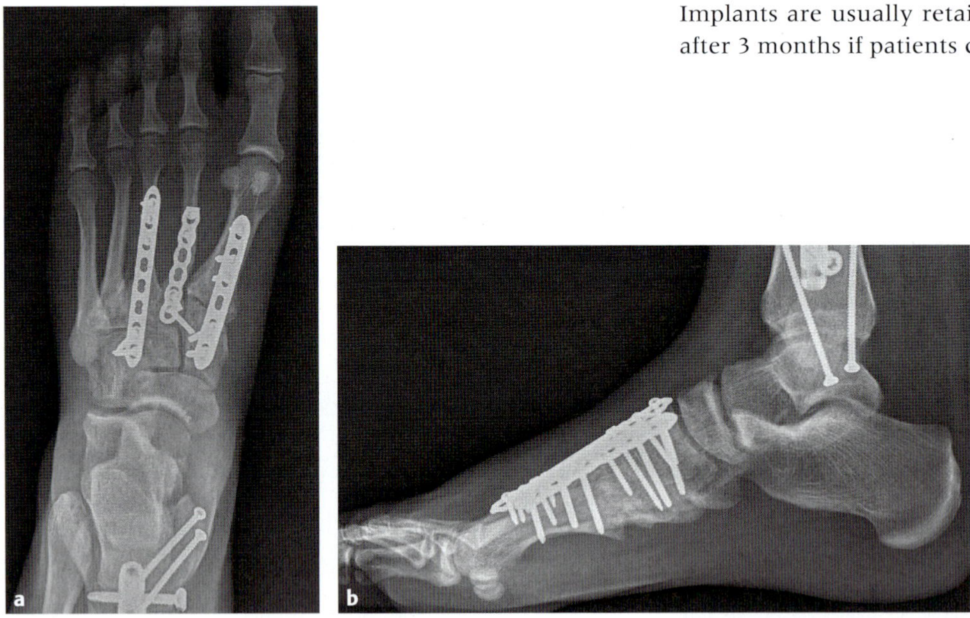

Fig 7.8-7a–b Postoperative x-rays at 2 months.
a Proper alignment and healing (AP view).
b Appropriate alignment (lateral view).

7 Postoperative management and rehabilitation

The foot is immobilized and elevated after surgical intervention to allow the soft tissues to heal following acute injury and surgical intervention. Surgical sutures are removed when the skin incision is appropriately healed, usually in 10–14 days.

Commonly, the patient is placed into a removable boot so that she or he can perform gentle active range-of-motion exercises of the ankle, hindfoot, and forefoot while maintaining nonweight bearing. Massage of the healed incision can assist in desensitization and skin mobility.

X-rays are taken to assess for bone healing and maintenance of the bony architecture of the midfoot (**Fig 7.8-7**). Weight bearing is not permitted until bone healing is documented radiographically, typically at 6–8 weeks after the injury, with resumption of full weight bearing at 3 months.

Implant removal

Implants are usually retained but they may be removed after 3 months if patients complain of painful hardware.

8 Recommended reading

Kestner CJ. Open reduction and fixation of unstable Lisfranc injuries using dorsal plates. *Techniques in Foot & Ankle Surgery.* 2015;14(4):181–187.
Seybold JD, Coetzee JC. Lisfranc injuries: when to observe, fix, or fuse. *Clin Sports Med.* 2015 Oct;34(4):705–723.
Welck MJ, Zinchenko R, Rudge B. Lisfranc injuries. *Injury.* 2015 Apr;46(4):536–541.

7.9 Fifth metatarsal base fracture (zone 1)

Vinod Kumar Panchbhavi

1 Case description

A 60-year-old man twisted his foot over an exposed tree root while walking his dog. He had immediate pain and swelling that improved to some extent with nonoperative management in a hard-soled shoe. However, he continued to experience pain 6 weeks after the injury. The pain limited his ability to walk and engage in day-to-day activities. The pain was localized to the fracture site. Dorsalis pedis pulse and sensation to light touch were intact. He had no other health problems.

Initial x-rays revealed a displaced fracture at the base of the fifth metatarsal (MT) at the distal end of zone 1 (AO/OTA 87.5.1.A) with a minimally displaced large tuberosity fragment (**Fig 7.9-1**). A control x-ray at 6 weeks showed further displacement at the fracture site and no bridging callus (**Fig 7.9-2**).

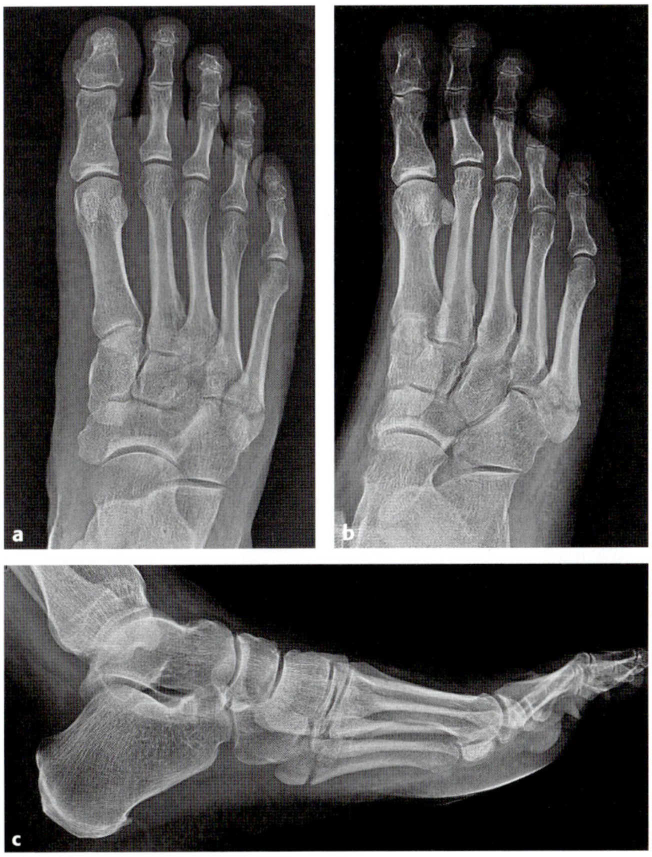

Fig 7.9-1a–c X-rays showing a minimally displaced fracture at the base of the fifth MT tuberosity.
- **a** AP view.
- **b** Oblique view.
- **c** Lateral view.

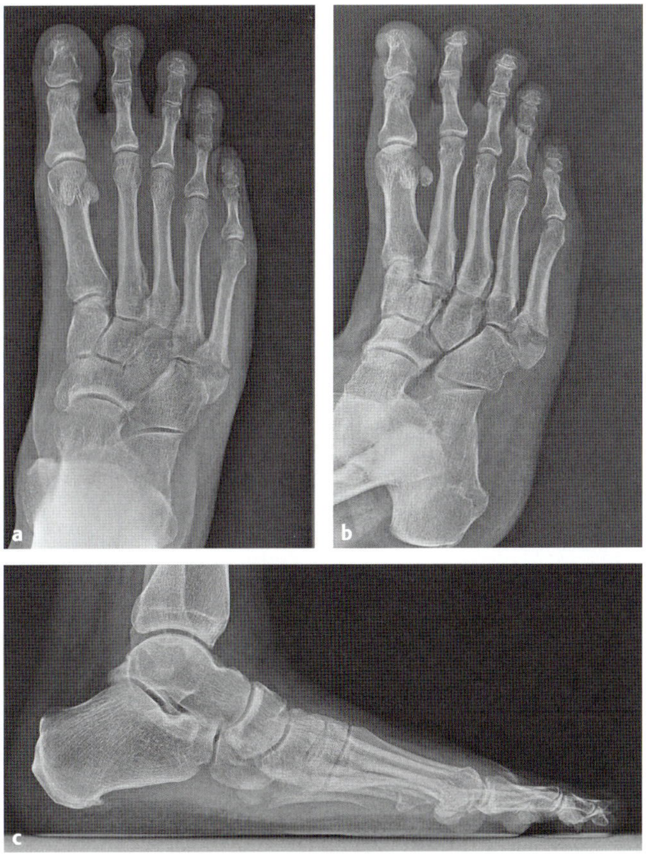

Fig 7.9-2a–c X-rays at a subsequent visit showing further displacement and absence of significant bone bridging at the fracture site.

2 Preoperative planning

Surgical intervention is indicated in a displaced, intraarticular fracture that is symptomatic and interferes with day-to-day activity. Surgical intervention can also be considered in individuals such as athletes who need to return to sport as soon as possible (**Fig 7.9-3**).

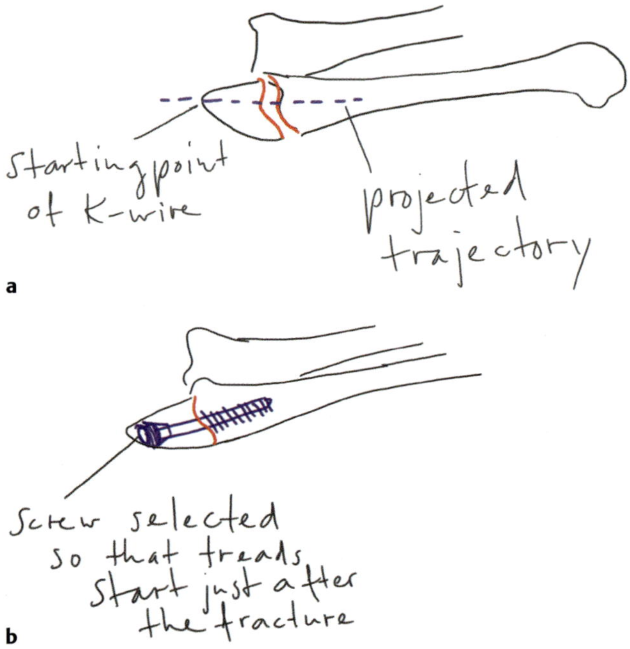

Fig 7.9-3a–b Preoperative planning sketches for the starting point of the K-wire and ideal trajectory.

3 Operating room setup

Patient positioning	• Supine with a bump under the ipsilateral hip to internally rotate the involved extremity. This enables an unhindered axial access to the base of the fifth MT and also allows an oblique view of the foot under C-arm imaging. • A supplemental bump under the chest and shoulder region
Anesthesia options	• Regional anesthesia, either ankle or popliteal block • General anesthesia may be considered in some cases.
C-arm location	• Ipsilateral, C-arm, or mini-C-arm are needed • Placed on the opposite side, perpendicular to the operative table
Tourniquet	• Not generally needed • Can be applied and not inflated

For illustrations and overview of anesthetic considerations, see chapter 1.

Equipment

General instruments:
- #15 scalpel blade, fine-tipped hemostats
- Periosteal elevator
- Curette
- Point-to-point reduction (Weber) clamp
- Screws (usually 3.5–5.0 mm)
- Guide wires

For tension band technique:
- 18-gauge stainless steel cerclage wire
- 1.6 mm K-wires
- Wire tensioner
- Pliers and wire cutters

4 Surgical procedure

The bone landmarks are drawn out with a sterile marker with accurate palpation of the base of the fifth MT and the tip of the fibula. The skin incision is marked. With the help of a radiopaque marker, the location of the fracture is marked out using the C-arm. The incision is along the lateral border of the foot positioned over the fifth MT tuberosity and the fracture, at the junction of the plantar and dorsal skin.

After the skin is incised, further dissection is carried out avoiding the sural nerve and its terminal branches. The interval between the peroneus brevis tendon and the lateral band of the plantar fascia is developed to gain exposure of the proximal end of the fifth MT. The dissection is carried distally to expose the fracture site. The fracture ends are cleaned of any intervening tissue. One end of the point-to-point reduction (Weber) clamp is placed at the tip of the avulsed tuberosity fragment and the other end distally gaining purchase on the shaft of the fifth MT and using the plantar curvature to prevent it from slipping. It may be necessary to make an indentation or a hole with a drill to allow the clamp to gain purchase in the distal fragment.

The fracture is then reduced under direct visualization and C-arm guidance and the reduction held with the clamp. The tip of the guide wire for the cannulated screw is used to locate the most proximal point of the tuberosity fragment under C-arm imaging (**Fig 7.9-4a**), then the guide wire is directed across the fracture into the distal fragment (**Fig 7.9-4b**). The placement of the guide wire is checked in different projections, including AP, oblique, and lateral to confirm that it is as perpendicular to the fracture plane as possible and located intraosseously (**Fig 7.9-4c**). If not correctly placed, the wire is withdrawn and redirected until a satisfactory location is confirmed on C-arm imaging.

The appropriate diameter and length of the screw required can now be determined. The diameter of the screw should be large enough to provide a stable and secure fixation and not split the tuberosity fragment. The length of the partially threaded screw should allow the threaded portion of the screw to start immediately distal to the fracture. The threaded portion should gain purchase within the canal when directed intramedullary or in the medial cortex when directed towards the medial wall (**Fig 7.9-4d**). The screw can be laid over the skin and aligned with the fifth MT using C-arm imaging to determine the diameter and the length. Alternatively, the screw length required can be determined or checked with a depth gauge. The path for the screw in the distal fragment need not be drilled if a self-drilling and self-tapping screw is used. An appropriately sized drill should be used.

The screw is then gently inserted by hand while the other hand continues to hold the point-to-point reduction (Weber) clamp temporarily maintaining the fracture reduction. This is done to monitor and minimize the torque imparted to the fracture fragments. The screw is advanced under C-arm guidance ensuring appropriate placement with no undue prominence proximally. After the screw reducing and compressing the fracture is satisfactorily placed, the final AP, oblique, and lateral C-arm images are reviewed (**Fig 7.9-4e–f**).

The wound is closed and a well-padded posterior splint is applied over sterile dressings with the ankle and foot held in neutral dorsiflexion.

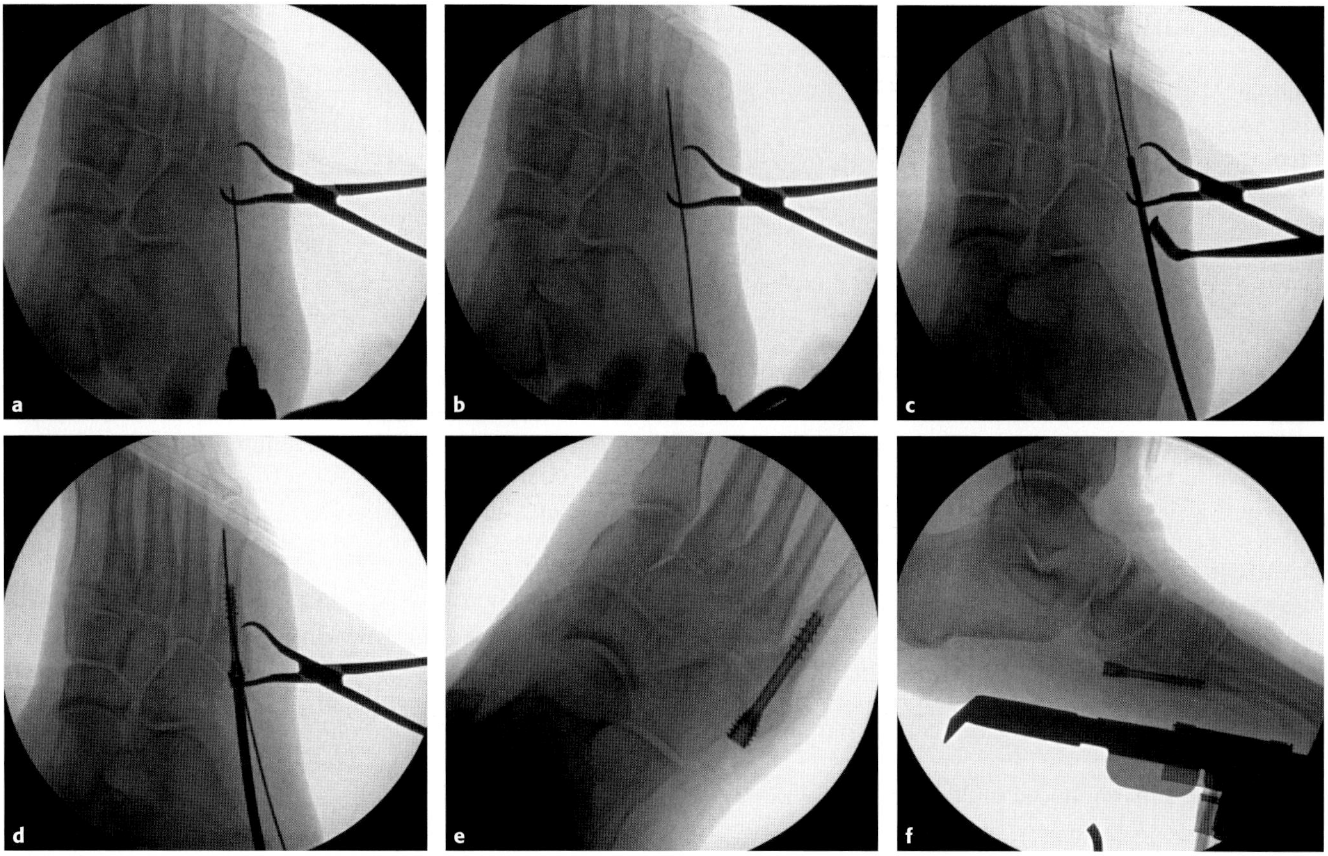

Fig 7.9-4a–f Intraoperative images.

a-b The fracture is held reduced with a point-to-point bone reduction clamp and the guide wire is introduced, starting at the tip of the tuberosity and advanced distally into the medullary canal.

c-d The drill in the proximal fragment and the screw is laid over to check the diameter and length.

e-f Final position of the screw.

5 Pitfalls and complications

Pitfalls

Identification of an older fracture

In an older fracture, the location of the fracture may not be immediately apparent after the dissection is carried down to the bone. A #15 scalpel blade can be used to check for its position. The tip of this blade can be walked down from a point where there is bony consistency along the length until a softer spot is reached. This is the fracture site. The scalpel blade can be used to excise the intervening consolidated fibrous tissue efficiently and without removing bone. Aggressive use of a bone curette to remove intervening scar tissue can result in removal of cancellous bone and should be avoided as this can leave a gap at the fracture site and minimize the surface area of bone apposition.

Clamp placement

There is usually some difficulty in securing fracture fragments with the bone reduction clamp. After opening the clamp, one tine of the clamp should be carefully guided and placed over the tip of the proximal fragment while avoiding the entry point for the screw and without compromising the grip that can be obtained by the clamp. Similarly, the other tine of the clamp may not get good purchase in the MT shaft, in which case a small notch or drill hole can be made in the cortical bone of the distal fragment so that the tip of the clamp can get a secure grip. Attention should be paid at the plantar aspect of the fracture site to prevent a gap in this location. If necessary, proximal and plantar flexion pressure can be applied manually to reduce the fracture, and the clamp can be used to further reduce and stabilize the fracture reduction.

Guide wire placement

The placement of the guide wire is critical. A guide wire that starts at the most proximal point of the proximal fragment gives the longest length the screw can traverse in this fragment and the best possible purchase. Checking the starting point for the guide wire and its trajectory in different C-arm projections before wire insertion avoids multiple attempts and enables optimal placement of this wire.

Selection of a screw that is too large for the fragment can potentially split the fragment. If this happens, the K-wire fixation with a tension band wire technique can be used as an alternative.

If tension band or hook plate are used, both are usually prominent under the skin and can be a source of discomfort requiring subsequent surgery for removal of hardware.

Complications

Failure of fixation

The internal fixation should be strong enough to counteract the displacing forces on the proximal fragment, especially through its attachment to the peroneus brevis muscle. If the screw size is small or the purchase of screw in bone fragments is poor, the screw can potentially pull out, displacing the fracture fragments. If this happens, the fixation can be revised using K-wires and a tension band technique or a hook plate.

Sural nerve injury

The sural nerve and its branches are in the vicinity and prone to injury. Injury can lead to problems such as numbness, neuroma formation, and hypersensitivity that may or may not be disabling. Careful dissection in planes deeper than skin and subcutaneous fascia helps to avoid such injuries.

6 Alternative techniques

If the proximal fragment is small, screws that are smaller in diameter can be used but may not provide strong enough fixation. Similarly, using screws in the presence of osteoporosis or fragmentation will not provide an optimal purchase or fixation. Therefore, in such circumstances alternative fixation techniques are used.

Internal fixation with K-wires using a tension band wire technique

Two parallel wires are used to traverse the fracture site perpendicular to the fracture plane. The distal tips of the K-wires can be driven into the medullary canal or the medial cortex in the distal fragment for a better purchase.

A cerclage wire is introduced through a drill hole in the distal fragment and in a figure-of-eight configuration passed underneath the proximal end of the two K-wires and then brought back to the starting point, twisted, then tensioned with a wire tensioner. The proximal ends are bent and cut to bury the sharp ends (**Fig 7.9-5**).

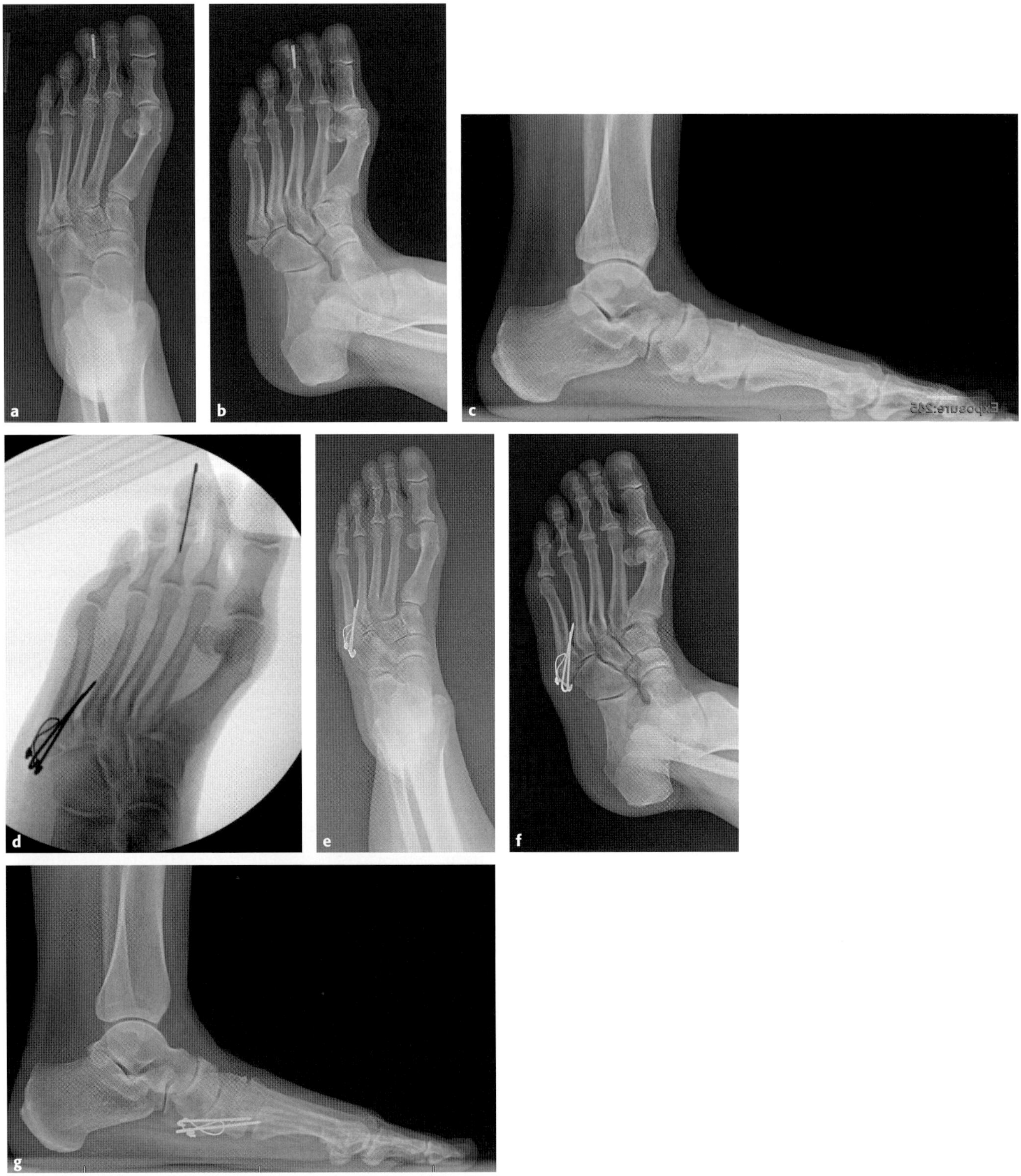

Fig 7.9-5a–g Example from a different case showing the technique using K-wires and tension band wiring.
a–c X-rays showing the displaced fracture in zone 1.
d Images taken after fixation.
e-g Radiographic union.

Hook plate

The hook plate can be used to secure the proximal fragment by applying a distally directed force; the distal end of the plate is secured with two or more screws.

Suture fixation

If the fragment is too small for internal fixation, it can be excised and a suture anchor used to secure the peroneus brevis tendon attachment in the cancellous base of the distal fragment.

Excision

If the proximal fragment is small or comminuted, it can be excised with repair of the peroneal brevis and plantar fascia.

7 Postoperative management and rehabilitation

Toe and knee exercises are encouraged.

After 7–10 days the splint is removed and the wound is checked.

A walking boot or removable cast is applied to allow gentle, intermittent mobilizing exercises and weight bearing as tolerated.

After 6 weeks, the fracture healing and implant integrity is checked with a weight-bearing x-ray. If there is satisfactory evidence of healing at the fracture site without complications such as implant failure or displacement at the fracture site, then the patient can be weaned off the boot or cast. The patient can be transitioned into a stiff-soled shoe which is recommended for a further 6-week period.

By 3 months, if the pain and tenderness is resolved and fracture consolidation is shown on x-rays, gradual return to full activities and use of regular footwear is permitted.

If further protection is necessary on the basis of continued pain, a carbon fiber insert and a rocker-soled shoe is provided until all symptoms resolve (**Fig 7.9-6**).

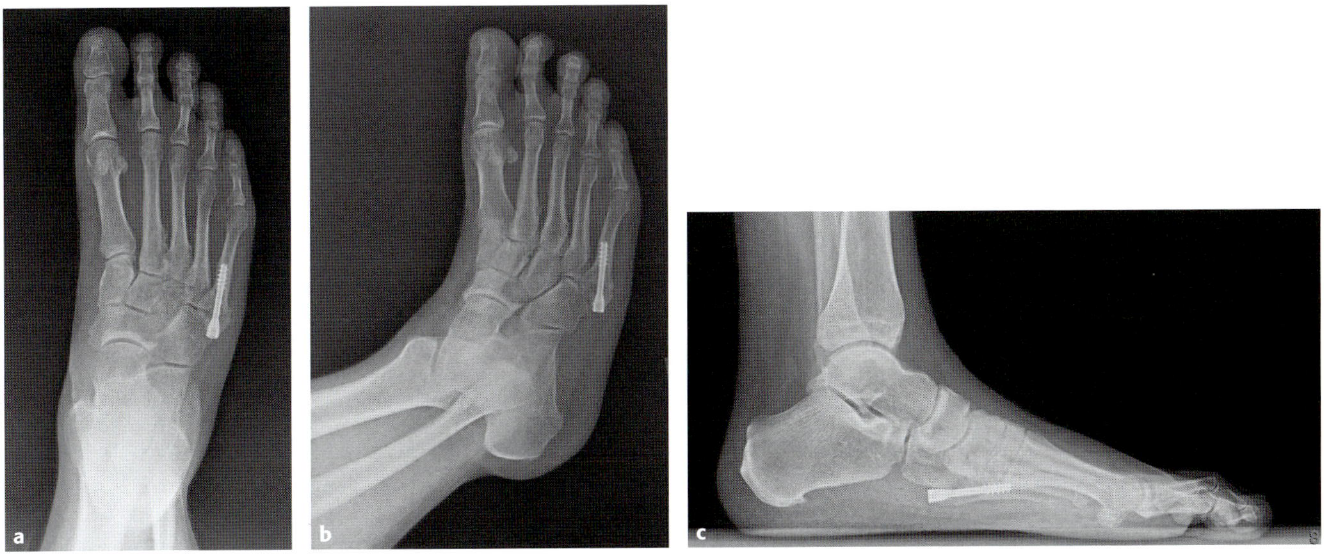

Fig 7.9-6a–c Radiographic consolidation at the fracture site.

Implant removal

The implant is removed if there is persistent pain or discomfort that can be located at the site of the hardware. This can be undertaken after 9–12 months if x-rays show bone healing (**Fig 7.9-7**).

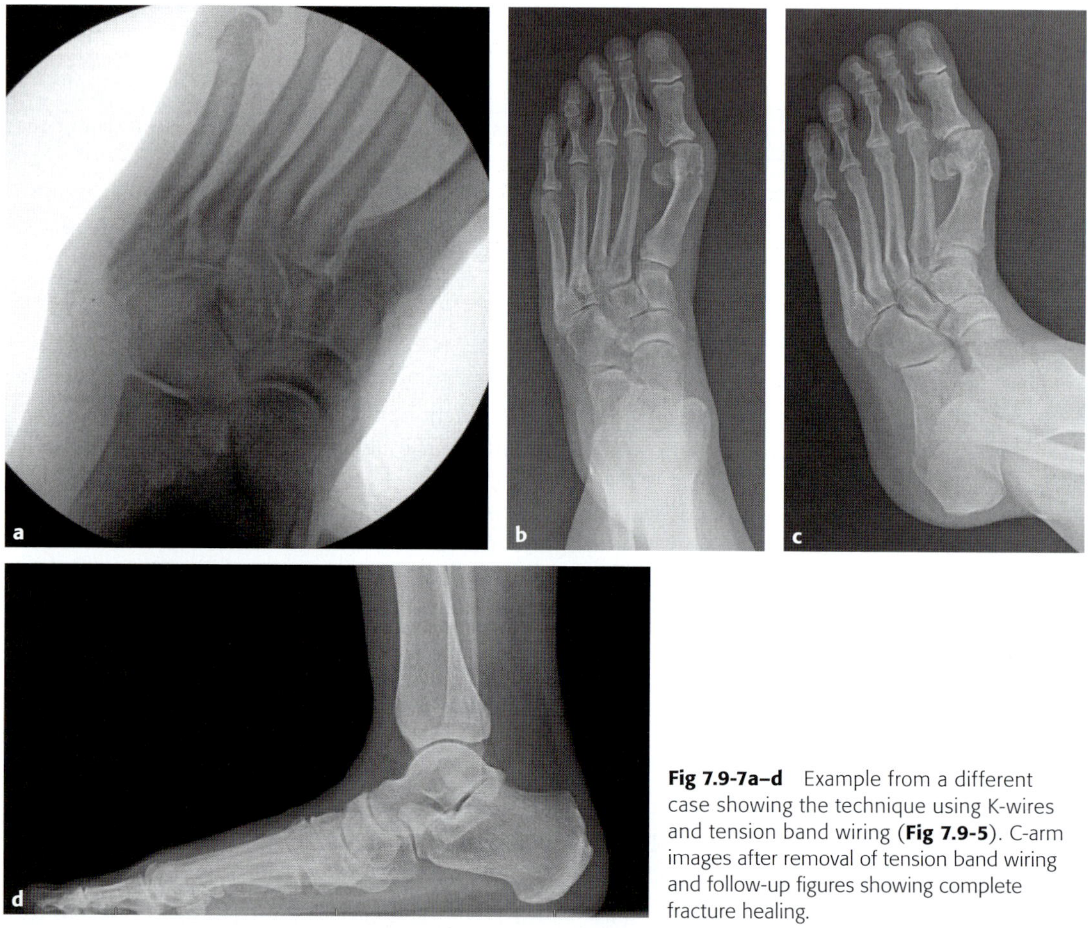

Fig 7.9-7a–d Example from a different case showing the technique using K-wires and tension band wiring (**Fig 7.9-5**). C-arm images after removal of tension band wiring and follow-up figures showing complete fracture healing.

8 Recommended reading

Den Hartog BD. Fracture of the proximal fifth metatarsal. *JAAOS.* 2009;17(7):458–464.

Heineck J, Wolz M, Haupt C, et al. Fifth metatarsal avulsion fracture: a rational basis for postoperative treatment. *Arch Orthop Trauma Surg.* 2009 Aug;129(8):1089–1092.

Lee SK, Park JS, Choy WS. LCP distal ulna hook plate as alternative fixation for fifth metatarsal base fracture. *Eur J Orthop Surg Traumatol.* 2013 Aug;23(6):705–713.

Morris PM, Francois AG, Marcus RE, et al. The effect of peroneus brevis tendon anatomy on the stability of fractures at the fifth metatarsal base. *Foot Ankle Int.* 2015 May;36(5):579–584.

Polzer H, Polzer S, Mutschler W, et al. Acute fractures to the proximal fifth metatarsal bone: development of classification and treatment recommendations based on the current evidence. *Injury.* 2012 Oct;43(10):1626–1632.

7.10 Fifth metatarsal base fracture (zone 2)

Andrew K Sands, Selene G Parekh, Joseph Tracey, Christopher E Gross

1 Case description

A 22-year-old man was skateboarding when he hit a rut and sustained a twisting injury to his left foot. He presented to the emergency department with pain along the lateral border of his right foot. There was swelling and ecchymosis. X-rays revealed a fracture of the fifth metatarsal (MT) (**Fig 7.10-1**) (AO/OTA 87.5.1.A).

The fracture was in the watershed zone of the blood supply distal to the metaphysis at the base of the shaft (cortical bone area). He was placed into a 3-sided ("AO") splint and discharged with instructions to keep his leg elevated.

The patient was subsequently seen in the outpatient orthopedic clinic where treatment options were discussed. The patient elected to have surgery.

2 Preoperative planning

While there is an excellent chance this fracture will heal nonoperatively with nonweight-bearing immobilization, the fracture is in an area of decreased blood supply, which makes healing slow with the possibility of nonunion. Additionally, in the case of a young athletic patient, internal fixation enhances the healing rate and promotes return to activity.

Screw insertion by minimally invasive osteosynthesis (MIO) is an excellent option for this kind injury as it neither disrupts the fracture site, nor damages the soft tissues which may further injure the blood supply to the MT.

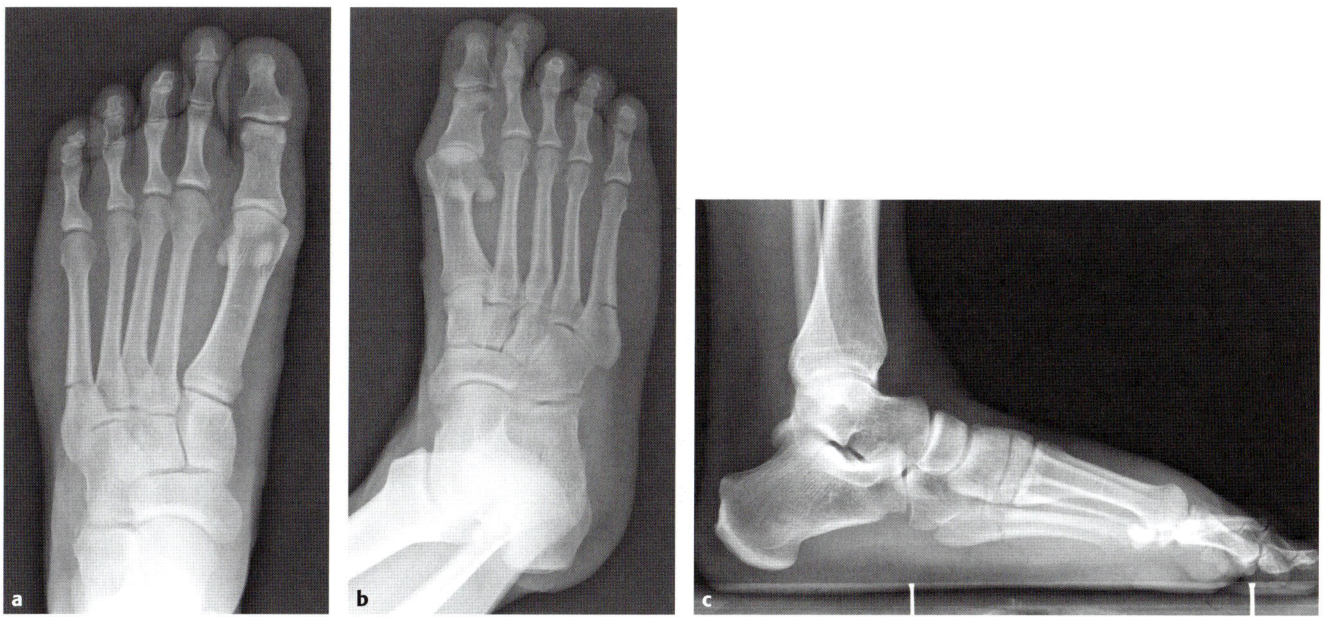

Fig 7.10-1a–c X-rays showing the proximal fifth MT fracture (zone 2).
a AP view.
b Oblique view
c Lateral view.

3 Operating room setup

Patient positioning	• Lateral on a radiolucent table • The affected leg is on top and should be free to move off the operative table onto the stage of the C-arm. • A towel bump can be placed under the medial malleolus to elevate the foot off the table.
Anesthesia options	• General with regional supplementation
C-arm location	• Along the posterior aspect of the laterally positioned patient • C-arm with the arm flipped with the imager inferior
Tourniquet	• Placed but not inflated unless necessary

For illustrations and overview of anesthetic considerations, see chapter 1.

Equipment

- Long drill bits (4.0 mm and 2.5 mm diameter)
- T-handle chuck and power drill
- Intramedullary (IM) tap
- IM screw set

4 Surgical procedure

The approach is made axially at the base of the fifth MT and extended toward the heel (**Fig 7.10-2**). The incision is deepened through the fascia with a #15 blade and spread bluntly until the base of the fifth MT is found. We make use of the "high and inside" approach (**Fig 7.10-3**), using the C-arm to locate the axis of the fifth MT is found using the C-arm.

Any screw may be used whether cannulated or solid. However, the solid 4.0 mm cortex screw is strong, inexpensive, and fits inside the fifth MT without difficulty.

Insertion of the 4.0 mm lag screw begins by using a 4.0 mm drill bit to open the proximal base of the fifth MT. The drill is advanced distally to just past the fracture site (**Fig 7.10-4**).

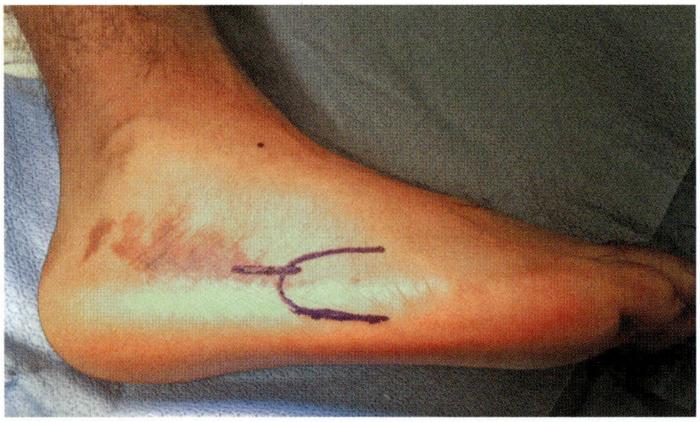

Fig 7.10-2 Incision planning. With direct palpation, a dorsomedial starting point (about 1.5 cm incision) is marked on the proximal fifth MT.

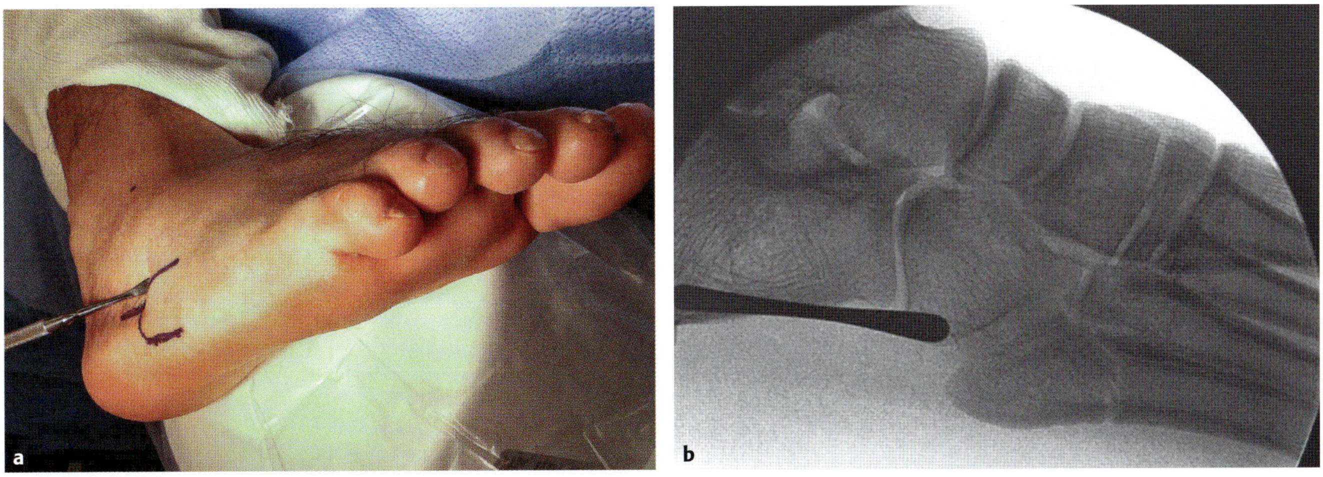

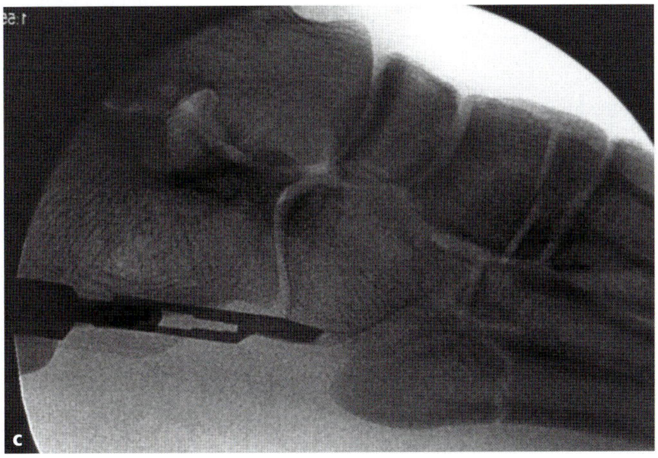

Fig 7.10-3a–c Incision placement under radiological guidance.
a–b A small (Freer) elevator is used to mark the exact spot for the guide wire or drill bit placement.
c Incision using a #15 blade with a "high and inside" approach.

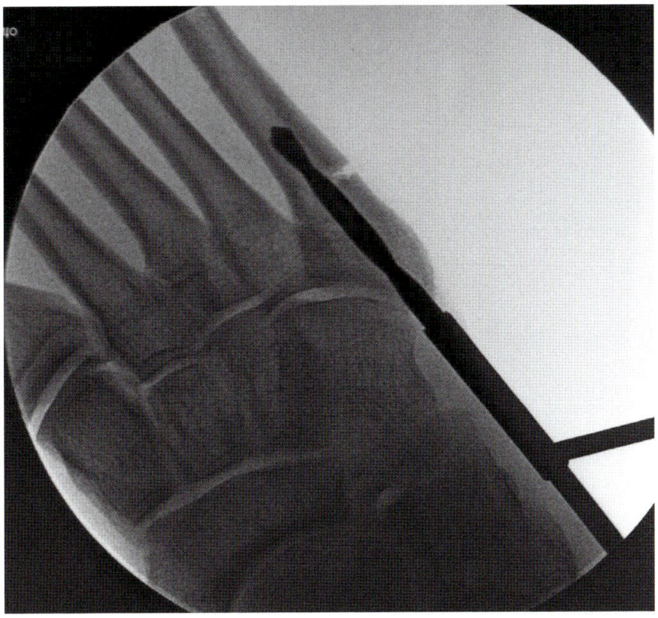

Fig 7.10-4 Opening drilling with a 4.0 mm drill bit and advancement under C-arm guidance.

Next, a long drill bit with a 2.5 mm diameter is inserted and advanced distally along the axis of the fifth MT on AP, oblique, and lateral C-arm views. These views are achieved either by rotating the mini-C-arm or by lifting the knee off the table, which rotates the foot into the proper view on the imaging base.

The distal 2.5 mm drill may be advanced by hand with the drill bit chucked into a T-handle device. As there is little resistance, this allows the surgeon to have excellent tactile feedback along the distal fifth MT (**Fig 7.10-5**). If the distal shaft is perforated, it will not negatively impact the results of screw insertion by MIO.

The depth gauge is then gently inserted to determine the appropriate screw length (**Fig 7.10-6**).

The screw is carefully inserted under C-arm view until the head abuts the cortex. It may be further gently turned to compress the fracture site (**Fig 7.10-7**).

Since the fracture site is not exposed, bone grafting is usually not done in conjunction with this technique. The drilling of the shaft is also thought to provide a measure of endosteal stimulation and some bone graft as the drill passes the fracture site.

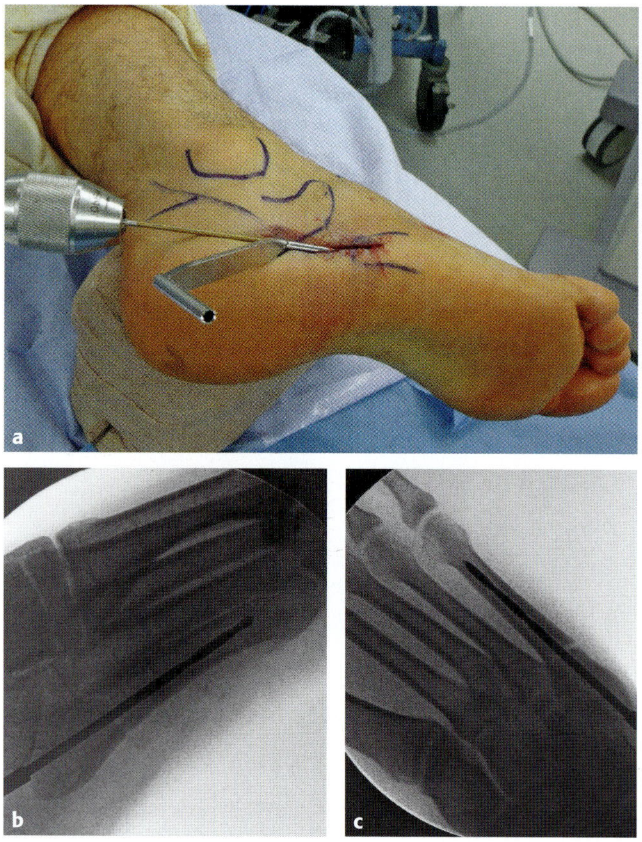

Fig 7.10-5a–c Drill (2.5 mm) advancement distally.

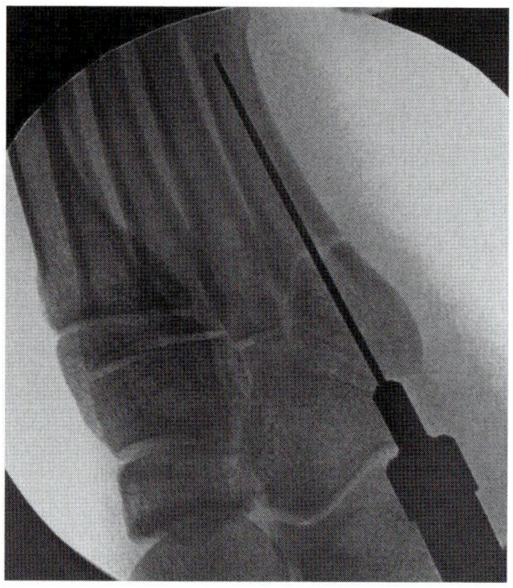

Fig 7.10-6 Measuring screw length with a depth gauge.

5 Pitfalls and complications

Pitfalls

- Overly long screws can distract the bone. Care should be taken during fixation as residual gapping may occur.
- Overly long screws can also pierce the distal medial cortex.
- Restoration of physiological length and rotation must also be considered during reduction and fixation as errors could lead to delayed union, nonunion, or higher rates of refracture.

Complications

- Loss of fixation
- Nonunion
- Infection
- Deformity with loss of proper weight-bearing alignment
- Damage to the sural nerve

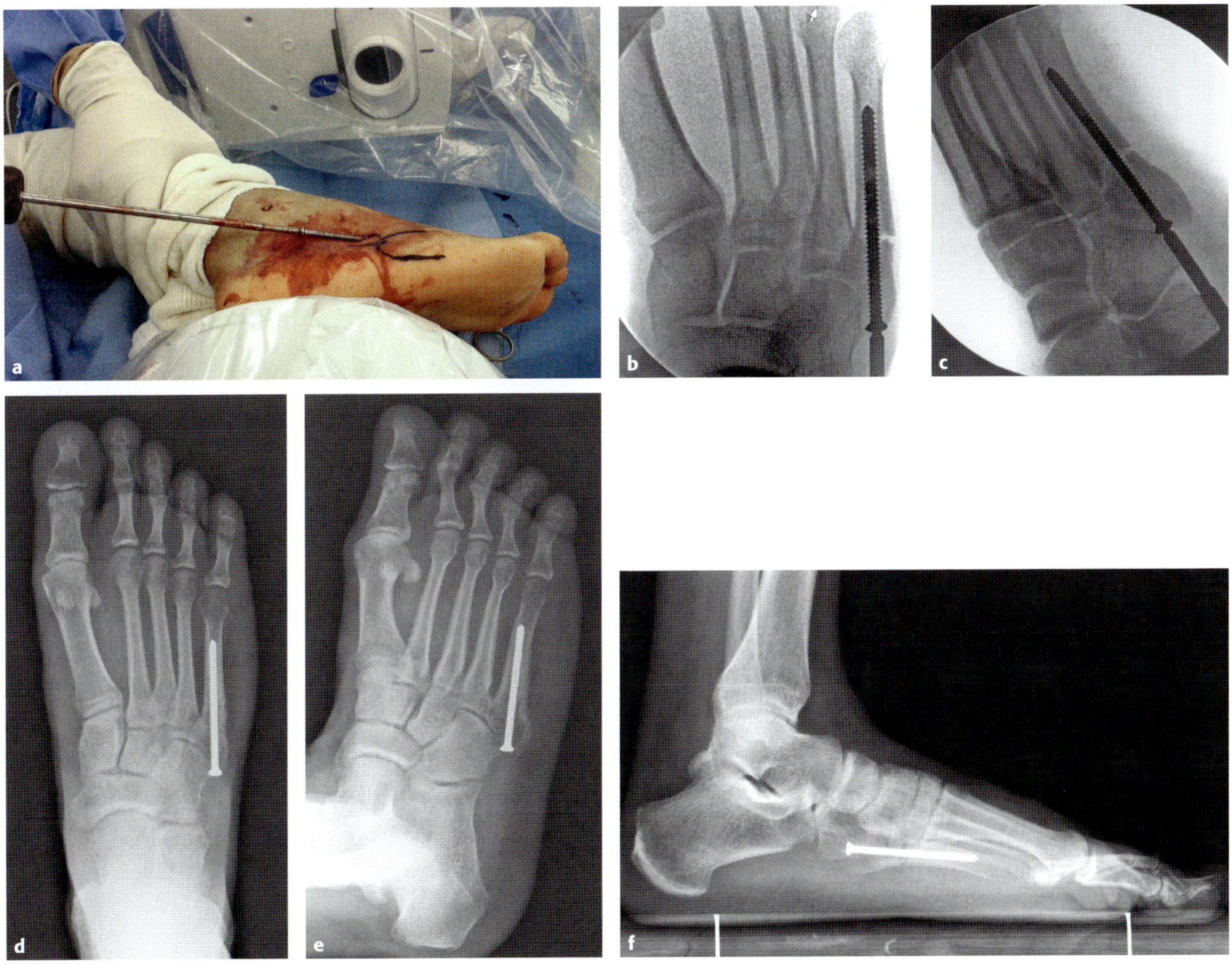

Fig 7.10-7a–f Insertion of noncannulated screw under image guidance.

6 Alternative techniques

Lateral plating

Lateral plating can be used in zone 2 fractures either acutely or with nonunions. Plating is recommended in cases of inadequate bone stock and severe comminution.

Case example: A 21-year-old male basketball player presented with residual pain after undergoing IM fixation of a Jones fracture (zone 2). The AP and lateral x-rays showed a fracture nonunion (**Fig 7.10-8a–c**).

C-arm guidance is used to identify the fracture, and a 4 cm incision is made over the fracture site, which can be extended posteriorly for hardware removal. Careful dissection is made to preserve the sural nerve as complications involving this nerve are a significant issue in proximal fifth MT plating. The abductor digiti minimi is also encountered and must be retracted. The fracture site is then mobilized and reduced with particular attention paid to maintaining or restoring length and rotation.

In cases of IM revision, the screw must first be removed, then the implant void should be corrected. Bone graft is tamped into the defect, followed by additional reduction of the nonunion site and bone graft application about the nonunion margins (**Fig 7.10-8d–e**). A clamp can be used for further compression, prior to placement of a (hook) plate along the lateral aspect of the fifth MT (**Fig 7.10-8f**). A screw is then placed proximally and inspected using the C-arm. A compression screw is then inserted distally. Additional locking screws are then placed proximal and distal to the fracture site under C-arm guidance (**Fig 7.10-8g–h**). Prior to closure, the fixation is inspected to confirm minimal prominence, adequate fracture reduction, and normal articulation with the cuboid. The wound was then closed with 4-0 nylon interrupted sutures. The patient had uneventful union.

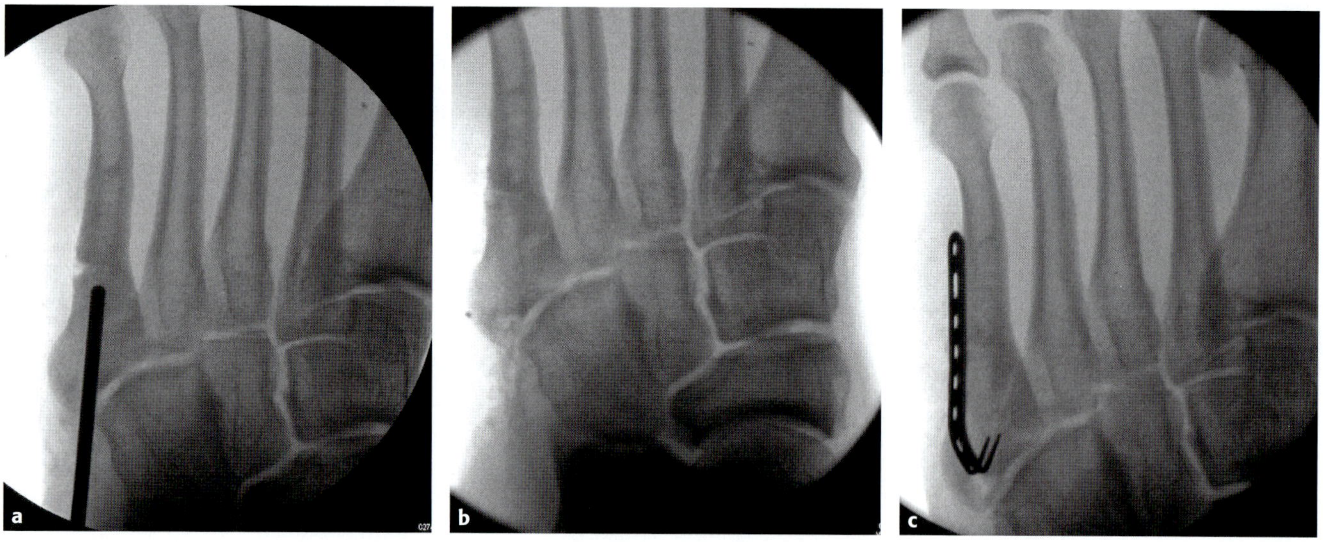

Fig 7.10-8a–h Technique of lateral plating after failed screw fixation.
a–b Intramedullary implant void after hardware removal. The void defect is filled with bone graft using a tamp (**a**). The nonunion site is further reduced, along with bone graft placement about the nonunion margins (**b**).
c Placement of lateral (hook) plate. Further compression may be used prior to lateral plate placement.

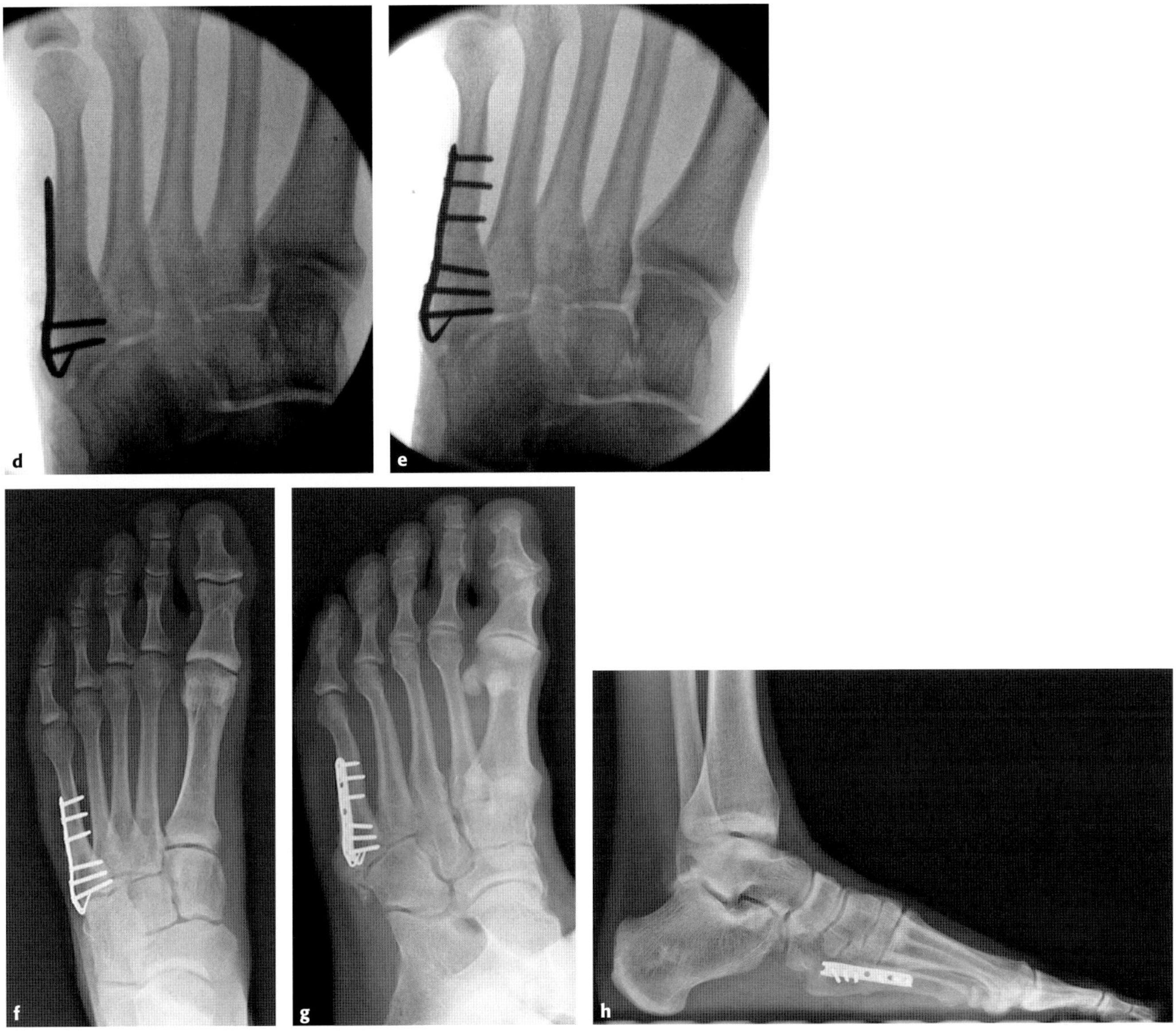

Fig. 7.10-8 a-h (cont) Technique of lateral plating after failed screw fixation.

d Placement of the proximal screw. Once the lateral plate is positioned, one or more proximal compression screws may be placed. Care must be taken to maintain plate alignment.

e Following the placement of a distal compression screw, locking screws may be placed proximally and distally.

f–h X-ray follow-up for Jones intramedullary revision. Proper placement and compression can be appreciated in the AP, oblique, and lateral x-rays. The patient returned to sports without complication.
(Images 8d–h courtesy of Mark E Easley, MD.)

7 Postoperative management and rehabilitation

Based on surgeon preference, patients are immediately placed into a short leg splint, cast, or boot. A period of nonweight bearing, typically for the first 2 weeks, is recommended. Following the initial 2 weeks, patients are transitioned into a controlled-ankle-motion (CAM) boot, strict nonweight-bearing, and range-of-motion exercises begin out of the CAM boot. At week 6, the patient is transitioned from the CAM boot to a cushioned heel rocker bottom shoe with gradual increased WB. For a professional athlete, low impact training activities can then begin. In the general population, low-impact physical therapy is continued. By week 9, athletes can return to athletic play and the general population can begin higher impact physical therapy.

8 Recommended reading

Huh J, Glisson RR, Matsumoto T, et al. Biomechanical comparison of intramedullary screw versus low-profile plate fixation of a jones fracture. *Foot Ankle Int.* 2016 Apr;37(4):411–418.

Hunt KJ, Anderson RB. Treatment of Jones fracture nonunions and refractures in the elite athlete: outcomes of intramedullary screw fixation with bone grafting. *Am J Sports Med.* 2011 Sep;39(9):1948–1954.

Le M, Anderson R. Zone II and III fifth metatarsal fractures in athletes. *Curr Rev Musculoskelet Med.* 2017 Mar;10(1):86–93.

Nunley JA. Fractures of the base of the fifth metatarsal: the Jones fracture. *Orthop Clin North Am.* 2001 Jan;32(1):171–180.

Torg JS, Balduini FC, Zelko RR, et al. Fractures of the base of the fifth metatarsal distal to the tuberosity. Classification and guidelines for non-surgical and surgical management. *J Bone Joint Surg Am.* 1984 Feb;66(2):209–214.

Varner KE, Harris JD. The proximal fifth metatarsal metadiaphyseal jones fracture: intramedullary screw vs plantar plate. *Operative Techniques in Sports Medicine.* 2017 Mar;25(2): 59–66.

8 Phalanges and sesamoids

Phalanges and sesamoids

8 Phalangeal and sesamoid fractures and dislocations

Stefan Rammelt

1 Introduction

Fractures of the phalanges are the most common injuries to the forefoot. The majority of these do not require surgery and can be safely treated with closed reduction and taping. However, several fractures will require more attention, such as open fractures, nail-bed lacerations, physeal injuries in children, and condylar fractures of the great toe. Likewise, while most toe dislocations are amenable to closed reduction, interposition of the capsule, ligaments, and tendons, the sesamoids, or the plantar plate may require open reduction.

2 Anatomy and pathomechanics

Anatomy

The great toe (hallux) has two phalanges, the second to fourth toes have three phalanges, and the fifth toe has three or two phalanges in approximately 50% of cases with considerable geographic variations.

The metatarsophalangeal (MTP) joints are shaped like ball and socket joints. However, motion in the horizontal plane is limited by the adjacent toes and the lack of individual muscles for each of the second, third, and fourth toes. Therefore, only the hallux and fifth toe can perform some abduction and adduction. The interphalangeal (IP) joints are simple hinge joints allowing flexion and extension only. The joint capsules are reinforced by strong medial and lateral collateral ligaments.

The two sesamoids beneath the first metatarsal (MT) head at the first MTP joint are the only constant sesamoids in the foot. They are embedded into a strong capsuloligamentous complex and the course of the two flexor hallucis brevis (FHB) tendon slips. In addition, through conjoint tendons the abductor hallucis tendon inserts at the medial sesamoid, and the adductor hallucis tendon at the lateral sesamoid (**Fig 8-1**). The medial sesamoid is bipartite in about 12% and lateral in 2.5% of the population. Both sesamoids can be tripartite and quadripartite in rare cases. Physiological partition must be distinguished from fractures and nonunions.

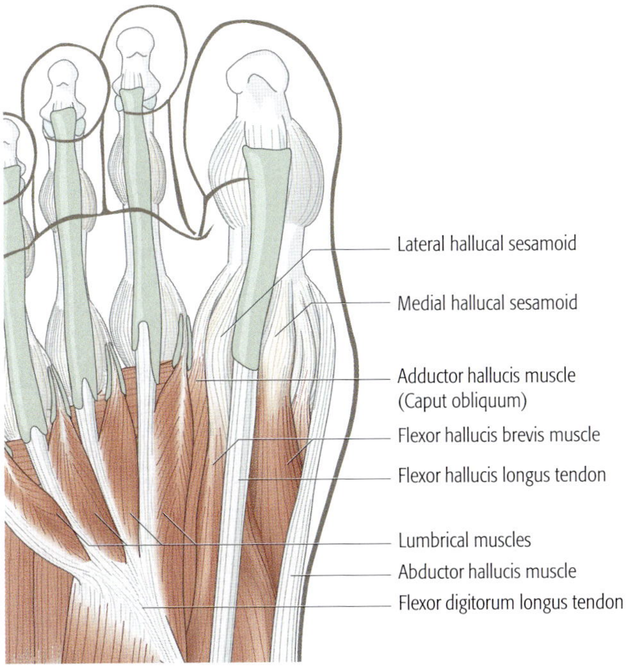

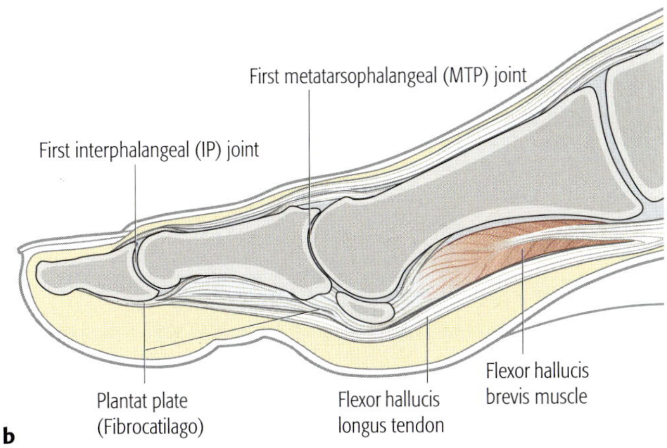

Fig 8-1a–b Anatomy of the extrinsic and intrinsic tendons and muscles to the sesamoids and toes from plantar (**a**) and lateral (**b**) views at the level of the first ray.

The sesamoids are held together by an intersesamoid ligament and are tightly associated with the fibrocartilaginous plantar plate. The latter is firmly attached to the base of the proximal phalanx and loosely attached at the neck of the first MT via the plantar capsule.

The dorsal capsule of all MTP joints is structurally weak, which predisposes it to dorsal dislocation of the toes in both traumatic and nontraumatic conditions. The plantar capsule is a strong specialized structure with a firm attachment to the base of the proximal phalanx where it blends with the plantar plate and a thinner, more flexible attachment to the undersurface of the MT head or neck junction.

The plantar fascia, which originates at the anterior weight-bearing (WB) tubercle of the calcaneus, spans the plantar aspect of the midfoot and attaches to the plantar skin beneath the toes and to the bases of the proximal phalanges. At the level of the MTP joints, the longitudinal fibers of the plantar fascia fan out to the five toes and contribute vertical fibers to the fibrous flexor sheaths and the subcutaneous tissue resulting in a digital cutaneous anchorage. These longitudinal and vertical fibers are reinforced by the transverse mooring ligaments and, more distally, the natatory webbing ligaments forming a three-dimensional network of small chambers containing adipose tissue providing cushioning during push-off.

The flexor hallucis longus (FHL) tendon attaches to the distal phalanx, while the FHB tendon attaches to the proximal phalanx of the great toe. At the lesser toes, the flexor digitorum longus tendon attaches to the distal phalanx, while the flexor digitorum brevis tendon attaches to the middle phalanx of the second to fifth toes. The long and short extensor tendons form a common extensor hood over the dorsal aspect of the toes.

The tendons of the intrinsic foot muscles pass dorsally (interossei) and plantarly (lumbricals) to the deep transverse intermetatarsal ligament. They reinforce the MTP joint capsule together with the transverse lamina (extending from the extensor tendon sheath) and the plantar plate forming a fibrous ring around the MTP joints (**Fig 8-2**).

Pathomechanics

Fractures

The mechanism of injury ranges from low-energy trauma resulting from direct or indirect forces, to high-energy trauma resulting from a heavy object or a direct impaction force following a fall from a height or motor vehicle accident.

Comminuted or displaced fractures through the lesser toes most commonly occur at the proximal phalanx since this is the longest of the phalanges and thus has the longest lever arm. The most common fracture mechanism is a stubbing

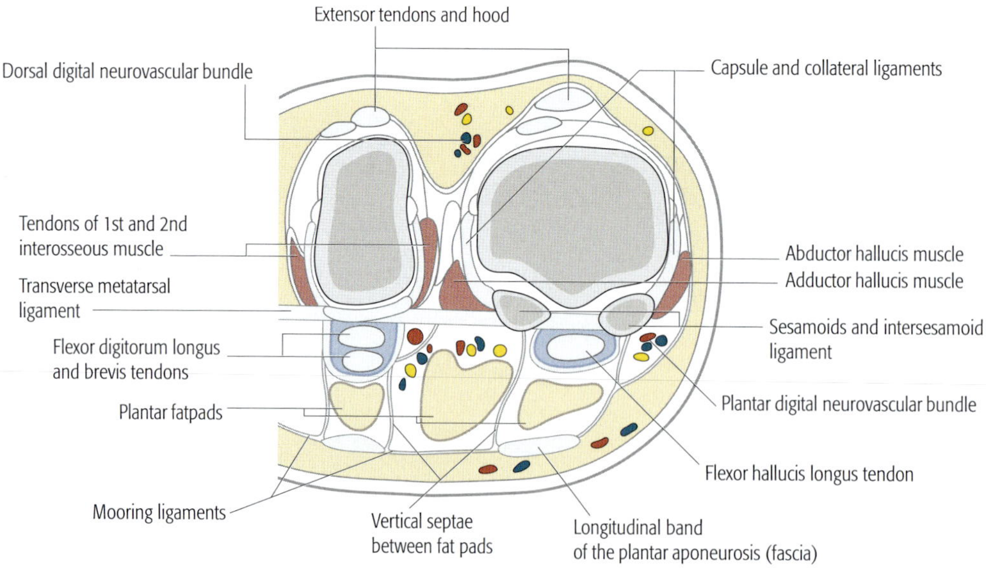

Fig 8-2 Cross-section of the first and second MT head at the MTP joints.

injury. One of the most common injuries is the so-called "bedroom" or "night-walker" fracture which involves abduction of the proximal phalanx of the fifth toe when catching a doorstep, door frame, or other object while walking barefoot.

Phalangeal fractures usually result in dorsiflexion and abduction secondary to the combined action of the long extensors and intrinsic muscles.

Stress fractures of the distal phalanx of the first toe have been described. Hallux valgus is thought to predispose to this condition.

Fractures in the sesamoids rarely occur by direct trauma. Acute sesamoid fractures are rather produced by indirect forces like forced dorsiflexion of the great toe in the wake of first MTP joint dislocations. More frequently, stress fractures due to repetitive overuse are seen. Predisposing deformities include the subtle cavus foot.

Progressive traumatic hyperextension of the first MTP joint leads to a lesion of the plantar capsule at the MT neck, since this attachment is weaker than the attachment at the proximal phalanx.

Dislocations

Dislocations most commonly occur at the first MTP joint. They are frequently caused by sporting injuries through an axial force acting on the hyperextended great toe (eg, "turf toe" in American football) or injury of the joint capsule of the MTP joint without dislocation (eg, the "en-pointe" position of ballet dancers). The majority of toe dislocations are dorsal because the dorsal capsule is substantially weaker than the plantar capsule. At the first MTP joint, the fibrocartilaginous-sesamoid complex can be dorsally dislocated over the neck of the first MT creating a buttonhole deformity that warrants open reduction.

Metatarsophalangeal dislocations of the lesser toes are typically produced by axial force on the extended toe resulting in a dorsal dislocation of the latter. However, in rare cases, the plantar plate or lumbrical muscles can be interposed, rendering closed reduction difficult or impossible. At the IP joints the medial collateral ligament can fold inwards with dislocation. Interposition of the flexor digitorum longus tendon has been described. Plantar and lateral subluxations are very rare and dislocations.

3 Fracture classification

Fractures and dislocations of the toes can be classified using the AO/OTA Fracture and Dislocation Classification (see appendix). According to the general principles of this classification, the phalanges represent the anatomical region 88. Each toe and phalangeal segment is further identified with numbers. The main distinction between types A, B, and C is the same as in the long-bone fractures:
Type A Extraarticular
Type B Partial articular
Type C Complete intraarticular

Dislocations at the forefoot (80E) are classified separately.

Jahss introduced a separate classification for dislocations of the first MTP joint to which further (sub)types were added later (**Fig 8-3**):
Type I Intersesamoid ligament intact
Type IIA Rupture of the intersesamoid ligament
Type IIB Transverse sesamoid fracture
Type IIC Rupture of the intersesamoid ligament and transverse sesamoid fracture
Type III Additional rupture of the FHB tendon

Rupture of the intersesamoid ligament becomes evident with widening of the intersesamoid interval on plain x-rays. With the intersesamoid ligament intact, the proximal phalanx dislocates with the attached sesamoids and plantar plate over the first MT head. The MT head may get stuck ("buttonhole effect") rendering closed reduction impossible. The plantar plate typically ruptures at its weaker proximal attachment to the MT neck and dislocates with attached sesamoids riding over the MT head.

Miki et al distinguish between two types of irreducible dislocations of the IP joint of the great toe (**Fig 8-4**):
Type I Interposition of the sesamoid
Type II Interposition of the plantar plate

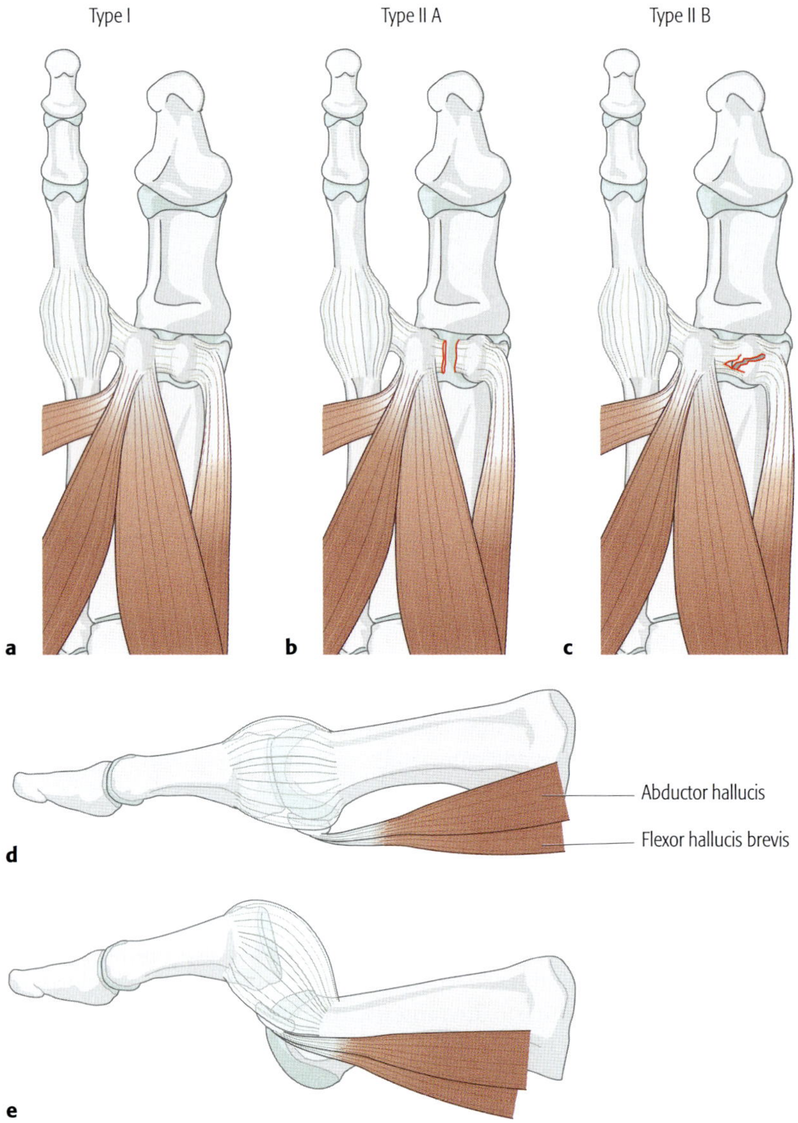

Fig 8-3a–e Classification of first MTP dislocations according to Jahss.

- **a** Type I with the intersesamoid ligament intact.
- **b** Type IIA with intersesamoid ligament rupture.
- **c** Type IIB with transverse sesamoid fracture.
- **d–e** With the intersesamoid ligament intact, the first MT head can get trapped creating a buttonhole deformity that is not amenable to closed reduction.

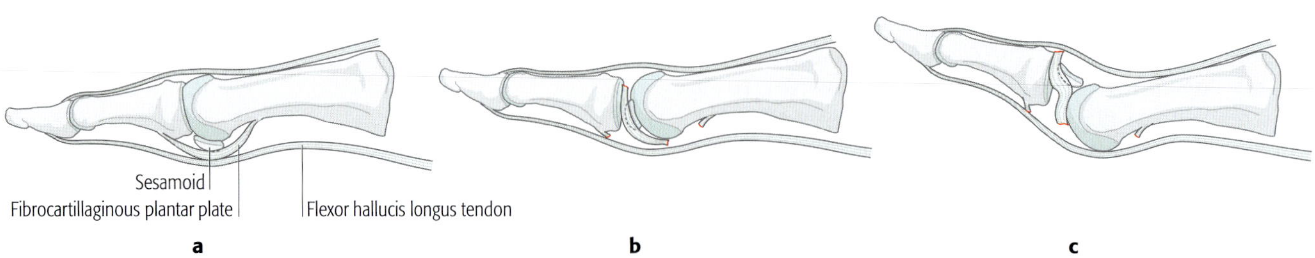

Fig 8-4a–c Classification of first MTP dislocations according to Miki et al.

- **a** Normal anatomy.
- **b** Type I with sesamoid interposition.
- **c** Type II with plantar plate interposition.

4 Preoperative assessment

Most deformities resulting from fractures and dislocations are evident from inspection of the bare foot (**Fig 8-5**). Physical examination focuses on the location of pain, tenderness, and swelling of the involved digit. Subungual hematoma is a hallmark of distal phalangeal fractures. The neurovascular status of the toes is documented.

In case of dislocation, there is typically an evident dorsal malposition of the phalanges with tension of the local soft tissues. The skin of the toes is pale on the plantar aspect and retracted dorsally. An exception is the dislocation of the IP joint of the great toe with interposition of the plantar plate or the sesamoid into the joint space. In these cases, the great toe only appears slightly longer. Also in these cases, loss of active motion in the IP joint definitely requires further diagnostic workup.

Imaging

Standard x-rays include AP, lateral, and 45° oblique views of the forefoot (**Fig 8-6**). Further imaging is usually not needed for acute injuries to the toes. However, computed tomography (CT) or magnetic resonance imaging (MRI) may be useful in differentiating between acute fractures and chronic conditions of the sesamoids (**Fig 8-7**), and adjacent soft tissues (such as congenital bipartition, stress fractures, sesamoiditis, avascular necrosis, tenosynovitis of the FHL or FHB, plantar plate avulsion, localized plantar keratosis, and impingement of the medial plantar digital nerve).

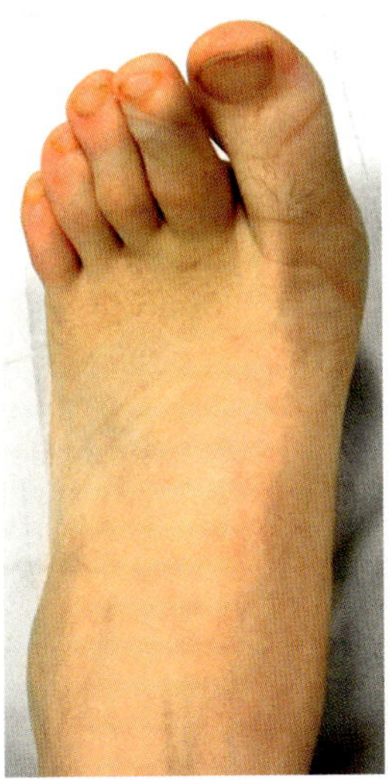

Fig 8-5 Clinical presentation of a displaced fracture with obvious hematoma, swelling, and deformity.

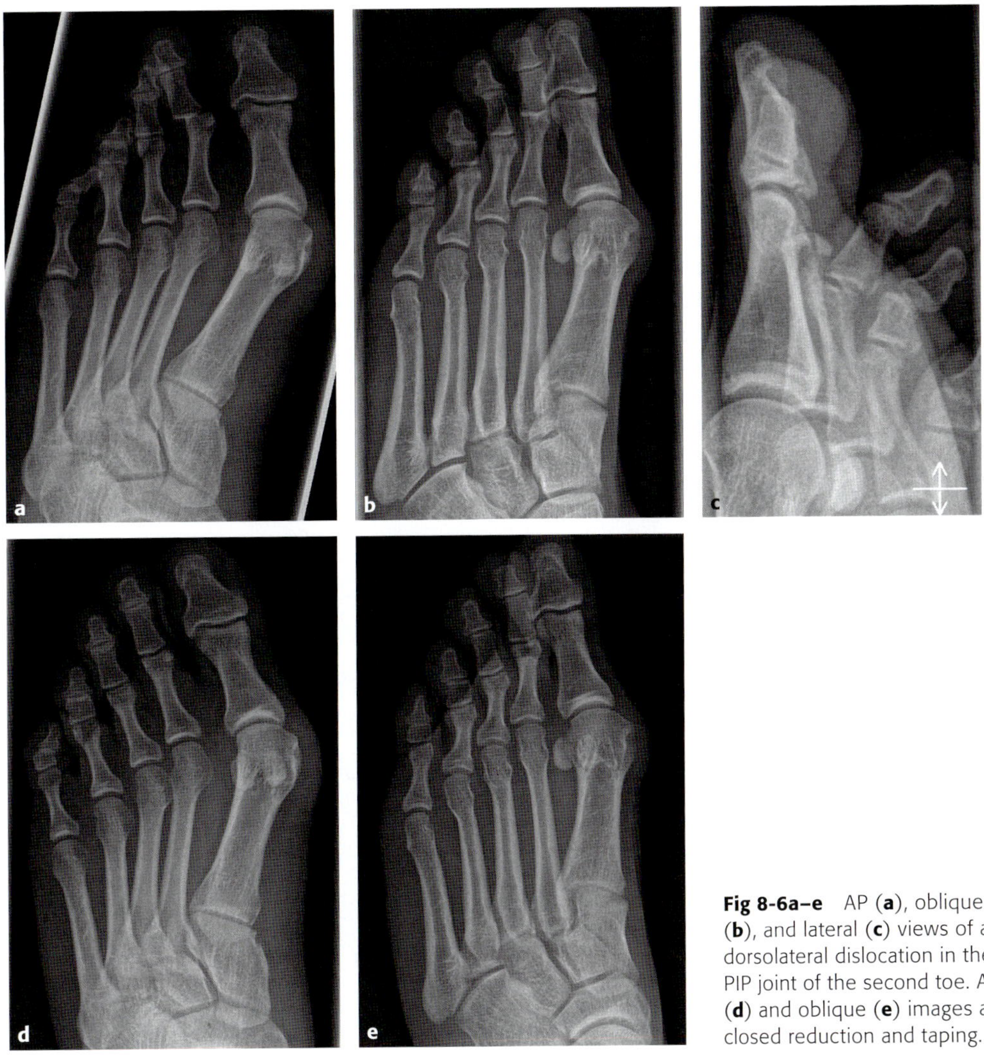

Fig 8-6a–e AP (**a**), oblique (**b**), and lateral (**c**) views of a dorsolateral dislocation in the PIP joint of the second toe. AP (**d**) and oblique (**e**) images after closed reduction and taping.

5 Nonoperative treatment

The majority of toe and sesamoid fractures are treated nonoperatively. Nondisplaced fractures of the great toe can be treated with offloading of the affected foot in a hard-soled cast or shoe for 6 weeks. Alternatively, a forefoot-offloading shoe or orthosis may be used. Follow-up x-rays are obtained at 1–2 weeks to rule out secondary displacement.

Nondisplaced fractures of the lesser toes undergo early functional treatment by taping to the adjacent toe (buddy taping) for 3–4 weeks and protected mobilization in a rigid soled shoe with a wide toe box. The interdigital space should be padded, to avoid maceration of the skin. Most displaced lesser toe fractures are treated with closed reduction under regional or local anesthesia. Reduction is achieved by longitudinal traction and simultaneous adduction or, less frequently, abduction followed by buddy taping for 4–5 weeks (**Fig 8-8**).

Dorsal MTP and IP dislocations are reduced promptly to avoid further soft-tissue damage. In most cases, closed reduction is achieved with longitudinal traction and simultaneous plantar flexion with plantar to dorsal pressure on the proximal phalanx (**Fig 8-6**). After successful reduction, the toe is protected with buddy taping. After first MTP or IP dislocations, a rigid-soled shoe is recommended for 3 weeks. Most patients with sesamoid fractures can be treated nonoperatively by protection, rest, ice, compression, and elevation (PRICE).

6 Operative treatment

Indications

Emergent surgery is indicated in open fractures or dislocations and traumatic amputation of one or more toes. Fractures of the distal phalanx associated with laceration injury to the nail bed must be treated like open fractures to prevent osteitis or recurrent nail-bed infections. Massive subungual hematomas are trephined under sterile conditions to prevent secondary infection or disturbance of nail growth.

Surgery is indicated for displaced intraarticular fractures and highly unstable, comminuted extraarticular fractures, particularly at the great toe (see chapters 8.1 and 8.2). In lesser toe fractures, open reduction and internal fixation (ORIF) is indicated for severe dislocation of the articular condyle(s), which are irreducible by closed manipulation (see chapter 8.3).

Open reduction is warranted for irreducible MTP or IP joint dislocations. The same applies to gross instability with recurrent dislocation after closed reduction (see chapter 8.4). Indications for operative intervention in first MTP dislocations ("turf toe" injuries) further include displaced sesamoid fractures (see chapter 8.5) and retraction (including diastasis of a bipartite sesamoid), loose bodies or chondral injury, large capsular or plantar plate avulsions, and gross vertical instability including after failed nonoperative treatment.

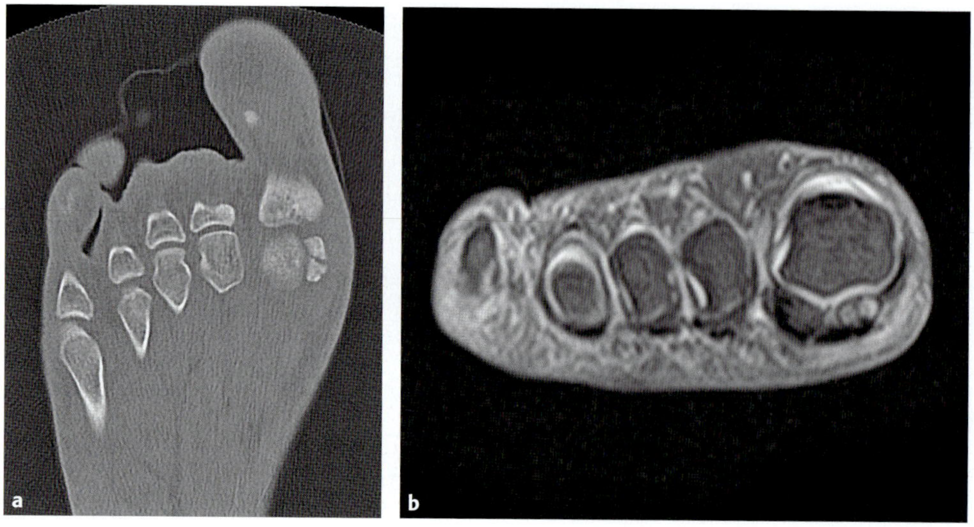

Fig 8-7a–b Imaging of a nonunion of the medial (tibial) sesamoid of the great toe.
- **a** CT imaging shows sclerosis.
- **b** MRI demonstrates avascular necrosis of the distal fragment.

Patient positioning

The patient is positioned supine on a radiolucent table. A tourniquet may be used during reduction at the surgeon's discretion.

Surgical approaches

The great toe is approached via a straight medial or lateral approach depending on the individual fracture anatomy (see chapters 8.1 and 8.2). A bilateral approach is rarely needed.

A dorsal approach is used for most lesser toe fractures and dislocations (see chapter 8.4). Fractures of the condyles are approached from medial or lateral, depending on the individual fracture location (see chapter 8.3).

A plantar approach is used for fractures, diastasis, and symptomatic nonunions of the lateral sesamoid. The medial sesamoid is approached from a low-lying medial approach at the first MT head (see chapter 8.5).

Considerations for surgery

Severe soft-tissue trauma

In compound injuries with total or subtotal amputation, replantation of a toe is rarely indicated with the exception of the great toe in children in the absence of life-threatening injuries. Following copious lavage and debridement of necrotic tissue, the definite level of amputation is defined by the intact plantar skin which should cover the stump of the remaining toe or the MT head. If possible, preservation of the stump of the proximal phalanx will be helpful in providing a buttress for the adjacent toes to prevent horizontal instability and secondary deformity.

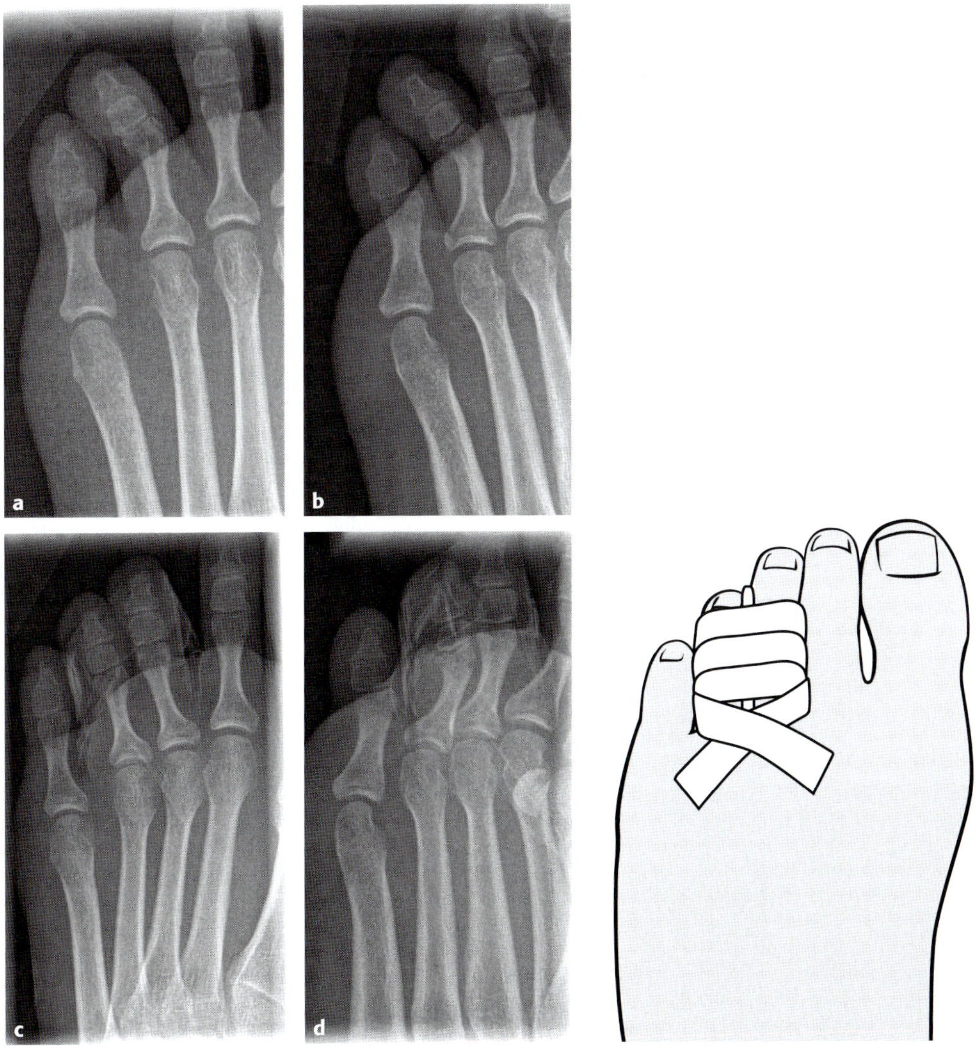

Fig 8-8a–e Nonoperative treatment of a closed displaced lesser toe fracture.
- **a–b** AP and oblique x-rays of a closed fracture of the proximal phalanx of the fourth toe with lateral deviation (abduction).
- **c–e** After successful closed reduction, the fractured toe was taped to the adjacent uninjured third toe (buddy taping).

Open fractures and dislocations of the toes are treated according to the general principles of open fracture treatment (**Fig 8-9**). The open wound is debrided and irrigated. Debridement is followed by open reduction of the fracture or dislocation via the existing wound, typically through longitudinal traction and direct manipulation of the fragment(s). Internal fixation is tailored to the individual pattern of injury. With severe soft-tissue trauma or even defect, minimally invasive K-wire fixation is preferred (chapter 8.4). Subungual hematomas are trephined under sterile conditions. Fractures associated with laceration injury to the nail bed must be treated like open fractures. This involves debridement, lavage, and temporary axial K-wire transfixation for unstable injuries.

Great toe fractures

Simple oblique fractures and unicondylar fractures can be treated with screw fixation (chapter 8.1). Alternatively, percutaneous crossed K-wires may be used for transverse extraarticular fractures, but they offer less stability than screws. K-wires should not cross at the fracture level.

Bicondylar fractures of the hallux are best treated with small fragment plates (chapter 8.2). In comminuted fractures or patients with osteoporotic bone, interlocking plates may be used as a more stable means of fixation.

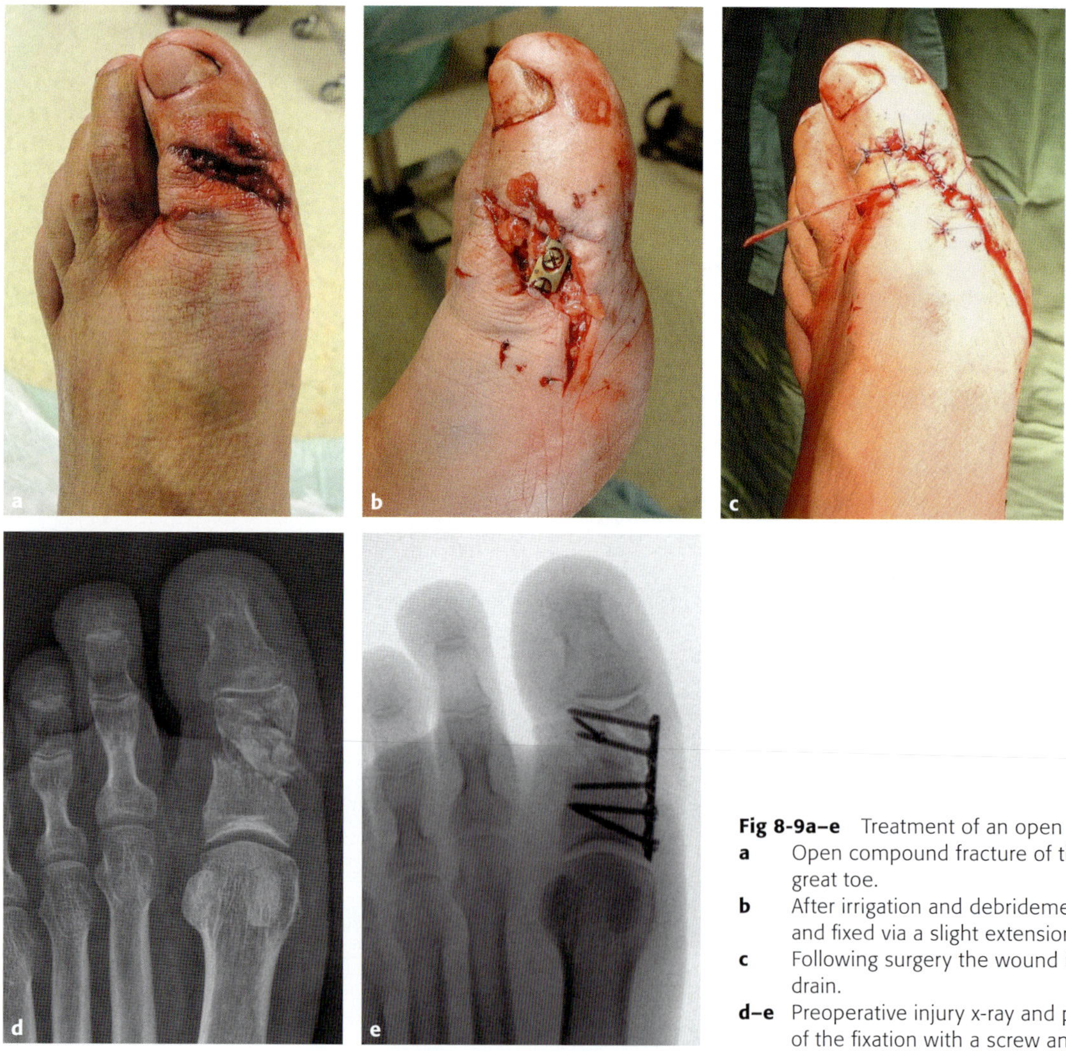

Fig 8-9a–e Treatment of an open fracture of the great toe.
- **a** Open compound fracture of the proximal phalanx of the great toe.
- **b** After irrigation and debridement, the fracture is reduced and fixed via a slight extension of the distal wound.
- **c** Following surgery the wound is closed over a capillary drain.
- **d–e** Preoperative injury x-ray and postoperative C-arm image of the fixation with a screw and medial plate.

Great toe dislocations

Irreducible first MTP dislocations (buttonhole deformity) are reduced via a dorsal approach. After splitting the dorsal capsule, the plantar plate is pushed back with a smooth elevator. The sesamoids are then pulled back below the first MT head.

In irreducible IP dislocations, an attempt can be made to push back the interposed plantar plate or sesamoid with a K-wire introduced percutaneously. If this is unsuccessful, open reduction is carried out via a dorsal or medial approach. If instability persists after open reduction, the toe is transfixed with a 1.8 mm K-wire for 4–5 weeks.

Lesser toe fractures and dislocations

Displaced condylar fractures are reduced via a direct approach (see chapter 8.3). Fixation is achieved with a minifragment screw, K-wire, or resorbable pin (if introduced through the joint cartilage). Dislocations not amenable to closed reduction are reduced via a dorsal approach (see chapter 8.4). If the toe remains unstable after open reduction, temporary fixation with a 1.6 mm K-wire for 4–5 weeks is indicated.

Sesamoid fractures

Displaced sesamoid fractures are fixed with one or two screws depending on the size and shape of the fragments (see chapter 8.5). Necrotic fragments are excised. Sesamoid nonunions or symptomatic bipartite sesamoids may be treated with either local bone grafting and screw fixation or resection of the smaller or incongruent fragment. The continuity of the plantar plate and FHB tendons has to be restored in both acute and chronic injuries. Complete excision of both sesamoids should be avoided whenever possible as it leads to muscular imbalance of the great toe.

7 Postoperative care

Postoperatively, the foot is immobilized in a splint or a hard-soled cast, and the lower leg is elevated. Active and passive range-of-motion (ROM) exercises of the foot and ankle with the toes protected are initiated on the first postoperative day, including continuous passive motion if such equipment is available.

A rigid-soled cast shoe is applied. For fractures of the hallux, the patient is restricted to partial weight bearing (WB) (up to 20 kg) on the injured leg for 6 weeks. Alternatively, a forefoot offloading shoe is used (**Fig 8-10**). WB is gradually increased at that point if x-rays demonstrate bone union. An active rehabilitation protocol is then initiated including ROM exercises of the great toe, muscular balancing, and gait training. With progressive WB, an athletic shoe with carbon fiber insert may be used for athletes who resume their training.

K-wires are typically removed 4–5 (or 6) weeks postoperatively. Other implants such as screws and small fragment plates are only removed if the patient feels prominent implants using the same approach after approximately 1 year.

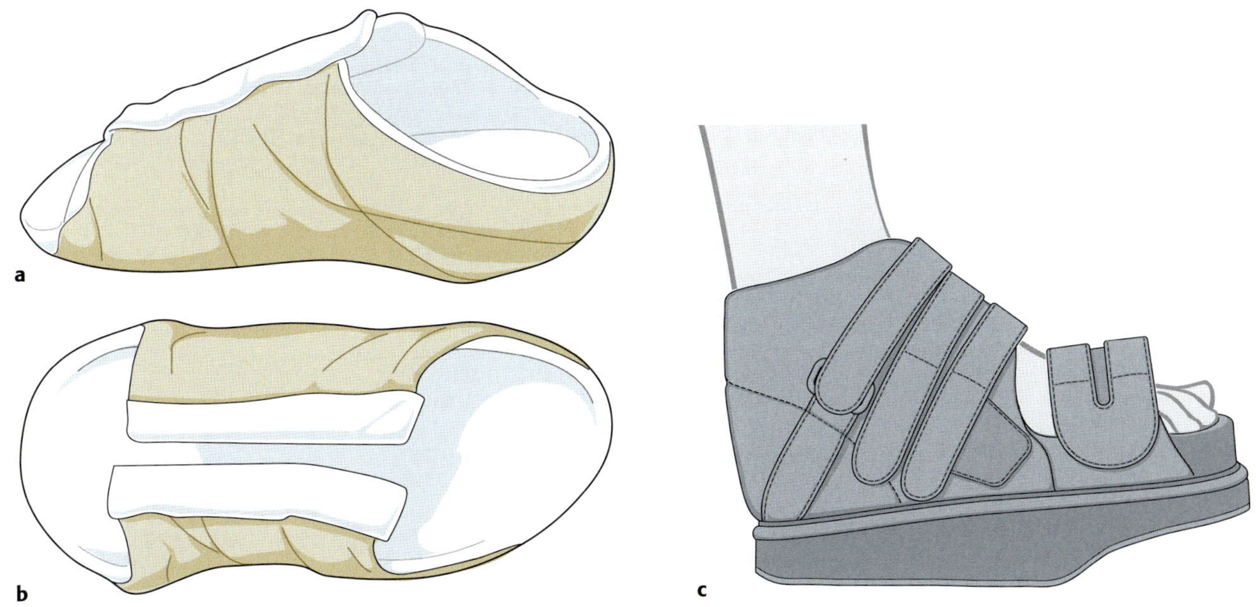

Fig 8-10a–c Hard-soled cast shoe (**a–b**) and forefoot-offloading shoe (**c**) for postoperative care.

8 Complications and outcomes

Overall, fractures of the toes generally have a good prognosis. However, the following complications may arise and result in persisting symptoms and functional restrictions:

- Relevant injuries to the toes may be overlooked if not perceived by patients with systemic metabolic disease (eg, diabetes mellitus) or neurological disorders leading to peripheral somatosensory deficits.
- The injury may be overlooked or underestimated if the initial clinical presentation of trauma is minimally symptomatic as in some physeal injuries of the distal phalanx of a stubbed toe in children. In these cases, subungual bleeding may be the only sign of an open fracture and later sequelae (such as osteomyelitis and growth arrest) may develop.
- Inadequate management of nail-bed trauma may lead to nail deformity, malalignment, splitting, or chronic infection.
- Malunions of the great toe with axial malalignment will lead to posttraumatic hallux valgus or varus. Malunited lesser toe fractures can lead to dorsal, plantar, or interdigital corns. Intraarticular fractures with or without malunion can lead to symptomatic posttraumatic arthritis and limitation of movement, above all at the great toe resulting in hallux rigidus (limitus).
- Decreased ROM at the MTP and IP joints can result from excessive scarring after fractures and dislocations. Particularly after turf toe injuries in athletes, about 50% report persisting symptoms 5 years later. Following surgical repair for severe turf toe injuries, good clinical outcomes with return to sports in professional players have been reported in several studies.
- Overlooked subluxations ad dislocations of the lesser toes may become symptomatic with persistent pain over the heads of the MTs and chronic clawing of the affected toe due to a subsequent imbalance of the intrinsic and extrinsic muscles.
- Chronic stress fractures, nonunions, and necrosis of the sesamoids may lead to chronic pain and sesamoiditis.

9 Recommended reading

Armagan OE, Shereff MJ. Injuries to the toes and metatarsals. *Orthop Clin North Am.* 2001 Jan;32(1):1–10.

Berkowitz M, Sanders R. Dislocations of the foot. In: Coughlin MJ, Saltzman CR, Anderson JB, eds. *Mann's Surgery of the Foot & Ankle.* 9th ed. Philadelphia: Elsevier Saunders; 2013:1905–1972.

Bojsen-Møller F, Jørgensen U. The Plantar Soft Tissues: Functional Anatomy and Clinical Applications. In: Jahss MH. *Disorders of the Foot and Ankle*: Medical and Surgical Management: Saunders; 1991:532–540.

Bowers KD, Jr., Martin RB. Turf-toe: a shoe-surface related football injury. *Med Sci Sports.* 1976 Summer;8(2):81–83.

Jahss MH. Stubbing injuries to the hallux. *Foot Ankle.* 1981 May;1(6):327–332.

Karadaglis D, Grace D. Morphology of the hallux sesamoids. *Foot Ankle Surg;* 2003 Dec;9(3):165–167.

Kensinger DR, Guille JT, Horn BD, et al. The stubbed great toe: importance of early recognition and treatment of open fractures of the distal phalanx. *J Pediatr Orthop.* 2001 Jan–Feb;21(1):31–34.

Klaue K. *The foot. From evaluation to surgical correction.* Berlin Heidelberg: Springer; 2015.

Lanz J, Wachsmuth W. Pes, der Fuß. In: Lanz J, Wachsmuth W. *Praktische Anatomie—Bein und Statik.* Vol1/4. Berlin Heidelberg New York: Springer; 1972:351–444. German.

Leung WY, Wong SH, Lam JJ, et al. Presentation of a missed injury of a metatarsophalangeal joint dislocation in the lesser toes. *J Trauma.* 2001 Jun;50(6):1150–1152.

Miki T, Yamamuro T, Kitai T. An irreducible dislocation of the great toe. Report of two cases and review of the literature. *Clin Orthop Relat Res.* 1988 May;(230):200–206.

Mittlmeier T, Haar P. Sesamoid and toe fractures. *Injury.* 2004 Sep;35 Suppl 2:Sb87–97.

Rammelt S. Verletzungen des Vorfußes. In: Sabo D, ed. *Vorfußchirurgie.* 2nd ed. Berlin Heidelberg New York: Springer; 2012:139–153. German.

Rammelt S. From prehistory to judgement day: Accessory bones and sesamoids of the foot. In: Rammelt S, Zwipp H, eds. *The Foot—Arts, Myths, and Secrets.* Davos: AO Foundation; 2016: 79–102.

Rein S, Tan KJ, Rammelt S, Zwipp H. Foot and Ankle Injuries. In: Oestern HJ, Trentz O, Uranues S, eds. *European Manual of Medicine, Trauma Surgery III: Bone and Joint Injuries.* Berlin Heidelberg New York: Springer, 2014: 357–432.

Richardson EG. Hallucal sesamoid pain: causes and surgical treatment. *J Am Acad Orthop Surg.* 1999 Jul-Aug;7(4):270–278.

Sanders R, Papp S. Fractures of the midfoot and forefoot. In: Mann RA, Coughlin MJ, Saltzman CL, eds. *Surgery of the Foot and Ankle.* 8th ed. St Louis: Mosby; 2007: 2199–2235.

Sarrafian SK. *Anatomy of the foot and ankle: descriptive, topographic, functional.* 2nd ed. Philadelphia: Lippincott; 1993.

Schnaue-Constantouris EM, Birrer RB, Grisafi PJ, et al. Digital foot trauma: emergency diagnosis and treatment. *J Emerg Med.* 2002 Feb;22(2):163–170.

Smith K, Waldrop N. Operative Outcomes of Grade 3 Turf Toe Injuries in Competitive Football Players. *Foot Ankle Int.* 2018 Sep;39(9):1076–1081.

Woon CY. Dislocation of the interphalangeal joint of the great toe: is percutaneous reduction of an incarcerated sesamoid an option? A report of two cases. *J Bone Joint Surg Am.* 2010 May;92(5):1257–1260.

Zwipp H, Rammelt S. *Tscherne Unfallchirurgie: Fuß.* Berlin: Springer; 2014:434–435. German.

8.1 Unicondylar proximal phalangeal fracture of the great toe

Konrad Kamin, Stefan Rammelt

1 Case description

A 30-year-old athlete stubbed his right great toe while practicing martial arts. The man immediately experienced a sharp pain and was unable to walk normally, with an antalgic gait pattern and a limp on the right side.

He presented to the emergency department with pain, swelling, ecchymosis, and a valgus deformity of the right great toe. X-rays revealed a displaced oblique shaft fracture of the proximal phalanx of the hallux (AO/OTA 88.1.2.2A) (**Fig 8.1-1**).

2 Preoperative planning

The indication for surgery was the marked dislocation of the proximal phalanx of the hallux in an otherwise healthy and active man.

An oblique extraarticular fracture is typically fixed with two screws via a small medial approach (**Fig 8.1-2**).

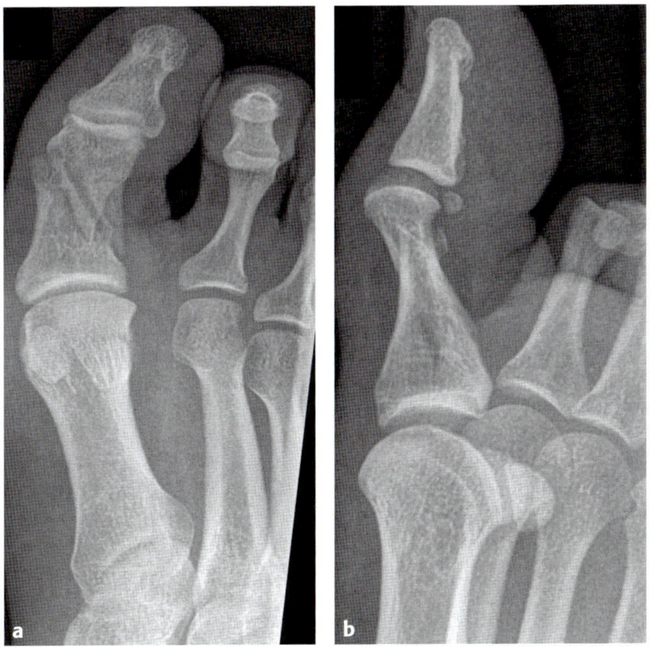

Fig 8.1-1a–b X-rays of a displaced shaft fracture of the proximal phalanx of the great toe.
a AP view.
b Oblique view.

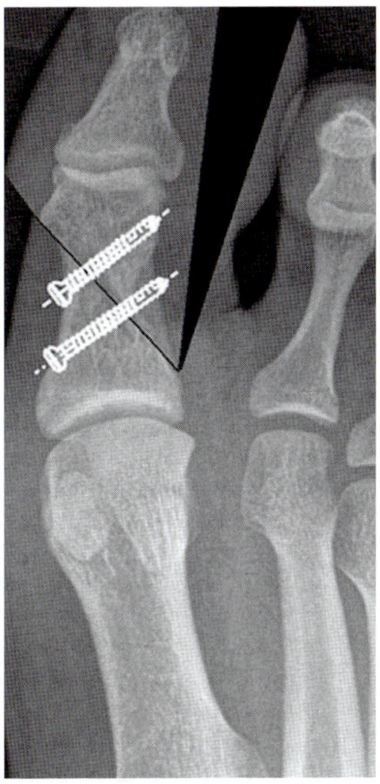

Fig 8.1-2 Preoperative plan.

3 Operating room setup

Patient positioning	• Supine on a radiolucent table
Anesthesia options	• Regional block, alternatively general or spinal anesthesia
• C-arm location	• Opposite side, toward the front side of the operative table
Tourniquet	• If needed, for the joint reduction, as per surgeon preference
Tips	• For dorsoplantar and oblique views, the knee is bent by an assistant and the foot is placed flat on the operative table

For illustrations and overview of anesthetic considerations, see chapter 1.

Equipment

- K-wires, resorbable pins
- 2.4–2.7 mm fully threaded solid cortex screws
- Interlocking plate 2.4 (if needed secondary to poor bone quality)
- Smooth and sharp elevators

Size of system, instruments, and implants may vary according to the anatomy of the patient.

4 Surgical procedure

For internal fixation according to the preoperative plan a small medial approach is used. The incision is carried out centrally on the medial aspect of the great toe, thus avoiding the dorsal and plantar neurovascular bundle (**Fig 8.1-3**). Dissection is carried directly to the bone without raising flaps.

The fragments are carefully cleared of fracture hematoma. If locked, the fragments may be loosened through manipulation with an elevator (**Fig 8.1-4a**). Reduction is achieved with longitudinal traction on the distal phalanx of the hallux. Placement of a sharp tip reduction bone holding clamp in the distal phalanx may facilitate axial traction and reduction (**Fig 8.1-4b**). After temporary K-wire fixation, anatomical reduction is checked with the C-arm. Definite fixation is achieved with small lag screws (**Fig 8.1-4c–e**).

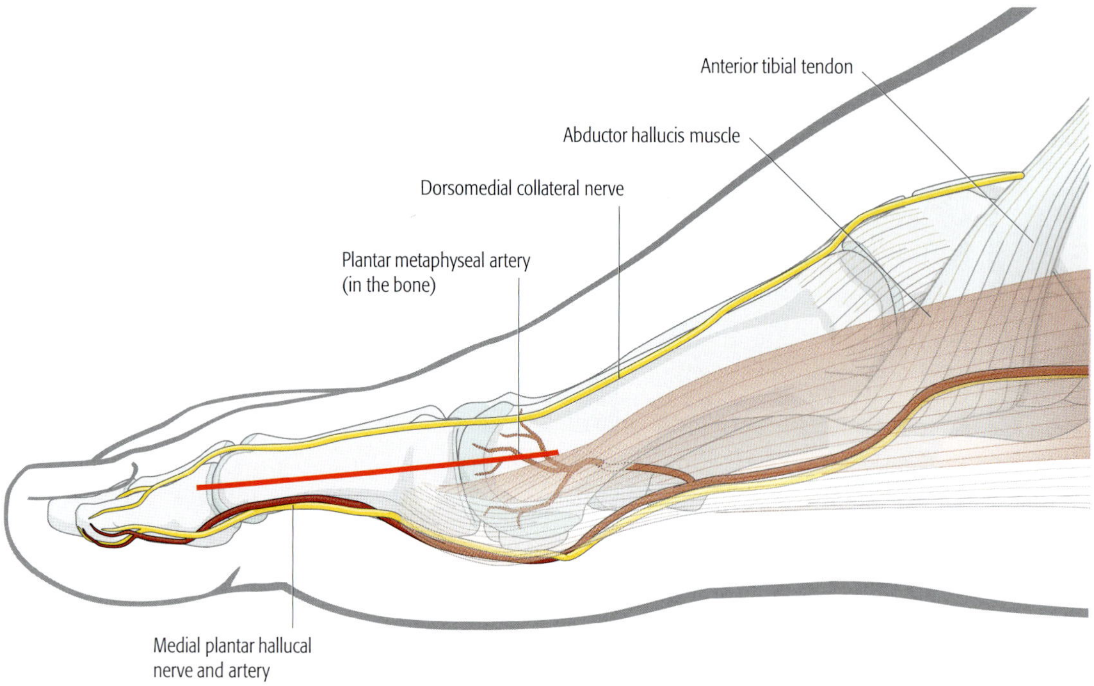

Fig 8.1-3 Direct medial approach to the proximal phalanx of the great toe.

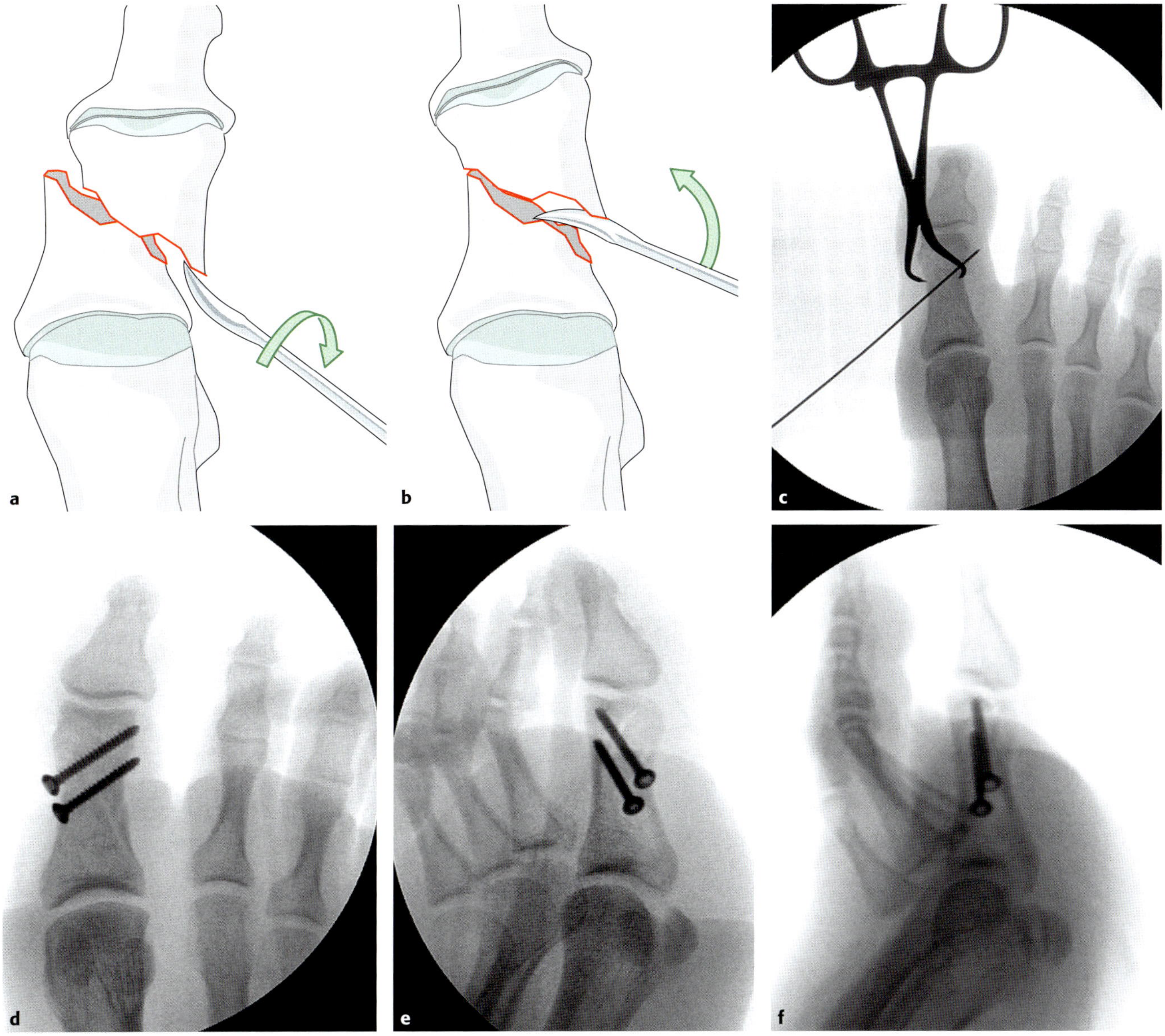

Fig 8.1-4a–f Manipulation of the fragments with a sharp elevator (**a–b**). Reduction of the displaced fracture of the proximal phalanx with a pointed reduction clamps under longitudinal traction combined with varus stress and temporary fixation with a K-wire (**c**). C-arm images in AP (**d**), oblique, (**e**), and lateral (**f**) views confirming anatomical reduction and definite fixation is achieved with 2.7 mm cortex screws.

5 Complications

- Loss of fixation
- Malunion
- Nonunion
- Posttraumatic arthritis

6 Alternative techniques

Nondisplaced fractures can be treated nonoperatively with offloading of the affected foot in a hard-sole cast, shoe or removable fracture boot for 6 weeks. Alternatively, a forefoot-offloading shoe or orthosis may be used. Repeated x-rays are obtained at 1 and 2 weeks to rule out secondary displacement, which may occur as a result of the strong pull and imbalance of the extensor hallucis longus and flexor hallucis longus.

If surgery is performed promptly, closed reduction and percutaneous screw fixation can be carried out. Crossed K-wires can be used alternatively but they offer less stability than screws (**Fig 8.1-5**). K-wires should not cross at the fracture level.

In comminuted fractures or patients with osteoporotic bone, interlocking plates can be used as a more stable means of fixation (see chapters 8 and 8.2).

7 Postoperative management and rehabilitation

Postoperatively, the foot is immobilized in a splint or hard-sole cast or a removable fracture boot. The leg is elevated. Active and passive range-of-motion (ROM) exercises of the foot and ankle are initiated on postoperative day 1 including continuous passive motion, if available. A rigid boot or foot orthosis is applied, and the patient is restricted to partial weight bearing (WB) (up to 20 kg) on the injured leg for 6 weeks. Alternatively, a forefoot-offloading shoe may be used. Weight bearing is gradually increased after 6 weeks if x-rays demonstrate fracture union. An active rehabilitation protocol is then initiated including ROM exercises of the hallux, muscular balancing, and gait training.

Implant removal

The screws are only removed if the patient feels prominent screw heads. The same surgical approach is used. Typically, removal is performed after 1 year.

8 Recommended reading

Mittlmeier T, Haar P. Sesamoid and toe fractures. *Injury.* 2004 Sep;35 Suppl 2:Sb87–97.
Sanders R, Papp S. Fractures of the midfoot and forefoot. In: Mann RA, Coughlin MJ, Saltzman CL, eds. *Surgery of the Foot and Ankle.* 8th ed. St Louis: Mosby; 2007: 2199–2235.
Zwipp H, Rammelt S. *Tscherne Unfallchirurgie: Fuß.* Berlin: Springer; 2014:434–435.

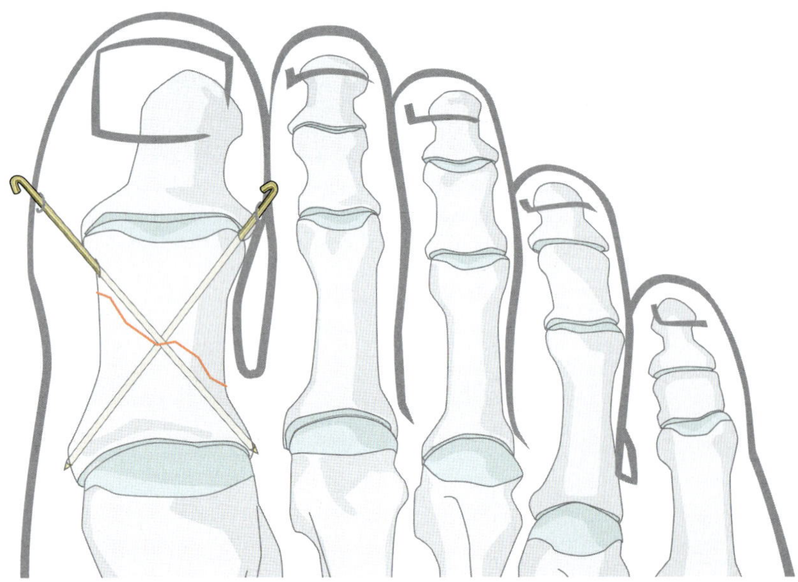

Fig 8.1-5 K-wire fixation of a simple fracture of the proximal phalanx. K-wires are removed after 4–6 weeks.

8.2 Bicondylar proximal phalangeal fracture of the great toe

Stefan Rammelt, Konrad Kamin

1 Case description

During a handball game, a 23-year-old athlete sustained a direct hit on his right foot, with subsequent immobilizing pain. The man presented to the emergency department with pain, swelling, ecchymosis, and a marked valgus and flexion deformity at the right great toe.

X-rays revealed a displaced bicondylar articular fracture of the proximal phalanx of the hallux (AO/OTA 88.1.2.3C) (**Fig 8.2-1**). Gross reduction was carried out under local anesthesia using longitudinal traction and a splint was applied.

2 Preoperative planning

Indication for surgery was axial deviation and intraarticular dislocation of the fracture in an otherwise healthy and active patient. A bicondylar fracture is typically fixed with a plate (**Fig 8.2-2**). For better access and manipulation, a medial approach is generally preferred.

3 Operating room setup

Patient positioning	• Supine on a radiolucent table
Anesthesia options	• Regional block, alternatively general or spinal anesthesia
C-arm location	• Opposite side, toward the front side of the operative table
Tourniquet	• Only at the time of joint reduction

For illustrations and overview of anesthetic considerations, see chapter 1.

Equipment

- K-wires, resorbable pins
- 2.0, 2.4, and 2.7 mm cortex screws
- Interlocking plate 2.0/2.4 (in case of poor bone quality)
- Smooth and sharp elevators
- Point-to-point reduction (Weber) clamps.

Size of system, instruments, and implants may vary according to the anatomy of the patient.

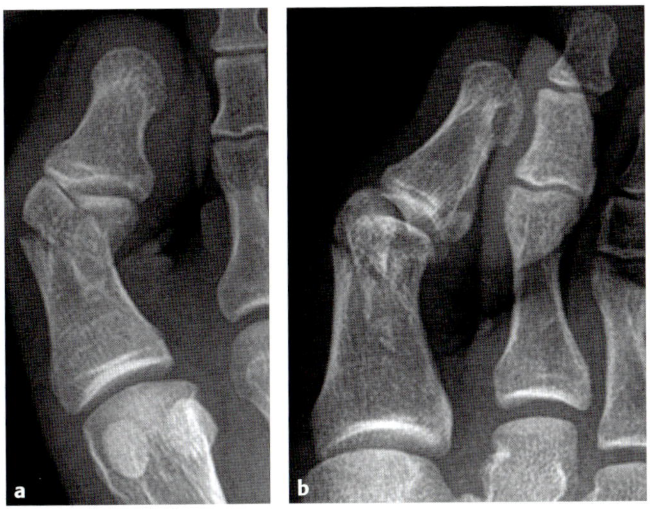

Fig 8.2-1a–b X-rays of a displaced bicondylar fracture of the proximal phalanx of the great toe.
a AP view.
b Oblique view.

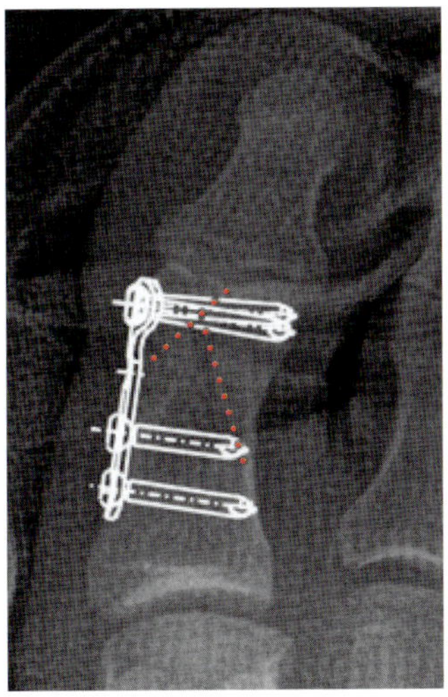

Fig 8.2-2 Preoperative plan.

4 Surgical procedure

For internal fixation according to the preoperative plan, the distal part of the straight medial utility incision or a slightly curved medial approach extending from the base of the distal phalanx to the metatarsal head is used. The incision is on the medial aspect of the great toe avoiding the dorsal and plantar neurovascular bundles (**Fig 8.2-3**). Dissection is carried directly to the bone and the interphalangeal joint capsule is opened medially. The fracture hematoma is carefully removed and the hemarthrosis is washed out of the IP joint.

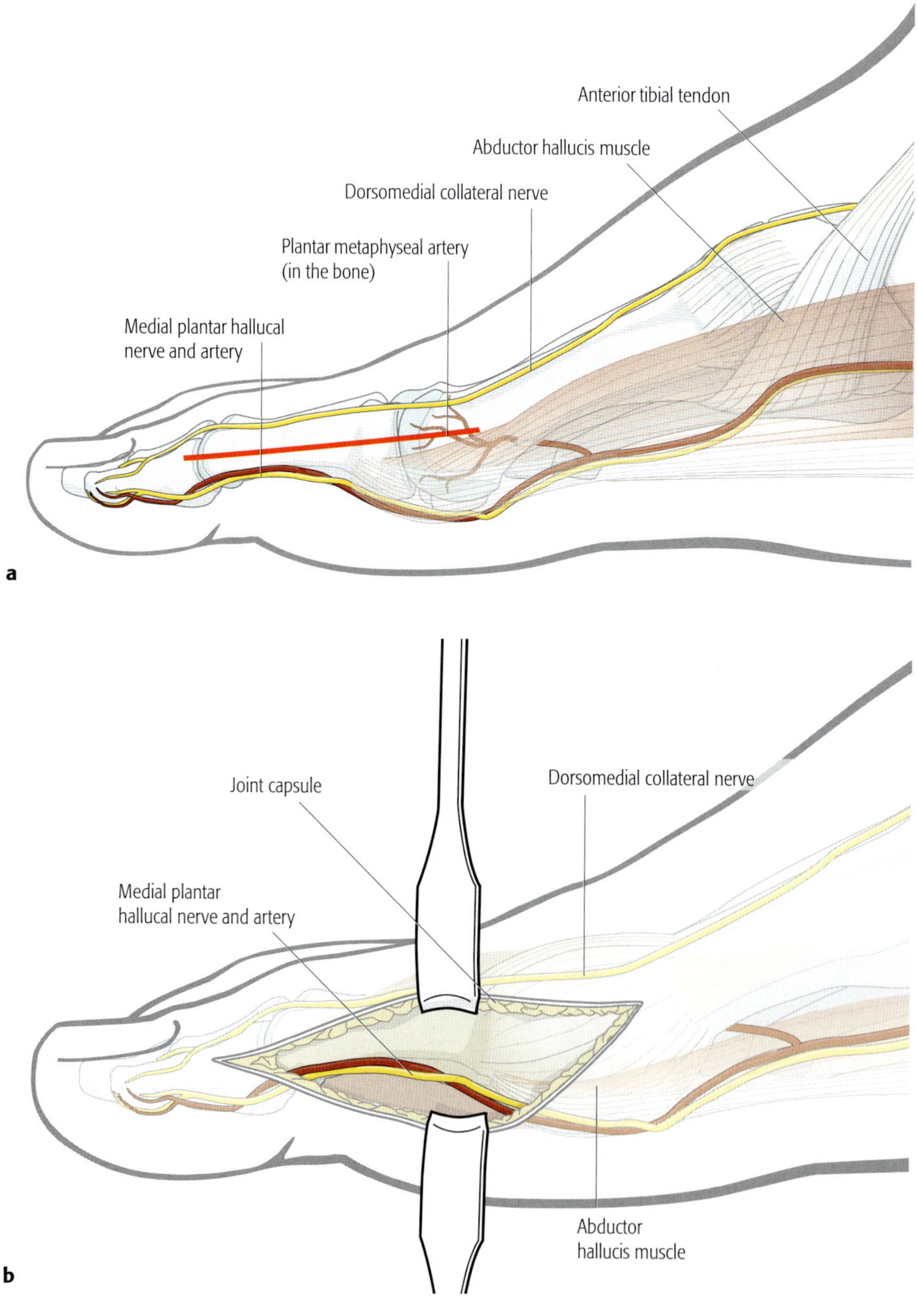

Fig 8.2-3a–b Medial approach to the proximal phalanx. The incision is carried out toward the distal phalanx and/or first metatarsal head depending on joint involvement.

Reduction starts with the articular fragments, which are reduced to each other under direct visualization and fixed temporarily with a K-wire. Reduction is facilitated with the use of a K-wire as joystick and/or a small point-to-point reduction (Weber) clamp. The reconstructed joint block is then reduced to the shaft under longitudinal traction of the great toe (**Fig 8.2-4a**).

Definite fixation is then achieved with a medial plate. The shape and size of the plate depend on the size of the fragment and the bone quality (**Fig 8.2-4b–c**). Standard postoperative x-rays demonstrate anatomical reduction.

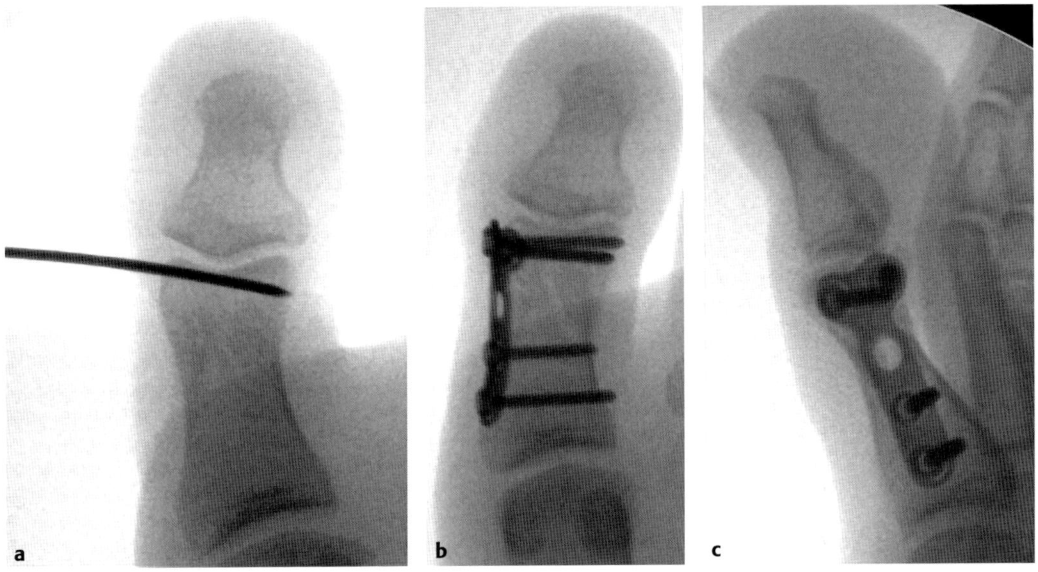

Fig 8.2-4a–c The articular condyles are reduced toward each other and fixed temporarily with a K-wire.
a The shaft fracture is then reduced by longitudinal traction.
b–c After anatomical reduction has been confirmed, definite fixation is achieved with a medial plate 2.4.

5 Complications

- Loss of fixation
- Malunion
- Nonunion
- Posttraumatic arthritis

6 Alternative techniques

Nondisplaced fractures can be treated nonoperatively with offloading of the affected foot in a hard-soled cast or shoe for 6 weeks. Alternatively, a forefoot-offloading shoe or orthosis may be used. X-rays are obtained both at 1 and 2 weeks to rule out secondary displacement.

Displaced unicondyar fractures are reduced under direct vision at the joint via a medial or lateral approach depending on the fracture location. Fixation is achieved with compression screws (**Fig 8.2-5**). The same postoperative management is used as described above for bicondylar fractures.

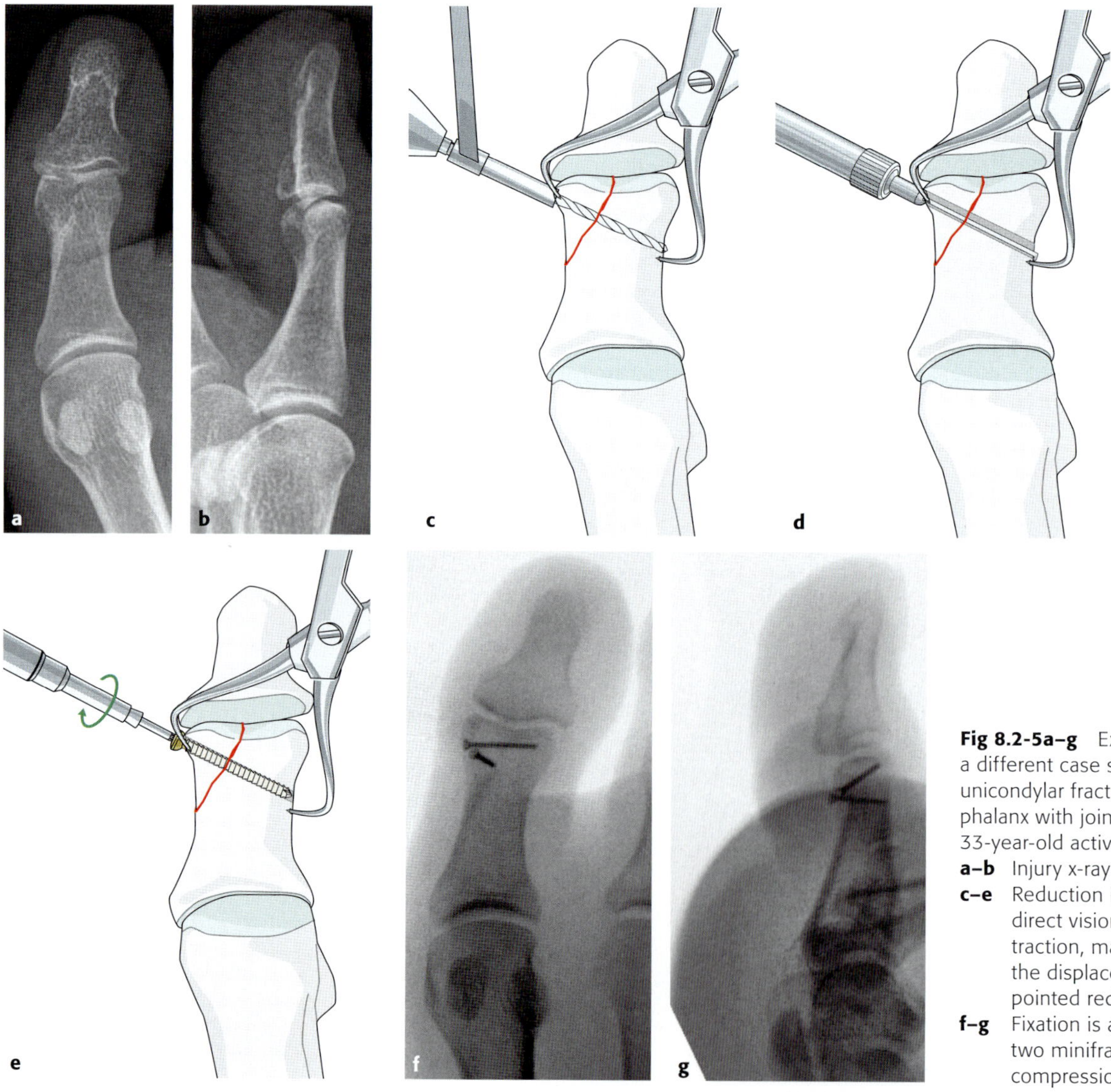

Fig 8.2-5a–g Example from a different case showing a unicondylar fracture of the proximal phalanx with joint displacement in a 33-year-old active woman
a–b Injury x-rays.
c–e Reduction is achieved under direct vision with longitudinal traction, manipulation of the displaced condyle and a pointed reduction forceps.
f–g Fixation is achieved with two minifragment 2.0 mm compression screws.

Interlocking plates may be used for fixation in osteoporotic bone or in case of comminuted fractures. Defects resulting from articular disimpaction can be filled with bone graft (**Fig 8.2-6**).

7 Postoperative management and rehabilitation

Postoperatively, the foot is immobilized in a splint or cast with a hard sole and the leg is elevated. Active and passive range-of-motion (ROM) exercises of the foot and ankle are initiated. A rigid boot or foot orthosis is applied, and the patient is restricted to partial weight bearing (up to 20 kg) on the injured leg for 6 weeks. Alternatively, a forefoot-offloading boot is applied (**Fig 1.13**). Weight bearing is gradually increased when x-rays demonstrate bony union (**Fig 8.2-7**). An active rehabilitation protocol is then initiated including ROM exercises of the great toe, muscular balancing, and gait training.

Implant removal

No standard implant removal is advised. Prominent implants are typically removed using the same approaches after 1 year.

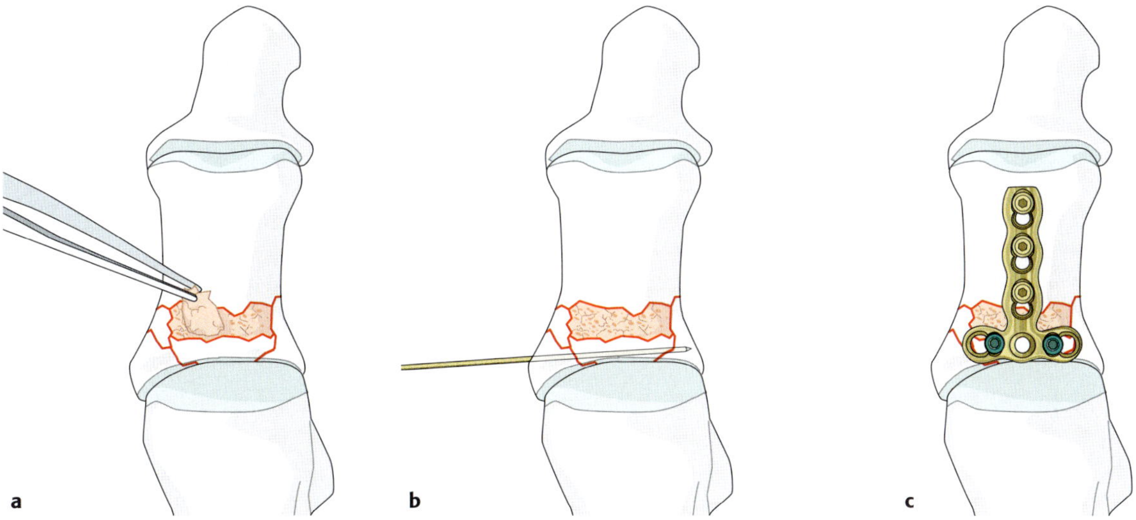

Fig 8.2-6a–c Alternative technique using bone graft and a locking plate.
a–b Defects resulting from articular disimpaction may be filled with bone graft from the calcaneus or distal tibia.
c Fixation is achieved with a locking plate bridging the defect.

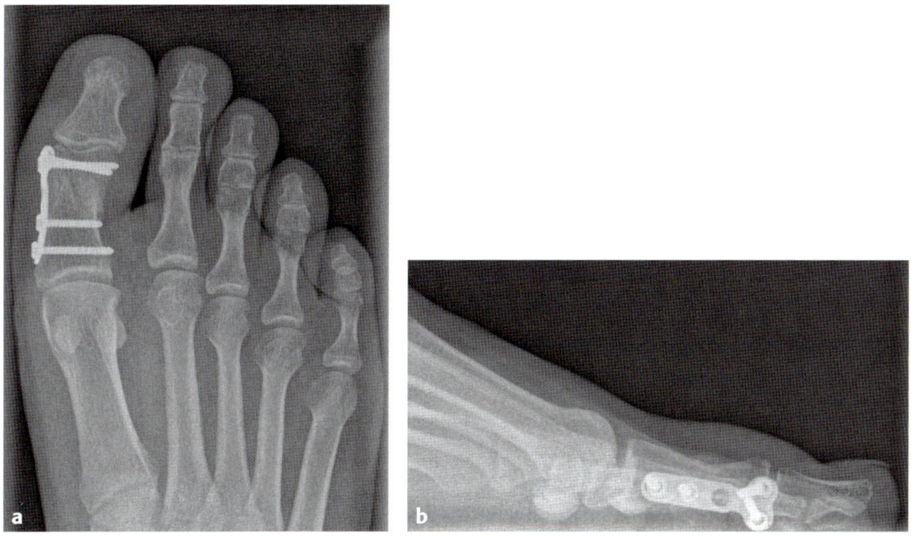

Fig 8.2-7a–b X-rays showing bony union.
a AP (dorsoplantar) view.
b Lateral view.

8 Recommended reading

Mittlmeier T, Haar P. Sesamoid and toe fractures. *Injury.* 2004 Sep;35 Suppl 2:Sb87–97.
Sanders R, Papp S. Fractures of the midfoot and forefoot. In: Mann RA, Coughlin MJ, Saltzman CL, eds. *Surgery of the Foot and Ankle.* 8th ed. St Louis: Mosby; 2007: 2199–2235.
Zwipp H, Rammelt S. *Tscherne Unfallchirurgie: Fuß.* Berlin: Springer; 2014:434–435. German.

8.3 Lesser toe fracture

Stefan Rammelt, Konrad Kamin

1 Case description

A 21-year-old man hit his bare left forefoot against a cupboard. He presented to the emergency department with second toe pain, swelling, ecchymosis, and deformity (**Fig 8.3-1**). No open wounds or neurovascular deficit were noted.

X-rays revealed a fracture dislocation of the lateral condyle of the proximal phalanx of the second toe (AO/OTA 88.2.1.3C) (**Fig 8.3-2**).

2 Preoperative planning

Closed reduction is the treatment of choice for most fractures and dislocations of the lesser toes. For this patient, the dislocation of the lateral condyle at the proximal interphalangeal (PIP) joint of the second toe, which was rotated more than 90° rendered the fracture irreducible by closed manipulation. Therefore, surgery with open reduction and internal fixation (ORIF) is indicated. After reduction of the condyle via a direct lateral approach over the PIP joint, the PIP joint will be transfixed with an axial K-wire.

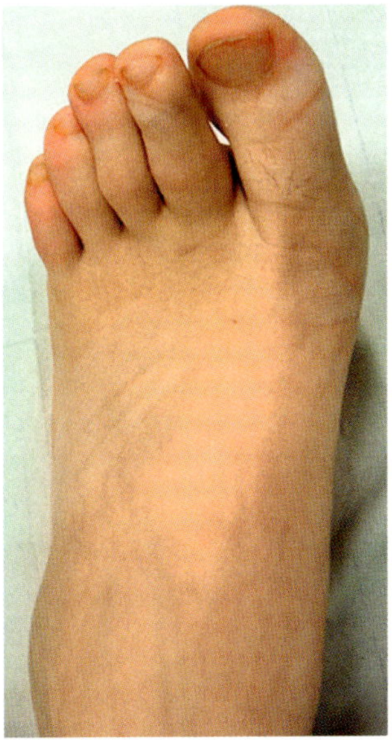

Fig 8.3-1 Clinical aspect of the left forefoot with swelling, ecchymosis, and visible deformity at the proximal interphalangeal joint of the second toe.

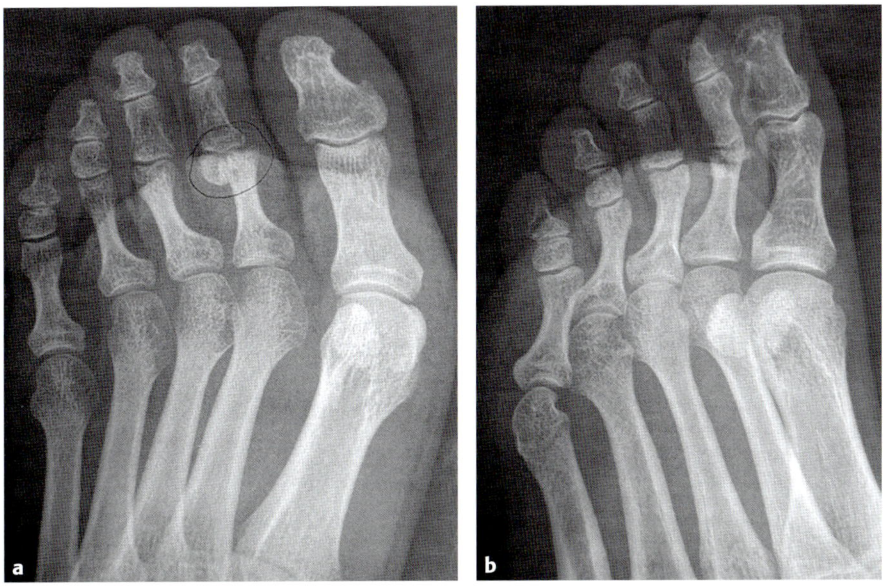

Fig 8.3-2a–b X-rays of the left forefoot showing a rotated fracture of the medial condyle of the proximal phalanx of the second toe.
a AP (dorsoplantar) view.
b Oblique view.

3 Operating room setup

Patient positioning	• Supine on a radiolucent table
Anesthesia options	• Regional block, alternatively general or spinal anesthesia
C-arm location	• Opposite side, toward the front side of the operative table
Tourniquet	• Only for joint reduction, if needed

For illustrations and overview of anesthetic considerations, see chapter 1.

Equipment

- K-wires of several sizes
- Wire driver
- Mini-C-arm
- Small fragment screws (2.0 mm) for alternative fixation

4 Surgical procedure

The PIP joint is approached directly from lateral. The dislocated and rotated lateral condyle of the proximal phalanx is seen through the skin incision (**Fig 8.3-3a**).

The condylar fragment is manipulated with a 1.4 mm K-wire used as a joystick (**Fig 8.3-3b–c**).

Fixation is achieved with a K-wire introduced percutaneously in a retrograde, axial manner from the tip of the second toe (**Fig 8.3-3d–f**). Alternatively, the wire may be drilled from the fracture site antegrade out through the tip of the toe, and then retrograde drilled back into the toe. This affords a better view of the fracture site and a more accurate direct reduction and fixation. Either way, the wire should exit the tip of the toe just plantar to the nail bed.

Any defects of the extensor tendon or capsule are reconstructed after bony stabilization. The wound is closed primarily.

5 Complications

- Loss of fixation
- Chronic instability
- Stiffness
- Posttraumatic arthritis
- Malreduction with varus/valgus deformity or malrotation

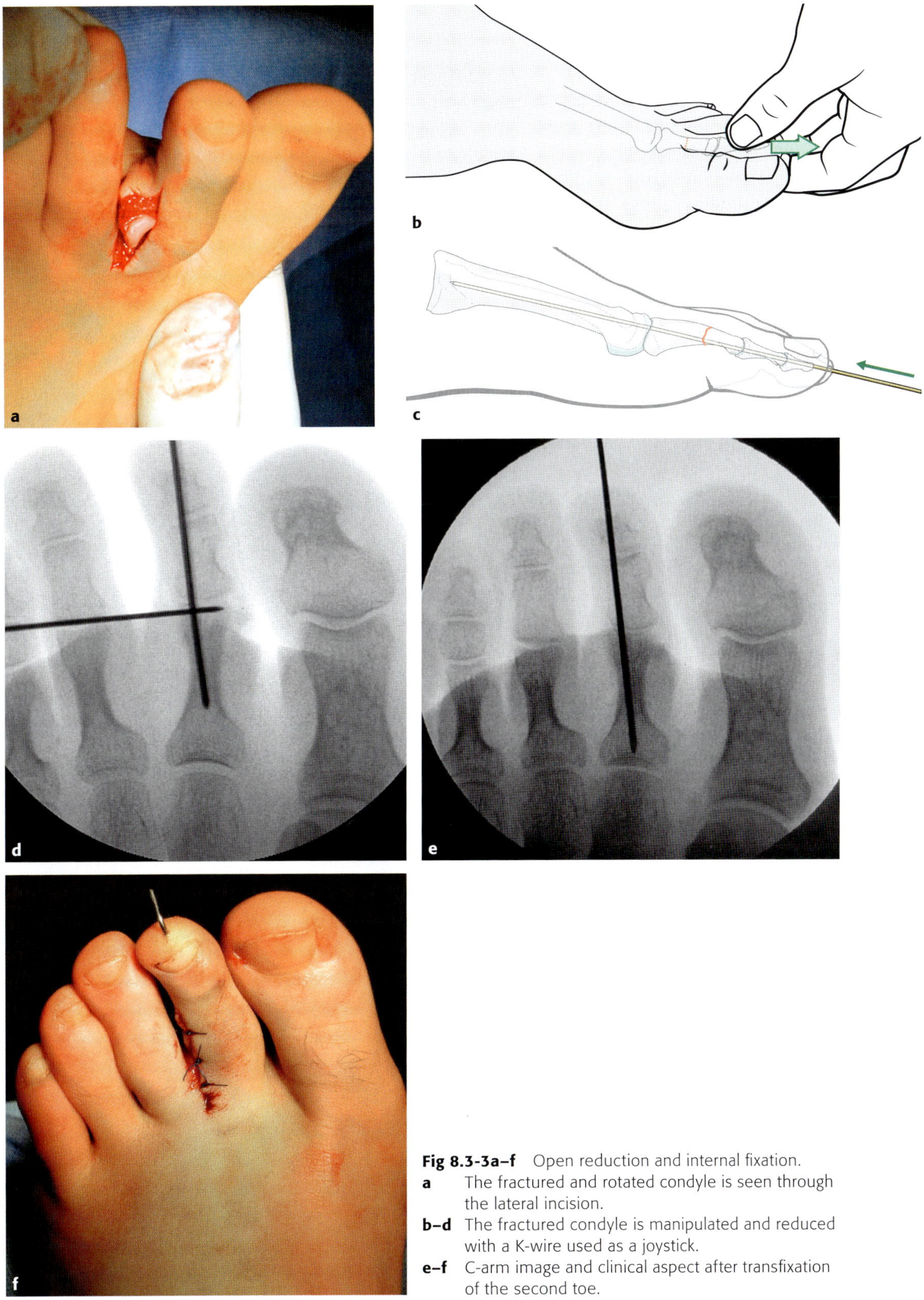

Fig 8.3-3a–f Open reduction and internal fixation.

- **a** The fractured and rotated condyle is seen through the lateral incision.
- **b–d** The fractured condyle is manipulated and reduced with a K-wire used as a joystick.
- **e–f** C-arm image and clinical aspect after transfixation of the second toe.

6 Alternative techniques

Most lesser toe fractures can be treated with closed reduction. Regional anesthetic block is applied at the toe base. Reduction is achieved through longitudinal traction and closed manipulation. The affected toe is then stabilized with tape or Velcro strapping to one intact neighboring toe. The intact toe acts as a stabilizing splint (buddy taping). Reduction is documented with x-rays after applying the strapping (**Fig 8.3-4**). A large condylar fragment can alternatively be fixed with a small fragment screw (2.0 mm).

Nondisplaced fractures can also be treated with strapping (**Fig 8.3-5**).

Tip: once the regional block is applied and the toe is numb, the surgeon can place a pencil in the web space at the base of the toe. This will serve as a fulcrum for reduction of varus or valgus displacement. The pencil is then removed, and a gauze is placed between the toes before the strapping is secured.

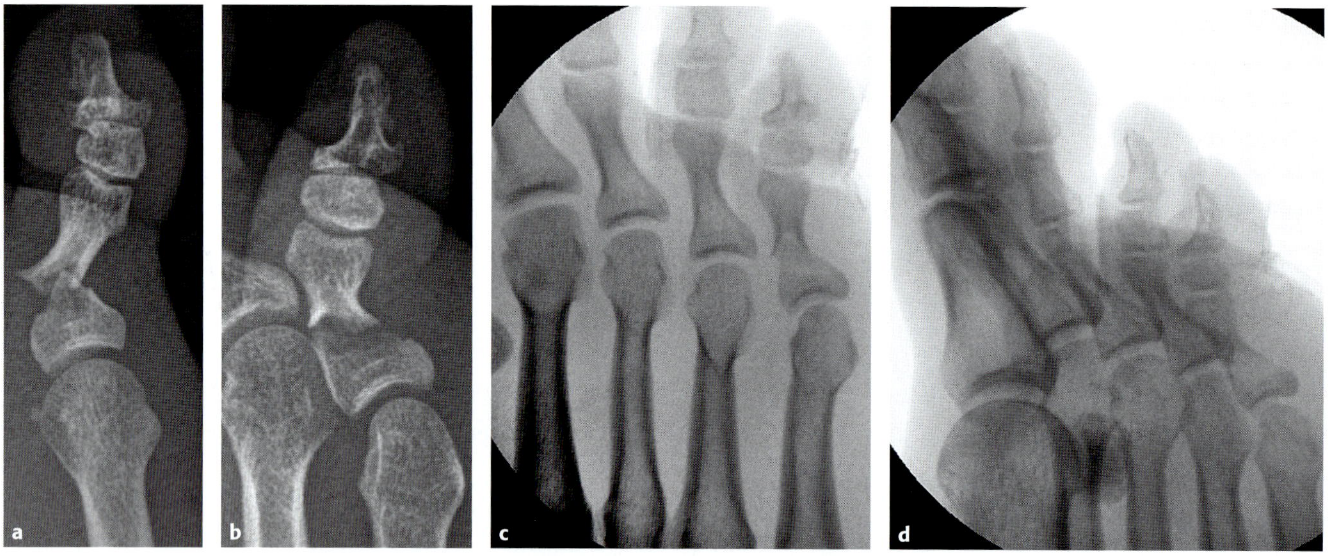

Fig 8.3-4a–d Example from a different case showing the alternative technique using strapping.
a–b Displaced fracture of the proximal phalanx of the fifth toe.
c–d X-rays after closed reduction and "buddy taping" to the fourth toe showing acceptable alignment.

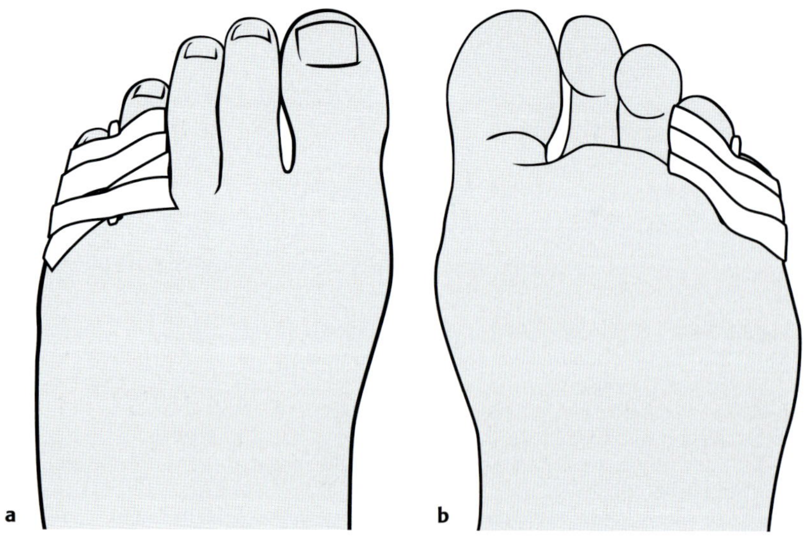

Fig 8.3-5a–b Alternative technique for stabilization of the fractured toe against the neighboring toe through strapping.

7 Postoperative management and rehabilitation

Postoperatively, the foot is immobilized in a forefoot-offloading shoe or a hard-sole cast and the leg is elevated. Reduction is confirmed on standard AP and lateral x-rays. The K-wire is removed after 6 weeks (**Fig 8.3-6**).

An active rehabilitation protocol is then initiated including range-of-motion exercises, muscular balancing, and gait training.

If it is necessary to place the wire across the metatarsophalangeal (MTP) joint, then it is important that the toe is fixed in a slightly plantar flexed position at the MTP joint. After the wire is removed, the toe will naturally drift back dorsal with gait. However, if the toe is fixed with the wire in dorsiflexion at the MTP joint, it may be difficult to regain proper toe position due to dorsiflexion contracture at the MTP joint. This may lead to transfer metatarsalgia and a deformity such a "floating toe".

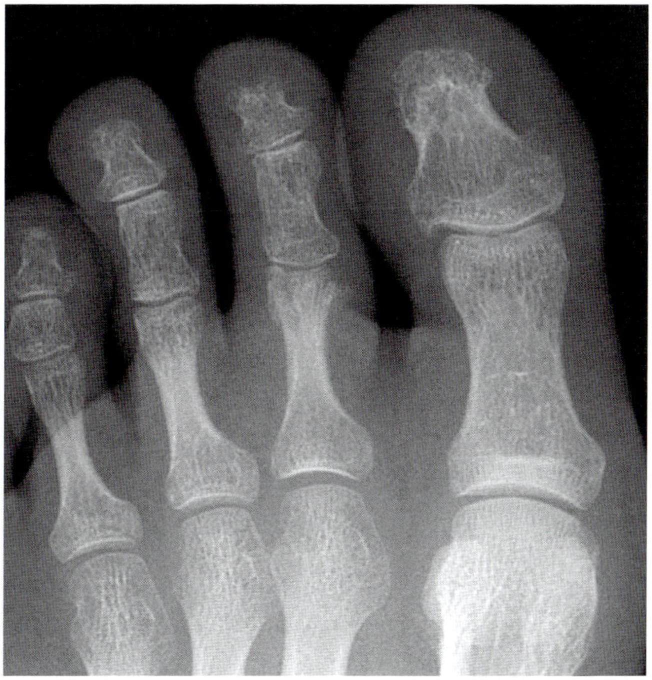

Fig 8.3-6 AP x-ray after removal of the K-wire demonstrating bony union at 6 weeks.

8 Recommended reading

Hughes J, Clark P, Klenerman L. The importance of the toes in walking. *J Bone Joint Surg Br.* 1990 Mar;72(2):245–251.
Mittlmeier T, Haar P. Sesamoid and toe fractures. *Injury.* 2004 Sep;35 Suppl 2:Sb87–97.
Zwipp H, Rammelt S. *Tscherne Unfallchirurgie: Fuß.* Berlin: Springer; 2014:434–435. German

8.4 Lesser toe dislocation

Konrad Kamin, Stefan Rammelt

1 Case description

A 23-year-old man hit his toe barefoot against a cupboard. He presented to the emergency department with a dislocated second toe and a 1 cm open wound at the medial proximal interphalangeal (PIP) joint. X-rays on admission revealed no bony injuries but a clear dislocation of the second toe in the PIP joint (**Fig 8.4-1**).

The injury was classified as a Gustilo-Anderson Grade II open dislocation of the second toe at the PIP joint (see the Gustilo-Anderson classification in the appendix).

2 Preoperative planning

Closed reduction is the treatment of choice for most fractures and dislocations of the lesser toes. In this case, the unstable, open dislocation of the second toe resulted in an indication for surgery.

3 Operating room setup

Patient positioning	• Supine on a radiolucent table
Anesthesia options	• Regional block, alternatively general or spinal anesthesia
C-arm location	• Opposite side, toward the front side of the operative table
Tourniquet	• Not needed

For illustrations and overview of anesthetic considerations, see chapter 1.

Equipment

- K-wires of several sizes

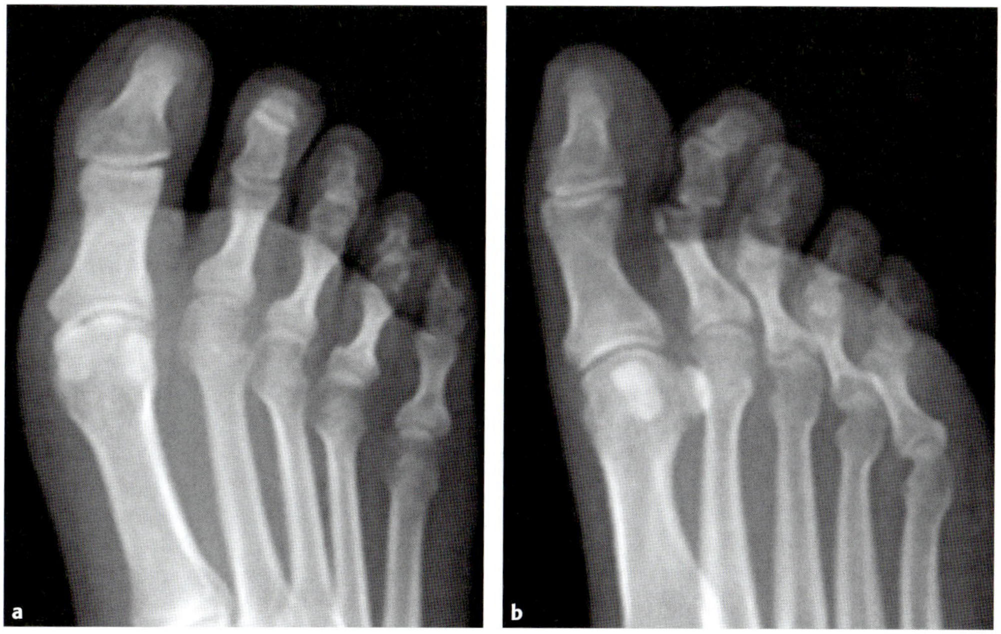

Fig 8.4-1a–b X-rays of the left forefoot.
a AP (dorsoplantar) view.
b Oblique view.

4 Surgical procedure

On rare occasions it is necessary to extend the traumatic wound to manage the injury.

The open wound is debrided and irrigated. The debridement is followed by open reduction via the existing wound, typically through longitudinal traction. Fixation is achieved with a K-wire introduced percutaneously in a retrograde, axial manner from the tip of the toe (**Fig 8.4-2**). Alternatively, the K-wire may be introduced in an antegrade manner through the open wound over the joint and then driven back retrograde across the fracture after exiting the tip of the toe.

Defects of the extensor tendon or capsule are reconstructed after bony stabilization. The wound is closed primarily by interrupted sutures.

5 Complications

- Loss of fixation
- Chronic instability
- Stiffness
- Posttraumatic arthritis

6 Alternative techniques

Most closed dislocations of the lesser toes can be treated with closed reduction. A toe block is performed at the toe base if there is significant pain or if manipulation is to be performed. Reduction is achieved through longitudinal traction and counteraction to the dislocating force. The affected toe is then stabilized by an intact neighboring toe with tape or Velcro strapping (buddy taping, see chapter 8.3). Adequate reduction is documented with x-rays after applying the tape or strap. Nondisplaced fractures can also be treated with buddy taping without attempts of reduction.

Temporary K-wire transfixation is only needed if the joint remains unstable after closed reduction. The same principles apply to the metatarsophalangeal (MTP) joint (**Fig 8.4-3**). If closed reduction is impossible, the joint is approached from dorsal and cleared of intervening tissue which is blocking reduction. Obvious tears in the capsule and plantar plate may be repaired.

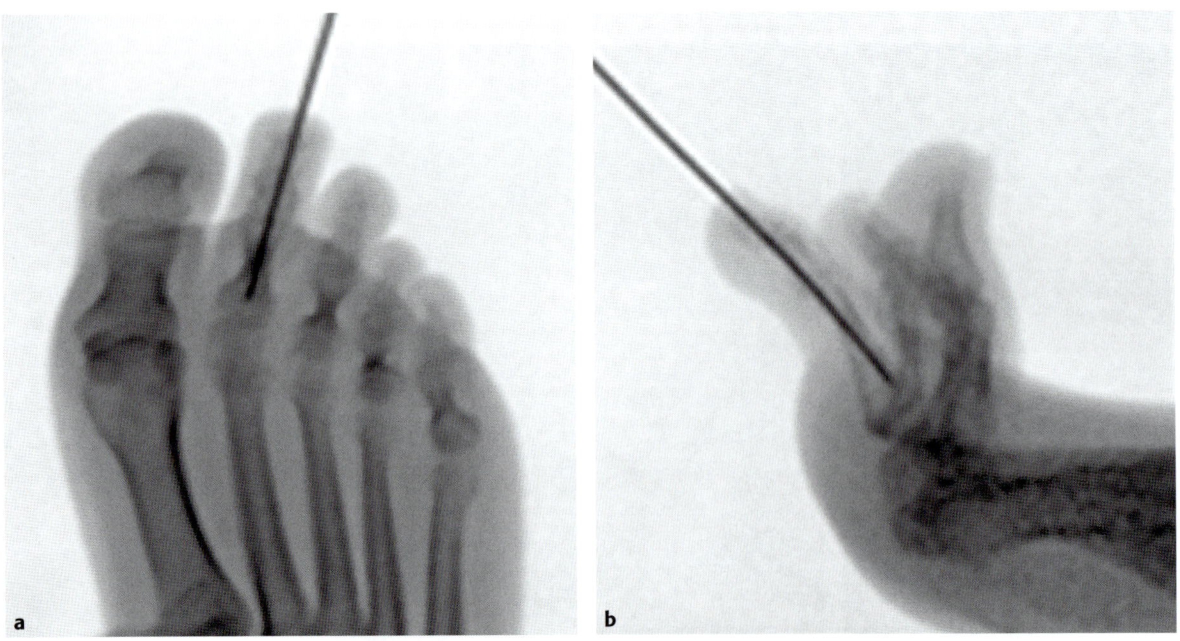

Fig 8.4-2a–b Intraoperative x-ray after open reduction and K-wire transfixation of the second toe.
a AP (dorsoplantar) view.
b Lateral view.

7 Postoperative management and rehabilitation

Postoperatively, the foot is immobilized in a forefoot-offloading shoe or a hard-soled cast and the leg is elevated. Standard postoperative x-rays should demonstrate anatomical reduction. The K-wire is removed after 5 weeks. As the wire should be a smooth wire, it usually comes out easily without the need for anesthesia of any type.

An active rehabilitation protocol is then initiated at 6 weeks postoperatively including range-of-motion exercises, muscular balancing, and gait training with progression of weight bearing on the forefoot as tolerated.

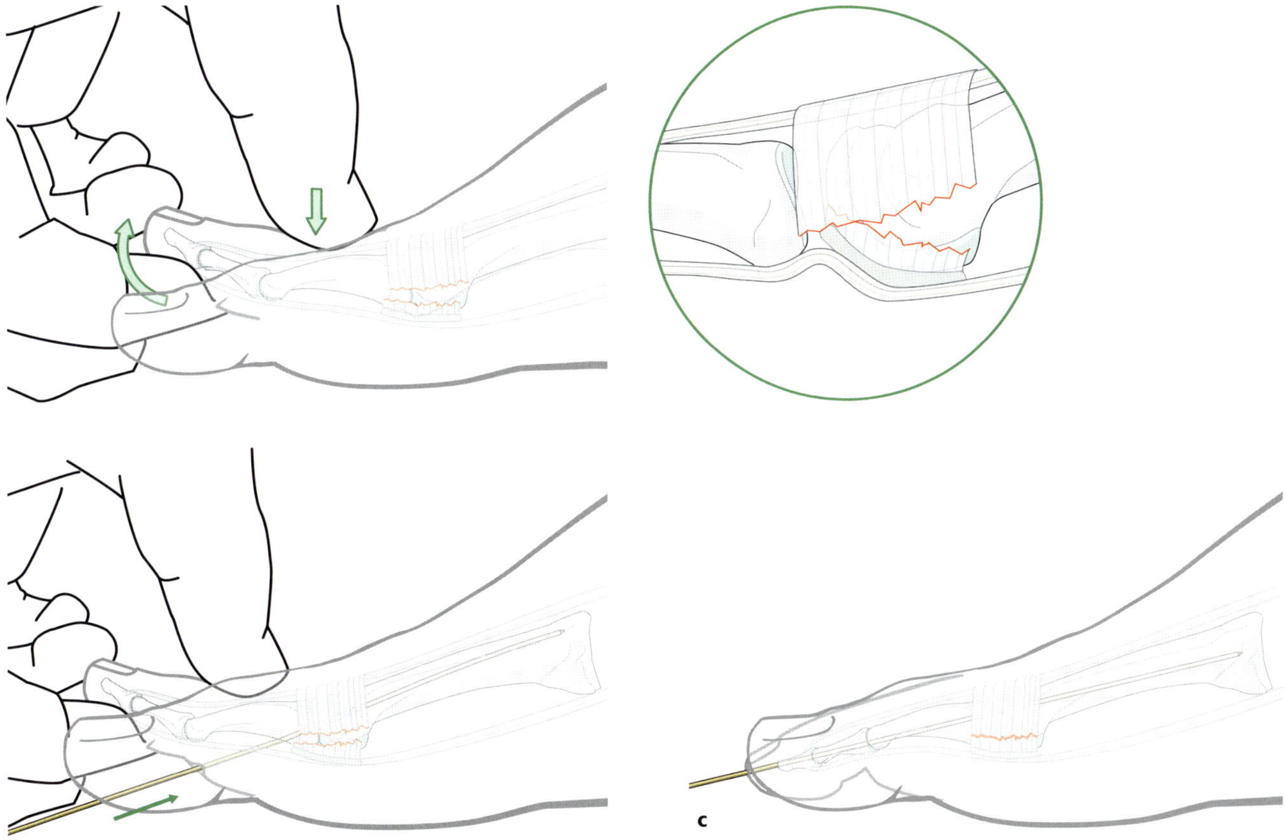

a b c

Fig 8.4-3a–c Closed reduction of a MTP dislocation (**a**) and temporary retrograde K-wire transfixation of the affected toe. The K-wire either catches the base of the proximal phalanx and is then driven across the joint into the shaft of the corresponding metatarsal while the reduction is maintained (**b**). Alternatively, an intramedullary K-wire is driven through the entire toe beginning just under the nail all the way to the shaft of the metatarsal (**c**).

8 Recommended reading

Gustilo RB, Anderson JT. Prevention of infection in the treatment of one thousand and twenty-five open fractures of long bones: retrospective and prospective analyses. *J Bone Joint Surg Am.* 1976 Jun;58(4):453–458.

Mittlmeier T, Haar P. Sesamoid and toe fractures. *Injury.* 2004 Sep;35 Suppl 2:Sb87–97.

Zwipp H, Rammelt S. *Tscherne Unfallchirurgie: Fuß.* Berlin: Springer; 2014:434–435. German.

8.5 Sesamoid fracture

Stefan Rammelt, Konrad Kamin

1 Case description

A 21-year-old female athlete presented with pain beneath the left great toe for 3 months following a jump with hyperdorsiflexion of the great toe. Nonoperative measures, such as temporary offloading, soft insoles, and physical therapy, provided no pain relief. X-rays at the time of presentation showed a bipartite medial sesamoid at the first metatarsophalangeal (MTP) joint. (**Fig 8.5-1**).

Computed tomographic (CT) scans revealed an irregular, ragged line between the two fragments of the medial sesamoid of the great toe. The distal fragment was slightly displaced laterally (**Fig 8.5-2**).

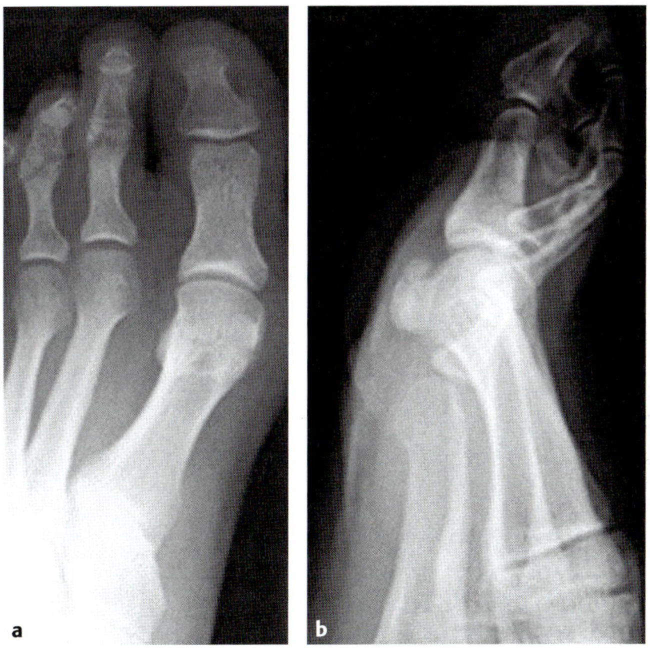

Fig 8.5-1a–b X-rays showing a bipartite medial sesamoid at the first MTP joint.
a AP (dorsoplantar) view.
b Lateral view.

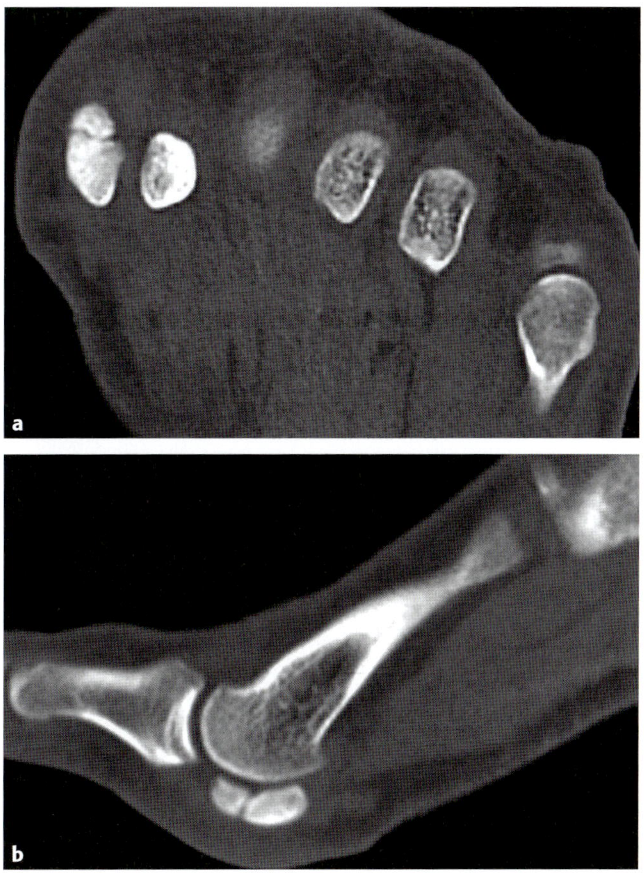

Fig 8.5-2a–b Computed tomographic images raising the suspicion of a 3-month-old fracture of the medial sesamoid at the first MTP joint.
a Axial view.
b Sagittal view.

Magnetic resonance imaging (MRI) showed edema of the medial sesamoid, and raised the suspicion of an acute injury (**Fig 8.5-3**). The findings were compatible with a 3-month-old fracture of the medial sesamoid. The differential diagnosis included a bipartite medial sesamoid that became symptomatic after the injury.

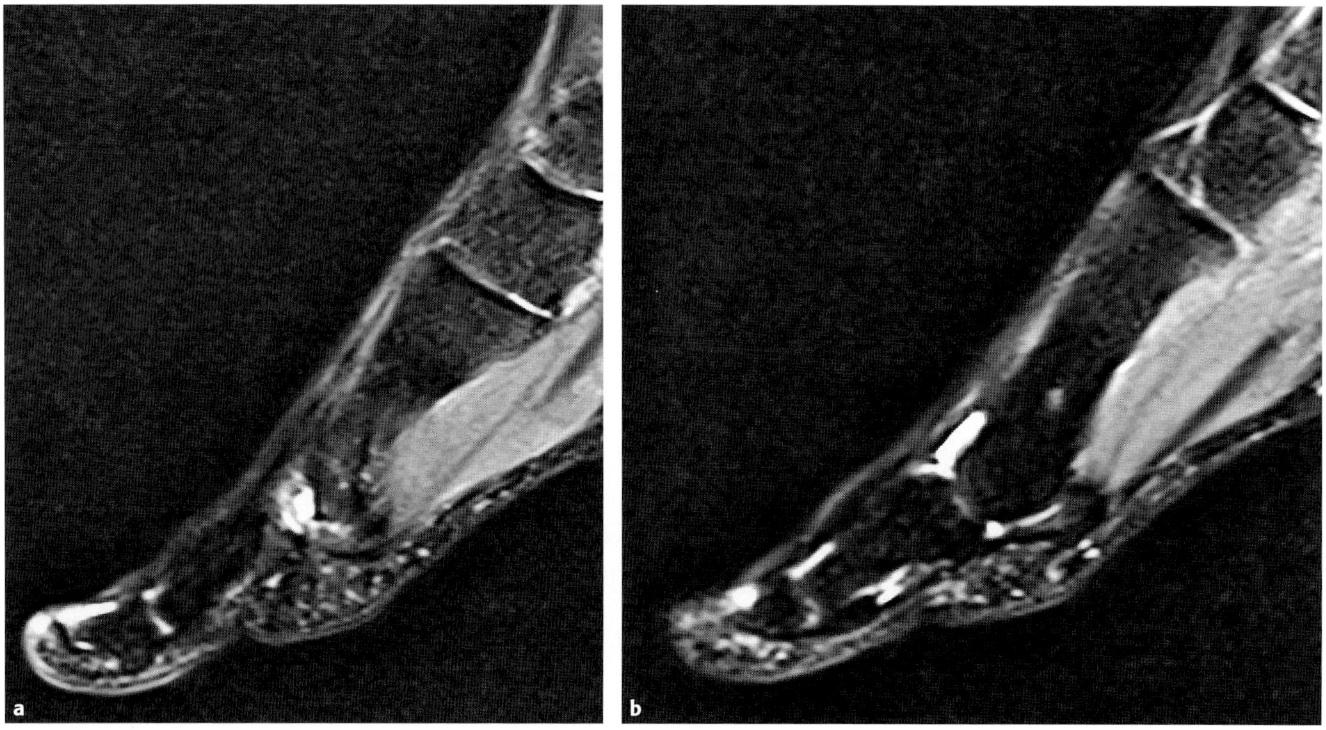

Fig 8.5-3 The MRI showing edema at the medial sesamoid at the first MTP joint indicating a subacute injury.

2 Preoperative planning

The decision for surgery was made after an attempt of nonoperative treatment failed for more than 3 months. Because an acute fracture with two relatively large fragments was suspected, the patient was scheduled for internal fixation. With multiple fragmentation, fragments that do not fit together, or necrosis of one or both parts, internal fixation could not be considered.

Forced hyperdorsiflexion as reported by the patient is an adequate fracture mechanism through a pull of the flexor hallucis brevis (FHB) tendon, with the first metatarsal head acting as a fulcrum (hypomochlion) (**Fig 8.5-4**). Because of the small size of the distal fragment, one minifragment screw was planned to be introduced from distal to proximal via a small medial approach (**Fig 8.5-5**). In case of a symptomatic bipartition through loosening of the formerly asymptomatic parts, treatment options should include debridement and fusion of the two parts. Removal of the smaller fragments with FHB repair and flexor hallucis longus transfer to the base of the proximal phalanx is also a possibility, particularly with multiple fragmentation or necrosis of the sesamoid.

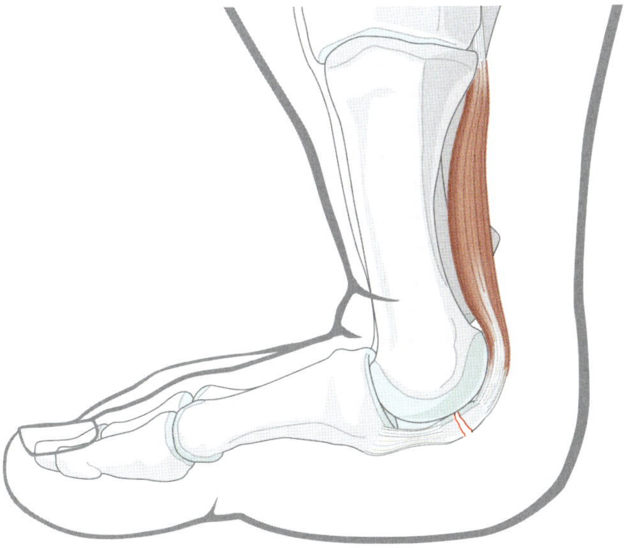

Fig 8.5-4 Trauma mechanism for sesamoid fracture through hyperextension. Acute sesamoid fractures also occur in the wake of first metatarsophalangeal joint dislocations.

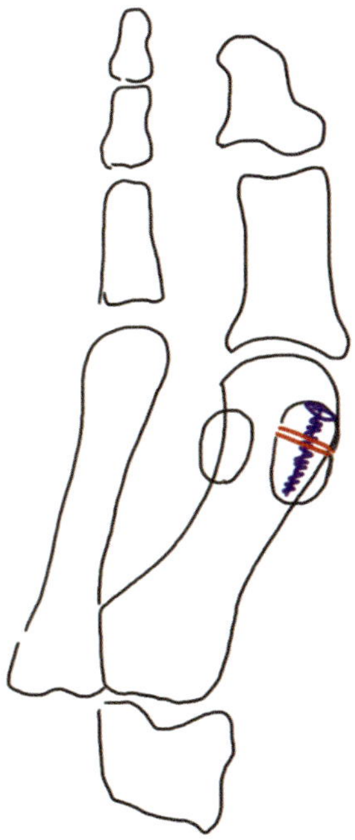

Fig 8.5-5 Preoperative plan for internal fixation.

3 Operating room setup

Patient positioning	• Supine, on a radiolucent table
Anesthesia options	• Regional block, alternatively general or spinal anesthesia
C-arm location	• Opposite side, toward the front side of the operative table
Tourniquet	• Only for the time of joint reduction

For illustrations and overview of anesthetic considerations, see chapter 1.

Equipment

- K-wires
- 1.5 or 2.0 mm cortex screws

Size of system, instruments, and implants may vary according to the anatomy of the patient.

4 Surgical procedure

The medial sesamoid is accessed via a medial approach at the border to the glabrous plantar skin. The skin and subcutaneous tissue are dissected, and the capsule of the first MTP joint is incised in a longitudinal fashion (**Fig 8.5-6**). For this patient, a subacute sesamoid fracture with cancellous fracture ends was seen on opening the fracture (**Fig 8.5-7a**). The fracture gap is cleared of fibrous tissue and the fragments are reduced anatomically under direct vision at the joint surface toward the first metatarsal head (**Fig 8.5-7b–c**). A 1.0 mm K-wire is used for temporary fixation. Internal fixation is achieved with one 1.5 mm screw (**Fig 8.5-7d–e**).

5 Complications

- Loss of fixation
- Malunion
- Nonunion
- Posttraumatic arthritis

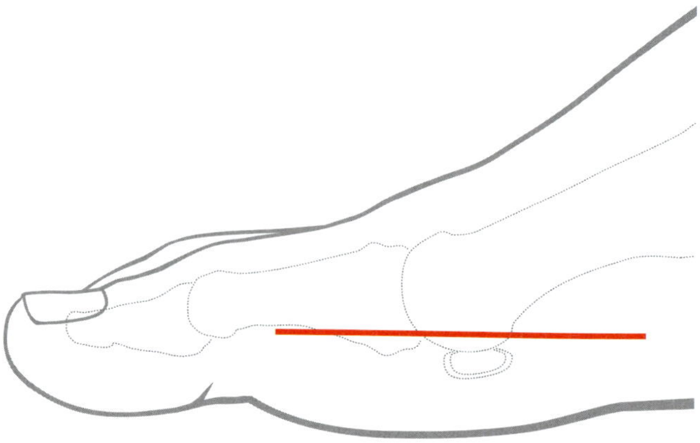

a

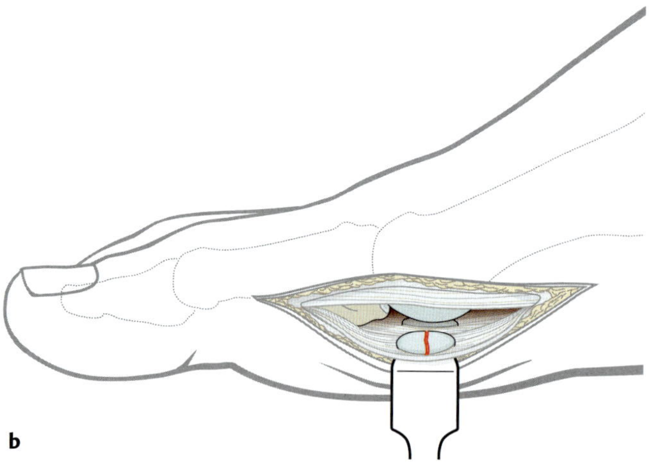

b

Fig 8.5-6a–b Medial approach to the medial hallucal sesamoid.

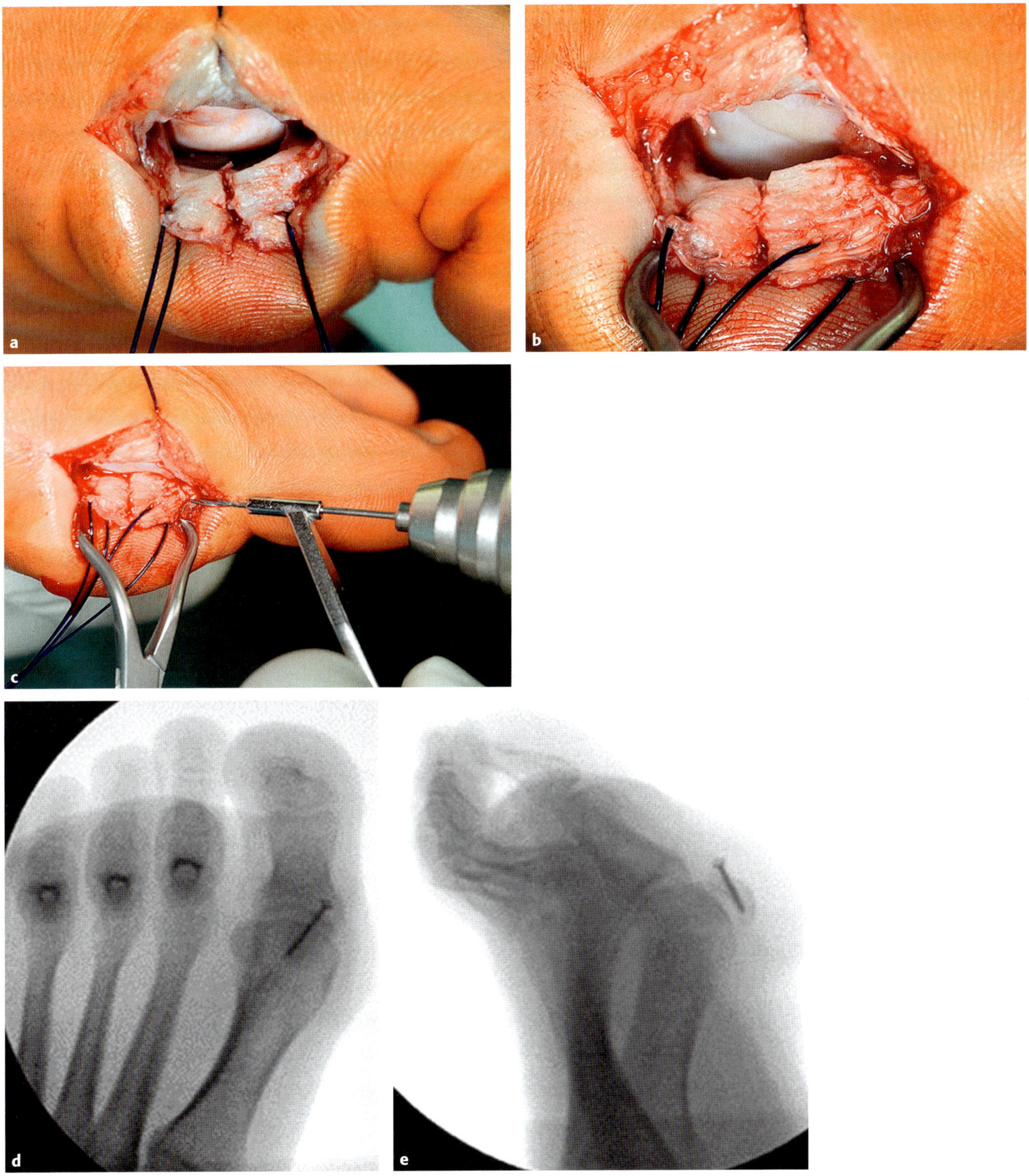

Fig 8.5-7a–e Upon direct inspection a subacute fracture with sharp cancellous edges is noted (**a**). The fragments are cleared of debris and reduced anatomically with a point-to-point reduction (Weber) clamps (**b**). A 1.0 mm hole is drilled (**c**) and internal fixation is achieved with a single 1.5 mm cortex screw introduced from distal through the smaller fragment as seen on the AP (**d**) and lateral (**e**) C-arm images. The fibers of the extensor hallucis brevis that are marked with resorbable sutures are reattached at the end of the surgery.

6 Alternative techniques

Nondisplaced fractures can be treated nonoperatively with a forefoot-offloading shoe for 6 weeks.

If the lateral sesamoid is injured, it is approached via a plantar incision in the skinfold between the first and second toes. The vascular bundle is thereby spared and the sesamoid can be approached from the lateral side (**Fig 8.5-8**).

Depending on the size of the fragments, two screws may be used for more rigid fixation. Alternatively, percutaneous screw fixation in hyperextension position of the great toe has been described. However, care must be taken not to displace the fracture with that maneuver.

If a nonunion or a symptomatic bipartition with traumatic loosening of the two fragments is detected, debridement of the fragments is followed by fusion of the two parts with local cancellous bone grafting (eg, from the middle cuneiform). If no congruent joint surface toward the first metatarsal head can be achieved or if the distal fragment is too small for internal fixation, the smaller distal fragment is excised. Care is taken to suture the fibers of the FHB tendon (**Fig. 8.5-4**). Complete sesamoidectomy is not encouraged, as it may lead to persistent symptoms.

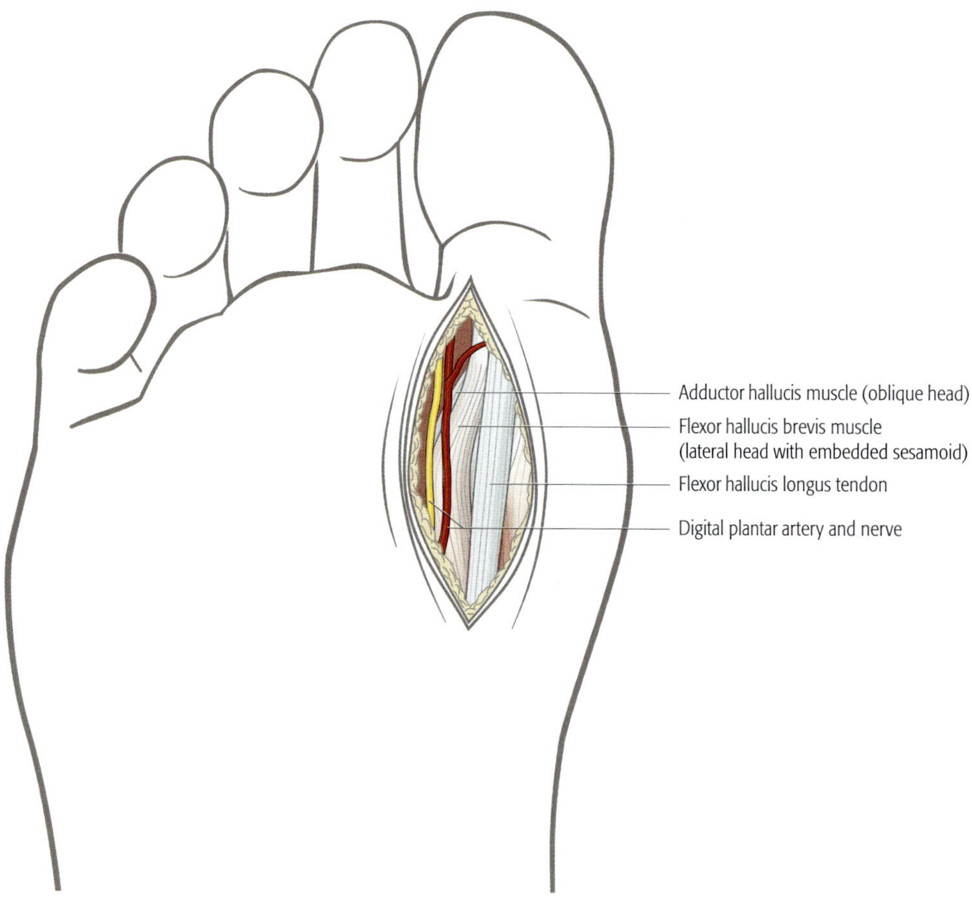

Fig 8.5-8 Plantar approach to the lateral hallucal sesamoid.

7 Postoperative management and rehabilitation

Postoperatively, the foot is immobilized in a splint with an extended toe plate and the leg is elevated. Active and passive range-of-motion (ROM) exercises are initiated 1 week postoperatively. A forefoot offloading fracture boot, an individually hard-soled cast or foot orthosis is applied, and the patient is restricted to partial weight bearing (up to 20 kg) on the injured leg for 6 weeks.

Standard postoperative x-rays demonstrate anatomical reduction. Weight bearing is gradually increased after 6 weeks if x-rays demonstrate bony union (**Fig 8.5-9** and **Fig 8.5-10**). An active rehabilitation protocol is then initiated including ROM exercises, muscular balancing, and gait training.

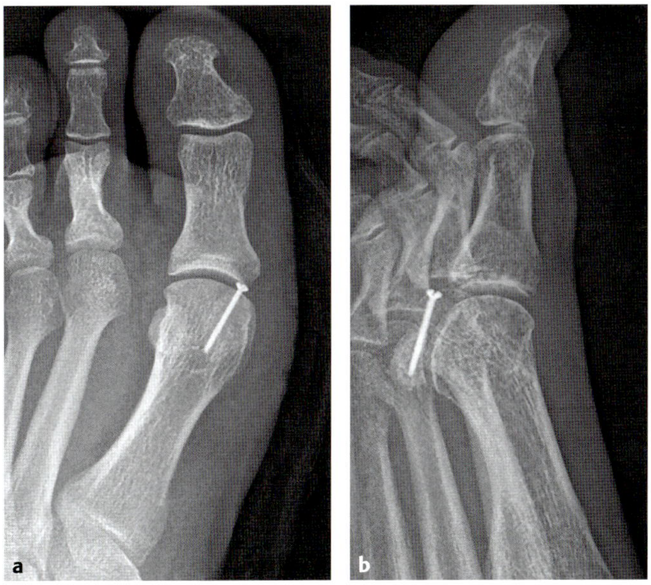

Fig 8.5-9a–b X-rays 2 months postoperatively demonstrating bony union.

a AP (dorsoplantar) view.

b Lateral view.

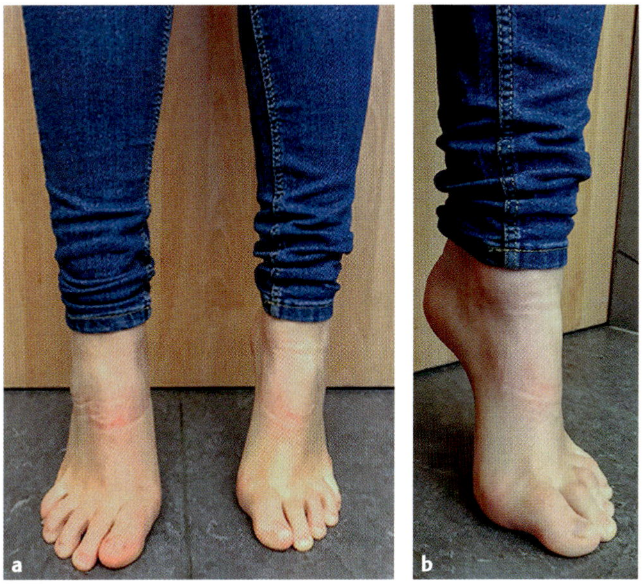

Fig 8.5-10a–b Two months postoperatively the patient has no pain on full weight bearing and when standing on toes.

8 Recommended reading

Anderson RB, McBryde AM Jr. Autogenous bone grafting of hallux sesamoid nonunions. *Foot Ankle Int.* 1997 May;18(5):293–296.

Aper RL, Saltzman CL, Brown TD. The effect of hallux sesamoid excision on the flexor hallucis longus moment arm. *Clin Orthop Relat Res.* 1996 Apr(325):209–217.

Blundell CM, Nicholson P, Blackney MW. Percutaneous screw fixation for fractures of the sesamoid bones of the hallux. *J Bone Joint Surg Br.* 2002 Nov;84(8):1138–1141.

Mittlmeier T, Haar P. Sesamoid and toe fractures. *Injury.* 2004 Sep;35 Suppl 2:Sb87–97.

Richardson EG. Hallucal sesamoid pain: causes and surgical treatment. *J Am Acad Orthop Surg.* 1999 Jul–Aug;7(4):270–278.

Rammelt S. From prehistory to judgement day: Accessory bones and sesamoids of the foot. In: Rammelt S, Zwipp H, eds. *The Foot—Arts, Myths, and Secrets.* Davos: AO Foundation; 2016: 79–102.

Zwipp H, Rammelt S. *Tscherne Unfallchirurgie: Fuß.* Berlin: Springer; 2014:434–435. German.

Appendix

For further educational material about the classification and access to the complete Fracture and Dislocation Classification Compendium, please use the QR code.

43

Location: Tibia, **distal end segment** 43

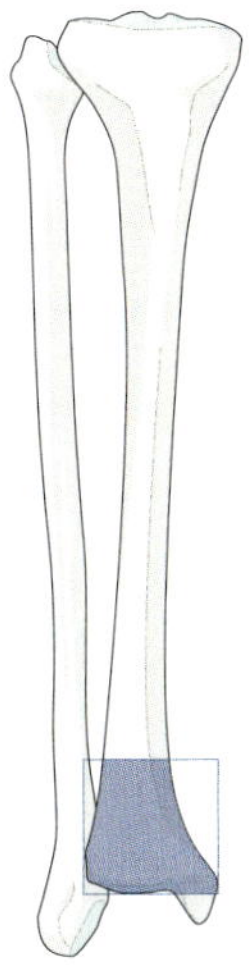

Types:

Tibia, distal end segment, **extraarticular fracture** 43A

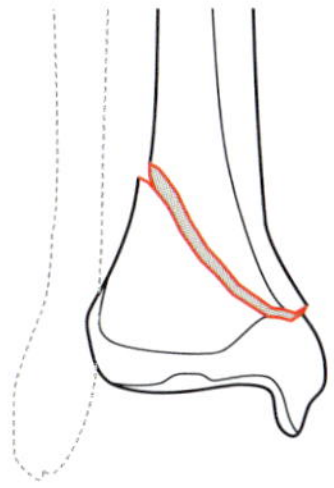

Tibia, distal end segment, **partial articular fracture** 43B

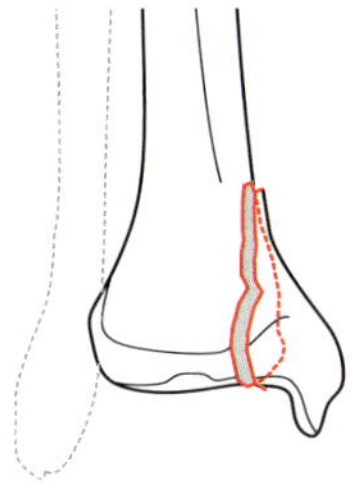

Tibia, distal end segment, **complete articular fracture** 43C

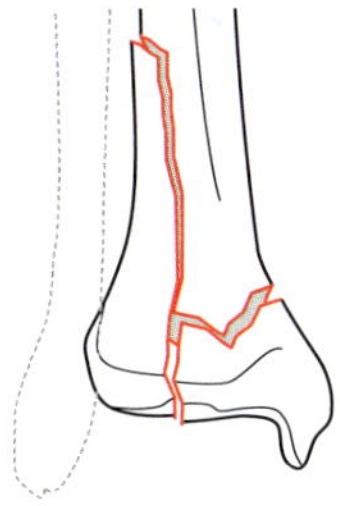

43A

Type: Tibia, distal end segment, **extraarticular fracture** 43A

Group: Tibia, distal end segment, extraarticular, **simple fracture** 43A1

Subgroups:

Spiral fracture
43A1.1

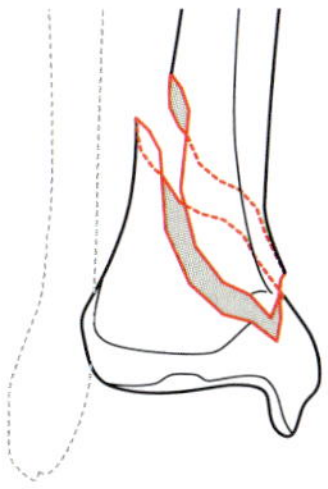

Oblique fracture
43A1.2

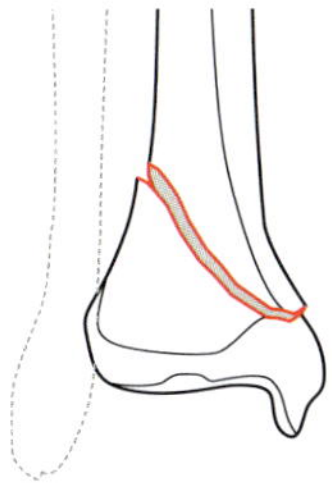

Transverse fracture
43A1.3

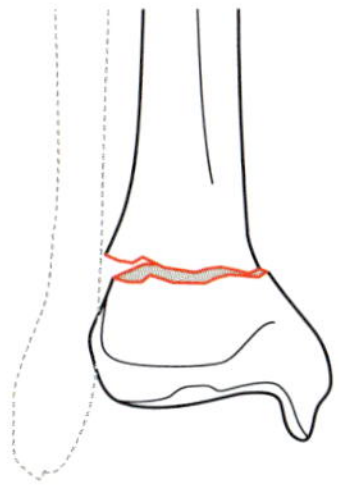

Group: Tibia, distal end segment, extraarticular, **wedge fracture** 43A2

Subgroups:

Posterolateral impaction fracture
43A2.1

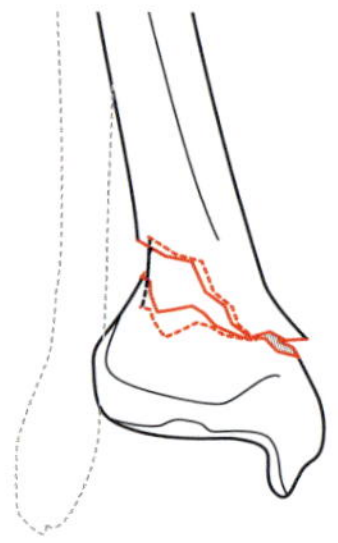

Anteromedial wedge fracture
43A2.2

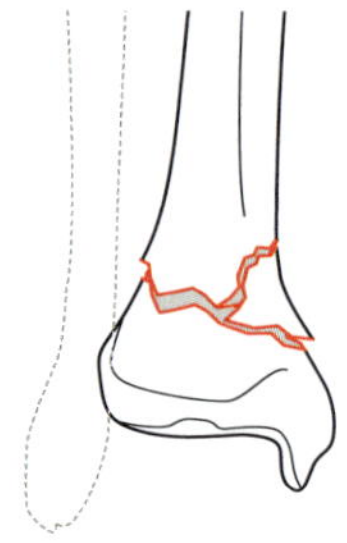

Fracture extending into diaphysis
43A2.3

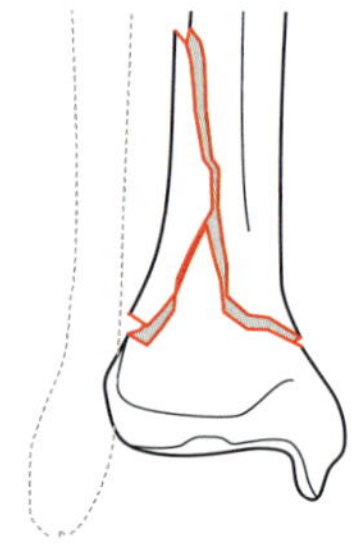

Group: Tibia, distal end segment, extraarticular, **multifragmentary fracture** 43A3

Subgroups:

With 3 intermediate fragments
43A3.1

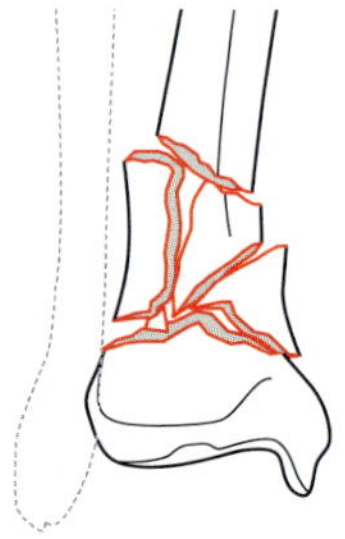

With more than 3 intermediate fragments
43A3.2

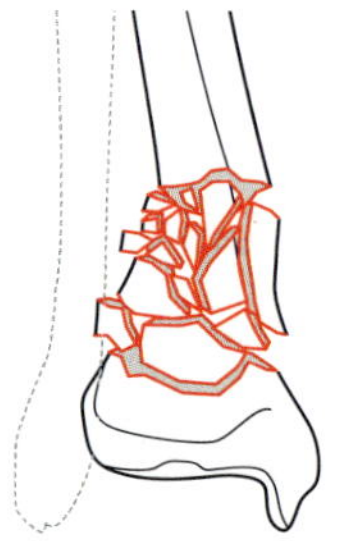

Extending into diaphysis
43A3.3

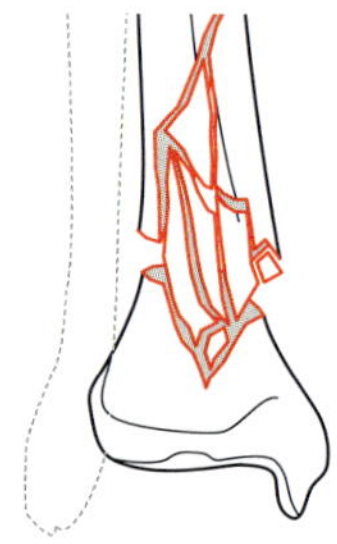

43B

Type: Tibia, distal end segment, **partial articular fracture** 43B

Group: Tibia, distal end segment, partial articular, **split fracture** 43B1

Subgroups:

Frontal/coronal fracture
43B1.1*

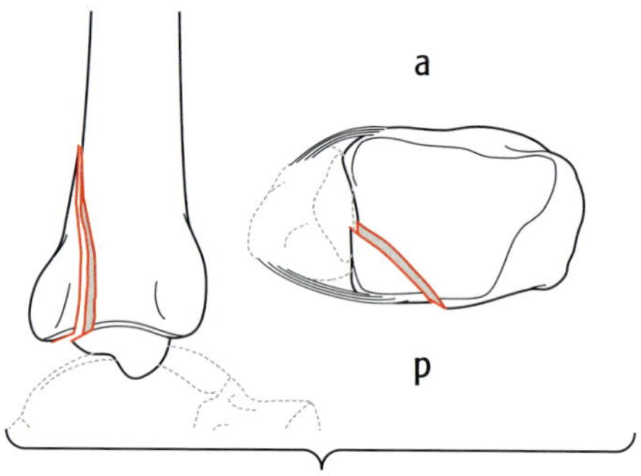

*Qualifications:
- o Anterior
- y **Posterior Volkmann**

Sagittal fracture
43B1.2*

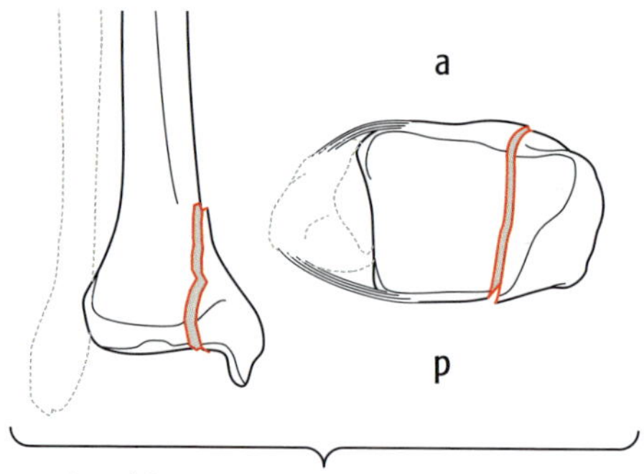

*Qualifications:
- f Lateral
- z **Medial articular surface including medial malleolus**

Fragmentary metaphyseal fracture
43B1.3

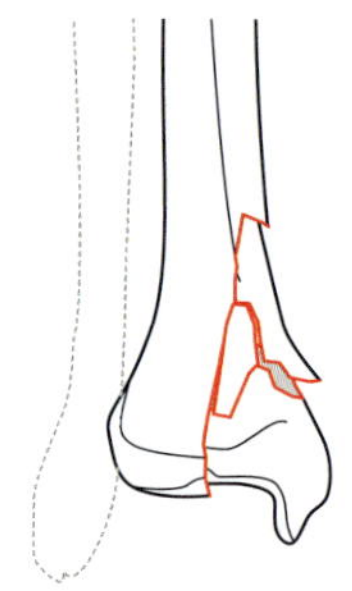

Group: Tibia, distal end segment partial articular, **split depression fracture** 43B2

Subgroups:

Frontal/coronal fracture
43B2.1*

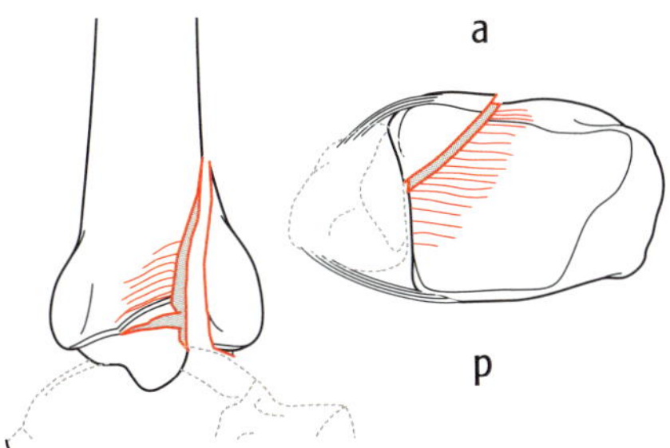

Sagittal fracture
43B2.2*

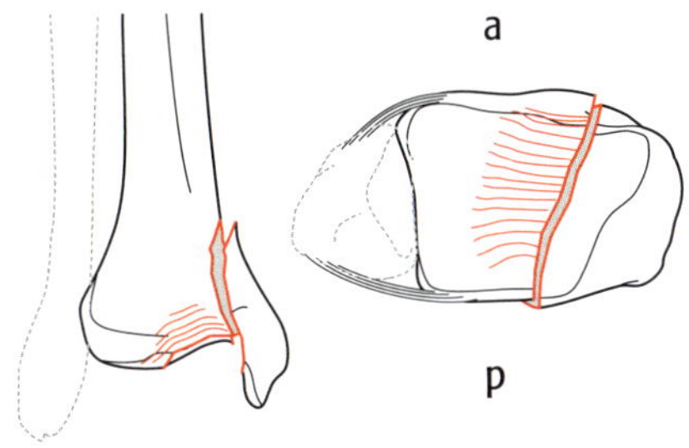

Central fragment fracture
43B2.3

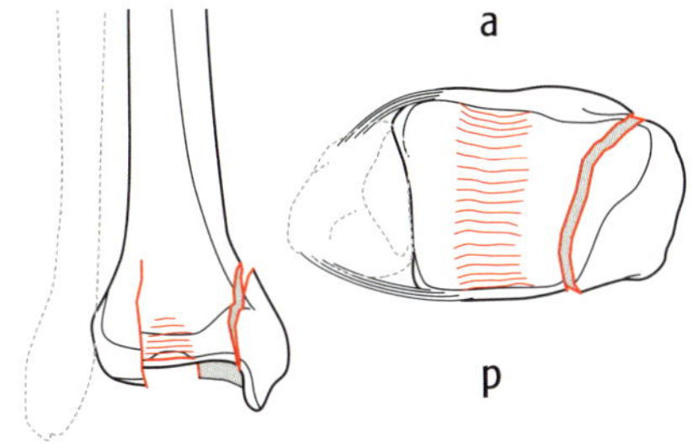

*Qualifications (43B2.1):
- o **Anterior**
- y Posterior Volkmann

*Qualifications (43B2.2):
- f Lateral
- h **Medial**

Group: Tibia, distal end segment, partial articular, **depression fracture** 43B3

Subgroups:

Frontal/coronal fracture
43B3.1*

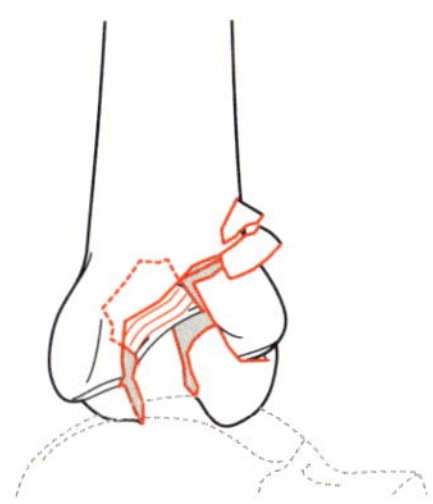

Sagittal fracture
43B3.2*

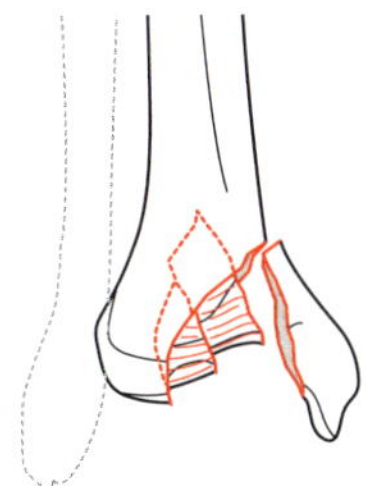

Fragmentary metaphyseal fracture
43B3.3

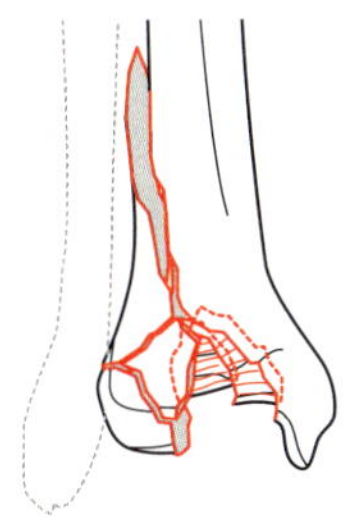

*Qualifications (43B3.1):
- o **Anterior**
- y Posterior Volkmann

*Qualifications (43B3.2):
- f Lateral
- h **Medial**

43C

Type: Tibia, distal end segment, **complete articular fracture** 43C

Group: Tibia, distal end segment, complete, **simple articular, simple metaphyseal fracture** 43C1

Subgroups:

Without impaction
43C1.1*

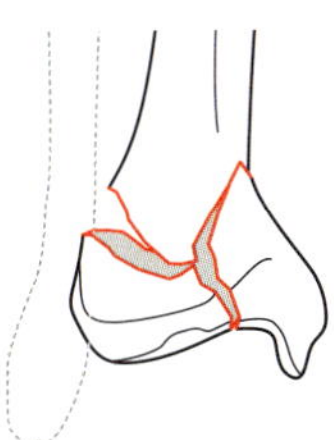

With epiphyseal depression
43C1.2

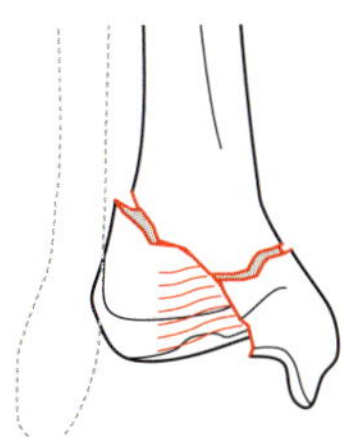

Extending into diaphysis
43C1.3

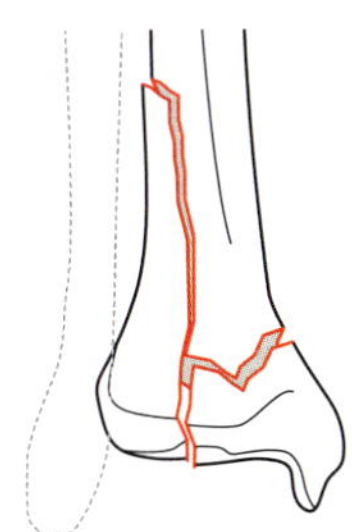

*Qualifications (43C1.1):
- q Frontal/coronal plane
- r **Sagittal plane**

Group: Tibia, distal end segment, complete, **simple articular, multifragmentary metaphyseal fracture** 43C2

Subgroups:

With asymmetric impaction
43C2.1*

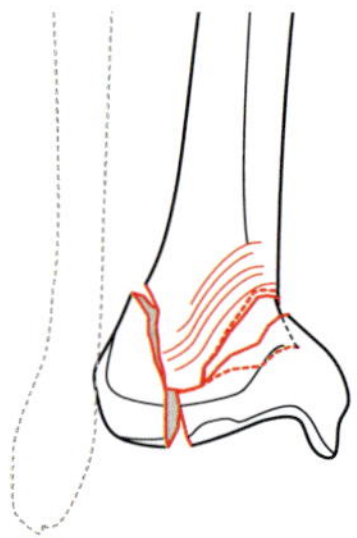

*Qualifications:
q Frontal/coronal plane
r **Sagittal plane**

Without asymmetric impaction
43C2.2

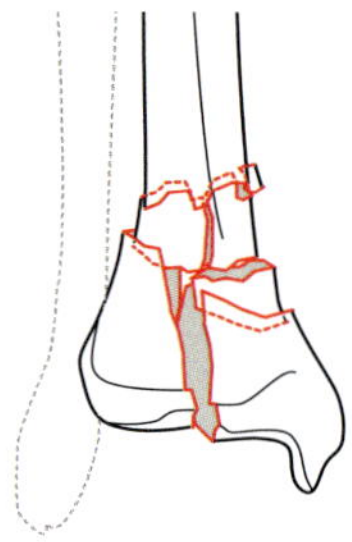

Extending into diaphysis
43C2.3

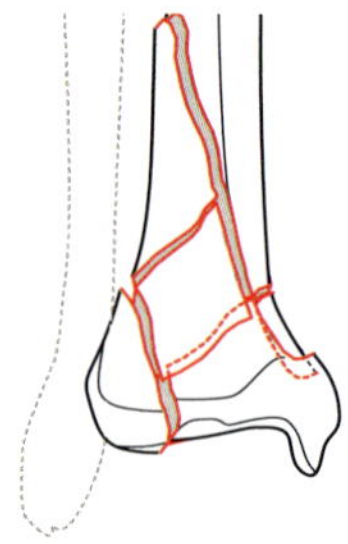

Group: Tibia, distal end segment, complete, **multifragmentary articular and metaphyseal fracture** 43C3

Subgroups:

Epiphyseal fracture
43C3.1

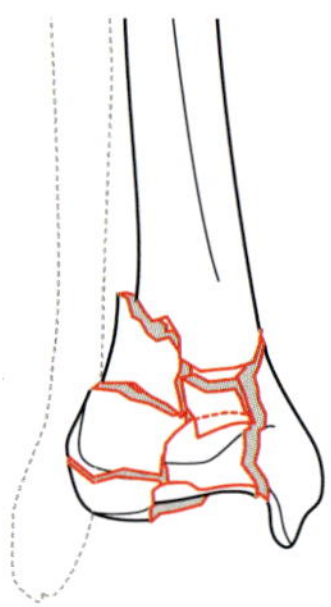

Epiphyseal-metaphyseal fracture
43C3.2

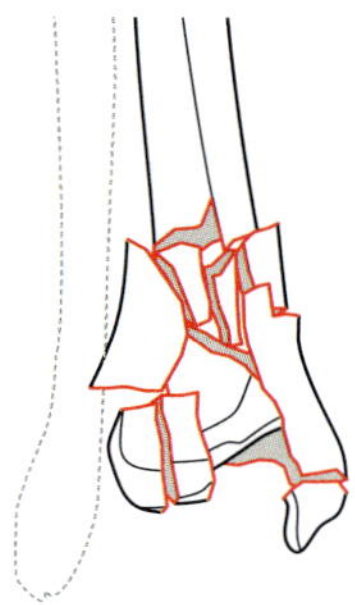

Epiphyseal-metaphyseal-diaphyseal fracture
43C3.3

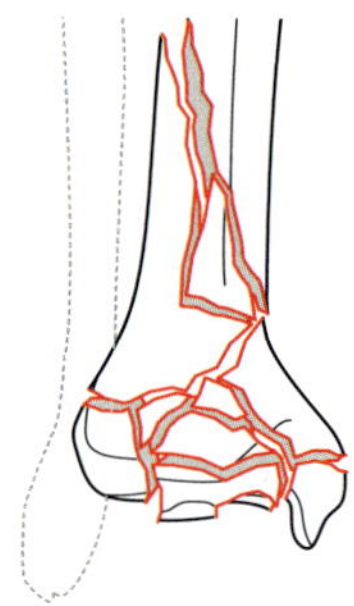

Qualifications *are optional and applied to the fracture code where the asterisk is located as a lower-case letter within rounded brackets. More than one qualification can be applied for a given fracture classification, separated by a comma. For a more detailed explanation, see the compendium introduction.*

4F3

Location: Fibula, **distal end segment**
(excluding lateral malleolar fractures 44) 4F3

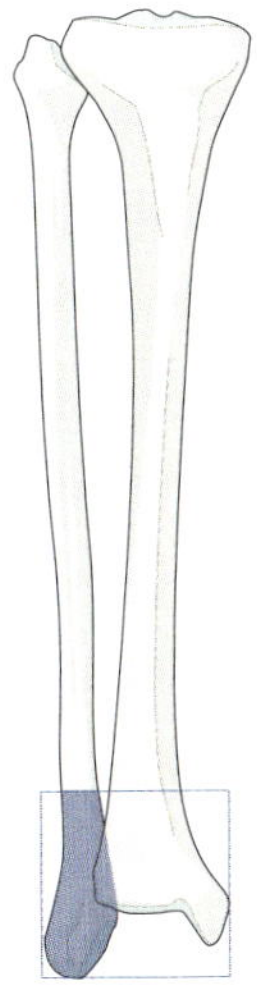

Types:

Distal end segment,
simple fracture
4F3A

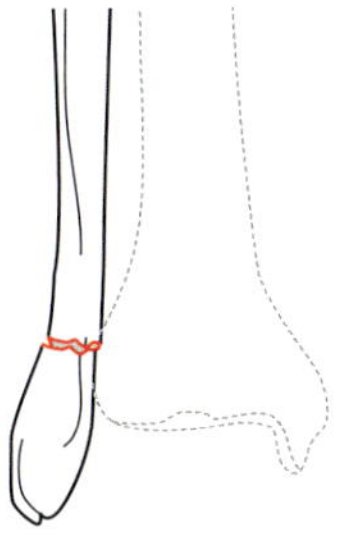

Distal end segment
wedge or multifragmentary fracture
4F3B

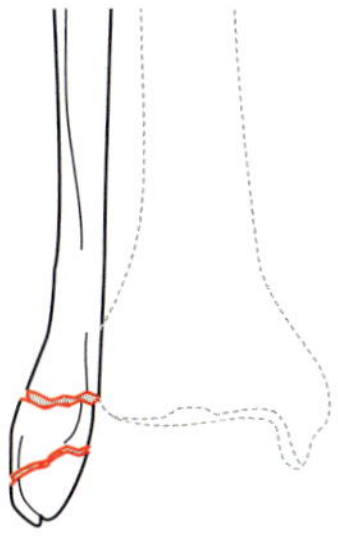

→ The fibular fracture code is used only if the distal fibula fracture is NOT part of a malleolar fracture (44). For further information, please refer to the Appendix.

Qualifications *are optional and applied to the fracture code where the asterisk is located as a lower-case letter within rounded brackets. More than one qualification can be applied for a given fracture classification, separated by a comma. For a more detailed explanation, see the compendium introduction.*

Malleolar segment

Location: Tibia/fibula, **malleolar segment** 44

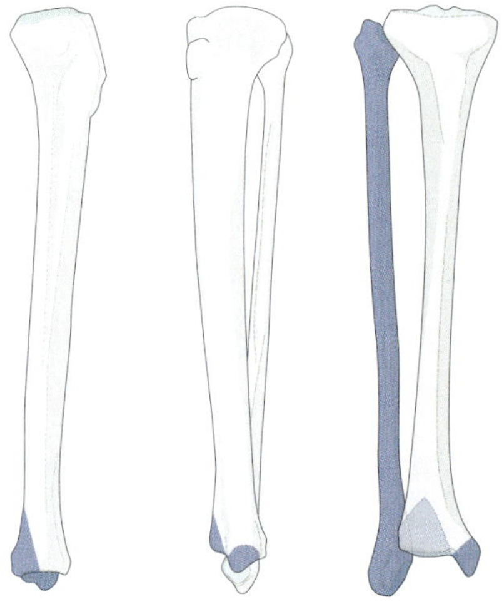

Types:

Tibia/ fibula, malleolar segment, **infrasyndesmotic fibula injury** 44A

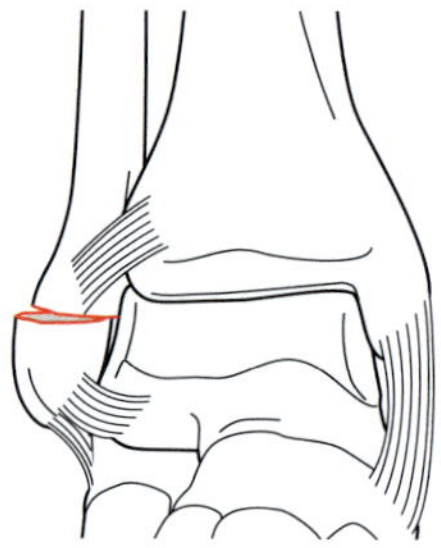

Tibia/fibula, malleolar segment, **transsyndesmotic fibula fracture** 44B

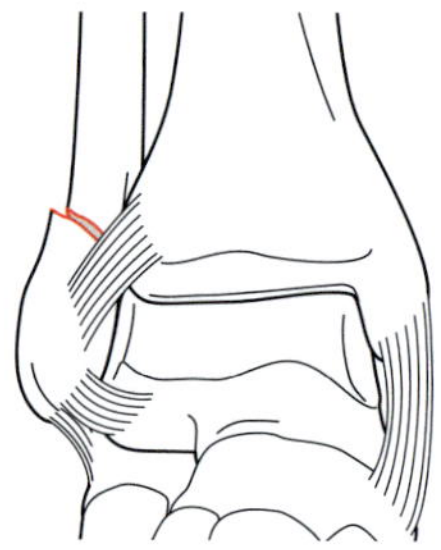

Tibia/fibula, malleolar segment, **suprasyndesmotic fibula fracture** 44C

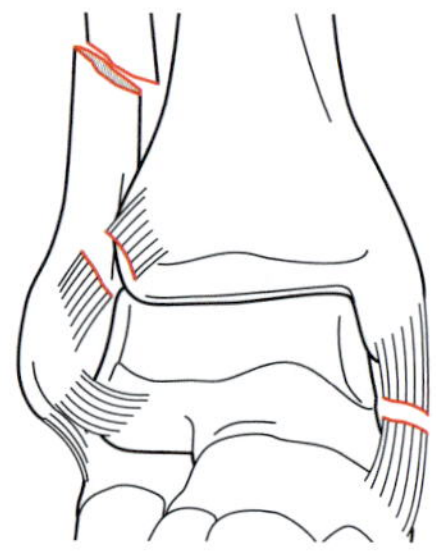

44A

Type: Tibia/fibula, malleolar segment, **infrasyndesmotic fibula injury** 44A

Group: Tibia/fibula, malleolar segment, infrasyndesmotic, **isolated fibula injury** 44A1

Subgroups:

Rupture of the lateral collateral ligament 44A1.1

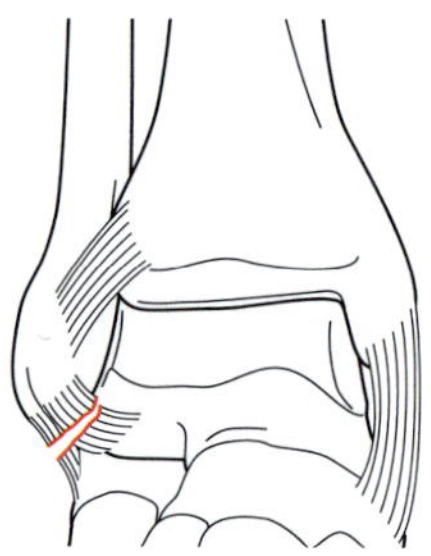

Avulsion fracture of the tip of the lateral malleolus 44A1.2

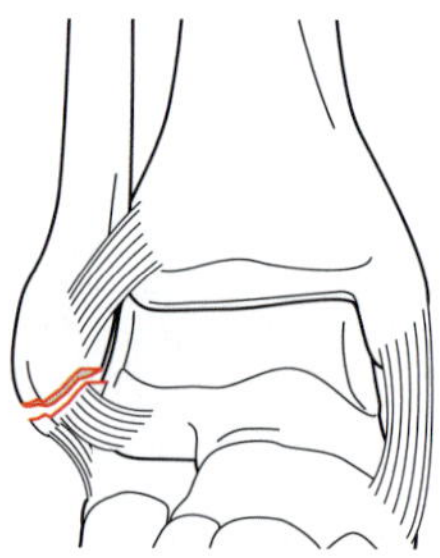

Transverse fracture of the lateral malleolus 44A1.3

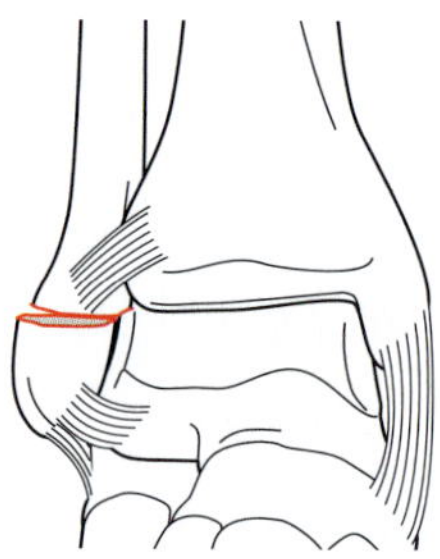

Qualifications *are optional and applied to the fracture code where the asterisk is located as a lower-case letter within rounded brackets. More than one qualification can be applied for a given fracture classification, separated by a comma. For a more detailed explanation, see the compendium introduction.*

Group: Tibia/fibula, malleolar, infrasyndesmotic fibula injury **with a medial malleolar fracture** 44A2

Subgroups:

Rupture of the lateral collateral ligament
44A2.1

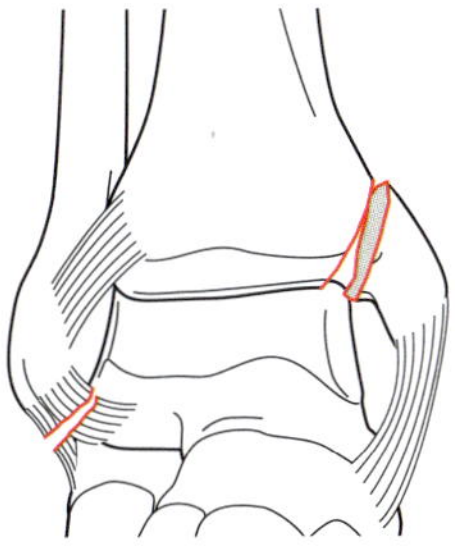

Avulsion fracture of the tip of the lateral malleolus
44A2.2

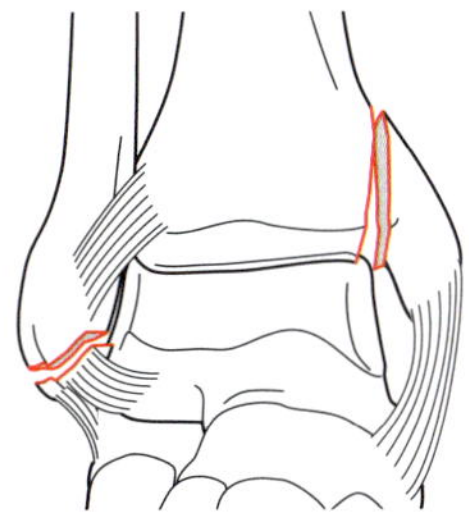

Transverse fracture of the lateral malleolus
44A2.3

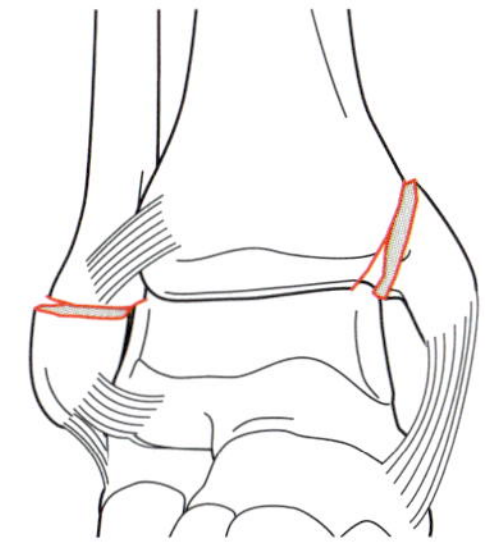

Group: Tibia/fibula, malleolar, infrasyndesmotic fibular injury **with a posteromedial fracture** 44A3

Subgroups:

Rupture of the lateral collateral ligament with a posteromedial fracture
44A3.1

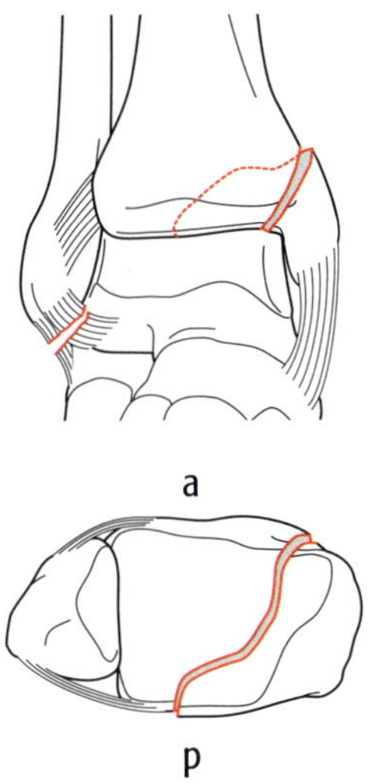

Avulsion fracture of the tip of the lateral malleolus with a posteromedial fracture
44A3.2

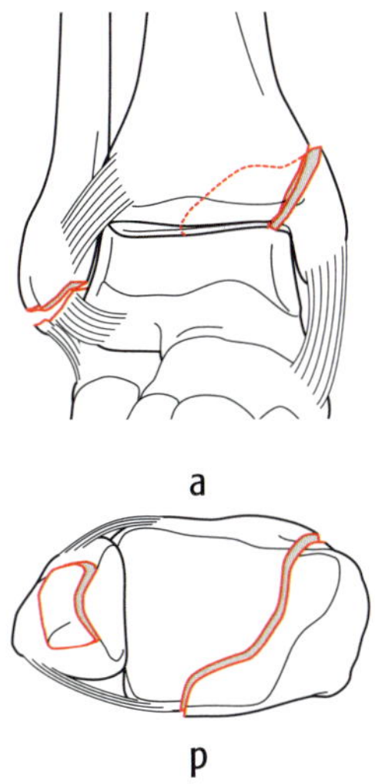

Transverse fracture of the lateral malleolus with a posteromedial fracture
44A3.3

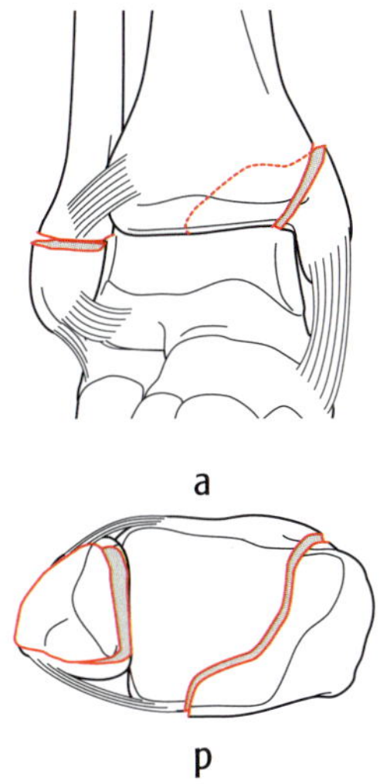

44B

Type: Tibia/fibula, malleolar segment, **transsyndesmotic fibula fracture** 44B

Group: Tibia/fibula, malleolar segment, transsyndesmotic **isolated fibula fracture** 44B1

Subgroups:

Simple fibula fracture
44B1.1*

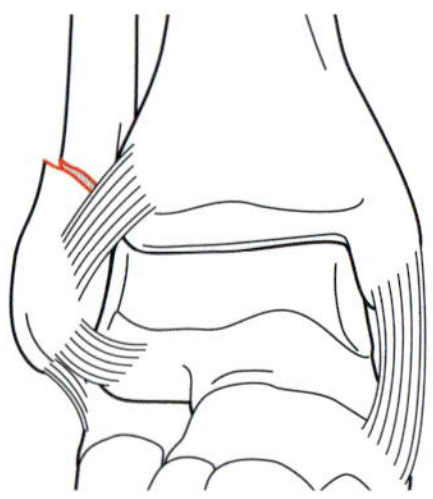

With a rupture of the anterior syndesmosis
44B1.2*

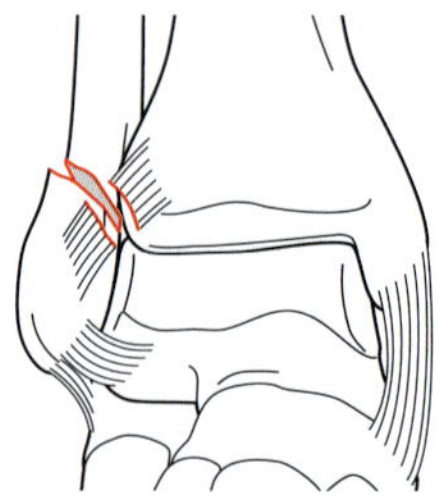

Wedge or multifragmentary fibula fracture
44B1.3*

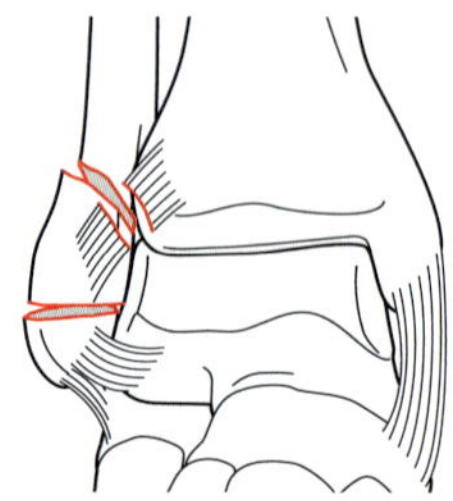

*Qualifications:
- n Tillaux-Chaput tubercle fracture
- o Wagstaffe-Le Fort avulsion fracture
- u Syndesmosis unstable

Group: Tibia/fibula, malleolar segment, transsyndesmotic fibula fracture **with a medial injury** 44B2

Subgroups:

With a rupture of the deltoid ligament and anterior syndesmosis
44B2.1*

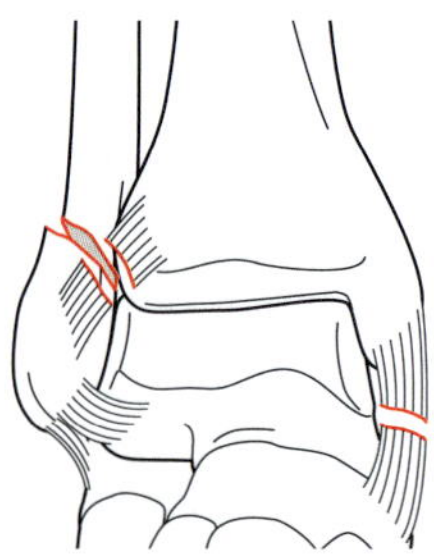

With a medial malleolus fracture and a rupture of the anterior syndesmosis
44B2.2*

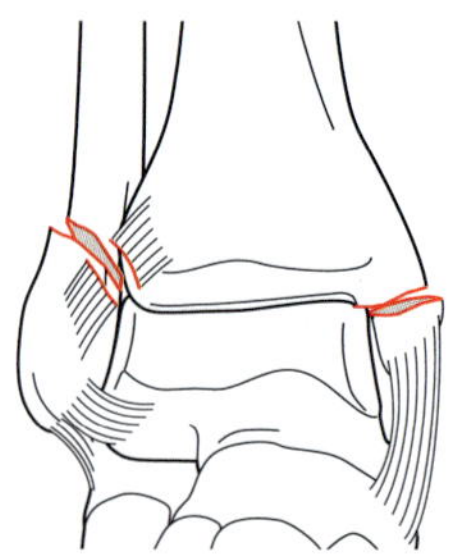

*Qualifications:
- n Tillaux-Chaput tubercle fracture
- o Wagstaffe-Le Fort avulsion fracture
- u Syndesmosis unstable

Wedge or multifragmentary fibula fracture with medial injury
44B2.3*

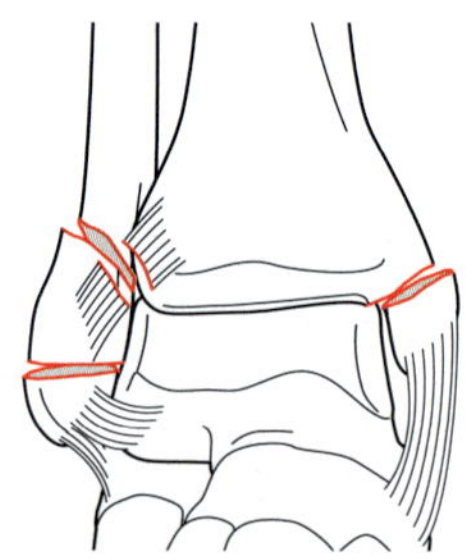

*Qualifications:
- r Rupture of deltoid ligament
- s **Fracture of medial malleolus**
- u Syndesmosis unstable

Group: Tibia/fibula, malleolar segment, **transsyndesmotic fibula fracture with a medial injury and fracture of the posterolateral rim (Volkmann's fragment)** 44B3

Subgroups:

Simple, with a deltoid ligament rupture
44B3.1*

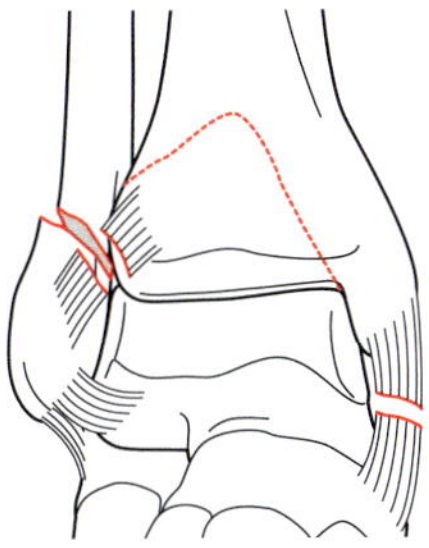

Simple medial malleolus fracture
44B3.2*

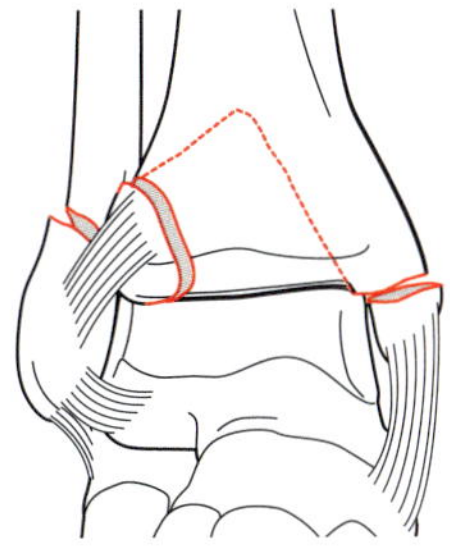

Wedge or multifragmentary fibular fracture with a fracture of the medial malleolus
44B3.3*

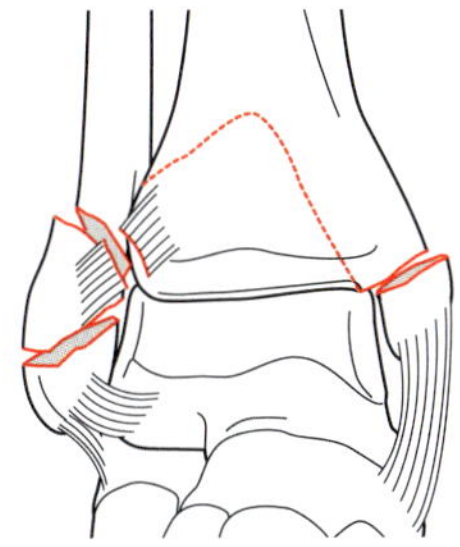

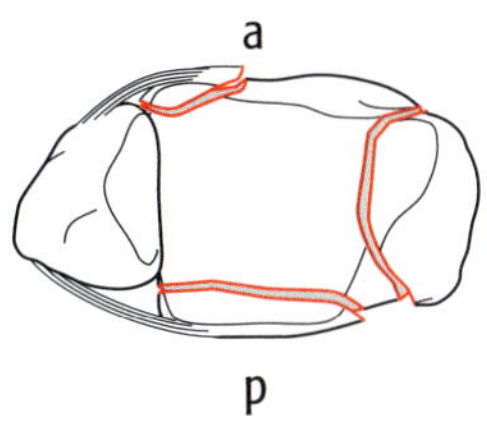

*Qualifications:
n Tillaux-Chaput tubercle fracture
o Wagstaffe-Le Fort avulsion fracture
u Syndesmosis unstable

44C

Type: Tibia/fibula, malleolar segment, **suprasyndesmotic fibula injury** 44C

Group: Tibia/fibula, malleolar segment, suprasyndesmotic, **simple diaphyseal fibula fracture** 44C1

Subgroups:

With a rupture of the deltoid ligament
44C1.1*

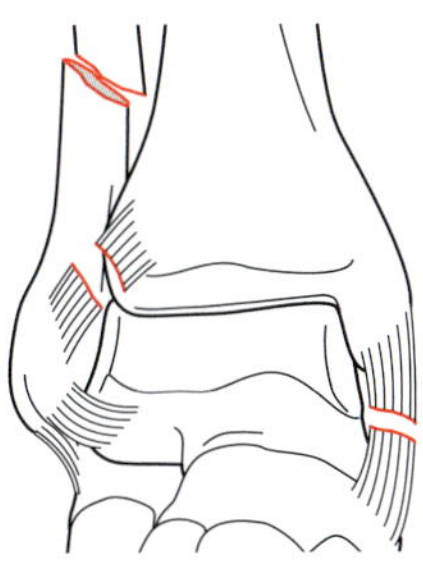

With a fracture of the medial malleolus
44C1.2*

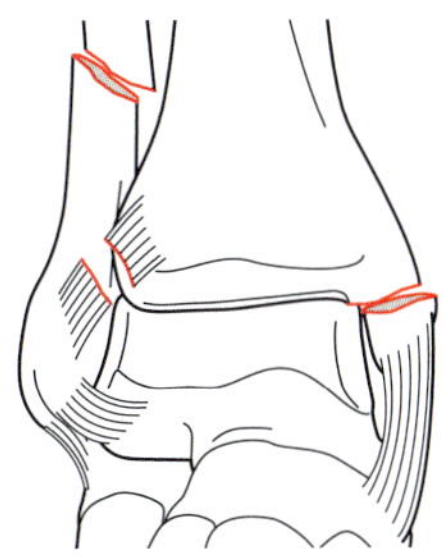

With a medial and a posterior malleolus fracture
44C1.3*

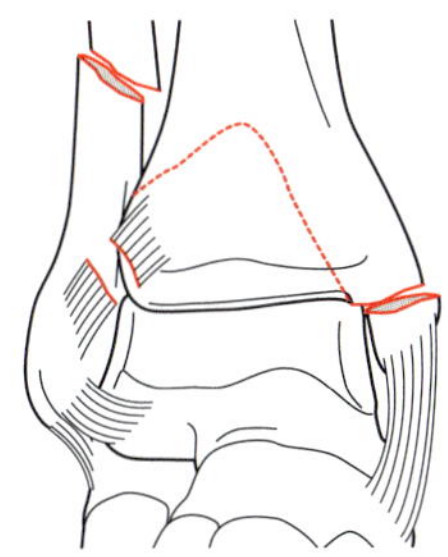

*Qualifications:
t Syndesmosis stable
u Syndesmosis unstable

Group: Tibia/fibula, malleolar segment, suprasyndesmotic, **wedge or multifragmentary diaphyseal fibula fracture** 44C2

Subgroups:

With a rupture of the deltoid ligament
44C2.1*

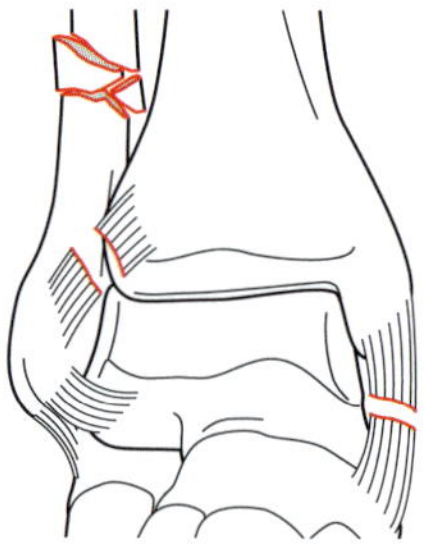

With a fracture of the medial malleolus
44C2.2*

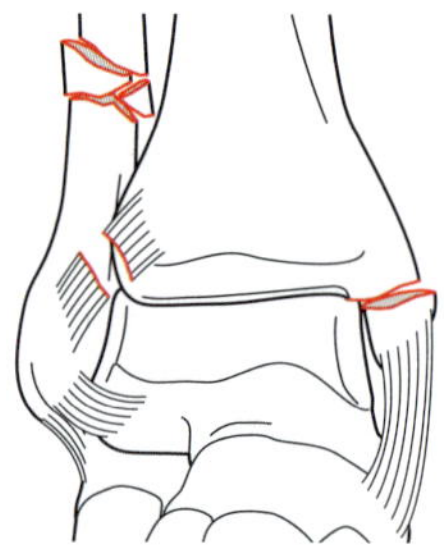

With a fracture of the medial malleolus and posterior malleolus
44C2.3*

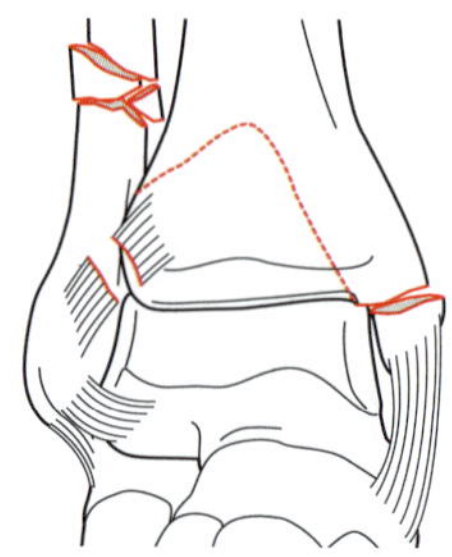

*Qualifications:
- t Syndesmosis stable
- u Syndesmosis unstable

Group: Tibia/fibula, malleolar segment, suprasyndesmotic, **proximal fibula injury** 44C3

Subgroups:

With a medial side injury
44C3.1*

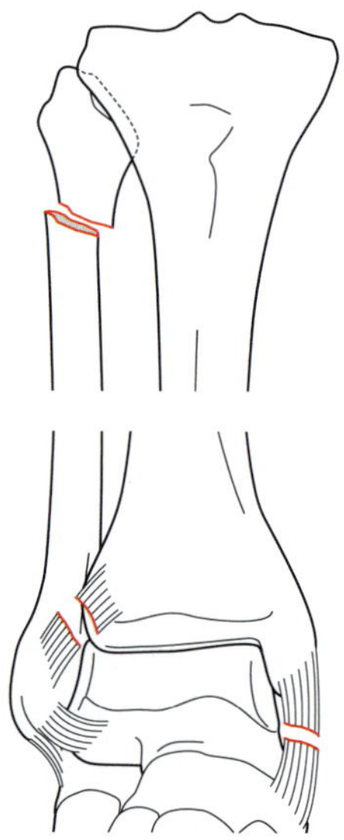

With shortening and a medial side injury
44C3.2*

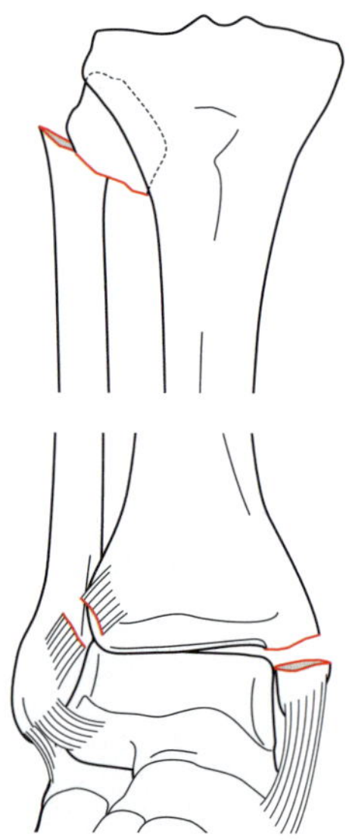

With a medial side injury and a posterior malleolus fracture
44C3.3*

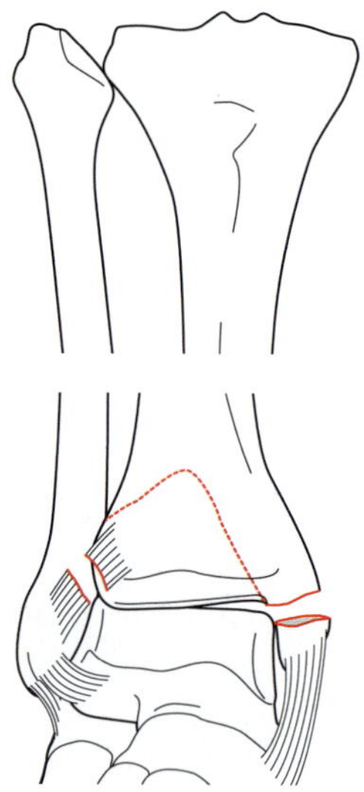

*Qualifications:
- p Fibula neck fracture
- q Proximal tibio-fibular joint dislocation
- r Rupture of deltoid ligament
- s Fracture of medial malleolus

Qualifications *are optional and applied to the fracture code where the asterisk is located as a lower-case letter within rounded brackets. More than one qualification can be applied for a given fracture classification, separated by a comma. For a more detailed explanation, see the compendium introduction.*

Foot

Anatomical region: Foot 8

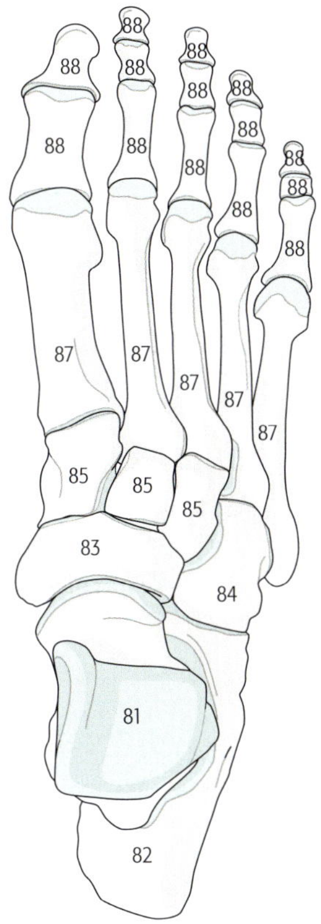

Bones:
Foot, **Talus** 81
Foot, **Calcaneus** 82
Foot, **Navicular** 83
Foot, **Cuboid** 84
Foot, **Cuneiforms** 85
Foot, **Metatarsals** 87
Foot, **Phalanges** 88
Foot, **Crush, multiple foot fractures** 89

Qualifications *are optional and applied to the fracture code where the asterisk is located as a lower-case letter within rounded brackets. More than one qualification can be applied for a given fracture classification, separated by a comma. For a more detailed explanation, see the compendium introduction.*

Talus 81

Bone: Foot, **talus** 81

Locations:

Foot, talus, **body**
81.1.

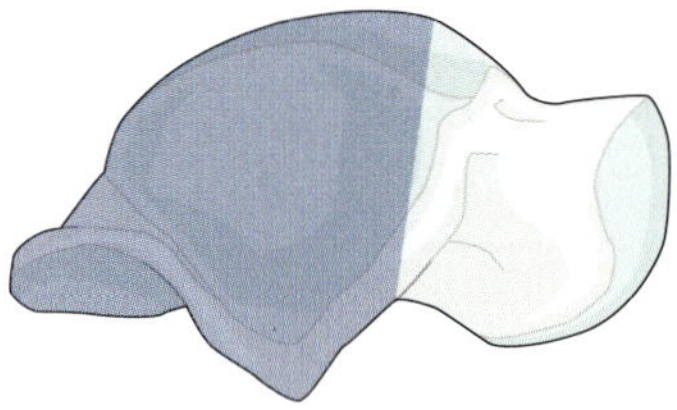

Foot, talus, **neck**
81.2.

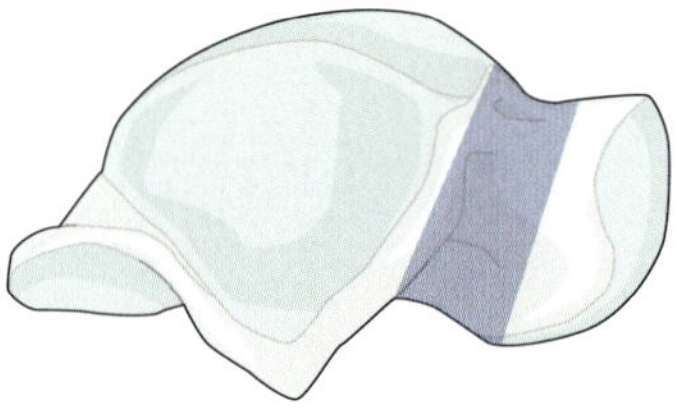

Foot, talus, **head**
81.3.

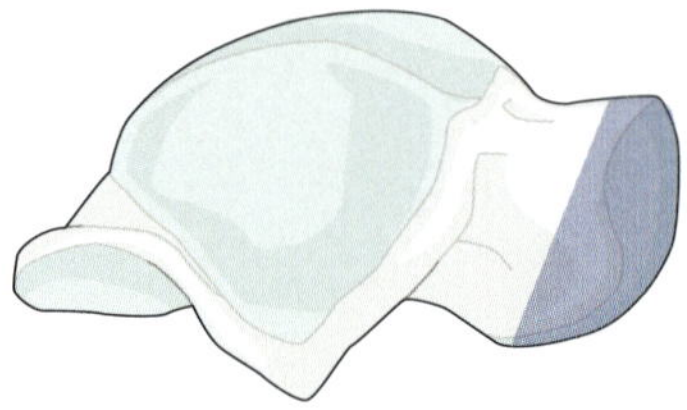

→ The talus is anatomically identified as follows: body = 1, neck = 2, and head = 3.
→ The talar anatomical divison is added (between two dots .__.) after the bone code.

81.1.

Location: Foot, talus, **body** 81.1.

Types:

Foot, talus, body, **avulsion fracture**
81.1.A

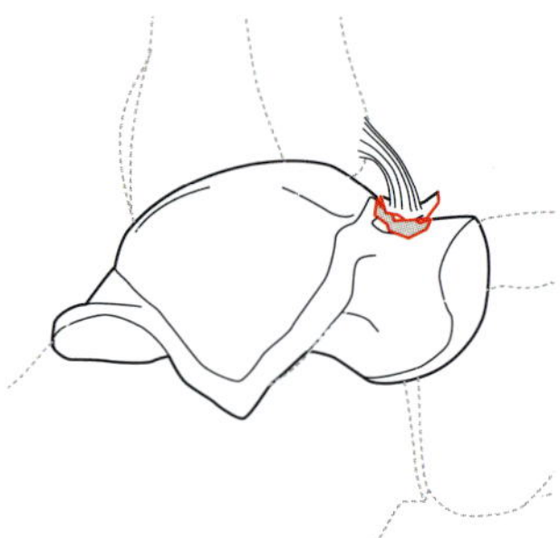

Foot, talus, body, **partial articular fracture**
81.1.B

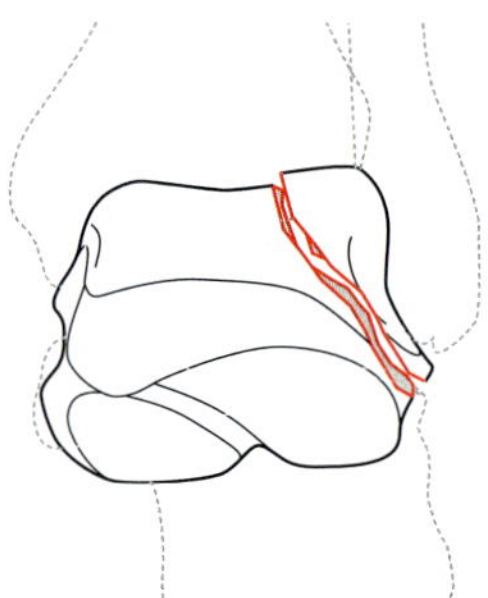

Foot, talus, body, **complete articular fracture**
81.1.C

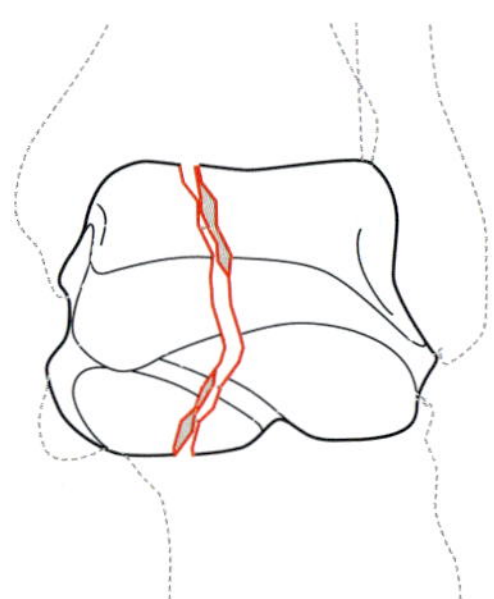

Type: Foot, talus, body, **avulsion fracture** 81.1.A

Groups:

Foot, talus, body, avulsion fracture,
anterior neck
81.1.A1

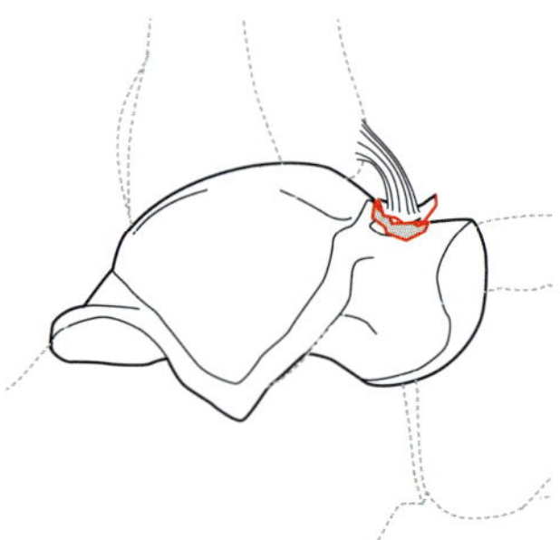

Foot, talus, body, avulsion fracture,
lateral process
81.1.A2

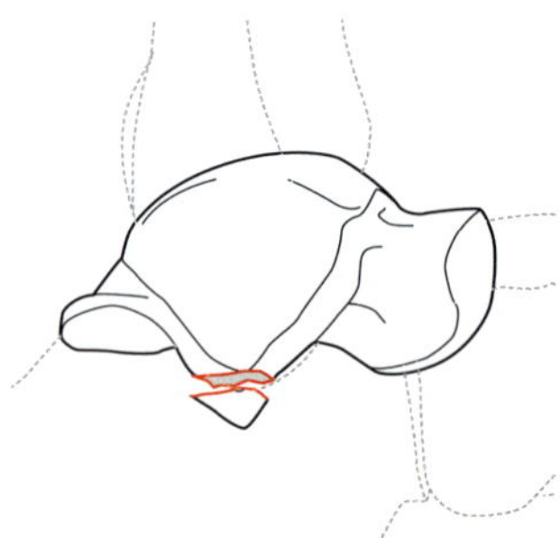

Foot, talus, body, avulsion fracture,
posterior process
81.1.A3

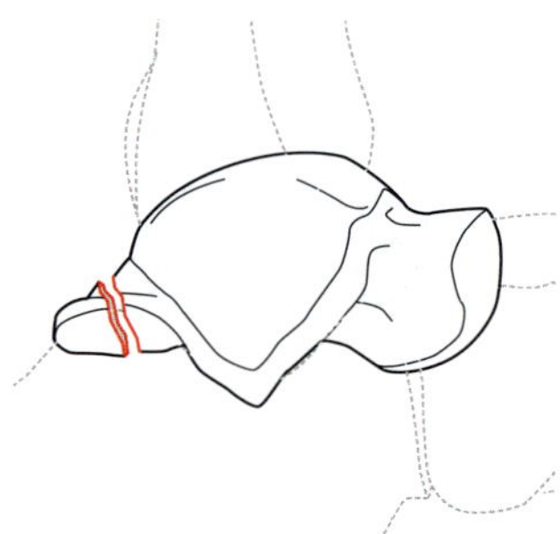

Type: Foot, talus, body, **partial articular fracture** 81.1.B

Groups:

Foot, talus, body, partial articular,
osteochondral fracture
81.1.B1

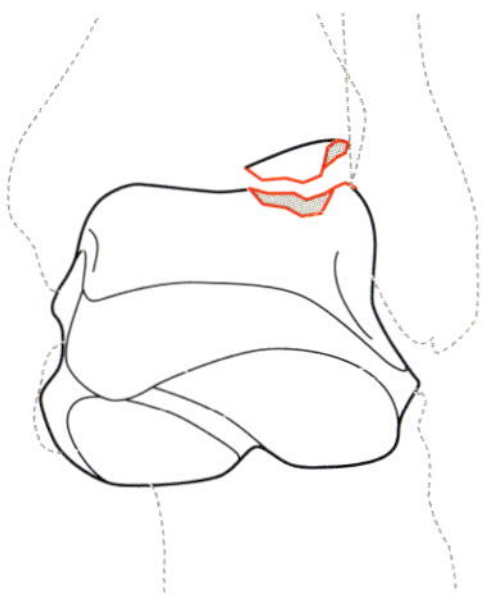

Foot, talus, body, partial articular,
simple fracture
81.1.B2

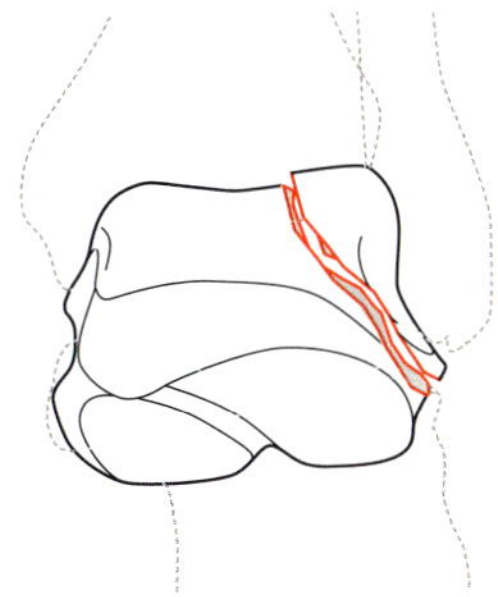

Talus, body, partial articular,
fragmentary fracture
81.1.B3

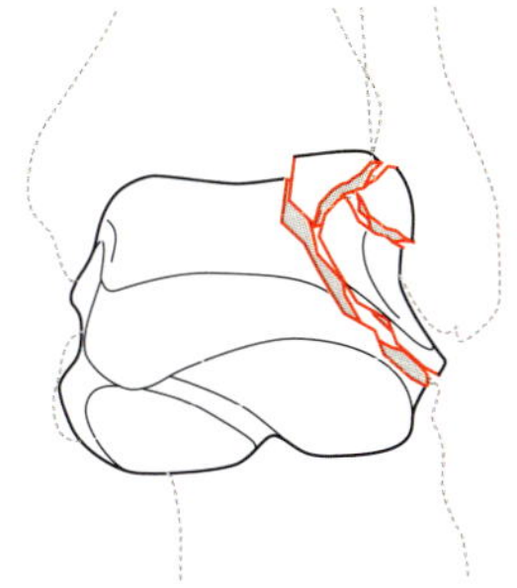

Type: Foot, talus, body, **complete articular fracture** 81.1.C

Groups:

Foot, talus, body, complete articular,
simple fracture
81.1.C1

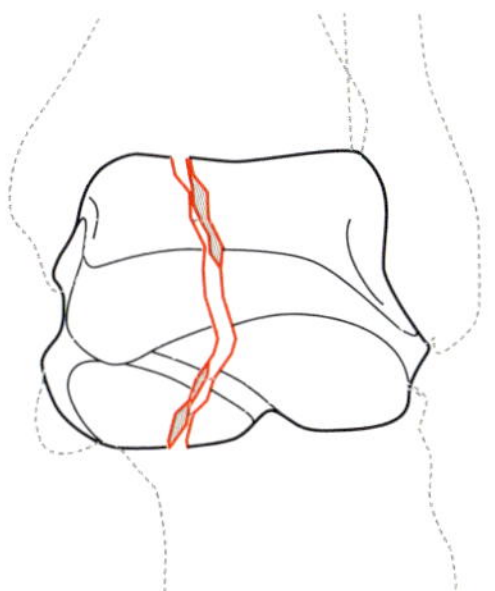

Foot, talus, body, complete articular,
multifragmentary fracture
81.1.C3

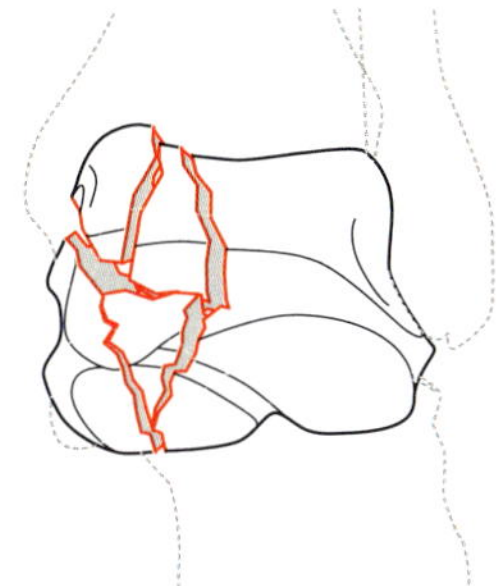

81.2.

Location: Foot, talus, **neck fracture** 81.2.

Types:

Foot, talus, neck, **nondisplaced (Hawkins 1)**
81.2.A

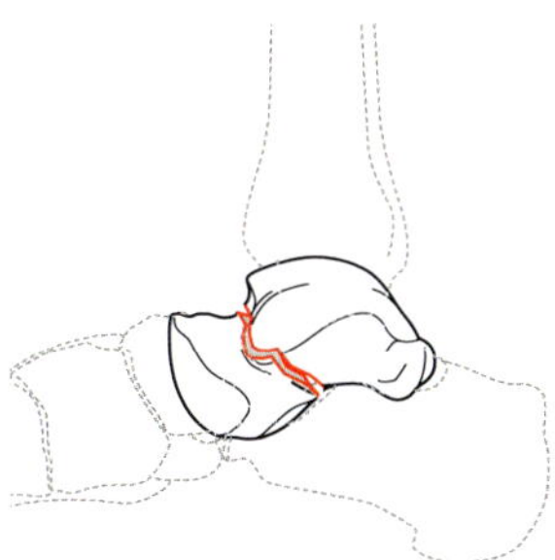

Foot, talus, neck, **displaced with subtalar joint subluxation/dislocation (Hawkins 2)**
81.2.B*

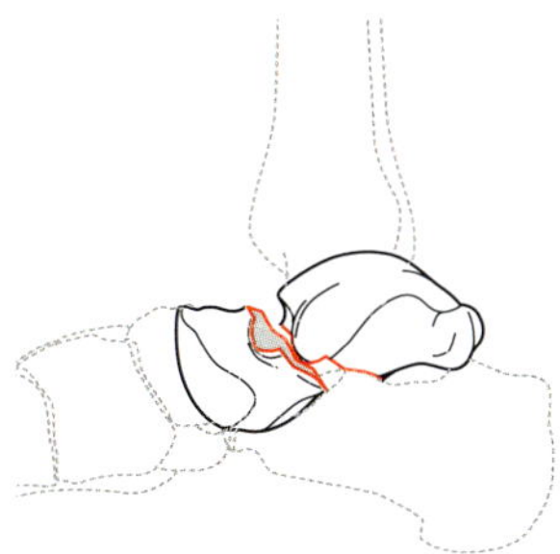

Foot, talus, neck, **displaced talar neck with talar body dislocation (Hawkins 3)**
81.2.C*

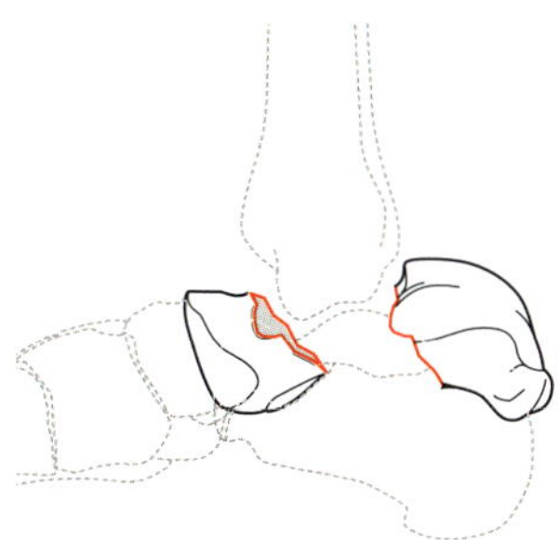

Foot, talus, neck, **displaced talar neck with talar body and head dislocation (Hawkins 4)**
81.2.D*

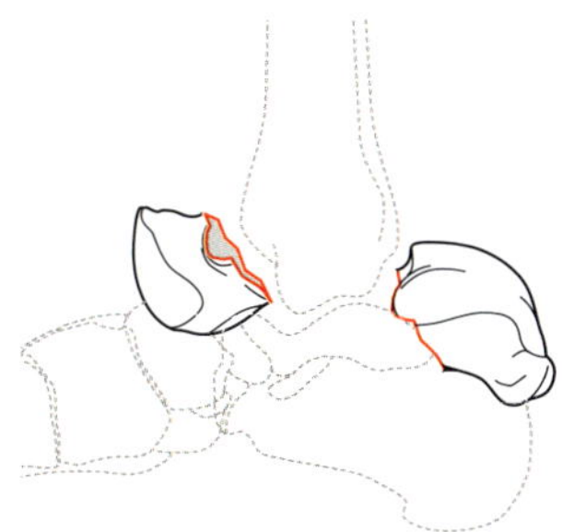

*Qualifications:
a **Simple**
b Multifragmentary

81.3.

Location: Talus, **head** 81.3.

Types:

Talus, head, **avulsion fracture**
81.3.A

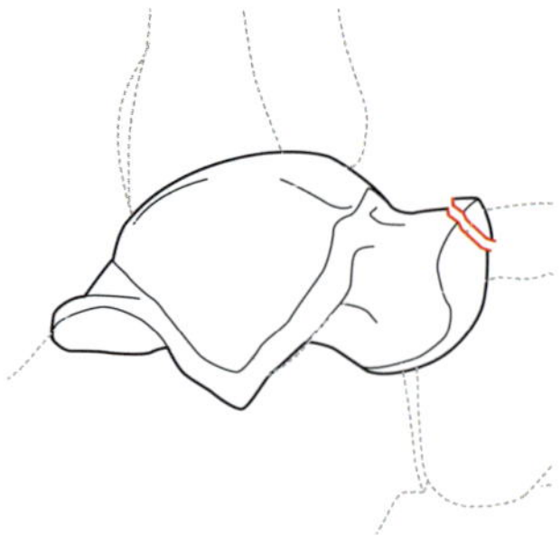

Talus, head, **partial articular fracture**
81.3.B*

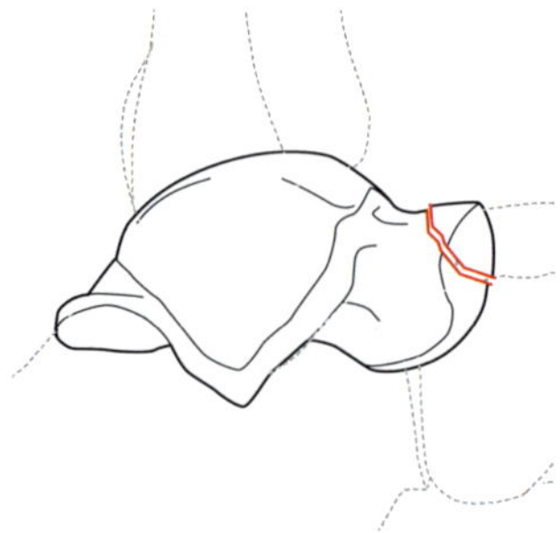

Talus, head, **complete articular fracture**
81.3.C*

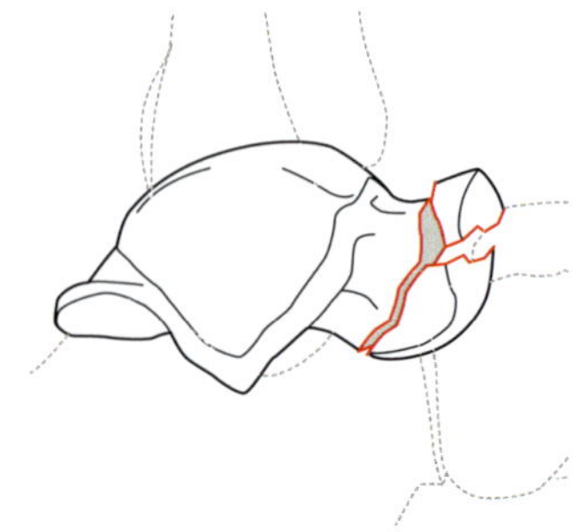

*Qualifications:
a Simple
b Multifragmentary

Calcaneus 82

Bone: Foot, **calcaneus** 82

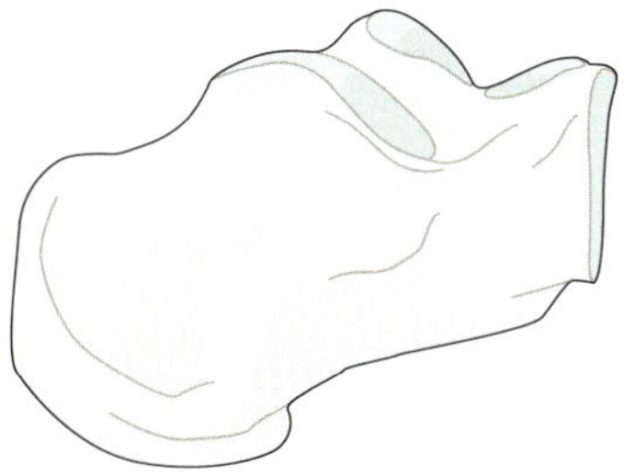

Types:

Foot, calcaneus, **extraarticular fracture**
82A

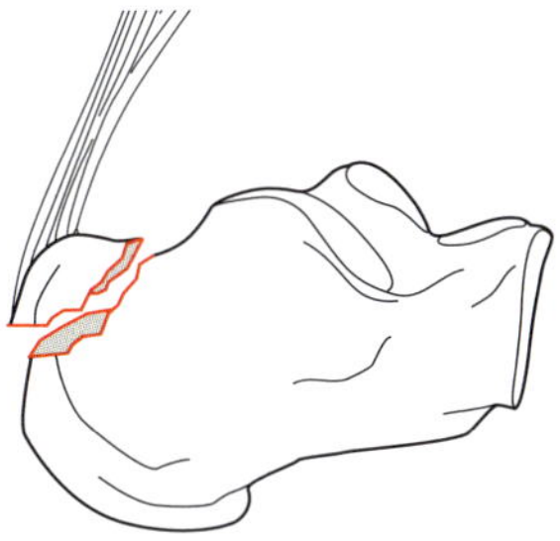

Foot, calcaneus, **tongue-type fracture exiting into posterior facet**
82B

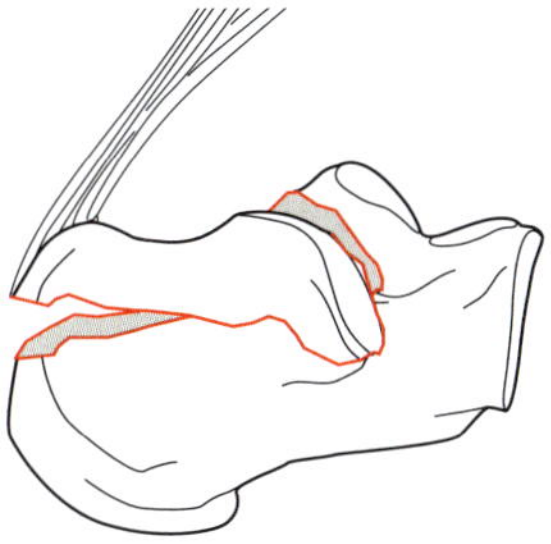

Foot, calcaneus, **complete articular joint depression**
82C

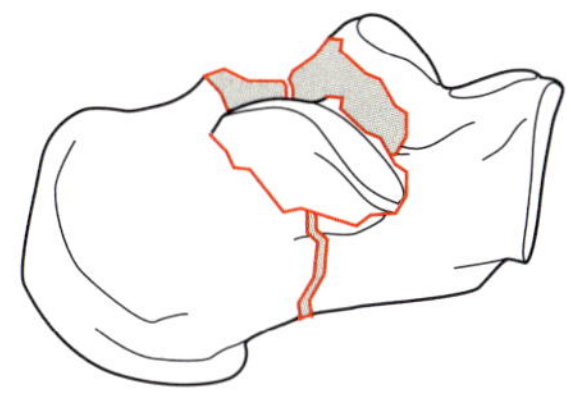

82A

Type: Foot, calcaneus, **extraarticular fracture** 82A

Groups:

Foot calcaneus, extraarticular, **avulsion, posterior tuberosity fracture or extraarticular tongue fracture**
82A1

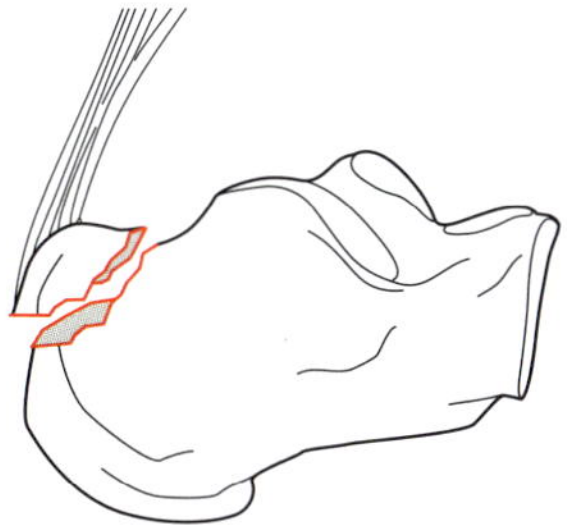

Foot calcaneus, extraarticular, **body fracture**
82A2

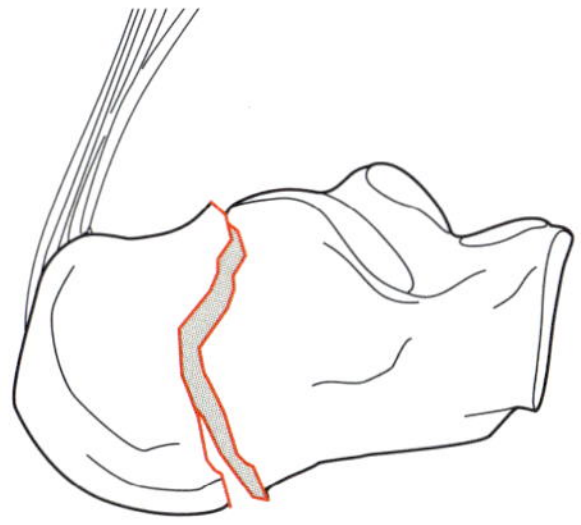

82B

Types: Foot, calcaneus, **tongue-type fracture exiting into posterior facet** 82B

Foot, calcaneus, tongue-type fracture exiting into posterior facet, **tongue-type, simple fracture**
82B1

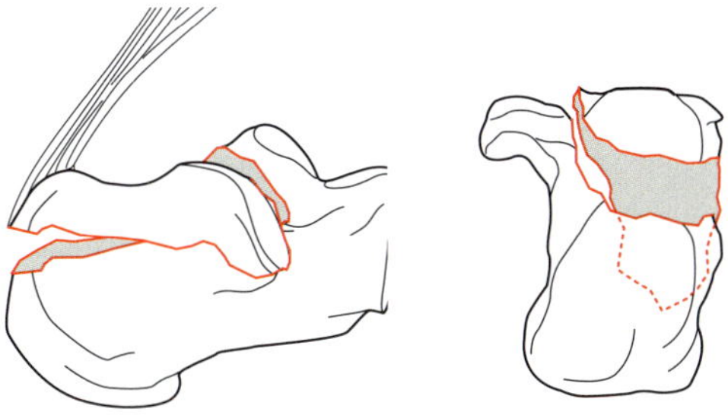

Foot, calcaneus, tongue-type fracture exiting into posterior facet, **multifragmentary fracture**
82B3

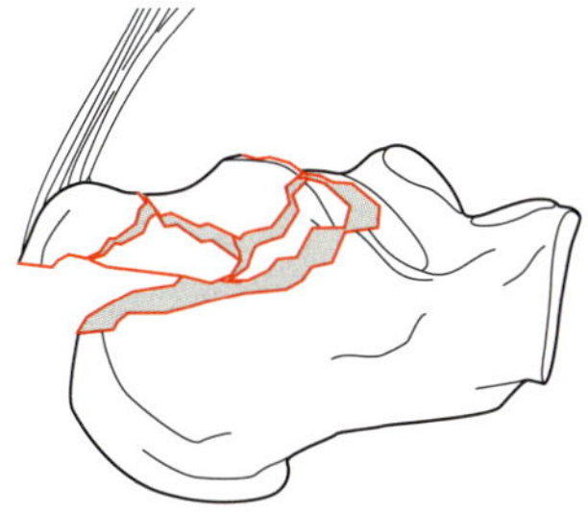

82C

Type: Foot, calcaneus, **complete articular joint depression fracture** 82C

Groups:

Foot, calcaneus, complete articular fracture, **with joint depression (Sanders 2)**
82C1

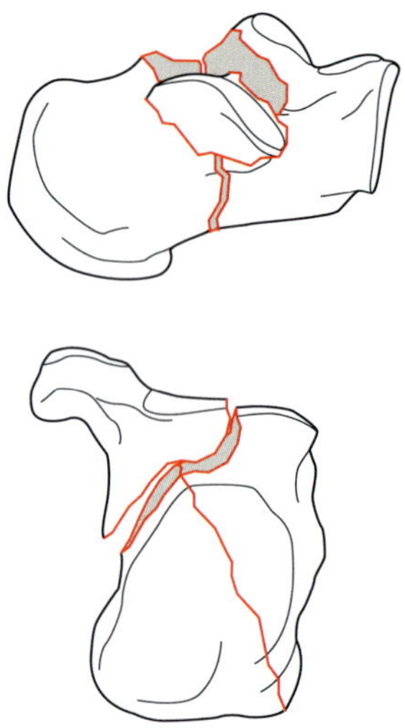

Foot, calcaneus, complete articular fracture, **with joint depression (Sanders 3)**
82C2

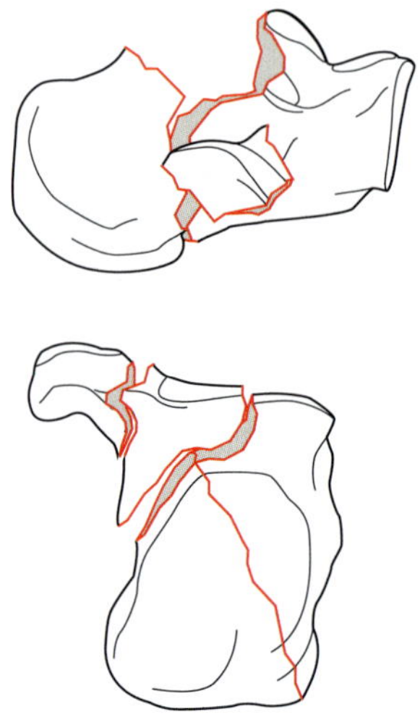

Foot, calcaneus, complete articular fracture, **multifragmentary fracture (Sanders 4)**
82C3

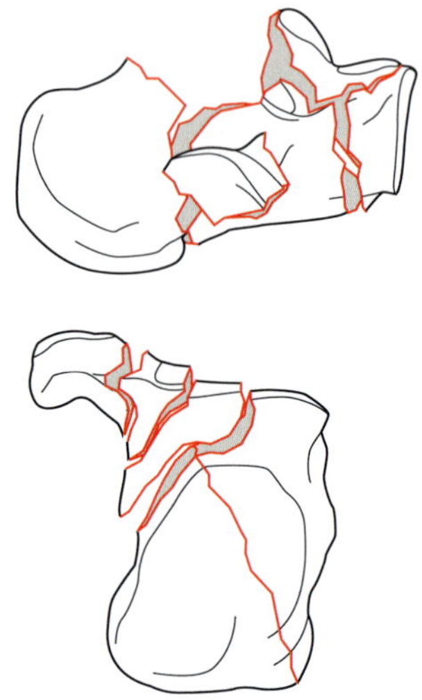

Navicular 83

Bone: Foot, **navicular** 83

Types:

Foot, navicular, **avulsion fracture**
83A

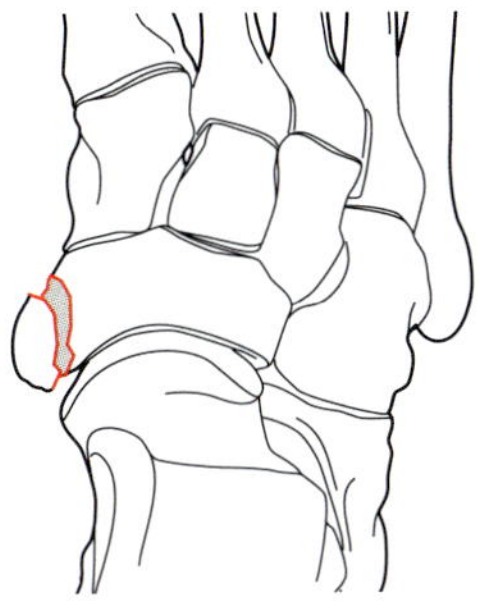

Foot, navicular, **partial articular fracture**
83B*

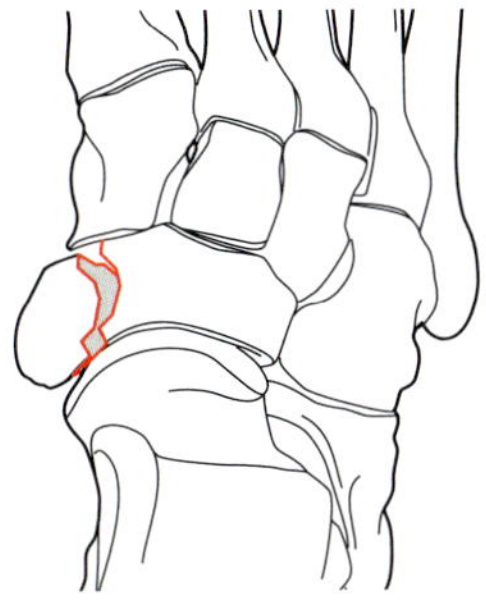

Foot, navicular, **complete articular fracture**
83C*

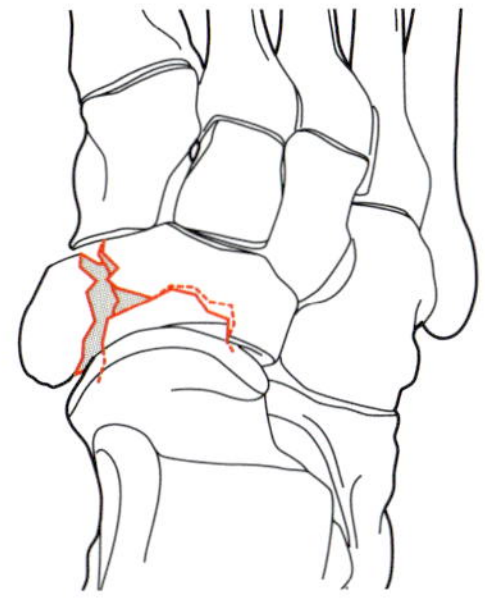

*Qualifications:
a Simple
b Multifragmentary

Cuboid 84

Bone: Foot, **cuboid** 84

Types:

Foot, cuboid, **avulsion fracture**
84A

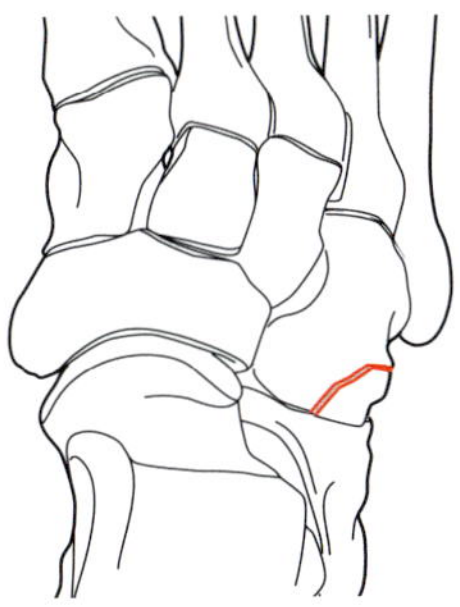

Foot, cuboid, **partial articular fracture**
84B*

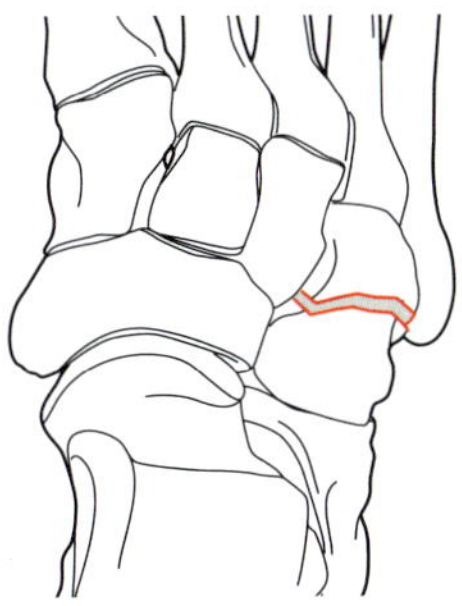

Foot, cuboid, **complete articular fracture**
84C*

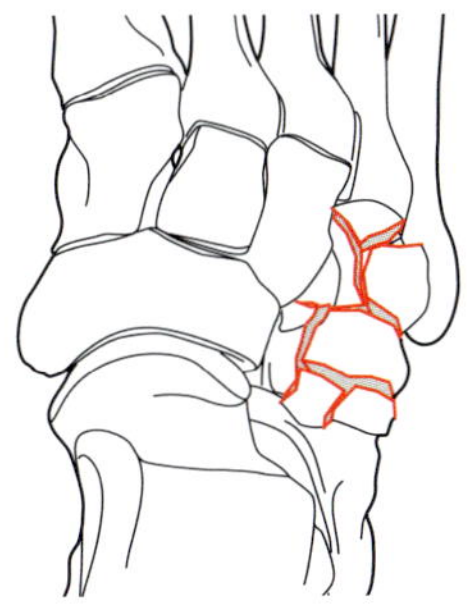

*Qualifications:
a Simple
b Multifragmentary

Cuneiform 85.__.

Bone: Foot, **cuneiform** 85.__.

Locations:

Foot, cuneiform, **medial**
85.1.

Foot, cuneiform, **middle**
85.2.

Foot, cuneiform, **lateral**
85.3.

→ The cuneiform locations are identified as follows: medial = 1, middle = 2, and lateral = 3.
→ The cuneiform location is added (between two dots .__.) after the bone code.

85.1.

Types:

Foot, cuneiform, medial,
avulsion fracture
85.1.A

Foot, cuneiform, medial,
partial articular fracture
85.1.B

Foot, cuneiform, medial,
complete articular fracture
85.1.C

85.2.

Types:

Foot, cuneiform, middle,
avulsion fracture
85.2.A

Foot, cuneiform, middle,
partial articular fracture
85.2.B

Foot, cuneiform, middle,
complete articular fracture
85.2.C

85.3.

Types:

Foot, cuneiform, lateral,
avulsion fracture
85.3.A

Foot, cuneiform, lateral,
partial articular fracture
85.3.B

Foot, cuneiform, lateral
complete articular fracture
85.3.C

Metatarsals 87

Bone: Foot, **metatarsal** 87

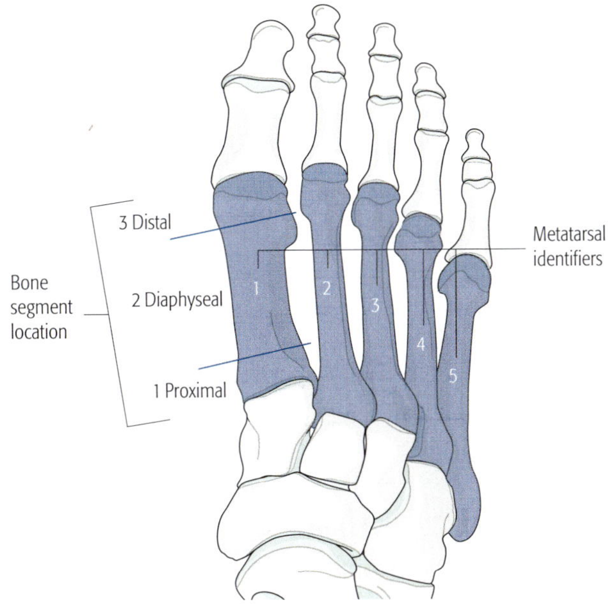

→ The metatarsal bones are identified as follows: First metatarsal = 1, second metatarsal = 2, third metatarsal = 3, fourth metatarsal = 4, fifth metatarsal = 5.
→ The metatarsal identifier is added (between two dots .__.) after the bone code.
→ The bone segment location is then added.
→ Example: Foot, third metatarsal, proximal end segment = 87.3.1

Locations:

Foot, metatarsal,
proximal end segment
87.__.1

Foot, metatarsal,
diaphyseal segment
87.__.2

Foot, metatarsal,
distal end segment
87.__.3

87.__.1

Location: Foot, metatarsal, **proximal end segment** 87.__.1
→ Example code for the third metatarsal is indicated with an underline 87.3.1

Types:

Foot, metatarsal, proximal end segment,
extraarticular fracture
87.3.1A*

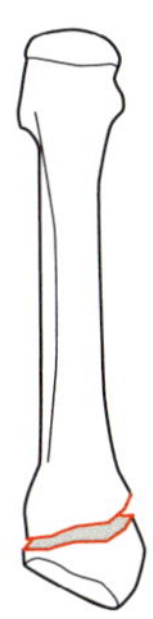

Foot, metatarsal, proximal end segment,
partial articular fracture
87.3.1B*

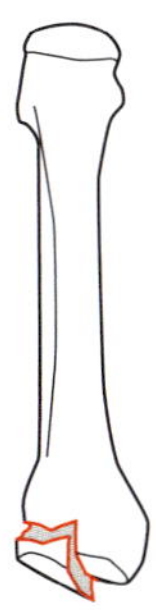

Foot, metatarsal, proximal end segment,
complete articular fracture
87.3.1C*

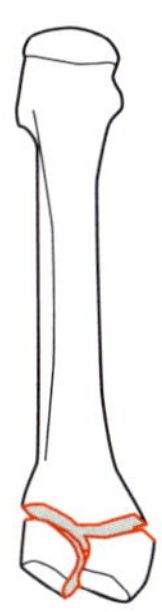

*Qualifications:
a **Simple**
b Multifragmentary

87.__.2

Location: Foot, metatarsal, **diaphyseal segment** 87.3.2
→ Example code for the third metatarsal is indicated with an underline 87.3.2

Types:

Foot, metatarsal, diaphyseal segment,
simple fracture
87.3.2A

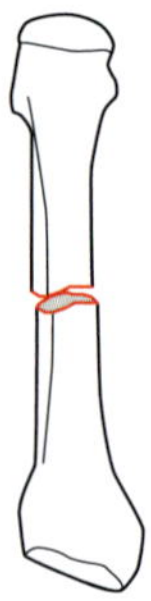

Foot, metatarsal, diaphyseal segment,
wedge fracture
87.3.2B

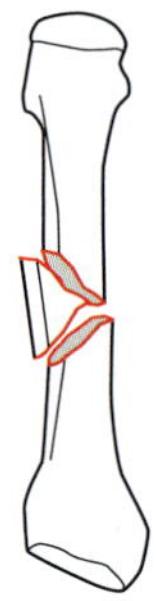

Foot, metatarsal, diaphyseal segment,
multifragmentary fracture
87.3.2C

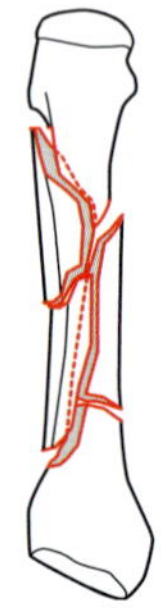

87.__.3

Location: Foot, metatarsal, **distal end segment** 87.__.3
→ Example code for the third metatarsal is indicated with an underline 87.3.3

Types:

Foot, metatarsal, distal end segment,
extraarticular fracture
87.3.3A*

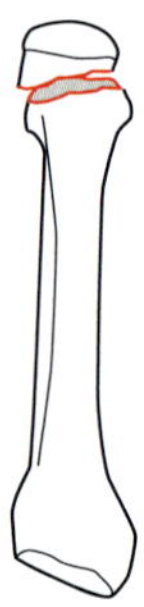

Foot, metatarsal, distal end segment,
partial articular fracture
87.3.3B*

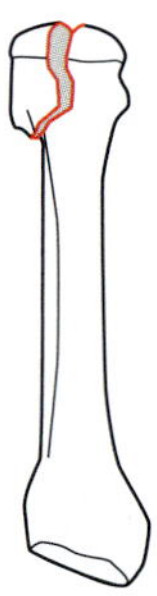

Foot, metatarsal, distal end segment,
complete articular fracture
87.3.3C*

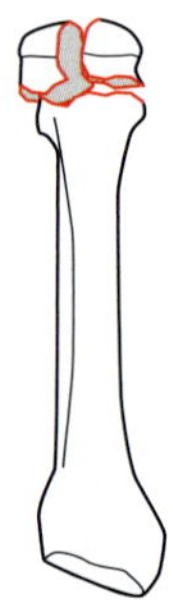

*Qualifications:
a **Simple**
b Multifragmentary

Phalanx 88

Bone: Foot, **phalanx** 88

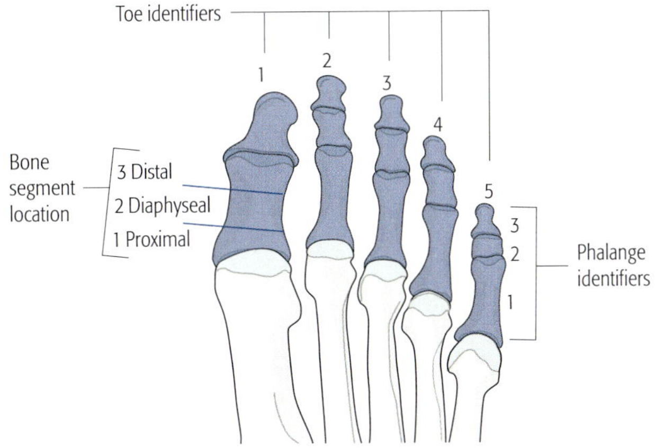

→ The toes and phalanges are identified as follows:
Toes: First or great toe = 1, second toe = 2, third toe = 3, fourth toe= 4, and fifth toe = 5.
Phalanges: Proximal phalanx = 1, middle phalanx = 2, and distal phalanx = 3.

→ The toe identifier plus phalanx identifier are added (between dots .__.__.) after the bone code.

→ Example: Great toe, middle phalanx fracture is 88.1.2.

→ The phalangeal bone segment location is then added.

→ **Anatomical region+bone.Toe.Phalanx.Bone segment location+Type**

→ Example: Great toe, middle phalanx, proximal end segment is 88.1.2.1

Locations:

Foot, phalanx .__.__.
proximal end segment
88.__.__.1

Foot, phalanx .__.__.
diaphyseal segment
88.__.__.2

Foot, phalanx .__.__.
distal end segment
88.__.__.3

88.__.__.1

Location: Foot, phalanx, **proximal end segment** 88.1.2.1
→ Example code for the proximal great toe is indicated with an underline 88.1.2.1

Types:

Foot, phalanx proximal end segment,
extraarticular fracture
88.1.2.1A

Foot, phalanx proximal end segment,
partial articular fracture
88.1.2.1B

Foot, phalanx proximal end segment,
complete articular fracture
88.1.2.1C

88.__.__.2

Location: Foot, phalanx, **diaphyseal segment** 88.1.2.2
→ Example code for the proximal great toe is indicated with an underline 88.1.2.2

Types:

Foot, phalanx, diaphyseal segment,
simple fracture
88.1.2.2A

Foot, phalanx, diaphyseal segment,
wedge fracture
88.1.2.2B

Foot, phalanx, diaphyseal segment,
multifragmentary fracture
88.1.2.2C

88.__.__.2

Location: Foot, phalanx, **distal end segment** 88.1.2.3
→ Example code for the proximal great toe is indicated with an underline 88.1.2.

Types:

Foot, phalanx, distal end segment,
extraarticular fracture
88.1.2.3A

Foot, phalanx, distal end segment,
partial articular fracture
88.1.2.3B

Foot, phalanx, distal end segment,
complete articular fracture
88.1.2.3C

89

Location: Foot, **crush, multiple fractures whole foot** 89

Types:

Foot, crush, multiple fractures, **hindfoot**
89A

Foot, crush, multiple fractures, **midfoot**
89B

Foot, crush, multiple fractures, **forefoot**
89C

Qualifications *are optional and applied to the fracture code where the asterisk is located as a lower-case letter within rounded brackets. More than one qualification can be applied for a given fracture classification, separated by a comma. For a more detailed explanation, see the compendium introduction.*

80

Anatomical region: Foot and ankle 80D

Locations:

Foot and ankle, **syndesmosis**
80A[5_]

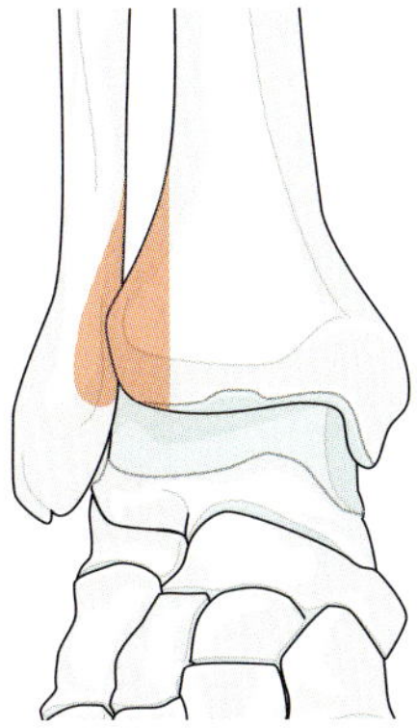

Foot and ankle, **ankle joint (tibiotalar/talocrural)**
80B[5_]

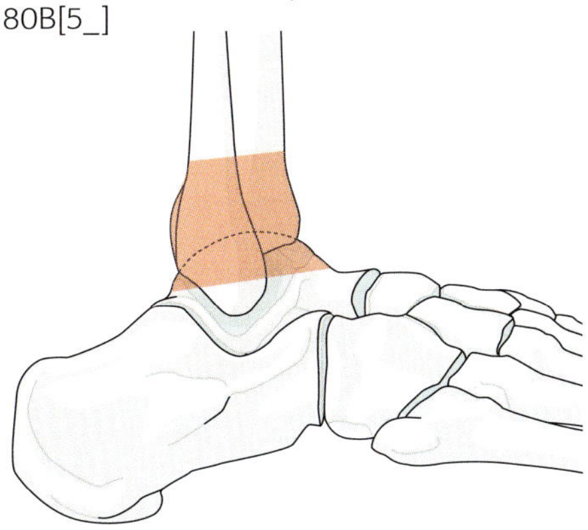

Foot and ankle, **hindfoot (subtalar joint)**
80C[5_]

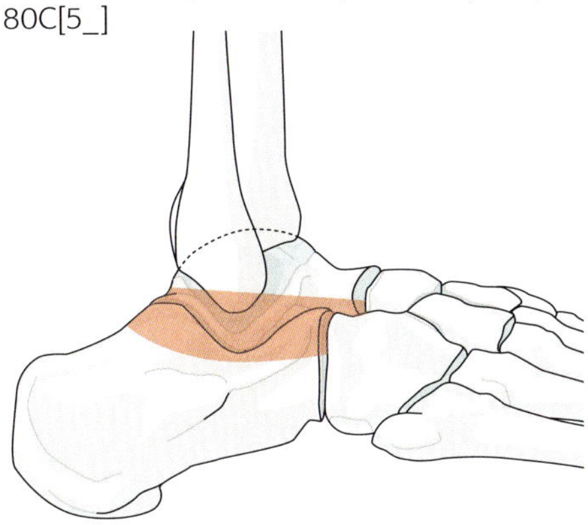

Foot and ankle, **midfoot**
80D

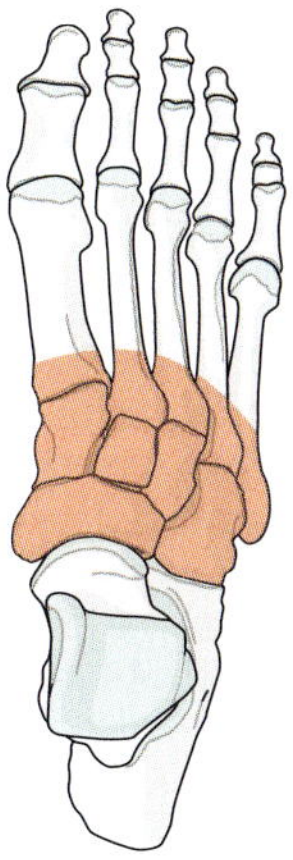

Foot and ankle, **forefoot**
80E

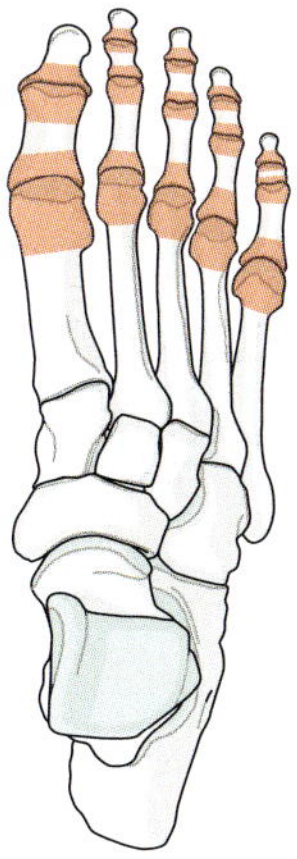

80D

Location: Foot and ankle, **midfoot** 80D

Types: Foot and ankle, midfoot, **talonavicular joint** 80D1[5_]
Foot and ankle, midfoot, **calcaneocuboid joint** 80D2[5_]
Foot and ankle, midfoot, **navicular-cuneiform joint** 80D3[5_]
Foot and ankle, midfoot, **intercuneiform joint** 80D4[5_]
Foot and ankle, midfoot, **tarsal-metatarsal joint** 80D5

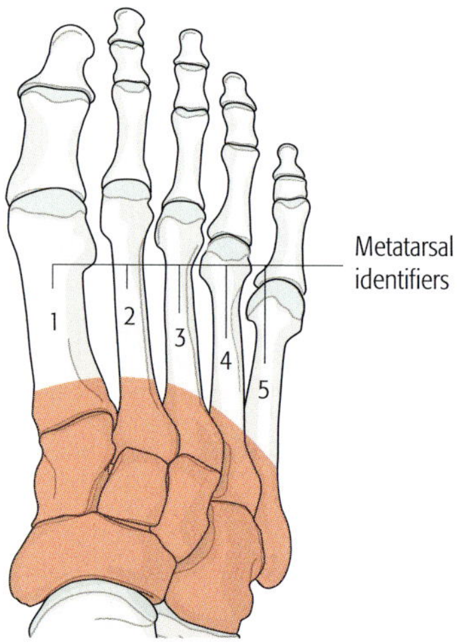

Groups: Foot and ankle, midfoot, tarsal-metatarsal joint, **1st metatarsal medial cuneiform** 80D5.1[5_]
Foot and ankle, midfoot, tarsal-metatarsal joint, **2nd metatarsal middle cuneiform** 80D5.2[5_]
Foot and ankle, midfoot, tarsal-metatarsal joint, **3rd metatarsal lateral cuneiform** 80D5.3[5_]
Foot and ankle, midfoot, tarsal-metatarsal joint, **4th metatarsal cuboid** 80D5.4[5_]
Foot and ankle, midfoot, tarsal-metatarsal joint, **5th metatarsal cuboid** 80D5.5[5_]
Foot and ankle, midfoot, tarsal-metatarsal joint, **multiple metatarsal-tarsal** 80D5.6[5_]
Foot and ankle, midfoot, **multiple joint dislocations** 80D6

Type: Foot and ankle, midfoot, **multiple joint dislocations** 80D6

80E

Location: Foot and ankle, **forefoot** 80E

Type: Foot and ankle, forefoot, **phalangeal joint** 80E1

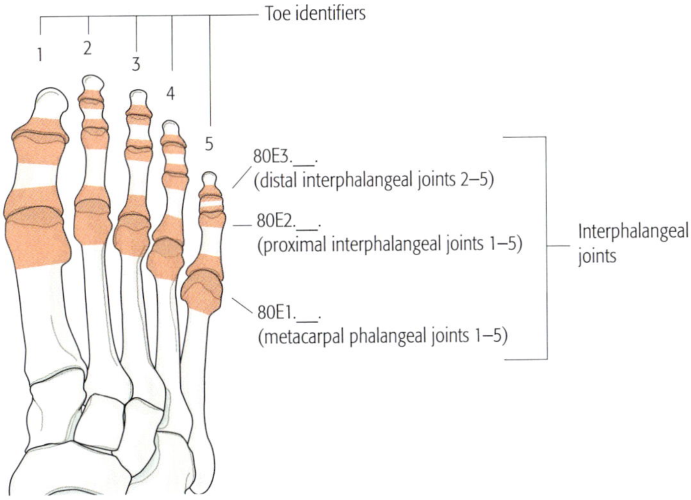

Groups (by joint medial to lateral): Foot and ankle, forefoot, phalangeal joint, **1st metatarsal phalangeal joint** 80E1.1.[5_]
Foot and ankle, forefoot, phalangeal joint, **2nd metatarsal phalangeal joint** 80E1.2.[5_]
Foot and ankle, forefoot, phalangeal joint, **3rd metatarsal phalangeal joint** 80E1.3.[5_]
Foot and ankle, forefoot, phalangeal joint, **4th metatarsal phalangeal joint** 80E1.4.[5_]
Foot and ankle, forefoot, phalangeal joint, **5th metatarsal phalangeal joint** 80E1.5.[5_]

Type: Forefoot, phalangeal joint, **proximal interphalangeal joint** 80E2

Groups (by joint medial to lateral): Forefoot, phalangeal joint, proximal interphalangeal joint, **1st toe** (IP joint as there is no DIP in great toe) 80E2.1[5_]
Forefoot, phalangeal joint, proximal interphalangeal joint, **2nd toe** 80E2.2.[5_]
Forefoot, phalangeal joint, proximal interphalangeal joint, **3rd toe** 80E2.3.[5_]
Forefoot, phalangeal joint, proximal interphalangeal joint, **4th toe** 80E2.4.[5_]
Forefoot, phalangeal joint, proximal interphalangeal joint, **5th toe** 80E2.5.[5_]

Type: Forefoot, phalangeal joint, **distal interphalangeal joint** 80E3

Groups (by joint medial to lateral): Forefoot, phalangeal joint, distal interphalangeal joint, **2nd toe** 80E3.2.[5_]
Forefoot, phalangeal joint, distal interphalangeal joint, **3rd toe** 80E3.3.[5_]
Forefoot, phalangeal joint, distal interphalangeal joint, **4th toe** 80DE3.4.[5_]
Forefoot, phalangeal joint, distal interphalangeal joint, **5th toe** 80DE3.5.[5_]

Type: Foot and ankle, forefoot, **sesamoid dislocation (any)** 80E4[5_]

Type: Foot and ankle, forefoot, **multiple dislocations** 80E5

References

1. **Schenck RC, Jr.** The dislocated knee. *Instr Course Lect.* 1994;43:127–136.
2. **Wascher DC.** High-velocity knee dislocation with vascular injury. Treatment principles. *Clin Sports Med.* 2000 Jul;19(3):457–477.

***Qualifications** are optional and applied to the fracture code where the asterisk is located as a lower-case letter within rounded brackets. More than one qualification can be applied for a given fracture classification, separated by a comma. For a more detailed explanation, see the compendium introduction.*

Universal modifiers

The universal modifiers are descriptive terms of fracture morphology, displacement, associated injury, or location that are generalizable to most fractures. They provide detail that are optional for users.

Universal modifiers may be added to the end of the fracture code within square brackets, eg, [1].

Multiple universal modifiers may be contained within the same set of squared brackets and separated by a comma.

Example: A proximal humerus fracture-dislocation with **displacement, anterior dislocation, cartilage injury, and osteopenia** = 11A1.2**[2,5a,8e,9]**

Example: Humerus, proximal end segment, articular or 4-part fracture, with multifragmentary metaphyseal fracture and articular fracture with an **anterior dislocation** = 11C3.2**[5a]**

List of universal modifiers

1		**Nondisplaced**	
2		**Displaced**	
3		**Impaction**	
	3a	Articular	
	3b	Metaphyseal	
4		**No impaction**	
5		**Dislocation**	
	5a	Anterior (volar, palmar, plantar)	
	5b	Posterior (dorsal)	
	5c	Medial (ulnar)	
	5d	Lateral (radial)	
	5e	Inferior (with hip is also obturator)	
	5f	Multidirectional	
6		**Subluxation/ligamentous instability**	
	6a	Anterior (volar, palmar, plantar)	
	6b	Posterior (dorsal)	
	6c	Medial (ulnar)	
	6d	Lateral (radial)	
	6e	Inferior (with hip is also obturator)	
	6f	Multidirectional	
7		**Diaphyseal extension**	
8		**Articular cartilage injury#**	
	8a	ICRS Grade 0	Normal
	8b	ICRS Grade 1	Superficial indentation (A) and /or superficial fissures and cracks (B)
	8c	ICRS Grade 2	Abnormal lesions extending down to 50% of cartilage depth
	8d	ICRS Grade 3	Severely abnormal with defects extending down >50% of cartilage depth (A); down to calcified layer (B); down to subchondral bone but not through (C); blisters included (D)
	8e	ICRS Grade 4	Severely Abnormal Cartilage loss through subchondral bone
9		**Poor bone quality**	
10		**Replantation**	
11		**Amputation associated with a fracture**	
12		**Associated with a nonarthroplasty implant**	
13		**Spiral type fracture**	
14		**Bending type fracture**	

#This grading system is used with the permission of the International Cartilage Repair Society.[38]

OTA Open Fracture Classification (OTA-OFC)

The open fracture classification was developed by the OTA classification committee to address the limitation of the Gustilo-Anderson classification. The OTA-OFC is designed to be used at the time of initial debridement by the treating surgeon. It is generic, usable on all anatomical areas, and focused on factors related to injury not treatment.

Skin	1. Laceration with edges that approximate. 2. Laceration with edges that do not approximate. 3. Laceration associated with extensive degloving.
Muscle	1. No appreciable muscle necrosis, some muscle injury with intact muscle function. 2. Loss of muscle but the muscle remains functional, some localized necrosis in the zone of injury that requires excision, intact muscle-tendon unit. 3. Dead muscle, loss of muscle function, partial or complete compartment excision, complete disruption of a muscle-tendon unit, muscle defect does not reapproximate.
Arterial	1. No major vessel disruption. 2. Vessel injury without distal ischemia. 3. Vessel injury with distal ischemia.
Contamination	1. None or minimal contamination. 2. Surface contamination (not ground in). 3. Contaminant embedded in bone or deep soft tissues or high-risk environmental conditions (eg, barnyard, fecal, dirty water).
Bone loss	1. None. 2. Bone missing or devascularized bone fragments, but still some contact between proximal and distal fragments. 3. Segmental bone loss.

Reference

Orthopaedic Trauma Association: Open Fracture Study Group. A new classification scheme for open fractures. *J Orthop Trauma.* 2010 Aug;24(8):457–464.

Gustilo-Anderson Classification of Open Fractures

Grade	Wound size	Contamination	Soft-tissue damage	Soft-tissue damage
I	< 1 cm	Clean	Minimal	Simple with minimal comminution
II	1–10 cm	Moderate	Moderate with some muscular damage	Moderate comminution
IIIA	> 10 cm	High	Severe with associated crush injury	Moderate–soft-tissue cover possible
IIIB	> 10 cm	High	Severe loss of cover	Requires reconstructive procedures
IIIC	> 10 cm	High	Severe vascular injury requiring repair	Requires reconstructive procedures

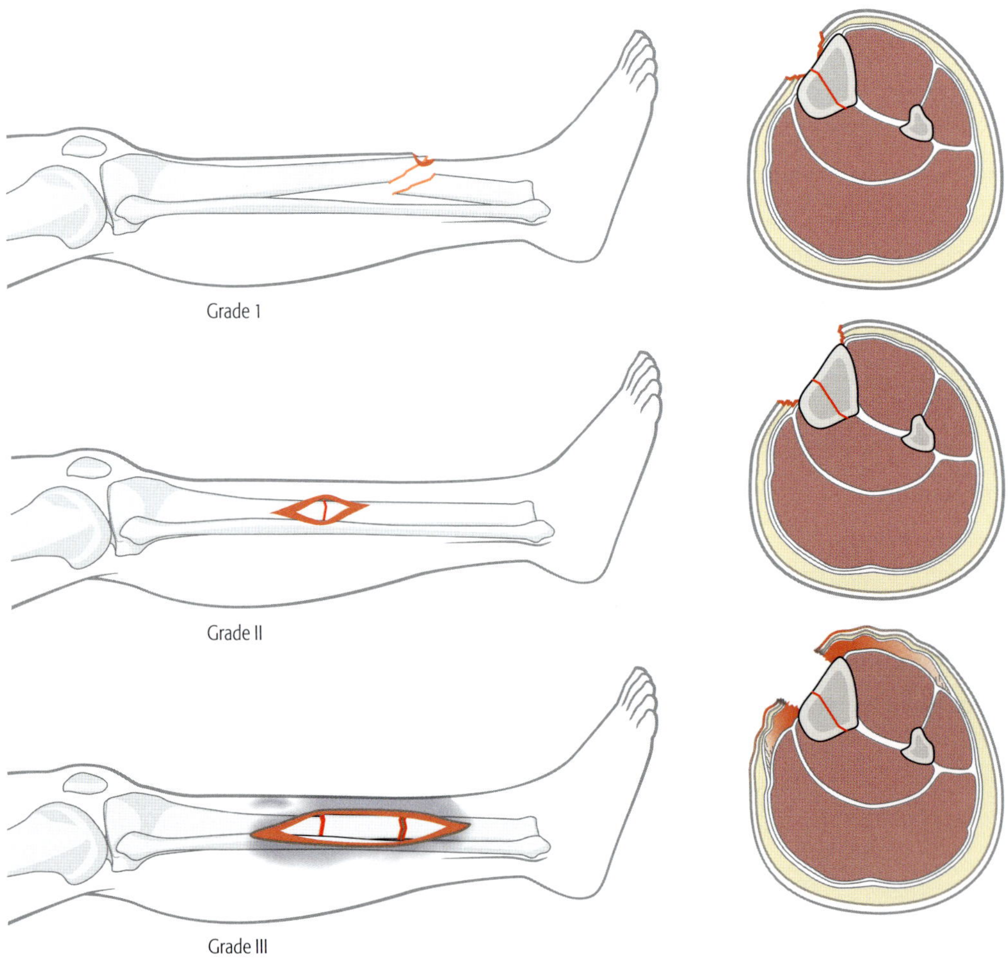

Gustilo RB, Anderson JT. Prevention of infection in the treatment of one thousand and twenty-five open fractures of long bones: retrospective and prospective analyses. *J Bone Joint Surg Am.* 1976 Jun;58(4):453–458.

Index

Page references with an "*f*" refer to figures.
Page references with a "*t*" refer to tables.

A

B

T

V

W